WITHDRAWN

KT-463-359

BRO

Staff

Si

Singleton Staff Library
S011033

Brook's Clinical Pediatric Endocrinology

Staff Library
Singleton Hospital
Tel: 01792 205666 Ext. 5281

Brook's Clinical Pediatric Endocrinology

EDITED BY

CHARLES G.D. BROOK MA MD FRCP FRCPCH
Emeritus Professor of Paediatric Endocrinology
University College London
London, UK

PETER E. CLAYTON MD MRCP FRCPCH
Professor of Child Health and Paediatric Endocrinology
University of Manchester
Manchester, UK

ROSALIND S. BROWN MD CM
Associate Professor of Pediatrics
Harvard Medical School
Director, Clinical Trials Research, Endocrine Division
Children's Hospital Boston
Boston, MA, USA

SIXTH EDITION

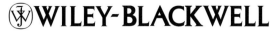
A John Wiley & Sons, Ltd., Publication

This edition first published 2009, © 1981, 1989, 1995, 2001, 2005, 2009 Blackwell Publishing Limited
Blackwell Publishing was acquired by John Wiley & Sons in February 2007. Blackwell's publishing program
has been merged with Wiley's global Scientific, Technical and Medical business to form Wiley-Blackwell.

Registered office: John Wiley & Sons Ltd, The Atrium, Southern Gate, Chichester, West Sussex, PO19 8SQ, UK

Editorial offices: 9600 Garsington Road, Oxford, OX4 2DQ, UK
 The Atrium, Southern Gate, Chichester, West Sussex, PO19 8SQ, UK
 111 River Street, Hoboken, NJ 07030-5774, USA

For details of our global editorial offices, for customer services and for information about how to apply for
permission to reuse the copyright material in this book please see our website at
www.wiley.com/wiley-blackwell

The right of the author to be identified as the author of this work has been asserted in accordance with the
Copyright, Designs and Patents Act 1988.

All rights reserved. No part of this publication may be reproduced, stored in a retrieval system, or transmitted,
in any form or by any means, electronic, mechanical, photocopying, recording or otherwise, except as
permitted by the UK Copyright, Designs and Patents Act 1988, without the prior permission of the publisher.

Wiley also publishes its books in a variety of electronic formats. Some content that appears in print may not
be available in electronic books.

Designations used by companies to distinguish their products are often claimed as trademarks. All brand
names and product names used in this book are trade names, service marks, trademarks or registered
trademarks of their respective owners. The publisher is not associated with any product or vendor mentioned
in this book. This publication is designed to provide accurate and authoritative information in regard to the
subject matter covered. It is sold on the understanding that the publisher is not engaged in rendering
professional services. If professional advice or other expert assistance is required, the services of a competent
professional should be sought.

The contents of this work are intended to further general scientific research, understanding, and discussion
only and are not intended and should not be relied upon as recommending or promoting a specific method,
diagnosis, or treatment by physicians for any particular patient. The publisher and the author make no
representations or warranties with respect to the accuracy or completeness of the contents of this work and
specifically disclaim all warranties, including without limitation any implied warranties of fitness for a
particular purpose. In view of ongoing research, equipment modifications, changes in governmental
regulations, and the constant flow of information relating to the use of medicines, equipment, and devices, the
reader is urged to review and evaluate the information provided in the package insert or instructions for each
medicine, equipment, or device for, among other things, any changes in the instructions or indication of
usage and for added warnings and precautions. Readers should consult with a specialist where appropriate.
The fact that an organization or Website is referred to in this work as a citation and/or a potential source of
further information does not mean that the author or the publisher endorses the information the organization
or Website may provide or recommendations it may make. Further, readers should be aware that Internet
Websites listed in this work may have changed or disappeared between when this work was written and when
it is read. No warranty may be created or extended by any promotional statements for this work. Neither the
publisher nor the author shall be liable for any damages arising herefrom.

Library of Congress Cataloging-in-Publication Data
Brook's clinical pediatric endocrinology / edited by Charles G.D. Brook, Peter E. Clayton, Rosalind S. Brown.
 – 6th ed.
     p. ; cm.
   Rev ed. of: Clinical pediatric endocrinology. 5th ed. 2005.
   Includes bibliographical references and index.
   ISBN 978-1-4051-8080-1 (alk. paper)
   1. Pediatric endocrinology. I. Brook, C. G. D. (Charles Groves Darville)   II. Clayton, Peter E.
III. Brown, Rosalind S.   IV. Clinical pediatric endocrinology.   V. Title: Clinical pediatric endocrinology.
   [DNLM: 1. Endocrine System Diseases. 2. Adolescent. 3. Child. 4. Infant. WS 330 B873 2009]
   RJ418.C567 2009
   618.92′4–dc22
                                                                                    2008043612

A catalogue record for this title is available from the British Library

Set in 9.25/12pt Minion by SNP Best-set Typesetter Ltd., Hong Kong
Printed and bound in Singapore by Fabulous Printers Pte Ltd

1   2009

Contents

Staff Library
Singleton Hospital
Tel: 01792 205666 Ext. 5281

List of Contributors

Kyriaki S. Alatzoglou MD
ESPE Clinical Fellow
Developmental Endocrinology Research Group
UCL Institute of Child Health
London, UK

Jeremy Allgrove MA, MD, FRCP, FRCPCH
Consultant Paediatric Endocrinologist
Royal London Hospital
Honorary Consultant Paediatric Endocrinologist
Great Ormond Street Hospital for Children
London, UK

Bart E.P.B. Ballieux PhD
Clinical Biochemist
Department of Clinical Chemistry
Leiden University Medical Center
Leiden, The Netherlands

Joanne C. Blair MB, ChB, MRCP, MRCPCH, MD
Consultant Endocrinologist
Alder Hey Children's NHS Foundation Trust
Liverpool, UK

Rosalind S. Brown MD, CM
Associate Professor of Pediatrics
Harvard Medical School
Director, Clinical Trials Research
Endocrine Division
Childrens' Hospital Boston
Boston, MA, USA

Tim D. Cheetham BSc, MD, MRCP, MRCPCH
Senior Lecturer in Paediatric Endocrinology
Department of Paediatrics
Royal Victoria Infirmary
Newcastle-upon-Tyne, UK

Steven D. Chernausek MD
Professor of Pediatrics
CMRI Edith Kinney Gaylord Chair
Department of Pediatrics
University of Oklahoma Health Sciences Center
Oklahoma City, OK, USA

Peter E. Clayton MD, MRCP, FRCPCH
Professor of Child Health and Paediatric
Endocrinology
Endocrine Science Research Group
University of Manchester
Manchester, UK

Andrew Cotterill MBBS, MRCP(UK), FRACP, MD
Director, Department of Paediatric Endocrinology
Mater Children's Hospital, Brisbane
Associate Professor
Department of Paediatrics and Child Health
University of Queensland
Brisbane, Queensland, Australia

David M. Cowley BSc(Hons), MBChB, FRCPA, FHGSA
Director of Chemical Pathology
Mater Health Services Brisbane Ltd
Brisbane, Queensland, Australia

Mehul T. Dattani MBBS, DCH, FRCPCH, FRCP, MD
Professor and Lead in Paediatric Endocrinology
Developmental Endocrinology Research Group
Clinical and Molecular Genetics Unit
UCL Institute of Child Health and Great Ormond
Street Hospital for Children
London, UK

I. Sadaf Farooqi PhD, FRCP
Wellcome Trust Senior Clinical Fellow
University of Cambridge Metabolic Research
Laboratories
Addenbrooke's Hospital
Cambridge, UK

Michael Freemark MD
Professor and Chief
Division of Pediatric Endocrinology and Diabetes
Duke University Medical Center
Durham, NC, USA

Evelien F. Gevers MD, PhD
Senior Research Investigator
MRC National Institute for Medical Research
Developmental Endocrinology Research Group
UCL Institute of Child Health
London, UK

Helena K. Gleeson MD, MRCP
Consultant in Adolescent Endocrinology
Department of Paediatric Endocrinology
Royal Manchester Children's Hospital
Manchester, UK

Ristan Greer PhD
Discipline of Paediatrics and Child Health
University of Queensland
Mater Children's Hospital
Brisbane, Queensland, Australia

M. Isabel Hernandez MD
Institute of Maternal and Child Research
Faculty of Medicine
University of Chile
Santiago, Chile

Peter C. Hindmarsh MD, FRCP
Professor of Paediatric Endocrinology
Developmental Endocrinology Research Group
Clinical and Molecular Genetics Unit
UCL Institute of Child Health
London, UK

Christopher P. Houk MD
Associate Professor of Pediatrics
Medical College of Georgia
Augusta, GA, USA

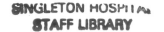
Ieuan A. Hughes MD, FRCP, FRCPCH, FMedSci
Professor of Paediatrics
University of Cambridge
Addenbrooke's Hospital
Department of Paediatrics
Cambridge, UK

Marcel Karperien PhD
Department of Tissue Regeneration
Biomedical Technology Institute
Twente University
Enschede, The Netherlands

Peter A. Kopp MD
Associate Professor
Director ad interim Center for Genetic Medicine
and Division of Endocrinology Metabolism and
Molecular Medicine
Northwestern University
Chicago, IL, USA

Peter A. Lee MD, PhD
Professor of Pediatrics
Penn State College of Medicine
The Milton S. Hershey Medical Center
Hershey, PA
Indiana University School of Medicine
The Riley Hospital for Children
Indianapolis, IN, USA

Ameeta Mehta DCH, DNBE, MRCP, MSc, MD
Clinical Editor BMJ Publishing Group
Hon. Consultant in Pediatric Endocrinology
Developmental Endocrinology Research Group
UCL Institute of Child Health
London, UK

Verónica Mericq MD
Institute of Maternal and Child Research
Faculty of Medicine
University of Chile
Santiago, Chile

Jakub Mieszczak MD
Indiana University School of Medicine
The Riley Hospital for Children
Indianapolis, IN, USA

Walter L. Miller MD
Professor of Pediatrics
Chief of Endocrinology
Department of Pediatrics
University of California
San Francisco, CA, USA

Andrew W. Norris MD, PhD
Assistant Professor of Pediatrics
The University of Iowa
Division of Endocrinology and Diabetes
University of Iowa Children's Hospital
Iowa City, IO, USA

Catherine J. Owen PhD, MRCP, MRCPCH
Institute of Human Genetics
Newcastle University
Newcastle upon Tyne, UK

Leena Patel MB BS, MD, MRCP, MHPE, MD
Senior Lecturer in Child Health
The University of Manchester
Department of Paediatric Endocrinology
Royal Manchester Children's Hospital
Manchester, UK

Simon H.S. Pearce MD, FRCP
Professor of Endocrinology
Institute of Human Genetics
Newcastle University
Newcastle upon Tyne, UK

David R. Repaske PhD, MD
Director, Division of Endocrinology, Metabolism
and Diabetes
Nationwide Children's Hospital
Ohio State University
Columbus, OH, USA

Stephen M. Shalet MD, FRCP
Professor of Endocrinology
Department of Endocrinology
Christie Hospital NHS Trust
Manchester, UK

Vaitsa Tziaferi MD, MRCPCH
Academic Clinical Fellow
Developmental Endocrinology Research Group
UCL Institute of Child Health
London, UK

Jerry K.H. Wales DM, MA, BM BCh, MRCP, FRCPCH
Senior Lecturer in Paediatric Endocrinology
Academic Unit of Child Health
Sheffield Children's Hospital
Sheffield, UK

Melissa Westwood BSc, PhD
Senior Lecturer in Endocrinology
Maternal and Fetal Health Research Group
The University of Manchester
Manchester, UK

Jan M. Wit MD, PhD
Emeritus Professor of Pediatrics
Department of Pediatrics
Leiden University Medical Center
Leiden, The Netherlands

Joseph I. Wolfsdorf MB, BCh
Clinical Director and Associate Chief
Director, Diabetes Program
Division of Endocrinology
Children's Hospital Boston
Professor of Pediatrics
Harvard Medical School
Boston, MA, USA

Preface

Four years have passed since the last edition of *Clinical Pediatric Endocrinology* and 28 since the first and still the emphasis remains on Clinical. The science has changed but the discipline of clinical medicine – history and clinical examination – has not and my co-editors and I make no apology for continually stressing the relevance of careful thought before reaching for the investigation pad. Advances in our understanding of molecular mechanisms has led to the introduction of many new tests but a diagnosis is seldom made by untargeted indiscriminate investigation.

We have been ably assisted on this occasion by the team at what used to be Blackwell and is now Wiley-Blackwell, and especially by Rob Blundell and Helen Harvey, but it is the authors delivering their commissions on time (and most of them did) that makes a book. Some of them are new to this book and some are trusty friends: we thank them all.

The contributions were edited by me so I take full responsibility for idiosyncrasies of spelling and punctuation as well as for errors and omissions. Commissions were solicited on the advice of Rosalind Brown and Peter Clayton with whom working has again been a pleasure. In launching this edition at the 2009 joint meeting of the world's pediatric endocrinology societies, we acknowledge the global spread of our discipline which happily thrives in the 21st century.

C.G.D. Brook
Hadspen Farm
Somerset, UK

1 Genetics and Genomics

Peter A. Kopp

Division of Endocrinology, Metabolism and Molecular Medicine, Northwestern University, Chicago, IL, USA

The understanding of the molecular basis of many endocrine and non-endocrine disorders has grown during the last decade (see OMIM, Online Mendelian Inheritance in Man, a comprehensive catalog of human genes and genetic disorders: http://www.ncbi.nlm.nih.gov/sites/entrez?db=omim) (Table 1.1). With the exception of simple trauma, every disease has a genetic component. In *monogenic disorders*, for example, congenital adrenal hyperplasia (CAH), the genetic component is the major etiologic factor. In *complex disorders*, multiple genes in conjunction with environmental and lifestyle factors contribute to the pathogenesis; hence their designation as *polygenic* or *multifactorial* disorders. In other instances, genetic factors influence the manifestation of disease indirectly by defining the host's susceptibility and resistance as, for example, in an environmental disease such as infection.

Genetics can be defined as the science of heredity and variation. *Medical genetics*, the clinical application of genetics, has historically focused on chromosomal abnormalities and inborn errors of metabolism, because of readily recognizable phenotypes and techniques to diagnose the conditions. Analysis of the transmission of human traits and disease within families, together with the study of the underlying molecular basis, has culminated in understanding many *monogenic* or *Mendelian* disorders, which has led to a significant modification in the diagnostic process for an increasing number of them. Many major health care problems, such as diabetes mellitus type 2, obesity, hypertension, heart disease, asthma and mental illnesses, are complex and we are at the early stages of unraveling the genetic alterations predisposing to these disorders, which are significantly influenced by exogenous factors. It is important to recognize that phenotype can also be influenced by genetic and environmental *modifiers* in monogenic disorders. For example, the expression of the phenotype in monogenic forms of diabetes mellitus due to mutations in the MODY (Maturity Onset of Diabetes in the Young) genes is influenced by factors such as diet and physical activity.

Brook's Clinical Pediatric Endocrinology, 6th edition. Edited by C. Brook, P. Clayton, R. Brown. © 2009 Blackwell Publishing, ISBN: 978-1-4051-8080-1.

Cancer can also be viewed as a genetic disease, because *somatic* mutations in genes controlling growth and differentiation are key elements in its pathogenesis. Many cancers are associated with a predisposition conferred by hereditary *germline* mutations.

The term *genome*, introduced before the recognition that DNA is the genetic material, designates the totality of all genes on all chromosomes in the nucleus of a cell. *Genomics* refers to the discipline of mapping, sequencing and analyzing genomes. Because of the rapidly growing list of sequenced genomes in numerous organisms, genomics is currently undergoing a transition with increasing emphasis on functional aspects.

Genome analysis can be divided into *structural* and *functional genomics*. The analysis of differences among genomes of individuals of a given species is the focus of *comparative genomics*. The complement of messenger RNAs (mRNAs) transcribed by the cellular genome is called the *transcriptome* and the generation of mRNA expression profiles is referred to as *transcriptomics*. Epigenetic alterations, chemical modifications of DNA or chromatin proteins, influence gene transcription. The sum of all epigenetic information defines the *epigenome* and is a current focus of high-throughput analyses (*epigenomics*).

The term *proteome* has been coined to describe all the proteins expressed and modified following expression by the entire genome in the lifetime of a cell. *Proteomics* refers to the study of the proteome using techniques of large-scale protein separation and identification. The field of *metabolomics* aims at determining the composition and alterations of the *metabolome*, the complement of low-molecular-weight molecules. The relevance of these analyses lies in the fact that proteins and metabolites function in *modular networks* rather than linear pathways. Hence, any physiological or pathological alteration may have many effects on the proteome and metabolome. *Metagenomics* refers to the analysis of the genomes of the microorganisms present in a specific compartment (e.g. the gut flora).

The growth of biological information has required computerized databases to store organize, annotate and index the data. This has led to the development of *bioinformatics*, the application of informatics to (molecular) biology. Computational and

Table 1.1 Selected databases relevant for genomic medicine.

Site	Content	URL
National Center for Biotechnology Information (NCBI)	Portal with extensive links to genomic databases, PubMed, OMIM. Links to educational online resources including guidelines for the use of genomic databases	http://www.ncbi.nlm.nih.gov/
Online Mendelian Inheritance in Man (OMIM)	Catalog of human genetic disorders	http://www.ncbi.nlm.nih.gov/omim/
National Human Genome Research Institute	Information about the human genome sequence, genomes of other organisms and genomic research	http://www.genome.gov/
European Bioinformatics Institute (EBI)	Portal to numerous databases and tools for the analysis of sequences and structures	http://www.ebi.ac.uk
DNA Database of Japan	Portal to numerous databases and tools for the analysis of sequences and structures	http://www.ddbj.nig.ac.jp/
University of California, Santa Cruz (UCSC) Genome Bioinformatics	Reference sequence of the human and other genomes. Multiple tools for sequence analysis	http://genome.ucsc.edu/
Swiss-Prot	Protein sequence database with description of protein function, domains structure, post-translational modifications and variants	http://www.ebi.ac.uk/swissprot/index.html
Protein Structure Database	Portal to Biological Macromolecular Structures	http://www.rcsb.org/pdb/home/home.do
American College of Medical Genetics	Access to databases relevant for the diagnosis, treatment and prevention of genetic disease	http://www.acmg.net/
Genecards	A database of human genes, their products and involvement in diseases	http://bioinformatics.weizmann.ac.il/cards/
GeneTests·GeneClinics	Directory of laboratories offering genetic testing	http://www.genetests.org/
Gene Ontology	The Gene Ontology project provides a controlled vocabulary to describe gene and gene product attributes in any organism	http://www.geneontology.org/
Chromosomal Variation in Man	Catalog of chromosomal disorders	http://www.wiley.com/legacy/products/subject/life/borgaonkar/access.html
Database of Chromosomal Imbalance and Phenotype in Humans using Ensembl Resources (DECIPHER)	Catalog of genomic and clinical information of patients with chromosomal disorders	http://www.sanger.ac.uk/PostGenomics/decipher
Mitochondrial disorders, DNA repeat sequences & disease	Catalog of disorders associated with mtDNA mutations and DNA repeats	http://neuromuscular.wustl.edu/
National Organization for Rare Disorders	Catalog of rare disorders including clinical presentation, diagnostic evaluation and treatment	http://www.rarediseases.org/

mathematical tools are essential for the management of nucleotide and protein sequences, the prediction and modeling of secondary and tertiary structures, the analysis of gene and protein expression and the modeling of molecular pathways, interactions and networks. Numerous continuously evolving databases provide easy access to the expanding information about the genome of humans and other species, genetic disease and genetic testing (Table 1.1). The integration of data generated by transcriptomic, proteomic, epigenomic and metabolomic analyses through informatics, *systems biology*, is an emerging discipline aimed at understanding phenotypic variations and creating comprehensive models of cellular organization and function. These efforts are based on the expectation that an understanding of the complex and dynamic changes in a biological system may provide insights into pathogenic processes and the development of novel therapeutic strategies and compounds.

DNA, genes and chromosomes

Structure of DNA

The recognition in 1944 that DNA carries the genetic information was followed by the deduction of its structure in 1953. DNA is a double-stranded helix. Each strand consists of a backbone formed

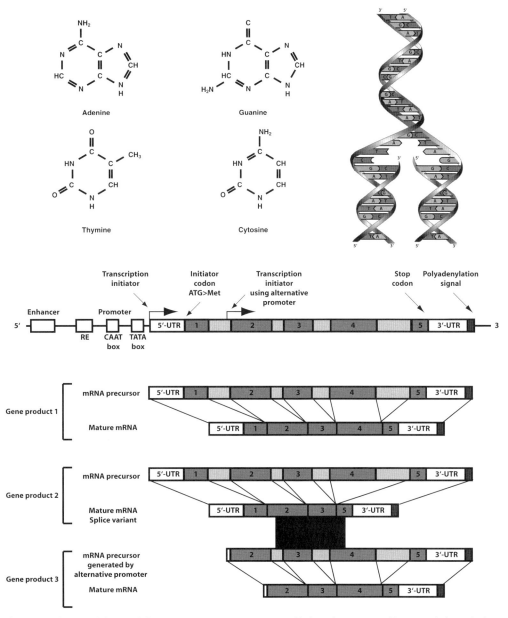

Figure 1.1 *Top*: The four bases of DNA and the DNA helix. Semiconservative replication generates two identical daughter molecules, each composed of one parental strand and one newly synthesized strand.
Bottom: General structure of a gene. The 5′ regulatory regions contain enhancer elements, response elements (RE) and often a CAAT box and a TATA box. The exons (dark gray) are separated by introns (light gray). Alternative splicing may generate distinct mRNA products from a given gene and is an important mechanism generating diversity at the protein level. ATG, start codon; Met, methionine; TATA box, TATA-binding protein box; UTR, untranslated region.

by a deoxyribose-phosphate polymer (Fig. 1.1). Four different nitrogen-containing bases are attached to the sugar ring: the purines, adenine (A) and guanine (G), and the pyrimidines, cytosine (C) and thymidine (T). The two strands of DNA are complementary and held together by hydrogen bonds pairing adenine with thymidine and guanine with cytosine. The double-stranded nature of DNA and its strict base pair complementarity permit faithful replication during cell division, as each strand can serve as a template for the synthesis of a new complementary strand referred to as *semiconservative* replication. The complementary

structure of the two strands is also of importance as a defense against DNA damage. Damage or loss of a base on the opposite strand can be repaired using the intact strand as a template.

The presence of four different bases provides surprising genetic diversity. In the protein-coding regions of genes, the DNA bases are arranged into codons, triplets of bases that encode one of the 20 different amino acids or a stop codon. Combinatorial arrangement of the four bases creates 64 different triplets (4^3). Many amino acids, as well as the stop of translation, can be specified by several different codons. Because there are more codons than amino acids, the genetic code is said to be degenerate. Arranging the codons in different combinations of various length permits the generation of a tremendous diversity of polypeptides.

The human genome

The *Human Genome Project*, launched in the 1980s, first led to the creation of genetic and physical maps. A *genetic map* describes the order of genes and defines the position of a gene relative to other loci on the same chromosome. It is constructed by assessing how frequently two markers are inherited together, i.e. *linked*, by linkage studies. Distances of the genetic map are expressed in recombination units or centimorgans (cM). One centimorgan corresponds to a recombination frequency of 1% between two polymorphic markers and corresponds to approximately 1 Mb of DNA. *Physical maps* indicate the position of a locus or gene in absolute values. Sequence-tagged sites (STSs), any site in a chromosome or genome that is identified by a known unique DNA sequence, have been widely used for physical mapping and, after cloning of DNA fragments, they have served as landmarks for arranging cloned DNA fragments in the same order as they occur in the genome. These overlapping clones then allowed the characterization of contiguous DNA sequences (*contigs*). This approach led to high-resolution physical maps by cloning the whole genome into overlapping fragments. The complete DNA sequence of each chromosome provides the highest resolution physical map and, after publication of a first draft of the whole genome in 2000, its sequence analysis was largely completed in 2003.

Human DNA consists of about 3 billion base pairs (bp) of DNA per haploid genome contained in the 23 chromosomes. The smallest chromosome (chromosome 21) contains approximately 47 million bp, the largest (chromosome 1) 247 million bp. The human genome is estimated to contain about 30 000–40 000 *genes*. This number is smaller than the original estimates (up to 100 000 genes), which were derived from the large diversity of proteins. This observation indicates that *alternative splicing* of genes and the use of various promoters are important mechanisms generating protein diversity (Fig. 1.1).

Historically, genes were identified because they conferred specific traits that are transmitted from one generation to the next. Genes can be defined as functional units that are regulated by transcription and encode RNA (Fig. 1.1). The majority of RNA transcripts consist of mRNA which is subsequently translated into protein. Other RNA transcripts exert specialized functions, such as transfer of amino acids for polypeptide synthesis (tRNA), contribute to ribosome structure (rRNA) or regulate transcription. MicroRNAs (miRNAs) are small non-coding RNAs that regulate gene expression by targeting mRNAs of protein coding genes or non-coding RNA transcripts. They have an important role in developmental and physiologic processes and can act as tumor suppressors or oncogenes in cancer development.

Genes account for 10–15% of the genomic DNA. Much of the remaining DNA consists of highly repetitive sequences, the func-

tion of which remains incompletely understood. These repetitive DNA regions, along with non-repetitive sequences that do not encode genes, are, in part, involved in the packaging of DNA into chromatin and chromosomes or in the regulation of gene expression. Genes are unevenly distributed across the various chromosomes and vary in size from a few hundred to more than 2 million base pairs. The vast majority of genes are located in nuclear DNA but a few are found in mitochondrial DNA (mtDNA).

A major goal of human genetics aims at understanding the role of common genetic variants in susceptibility to common disorders. This involves identifying, cataloging and characterizing gene variants, followed by performing *association studies*. The variants include short repetitive sequences in regulatory or coding regions and single-nucleotide polymorphisms (SNPs), changes in which a single base in the DNA differs from the usual base at that position (Fig. 1.2). SNPs occur roughly every 300 bp and most are found outside coding regions. SNPs within a coding sequence can be synonymous (i.e. not altering the amino acid code) or nonsynonymous. There are roughly 3 million differences between the DNA sequences of any two copies of the human genome. The identification of approximately 10 million SNPs that occur commonly in the human genome through the International HapMap Project is of great relevance for genome-wide association studies (GWAS).

Structure and function of genes

The structure of a typical gene consists of regulatory regions followed by exons and introns and downstream untranslated regions (Fig. 1.1). The regulatory regions controlling gene expression most commonly involve sequences upstream (5′) of the transcription start site, although there are examples of control elements located within introns or downstream of the coding region of a gene. Exons designate the regions of a gene that are eventually spliced together to form the mature mRNA. Introns refer to the intervening regions between the exons that are spliced out of precursor RNAs during RNA processing. A gene may generate various transcripts through the use of alternative promoters and/or alternative splicing of exons (Fig. 1.1). These mechanisms contribute to the diversity of proteins and their functions.

The regulatory DNA sequences of a gene, which are typically located upstream of the coding region, are referred to as the *promoter*. The promoter region contains specific sequences, *response elements* that bind transcription factors. Some transcription factors are ubiquitous; others are cell-specific. Gene expression is controlled by additional regulatory elements, *enhancers* and *locus control regions*, which may be located far away from the promoter region. The transcription factors that bind to the promoter and enhancer sequences provide a code for regulating transcription that is dependent on developmental state, cell type and endogenous and exogenous stimuli. Transcription factors interact with other nuclear proteins, *co-activators* and *co-repressors* and generate large regulatory complexes that ultimately activate or repress transcription.

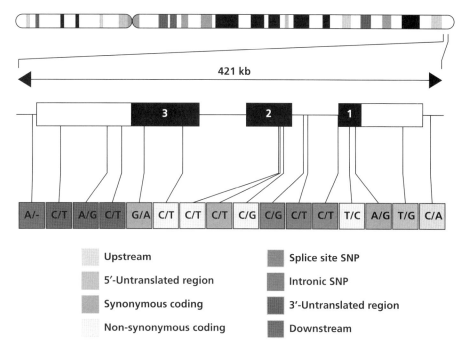

Figure 1.2 Single-nucleotide polymorphisms in the *PROP1* gene, which encodes a homeodomain transcription factor involved in programing the development of the anterior pituitary gland. The gene is located on chromosome 5q. The transcription of this gene, which contains three exons, occurs from right to left. SNPs are found in all regions of the gene, the 5′-untranslated region, the exons, splice sites, introns and the 3′-untranslated region. In the coding region, the SNPs may be synonymous, i.e. the encoded amino acid remains unchanged; non-synonymous SNPs result in an amino acid substitution. SNPs are found about every 300 bp throughout the genome.

Upstream · 5′-Untranslated region · Synonymous coding · Non-synonymous coding · Splice site SNP · Intronic SNP · 3′-Untranslated region · Downstream

In the eukaryotic cell nucleus, DNA is packaged by histones into nucleosomes. This packaging inhibits transcription by impeding the binding of transcriptional activators to their cognate DNA sites. Therefore, alterations in chromatin structure typically precede gene transcription. Repression is often associated with histone deacetylation. Conversely, activation of transcription may involve histone acetylation, which results in the remodeling of chromatin and subsequent binding of *trans*-acting factors to DNA (Fig. 1.3). Once bound to DNA, the transcription factor complexes recruit proteins that form the basal transcription complex including RNA polymerase. Gene transcription occurs with the synthesis of RNA from the DNA template by RNA polymerase. mRNA is encoded by the coding strand of the DNA double helix and is translated into proteins by ribosomes. The transcriptional termination signals reside in the 3′ region of a gene. A polyadenylation signal encodes a poly-A tail, which influences mRNA export to the cytoplasm, stability and translation efficiency.

Transcription factors account for about 30% of all expressed genes. Mutations in transcription factors cause a significant number of endocrine and non-endocrine genetic disorders. Because a given set of transcription factors may be expressed in various tissues, it is not uncommon to observe a syndromic phenotype. The mechanism by which transcription factor defects cause disease often involves *haploinsufficiency*, a situation in which a single copy of the normal gene is incapable of providing sufficient protein production to assure normal function. Biallelic mutations in such a gene may result in a more pronounced phenotype. For example, monoallelic mutations in the transcription factor HESX1 (RPX) result in various constellations of pituitary hormone deficiencies and the phenotype is variable among family members with the same mutation. Inactivating mutations of both alleles of HESX1 cause familial septo-optic dysplasia and combined pituitary hormone deficiency.

Gene expression is also influenced by *epigenetic events*, such as X-inactivation and imprinting, i.e. a marking of genes that results in monoallelic expression depending on their parental origin. In this situation, DNA methylation leads to silencing, i.e. suppression of gene expression on one of the chromosomes. Genomic imprinting has an important role in the pathogenesis of several genetic disorders [e.g. Prader–Willi syndrome and Albright hereditary osteodystrophy (AHO)].

Chromosomes

The normal diploid number of chromosomes in humans is 46, consisting of two homologous sets of 22 autosomes (chromosomes 1 to 22) and a pair of sex chromosomes. Females have two X chromosomes (XX), whereas males have one X and one Y chromosome (XY). As a consequence of *meiosis*, germ cells – sperm or oocytes – are haploid and contain one set of 22 autosomes and one of the sex chromosomes. At the time of fertilization, the pairing of the homologous chromosomes from the mother and father results in reconstitution of the diploid genome. With each cell division, i.e. *mitosis*, chromosomes are replicated, paired, segregated and divided into two daughter cells.

The normal human genome contains large blocks (>1 kb) of DNA sequences, often containing numerous genes, that can be duplicated one or several times or missing on a given chromosome. These *copy number variants* (CNV) tends to vary in a specific manner among different populations. CNVs are associated with hot spots of chromosomal rearrangements. Because CNVs can result in differential levels of gene expression, they are thought

Repression in presence of thyroid hormone receptor and T3

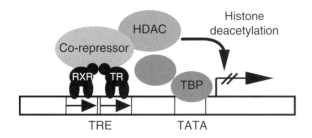

Relief of repression after binding of T3

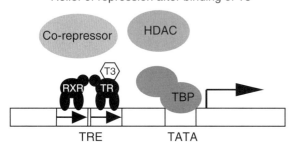

Activation in presence of T3

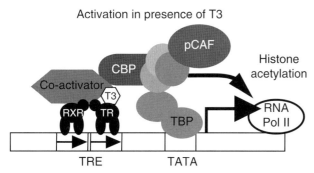

Figure 1.3 Control of gene transcription by the ligand-dependent thyroid hormone receptor (TR) interacting with co-repressors and co-activators. In the absence of triiodothyronine (T3), the TR binds to a thyroid hormone response element (TRE) in conjunction with the retinoid X receptor (RXR). Co-repressors associated with the TR recruit histone deacetylases (HDAC) and transcription is silenced. After binding of T3, the TR undergoes a conformational alteration, the co-repressors dissociate and co-activators can interact with the receptor. This, in turn, leads to binding of histone acetylases such as pCAF that modify chromatin structure and enable transcription. In the case of resistance to thyroid hormone, mutations in TRβ do not permit release of the co-repressors and lead to silencing of gene transcription in target genes. CBP, CREB-binding protein; CREB, cyclic AMP response element-binding protein; RNA Pol II, RNA polymerase II; TBP, TATA-binding protein.

to contribute significantly to normal phenotypic variation. Genomic imbalances resulting from CNVs are also causally involved in numerous disorders; for example, Williams syndrome (short stature, elfin facies, supravalvular aortic stenosis and hypercalcemia).

Replication of DNA, mitosis and meiosis

Genetic information in DNA is transmitted to daughter cells during two different types of cell division: *mitosis* and *meiosis*. Somatic cells divide by mitosis, allowing the diploid ($2n$) genome to replicate itself during cell division. The formation of germ cells, sperm and ova, requires meiosis, a process that leads to the reduction of the diploid ($2n$) set of chromosomes to the haploid state ($1n$).

Before mitosis, cells exit the resting or G_0 state and enter the cell cycle. After traversing a critical checkpoint in G_1, cells undergo DNA synthesis (S phase), during which the DNA in each chromosome is replicated, yielding two pairs of sister chromatids ($2n$ to $4n$). The process of DNA synthesis requires strict fidelity in order to avoid transmitting errors to subsequent generations of cells. Therefore, genetic abnormalities of enzymes that are involved in DNA mismatch repair predispose to neoplasia because of the rapid acquisition of additional mutations (e.g. xeroderma pigmentosa, Bloom syndrome, ataxia telangiectasia and hereditary non-polyposis colon cancer). After completion of DNA synthesis, cells enter G_2 and progress through a second checkpoint before entering mitosis. Subsequently, the chromosomes condense and are aligned along the equatorial plate at metaphase. The two identical sister chromatids, held together at the centromere, divide and migrate to opposite poles of the cell. After the formation of a nuclear membrane around the two separated sets of chromatids, the cell divides forming two daughter cells with a diploid ($2n$) set of chromosomes.

Meiosis occurs only in germ cells of the gonads. It involves two steps of cell division that reduce the chromosome number to the haploid state. *Recombination*, the exchange of DNA between homologous paternal and maternal chromosomes during the first cell division, is essential for generating genetic diversity. Each chromosome pair forms two sister chromatids ($2n$ to $4n$). This is followed by an exchange of DNA between homologous chromosomes through the process of *crossover*. In most instances, there is at least one crossover on each chromosomal arm. This recombination process occurs more frequently in female meiosis than in male meiosis. Subsequently, the chromosomes segregate randomly. As there are 23 chromosomes, this can generate 2^{23} (>8 million) possible combinations of chromosomes. Together with the genetic exchanges that occur during recombination through crossover, chromosomal segregation generates tremendous diversity and therefore each gamete is genetically unique. The processes of recombination and independent segregation of chromosomes provide the foundation for performing linkage analyses, in which the inheritance of *linked* genes is correlated with the presence of a disease or genetic trait. After the first meiotic division, which results in two daughter cells ($2n$), the two chromatids of each chromosome separate during a second meiotic division to yield four gametes with a haploid chromosome set ($1n$). Through fertilization of an egg by a sperm, the two haploid sets are combined, thereby restoring the diploid state ($2n$) in the zygote.

Analysis of chromosomes, DNA and RNA

Analyses of large alterations in the genome are possible using cytogenetics, fluorescence *in situ* hybridization (FISH), Southern blotting, high-throughput genotyping and sequencing. More discrete sequence alterations rely heavily on the use of the *polymerase chain reaction* (PCR). PCR permits rapid genetic testing and mutational analysis with small amounts of DNA extracted from solid tissues, nucleated blood cells, leukocytes, buccal cells or hair roots. Reverse transcription PCR (RT-PCR) transcribes RNA into a complementary DNA strand, which can then be amplified by PCR. RT-PCR can be used for sequence analyses of the coding regions and to detect absent or reduced levels of mRNA expression resulting from a mutated allele.

Screening for point mutations can be performed by numerous methods, such as sequencing of DNA fragments amplified by PCR, recognition of mismatches between nucleic acid duplexes or electrophoretic separation of single- or double-stranded DNA. Most traditional diagnostic methods are gel-based and focus on single genes. Novel techniques for the analysis of mutations, genetic mapping and mRNA expression profiles are rapidly evolving. Chip techniques allow hybridization of DNA or RNA to hundreds of thousands of probes simultaneously. Microarrays are being used clinically for mutational analysis of several human disease genes, for the identification of viral sequence variations and for large-scale analyses of mRNA transcripts. Comprehensive genotyping of SNPs can be performed with microarray and beadarray technologies or mass spectrometry. These technologies are widely used for genotyping in GWAS, analyses of copy number variations and characterization of genomic DNA methylation. While traditional sequencing technologies are still of importance and widely used, particularly for the sequencing of PCR products, high-throughput sequencing technologies are rapidly evolving and several platforms have become commercially available in the recent past. These techniques provide the foundation to expand from a focus on single genes to analyses at the scale of the genomes of prokaryotes and eukaryotes. It is anticipated that sequencing of the whole human genome of an individual for a cost of $1000 or less will soon become a reality. In addition to sequencing DNA, high-throughput sequencing technologies can be used for the characterization of RNA expression, non-coding and microRNAs, protein–DNA interactions, epigenomic alterations and metagenomic analyses.

The availability of comprehensive individual sequence information is expected to have a significant impact on medical care and preventative strategies but it also raises ethical and legal concerns how such information may be used by insurers and employers. Protection against discrimination based on genetic information for health insurance and employment is needed; for example, the recently introduced Genetic Information Nondiscrimination Act (GINA) in the USA is an important first step to avoid misuse of genetic information.

Concerns that the exclusive protection of genetic risks results in an increasing discrimination against lifestyle risks persist. The impact of genetic testing on health care costs has not been addressed in detail and probably depends on the specific disorder and the availability of effective therapeutic modalities. In certain instances it can be cost-effective; for example, in carrier detection in family members of individuals affected by multiple endocrine neoplasia type 2 (MEN2). The marketing of genetic testing directly to consumers (consumer genomics) through the Internet by commercial companies raises numerous questions about the accuracy and confidentiality of the information, how the results should be handled and how to ensure appropriate regulatory oversight.

Genetic linkage and association

There are two primary strategies for mapping genes that cause or increase susceptibility to human disease: *linkage* and *association* studies.

Genetic linkage refers to the fact that genes and polymorphic DNA markers such as microsatellites and SNPs are physically connected, i.e. *linked*, to one another along the chromosomes (Fig. 1.4). Two principles are essential for understanding the concept of genetic linkage. First, when two genes are close together on a chromosome, they are usually transmitted together, unless a recombination event separates them. Secondly, the odds of a crossover or recombination event between two linked genes are proportional to the distance that separates them. Thus, genes that are further apart are more likely to undergo a recombination event than genes that are very close together. The detection of chromosomal loci that segregate with a disease by linkage has been widely used to identify the gene responsible for the disease by *positional cloning*, a technique of isolating a gene from the knowledge of its map location. It has also been used to predict the odds of disease gene transmission in genetic counseling.

Polymorphisms are essential for linkage studies because they provide a means to distinguish the maternal and paternal chromosomes in an individual. On average, one out of every 300 bp varies from one person to the next. Although this degree of variation seems low (99.9% identical), it means that more than 3 million sequence differences exist between any two unrelated individuals and the probability that the sequence at such loci will differ on the two homologous chromosomes is high (often, >70–90%). These sequence variations include a variable number of tandem repeats (VNTRs), microsatellites [also referred to as short tandem repeats (STRs)] and SNPs. Most microsatellite markers consist of di-, tri- or tetranucleotide repeats that can be measured readily using PCR and primers that reside on either side of the repeat sequences (Fig. 1.4). Automated analysis of SNPs with microarrays, beadarrays or mass spectrometry are now the methods of choice for determining genetic variation for linkage and association studies.

In order to identify a chromosomal locus that segregates with a disease, it is necessary to determine the genotype or *haplotype* of DNA samples from one or several pedigrees. A haplotype

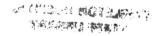

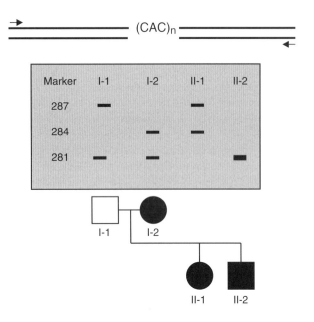

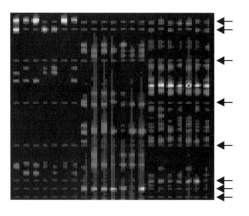

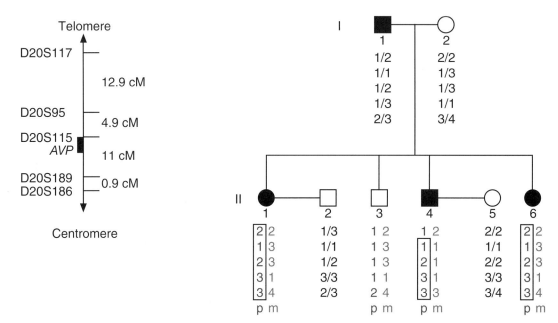

Figure 1.4 Analysis of polymorphic microsatellite markers and linkage analysis. *Upper panel:* The example depicts a CAC trinucleotide repeat with three alleles in a nuclear family. PCR with primers flanking the polymorphic region results in products of variable length, depending on the number of CAC repeats. After characterization of the alleles in the parents, transmission of the paternal and maternal alleles can be determined in the offspring. The gel on the right shows the concomitant analysis of multiple microsatellites. The PCR products reflecting the different alleles can be distinguished by differences in length and fluorescent labels. The red marker (arrowed) included in every lane is a size standard. *Lower panel:* Determination of polymorphic microsatellite markers flanking the arginine vasopressin (*AVP*) gene located on chromosome 20p13 in a family with autosomal dominant neurohypophyseal diabetes insipidus. The parental origin of the alleles can be determined in generation II (p, paternally inherited; m, maternally inherited). The three affected individuals II-1, II-4, II-6 share the same alleles for the markers D20S95/115/189/186. In individual II-4, a recombination has occurred between markers D20S117 and 95 of the paternal chromosome. The unaffected individual II-3 has inherited the alternate paternal alleles. Although individual II-5 is homozygous for the alleles segregating with the phenotype in this family, she is not related to I-1 and she does not have diabetes insipidus. The haplotype of these markers is only associated with the phenotype in the original family but not in the general population.

SINGLETON HOSPITAL
STAFF LIBRARY

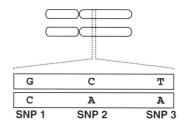

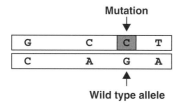

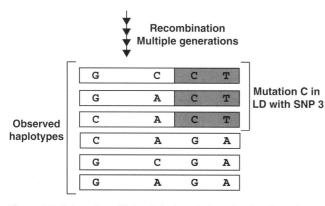

Figure 1.5 Linkage disequilibrium (LD). Three single nucleotide polymorphisms are shown in the selected genomic region. The combinations G, C, T and C, A, A form the original haplotypes. A mutation G > C then occurs in the chromosome with haplotype G, C, T. With time, multiple recombinations occur and lead to the formation of new haplotypes. However, the mutation remains linked to the T variant of SNP 3 and is therefore said to be in linkage disequilibrium.

designates a group of alleles that are closely linked, i.e. in close proximity on a chromosome and that are usually inherited as a unit. After characterizing the alleles, one can assess whether certain marker alleles co-segregate with the disease. Markers closest to the disease gene are less likely to undergo recombination events and therefore receive a higher linkage score. Linkage is expressed as a *logarithm of odds (lod) score*, i.e. the ratio of the probability that the disease and marker loci are linked rather than unlinked. Lod scores of +3 (1000:1) are generally accepted as supporting linkage.

Allelic association refers to a situation in which the frequency of an allele is significantly increased or decreased in a particular disease. Linkage and association differ in several respects. Genetic linkage is demonstrable in families or sibships. Association studies compare a population of affected individuals with a control population. Association studies are often performed as case–control studies that include unrelated affected individuals and matched controls or as family-based studies that compare the frequencies of alleles that are transmitted to affected children. Allelic association studies are useful for identifying susceptibility genes in complex disorders. When alleles at two loci occur more frequently in combination than would be predicted based on known allele frequencies and recombination fractions, they are said to be in *linkage disequilibrium* (Fig. 1.5).

The HapMap project and its impact on association studies

After the identification of the approximately 10 million SNPs that are commonly found in the human genome, the International HapMap Project has generated a catalog of common genetic variants that occur in individuals from distinct ethnic backgrounds (http://www.hapmap.org/). SNPs that are in close proximity are inherited together as blocks referred to as haplotypes, hence the name HapMap. These blocks can be identified by genotyping selected SNPs, so called *Tag SNPs*, an approach that greatly reduces cost and workload (Fig. 1.6). This permits one to char-

Figure 1.6 Haplotype blocks. The figure shows 10 SNPs in the selected genomic region. The associations between these SNPs has been determined and is shown graphically. Dark gray indicates the strongest association, white the lowest association. This analysis reveals that three blocks of associated SNPs occur in this region. In order to characterize the region through genotyping, one can rely on so-called Tag SNPs (SNP 2, 5, 8) as representatives of the three blocks, rather than genotyping all SNPs. Such information is available for the whole genome and for different ethnic groups. It now allows performing genome-wide associations studies more efficiently and at lower cost.

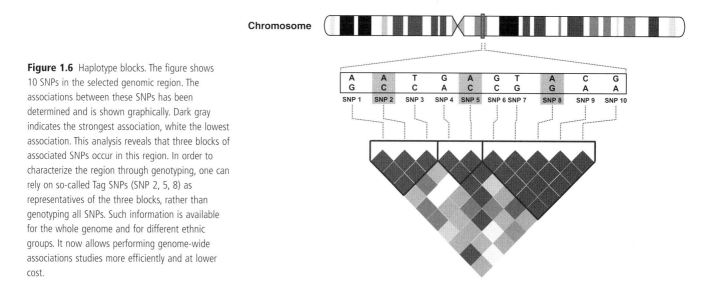

acterize a limited number of SNPs in order to identify the set of haplotypes present in an individual and greatly facilitates performing GWAS aiming at the elucidation of the complex interactions among multiple genes and lifestyle factors in multifactorial disorders.

Medical genetics

Mutations and human disease

Structure of mutations

Mutations are an important cause of genetic diversity as well as disease. A *mutation* can be defined as any change in the nucleotide sequence of DNA regardless of its functional consequences (Fig. 1.7). Mutations are structurally diverse. They can affect one or a few nucleotides, consist of gross numerical or structural alterations in individual genes or chromosomes or involve the entire genome. Mutations can occur in all domains of a given gene. Large deletions may affect a portion of a gene or an entire gene or, if several genes are involved, they may lead to a *contiguous*

gene syndrome. Occasionally, mispairing of homologous sequences leads to *unequal crossover.* This results in gene duplication on one of the chromosomes and gene deletion on the other chromosome.

For example, a significant fraction of growth hormone (*GH*) gene deletions involves unequal crossing-over. The *GH* gene is a member of a large gene cluster that includes a growth hormone variant gene as well as several structurally related chorionic somatomammotropin genes and *pseudogenes*, which are highly homologous but functionally inactive relatives of a normal gene. Because such gene clusters contain multiple homologous DNA sequences arranged along the same chromosome, they are particularly prone to undergo recombination and, consequently, gene duplication or deletion.

Unequal crossing-over between homologous genes can result in fusion gene mutations, as illustrated, for example, by glucocorticoid-remediable aldosteronism (GRA). GRA is caused by a rearrangement involving the genes that encode aldosterone synthase (*CYP11B2*) and steroid 11β-hydroxylase (*CYP11B1*), normally arranged in tandem on chromosome 8q. Because these two genes are 95% identical, they are predisposed to undergo unequal recombination. The rearranged gene product contains the regulatory regions of 11β-hydroxylase upstream to the coding sequence of aldosterone synthetase. The latter enzyme is then expressed in the adrenocorticotropic hormone (ACTH) dependent zona fasciculata of the adrenal gland, resulting in overproduction of mineralocorticoids and hypertension.

Gene conversion refers to a non-reciprocal exchange of homologous genetic information by which a recipient strand of DNA receives information from another strand having an allelic difference. The original allele on the recipient strand is converted to the new allele as a consequence of this event. These alterations may range from a few to several thousand nucleotides. Gene conversion often involves exchange of DNA between a gene and a related pseudogene. For example, the 21-hydroxylase gene (*CYP21A*) is adjacent to a non-functional pseudogene. Many of the nucleotide substitutions found in the *CYP21A* gene in patients with CAH correspond to sequences present in the pseudogene, suggesting gene conversion as the underlying mechanism of mutagenesis. In addition, mitotic gene conversion has been suggested as a mechanism to explain revertant mosaicism in which an inherited mutation is "corrected" in certain cells.

Trinucleotide repeats may be unstable and expand beyond a critical number. Mechanistically, the expansion is thought to be caused by unequal recombination and slipped mispairing. A premutation represents a small increase in trinucleotide copy number. In subsequent generations, the expanded repeat may increase further in length. This increasing expansion is referred to as *dynamic mutation*. It may be associated with an increasingly severe phenotype and earlier manifestation of the disease (*anticipation*). Trinucleotide expansion was first recognized as a cause of the fragile X syndrome, one of the most common causes of mental retardation. Malignant cells are also characterized by

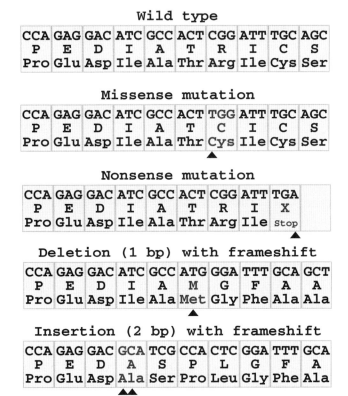

Figure 1.7 Examples of mutations. The coding strand is shown with the encoded amino acid sequence in the one-letter code and the three-letter code.

genetic instability, indicating a breakdown in mechanisms that regulate DNA repair and the cell cycle.

Mutations involving single nucleotides are referred to as *point mutations* (Fig. 1.7). Substitutions are called *transitions* if a purine is replaced by another purine base (A to G) or if a pyrimidine is replaced by another pyrimidine (C to T). Changes from a purine to a pyrimidine or vice versa are referred to as *transversions*. Certain DNA sequences, such as successive pyrimidines or CG dinucleotides, are particularly susceptible to mutagenesis. Therefore, certain types of mutations (C to T or G to A) are relatively common. Moreover, the nature of the genetic code results in overrepresentation of certain amino acid substitutions. If the DNA sequence change occurs in a coding region and alters an amino acid, it is called a *missense mutation*. Depending on the functional consequences of such a missense mutation, amino acid substitutions in different regions of the protein can lead to distinct phenotypes. Small deletions and insertions alter the reading frame if they do not represent a multiple of three bases. Such "*frameshift*" mutations lead to an entirely altered carboxy-terminus. Mutations may also be found in the regulatory sequences of genes and result in reduced gene transcription. Mutations in intronic sequences or in exon junctions may destroy or create splice donor or splice acceptor sites.

Some mutations are lethal, some have less deleterious yet recognizable consequences and some confer evolutionary advantage. Mutations occurring in germ cells can be transmitted to the progeny. Alternatively, mutations can occur during embryogenesis or in somatic tissues. Mutations that occur during development lead to *mosaicism*, a situation in which tissues are composed of cells with different genetic constitutions, as illustrated by Turner syndrome or McCune–Albright syndrome. If the germline is mosaic, a mutation can be transmitted to some progeny but not others, which sometimes leads to confusion in assessing the pattern of inheritance. Other somatic mutations are associated with neoplasia because they confer a growth advantage to cells by activating (proto)oncogenes or inactivating tumor suppressor genes. Epigenetic events, heritable changes that do not involve changes in gene sequence (e.g. altered DNA methylation), may also influence gene expression or facilitate genetic damage.

Polymorphisms are sequence variations that have a frequency of at least 1% and do not usually result in an overt phenotype. Often they consist of single base pair substitutions that do not alter the protein coding sequence because of the degenerate nature of the genetic code, although some might alter mRNA stability, translation or the amino acid sequence. Silent base substitutions and SNPs are encountered frequently during genetic testing and must be distinguished from true mutations that alter protein expression or function. However, some SNPs or combinations of SNPs may have a pathogenic role in complex disorders by conferring susceptibility for the development of the disease.

Functional consequences of mutations

Mutations can broadly be classified as gain-of-function and loss-of-function mutations. The consequences of an altered protein sequence often need experimental evaluation *in vitro* to determine that the mutation alters protein function. The appropriate assay depends on the properties of the protein and may, for example, involve enzymatic analyses, electromobility shift experiments or reporter gene assays (Fig. 1.8).

Gain-of-function mutations are typically dominant and result in phenotypic alterations when a single allele is affected. Inactivating mutations are usually recessive and an affected individual is homozygous or compound heterozygous (i.e. carrying two different mutant alleles) for the disease-causing mutations. Mutation in a single allele can result in *haploinsufficiency*, a situation in which one normal allele is not sufficient to maintain a normal phenotype. Haploinsufficiency is a commonly observed mechanism in diseases associated with mutations in transcription factors. For example, monoallelic mutations in the transcription factor TTF1 (NKX2.1) are associated with transient congenital hypothyroidism, respiratory distress and ataxia.

The clinical features among patients with an identical mutation in a transcription factor often vary significantly. One mechanism underlying this variability consists of the influence of modifying genes. Haploinsufficiency can affect the expression of rate-limiting enzymes. For example, in MODY2 heterozygous glucokinase mutations result in haploinsufficiency with a higher threshold for glucose-dependent insulin release and mild hyperglycemia.

Mutation of a single allele can result in loss-of-function due to a dominant-negative effect. In this case, the mutated allele interferes with the function of the normal gene product by several different mechanisms. The mutant protein may interfere with the function of a multimeric protein complex, as illustrated by Liddle syndrome, which is caused by mutations in the β- or γ-subunit (SCCN1B, SCCN1G) of the renal sodium channel. In thyroid hormone resistance, mutations in the thyroid hormone receptor β (TRβ, THRB) lead to impaired T3 binding; the receptors cannot release co-repressors and they silence transcription of target genes. The mutant protein can be cytotoxic, as in autosomal-dominant neurohypophyseal diabetes insipidus, in which abnormal folding leads to retention in the endoplasmic reticulum and degeneration of neurons secreting arginine vasopressin (AVP).

An increase in dosage of a gene product may also result in disease. For example, duplication of the *DAX1* (*NR0B1*) gene results in dosage-sensitive sex reversal.

Genotype and phenotype

An observed trait is referred to as a *phenotype*. The genetic information defining the phenotype is called the *genotype*. Alternative forms of a gene or a genetic marker are referred to as alleles, which may be polymorphic variants of nucleic acids that have no apparent effect on gene expression or function. In other instances, these variants may have subtle effects on gene expression, thereby conferring adaptive advantages or increased susceptibility. Commonly occurring allelic variants may reflect mutations in a gene that clearly alter its function, as illustrated, for example, by the ΔF508 deletion in the cystic fibrosis conductance regulator (CFTR).

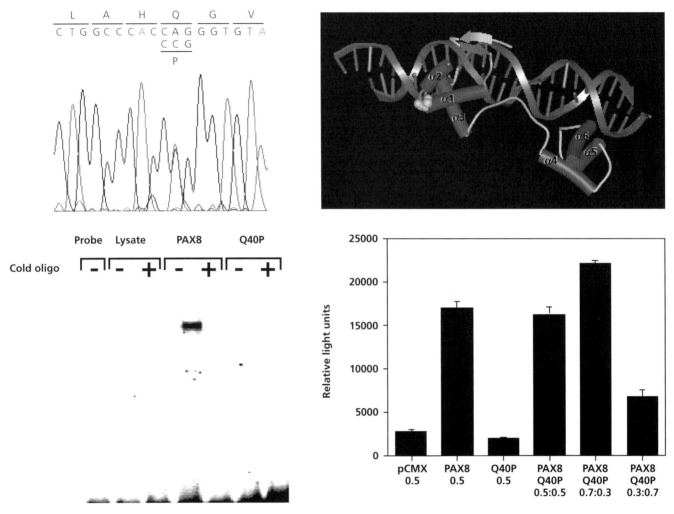

Figure 1.8 Functional analysis of a mutation in the transcription factor PAX8 found in a child with thyroid hypoplasia and congenital hypothyroidism.
Upper panels: The point mutation 119A > C leads to a substitution of glutamine 40 by proline (Q40P) in the DNA binding domain of the transcription factor.
Left lower panel: Gel shift experiment. A radiolabeled DNA response element migrates very fast through the gel in the absence of a protein-DNA interaction (lanes 1–3). The wild type PAX8 protein binds to the responses element and this leads to an electomobility shift (lane 4). Cold oligo in excess can compete for the labeled oligo documenting that the interaction is specific (lane 5). The mutated protein is unable to bind to this response element (lane 6).
Right lower panel: Plasmid vectors encoding wild type or mutated PAX8 were transfected into embryonic kidney cells together with a luciferase reporter gene. The reporter gene consists of a plasmid containing a PAX8 response element upstream of the coding sequence for luciferase. The transcriptional stimulation of the luciferase gene can be determined by measuring the light emission of cell lysates incubated with the substrate luciferin. The example shows that the wild type protein stimulates transcription of the luciferase reporter gene (pCMX = control vector). In contrast, there is no significant induction by the mutant. Co-transfection of wild type and mutant plasmids in different ratios shows that the mutant does not have a dominant negative effect. (After Congdon *et al.* 2001 with permission.)

Because each individual has two copies of each chromosome, an individual can have only two alleles at a given locus. However, there can be many different alleles in the population. The normal or common allele is usually referred to as *wild type*. When alleles at a given locus are identical, the individual is *homozygous*. Inheriting such identical copies of a mutant allele occurs in many autosomal-recessive disorders, particularly in circumstances of consanguinity. If the alleles are different, the individual is *heterozygous* at this locus. If two different mutant alleles are inherited at a given locus, the individual is referred to as a *compound heterozygote*. *Hemizygous* is used to describe males with a mutation

in an X-chromosomal gene or a female with a loss of one X-chromosomal locus.

A *haplotype* refers to a group of alleles that are closely linked together at a genomic locus. Haplotypes are useful for tracking the transmission of genomic segments within families and for detecting evidence of genetic recombination, if the crossover event occurs between the alleles.

Allelic and phenotypic heterogeneity
Allelic heterogeneity refers to the fact that different mutations in the same genetic locus can cause an identical or similar pheno-

type. *Phenotypic heterogeneity* occurs when more than one phenotype is caused by allelic mutations. For example, different mutations in the androgen receptor can result in a wide phenotypic spectrum. In some cases, the receptor is deleted or mutated in a manner that inactivates it completely. In a karyotypic male, this leads to *testicular feminization*. In contrast, the phenotype may be milder if the androgen receptor is only partially inactivated. In these patients, the phenotype may include infertility, gynecomastia or epispadias. Allelic heterogeneity is explained by the fact that many different mutations are capable of altering protein structure and function. Allelic heterogeneity creates a significant problem for genetic testing because one must often examine the entire genetic locus for mutations, because these can differ in each patient.

Locus or non-allelic heterogeneity and phenocopies

Non-allelic or *locus heterogeneity* refers to the situation in which a similar disease phenotype results from mutations at different genetic loci. This often occurs when more than one gene product produces different subunits of an interacting complex or when different genes are involved in the same genetic cascade or physiological pathway. For example, congenital hypothyroidism associated with dyshormonogenesis can arise from mutations in several genes (*NIS, TG, TPO, PDS/SLC26A4, DUOX2, DUOXA2, DEHAL1*) located on different chromosomes. The effects of inactivating mutations in these genes are similar because the protein products are all required for normal hormone synthesis. Similarly, the genetic forms of diabetes insipidus can be caused by mutations in several genes. Mutations in the AVP-NPII gene cause autosomal-dominant or -recessive forms of neurohypophyseal diabetes insipidus. The nephrogenic forms can be caused by mutations in the X-chromosomal *AVPR2* receptor gene, whereas mutations in the aquaporin 2 (*AQP2*) gene cause either autosomal-recessive or -dominant nephrogenic diabetes insipidus.

Recognition of non-allelic heterogeneity is important because the ability to identify disease loci in linkage studies is reduced by including patients with similar phenotypes but different genetic disorders. Genetic testing is more complex because several different genes need to be considered along with the possibility of different mutations in each of the candidate genes.

Phenocopies designate a phenotype that is identical or similar but results from non-genetic or other genetic causes. For example, obesity may be caused by several rare Mendelian defects, the result of a complex disorder or have a primarily behavioral origin. As in non-allelic heterogeneity, the presence of phenocopies has the potential to confound linkage studies and genetic testing. Patient history, subtle differences in clinical presentation and rigorous clinical testing are key in assigning the correct phenotype.

Variable expressivity and incomplete penetrance

Penetrance and *expressivity* are two different yet related concepts which are often confused. Penetrance is a qualitative notion designating whether a phenotype is expressed for a particular geno-type. Expressivity is a quantitative concept describing the degree to which a phenotype is expressed. It is used to describe the phenotypic spectrum in individuals with a particular disorder. Thus, expressivity is dependent on penetrance.

Penetrance is complete if all carriers of a mutant express the phenotype, whereas it is said to be *incomplete* if some individuals do not have any features of the phenotype. Dominant conditions with incomplete penetrance are characterized by skipping of generations with unaffected carriers transmitting the mutant gene. For example, hypertrophic obstructive cardiomyopathy (HOCM) caused by mutations in the *myosin-binding protein C* gene is a dominant disorder with clinical features in only a subset of patients who carry the mutation. Incomplete penetrance in some individuals can confound pedigree analysis. In many conditions with postnatal onset, the proportion of gene carriers affected varies with age. Therefore, it is important to specify age when describing penetrance. Variable expressivity is used to describe the phenotypic spectrum in individuals with a particular disorder.

Some of the mechanisms underlying expressivity and penetrance include modifier genes (*genetic background*), gender and environmental factors. Thus, variable expressivity and penetrance illustrate that genetic and/or environmental factors do not influence only complex disorders but also "simple" Mendelian traits. This has to be considered in genetic counseling, because one cannot always predict the course of disease, even when the mutation is known.

Sex-influenced phenotypes

Certain mutations affect males and females quite differently. In some instances, this is because the gene resides on the X or Y sex chromosomes. As a result, the phenotype of mutated X-linked genes will usually be expressed fully in males but variably in heterozygous females, depending on the degree of X-inactivation and the function of the gene. Because only males have a Y chromosome, mutations in genes such as *SRY* (which causes male-to-female sex reversal) or *DAZ* (*deleted in azoospermia*), which causes abnormalities of spermatogenesis, are unique to males.

Other diseases are expressed in a sex-limited manner because of the differential function of the gene product in males and females. Activating mutations in the luteinizing hormone receptor (LHR) cause dominant male-limited precocious puberty in boys. The phenotype is unique to males because activation of the receptor induces testosterone production in the testis, whereas it is functionally silent in the immature ovary. Homozygous inactivating mutations of the follicle-stimulating hormone (FSH) receptor cause primary ovarian failure in females because the follicles do not develop in the absence of FSH action. Affected males have a more subtle phenotype, because testosterone production allowing sexual maturation is preserved and spermatogenesis is only partially impaired. In congenital adrenal hyperplasia, most commonly caused by 21-hydroxylase deficiency, cortisol production is impaired and ACTH stimulation of the adrenal gland leads to increased production of androgenic precursors. In females, the increased androgen concentration causes ambiguous genitalia, which can be recognized at birth. In males, the diagnosis may be made on the basis of adrenal insufficiency at birth because the increased adrenal androgen level does not alter sexual differentiation or later in childhood because of the development of precocious puberty.

Approach to the patient

Clinical and biochemical evaluation is the first step in any attempt to unravel underlying pathogenic mechanisms. The family history is important to recognize the possibility of a hereditary component. For this purpose, it is extremely useful to draw a pedigree of the nuclear and, in some cases, of the extended family. This should include information about ethnic background, age, health status and deaths, particularly deaths in infancy which may have been forgotten. The physician should explore whether other individuals within the family are affected by the same or a related illness as the index patient. This should be followed by a survey for the presence of commonly occurring disorders.

Because of the possibility of age-dependent expressivity and penetrance, the family history may need updating on subsequent encounters. If the family history or other findings suggest a genetic disorder, the clinician has to assess whether some of the patient's relatives may be at risk of carrying or transmitting the disease. This information may become of practical relevance for carrier detection, genetic counseling or early intervention and prevention of a disease in relatives.

Where a diagnosis at the molecular level may be available, the physician faces several challenges. Genetic testing in children poses distinct ethical issues. In general, it should be limited to situations in which it has an immediate impact on the medical management of that child; it requires informed consent by the parents. If there is no apparent benefit, testing should usually be deferred until the patient can consent independently. This is particularly relevant in devastating disorders that manifest only later in life, such as Huntington disease.

If genetic testing is considered an option, the physician will have to identify an appropriate laboratory to perform the test. The *GeneTests* web site (http://www.genetests.org/servlet/access), a publicly funded medical genetics resource, contains an international Laboratory Directory which is useful for identifying approved laboratories offering testing for inherited disorders (Table 1.1). For rare disorders, the test may only be available through research laboratories.

If a disease-causing mutation is expected in all cells as a result of germline transmission, DNA can be collected from any tissue, most commonly nucleated blood cells or buccal cells, for cytogenetic and mutational analyses. In the case of somatic mutations, which are limited to neoplastic tissue, an adequate sample of the lesion will serve for the extraction of DNA or RNA. For the detection of pathogens, the material to be analyzed will vary and may include blood, cerebrospinal fluid, solid tissues, sputum or fluid obtained through bronchoalveolar lavage.

New findings on the genetic basis of endocrine disorders are published in numerous scientific journals, books and databases.

The continuously updated OMIM catalog lists several thousand genetic disorders and provides information about the clinical phenotype, molecular basis, allelic variants and pertinent animal models (Table 1.1). Hyperlinks to other electronic resources (e.g. PubMed, GenBank or databases compiling gene mutations) provide access to useful information that is relevant for both clinicians and basic scientists.

Chromosomal disorders

Chromosomal (cytogenetic) disorders are caused by numerical or structural aberrations in chromosomes. Large duplications and deletions are well recognized as cause of specific genetic disorders. Molecular cytogenetics has led to the identification of more subtle chromosome abnormalities such as microdeletions and duplications, imprinting syndromes and genomic imbalances brought about by CNVs.

Errors in meiosis and early cleavage divisions occur frequently. Ten to 25% of all conceptions harbor chromosomal abnormalities, which often lead to spontaneous abortion in early pregnancy. Numerical abnormalities, especially trisomy, which is found in about 25% of spontaneous abortions and 0.3% of newborns, are more common than structural defects. Trisomy 21, the most frequent cause of Down syndrome, occurs in 1:600–1000 live births. Trisomies 13 and 18 are also frequent.

Numerical abnormalities in sex chromosomes are relatively common. Males with a 47,XXY karyotype have Klinefelter syndrome and females with trisomy 47,XXX may be subfertile. Autosomal monosomies are usually incompatible with life but 45,XO is present in 1–2% of all conceptuses but leads to spontaneous abortion in 99% of cases. Mosaicism (e.g. 45,XO/45,XX, 45,XO/45,XXX), partial deletions, isochromosomes and ring chromosomes can also cause Turner syndrome. Sex chromosome monosomy usually results from loss of the paternal sex chromosome. 47,XXY can result from paternal or maternal non-disjunction, while the autosomal trisomies are most commonly caused by maternal non-disjunction during meiosis I, a defect that increases with maternal age. Trisomies are typically associated with alterations in genetic recombination.

Structural rearrangements involve breakage and reunion of chromosomes. Rearrangements between different chromosomes, *translocations*, can be *reciprocal* or *Robertsonian*. Reciprocal translocations involve exchanges between any of the chromosomes; Robertsonian rearrangements designate the fusion of the long arms of two acrocentric chromosomes. Other structural defects include deletions, duplications, inversions and the formation of rings and isochromosomes. Deletions affecting several tightly clustered genes result in *contiguous gene syndromes*, disorders that mimic a combination of single gene defects. They have been useful for identifying the location of new disease-causing genes. Because of the variable size of gene deletions in different patients, a systematic comparison of phenotypes and locations of deletion breakpoints allows the positions of particular genes to be mapped within the critical genomic region. Structural chromosome defects can be present in a "balanced" form without an abnormal phenotype. However, they can be transmitted in an "unbalanced" form to offspring and thus cause an hereditary form of chromosome abnormality.

Paternal deletions of chromosome 15q11-13 cause Prader–Willi syndrome (PWS), while maternal deletions are associated with Angelman syndrome. The difference in phenotype results from the fact that this chromosomal region is imprinted, i.e. differentially expressed on the maternal and paternal chromosome.

Traditional karyotype analysis usually identifies chromosomal rearrangements and/or aberrations of 3–5 Mb and larger. Comparative genomic hybridization and other techniques now permit the detection of more subtle, submicroscopic chromosomal imbalances such as CNVs. The clinical relevance of these alterations is not always known. The *Database of Chromosomal Imbalance and Phenotype in Humans using Ensembl Resources* (DECIPHER, http://www.sanger.ac.uk/PostGenomics/decipher) catalogs pertinent genomic and clinical information of such patients and can assist in the interpretation of genome-wide, high-resolution tests.

Acquired somatic abnormalities in chromosome structure are often associated with malignancies and are important for diagnosis, classification and prognosis. Deletions can lead to loss of tumor suppressor genes or DNA repair genes. Duplications, amplifications and rearrangements, in which a gene is put under the control of another promoter, can result in gain-of-function of genes controlling cell proliferation. For example, rearrangement of the 5′ regulatory region of the *parathyroid* (*PTH*) gene located on chromosome 11q15 with the *cyclin D1* gene from 11q13 creates the *PRAD1* oncogene, resulting in overexpression of cyclin D1 and the development of parathyroid adenomas.

Monogenic Mendelian disorders

Monogenic human diseases are often called *Mendelian disorders* because they obey the rules of genetic transmission defined by Gregor Mendel. The mode of inheritance for a given phenotype or disease is determined by pedigree analysis. About 65% of human monogenic disorders are autosomal dominant, 25% are autosomal recessive and 5% are X-linked. Genetic testing now available for many of these disorders has an increasingly important role in clinical medicine.

Autosomal-dominant disorders

In autosomal-dominant disorders, mutations in a single allele are sufficient to cause the disease; recessive disorders are the consequence of biallelic loss-of-function mutations. Various disease mechanisms are involved in dominant disorders, which include gain-of-function, a dominant-negative effect, and haploinsufficiency. In autosomal-dominant disorders, individuals are affected in successive generations and the disease does not occur in the offspring of unaffected individuals. Males and females are affected with equal frequency because the defective gene resides on one of the 22 autosomes. Because the alleles

segregate randomly at meiosis, the probability that an offspring will be affected is 50%. Children with a normal genotype do not transmit the disorder. The clinician must be aware that an autosomal-dominant disorder can be caused by *de novo* germline mutations, which occur more frequently during later cell divisions in gametogenesis, explaining why siblings are rarely affected. New germline mutations occur more frequently in fathers of advanced age. The clinical manifestations of autosomal-dominant disorders may be variable as a result of differences in *penetrance* or *expressivity*. Because of these variations, it is sometimes difficult to determine the pattern of inheritance.

Autosomal-recessive disorders

The clinical expression of autosomal-recessive disorders is usually more uniform than in autosomal-dominant disorders. Most mutated alleles lead to a partial or complete loss-of-function. They frequently involve receptors, proteins in signaling cascades or enzymes in metabolic pathways. The affected individual, who can be of either sex, is homozygous or compound heterozygous for a single gene defect. In most instances, an affected individual is the offspring of heterozygous parents. In this situation, there is a 25% chance that the offspring will have a normal genotype, a 50% probability of a heterozygous state and a 25% risk of homozygosity for the recessive alleles. In the case of one unaffected heterozygous and one affected homozygous parent, the probability of disease increases to 50% for each child. In this instance, the pedigree analysis mimics an autosomal-dominant mode of inheritance (*pseudodominance*). In contrast to autosomal-dominant disorders, new mutations in recessive alleles usually result in an asymptomatic carrier state without apparent clinical phenotype.

Many autosomal-recessive diseases are rare and occur more frequently in isolated populations in the context of parental consanguinity. A few recessive disorders, such as sickle cell anemia, cystic fibrosis and thalassemia, are relatively frequent in certain populations, perhaps because the heterozygous state may confer a selective biological advantage. Although heterozygous carriers of a defective allele are usually clinically normal, they may display subtle differences in phenotype that become apparent only with more precise testing or in the context of certain environmental influences.

X-linked disorders

Because males have only one X chromosome, a female individual always inherits her father's X chromosome in addition to one of the two X chromosomes of her mother. A son inherits the Y chromosome from his father and one maternal X chromosome. The characteristic features of X-linked inheritance are therefore the absence of father-to-son transmission and the fact that all daughters of an affected male are obligate carriers of the mutant allele. The risk of developing disease caused by a mutant X-chromosomal gene differs in the two sexes. Because males have only one X chromosome, they are hemizygous for the mutant allele. Consequently, they are more likely to develop the mutant phenotype, regardless of whether the mutation is dominant or recessive. A female may be either heterozygous or homozygous for the mutant allele, which may be dominant or recessive, and the terms *X-linked dominant* or *X-linked recessive* apply only to the expression of the mutant phenotype in women. In females, the expression of X-chromosomal genes is influenced by X chromosome inactivation. This can confound the assessment because skewed X-inactivation may lead to a partial phenotype in female carriers of an X-linked recessive defect, such as inactivating mutations of the AVPR2 receptor, the cause of X-linked nephrogenic diabetes insipidus.

Y-linked disorders

The Y chromosome harbors relatively few genes. Among them, the sex region-determining Y factor (*SRY*), which encodes the testis-determining factor (TDF), is essential for normal male development. Because the *SRY* region is closely adjacent to the pseudoautosomal region, a chromosomal segment on the X and Y chromosomes with a high degree of homology, crossing-over can occasionally involve the *SRY* region. Translocations can result in XY females, with the Y chromosome lacking the *SRY* gene, or XX males harboring the *SRY* gene on one of the X chromosomes. Point mutations in the *SRY* gene may result in individuals with an XY genotype and an incomplete female phenotype. Men with oligospermia or azoospermia frequently have microdeletions of the AZF (azoospermia factor) regions on the long arm of the Y chromosome, which contain several genes involved in the control of spermatogenesis. They may have point mutations in the transcription factor DAZ (deleted in azoospermia), which is located in this chromosomal region.

Exceptions to simple Mendelian inheritance
Mitochondrial disorders

Mendelian inheritance refers to the transmission of genes encoded by DNA in nuclear chromosomes but each mitochondrion contains several copies of a circular chromosome. mtDNA is small (16.5 kb) and encodes transfer and ribosomal RNAs and 13 proteins that are part of the respiratory chain involved in oxidative phosphorylation and ATP generation. In contrast to the nuclear chromosomes, the mitochondrial genome does not recombine and is inherited through the maternal line because sperm does not contribute significant cytoplasmic components to the zygote. The D-loop, a non-coding region of the mitochondrial chromosome, is highly polymorphic. This property, together with the absence of recombination of mtDNA, makes it a helpful tool for studies tracing human migration and evolution and for specific forensic applications.

Inherited mitochondrial disorders are transmitted in a matrilineal fashion. All children from an affected mother inherit the disease but it will never be transmitted from an affected father to his offspring except by intracytoplasmic sperm injection (ICSI). Alterations in the mtDNA affecting enzymes required for oxidative phosphorylation lead to reduction of ATP supply, generation

of free radicals and induction of apoptosis. Several syndromic disorders arising from mutations in the mitochondrial genome are known in humans and they affect both protein-coding and tRNA genes. The pleiotropic clinical spectrum often involves (cardio)myopathies and encephalopathies because of the high dependence of these tissues on oxidative phosphorylation.

Many may present with endocrine features. For example, the mitochondrial DIDMOAD syndrome consists of diabetes insipidus, diabetes mellitus, optic atrophy and deafness. The age of onset and the clinical course are variable because of the unusual mechanisms of mtDNA replication. mtDNA replicates independently from nuclear DNA and, during cell replication, the proportion of wild type and mutant mitochondria can drift among different cells and tissues. The resulting heterogeneity in the proportion of mitochondria with and without a mutation is referred to as *heteroplasmia* and underlies the phenotypic variability that is characteristic of mitochondrial diseases. Nuclear genes that encode proteins that are important for normal mitochondrial function can cause mitochondrial dysfunctions associated with autosomal-dominant or -recessive forms of inheritance.

Acquired somatic mutations in mitochondrial genes are thought to be involved in several age-dependent degenerative disorders involving muscle and the peripheral and central nervous systems. Because of the high degree of polymorphisms in mtDNA and the phenotypic variability of these disorders, it is difficult to establish that an mtDNA alteration is causal for a clinical phenotype.

Trinucleotide expansion disorders

Several diseases are associated with an increase in the number of trinucleotide repeats above a certain threshold. In some instances, the repeats are located within the coding region of the genes. For example, an expansion in a CAG repeat in the androgen receptor, which encodes a polyglutamine motif in its amino-terminus, leads to the X-linked form of spinal and bulbar muscular atrophy (SBMA, Kennedy syndrome) and can be associated with partial androgen insensitivity. Similarly, an expansion in the *huntingtin* (*HD*) gene is the cause of Huntington disease. In other instances, the repeats are located in regulatory sequences. If an expansion is present, the DNA fragment is unstable and tends to expand further during cell division; hence the designation *dynamic mutation*. The length of the nucleotide repeat often correlates with the severity of the disease. When repeat length increases from one generation to the next, disease manifestations may worsen or appear at an earlier age, a phenomenon referred to as *anticipation*. In Huntington disease, for example, there is a correlation between age of onset and length of the triplet codon expansion.

Mosaicism

Mosaicism refers to the presence of two or more genetically distinct cell lines in the tissues of an individual. It results from a mutation that occurs during embryonic, fetal or extrauterine development. The developmental stage at which the mutation arises will determine whether germ cells and/or somatic cells are involved. Chromosomal mosaicism results from non-disjunction at an early embryonic mitotic division, leading to the persistence of more than one cell line, as exemplified by some patients with Turner syndrome. Somatic mosaicism is characterized by a patchy distribution of genetically altered somatic cells that occurs early in development. This is best illustrated by the McCune–Albright syndrome, which is caused by activating mutations in the *GNAS1* gene encoding the stimulatory G-protein α (Gsα). The clinical phenotype varies depending on the tissue distribution of the mutation. Manifestations include ovarian cysts that secrete sex steroids and cause precocious puberty, polyostotic fibrous dysplasia, café-au-lait skin pigmentation, growth hormone-secreting pituitary adenomas and, among others, hypersecreting autonomous thyroid nodules.

Epigenetic modifications, X-inactivation, imprinting and uniparental disomy

According to traditional Mendelian principles, the parental origin of a mutant gene is irrelevant for the expression of the phenotype, although there are important exceptions to this rule. X-inactivation prevents the expression of most genes on one of the two X chromosomes in every cell of a female (*Lyonization*). Gene inactivation also occurs on selected chromosomal regions of autosomes. This phenomenon, *genomic imprinting*, leads to preferential expression of an allele depending on its parental origin. It is of importance in disorders in which the transmission of disease is dependent on the sex of the transmitting parent and has an important role in the expression of certain genetic disorders.

The two classic examples are the Prader–Willi and Angelman syndromes. PWS is characterized by diminished fetal activity, obesity, hypotonia, mental retardation, short stature and hypogonadotrophic hypogonadism. Deletions in PWS occur exclusively on the paternal chromosome 15. Patients with Angelman syndrome present with mental retardation, seizures, ataxia and hypotonia and have deletions at the same site of chromosome 15 but they are located on the maternal chromosome 15. These two syndromes may also result from *uniparental disomy*, i.e. by the inheritance of either two maternal chromosomes 15 (PWS) or two paternal chromosomes (Angelman syndrome).

Another example of importance for pediatric endocrinology concerns the *GNAS1* gene encoding the Gsα subunit. Heterozygous loss-of-function mutations in the *GNAS1* gene lead to Albright hereditary osteodystrophy (AHO) with its characteristic features including short stature, obesity, round face, brachydactyly, subcutaneous ossifications and mental deficits. Paternal transmission of *GNAS1* mutations leads to the AHO phenotype alone (*pseudo*pseudohypoparathyroidism), while maternal transmission leads to AHO in combination with resistance to several hormones such as PTH, thyroid-stimulating hormone (TSH) and gonadotropins, which act through transmembrane receptors coupling to Gsα (pseudohypoparathyroidism type IA). These phenotypic differences result from a tissue-specific imprinting of *GNAS1*, which is expressed primarily from the maternal allele in tissues such as the proximal renal tubule and the thyroid. In most other tissues, however, it is expressed biallelically. Disrupting mutations in the maternal allele lead to loss of Gsα expression in proximal tubules and loss of PTH action in the kidney, while mutations in the paternal allele have little effect on PTH action. In patients with isolated renal resistance to PTH (pseudohypoparathyroidism type IB), an imprinting defect of GNAS1 leads to decreased Gsα expression in the proximal renal tubules.

Somatic mutations

Acquired mutations that occur in somatic rather than germ cells are called *somatic mutations*. This creates a chimeric situation and, if the cells proliferate, a neoplastic lesion. Therefore, cancer can be defined as a genetic disease at the cellular level. Cancers are monoclonal, indicating that they have arisen from a single precursor cell that has acquired one or several mutations in genes controlling growth and/or differentiation. These mutations are somatic, i.e. restricted to the tumor and its metastases, but not found in surrounding normal tissue. The molecular alterations include dominant gain-of-function mutations in oncogenes, recessive loss-of-function mutations in tumor suppressor genes and DNA repair genes, gene amplification and chromosome rearrangements. Rarely, a single mutation in certain genes may be sufficient to transform a normal cell into a malignant cell but the development of a malignant phenotype in most cancers requires several genetic alterations for the gradual progression from a normal to a cancerous cell, a process termed *multistep carcinogenesis*.

In many cancer syndromes, there is an inherited *predisposition* to tumor formation. In these instances, a germline mutation is inherited in an autosomal-dominant fashion. This germline alteration affects one allele of an autosomal tumor suppressor gene. If the second allele is inactivated by a somatic mutation in a given cell, this will lead to neoplastic growth (*Knudson two-hit model*). In this instance, the defective allele in the germline is transmitted in a dominant way, whereas the tumorigenic mechanism results from a recessive loss of the tumor suppressor gene in affected tissues.

The classic example to illustrate this phenomenon is retinoblastoma, which can occur as a sporadic or hereditary tumor. In sporadic retinoblastoma, both copies of the retinoblastoma (*RB*) gene are inactivated through two somatic events. In hereditary retinoblastoma, one mutated or deleted *RB* allele is inherited in an autosomal-dominant manner and the second allele is inactivated by a subsequent somatic mutation. This "two-hit" model applies to other inherited cancer syndromes, such as multiple endocrine neoplasia type 1 (MEN1), which is caused by mutations in the tumor suppressor gene menin.

Inherited defects in enzymes involved in DNA replication and repair can lead to a significant increase in mutations and are associated with several disorders predisposing to cancer.

Complex disorders

Many disorders have a complex etiology involving multiple genes (*polygenic disorders*), often in combination with environmental and lifestyle factors (*multifactorial disorders*). The major health care problems, cardiovascular disease, hypertension, diabetes, obesity, asthma and psychiatric disorders, fall into this category but it also includes certain developmental abnormalities, such as cleft palate, congenital heart defects and neural tube defects.

Compared with single gene defects, complex disorders have a low heritability and do not fit a Mendelian pattern of inheritance. Twin studies are particularly helpful in demonstrating the importance of genetic and environmental factors. For example, first-degree relatives of patients with diabetes mellitus type 1 are about 15 times more likely to develop diabetes. The concordance rate for developing diabetes is about 50% in monozygotic twins and about 8% in dizygotic twins. The discordance rate in monozygotic twins illustrates the significant requirement for environmental factors. In addition, some of the susceptibility genes, a designation indicating that the carrier is susceptible to develop the disease, have a low penetrance. Susceptibility genes or loci can be mapped using several methods, including linkage analyses, association studies and affected sib-pair analyses. Current efforts aim to identify these genes by establishing correlations between SNPs or SNP haplotypes and complex disorders in large populations through GWAS. The HapMap data are significantly facilitating this type of study because they allow genotyping a reduced number of tag SNPs reflecting certain haplotypes (Fig. 1.6). The results of GWAS may, in part, depend on ethnicity and ascertainment criteria.

The study of rare monogenic diseases may also provide insights into genetic and molecular mechanisms important for the understanding of complex disorders. For example, the identification of the genetic defects underlying the various autosomal-dominant forms of MODY have defined them, in part, as candidate genes contributing to the pathogenesis of diabetes mellitus type 2.

Genomics and post-genomic techniques

Broadly defined, genomics designates the discipline of mapping, sequencing and analyzing genomes. The completion of the structural analysis of the human genome (*structural genomics*) has been followed by a rapid emergence of "postgenomic" disciplines focusing on biological function of the gene products (*functional genomics*). These disciplines are concerned with analyses of gene transcripts (*transcriptomics*), proteins and their secondary modifications and interactions (*proteomics*), epigenetic modifications of DNA and chromatin proteins (*epigenomics*), metabolites and their networks (*metabolomics*) and comprehensive analyses of the genomes of microorganisms populating specific compartments (*metagenomics*). The ultimate goal is the integration of these complementary data into a *systems biology* that permits a comprehensive definition of the phenotype and pathophysiological perturbations.

What can be expected from these developments? Genotyping may become important for stratifying patients according to disease risk and for predicting the response to certain drugs. Gene expression studies can be used for the assessment of prognosis and for guiding therapy. Proteomic studies may allow diagnosis of early stages of malignancy. Because most drug targets are proteins, proteomics will be important for drug discovery and development. These technologies, individually and in combination, permit first insights into the pathogenesis of complex disorders. Genomic approaches may have further impact on health care as a result of a thorough understanding of the genomes and proteins of infectious agents (e.g. *Plasmodium falciparum* or *Mycobacterium tuberculosis*), which may lead to the development of novel therapeutic strategies and compounds. Comprehensive genomic analyses of the metagenome are expected to provide new insights in the interactions between the host and the microbial environment in health and disease.

Comparative genomics

Comparative genomics involves the analysis of two or more genomes to identify the extent of similarity or large-scale screening of a genome to identify sequences present in another genome. Applications involve comparisons of prokaryotic and eukaryotic genomes to infer evolutionary relationships. The detection of high evolutionary conservation can be used as a screen for regulatory elements within otherwise poorly conserved non-coding DNA. Electronic screening of expressed sequence tags (EST) databases can identify homologs of genes in other species. For example, systematic screening of the *dbEST* database of ESTs has revealed many relevant human homologs of *Drosophila* genes known to be loci for mutant phenotypes.

Pharmacogenomics

Broadly defined, the scope of pharmacogenetics and pharmacogenomics is to define how the genome influences the response of an individual to a drug. Although many non-genetic factors influence the effects of medications, genetic polymorphisms in receptors, transporters, channels and enzymes can result in variable absorption, distribution, metabolism and excretion of a drug that ultimately lead to differential response or toxic concentrations. For example, a polymorphism in thiopurine methyltransferase (TMT) inactivates the enzyme and is associated with hematopoietic toxicity of mercaptopurine. Determination of the TMT genotype is therefore important for choosing a safe dose of the medication. In other instances, drug effects will be influenced by polymorphisms in multiple genes.

Further development of genotyping and pharmacogenomics may improve the safety of medical therapy by choosing appropriate medications and dose levels, thereby decreasing the number of adverse drug reactions. It is also expected that this discipline will have an impact on drug development because screenings of SNPs can be used to enroll or exclude subgroups of patients.

Transcriptomics

mRNA expression of one or a few genes has usually been determined by Northern blot analysis, a technique that has been largely replaced by semiquantitative RT-PCR, but both techniques permit only the analysis of the expression pattern of a limited number of genes. Paralleling the characterization of the genomic sequences of humans and other organisms, as well as the genes that they encode, various *expression profiling* techniques have been developed. These analyses enable surveys of gene expression patterns for thousands of genes in a single assay (Fig. 1.9). Such profiles are useful for the understanding of gene regulation and interactions in normal and pathologic tissues. As the complement of mRNAs transcribed by the cellular genome is also referred to as the *transcriptome*, the generation of mRNA expression profiles is now also referred to as *transcriptomics*.

The most widely used techniques for expression profiling include microarrays and serial analysis of gene expression (SAGE). After hybridization with the labeled probes, the microarrays are scanned and special software allows analysis of the fluorescence intensities for each spot (Fig. 1.9). The limitations of microarray technology include relatively high cost, special equipment and the inability to detect novel transcripts but SAGE is a powerful tool that allows a comprehensive analysis of gene expression patterns without the requirement of pre-existing probes or sophisticated equipment.

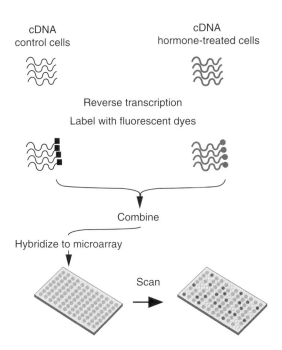

Figure 1.9 Principle of a microarray experiment. A large number of probes, cDNA sequences or DNA oligonucleotides are spotted on a glass slide. RNA is extracted from a control sample and a test sample, for example a tumor or treated cells. After differential labeling of the two RNA populations with fluorescent probes, the samples are mixed and hybridized to the probes on the slide. The slide is then scanned once for each fluorophore. The intensity of the emitted signal on each spot permits calculation of the ratios of each RNA that binds to the respective probe.

The simplest way to identify genes of potential interest by expression profiling is to search for those that are consistently upregulated or downregulated. The identification of *patterns* of gene expression and regulated *classes* of genes may, however, provide more informative insights into their biological function and relevance. Genes that are part of a particular pathway or that respond to a common endogenous or exogenous stimulus are expected to be co-regulated and should consequently show similar patterns of expression. Several computational techniques, such as hierarchical clustering, self-organizing maps and mutual information, are used for the analysis of gene expression data. The choice of the appropriate algorithm(s) for these analyses is a crucial element of the experimental design and the methods that are used to analyze the data can have a profound influence on the interpretation of the results.

Epigenomics

Eukaryotic genomes contain modifications of DNA or chromatin proteins. The totality of these epigenetic marks is designated as an *epigenome*. In contrast to the genome, the epigenome is highly variable between cells and changes within a single cell over time. Epigenetic modifications vary among different regions throughout the genome and result in alterations in levels of gene transcription. Thus, epigenetic changes and inheritance result in phenotypic consequences without changing the DNA sequence. Importantly, epigenetic marks can be heritable. They are propagated to the daughter cells during cell division and certain loci within the genome are paternally or maternally imprinted.

Epigenetic modifications consist of methylation of DNA, acetylation or methylation of histone proteins and interaction of proteins with histones. In eukaryotes, DNA methylation is found exclusively at cytosine residues. DNA methylation is involved in the repression of genes in the inactivated X chromosome (increased methylation in promoter regions, decreased methylation in intragenic regions) and it has an important role in imprinting, the establishment and maintenance of the allele-specific expression of maternally or paternally inherited genes. In mammalian genomes, the majority of the genome is methylated and all categories of DNA sequences, such as genes, intergenic regions and transposons (segments of DNA capable of independent replication and insertion of a copy into a new position within the same or another chromosome), can be the target of methylation. Unmethylated domains account for only about 2% of the genome and often consist of so-called CpG islands, DNA regions of ~1000 bp with a high occurrence of the dinucleotide CG. CpG islands are very frequently found in promoters and they are usually unmethylated, at least in germline DNA.

Although most CpG islands remain unmethylated, independent of expression state, a minority become methylated during development resulting in silencing of the associated gene. During mitosis, the DNA replication results in the generation of a methylated and an unmethylated strand; the hemimethylated DNA is subsequently converted to a fully methylated state by methyltransferases and the methylation status is therefore maintained.

The importance of conserving the methylation status is illustrated by the fact that mutations in methyltransferases result in disease. Mutations in the MECP2 result in Rett syndrome (autism, dementia, ataxia) and mutations in the DNMT3B cause the immunodeficiency–centromeric instability–facial anomalies syndrome.

On the inactive X chromosome, a large number of CpG islands become heavily methylated and the associated genes are no longer expressed. Without inactivation of one X chromosome in every cell of a female, the differences in the number of X chromosomes between females and males would result in the expression of the double amount of each gene product in females. In order to avoid this, dosage compensation is required. The inactivation of one X chromosome is dependent on the *X inactivation center* (Xic). The Xic locus is necessary to count the number of X chromosomes and it ensures that all but one X chromosome are inactivated. It also contains a gene called *Xist*. The *Xist* gene codes for an RNA that is not translated into a protein. The *Xist* RNA binds to one of the X chromosomes, which results in secondary events that silence the chromosome through methylation and deacetylation of histones. Once the inactivation of one of the X chromosomes has occurred, the pattern is passed on to descendant cells during mitosis.

Differential methylation of paternal and maternal alleles results in *imprinting* and results in a difference in the expression between the alleles inherited from each parent. Methylation is usually associated with inactivation of the imprinted gene. Remarkably, the imprinting pattern is inherited. Because one chromosome is imprinted, a lack of the other chromosome or the inheritance of two copies from the same parent can result in disease if it involves an imprinted chromosome or locus (e.g. PWS and Angelman syndrome). The faithful inheritance of the methylation pattern in germ cells involves a two-step process during gametogenesis (Fig. 1.10). First, the methylation is erased by a genome-wide demethylation and then the pattern specific for each sex is imposed on both alleles. This ensures that the pattern in the zygote is identical to the one originally present in the paternal and maternal somatic cells (Fig. 1.10).

Overall, the understanding of how epigenetic variation impacts health and disease is in its early stages. It is established that aberrant DNA methylation is involved in the development of malignancies. Deletion of imprinted loci or uniparental disomy are well recognized as a cause of a series of syndromic phenotypes. Significant differences in DNA methylation have also been reported in monozygotic twins. Epigenetic phenomena may also be of importance in the pathogenesis of complex disorders. Further insights into the contribution of epigenetic modifications in the development of disease are expected to be gained in the near future through comprehensive analyses at the level of the whole genome with the newly available high-throughput technologies.

Proteomics

The term *proteome* designates the complete set of proteins expressed by the genome. *Proteomics* includes studies focusing on the expression and function of the proteome, as well as aspects of structural biology. The study of the proteome is difficult because it is so dynamic. Apart from the expression of isoforms, proteins undergo a plethora of secondary modifications and protein–protein interactions (*interactome*) and they form higher order complexes.

Comprehensive analyses of the proteome relied initially on protein separation by two-dimensional gel electrophoresis with subsequent mass spectrometric identification of protein spots. This approach is constrained to the most abundant proteins in the sample. Studies of the proteome are now performed predominantly with direct mass spectrometric analyses, which have undergone technological refinement and can identify ever smaller amounts of proteins from complex mixtures.

The classic methodology for studying protein–protein interactions was the yeast two-hybrid system. Currently, various protein- and antibody-based arrays are emerging to study protein activities, secondary modifications and interactions. *Structural proteomics* has the ambitious goal of systematically understanding the structural basis for protein interactions and function.

Clinical proteomics aims to use proteomic patterns for disease detection and surveillance. In this approach, high-throughput mass spectrometry generates a proteomic fingerprint of a diagnostic sample, such as serum, fine-needle or nipple fluid aspirate. Bioinformatic pattern recognition algorithms can then be applied to identify patterns of protein alterations that can discriminate benign from malignant tissues. Importantly, the specific pattern itself could be diagnostic and the underlying identities of the proteins that comprise the patterns do not need to be known. As well as identifying novel diagnostic and prognostic biomarkers for human cancer, proteomics is also expected to have an impact on drug discovery and action, given that most drugs target proteins and subsequently modify intracellular networks.

Inspired by the success of the Human Genome Project, the Human Proteome Organization (HUPO) aims at coordinating proteomic research (http://www.hupo.org/). Major current goals in proteomics include definition of the plasma proteome, analyses of specific cell types, mapping of organelle compositions, generation of antibodies to all human proteins, generation of protein interaction maps and analyses of important model and pathogenic organisms.

Metabolomics

The *metabolome* can be defined as the quantitative complement of all the low-molecular-weight molecules present in cells in a particular physiological or developmental state. While metabolomics is complementary to transcriptomics and proteomics, there are several attractive reasons for analyzing the metabolome. Relative to alterations in the transcriptome and the proteome, changes in the metabolome are often amplified. Moreover, alterations in metabolic fluxes are not regulated by gene expression alone and, reflecting the activities of the cell at a functional level, affect the concentrations of numerous individual metabolites. High-throughput analyses of metabolites can be performed with tools such as nuclear magnetic resonance spectroscopy and mass spec-

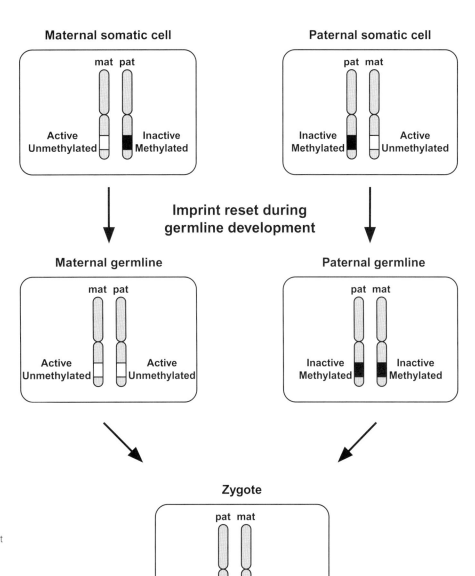

Maternal somatic cell

mat pat

Active
Unmethylated

Inactive
Methylated

Paternal somatic cell

pat mat

Inactive
Methylated

Active
Unmethylated

**Imprint reset during
germline development**

Maternal germline

mat pat

Active
Unmethylated

Active
Unmethylated

Paternal germline

pat mat

Inactive
Methylated

Inactive
Methylated

Zygote

pat mat

Inactive
Methylated

Active
Unmethylated

Figure 1.10 Imprint reset. Certain genomic regions are imprinted in a parent-specific fashion. The unmethylated chromosomal region is actively expressed, the methylated region is silenced and not expressed. In the germline, the imprint is reset. In this case, both chromosomes are unmethylated in the maternal germline and methylated in the paternal germline. In the zygote, the imprinting pattern is again identical with the situation in the somatic cells of the parents.

troscopy. Because of the complexity and heterogeneity of metabolites and the fact that the metabolic complement is even more dynamic than the proteome, the technical and computational challenges are substantial and this discipline is still in its early stages. However, it has already had a profound conceptual impact because of the ongoing shift from simple *metabolic pathways* to *metabolic networks*.

Bioinformatics

The enormous amounts of diverse biological data generated by recent biotechnological advances have led to the development and evolution of *bioinformatics*, in which biology and information technology converge. Initially, bioinformatics focused on the development and creation of nucleotide and protein databases

and methods for the analysis of the deposited sequences. The application of bioinformatics for analysis of nucleotide and polypeptide sequences is well established and widely used. The largest of these sequence databases include GenBank at the National Center for Biotechnology Information (NCBI), Ensembl at the European Molecular Biology Laboratory (EMBL), the DNA Data Bank of Japan and SwissProt, among others (Table 1.1). They permit rapid retrieval of sequence information of genomic DNA, mRNA, ESTs, SNPs or polypeptides for a rapidly growing number of species. The evolution of these databases has been accompanied by expanding capabilities to annotate sequences, linking the data with other electronic resources and more sophisticated tools for analysis of nucleotide and protein sequences. It is crucial that bioinformatics software development is linked at an early stage through agreed documentation, standardized rules for structuring web forms [eXtensible Markup Language (XML)] and controlled vocabularies that allow different tools to exchange primary data sets.

Navigation in this web of continuously evolving databases is often intimidating but the high degree of interconnection between the multitude of databases permits relatively easy exploration of this knowledge. User guides and the online NCBI handbook (Table 1.1) provide helpful instructions to questions such as the following:

1 How does one find a gene of interest and determine the structure of this gene?

2 How can one find information about SNPs?

3 How can one find all the members of a human gene family?

4 For a given protein, how can one determine whether it contains any functional domains of interest?

5 What other proteins contain the same functional domains as this protein?

6 How can one determine whether there is a similarity to other proteins, not only at the sequence level but also at the structural level?

Sequence alignments are performed most easily with the Basic Local Alignment Search Tool (BLAST), which compares a DNA or polypeptide sequence of interest with nucleotide or protein databases. In addition to determining the identity of an isolated nucleotide or protein fragment, this approach can detect similar related sequences in one or several organisms. This type of comparison is the basis for the development of gene and protein families and unravels evolutionary relationships. The sensitivity and specificity of a BLAST search can be modified in such a way that even discrete homologies can be unraveled. By referring to databases of known regulatory element sequences, computer programs can inspect genomic sequences for the presence of regulatory elements. Motifs (i.e. specific amino acid patterns associated with defined functions) can be identified by submitting a polypeptide to computational analysis. This may permit assignment of a protein to functional and structural families and making predictions on the functional role of newly isolated proteins.

As more protein structures are identified, the relationship between structure and function becomes easier to predict. The development of more accurate algorithms for predicting and modeling secondary and tertiary structures is, in part, moving out of the laboratory and into the hands of bioinformaticists.

The field of bioinformatics is now challenged to integrate the data generated by the various "-omic" techniques with the hope of elucidating the functional relationships between genotype and observed phenotype, thereby permitting a system-wide analysis from genome to phenome.

Acknowledgments

This work has, in part, been supported by 1R01DK63024-01 from NIH/NIDDK.

Bibliography

A user's guide to the human genome. *Nat Genet* 2003; **35**: 1–79.

Alberts B, Bray D, Lewis J, *et al.* (eds). *Molecular Biology of the Cell*, 4th edn. New York: Garland, 2002.

Antonarakis SE. Recommendations for a nomenclature system for human gene mutations. Nomenclature Working Group. *Hum Mutat* 1998; **11**: 1–3.

Beckmann JS, Estivill X, Antonarakis SE. Copy number variants and genetic traits: closer to the resolution of phenotypic to genotypic variability. *Nat Rev Genet* 2007; **8**: 639–646.

Bejjani BA, Shaffer LG. Clinical utility of contemporary molecular cytogenetics. *Annu Rev Genomics Hum Genet* 2008; **9**: 71–86.

Clayton EW. Ethical, legal and social implications of genomic medicine. *N Engl J Med* 2003; **349**: 562–569.

Collins FS, Green ED, Guttmacher AE, Guyer MS. A vision for the future of genomics research. *Nature* 2003; **422**: 835–847.

Collins FS. Shattuck Lecture: medical and societal consequences of the Human Genome Project. *N Engl J Med* 1999; **341**: 28–37.

Congdon T, Nguyen LQ, Nogueira CR, *et al.* A novel mutation (Q40P) in PAX8 associated with congenital hypothyroidism and thyroid hypoplasia: evidence for phenotypic variability in mother and child. *J Clin Endocrinol Metab* 2001; **86**: 3962–3967.

De Bakker PIW, Yelensky R, Pe'er I, *et al.* Efficiency and power in genetic association studies. *Nature Genetics* 2005; **37**: 1217–1223.

Den Dunnen JT, Antonarakis SE. Mutation nomenclature extensions and suggestions to describe complex mutations: a discussion. *Hum Mutat* 2000; **15**: 7–12.

Emery AEH, Mueller R, Young I, *et al. Emery's Elements of Medical Genetics*, 13th edn. New York: Churchill Livingston, 2007.

Feuk L, Carson AR, Scherer SW. Structural variation in the human genome. *Nat Rev Genet* 2006; **7**: 85–97.

Florez JC, Hirschhorn J, Altshuler D. The inherited basis of diabetes mellitus: implications for the genetic analysis of complex traits. *Annu Rev Genomics Hum Genet* 2003; **4**: 257–291.

Foster MW, Sharp RR. Out of sequence: how consumer genomics could displace clinical genetics. *Nat Rev Genet* 2008; **9**: 419.

Freeman JL, Perry GH, Feuk L, *et al.* Copy number variation: New insights in genome diversity. *Genome Res* 2006; **16**: 949–961.

Goldstein DB, Cavalleri GL. Genomics: Understanding human diversity. *Nature* 2005; **437**: 1241–1242.

Guttmacher AE, Collins FS. Genomic medicine: a primer. *N Engl J Med* 2002; **347**: 1512–1520.

Harper PS. *Practical Genetic Counseling*, 6th edn. Stoneham, MA: Butterworth-Heinemann, 2004.

Hinds, DA, Stuve LL, Nilsen GB, *et al.* Whole genome patterns of common DNA variation in three human populations. *Science* 2005; **307**: 1072–1079.

Hoedemaekers R, Gordijn B, Pijnenburg M. Solidarity and justice as guiding principles in genomic research. *Bioethics* 2007; **21**: 342–350.

HUGO Mutation Database Initiative. Issues, databases and perspectives for the new millennium. *Hum Mutat* 2000; **15**: 1.

International HapMap Consortium. A second generation human haplotype map of over 3.1 million SNPs. *Nature* 2007; **449**: 851–861.

International Human Genome Mapping Consortium. A physical map of the human genome. *Nature* 2001; **409**: 934–941.

Jones PA, Baylin SB. The epigenomics of cancer. *Cell* 2007; **128**: 683–692.

Kelsey G. Genomic imprinting: roles and regulation in development. *Endocr Dev* 2007; **12**: 99–112.

Kopp P. Genetics. In: Camacho PM, Gharib H, Sizemore GW, eds. *Evidence-based Endocrinology*, 2nd edn. Philadelphia: Lippincott Williams & Wilkins, 2006: 261–276.

Kopp P, Jameson JL. Principles of human genetics. In: Braunwald E, Fauci AS, Kasper DL, Hauser SL, Longo DL, Jameson JL, eds. *Harrison's Principles of Internal Medicine*, 17th edn. New York: McGraw-Hill, 2008: 385–406.

Korf BR. *Human Genetics and Genomics*, 3rd edn. Wiley-Blackwell, 2006.

Lewin B. *Genes IX*. Oxford: Jones and Bartlett Publishers, 2008.

Manolio TA, Bailey-Wilson JE, Collins FS. Genes, environment and the value of prospective cohort studies. *Nat Rev Genet* 2006; **7**: 812–820.

Manolio TA, Brooks LD, Collins FS. A HapMap harvest of insights into the genetics of common disease. *J Clin Invest* 2008; **118**: 1590–1605.

Mardis ER. Next-generation DNA sequencing methods. *Annu Rev Genomics Hum Genet* 2008; **9**: 387–402.

Nielsen R, Williamson S, Kim Y, *et al.* Genomic scans for selective sweeps using SNP data. *Genome Research* 2005; **15**: 1566–1575.

Nussbaum RL, Thompson MW, McInnes RR, *et al.* (eds). *Thompson and Thompson Genetics in Medicine*, 7th edn. New York: Elsevier Science, 2007.

Rimoin DL, Connor M, Pyeritz RE, *et al.* (eds). *Emery and Rimoin's Principles and Practice of Medical Genetics*, 5th edn. New York: Churchill Livingstone, 2006.

Scriver CR, Beaudet A, Sly W *et al.* (eds). *The Metabolic and Molecular Bases of Inherited Disease*, 8th edn. New York: McGraw-Hill, 2000.

Suzuki MM, Bird A. DNA methylation landscapes: provocative insights from epigenomics. *Nat Rev Genet* 2008; **9**: 465–476.

Tringe SG, Rubin EM. Metagenomics: DNA sequencing of environmental samples. *Nat Rev Genet* 2005; **6**: 805–814.

Tyers M, Mann M. From genomics to proteomics. *Nature* 2003; **422**: 193–197.

Weinshilboum R. Inheritance and drug response. *N Engl J Med* 2003; **348**: 529–537.

2 Principles of Hormone Action

Melissa Westwood

Maternal and Fetal Health Research Group, University of Manchester, Manchester, UK

Introduction

Hormones elicit their effects on target cell function by interacting with specific receptors. These are located either at the cell surface or within intracellular compartments, such as the cytoplasm and nucleus. Receptor location, which forms the basis of their classification into subgroups (Fig. 2.1), reflects ligand characteristics. Receptors for hydrophilic hormones, such as the pituitary-derived proteins, insulin and the catecholamines, are present at the plasma membrane; lipid-soluble steroid and thyroid hormones cross this barrier to access intracellular binding sites.

Receptors are specific and usually have a high affinity for their particular ligand but the forces involved in ligand–receptor binding (ionic attractions, van der Waals forces, hydrogen bonding or hydrophobic interactions) are weak. The reaction is therefore reversible and the receptor can be reused. K_d values, the concentration of ligand at which half the receptors are occupied, approximate the physiological concentration of the hormone (usually ranging between pico- and nanomolar concentrations), so that the receptor is sensitive to changes in hormone concentrations.

The concentration of each receptor can vary and a cell may become more or less sensitive to a given extracellular concentration of ligand. Sensitization can occur by increasing the number of binding sites available. This is achieved through a combination of increased receptor synthesis and decreased degradation. Cells can become refractory (desensitized) to ligand by altering receptor localization (e.g. by internalizing cell surface receptors), reducing receptor levels or recruiting molecules that deactivate intracellular signaling pathways. Internalization of cell-surface receptors involves endocytosis: the receptors relocate into clusters within the membrane, which then invaginates to form first a pit and then an endosomic vesicle. Once part of an endosome, the

Brook's Clinical Pediatric Endocrinology, 6th edition. Edited by C. Brook, P. Clayton, R. Brown. © 2009 Blackwell Publishing, ISBN: 978-1-4051-8080-1.

signal is terminated because the receptor–ligand complex dissociates as a result of the acidic pH within this compartment. Degradation usually involves the ubiquitin–proteosome pathway.

Cell-surface receptors

There are two major groups of cell-surface receptors linked to intracellular signals. The first relies upon tyrosine kinase for the initiation of signaling. The second tends to activate serine or threonine kinases by coupling to G-proteins. However, there is an underlying structural unity in all cell-surface receptors because each is made up of three segments: an extracellular domain, a transmembrane region and a cytoplasmic domain (Fig. 2.2).

The N-terminus of the protein forms the extracellular component of the receptor and this domain is responsible for hormone recognition and binding. The extracellular domain is heavily glycosylated and comparatively rich in cysteine residues. These are necessary for disulfide bond formation and correct protein folding but the functional significance of the oligosaccharide moieties is not known. The extracellular domain of some receptors [e.g. the growth hormone receptor and the receptor for thyroid-stimulating hormone (TSH)] can be cleaved from the plasma membrane so that it forms a separate entity that can be detected in the circulation, where it may function as hormone-binding proteins.

The transmembrane region varies in structure from a simple linear stretch of approximately 25 hydrophobic amino acids to a more complex arrangement that crosses the plasma membrane seven times. This segment of the receptor is often regarded as a passive lipid anchor but there is evidence to suggest that it can influence receptor function; for example, mutations in the transmembrane region of the fibroblast growth factor (FGF) receptor are associated with achondroplasia.

The cytoplasmic C-terminus of the receptor generally forms the effector region of the molecule because it initiates an intracellular signaling cascade, often involving protein phosphorylation, that eventually results in the cellular response.

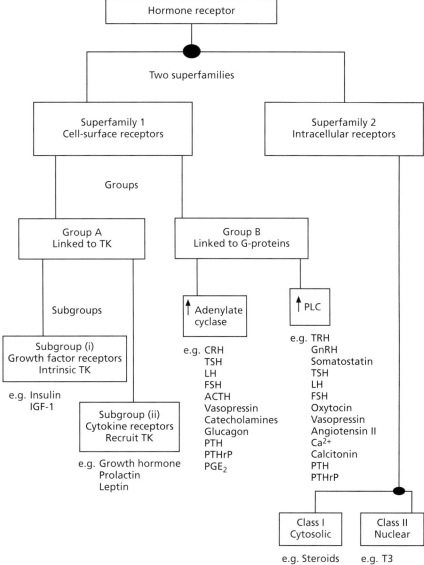

Figure 2.1 A composite diagram showing the different classes of hormone receptors. Receptors for some hormones can occur in more than one grouping. For example, different types of PTH receptors link to different G-proteins and therefore couple to either adenylate cyclase or phospholipase C (PLC). ACTH, adrenocorticotropin hormone ; CRH, corticotropin- releasing hormone; FSH, follicle-stimulating hormone; GnRH, gonadotropin-releasing hormone; IGF-1, insulin-like growth factor 1; LH, luteinizing hormone; PGE$_2$, prostaglandin E$_2$; PTH, parathyroid hormone, PTHrP, parathyroid hormone related peptide; TK, tyrosine kinase; TRH, thyrotropin-releasing hormone; TSH thyroid-stimulating hormone.

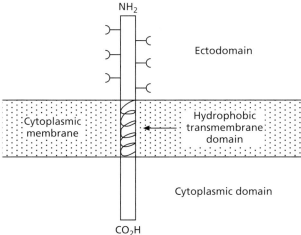

Figure 2.2 Schematic representation of a membrane-spanning cell-surface receptor with three clearly identifiable domains: the extracellular domain is bridged by a membrane-spanning component to the intracellular cytoplasmic domain. Each domain has characteristic structural features that reflect its location and function.

Protein phosphorylation

The amino acids serine, threonine and tyrosine each carry a polar hydroxyl group that can be exchanged for a phosphate group from adenosine triphosphate (ATP) by protein kinases. The energy generated during this reaction leads to a conformational change in the tertiary structure of the phosphorylated protein and, once activated in this way, many molecules within signaling pathways relay the signal by acting as protein kinases themselves. Each protein may be phosphorylated on more than one residue and a protein may be the substrate for more than one kinase, in many cases allowing the convergence of several signaling molecules. The target sequence of most kinases has been identified, although the presence of a consensus motif within a protein's primary sequence does not mean that the protein will automatically be phosphorylated because the tertiary structure may prevent kinase access.

Kinases are grouped according to which amino acid they target. Serine/threonine kinases account for approximately 350 of the known phosphorylating enzymes and are responsible for the majority of the 10% of proteins that are phosphorylated at any given time in a mammalian cell.

Tyrosine kinases account for only 0.05% of the phosphoamino acid content of a cell but they are key regulators of many cellular signaling pathways. In addition to protein activation, phosphorylation of tyrosine residues generates binding sites necessary for subsequent protein–protein interactions. The relatively long side-chain of phosphotyrosine enables it to dock with proteins containing "deep pockets" resulting from the presence of one or more consensus sequences (approximately 100 amino acids) known as the Src homology (SH2 or SH3) domain. Phosphorylation is a reversible process and this molecular switch can be rapidly overturned through the action of enzymes termed phosphatases.

Tyrosine kinase-linked cell-surface receptors

These have a relatively simple transmembrane domain and either possess intrinsic tyrosine kinase activity or recruit such enzymes after activation by ligand binding.

Receptors with intrinsic tyrosine kinase activity

This family contains the insulin receptor, the structurally related type 1 insulin-like growth factor (IGF-1) receptor and the receptors for epidermal growth factor (EGF), fibroblast growth factor (FGF) and platelet-derived growth factor (PDGF). They are often referred to as growth factor receptors or receptor tyrosine kinases (RTKs).

The structure of these receptors is shown in Figure 2.2. Some ligands (e.g. FGF and EGF) stimulate dimerization of two adjacent monomeric receptors, whereas others (e.g. insulin and IGF-1) bind to receptors that exist as dimers in their unoccupied state. Either way, ligand–receptor coupling results in activation of the tyrosine kinase located in the cytosolic domain of the receptor.

Insulin/type 1 IGF receptors

Both receptors are heterotetrameric structures comprising two extracellular α-subunits linked to two membrane-spanning β-subunits by disulfide bonds (Fig. 2.3) [1,2]. The α-subunits confer specificity for their cognate ligand, whereas the β-subunits possess the motifs required for recruiting the major signaling adaptor proteins and a tyrosine kinase domain, which is essential for the catalytic activity of the receptor. As a result of the consid-

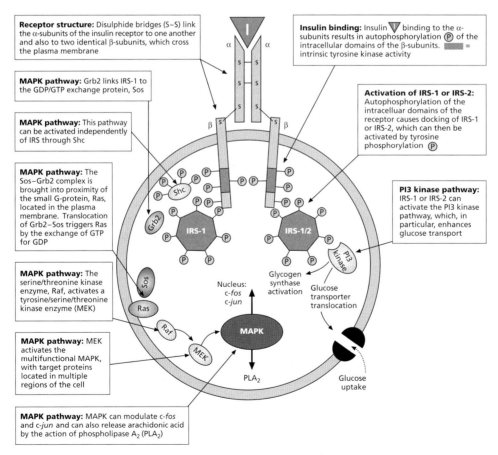

Figure 2.3 Signaling pathways initiated in response to activation of the insulin receptor, an example of a receptor with intrinsic tyrosine kinase activity. The type 1 IGF receptor shares many of these pathways.

erable homology between the insulin and type 1 IGF receptors, cells expressing both can form a hybrid of an insulin αβ-hemireceptor coupled to an IGF-1 αβ-hemireceptor [3]. The functional significance of this phenomenon has yet to be determined, although it is known that the hybrid receptors bind IGF-1 with a 50-fold higher affinity than that for insulin [4].

Insulin signaling pathways

Following autophosphorylation of tyrosine residues on the receptor β-subunit, a cascade involving more than 50 enzymes is activated; this includes primarily members of the insulin receptor substrate (IRS) family of proteins (Fig. 2.3) [5]. Four mammalian IRS proteins have been identified and evidence from transgenic mice suggests that they may display tissue and functional specificity [5,6], as IRS-1 seems to be important for somatic cell growth and insulin action in muscle and adipose tissue, whereas IRS-2 appears to be the main signaling molecule in the liver and is necessary for β-cell survival. Regulation of IRS protein levels may provide an additional mechanism for modulating insulin action as recent data suggest that the translation of IRS-1 is subject to negative regulation by endogenous microRNAs (miRNAs) with consequent effects on cellular function [7]. Indeed post-transcriptional regulation of proteins by miRNAs may prove to be relevant to numerous hormone/receptor signaling pathways as the expression of the angiotensin II type 1 receptor can be reduced by miR-155 [8]. Phosphorylation of IRS creates docking sites for proteins with Src homology 2 (SH2) domains. These include the regulatory (P85) subunit of phosphatidylinositol (PI) 3-kinase and growth factor receptor-binding protein 2 (Grb2). The effect of insulin depends on which of these effector molecules are expressed and recruited and which signaling pathways are activated as a result.

Stimulation of PI 3-kinase leads to the generation of PI 3-phosphate, by phosphorylation of phosphatidylinositol lipids at the D-3 position of the inositol ring and then activation of PI 3-dependent kinases (PDK) [9]. PDKs activate protein kinase B (PKB; also known as Akt) via phosphorylation of a critical serine and threonine residue, which results in the translocation of glucose transporters, predominantly GLUT-4, to the plasma membrane and the initiation of glycogen synthesis through activation of glycogen synthase (Fig. 2.3).

The mitogenic effects of insulin are mediated via Grb2. This adaptor protein links tyrosine-phosphorylated receptors or cytoplasmic tyrosine kinases to the guanine nucleotide exchange factor, SOS (son of sevenless protein) and, along with Ras, Raf and MEK, is part of the pathway that leads to the activation of mitogen-activated protein kinase (MAPK; Fig. 2.3) [9]. This acts on multiple proteins to result in cytoplasmic and nuclear responses. The latter lead to stimulation of gene expression, protein synthesis and cell growth. The MAPK pathway can be stimulated independently of IRS, because Shc, which is a substrate of the activated insulin receptor, can also associate with Grb2 (Fig. 2.3) [9].

IGF-1 signaling pathways

Insulin and IGF-1 have overlapping roles in metabolism, cell growth, differentiation and cell survival and their receptors have structural similarity, so it is not surprising that activation of the type 1 IGF receptor activates many of the intracellular signaling events described above. IRS proteins, Grb2 and Shc are all involved in the cellular response to IGF-1 (Fig. 2.3). However, it is thought that the two receptors can elicit distinct biological responses by using specific or preferential substrates, adaptor molecules or signaling pathways. For example, insulin activates protein kinase C (PKC) to stimulate proliferation of murine keratinocytes through PI 3-kinase and generation of PI 3-phosphate, whereas PKC is not involved in the proliferative response to IGF-1 in these cells [10].

Desensitization

A family of enzymes known as protein tyrosine phosphatases (PTPs), which includes PTPa, SHP2, LAR and PTP1B, has a key role in terminating the signal generated through the insulin or type 1 IGF receptor [11]. PTP1B is thought to be particularly important in relation to the negative regulation of insulin signaling pathways [12] because PTP1B *in vitro* dephosphorylates activated insulin receptors, IRS proteins and possibly other downstream molecules as well. PTP1B-deficient mice display enhanced insulin sensitivity and increased insulin-stimulated phosphorylation of the insulin receptor in muscle and glucose. PTP1B gene variants in humans are associated with changes in insulin sensitivity, which has prompted an interest in developing specific PTP1B inhibitors for the treatment of type 2 diabetes. PTP inhibitors may also prove to be useful in cancer therapy as inappropriate activation of the type 1 IGF receptor signaling pathway has been linked to cellular transformation [13] and, for example, loss of the PTP PTEN causes a reduction in IGF signaling [14].

Defects

Mutations in the gene coding for the insulin receptor are associated with syndromes of severe insulin resistance: type A insulin resistance, Rabson–Mendenhall syndrome and leprechaunism. All have impaired glucose metabolism in association with raised insulin concentrations but only patients with leprechaunism completely lack functional insulin receptors and they rarely survive beyond the first year of life [6]. Some patients with type A insulin resistance are reported to have normal insulin receptors and these may harbor as yet unidentified mutations in any of the other critical insulin signaling molecules described above. Mice deficient in the gene for IRS-1 display marked pre- and postnatal growth failure, insulin resistance, impaired glucose tolerance and other features of the metabolic syndrome but they do not develop diabetes, unlike the IRS-2 knockout animals [6]. This has led to the suggestion that IRS-2 is a diabetes-predisposing gene, although this has not been substantiated by clinical studies.

There have been no reports of humans completely lacking the gene for the type 1 IGF receptor; however, mutations associated with reduced receptor number and function have been documented in children with intrauterine and/or postnatal growth restriction [15] and *igfr1* null mice show severe growth failure, widespread developmental defects and usually die at birth as a result of respiratory failure [16].

Receptors that recruit tyrosine kinase activity

This group of receptors is referred to as the cytokine receptor superfamily. From an endocrine perspective, the most important members are the receptors for growth hormone (GH) and prolactin (PRL), which form the class 1 subgroup along with the receptors for erythropoietin, granulocyte-macrophage colony-stimulating factor (GM-CSF), leptin and the interleukins (IL) 2-7, IL-9, IL-11 and IL-12 [17].

Like the tyrosine kinase receptors, cytokine receptors are expressed at the cell surface and are composed of a ligand-binding extracellular domain, a transmembrane region and an intracellular carboxy tail (Fig. 2.2). Here the similarity ends, because members of the cytokine receptor superfamily do not possess enzymatic activity in their cytoplasmic domain. Instead, these receptors couple physically and functionally with non-receptor tyrosine kinases.

GH receptor activation

Early crystallographic studies revealed that ligand and receptor exist in a complex of one GH molecule and two molecules of receptor [18]. Subsequent work involving mutational analysis of residues within the ligand demonstrated that each molecule of GH has two distinct sites, a high-affinity "site 1" and a lower affinity "site 2," both of which are capable of binding to the extracellular domain of a GH receptor. The unoccupied receptor has not been crystallized and so there has been much speculation about whether dimerization occurs before or after GH binding. Initial studies supported the latter paradigm but more recent work suggests that GH receptor dimerization occurs in the absence of hormone [19] and that the dimer undergoes a conformational change upon GH binding that enables tyrosine kinase recruitment [19].

The receptors for PRL and erythropoietin also form homodimers and again, recent work challenges the accepted view that ligand is needed to induce dimerization [20,21] but members of the other subgroups of the cytokine receptor superfamily form heterodimers and oligomers.

Tyrosine kinase recruitment

Thirty-two mammalian non-receptor tyrosine kinases have been identified, which are classified into 11 groups based on sequence similarity in their SH1, SH2 and SH3 domains. Each has the ability to bind to the intracellular motif of different receptor molecules. Early studies of GH signaling pathways used cross-linking and immunoprecipitation techniques to demonstrate that the activated GH receptor recruits predominantly members of the Janus family of tyrosine kinases [22].

Janus-associated kinases (JAK)

Four evolutionarily conserved members of the JAK family have been identified: JAK1, JAK2, JAK3 and Tyk2. JAK3 is expressed primarily in hematopoietic cells, although the others are found in most cell types. GH and PRL usually recruit JAK2 [23], although GH-induced phosphorylation of JAK1 and JAK3 has also been reported. They all possess seven conserved JH regions (JH1–7), of which JH1 is the functional domain and JH2 a pseudokinase domain necessary to regulate the catalytic domain negatively so that the enzyme is inactive in the absence of a stimulus [24].

Although JAKs associate constitutively with the receptor through a proline-rich site known as Box 1 in the receptor's intracellular domain, they are spatially positioned and/or conformationally modified upon receptor activation so that transphosphorylation and activation of the kinase domain occur. This results in phosphorylation of the intracellular domain of the GH/PRL receptors and provision of docking sites for a variety of signaling molecules that contain SH2 or other phosphotyrosine-binding (PTB) motifs. These include SHC, IRS and members of the signal transducer and activator of transcription (STAT) family of proteins (Fig. 2.4) [25].

STATs

In mammals, there are seven STAT family members, STAT1–4, STAT5A, STAT5B and STAT6. Only STAT1, STAT3 and the STAT5 molecules are usually recruited in response to GH/PRL-induced JAK2 activation.

STAT proteins are localized in the cytoplasm in unstimulated cells but they are rapidly recruited to the intracellular domain of the receptor after ligand–receptor coupling through binding between STAT SH2 domains and phosphorylated tyrosine residues on the receptor [26]. This interaction is highly specific and represents a critical step in determining the specificity of receptor-mediated STAT activation. Once bound, the STATs become phosphorylated. This leads to the formation of STAT homo- and heterodimers, which translocate rapidly to the nucleus for DNA binding (Fig. 2.4). Most STAT dimers recognize an 8- to 10-bp inverted repeat DNA element with a consensus sequence of 5′-TT(N_{4-6})AA-3′, usually referred to as a GAS element as a result of its initial characterization as a γ-interferon activation sequence recognized by STAT1 homodimers.

Following DNA binding, activated STAT dimers initiate the transcription of immediate early response genes that regulate proliferation of more specific genes that determine the functional status of the cell [26].

Desensitization

Following activation, there is a rapid attenuation of receptor responsiveness to ligand. This process is achieved by removal of the receptor from the cell surface (internalization) and ubiquitin-dependent degradation of the receptor–JAK complex [27,28]. In addition, JAK/STAT signaling pathways are inhibited by at least three families of proteins: phosphatases, suppressors of cytokine

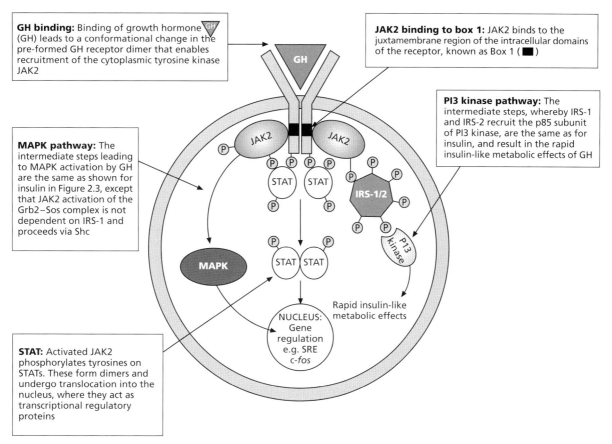

GH binding: Binding of growth hormone (GH) leads to a conformational change in the pre-formed GH receptor dimer that enables recruitment of the cytoplasmic tyrosine kinase JAK2

JAK2 binding to box 1: JAK2 binds to the juxtamembrane region of the intracellular domains of the receptor, known as Box 1 (■)

PI3 kinase pathway: The intermediate steps, whereby IRS-1 and IRS-2 recruit the p85 subunit of PI3 kinase, are the same as for insulin, and result in the rapid insulin-like metabolic effects of GH

MAPK pathway: The intermediate steps leading to MAPK activation by GH are the same as shown for insulin in Figure 2.3, except that JAK2 activation of the Grb2–Sos complex is not dependent on IRS-1 and proceeds via Shc

STAT: Activated JAK2 phosphorylates tyrosines on STATs. These form dimers and undergo translocation into the nucleus, where they act as transcriptional regulatory proteins

Figure 2.4 Signaling pathways initiated in response to activation of the growth hormone receptor, an example of a receptor that recruits tyrosine kinase activity.

signaling (SOCS) and protein inhibitors of activated STATs (PIAS) [23].

In vitro evidence for the involvement of protein tyrosine phosphatases (PTP) comes from the demonstration of prolonged GH-stimulated JAK2 and STAT5 phosphorylation in the presence of phosphatase inhibitors. Furthermore, in mice deficient in the enzyme SHP1, these signaling molecules are superactivated in response to GH [29] and mice lacking functional PTP-H1 are significantly larger than their wild-type littermates, suggesting that this enzyme has a role in regulating signaling through the GH receptor [30].

Activation of the JAK/STAT pathway also induces expression of the SOCS proteins; these interact with JAK and also with the GH receptor to result in proteosomal degradation [31]. Finally, PIAS have been shown to regulate signal transduction negatively in response to prolactin, although less is known about the involvement of PIAS in GH regulation of STAT-mediated transcription [32].

Alternative pathways
JAK/STAT pathways are important in the cellular response to GH and prolactin but there is evidence to suggest that other non-receptor tyrosine kinases may also mediate signal transduction of the cytokine receptor superfamily [23].

Members of the Src family of kinases (s-Src and c-Fyn) are activated by GH–receptor coupling and this may lead to phosphorylation of focal adhesion kinase (FAK), recruitment of Grb2 and stimulation of the MAPK pathway. c-Fyn has also been implicated in the activation of PI 3-kinase by prolactin. Furthermore, Src kinases can associate with STAT1, STAT3 and STAT5 and so it is possible that this pathway is also involved in the transcriptional events regulated by GH or PRL. The use of signaling molecules from the transduction pathways associated with insulin may explain the acute insulin-like effects of GH. In addition, GH and prolactin have been reported to increase intracellular free calcium through activation of phospholipase C.

Defects in GH and PRL signaling
Abnormalities in GH signal transduction result in GH resistance and severe growth impairment despite normal or elevated levels of circulating GH (Laron syndrome). Such patients have exceptionally low levels of IGF-1 and its principal carrier protein, IGF binding protein-3 (IGFBP3), and these cannot be elevated by the administration of exogenous GH. This observation gave the first clue that GH resistance resulted from non-responsive receptor or signaling pathways [33].

Deletions, nonsense, missense, splice and frameshift mutations have all been detected in the exons of the GH receptor that code for the extracellular domain (exons 2–7). Some affect the ability of the receptor to bind GH, whereas others result in reduced GH-stimulated dimerization. Mutations in exons 8–10, which code for the transmembrane and intracellular domains, can lead to defective GH receptor–JAK/STAT coupling [34]. However, some patients have no apparent defect in their GH receptor, suggesting that the problem must lie in genes further downstream. Indeed, STAT5b knockout mice fail to respond effectively to GH and mutations in the gene for STAT5b have been identified as the cause of GH insensitivity in a number of patients [35,36]. In addition, abnormalities in the intracellular phosphatases involved in regulating GH signaling may also cause GH resistance because mutations in the gene for the PTP SHP-2 (Noonan syndrome) are associated with GH insensitivity [37,38]. There have now been a number of demonstrations that defects (e.g. partial deletions and missense mutations) in the gene coding for IGF-1 [15] also lead to pre- and postnatal growth failure because this would clearly render the GH–IGF-1 axis ineffective.

There have been no reports of human disease resulting from gene defects in the prolactin receptor. This suggests that either mutations of the PRL receptor have no detectable effect *in vivo* or such mutations are lethal [39]. Evidence from PRL receptor knockout mice supports the former hypothesis: these animals are viable but they do display a number of reproductive, behavioral and bone abnormalities.

Circulating receptors

The extracellular domain of some class I cytokine receptors, including the GH receptor, can be cleaved by an enzyme thought to be the metalloprotease TACE (tumor necrosis factor α converting enzyme) to form a circulating binding protein with high affinity for GH (GHBP) [40]. The physiological significance of GHBP is poorly understood but "receptor decapitation" presents an alternative mechanism for receptor desensitization. The binding protein itself has the potential to modulate GH function either by prolonging its half-life and providing a circulating reservoir or by competing with GH for GH binding and inhibiting GH signaling through the formation of non-functional GHBP/GH receptor heterodimers.

Serum GHBP concentrations approximate GH receptor expression and are therefore used as a reflection of GH receptor status: for example, 75–80% of patients with Laron syndrome have low or undetectable levels of GHBP.

G-protein-coupled receptors

G-protein-coupled receptors (GPCRs) form a superfamily of more than 1000 membrane proteins which accounts for approximately 1% of the genes found within mammalian genomes. These receptors have a diverse range of ligands and, in addition to transducing hormonal signals, they also mediate the cellular response to neurotransmitters, lipids, including prostaglandins and leukotrienes, nucleotides, ions and sensory stimuli, such as light, smell and taste [41].

As their name suggests, activation of GPCRs generally leads to the recruitment of intracellular G (guanine) proteins and the generation of second messengers, for example, cyclic adenosine monophosphate (cAMP) and inositol 1,4,5-triphosphate (IP_3). Some of these receptors can signal through G-protein-independent pathways.

Structure

Although GPCRs have the same basic design as the tyrosine kinase-linked receptors, in that they possess extracellular, transmembrane and intracellular domains, they can be defined structurally by their more elaborate "serpentine" transmembrane region [41]. This contains seven α-helices linked by alternating intracellular and extracellular loops, which can be arranged to form a hydrophobic pore (Fig. 2.5). In general, each of the transmembrane segments consists of 20–27 amino acids. The extracellular N-terminal segment, loops and intracellular C-terminal domain are much more variable in size; consequently, GPCRs range from the gonadotropin-releasing hormone receptor, with only 337 amino acid residues, to the calcium-sensing receptor, which has 1085 residues. The latter has a disproportionately long N-terminus (>600 amino acids), because, in general, the length of the N-terminal segment is weakly correlated with ligand size. It has been suggested that this domain, along with the extracellular loops and transmembrane pore, has an important role in ligand recognition. Like the tyrosine kinase-linked receptors, the intracellular domains (both loops and C-terminus) are necessary for interaction with intracellular signaling partners.

GPCRs exist and function as homo- and heterodimers [42]. This process may be important for targeting functional receptors to the cell surface and it is possible that heterodimerization could generate novel ligand binding and signal transduction pathways to result in functional properties distinct from those of either of the receptors. However, the physiological significance of homo- and heterodimers remains to be determined.

GPCRs can be grouped into three families, A, B and C (Table 2.1), on the basis of sequence similarity within the transmembrane region. There is little similarity between the groups, apart from the characteristic tertiary structure facilitated by the seven transmembrane helices [41]. Group A, which is the largest family and contains the receptors for light and adrenaline, has a putative fourth intracellular loop resulting from palmitoylation of cysteine residues in the C-terminal domain. Group B includes receptors for a variety of hormones and neuropeptides and is characterized by a long amino-terminus containing several cysteine residues, which presumably form a network of disulfide bridges. Group C includes the receptors for glutamate, γ-aminobutyric acid and calcium.

G-proteins

Upon binding ligand, the conformation of the transmembrane domain, particularly the third and sixth helices, is altered. This leads to a conformational change in the intracellular domains to uncover previously masked binding sites for heterotrimeric G-

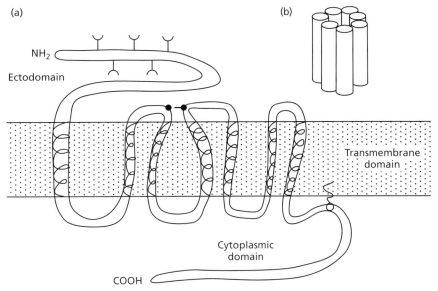

Figure 2.5 A schematic representation of G-protein-coupled receptors (GPCRs) showing the seven transmembrane domains. (a) The structure is an elaborate variation of the three-segment design depicted in Figure 2.2. The size of the N-terminal extracellular domain is generally in proportion to the size of the cognate ligand. Homology of this region, which is obviously important for ligand binding, is less than that of the transmembrane and cytoplasmic domains. This region can be heavily glycosylated and the carbohydrate moieties may contribute as much as 40% of its mass. The transmembrane domain has a characteristic heptahelical structure, most of which is embedded in the plasma membrane and provides a hydrophobic core. Conserved cysteine residues may form a disulfide bridge between the second and third extracellular loops. The cytoplasmic domain links the receptor to the signal-transducing G-proteins. Evidence from the β-adrenergic receptor suggests that specific regions in the third intracellular loop and sections of the C-terminal tail are critical for G-protein coupling. A fourth intracellular loop may be formed by a cysteine residue in the C-terminal tail, which could be palmitoylated in some GPCRs. (b) The hydrophobic pore formed by the seven transmembrane α-helices of the GPCR.

Table 2.1 Examples of GPCRs and their associated G-proteins/second messengers (AC, adenylate cyclase; PLC, phospholipase C). For somatostatin, vasopressin, calcitonin and PTH/PTHrP, different receptor subtypes determine α-subunit specificity and there may be differential tissue distributions of these receptor subtypes. This phenomenon provides opportunities to develop selective therapeutic antagonists.

Family	Characteristics	Examples	G-protein	Second messenger
A	Disulfide bridge connecting second and third extracellular loop Putative fourth intracellular loop	TRH receptor		
		GnRH receptor	$G\alpha_q$	PLC
		Oxytocin		
		Biogenic amine receptors		
		FSH receptor		
		LH receptor	$G\alpha_s/G\alpha_q$	AC/PLC
		TSH receptor		
		Vasopressin		
		Somatostatin	$G\alpha_i/G\alpha_q$	AC/PLC
		Melanocortin receptor	$G\alpha_s$	AC
B	Disulfide bridge connecting second and third extracellular loop Long amino-terminus containing several cysteine residues	Calcitonin receptor	$G\alpha_s/G\alpha_i/G\alpha_q$	AC/PLC
		CRH receptor		
		Glucagon receptor	$G\alpha_s$	AC
		PTH receptor		
		PTHrP receptor	$G\alpha_s/G\alpha_q$	AC/PLC
C	Very long (>600 amino acids) amino-terminus Very short and highly conserved third intracellular loop	Calcium receptors	$G\alpha_q/G\alpha_i$	AC/PLC
		Glutamate receptors	$G\alpha_s/G\alpha_q$	AC/PLC

CRH, corticotropin-releasing hormone; FSH, follicle-stimulating hormone; GnRH, gonadotropin-releasing hormone; LH, luteinizing hormone; PTH, parathyroid hormone; PTHrP, parathyroid hormone related peptide; TSH, thyroid-stimulating hormone.

proteins. G-proteins consist of α-, β- and γ-subunits. The β- and γ-subunits associate with such high affinity that G-proteins are usually described as having two functional units, Gα and Gβγ; 21 α-subunits, six β- and 12 γ-subunits have been described [43].

Activation by GPCRs induces a conformational change in the α-subunit, which results in the exchange of a molecule of GDP for a molecule of GTP and dissociation of the α-subunit from both the receptor and the βγ-dimer. Both the GTP-bound α-subunit and the βγ-dimer independently regulate a number of downstream signaling pathways.

Based on their primary effector molecules, the α-subunits can be grouped into four families. $G\alpha_s$ and $G\alpha_i$ activate or inhibit adenylate cyclase (AC) respectively. $G\alpha_q$ activates phospholipase C (PLC). Less is known about the $G\alpha_{12}$-subunits, although it appears that their effects are mediated through members of the Rho family of GTPases [44]. In addition to the effectors used by the α-subunits, Gβγ-dimers are known to target ion channels and protein kinases and the list continues to increase [44].

The existence of numerous G-protein subunits in combination with a variety of downstream effectors enables the diversity and selectivity of intracellular signals in response to GPCR activation. Each receptor has the possibility of interacting with many G-proteins (Table 2.1). Recruitment of a particular Gα-subunit depends on many factors [45], including receptor subtype (Fig. 2.6a), structural features of the cytoplasmic domain and the concentration of the ligand. For example, at low concentrations, TSH, calcitonin and luteinizing hormone (LH)/human chorionic gonadotropin (hCG) receptors activate adenylate cyclase through $G\alpha_s$, whereas at higher concentration, $G\alpha_q$ is recruited to activate PLC. Further complexity is introduced by the potential for receptors simultaneously or successively to couple with distinct G-proteins (Fig. 2.6b) and the ability of a particular G-protein to activate multiple intracellular signaling cascades (Fig. 2.6c).

Intracellular second messengers
cAMP
Activation of membrane-bound adenylate cyclase catalyzes the conversion of ATP to the potent second messenger cAMP (Fig. 2.7) [46]. This cyclic nucleotide activates the heterotetrameric protein kinase A (PKA) by binding to repressive regulatory subunits (R), which then dissociate from the two catalytic subunits (C) so that phosphorylation of serine/threonine residues in proteins containing the consensus sequence Arg-Arg-X-Ser/Thr-X can occur. These include intermediaries of lipolysis, glycogenolysis and steroidogenesis (e.g. glycogen synthase, hormone-sensitive lipase, cholesterol ester hydrolase) as well as the transcription factor CREB (cAMP response element binding protein). Phosphorylated CREB translocates to the nucleus where it binds to a short palindromic sequence, the CRE or cAMP response element, of cAMP-regulated genes (e.g. somatostatin). In this way, the generation of cAMP can have a direct effect on gene transcription.

cAMP does not act exclusively through PKA and there is a growing list of alternative cAMP targets [47]. The physiological effects of cAMP are also produced by direct regulation of monovalent and divalent cation channels and the ubiquitous guanine exchange factors Epac 1 and 2.

The cAMP-mediated signal is terminated by members of the phosphodiesterase (PDEs) family of proteins. These hydrolyze cAMP rapidly to the inactive 5′-AMP in response to phosphorylation by PKA and other mechanisms.

Diacylglycerol and Ca^{2+}
Occupancy of numerous GPCRs, including thyrotropin-releasing hormone (TRH), gonadotropin-releasing hormone (GnRH) and oxytocin, results in G-protein activation of the enzyme phospholipase C (PLC; Fig. 2.8) [48]. This leads to the hydrolysis of phospholipids, specifically phosphatidylinositol-4,5-bisphosphate (PIP_2), which resides in the inner leaflet of the plasma membrane, to yield diacylglycerol (DAG) and inositol-

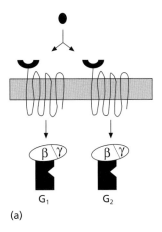

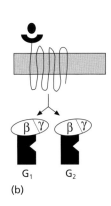

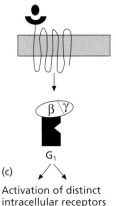

(a)

(b)

(c)

Activation of distinct intracellular receptors

Figure 2.6 Various mechanisms of G-protein selection and subsequent activation of intracellular second messengers. After Hermans [45], with permission.

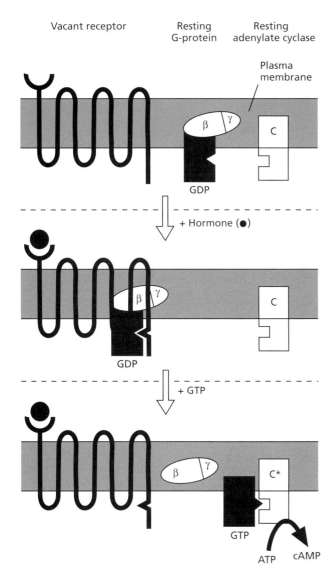

Figure 2.7 A representation of G-protein-modulated activation of a membrane-bound enzyme such as adenylate cyclase. A hormone (e.g. adrenaline) binds to the extracellular region of the receptor. The third intracellular loop and the C-terminus of the receptor associate with a G-protein (e.g. $G\alpha_s\beta\gamma$). This leads to displacement of GDP by GTP and dissociation of $G\alpha_s$ from the $\beta\gamma$-dimer. The α-subunit diffuses in the lipid bilayer and activates the catalytic subunit (C^*) to generate many molecules of cyclic adenosine monophosphate (cAMP).

1,4,5-triphosphate (IP_3). DAG, together with a cofactor phosphatidylserine, recruits another protein kinase, the membrane-bound PKC, which, in the presence of calcium, phosphorylates a wide variety of proteins and peptides to bring about the cellular response. Ca^{2+} is provided by IP_3, which diffuses through the cytoplasm to bind receptors on the endoplasmic reticulum, causing Ca^{2+} mobilization and a rapid increase in cytosolic free Ca^{2+}. In addition to PKC, the rise in intracellular Ca^{2+} also activates the protein kinase calmodulin and phospholipase A_2. Phospholipase A_2 liberates arachidonate from phospholipids and thereby generates potent local tissue activators known collectively as eicosanoids. These include thromboxanes, leukotrienes and prostaglandins. Prostaglandins are well-recognized paracrine and autocrine mediators that may amplify or prolong the response to the original hormone stimulus. Intracellular Ca^{2+} concentrations are restored to resting levels by several mechanisms including Ca^{2+} pumps and deactivation of G-proteins.

Non-G-protein pathways

GPCRs do not always signal through G-proteins and the list of GPCR effector molecules is growing apace. In some cases, these are known receptor-interacting proteins, such as the arrestins, which, in addition to their well-established role in receptor desensitization, appear to link GPCRs into MAP kinase pathways [49], although novel binding partners have also been identified. GPCRs can also elicit their effects through the "transactivation" of receptor tyrosine kinases both in the presence and absence of the RTK's cognate ligand [50] and the reverse situation might occur because there is growing evidence for RTKs using GPCRs as signaling intermediaries [50]. Another paradigm in GPCR signaling involves the translocation of GPCRs to the nucleus in order to directly regulate transcriptional activity [51]. The challenge now is to understand how the classic and new effector pathways are integrated to achieve specificity of GPCR signal transduction.

GPCR desensitization

GPCR desensitization results from changes to either the receptor [52] or the intracellular G-proteins [53]. The extent varies from complete termination of signaling, which occurs in the sensory systems, to a reduction in the potency of ligand, as is observed with the β-adrenergic receptors.

Internalization of receptors to intracellular compartments and reduced expression as a result of decreased mRNA and protein synthesis both lead to desensitization but this can be achieved more rapidly (in seconds rather than minutes or hours) by uncoupling the receptor from G-protein-mediated signaling pathways. It is widely accepted that both second messenger-dependent protein kinases [e.g. PKA and PKC] and G-protein-coupled receptor kinases (GRK) are responsible for uncoupling GPCRs from G-proteins by phosphorylating serine and threonine residues within the intracellular loop and carboxy-terminal tail domains of the receptor. GRK phosphorylation of GPCRs also promotes the binding of cytosolic cofactor proteins known as arrestins, which target GPCR for endocytosis by clathrin-coated vesicles.

GPCR signals can be terminated at the G-protein level. $G\alpha$-subunits possess intrinsic GTPase activity, which can cleave phosphate from GTP to result in GaGDP. This process can be enhanced by a family of proteins called regulators of G-protein signaling (RGS), which accelerate the rate of hydrolysis of GTP bound to both $G\alpha_i$ and $G\alpha_q$ to dampen $G\alpha_i$- and $G\alpha_q$-mediated signaling pathways. Hydrolysis of GTP allows the $G\alpha$-subunit to associate with a $G\beta\gamma$-dimer again and the heterotrimeric complex returns to the G-protein pool so that it can be activated by subsequent receptor occupation by ligand.

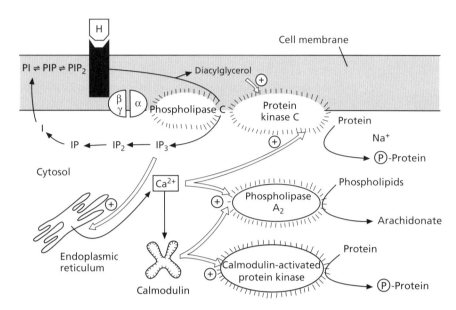

Figure 2.8 A representation of hormone-stimulated phospholipid turnover and calcium metabolism as a result of G-protein-coupled receptors activating phospholipase C.

Defects

Given their numerous and varied ligands, it is not surprising that mutations in GPCRs or their interacting G-proteins are associated with endocrine disease [54]. Mutations that alter the extracellular (ligand-binding) domains of the receptor lead to hormone resistance (e.g. the TSH receptor), whereas aberrations in the transmembrane region of the receptor can result in altered receptor function. Germline mutations in Xq28, which codes for the vasopressin V2 receptor, cause receptor misfolding and loss of receptor function so that circulating vasopressin, despite being present at very high concentrations, cannot increase urine concentration and nephrogenic diabetes insipidus results. Familial glucocorticoid deficiency and some cases of early-onset severe obesity may be explained by functional defects in the melanocortin-2 and melanocortin-4 receptors respectively.

Activating mutations are also detrimental, presumably by altering crucial helix–helix interactions so that the receptor is active even in the absence of ligand. Familial male precocious puberty (testotoxicosis) is the result of such a mutation in the gene coding for the LH receptor and activating mutations in the transmembrane domain of the TSH receptor have been reported in association with neonatal hyperthyroidism and toxic thyroid adenomas in adults.

Mutations resulting in the loss of $G\alpha_s$ function are linked to pseudohypoparathyroidism (Albright hereditary osteodystrophy). If the mutation is maternally transmitted, resistance to the multiple hormones that activate $G\alpha_s$ in their target tissues occurs. Mutations resulting in the constitutive activation of $G\alpha_s$ cause McCune–Albright syndrome and some cases of acromegaly.

Intracellular receptors

Receptors for hydrophobic hormones such as the sex steroids, glucocorticoids, thyroxine and aldosterone are part of a large family of receptors (>150 members) that are located inside the cell (Fig. 2.1). These receptors function as hormone-regulated transcription factors and control the expression of specific target genes by interacting with regions close to the gene promoters. Consequently, the cellular response to these hormones takes longer than the quickfire cell surface receptor/second-messenger systems described above.

Receptor structure

All intracellular receptors consist of three major regions (Fig. 2.9a) [55]. There is a highly variable N-terminal domain, which has a role in transcription activation because of a region known as AF1 (activation function) in some receptors. There is also a DNA-binding domain (DBD) and a C-terminal ligand-binding domain (LBD), although their molecular weights vary from 46 to 100 kDa. The DNA-binding domain shows the highest degree of homology across the receptor family. It is characterized by two polypeptide loops, each of approximately 20 amino acids, which are known as "zinc fingers" as a result of their formation from the coordination of four cysteine or two cysteine and two histidine residues by a single atom of zinc (Fig. 2.9b). These distinctive fingers are necessary for interlocking with target DNA sequences in the nucleus.

Based on the crystal structure reported for the LBD of the estrogen and progesterone receptors, this region is thought to be composed of 12 α-helices that are folded to create a hydrophobic pocket for the ligand. Following occupation by ligand, there is a conformational change such that the 12th helix is repositioned to "seal" the pocket like a lid [55].

Receptor activation and DNA binding

Unoccupied "class I" receptors (Fig. 2.1) shuttle between the cytoplasm and the nucleus. Although some reside mainly in the former (e.g. the glucocorticoid receptor), others (e.g. the androgen receptor) are predominantly nuclear. In either case, the

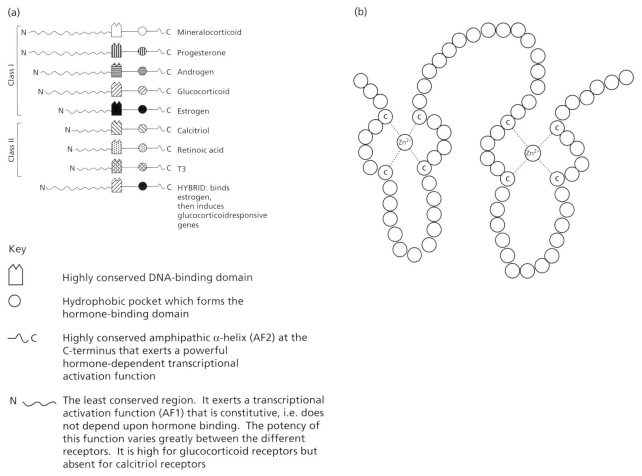

(a)

Class I
N ⌇⌇⌇ C Mineralocorticoid
N ⌇⌇⌇ C Progesterone
N ⌇⌇ C Androgen
N ⌇⌇⌇ C Glucocorticoid
N ⌇⌇ C Estrogen

Class II
N ⌇⌇ C Calcitriol
N ⌇⌇ C Retinoic acid
N ⌇ C T3
N ⌇⌇ C HYBRID: binds estrogen, then induces glucocorticoidresponsive genes

Key

⌂ Highly conserved DNA-binding domain

○ Hydrophobic pocket which forms the hormone-binding domain

—⌒C Highly conserved amphipathic α-helix (AF2) at the C-terminus that exerts a powerful hormone-dependent transcriptional activation function

N ⌇ The least conserved region. It exerts a transcriptional activation function (AF1) that is constitutive, i.e. does not depend upon hormone binding. The potency of this function varies greatly between the different receptors. It is high for glucocorticoid receptors but absent for calcitriol receptors

(b)

Figure 2.9 The intracellular receptor superfamily. Diagrammatic representation showing (a) the domain structure and relative sizes of these evolutionary related proteins and (b) the zinc fingers characteristic of the DNA-binding domain.

receptors are associated with "chaperone" molecules, such as heat shock protein 90 (hsp90), in a large heteromeric complex that obscures the zinc fingers of the DBD, thereby preventing the interaction with target sequences in the nucleus [56]. As a result of hormone binding, the inhibitory complex dissociates, the receptor becomes hyperphosphorylated and, if necessary, hormone–receptor complexes translocate to the nucleus. Activated receptors homodimerize here and then bind through the zinc fingers to DNA sequences that are specific for each receptor and known as the hormone response element (HRE; Fig. 2.10a). The glucocorticoid receptor binds to genes containing a glucocorticoid response element (GRE), the estrogen receptor to the estrogen response element (ERE) and so on. Targeting of the hormone–receptor complex to the HRE is directed by remarkably few amino acids in the DBD. These occur in a region called the P-box, which is usually located at the base of the first zinc finger. Each zinc finger recognizes a sequence of approximately six nucleotide basepairs and the HRE often consists of a palindromic or tandemly repeated sequence. The four steroid hormone receptors (glucocorticoid, mineralocorticoid, androgen and progesterone) bind to an imperfect palindrome that consists of two hexamers repeated in reverse orientation and separated by three nucleotides (5′-GGTACAnnnTGTTCT-3′) [57]. Despite the receptors recognizing the same target sequence, a specific hormonal response is achieved by the recruitment of auxiliary molecules known as co-activators or co-repressors.

Class II receptors (Fig. 2.1), for example the receptors for the thyroid hormones, are located exclusively in the nucleus where they are constitutively bound as homodimers or heterodimers [usually with an unoccupied retinoid X receptor (RAR)] to their DNA target sequence (Fig. 2.11b). In general, unoccupied receptors "silence" basal promoter activity, probably by associating with a co-repressor; ligand binding leads to a conformational change in the receptor and exchange of the inhibitory molecules for proteins necessary for the activation of transcription [58].

Co-activators and co-repressors

The hormone response element is usually upstream of the promoter region for the target gene. The promoter region also contains a consensus sequence, the TATA-box, for RNA polymerase. Through the recruitment of co-activators or co-repressors, which may be dependent on the phosphorylation status of the receptor

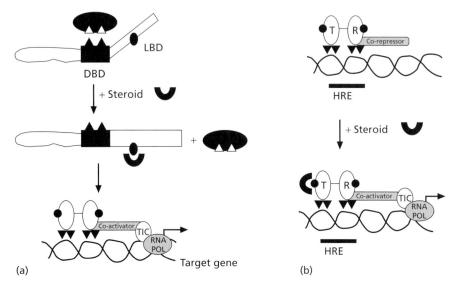

Figure 2.10 Activation of steroid hormone receptors. (a) Unoccupied class I receptors are associated with inhibitory molecules such as hsp90. Following hormone binding to the ligand-binding domain (LBD), the inhibitory protein dissociates and the two zinc fingers characteristic of the DNA-binding domain (DBD) are exposed. The receptor forms homodimers, interacts with the hormone response element (HRE) of target genes and, with the help of co-activator proteins, initiates transcription. TIC, transcriptor initiation complex; POL, polymerase. (b) Class II receptors, e.g. T3 receptor (T), are constitutively bound to DNA target sequences, usually as heterodimers with the retinoid X receptor (R). In the unoccupied state, they are transcriptionally inactive as a result of interaction with co-repressor molecules. Following ligand binding, the co-repressors are replaced by co-activators and RNA polymerase is activated.

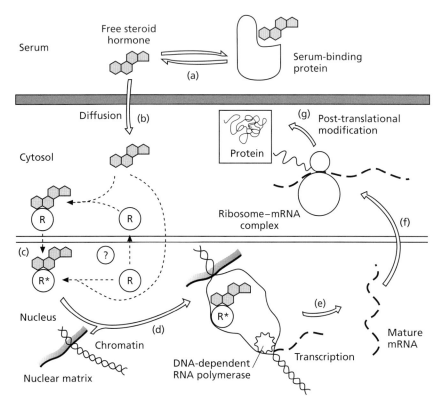

Figure 2.11 Classic mechanism of steroid hormone action. Free steroid hormone in equilibrium with bound hormone (a) diffuses across the target cell membrane (b) and binds to the steroid hormone receptor protein in the cytoplasm or in the cell nucleus. The hormone–receptor complex (c) interacts with chromatin and binds to a receptor site of one DNA strand associated with a particular gene (d). This region is the hormone response element (HRE). The promoter region permits DNA-dependent RNA polymerase to start transcription to yield messenger RNA (e), which passes out of the nucleus (f) after post-transcriptional modification. Peptides are formed by translation of the message on ribosomes attached to the endoplasmic reticulum and modification of the proteins gives the final gene product (g).

[59], the hormone–receptor complex can direct the binding and activity of this enzyme to enhance or suppress transcription [60]. Following transcription, the "genomic" pathway is completed by translation of the newly generated mRNA into the proteins that ultimately result in the cellular response to hormone stimulation (Fig. 2.11).

Co-activator proteins facilitate transcription by remodeling the chromatin environment so that it is more accessible to RNA polymerase or by coupling ligand-occupied receptors to the basal transcription apparatus [61]. They include CREB binding protein (CBP/p300) and steroid receptor co-activator-1 (SRC-1), both of which possess histone acetyltransferase activity. Co-repressors such as NcoR (nuclear receptor co-repressor) and SMRT (silencing mediator of retinoid and thyroid hormone receptors) also function by modifying chromatin, usually by recruiting histone deacetylase to the vicinity of the receptor [62].

Desensitization

As with the receptors expressed at the cell surface, ligand binding of intracellular receptors results in rapid desensitization. A ligand-

Table 2.2 Examples of defects in intracellular receptors that are associated with endocrine disease.

Receptor	Clinical effects	Molecular defects reported to date	Reference
Androgens (ARs)	Partial or complete androgen insensitivity syndromes	↓ Receptor number ↓ Androgen binding ↓ AR dimerization	[69]
	Kennedy syndrome	Expanded CAG repeat in N-terminus	[70]
	Breast cancer	Altered AR transcriptional activity	[71]
	Prostate cancer	↑ AR receptor number Altered interaction with co-regulators	[72]
Glucocorticoid	Generalized inherited glucocorticoid resistance	↓ Hormone binding ↓ GR number ↓ DNA binding	[73]
Oestrogen (ER)	Usually lethal Estrogen resistance	↓ Hormone binding ↓ DNA binding	[74]
T3 (TR)	Resistance to thyroid hormone	TRβ gene defects ↓ T3 binding	[75]
Calcitriol (VDR)	Calcitriol-resistant rickets	↓ VDR dimerization	[76]

dependent reduction in mRNA levels has been demonstrated for many of the steroid receptors. Other mechanisms for limiting hormone responsiveness include diminished receptor half-life, degradation via the ubiquitin/proteosome pathway and transfer to alternative intracellular compartments.

Non-genomic actions of steroids

The ability of intracellular receptors to act as hormone-regulated transcription factors is commonly accepted as the mechanism of steroid hormone action. However, steroids have a number of physiological effects, e.g aldosterone activation of the Na^+/H^+ exchanger, that cannot be attributed to activation of the genome because they occur over too short a timeframe.

Some hormones (e.g. estrogen) appear to mediate their "non-genomic" effects via classic estrogen receptors that are located at the cell membrane or cytoplasm [63,64]. However, evidence from knockout mice and pharmacological studies suggests that non-classic steroid receptors must also exist; for example, animals lacking the mineralocorticoid receptor have a similar aldosterone-stimulated rise in intracellular calcium and cAMP levels to their wild-type littermates and many of the effects of aldosterone cannot be blocked by spironolactone, a known inhibitor of the mineralocorticoid receptor.

Uncovering the mechanisms involved in mediating the non-genomic actions of steroids is an emerging focus of research, even though it seems that many of the intracellular receptors can activate the signaling molecules more typically associated with the superfamily of cell-surface receptors [64]. Understanding the relative contribution of genomic versus non-genomic pathways in determining the overall cellular response to a particular hormone will be important in unraveling normal hormone function.

Defects

Mutations in the genes coding for intracellular receptors are responsible for numerous endocrinopathies because they can result in hormone resistance resulting from reduced ligand binding, impaired receptor dimerization and decreased interaction with the HRE (summarized in Table 2.2). There is also evidence that defects resulting in abnormal receptor–co-activator interactions, and indeed problems with the co-activators themselves, may also be the cause of hormone resistance syndromes [60].

Target tissue metabolism

Some of the hormones that work through intracellular receptors are converted by enzymes expressed in their target cells to metabolites that are more potent because of their higher affinity for the receptor. For example, tissue-specific 5′-deiodinases convert T4 to T3 [65], 5α-reductase metabolizes testosterone to dihydrotestosterone [66] and 1α-hydroxylase in the mitochondria of cells in the renal tubule converts 25-OH-vitamin D to calcitriol [67]. These "activation" steps offer a way of achieving a range of effects and various disorders can result from defects in target tissue metabolism. The best known example is androgen insensitivity. Conversely, 11β-hydroxysteroid dehydrogenase (11β-HSD), which is expressed by aldosterone-responsive cells in the kidney, converts cortisol to cortisone to prevent the overstimulation of the mineralocorticoid receptor that would otherwise occur as a result of the high concentration of cortisol in relation to the

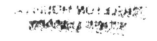

circulating levels of aldosterone [68]. Deficiency or impaired function of this enzyme leads to the hypertension and hypokalemia characteristic of the apparent mineralocorticoid excess (AME) syndrome.

References

1 Hubbard SR, Wei L, Ellis L, Hendrickson WA. Crystal structure of the tyrosine kinase domain of the human insulin receptor. *Nature* 1994; **372**: 746–754.

2 Ward CW, Garrett TP, McKern NM, *et al*. The three dimensional structure of the type I insulin-like growth factor receptor. *Mol Pathol* 2001; **54**: 125–132.

3 Bailyes EM, Nave BT, Soos MA, *et al*. Insulin receptor/IGF-1 receptor hybrids are widely distributed in mammalian tissues: quantification of individual receptor species by selective immuno-precipitation and immunoblotting. *Biochem J* 1997; **327** (Pt 1): 209–215.

4 Slaaby R, Schaffer L, Lautrup-Larsen I, *et al*. Hybrid receptors formed by insulin receptor (IR) and insulin-like growth factor I receptor (IGF-IR) have low insulin and high IGF-1 affinity irrespective of the IR splice variant. *J Biol Chem* 2006; **281**: 25869–25874.

5 Giovannone B, Scaldaferri ML, Federici M, *et al*. Insulin receptor substrate (IRS) transduction system: distinct and overlapping signaling potential. *Diabetes Metab Res Rev* 2000; **16**: 434–441.

6 Rhodes CJ, White MF. Molecular insights into insulin action and secretion. *Eur J Clin Invest* 2002; **32**: 3–13.

7 Shi B, Sepp-Lorenzino L, Prisco M, *et al*. Micro RNA 145 targets the insulin receptor substrate-1 and inhibits the growth of colon cancer cells. *J Biol Chem* 2007; **282**: 32582–32590.

8 Martin MM, Lee EJ, Buckenberger JA, Schmittgen TD, Elton TS. MicroRNA-155 regulates human angiotensin II type 1 receptor expression in fibroblasts. *J Biol Chem* 2006; **281**: 18277–18284.

9 Bevan P. Insulin signaling. *J Cell Sci* 2001; **114**: 1429–1430.

10 Dupont J, Dunn SE, Barrett C, LeRoith D. Microarray analysis and identification of novel molecules involved in insulin-like growth factor-1 receptor signaling and gene expression. *Rec Prog Horm Res* 2003; **58**: 525–542.

11 Stoker AW. Protein tyrosine phosphatases and signaling. *J Endocrinol* 2005; **185**: 19–33.

12 Cohen P. The twentieth century struggle to decipher insulin signaling. *Nat Rev Mol Cell Biol* 2006; **7**: 867–873.

13 Samani AA, Yakar S, LeRoith D, Brodt P. The role of the IGF system in cancer growth and metastasis: overview and recent insights. *Endocr Rev* 2007; **28**: 20–47.

14 Lackey J, Barnett J, Davidson L, *et al*. Loss of PTEN selectively desensitizes upstream IGF1 and insulin signaling. *Oncogene* 2007; **26**: 7132–7142.

15 Walenkamp MJ, Wit JM. Genetic disorders in the growth hormone–insulin-like growth factor-I axis. *Horm Res* 2006; **66**: 221–230.

16 Liu JP, Baker J, Perkins AS, Robertson EJ, Efstratiadis A. Mice carrying null mutations of the genes encoding insulin-like growth factor I (Igf-1) and type 1 IGF receptor (Igf1r). *Cell* 1993; **75**: 59–72.

17 Touw IP, De Konig JP, Ward AC, Hermans MH. Signaling mechanisms of cytokine receptors and their perturbances in disease. *Mol Cell Endocrinol* 2000; **160**: 1–9.

18 de Vos AM, Ultsch M, Kossiakoff AA. Human growth hormone and extracellular domain of its receptor: crystal structure of the complex. *Science* 1992; **255**: 306–312.

19 Waters MJ, Hoang HN, Fairlie DP, Pelekanos RA, Brown RJ. New insights into growth hormone action. *J Mol Endocrinol* 2006; **36**: 1–7.

20 Gadd SL, Clevenger CV. Ligand-independent dimerization of the human prolactin receptor isoforms: functional implications. *Mol Endocrinol* 2006; **20**: 2734–2746.

21 Constantinescu SN, Keren T, Socolovsky M, *et al*. Ligand-independent oligomerization of cell-surface erythropoietin receptor is mediated by the transmembrane domain. *Proc Natl Acad Sci U S A* 2001; **98**: 4379–4384.

22 Argetsinger LS, Campbell GS, Yang X, *et al*. Identification of JAK2 as a growth hormone receptor-associated tyrosine kinase. *Cell* 1993; **74**: 237–244.

23 Chilton BS, Hewetson A. Prolactin and growth hormone signaling. *Curr Top Dev Biol* 2005; **68**: 1–23.

24 Schindler CW. JAK-STAT signaling in human disease. *J Clin Invest* 2002; **109**: 1133–1137.

25 Aaronson DS, Horvath CM. A road map for those who don't know JAK-STAT. *Science* 2002; **296**: 1653–1655.

26 O'Shea JJ, Gadina M, Schreiber RD. Cytokine signaling in 2002: new surprises in the Jak/Stat pathway. *Cell* 2002; **109** (Suppl): S121–S131.

27 Strous GJ, dos Santos CA, Gent J, *et al*. Ubiquitin system-dependent regulation of growth hormone receptor signal transduction. *Curr Top Microbiol Immunol* 2004; **286**: 81–118.

28 Li Y, Kumar KG, Tang W, Spiegelman VS, Fuchs SY. Negative regulation of prolactin receptor stability and signaling mediated by SCF(beta-TrCP) E3 ubiquitin ligase. *Mol Cell Biol* 2004; **24**: 4038–4048.

29 Hackett RH, Wang YD, Sweitzer S, *et al*. Mapping of a cytoplasmic domain of the human growth hormone receptor that regulates rates of inactivation of Jak2 and Stat proteins. *J Biol Chem* 1997; **272**: 11128–11132.

30 Pilecka I, Patrignani C, Pescini R, *et al*. Protein-tyrosine phosphatase H1 controls growth hormone receptor signaling and systemic growth. *J Biol Chem* 2007; **282**: 35405–35415.

31 Rico-Bautista E, Flores-Morales A, Fernandez-Perez L. Suppressor of cytokine signaling (SOCS) 2, a protein with multiple functions. *Cytokine Growth Factor Rev* 2006; **17**: 431–439.

32 Wormald S, Hilton DJ. Inhibitors of cytokine signal transduction. *J Biol Chem* 2004; **279**: 821–824.

33 Laron Z. Natural history of the classical form of pituitary growth hormone (GH) resistance (Laron syndrome). *J Pediatr Endocrinol Metab* 1999; **12** (Suppl 1): 231–249.

34 Rosenfeld RG, Belgorosky A, Camacho-Hubner C, *et al*. Defects in growth hormone receptor signaling. *Trends Endocrinol Metab* 2007; **18**: 134–141.

35 Kofoed EM, Hwa V, Little B, *et al*. Growth hormone insensitivity associated with a STAT5b mutation. *N Engl J Med* 2003; **349**: 1139–1147.

36 Hwa V, Little B, Adiyaman P, *et al*. Severe growth hormone insensitivity resulting from total absence of signal transducer and activator of transcription 5b. *J Clin Endocrinol Metab* 2005; **90**: 4260–4266.

37 Binder G, Neuer K, Ranke MB, Wittekindt NE. PTPN11 mutations are associated with mild growth hormone resistance in individuals

SINGLETON HOSPITAL
STAFF LIBRARY

with Noonan syndrome. *J Clin Endocrinol Metab* 2005; **90**: 5377–5381.

38 Limal JM, Parfait B, Cabrol S, *et al.* Noonan syndrome: relationships between genotype, growth and growth factors. *J Clin Endocrinol Metab* 2006; **91**: 300–306.

39 Goffin V, Binart N, Touraine P, Kelly PA. Prolactin: the new biology of an old hormone. *Annu Rev Physiol* 2002; **64**: 47–67.

40 Fisker S. Physiology and pathophysiology of growth hormone-binding protein: methodological and clinical aspects. *Growth Horm IGF Res* 2006; **16**: 1–28.

41 Kristiansen K. Molecular mechanisms of ligand binding, signaling and regulation within the superfamily of G-protein-coupled receptors: molecular modeling and mutagenesis approaches to receptor structure and function. *Pharmacol Ther* 2004; **103**: 21–80.

42 Bulenger S, Marullo S, Bouvier M. Emerging role of homo- and heterodimerization in G-protein-coupled receptor biosynthesis and maturation. *Trends Pharmacol Sci* 2005; **26**: 131–137.

43 Oldham WM, Hamm HE. Heterotrimeric G protein activation by G-protein-coupled receptors. *Nat Rev Mol Cell Biol* 2008; **9**: 60–71.

44 Wettschureck N, Offermanns S. Mammalian G proteins and their cell type specific functions. *Physiol Rev* 2005; **85**: 1159–1204.

45 Hermans E. Biochemical and pharmacological control of the multiplicity of coupling at G-protein-coupled receptors. *Pharmacol Ther* 2003; **99**: 25–44.

46 Antoni FA. Molecular diversity of cyclic AMP signaling. *Front Neuroendocrinol* 2000; **21**: 103–132.

47 Kopperud R, Krakstad C, Selheim F, Doskeland SO. cAMP effector mechanisms: novel twists for an 'old' signaling system. *FEBS Lett* 2003; **546**: 121–126.

48 Kiselyov K, Shin DM, Muallem S. Signaling specificity in GPCR-dependent Ca²⁺ signaling. *Cell Signal* 2003; **15**: 243–253.

49 Lefkowitz RJ, Shenoy SK. Transduction of receptor signals by beta-arrestins. *Science* 2005; **308**: 512–517.

50 Delcourt N, Bockaert J, Marin P. GPCR-jacking: from a new route in RTK signaling to a new concept in GPCR activation. *Trends Pharmacol Sci* 2007; **28**: 602–607.

51 Goetzl EJ. Diverse pathways for nuclear signaling by G protein-coupled receptors and their ligands. *FASEB J* 2007; **21**: 638–642.

52 Moore CA, Milano SK, Benovic JL. Regulation of receptor trafficking by GRKs and arrestins. *Annu Rev Physiol* 2007; **69**: 451–482.

53 Neitzel KL, Hepler JR. Cellular mechanisms that determine selective RGS protein regulation of G protein-coupled receptor signaling. *Semin Cell Dev Biol* 2006; **17**: 383–389.

54 Lania AG, Mantovani G, Spada A. Mechanisms of disease: mutations of G proteins and G-protein-coupled receptors in endocrine diseases. *Nat Clin Pract Endocrinol Metab* 2006; **2**: 681–693.

55 Bain DL, Heneghan AF, Connaghan-Jones KD, Miura MT. Nuclear receptor structure: implications for function. *Annu Rev Physiol* 2007; **69**: 201–220.

56 Beato M, Klug J. Steroid hormone receptors: an update. *Hum Reprod Update* 2000; **6**: 225–236.

57 Geserick C, Meyer HA, Haendler B. The role of DNA response elements as allosteric modulators of steroid receptor function. *Mol Cell Endocrinol* 2005; **236**: 1–7.

58 Oetting A, Yen PM. New insights into thyroid hormone action. *Best Pract Res Clin Endocrinol Metab* 2007; **21**: 193–208.

59 Weigel NL, Moore NL. Steroid receptor phosphorylation: a key modulator of multiple receptor functions. *Mol Endocrinol* 2007; **21**: 2311–2319.

60 Lonard DM, Lanz RB, O'Malley BW. Nuclear receptor coregulators and human disease. *Endocr Rev* 2007; **28**: 575–587.

61 Lonard DM, O'Malley BW. The expanding cosmos of nuclear receptor coactivators. *Cell* 2006; **125**: 411–414.

62 Kumar R, Gururaj AE, Vadlamudi RK, Rayala SK. The clinical relevance of steroid hormone receptor corepressors. *Clin Cancer Res* 2005; **11**: 2822–2831.

63 Wehling M, Losel R. Non-genomic steroid hormone effects: membrane or intracellular receptors? *J Steroid Biochem Mol Biol* 2006; **102**: 180–183.

64 Hammes SR, Levin ER. Extranuclear steroid receptors: nature and actions. *Endocr Rev* 2007; **28**: 726–741.

65 Bianco AC, Kim BW. Deiodinases: implications of the local control of thyroid hormone action. *J Clin Invest* 2006; **116**: 2571–2579.

66 Sultan C, Paris F, Terouanne B, *et al.* Disorders linked to insufficient androgen action in male children. *Hum Reprod Update* 2001; **7**: 314–322.

67 Ebert R, Schutze N, Adamski J, Jakob F. Vitamin D signaling is modulated on multiple levels in health and disease. *Mol Cell Endocrinol* 2006; **248**: 149–159.

68 White PC. 11beta-hydroxysteroid dehydrogenase and its role in the syndrome of apparent mineralocorticoid excess. *Am J Med Sci* 2001; **322**: 308–315.

69 McPhaul MJ. Androgen receptor mutations and androgen insensitivity. *Mol Cell Endocrinol* 2002; **198**: 61–67.

70 Eder IE, Culig Z, Putz T, *et al.* Molecular biology of the androgen receptor: from molecular understanding to the clinic. *Eur Urol* 2001; **40**: 241–251.

71 Nicolas Diaz-Chico B, German RF, Gonzalez A, *et al.* Androgens and androgen receptors in breast cancer. *J Steroid Biochem Mol Biol* 2007; **105**: 1–15.

72 Dehm SM, Tindall DJ. Androgen receptor structural and functional elements: role and regulation in prostate cancer. *Mol Endocrinol* 2007; **21**: 2855–2863.

73 Charmandari E, Kino T. Novel causes of generalized glucocorticoid resistance. *Horm Metab Res* 2007; **39**: 445–450.

74 Mueller SO, Korach KS. Estrogen receptors and endocrine diseases: lessons from estrogen receptor knockout mice. *Curr Opin Pharmacol* 2001; **1**: 613–619.

75 Olateju TO, Vanderpump MP. Thyroid hormone resistance. *Ann Clin Biochem* 2006; **43**: 431–440.

76 Koren R. Vitamin D receptor defects: the story of hereditary resistance to vitamin D. *Pediatr Endocrinol Rev* 2006; **3** (Suppl 3): 470–475.

3 Measuring Hormones, Molecular Tests and their Clinical Application

Jan M. Wit[1], Marcel Karperien[2] & Bart E.P.B. Ballieux[3]

[1] Department of Pediatrics, Leiden University Medical Center, Leiden, The Netherlands
[2] Biomedical Technology Institute, Twente University, Enschede, The Netherlands
[3] Department of Clinical Chemistry, Leiden University Medical Center, Leiden, The Netherlands

Principles of diagnostic procedures

The aim of investigation is to increase or decrease the probability of a diagnosis and to monitor the natural history of a condition or the response to treatment. It can thus reshuffle the order of likelihood of the differential diagnosis based on the clinical presentation. The definition of a diagnosis is arbitrary and subject to changing views. For example, it is open to discussion whether symptoms and signs should define it or whether it is defined by biochemical, anatomical or pathological similarities or by genetic markers. Furthermore, in each patient, a medical condition has a somewhat different expression, probably because of variation in genetic and environmental influences [1].

Part of the fuzziness of diagnostic labels in endocrinology is caused by the uncertainty about the biological effect of circulating hormones. Endocrinology has traditionally focused on hormone concentrations in serum and urine but little is known about sensitivity to hormones. In the field of growth, the variation in growth patterns is determined not only by growth hormone (GH) secretion but also by GH sensitivity (Fig. 3.1) [2]. Sensitivity to hormones can vary greatly, which is important to consider if hormone concentrations are used as indicators of a diagnosis.

For common clinical presentations, like short stature, evidence-based guidelines for diagnosis can be developed. In cases with an unusual presentation, diagnostic procedures are used not only for detecting or excluding known disorders but also for seeking novel causes of disease through investigations for pathophysiological mechanisms. In most instances, establishing the diagnosis leads to decisions on management.

Value of a diagnostic test

A diagnostic test should not be used before its value is clearly documented. For a proper assessment of the value of a diagnostic test, its validity, importance and applicability have to be considered (Table 3.1) [3,4].

Validity

A number of points have to be established for test validity:
1 The test should be compared with a "gold standard" test that can demonstrate a disease with maximal certainty. Gold standards are often lacking in pediatric endocrinology.
2 The index and reference tests should be assessed blindly (independently). If this is not done, it will usually cause an artificially increased agreement between the two tests (review bias).
3 Both tests should be carried out in all patients. If, for example, only the index test-positive patients were referred for the reference test, this would lead to so-called workup bias.
4 The index test should be independent of other relevant information about the clinical condition of the patient.
5 The value of the index test should be investigated in a population that is relevant to the situation in which the test is to be carried out. In general, the spectrum of disease characteristics should be broad. The group that does not have the pertinent disorder should consist of persons with medical conditions that can easily be confused with the disorder and who are similar to those in whom one would use it in practice.
6 The test should be validated in a second, independent group of patients.

Importance

If the test is valid, the extent and how precisely the index test can predict the presence or absence of the suspected condition have to be determined. The key principle is probability (likelihood) as an (inverse) expression of diagnostic uncertainty. In order to quantify this, it is necessary first to decide whether the test result can be treated as dichotomous (positive or negative) or continuous. In the latter, an analysis including a series of cutoff points resulting in a so-called receiver operating characteristic (ROC) curve (see below) has to be performed.

Various parameters are available for measuring the power of a test. An example of the general scheme, a hypothetical

Brook's Clinical Pediatric Endocrinology, 6th edition. Edited by C. Brook, P. Clayton, R. Brown. © 2009 Blackwell Publishing, ISBN: 978-1-4051-8080-1.

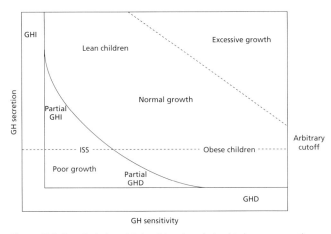

Figure 3.1 Hypothetical model describing the relationship between growth hormone (GH) secretion and GH sensitivity in growth regulation. GHD, growth hormone deficiency; GHI, growth hormone insufficiency; ISS, idiopathic short stature. From Kamp [2] with permission.

Table 3.1 Criteria for evaluating the value of a diagnostic test. After Sackett *et al.* [3] and Offringa *et al.* [4].

Validity

1 Was there a valid reference test (gold standard)?
2 Was there an independent (blind) comparison of the index test with the reference test?
3 Was the reference test applied regardless of the diagnostic test result?
4 Was the index test carried out independently of other relevant information about the health status of the patient?
5 Was the test evaluated in an appropriate spectrum of patients (like those in whom one would use it in practice)?
6 Was the test validated in a second, independent group of patients?

Importance

1 Diagnostic value of the index test
2 Precision of the estimated diagnostic parameters

Applicability

1 Is the diagnostic test available, affordable, accurate and precise in one's own setting?
2 Can one generate a clinically sensible estimate of the patient's pretest probability? (from personal experience, prevalence statistics, practice databases or primary studies; from an estimation of the similarity of the described patients to one's own practice; from an estimate of whether the disease possibilities have changed since the evidence was gathered)
3 Will the resulting post-test probabilities affect one's management and help one's patient? (Could it move us across the test-treatment threshold? Would the patient be a willing partner in carrying it out? Would the consequences of the test help our patient reach his or her goals in all of this?)
4 Does the severity of the disease and the possibilities for treatment, as well as the possible hazards and side-effects of the test and the risk of false-positive and false-negative results warrant the use of this test?

diagnostic test for GH deficiency and a definition of the various test characteristics is shown in Table 3.2 (the 2 × 2 table) [5].

The best known parameters are sensitivity and specificity. The sensitivity of a test is the proportion of positive index test results among the diseased (20 of 25). In the remaining patients (5 of 25), the test result is negative (a false-negative result). The specificity of a test is the proportion of negative index test results among the non-diseased. In the remaining persons (in our example 13%), the positive test would wrongly suggest disease (a false-positive result). When a test has a high sensitivity, a negative result rules *out* the diagnosis. Similarly, when a test has a high specificity, a positive result rules *in* the diagnosis. Because testing normal children is difficult, sufficient data are rarely available for an accurate assessment of specificity.

Sensitivity and specificity have only limited value for the practicing clinician. What is needed are the positive and negative predictive values of the test, i.e. the proportion of patients with the condition among patients with a positive test result and the proportion without the condition among the patients with a negative test result. These values can be considered as post-test probabilities of the presence or absence of disease.

In this example, the pretest probability of GH deficiency (prevalence) was 25%; with a positive test result, the post-test probability increased to 67%. The pretest probability of an absence of GH deficiency was 75%; with a negative test result, the post-test probability of absence of GH deficiency increased to 93%.

The predictive value depends on the prevalence of the condition. For example, if the data in Table 3.2 are reworked with a lower presumed prevalence, a positive test result increased the probability of GH deficiency from 5% to 25% and a negative test result increased the probability of non-GH deficiency from 95% to 99% (Table 3.3). The relationship between pretest probability (prevalence) and post-test probability is shown in Figure 3.2. The largest diagnostic benefit can be obtained in situations where the prevalence is between 30% and 70%. If the prevalence is lower or higher, a test result does not add much to the clinical (un)certainty.

A test characteristic independent of the prevalence is the likelihood ratio (LR) for a positive (LR+) or negative (LR−) test. The LR+ is the proportion between the probability of a positive test result in people with or without the condition. A test with a LR+ of 1 is not informative but gets more informative as the LR+ increases: an infinite LR+ is pathognomonic for the disease. The LR− is the proportion between the probability of a negative test result in people with or without the condition, so a test with a LR− of 0 excludes the condition. With the LR, a pretest probability (prevalence) can be transformed to a post-test probability. This transformation goes via the ratio between the probability of the occurrence of something and the probability that it does not occur. The equations were first described by Bayes (Bayes' theorems). For this calculation, one needs the following equations:

Table 3.2 The classic 2 × 2 table (a), a hypothetical example of test results in 100 individuals with respect to a diagnosis of growth hormone (GH) deficiency (b) and calculation of parameters for quantitating the value of a diagnostic test (c). After [3–5].

(a)

		Target disorder		
		Present	Absent	Totals
Test result	Positive	a	b	a + b
	Negative	c	d	c + d
Totals		a + c	b + d	a + b + c + d

(b)

		GH deficiency		
		Present	Absent	Totals
GH test result	Positive	20	10	30
	Negative	5	65	70
Totals		25	75	100

(c)

Parameter	Calculation	Outcome in example
Sensitivity (se) = proportion of positive index test results (true positives) among the diseased	a/(a + c)	20/25 = 0.80
Specificity (sp) = proportion of negative index test results (true negatives) among the non-diseased	d/(b + d)	65/75 = 0.87
Prevalence of disease (pretest probability of disease)	(a + c)/(a + b + c + d)	25/100 = 0.25
Prevalence of non-disease (pretest probability of non-disease)	(b + d)/(a + b + c + d)	75/100 = 0.75
Positive predictive value = proportion diseased among the persons with a positive result on the index test = post-test probability of disease	a/(a + b)	20/30 = 0.67
Negative predictive value = proportion non-diseased among the persons with a negative result on the index test = post-test probability of non-disease	d/(c + d)	65/70 = 0.93
Likelihood ratio for a positive result (LR+) = the ratio between the probability of a positive test result in diseased and in non-diseased	(a/(a + c))/(b/(b + d)) = se/(1−sp)	0.8/0.133 = 6.0
Likelihood ratio for a negative result (LR−) = the ratio between the probability of a negative test result in diseased and in non-diseased	(c/(a + c))/(d/(b + d)) = (1−se)/sp	0.20/0.87 = 0.23
Pretest odds = prevalence/(1 − prevalence)		0.25 : 0.75 = 0.33
Post-test odds = pretest odds × likelihood ratio		0.33 × 6 = 2 : 1 = 2
Post-test probability = post-test odds/(post-test odds + 1)		2/(2 + 1) = 0.67

Note: for calculating test characteristics and their 95% confidence intervals, see for example http://www.cebm.net/toolbox.asp or http://araw.mede.uic.edu/cgi-alansz/testcalc.pl.

Pretest odds = pretest probability/(1 − pretest probability)

Post-test odds = LR × pretest odds

Post-test probability = post-test odds/(post-test odds + 1)

Alternatively, the nomogram in Figure 3.3 can be used.

Dividing test results into normal and abnormal is a gross simplification. In reality, the test result is assessed and interpreted in more detail; some abnormal results are pathognomonic for disease, while a less extreme value is not. For example, the interpretation of a serum thyroid-stimulating hormone (TSH) of 6 is quite different from the interpretation of a serum TSH of >500 mU/L, although both are above the cutoff level of approximately 5 mU/L (depending on the laboratory method).

In most cases, there is an overlap of test results in diseased and non-diseased persons, which obviously leads to imperfect sensitivity and specificity. In Table 3.4, data are shown for various ranges of serum glucose in 300 persons with and 700 persons without diabetes mellitus [4]. If the cutoff point were set at 10.5 mmol/L, there would be no non-diabetic persons above that limit (specificity 100%) but a considerable number of diabetic patients would not be detected (low sensitivity, high percentage of false-negative results). Within the zone of overlap, each cutoff would be associated with a certain sensitivity and specificity. In

Table 3.3 Results of a test with identical test characteristics as the test in Table 3.2 but with a prevalence of 5% instead of 25%. From Hindmarsh & Brook [5].

		GH deficiency		
		Present	Absent	Totals
GH test result	Positive	20	63	83
	Negative	5	412	417
Totals		25	475	500

Sensitivity = 20/25 = 80%.
Specificity = 412/475 = 87%.
Pretest probability of GH deficiency = 25/500 = 0.05.
Pretest probability of absence of GH deficiency = 475/500 = 0.95.
Positive predictive value = post-test probability of disease = 20/83 = 0.24.
Negative predictive value = post-test probability of non-disease = 412/417 = 0.99.
Likelihood ratio for a positive test result = se/(1-sp) = 0.80/0.133 = 6.0.
Likelihood ratio for a negative test result = (1-se)/sp = 0.20/0.87 = 0.23.

Table 3.4 Serum glucose concentrations (mmol/L) in 300 persons with and 700 persons without diabetes and sensitivity and specificity of serum glucose for diabetes mellitus for various cutoff points. From Offringa et al. [4].

Serum glucose	Diabetes	No diabetes	Sensitivity	Specificity
≥11.0	66	0	0.22	1.00
10.5–10.9	31	0	0.32	1.00
10.0–10.4	29	1	0.42	1.00
9.5–9.9	25	1	0.50	1.00
9.0–9.4	16	3	0.56	0.99
8.5–8.9	19	4	0.62	0.99
8.0–8.4	10	5	0.65	0.98
7.5–7.9	16	20	0.71	0.95
7.0–7.4	20	30	0.77	0.91
6.5–6.9	18	52	0.83	0.83
6.0–6.4	13	111	0.88	0.68
5.0–5.9	16	166	0.93	0.44
4.0–4.9	11	155	0.97	0.22
<4.0	10	152		
Total	300	700		

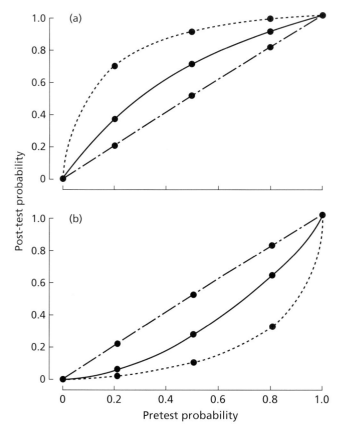

Figure 3.2 The relation between pretest and post-test probability of disease. The data were constructed using Bayes' theorem with a test sensitivity and specificity of either ———, 70% or ------, 90%. (a) The post-test probability if the test were positive; (b) the post-test probability if the test were negative. If the post-test probability were the same as the pretest probability, then the relation would be given by the 45° line.

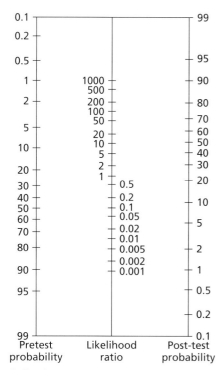

Figure 3.3 A likelihood ratio nomogram. With this nomogram, the post-test probability for a disease can be calculated from the likelihood ratio and the pretest probability. Draw a line from the pretest probability on the left axis to the likelihood ratio on the middle axis. Extrapolate this line toward the right axis to indicate the post-test probability. From Offringa et al. [4] with permission.

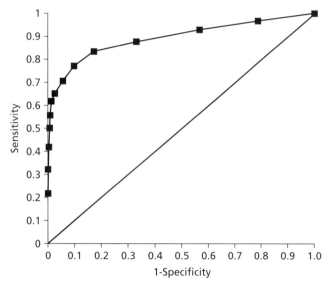

Figure 3.4 Receiver operating characteristic (ROC) curve of the relationship between sensitivity and (1 – specificity) of serum glucose determinations for the diagnosis of diabetes mellitus at 14 different cutoff points (data from Table 3.4). Each dot represents a cutoff point. From Offringa *et al.* [4] with permission.

this example, there is no range where there would be no diabetic patients, so the sensitivity never reaches 100%.

The ROC curve can express the relationship between sensitivity and specificity. The ROC curve belonging to the data in Table 3.4 is shown in Figure 3.4. Sensitivity is plotted on the *y*-axis and 1-specificity on the *x*-axis. The optimal cutoff point, the best combination of sensitivity and specificity, is the point located as close as possible to the upper left corner of the diagram. Using this cutoff point, the number of false-positive and false-negative values is minimal. The better the diagnostic power of the test, the bigger are the surface between the curve and the diagonal (area under the curve). Thus, a test with a ROC curve close to the diagonal is not discriminative.

The precision of the estimated diagnostic parameters is usually expressed as the 95% confidence interval. The bigger the number of patients, the smaller the 95% confidence interval gets. Equations can be found in books on evidence-based medicine [3] and on the Internet (see footnote to Table 3.2).

Applicability

Before using a test, four conditions should be met: first, whether the test is available, affordable, accurate and precise and whether the characteristics of the patient(s) in whom the test is to be used are sufficiently similar to the patients in whom the test has been described. Secondly, the pretest probability (prevalence) of the condition should be estimated. Thirdly, using the nomogram in Figure 3.3, it can be seen whether the test results may cause a substantial change in the probability of disease and thereby change decisions on treatment. In this context, the concepts of "test threshold" and "treatment threshold" are helpful [3]. If the probability of disease is (or would become) lower than the test

Table 3.5 Results of applying two tests assessing growth hormone (GH) secretion (insulin-induced hypoglycemia and clonidine) to patients with or without GH insufficiency (assuming the availability of a gold standard). From Hindmarsh & Brook [5].

(a)

		GH deficiency		
		Present	Absent	Totals
Insulin-induced	Positive	70	35	105
hypoglycemia	Negative	30	65	95
Totals		100	100	200

Sensitivity = 70/100 = 0.70.
Specificity = 65/100 = 0.65.
Pretest probability of GH deficiency = 100/200 = 0.50.
Pretest probability of absence of GH deficiency = 100/200 = 0.50.
Positive predictive value = post-test probability of disease = 70/105 = 0.67.
Negative predictive value = post-test probability of non-disease = 65/95 = 0.68.
Likelihood ratio for a positive test result = se/(1-sp) = 0.70/0.35 = 2.0.
Likelihood ratio for a negative test result = (1-se)/sp = 0.30/0.65 = 0.46.

(b)

		GH deficiency		
		Present	Absent	Totals
Clonidine test	Positive	65	15	80
	Negative	35	85	120
Totals		100	100	200

Sensitivity = 65/100 = 0.65.
Specificity = 85/100 = 0.85.
Positive predictive value = post-test probability of disease = 65/80 = 0.81.
Negative predictive value = post-test probability of non-disease = 85/120 = 0.71.
Likelihood ratio for a positive test result = se/(1-sp) = 0.65/0.15 = 4.3.
Likelihood ratio for a negative test result = (1-se)/sp = 0.35/0.85 = 0.41.

(c)

		GH deficiency		
		Present	Absent	Totals
Both tests	Both positive	55	10	65
combined	One positive	25	30	55
	Both negative	20	60	80
Totals		100	100	200

If one demands that both tests are positive:
Sensitivity = 55/100 = 0.55.
Specificity = 90/100 = 0.90.
Positive predictive value = post-test probability of disease = 55/65 = 0.85.
Negative predictive value = post-test probability of non-disease = 90/135 = 0.67.
Likelihood ratio for a positive test result = se/(1-sp) = 0.55/0.10 = 5.5.
Likelihood ratio for a negative test result = (1-se)/sp = 0.45/0.90 = 0.5.
If one demands that one or two tests are positive:
Sensitivity = 80/100 = 0.80.
Specificity = 60/100 = 0.60.
Positive predictive value = post-test probability of disease = 80/120 = 0.67.
Negative predictive value = post-test probability of non-disease = 60/80 = 0.75.
Likelihood ratio for a positive test result = se/(1-sp) = 0.80/0.40 = 2.0.
Likelihood ratio for a negative test result = (1-se)/sp = 0.20/0.60 = 0.3.

threshold, no more testing is needed. If the probability of disease is or gets higher than the treatment threshold, further testing would be abandoned and treatment started. Only if the diagnostic test result left the clinician stranded between the test and the treatment thresholds would other tests be performed. Finally, the decision to use a test should depend not only on the expected change in probability and its consequences for treatment but also on the severity of the disease and the possibilities for treatment, as well as the possible hazards and side effects of the test and the risk of false-positive and false-negative results.

The decision to stop investigation and to treat or not depends on how convinced the clinician is of the diagnosis, the benefits and risks of therapy and the potential yield and risks of further tests. In such circumstances, the clinician can conduct another test or use a more sophisticated analysis rather than a simple positive or negative. The strategy of using two tests for the diagnosis of GH deficiency is common. The additional value of a second test is illustrated in Table 3.5. The highest positive predictive value and the highest likelihood ratio for a positive test result can be reached with the combination of two tests if both tests are positive. The highest negative predictive value and lowest likelihood ratio for a negative test result can be reached when neither test is positive. The next step is to decide the level of probability required for the decision to start treatment.

Diagnostic strategy

Confronted with a child with a given set of symptoms and signs, an experienced clinician will summarize the problems, make a differential diagnosis and list the diagnostic procedures. The list is usually a compromise of rational, economic and social considerations. The rational approach would dictate that laboratory tests should aim to confirm or refute the most likely condition(s) in a stepwise manner and, at the same time, check for rarer conditions for which timely diagnosis and intervention are important. Economic considerations would urge the clinician only to use tests that offer a reasonable chance of shedding light on the diagnosis at a minimum cost. Social considerations would lead to minimizing the burden for the child by limiting the number of venepunctures, preferably to one. In many cases, it is useful to store part of the serum from the first venepuncture so that additional tests can be performed based on the findings from initial analyses. For this purpose, however, a well-organized storage system is needed.

An often overlooked aspect of diagnostic tests is the timing of blood sampling. Some hormone concentrations show a strong diurnal variation (e.g. cortisol) but plasma testosterone and estradiol also show diurnal variation in early puberty.

Measurements of hormones in blood, urine and other body fluids

The pediatric endocrinologist is heavily dependent on the laboratory to make a diagnosis for patient management. Therefore, some basic knowledge of hormone assays and a good relationship with the pathologist or clinical chemist is essential. In this collaboration, it is important to acknowledge that the physician is responsible for the choice of laboratory parameters to be examined and the test circumstances (e.g. timing, influence of nutrition, medication), for the appropriate transport of the sample to the laboratory and for the clinical interpretation. The laboratory is responsible for the technical validity and reproducibility of the hormone measurements through standardized laboratory procedures and quality control [6,7] but in many hospital settings the laboratory is also responsible for venepuncture and transport.

The concentration of hormones in biological fluids is low, down to the lower pmol/L range for free thyroxine so assays used to measure hormones must be exceptionally sensitive. Most hormones are easily detected with fast and sensitive immunoassays but other methods, such as bioassays, radioreceptor assays and *in situ* methods, are used in some specific situations.

Before the introduction of radioimmunoassay, bioassays were the only methods to determine hormone concentrations. These are now used only for the standardization of hormone preparations (e.g. by reference laboratories of the World Health Organization), for testing the biological effectiveness of newly developed drugs and to test the biological activity of hormones in the serum of patients in whom there appears to be a discrepancy between the immunoassayable concentration and the biological effect. Example of the last are tests of biological activity of insulin-like growth factor type 1 (IGF-1) [8] and TSH receptor stimulating immunoglobulins [9].

With radioreceptor assays (RRAs), the specific binding of the hormone to a membrane receptor is examined, which obviously does not need to be identical to the biological activity. For this purpose, lymphocytes are mostly used. Immunofunctional assays (IFAs) involve binding of the ligand to the binding site of its natural receptor and subsequent recognition of the ligand bound by a specific monoclonal antibody that serves for quantitative detection [7,10].

In situ methods are mainly used in basic research. They use labeled antibodies and antibody sandwiches for detecting immobilized antigens in microtome sections of tissues (immunohistochemistry), in cells (cytochemistry) and after transfer (blotting) on to carrier membranes (dot-blot, Western immunoblot) [7].

Immunoassays

Immunoassays make use of specific, high-affinity bonding between antibodies and their antigens and are usually divided into competitive (reagent-limited) and non-competitive (reagent-excess) assays [6,7].

The principle of the competitive immunoassay (IA) is that, after mixing the antigen (the hormone in the sample) with antibodies and a labeled antigen (tracer), an equilibrium is created between the bound tracer and the bound antigen that reflects their relative concentrations in the assay mixture (Fig. 3.5). By subsequently removing the unbound component, the amount of bound antigens can be estimated. Using a calibration curve

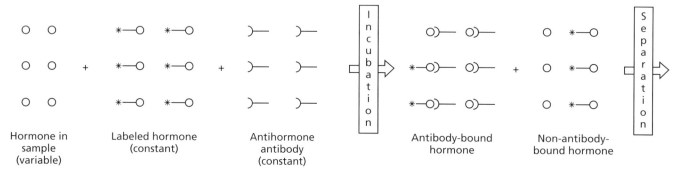

Figure 3.5 A schematic representation of a competitive immunoassay. Hormone in the patient sample and a fixed amount of labeled hormone compete for a fixed, limited number of antibody binding sites. A variety of methods are used to separate antibody-bound hormone and unbound hormone. The amount of bound labeled hormone is then determined. From Wheeler [6] with permission.

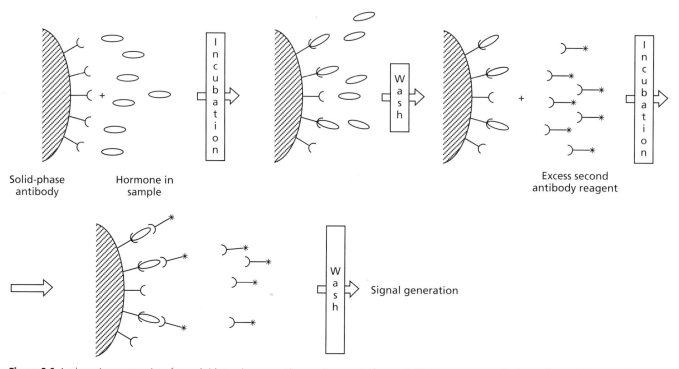

Figure 3.6 A schematic representation of a sandwich-type immunometric assay. Hormone in the sample binds to a capture antibody, usually attached to a solid phase. Excess hormone is aspirated away and a second labeled antibody is added in excess. After a short incubation time, excess labeled antibody is aspirated away. The amount of labeled antibody bound is then measured. From Wheeler [6] with permission.

describing the strength of the signal as a function of the analyte concentration, the concentration in the sample is calculated. The initial amount of antigen in the sample is inversely proportional to the signal of the bound tracer. Competitive assays are most commonly used for the measurement of steroids and other very small molecules with only one epitope available for antibody binding [7].

Non-competitive immunometric assays (IMAs) use a labeled antibody for signal generation. The most common format is the sandwich technique, which uses a solid-phase bound antibody as a capture antibody (Fig. 3.6) [11]. This antibody binds a propor-

tion of the hormone in the serum. The second antibody (tracer), to which the signal-generating label is attached, is added in excess so that it quickly binds to the captured hormone. Reactions can be quite short because only enough hormone, sufficient to produce a detectable signal when the tracer is bound, is required. In IMAs, the bound signal is proportional to the amount of antigens in the sample.

Over the years, many improvements have been implemented. Originally, the tracer (in IA and IMA) was labeled with radionuclides but enzymes, fluorescent and chemoluminescent labels are now used. These labels may be coupled directly or indirectly through biotin–streptavidin coupling. Owing to the catalytic effect in enzyme-based assays, it is possible for small amounts of bound enzyme to metabolize large quantities of substrate [7]. The most common endpoint used in both IAs and IMAs is chemoluminescence.

The separation of the unbound components in IA was mostly carried out by precipitation and subsequent centrifugation of the antigen–antibody complex with the help of a secondary antibody and/or the addition of a precipitation reagent. An improvement comes from the use of solid-phase bound capture antibodies. Usually, this solid phase is the wall of a polystyrene tube but polystyrene beads or magnetic particles are also used. Excess tracer can thus be removed easily by decanting or suction and washing away a specifically bound tracer is also achieved in the same way. Examples include the magnetic microparticle-based electrochemiluminescence immunoassay (ECLIA) and the enzyme-linked immunosorbent assay (ELISA), in which immobilization takes place mostly on 96-well microtitration plates.

Polyclonal antibodies are raised by repeated immunizations of animals with biomaterials. Specificity of the antiserum is subsequently improved by extracting cross-reacting immunoglobulins on immunoaffinity columns. Improvements were found in using recombinant antigens of high purity for immunization and polyclonal antibodies are being substituted by monoclonal antibodies.

One of the most significant changes in immunoassay technology has been the development of fully automated analyzers drastically increasing throughput of endocrinological laboratories [6]. In the near future, new measuring techniques based on biosensorics are expected. In these techniques, binding of the analyte to the immobilized biosensor on a chip directly produces a physical signal that can be detected and processed electronically [7]. Similarly, various physical, biosensor-based measuring techniques are being developed using amperometric, potentiometric, mass detection or optical biosensors. The microarray chip technology, which is currently mainly used for DNA analysis, is now also available for hormone measurements in protein arrays.

Besides immunoassays, high throughput gas or liquid chromatography linked to mass spectrometry is rapidly gaining importance for the measurement of small molecules such as steroids. The main use of this technique in routine hormone analysis is in the measurement of steroids in urine [12] and low concentrations of testosterone in blood [13]. Hormone concentrations can also be measured in body fluids other than blood and urine. In pediatrics, hormone measurements in saliva specimens, which can be obtained non-invasively, are used increasingly, for example for cortisol, 17α-hydroxyprogesterone and androstenedione.

There are four requirements for a good assay. It must be specific (i.e. measure only the particular analyte of interest and not others), sensitive (so that even low concentrations can be measured), accurate (i.e. the result should be close to the target value) and precise (i.e. the result should be reproducible). The result should be compared with an appropriate reference range.

Specificity

A constant challenge to the immunoassayist is specificity. The structures of steroid hormones are very similar and it may be difficult to differentiate one steroid from another. Protein hormones circulate in different forms, as fragments with small pieces of protein removed, as subunits or as macromolecular forms [14]. The measurement of the biologically active form may be very difficult because more than one form of the hormone may bind to the hormone receptor. Many protein and steroid hormones circulate in blood bound to a binding protein and decisions have to be made whether the total hormone or the non-protein-bound hormone is measured. If the non-protein-bound fraction is measured, the concentration may only be 1/100th of the concentration of the total hormone (e.g. T4, T3, testosterone) [6]. The ectodomain of receptors may circulate as a binding protein [e.g. GH binding protein (GHBP), TSH receptor fragments, leptin-soluble receptor]. Intracellular conversion of some hormones takes place to a more potent metabolite, for example T4 to T3, T to DHT and 25-OH-vitamin D to calcitriol. Local conversion of a potent hormone to a less potent one (cortisol to cortisone in the kidney by 11β-hydroxylase) also occurs.

The ability to produce monoclonal antibodies [15] has led to increased specificity, particularly for peptide hormones. A monoclonal antibody recognizes a single epitope on a molecule. This may not be enough to provide absolute specificity because that epitope may also be present on circulating subunits and fragments of the same hormone or even a different hormone. Greater specificity is imbued by the use of a second monoclonal antibody that recognizes another unique epitope on the hormone. If the two monoclonal antibodies bind to epitopes at different ends of the molecule, then only the intact molecule will be captured and fragments and subunits are excluded.

Another way to increase specificity (and to remove interference) is to carry out a purification or separation step before immunoassay. Common examples are adsorption, solvent extraction and high-performance liquid chromatography (HPLC). Alternatively, for protein assays, large concentrations of a substance that has minimal or no cross-reaction with the antibody but binds to the binding protein can be added to the assay reagents to displace the hormone from the binding proteins.

An objective parameter of specificity is cross-reaction, which describes the amount of an analyte similar to the one being measured that will be measured in an assay in percentage terms. The cross-reaction is usually calculated from the virtual analyte concentrations that are detected in samples containing the cross-reacting analyte expressed as a percentage of the given concentration of the cross-reacting analyte.

Sensitivity

Sensitivity may be described as either analytical or functional sensitivity. Analytical sensitivity is the lowest concentration of analyte that is significantly different from zero and is usually the sensitivity quoted for an assay if the two terms are not used separately. Twenty replicate analyses of the zero standard are usually carried out and the standard deviation (SD) of the responses is calculated. The concentration on the standard curve equivalent to either 2 or 2.5 SD from the zero response is taken as the sensitivity of the assay. Because of variation in the determination of analytical sensitivity and criticism of its usefulness [16], functional sensitivity is more meaningful. The functional sensitivity is defined as the lowest concentration above the analytical sensitivity threshold at which the interassay precision is <20%, which can be determined from the between-assay precision profile (see below) [6].

Accuracy

Accuracy or the absence of bias relate to the closeness of a result to a target value or the systematic error of measurement. This is probably of more concern to the laboratory professional than to the clinician because, as long as reference ranges have been determined properly for the assay in use and no change in the assay occurs, the clinician can determine whether or not a patient has a "normal" result. In the case of assays intended to measure hormones at the lower level of detection (i.e. testosterone in females and children), systematic bias is hard to establish due to the disproportionately large imprecision. Differences between manufacturers may also be substantial. More specific assay methods, such as LC-tandem-mass-spectrometry, will probably prove to be more suitable not only as reference methods but also in clinical practice

Precision

Precision represents the reproducibility of the measurement of an analyte at different concentrations. The intra-assay or within-assay precision (reproducibility of measurement in a single assay) and the interassay or between-assay precision (reproducibility of measurement between separate assays) are usually quoted for assays. However, precision is affected by differences between operators, the lot numbers of kits and temperature and it varies also with analyte concentration so that a single figure for precision is not possible. Instead, the precision of an assay can be cal-

culated across a wide range of concentrations and the data are plotted to give a precision profile (Fig. 3.7). The intra-assay precision will usually be better than the interassay precision. Therefore, specimens from studies examining changes in one individual on several occasions should be analyzed in a single assay to improve the detection of small but important changes in concentration.

The standard procedure to monitor stability of an assay over time is to include QC samples. These are often commercially produced preparations, usually provided in lyophilized form, that are included in every assay. A common approach is to run QC specimens at the beginning of the day to check that the machine is operating properly and that the calibration curve is giving the correct results. The QC specimens are then analyzed again at the end of the day. In manual assays run in batches, QC samples are usually included in the beginning and at the end of a series of samples. No matter what system is used, the results of the QC specimens must meet predetermined criteria. The most common approach is to plot the results on a Shewart or Levy Jennings graph (Fig. 3.8). To set up this chart, the QC specimens should be analyzed in 20 separate assays. The mean and SD are calculated and plotted. The SD should reflect the interassay precision of the assay determined during the development of the assay or as stated by the manufacturer. Examining the QC plot will indicate whether the assay is acceptable. However, the SD calculated from QC specimens may overestimate true precision, as lyophilization and reconstitution may introduce additional imprecision.

The working range of an assay is derived from the precision profile and is the range of concentration over which the intra-assay precision is less than a chosen amount, usually <10%. Examination of Figure 3.7 shows that, using this convention, method A has a working range of 1–30 nmol/L and method B a working range of 5 to >35 nmol/L. Method A thus shows greater sensitivity and is better suited to measure low concentrations but method B is superior to method A over the range 10–30 nmol/L because it achieves a precision of <5%. It also shows better precision than method A at higher concentrations.

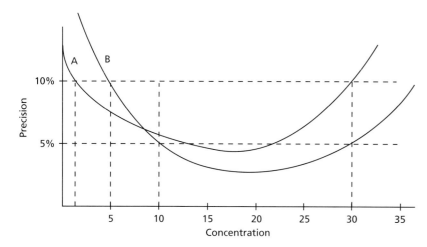

Figure 3.7 The precision profiles for two methods, A and B. Method A has a greater precision (<10%) at low concentrations, whereas method B shows better precision than method A at higher concentrations. Choice of method would depend on the range of concentration to be encountered in clinical samples. From Wheeler [6].

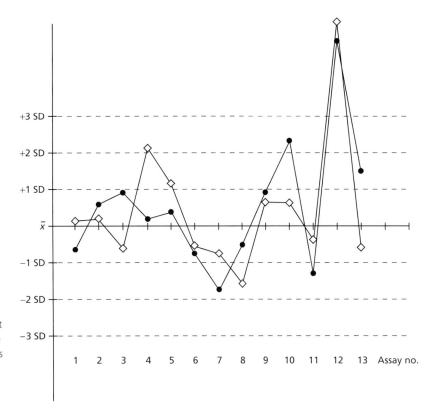

Figure 3.8 A typical plot of a quality control (QC) specimen run at the beginning (●) and at the end (◇) of the assay. Drift would be indicated by the latter having a constant bias to the former. Assay 12 should be rejected and the patient specimens reanalyzed. There would be at least two and often three, QCs of different concentrations run in every assay. From Wheeler [6] with permission.

The most important information of an assay for the clinician is the between-assay precision (representing 1 SD) because specimens are usually sent over a period of days, weeks or months. As a rough guide, within-assay precision is usually about 1–2% less than between-assay imprecision, so that an assay with a between-assay precision of 5% will have a within-assay precision of 3–4%.

Reference range

Having developed an assay capable of measuring the hormone of interest in its clinically most relevant form, interpretation of results is complicated by physiological variables (Table 3.6). Some hormones demonstrate a marked circadian rhythm, which may develop during puberty [e.g. luteinizing hormone (LH)] [17,18], and this has been examined as a possible diagnostic tool in the investigation of delayed puberty in children. Many hormones, both steroids and proteins, are increased during times of stress, which may confuse the interpretation of a result but, again, has been exploited clinically (e.g. the GH response to exercise in the investigation of GH deficiency in children) [19].

The *reference range* or reference interval is the range of concentrations of an analyte found in 95% of a defined population with no apparent pathology. Therefore, by definition, 5% of this population has analyte concentrations outside this range. Ideally, a reference range is determined by analyzing samples using the same laboratory assay and it should be established in a population clearly defined by sex, age range and time of day. If using a com-

Table 3.6 Physiological parameters associated with changes in hormone concentration. After Wheeler [6].

Parameter	Hormones
Circadian rhythm	Growth hormone, adrenal steroids
Sleep	Growth hormone, prolactin
Puberty	LH, FSH, gonadal steroids, adrenal steroids, growth hormone
Stress and exercise	Growth hormone, cortisol, prolactin
Food	Insulin, glucagon
Age	Estradiol, testosterone, SHBG, IGF-1, DHEAS
Sex	Estradiol, testosterone, SHBG
Menstrual cycle	LH, FSH, estradiol, progesterone
Low and high body weight	Reproductive hormones, growth hormone, leptin

DHEAS, dehydroepiandrosterone sulfate; FSH, follicle-stimulating hormone; IGF-1, insulin-like growth factor type 1; LH, luteinizing hormone; SHBG, sex hormone-binding globulin.

mercial kit, laboratories may use the range quoted by a manufacturer although they usually state that the reference range data are provided only as a guide. If sufficient details on the method of establishment are given it is often sufficient to check the validity of the given reference range for the local population with a limited number of samples. Alternatively, a range quoted in the literature can be used but using a reference range established using another method should be avoided. As shown in Table 3.7, the concentration of a number of hormones changes throughout life. In addition, the investigation of some diseases requires dynamic tests and reference ranges for the response are also required. Reference ranges do not necessarily reflect health or disease. For example, high insulin values within the reference range for the general population may reflect subclinical insulin resistance in obese individuals. Therefore, evidence-based target values may sometimes be more appropriate.

Reference values of some analytes display a considerable nonlinear relation with age (e.g. IGF-1, IGFBP3, adrenal androgens). In addition, many analytes show a markedly asymmetrical (non-Gaussian) distribution over the whole age range. These complex relationships are not adequately reflected by reference ranges expressed in mean ±2 SD provided for discrete age intervals. Smoothed reference curves can be produced with the LMS method, which produces continuous values for skewness (L), mean (M) and standard deviation (SD) for age [20,21].

Table 3.7 Situations that require separate reference ranges for the hormones affected. From Wheeler [6].

Parameter	Hormones affected	Changes encountered
Neonate dctlpar	17α-Hydroxyprogesterone	Rapid changes after delivery
	Testosterone in males	Rises after first 2 weeks of life and then falls at about 8–10 weeks
Children	Reproductive hormones	Low prepubertally and increase during puberty
	Adrenal androgens	
	IGF-1	
Aging adult	Gonadotrophins in women	Increase in post-menopausal women
	IGF-1	
	DHEAS and DHEA	Decrease with age
	Testosterone in men	
	SHBG	Increase as age increases
Menstrual cycle	Gonadotrophins	Concentrations are different in the follicular, mid-cycle and luteal phases
	Estradiol	
	Progesterone	
	Inhibins	
	17α-Hydroxyprogesterone	
Circadian rhythm	ACTH	Higher concentrations in the morning than in afternoon and evening
	Cortisol and other adrenal steroids	
	Testosterone in men	
Sleep	GH	Higher concentrations at night
	Prolactin	
Posture	Renin	Increase in concentrations moving from supine to standing
	Aldosterone	

ACTH, adrenocorticotropic hormone; DHEA, dehydroepiandrosterone; DHEAS, dehydroepiandrosterone sulfate; GH, growth hormone; IGF-1, insulin-like growth factor type 1; SHBG, sex hormone-binding globulin.

After diagnosis, laboratory support in patient management is often characterized by repeated measurements over time in order to evaluate disease recurrence or progression, the effect of therapy and patient adherence to a therapeutic regimen. Interpretation of these results is dependent on the knowledge of both analytical variance (CV_a) of the requested assay and the within-subject biological variation (CV_i) of the measured hormone. CV_a is known for most assays from internal quality control data at the local laboratory. The first evidence-based database of biological variation in clinical chemistry was published in 1999 [22]. Since then this list is constantly updated and freely available on the "Westgard QC" website (http://www.westgard.com/biodatabase1.htm).

Reference change value

Clinical decisions derived from changes in laboratory results are often based on clinical experience. A more objective guide is provided by the reference change value (RCV), which is the minimal difference between two successive measurements in one subject exceeding the random difference derived from assay and biological variations. The RCV is calculated as $\sqrt{2} \times Z \times \sqrt{[CV_a^2 + CV_i^2]}$, where Z is the number of standard deviations appropriate to the probability selected (i.e. Z = 1.96 for $P < 0.05$ and 2.56 for $P < 0.01$).

For example, for thyroid stimulating hormone (TSH), the given biological variation (CV_i) is 19.3% and a realistic assay variation (CV_a) is 4%. Thus, the calculated RCV is $\sqrt{2} \times 1.96 \times \sqrt{[4.0^2 + 19.3^2]} = 2.77 \times \sqrt{[16 + 372.5]} = 54.6\%$. If thyroxine therapy is adjusted between two successive TSH measurements in a single subject and the difference exceeds 54.6%, the likelihood that this difference is the consequence of random variation is less than 5%. Thus it is reasonable to assume that this change is the result of therapeutic intervention.

For HbA1c, the effect of adjustment of insulin therapy is reflected by a RCV of $2.77 \times \sqrt{[1.9^2 + 2.0^2]} = 7.6\%$ of the previous HbA1c result. If the first HbA1c result is 7, the RCV is $0.076 \times 7 = 0.5$, so a HbA1c <6.5 or >7.5 reflects a statistically significant change.

Endocrine tests (profiles, stimulation tests, suppression tests)

Assessment of endogenous secretion

Many hormones are secreted in pulses or have specific oscillatory activity. The time course over which these cycles take place is variable. For example, while insulin has a dominant periodicity of 13 min, GH pulses appear on average once every 3 h and cortisol has a diurnal rhythm with superimposed smaller pulses. In the case of a diurnal rhythm, at least two blood samples have to be drawn, as is often used to estimate diurnal variation of cortisol secretion.

From a clinical perspective, the main reason for performing multiple measurements of a hormone over time is to estimate its secretion. In pediatric endocrinology, this applies primarily to GH profiles [23]. A second reason is to assess the pulsatile pattern, either for diagnostic reasons (e.g. a nocturnal LH profile to estimate whether puberty has started) or to improve our understanding of the physiological role of pulsatile patterns. There is strong evidence that pulsatile secretion in animals may act as a biological signal for tissue-specific responses [24].

In discussing pulse analysis, it is worth considering why we should analyze them. From a clinical point of view, a glance at an individual data array is enough to demonstrate the existence of oscillation. However, where multiple data sets are available and when statements need to be made about group data, it becomes important to be able to extract attributes of pulsatility, which can then be pooled to provide a generic description.

Blood sampling

Two methods have been devised to obtain hormone profiles, discrete (single spot samples) and integrated sampling, where blood is withdrawn continuously over periods of varying length. Both techniques have advantages and disadvantages but, as long as the proper time interval is chosen (e.g. 20 min for GH), the results are similar [23].

To define rhythm, sampling must take place over more than one cycle. It is important with any sampling technique to consider also the effect of the sampling interval on the results obtained. Inappropriately long sampling intervals can lead to spurious results and failure to detect the oscillation of a hormone concentration. A minimum of five or six samples per cycle is required to prevent the mismatching of infrequent sampling intervals to the predominant period of pulsatility that is being observed. This mismatching is known as aliasing and is illustrated in Figure 3.9 [25].

The sampling interval determines the cycle frequency that can be detected. The lower the frequency of interest, the longer the time period over which measurements can be taken; conversely, the higher the frequency, the more frequently observations must be made.

Analysis of profiles

For clinical purposes, a single profile requires little analysis. Routine parametric statistics can be used to establish the mean and SD of the data. There is no advantage in calculating the area under the curve, because it is identical to the mean multiplied by the total duration of the sampling. Other parameters that can be read directly from the raw data include the number and amplitude of the peaks and the maximum peak.

Where statements need to be made about populations or subpopulations or the changes within pathological states or following treatment intervention or when other attributes of pulsatile systems (such as periodicity, regularity, trough values, shape of peaks, rate of change of hormone concentrations, frequency and/ or amplitude modulation) are to be investigated, more sophisticated techniques are required. These techniques fall under the general heading of "time series analysis," which involves tech-

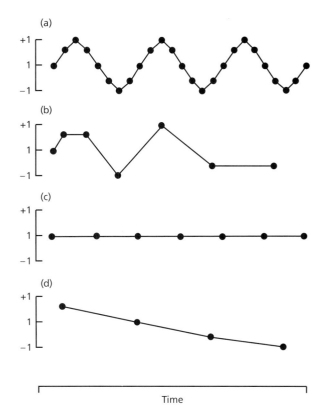

Figure 3.9 For a real oscillation (a), an incorrect assessment of its period can be made using inappropriate sampling intervals (b, c and d). From Matthews & Hindmarsh [25] with permission.

niques for analyzing regularly sampled data [25]: all use a form of pulse detection. Several computerized peak detection algorithms have been developed for this purpose, each trying to pinpoint criteria of what constitutes a peak and what is biological noise. Two programs, PULSAR [26] and Cluster [27], have been used most widely. An estimate of the secretion can be made with deconvolution analysis, for example with the program Deconv/ Pulse [28]. Furthermore, approximate entropy, a measure that attempts to quantitate regularity in data [29], can be assessed. The greater the entropy, the more the randomness and the less the system order. Other mathematical procedures that have been used in the analysis of hormone profiles include autocorrelation, Fourier analysis and distribution methods [25].

Clinical implications

Sequential hormone measurements are mostly performed for GH. In theory, it should be the gold standard for endogenous GH secretion in a particular child but it is assessed in only a minority of patients because it is time-consuming and burdensome both for the patient and for medical and nursing staff. Other problems are that the amount of blood drawn must be small in relation to the patient's blood volume and it may be difficult in small children to establish a peripheral catheter large enough to draw blood and remain patent.

A further problem is that it is almost impossible to obtain control data. In addition, in the rare studies in which healthy children have undergone 24-h sampling, a remarkably large variation in 24-h GH secretion was observed [30]. Part of this large variation appears to result from day-to-day variability, which further decreases the value of the test [31]. Another part of the variation may be due to interindividual differences in GH sensitivity.

A 12- or 24-h GH profile may deserve a place in the diagnostic armamentarium in those patients in whom a clinical suspicion of GH deficiency in combination with low plasma IGF-1 and IGF binding protein 3 (IGFBP-3) values is not confirmed by a low GH peak at a provocation test. If a discrepancy between a low spontaneous secretion and a normal GH peak after provocation is found, this may be labeled neurosecretory dysfunction [32], although obviously the low spontaneous secretion may also be a false-positive result.

Another hormone with a strong pulsatile character is LH. In the early phases of puberty the first sign is pulsatile secretory LH activity during sleep [33]. As puberty progresses, the amplitude and frequency of LH pulses increase, initially only during the night but, when puberty progresses, also during the day, leading ultimately to the adult pattern of LH bursts [18]. If a gonadotropin-releasing hormone (GnRH) test and GnRH analog test still leave the clinician in doubt as to whether puberty has started, night-time sampling of LH and follicle-stimulating hormone (FSH) can be performed, with an interval of not more than 20 min. Besides GH, LH and FSH, secretion of ACTH, TSH and prolactin also show pulsatile patterns.

Stimulation and suppression tests

Stimulation tests are used to assess the maximum secretion of a hormone. In principle, the tests measure the responsiveness to the stimulus and the hormonal reserve in the target cells, which is not necessarily identical to the endogenous secretion. There is only a moderate correlation between a 24-h profile and GH stimulation test results [34,35], which is probably due to considerable intraindividual variation in both tests. Still, for practical reasons, GH stimulation tests are generally used as a proxy parameter of endogenous secretion.

Theoretically, a stimulation test should more sensitively pick up deficiencies that would be missed by assessing spontaneous hormone concentrations as compared with baseline hormone concentrations. For example, subclinical (compensated) hypothyroidism may become apparent only by elevated stimulated TSH values after a thyrotrophin-releasing hormone (TRH) bolus. Similarly, partial deficiency or heterozygosity of one of the adrenal enzymes or partial (compensated) primary or secondary hypocortisolism may become apparent only after stimulation with ACTH.

A problem with every stimulation test is that standardization is poor. As with all tests in pediatrics, there are considerable difficulties obtaining age-matched controls. Protocols are usually based on historical precedents, for example the first reported protocol.

Suppression tests are performed to study whether the hormone production remains under physiological control: examples include the oral glucose tolerance test to check whether GH secretion can be suppressed and the administration of dexamethasone to check whether cortisol or adrenal androgens can be suppressed.

Chromosomal analysis and molecular tests

Chromosomal analysis and molecular (DNA) tests have become increasingly important in pediatric endocrinology because many of the diseases encountered in clinical practice have a genetic cause. Chromosomal analysis and molecular/DNA tests are usually performed to confirm a diagnosis and make it more precise in terms of the molecular defect. For example, chromosomal analysis is a crucial part of diagnosis of girls with short stature. Short girls without the classic stigmata may have Turner syndrome which can be confirmed only by assessing the karyotype. This technique usually requires mononuclear cells but when the karyotype of the leukocytes is reported as normal, Turner syndrome still cannot be completely excluded because mosaicism may occur (although rarely), when the chromosomal abnormality is absent in leukocytes but present in other cell types, such as skin fibroblasts. Chromosomal analysis is also crucial in children with ambiguous genitalia and in boys suspected of Klinefelter syndrome (XXY) or an XYY karyotype and is helpful in children with dysmorphic features. Although karyotyping allows a genome-wide detection of numerical and larger structural chromosomal abnormalities, the resolution of the conventional chromosome analysis is limited to 5–10 Mb.

Fluorescence *in situ* hybridization (FISH) analysis is a valuable addition to conventional chromosomal analysis. Smaller deletions and translocations that are not detectable in a karyogram can be visualized but the technique does not have the sensitivity to detect very small deletions of, for example, a few exons or a few nucleotides. FISH can be used to demonstrate whether two copies of a gene are present (the normal situation) or one (haplodeficiency) or three (duplication).

It is based on the principle that DNA consists of two complementary DNA strands packed in a double helix. The strands of the DNA can be separated by a process called denaturing. Denatured DNA can be mixed with a set of single-stranded DNA probes. One probe has a DNA sequence complementary to the gene or critical region of the suspected disorder and is labeled with a unique fluorescent marker (fluorochrome). Another probe is used as a control and contains a DNA sequence that is located on the same chromosome on which the defect is suspected. This probe is labeled with a different fluorochrome. A chromosome preparation is made of cells of the patient. After denaturing the DNA, this cell fraction is mixed with the single-stranded DNA probes under conditions that allow hybrization of the labeled probes with the complementary chromosomal DNA. The hybridized probes are subsequently visualized using fluorescence techniques.

In normal circumstances, one dot for the critical region and one for the control gene are visible on each of the two homologous chromosomes. In the case of a deletion of the gene on one chromosome, only one colored dot is detected in comparison to two dots on the control gene. Duplication of the gene on one of the chromosomes is detected by three dots (Fig. 3.10).

Although FISH is far more sensitive than a karyogram, the chromosomal defect that can be detected has to be a few tens of thousands of base pairs long. Smaller intergenic deletions or amplifications of a few exons cannot be detected. Techniques such as Multiplex Ligation-dependent Probe Amplification (MLPA) are available for the detection of such defects [36]. Smaller defects, such as point mutations in the DNA sequence, require still more sensitive detection techniques. In contrast to karyotyping or FISH, which require the presence of intact cells for the analysis, the latter techniques all rely on the presence of genomic DNA and are invariably based on the application of one particular technique, polymerase chain reaction (PCR). The isolation of genomic DNA and the PCR is described in detail below.

Indications for molecular tests

The purpose of genetic testing is to find a DNA mutation responsible for the disorder of the patient. A mutation is a change in the primary nucleotide sequence of DNA. Mutations can occur in the germline, during embryogenesis or in somatic tissues. Mutations that occur during development lead to mosaicism: a mutation can influence the function of a gene and thus the protein it encodes but whether this occurs is dependent on the location of the mutation and its nature. Polymorphisms are defined either in terms of prevalence (a mutation that occurs in more than 1% or 5% of the population) or in terms of functionality (a mutation that has no effect). In contrast to a mutation that affects the function of a gene, which is often the cause of the disease, polymorphisms are not disease-causing although they may be associated with disease.

For the practicing pediatric endocrinologist, family history is an essential step in recognizing the possibility of hereditary disorders, so a detailed pedigree of the first-degree relatives is required. In patients suspected of a genetic disorder with no family history, it is useful to collect DNA from the index case and the parents to check whether a mutation has occurred *de novo* (present in the index case but not in the parents). In such cases, a *de novo* mutation provides convincing evidence of pathogenicity. If no candidate gene is known, it is helpful to obtain material from as many family members, affected and unaffected, as possible.

In patients suspected of a disorder of which the genetic cause is known (e.g. achondroplasia, hypochondroplasia) or in a family where an index case with a genetic disorder is known, direct investigation of the expected affected gene or mutation is performed. In some disorders, one particular mutation or just a few are observed in a disease (e.g. the different mutations in the FGFR-3 gene in achondroplasia and hypochondroplasia). In other disorders, an almost unlimited number of different mutations is found (e.g. in congenital adrenal hyperplasia due to 21-hydroxylase deficiency [37]). The additional information on the exact genetic defect is of value for the patient because it can provide certainty about the diagnosis and, in some cases, it provides more reliable information about the clinical course and prognosis of the disorder.

It can serve as a basis for genetic counseling and prenatal diagnosis and is also of value in terms of clinical research, because an analysis of the phenotype and genetic defects of a group of patients provides better insight into the genotype–phenotype correlation. In turn, this will be of use for a firmer diagnosis of and information for future patients. Examples of this are the genotype–phenotype studies in patients with congenital adrenal hyperplasia due to a 21-hydroxylase defect, which have led to a better understanding of which mutations lead to a severe clinical phenotype and which to the non-classic presentation [37].

While this form of genetic testing is still in line with classic biochemical tests and is in fact an extension of them, molecular tests can also be used to unravel the causes of a disorder different from ones described before. The clinician should always keep an open mind in such cases and try to find the genetic explanation in collaboration with clinical geneticists and molecular biologists. There could be a new mutation in a known gene or an abnormality in a gene that was not associated with disease before. The number of disorders of which the genetic etiology has been resolved is steadily increasing. Most of this information is available in the Online Mammalian Inheritage in Man (OMIM) website (http://www.ncbi.nlm.nih.gov).

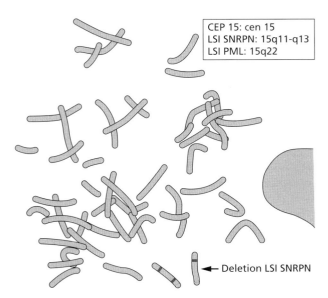

CEP 15: cen 15
LSI SNRPN: 15q11-q13
LSI PML: 15q22

← Deletion LSI SNRPN

Figure 3.10 Fluorescence *in situ* hybridization (FISH) of a patient with a deletion of the critical region for the Prader–Willi–Labhart syndrome (PWS). The LSI SNRPN probe is specific for the critical region of PWS located within 15q11-q13. The CEP15 (15p11.2) and LSI PML (15q22) serve as control probes for chromosome 15. Courtesy of Drs K. Hansson and C. Ruivenkamp, Department of Clinical Genetics, Leiden University Medical Center, Leiden, The Netherlands.

The elucidation of many genetic disorders has been greatly facilitated by the Human Genome Project, which has generated genetic and physical maps of the majority of the human genome. Thus, an important advantage of techniques of molecular biology applied in genetic research is that they enable the detection of disorders that do not lend themselves to conventional hormone measurements or have not been defined in their pathophysiology [38]. In this way, the identification of defective genes can pinpoint cellular pathways involved in key physiological processes.

Sample preparation and isolation of DNA

Most standard techniques used for mutation detection rely on the isolation of high-quality genomic DNA from whole blood. Sample preparation must be performed according to the instructions of the laboratory where the DNA analysis will take place. In most cases, a blood sample (5–10 mL) is taken into a tube treated with EDTA (ethylene diamine tetra-acetic acid) or heparin and mailed to the laboratory at room temperature. High-quality DNA can be isolated from these samples, even when they have been stored for more than 2 weeks at room temperature. The first step is then to isolate DNA, which can be stored for prolonged periods of time at 4°C without quality reduction until appropriate tests are available for a genetic disorder of as yet unknown origin.

In some situations, it may be advisable to obtain RNA instead of DNA. The handling of RNA is more complicated because RNA degrades rapidly and must be extracted directly from fresh tissue and stored at −80°C for later processing. To ensure RNA for future testing, it is useful to perform a skin biopsy from which a dermal fibroblast culture is established. Patient lymphocytes can also be Epstein–Barr virus (EBV) immortalized. Both fibroblasts and immortalized lymphocytes can be stored indefinitely in liquid nitrogen. In the case of possible somatic mutations, which are limited to a neoplastic tissue (e.g. in McCune–Albright syndrome), a sample of this lesion can be used for extraction of DNA or RNA.

Techniques commonly used for mutation detection

At the start of nearly all procedures currently used for the detection of mutations in DNA is the PCR, an *in vitro* method for copying a given DNA sequence exponentially. PCR has simplified and accelerated the isolation and cloning of DNA fragments dramatically. The components of a PCR include:

1 A DNA template (usually genomic DNA but also cDNA obtained after reverse transcription of mRNA; see below);

2 Oligonucleotide primers: short (about 20 nucleotides long), biochemically synthesized, single-stranded DNA molecules complementary to the DNA sequences that bracket the target DNA sequence of the template, present in great excess;

3 The nucleotides dATP, dGTP, dTTP and dCTP (dNTPs) as substrate for the DNA copies and energy donors for the polymerization process;

4 A heat-resistant DNA polymerase; and

5 Buffers that create an optimal environment for both polymerase activity and primer annealing.

There are three stages in a PCR cycle. At high temperature, the double-stranded DNA template is denatured (made single-stranded). The temperature is then lowered to enable the primers to bind to their complementary DNA sequence (annealing). Thereafter, the temperature is raised again to create the optimal temperature for the action of DNA polymerase, whereby the new DNA strand is made (extension). Then a new cycle starts, usually 20–30 times. The nucleotide sequence of the amplified PCR product is confirmed by sequencing.

PCR can also be used for the amplification of mRNA. To accomplish this, one has first to transcribe the mRNA into complementary DNA (cDNA) using the enzyme reverse transcriptase. This process is called reverse transcription. mRNA is incubated with an oligonucleotide primer of thymidine residues complementary to the poly-A tail of the mRNA. After annealing of the primer sequence to the mRNA, the primer sequence is extended by the enzyme reverse transcriptase, for which the mRNA serves as a template. Alternatively, random priming can be performed using hexanucleotides, which facilitate the amplification of 5′ regions of the mRNA. The result of the activity of the reverse transcriptase is a double-stranded RNA-DNA duplex, the cDNA, which can be used as input in a PCR. This procedure is called reverse transcription PCR (RT-PCR) and is useful as a qualitative or, with some modifications, a quantitative measure of gene expression.

For the detailed analysis of a piece of DNA, frequently obtained by PCR, the nucleotide sequence is determined by sequencing [39]. The present form of this technique is a unidirectional PCR (instead of two primers necessary for exponential amplification, only one primer is added to the reaction resulting in linear amplification). On top of the natural nucleotides, abnormal nucleotides [dideoxynucleotide triphosphate (ddNTP)] labeled with different fluorochromes are added. In each tube, a different one is used representing each of the four ddNTPs that stop the PCR randomly at a certain point. The resulting mixture consists of fluorescently labeled fragments of various lengths that are separated by gel electrophoresis. The sequence is subsequently read using the fluorochromes.

This method can be automated and sequences of various DNA templates can be determined simultaneously. Sequence analysis of PCR-amplified DNA fragments representing a candidate disease gene is the method of choice in the search for pathogenic mutations. It is simple, cheap, reliable and has a high sensitivity for the detection of mutations. Developments in this area, including the automation of the procedure and the use of PCR and sequencing robots, have reduced the use of various other more time-consuming and laborious screening techniques, such as single-strand conformation polymorphism (SSCP) [40], denaturing gradient gel electrophoresis (DGGE) [41], temperature gradient gel electrophoresis [TGGE] and heteroduplex detection by denaturing HPLC (dHPLC) [38,42].

PCR and the Human Genome Project have replaced many of the molecular biological techniques, such as traditional cloning techniques, that were formerly used in identifying disease-causing genes. Cloning refers to the creation of a recombinant DNA molecule that can be propagated indefinitely, most often using the bacterium strain *Escherichia coli* K-12 as a carrier. Computational methods and bioinformatics can now be used to predict gene function of previously uncharacterized genes and to test directly hypotheses about gene function in experimental models. Cloning techniques still have an important role in biological tests to prove pathogenicity of a new mutation in a particular gene. An example of a hormone receptor that is cloned by conventional strategies is the PTH receptor, the rat homolog of which was cloned by expression cloning, using radiolabeled PTH as bait. Subsequently, the rat cDNA was used for isolation of the mouse and human homologs [43,44].

Mutation detection in case of certainty about the gene involved

Knowledge of the identity of a disease-causing gene is fundamental for the detection of a pathogenic mutation. When the genetic defect of a particular disorder is known, mutation analysis is straightforward. If the disease is caused by a deletion or amplification of a gene, FISH analysis or MLPA are the methods of choice to start the search for the genetic defect (e.g. in mutation screening for Sotos syndrome and in patients with short stature suspected of a defect in the IGF-1R [45,46]). The genetic screen can be extended by direct sequencing of the DNA of the affected gene to identify a disease-causing point mutation. The mutations in the FGFR3 causing hypochondroplasia or achondroplasia can only be revealed by sequencing. If information on the gene involved is lacking, various approaches can be followed to localize and identify the genetic defect as discussed below.

Figure 3.11 shows the steps in the identification of a pathogenic mutation by sequencing in a disorder of which the gene defect is known. After isolation of genomic DNA from the index case, overlapping fragments of the candidate gene covering all coding exons and approximately 50 bp of flanking intron sequences are amplified by PCR. The required oligonucleotide primers can be derived either from the literature or be designed using software programs freely available on the Internet and the sequence information of the gene provided by the Human Genome Project. The nucleotide sequence of the PCR products is determined and compared with a reference sequence. In this way, heterozygous or homozygous nucleotide alterations can be detected with high specificity. The alterations have subsequently to be classified as either disease-causing (pathogenic) or non-functional.

A variety of point mutations can be found using sequencing: these include small insertions or deletions of one or a few nucleotides or single-nucleotide alterations, which can be divided into neutral, nonsense and missense mutations that are located either in the coding exon or the non-translated intronic parts of the gene that are amplified in the PCR reaction. The addition or removal of one (or a number that cannot be divided by three) nucleotide(s) leads to a frameshift which means that the code of all consequent codons changes and an abnormal protein is formed. Usually, one of the codons changes into a stop codon, so that the formation of the protein stops prematurely. This is almost invariably associated with disease. A nonsense mutation also leads to a premature stop codon and thus to a truncated protein. A neutral mutation indicates a nucleotide alteration that does not result in a change of amino acid in the translated protein. This usually has no functional relevance, unless the nucleotide alteration affects mRNA stability or protein translation.

If the mutated codon codes for another amino acid, a so-called missense mutation, it is not always clear whether the mutation causes disease. The protein may still retain its full function or part of it. The phenotype can thus vary from a complete deficiency to no signs at all. Additional functional tests may be needed in such cases before the mutation is causally associated with the disease.

If the mutation results in a protein with an amino acid with a different charge, particularly if it is located in a functional domain of the protein crucial for protein–protein interactions, folding or other aspects of secondary and tertiary structure, one can be almost sure that the mutation is functional. If a mutation leads to less clear changes in the protein, one can check whether the mutation is found in control subjects. If it is not, the likelihood of a mutation being functional increases and the next step is to check whether the mutation is present in family members with or without the disease. If the mutation segregates with the disease, it provides additional evidence and, depending on the number of family members available for analysis, can even prove causality. Finally, biochemical tests in cellular models or knockout models may be necessary to clarify the functional importance of the mutation and its relation to disease.

The great majority of mutations in non-coding regions have no functional relevance but there are three exceptions: a mutation in the promoter region or a response element of the promoter can cause diminished transcription and therefore less protein production [47]; a mutation at the boundary between an exon and an intron or in its close vicinity can disturb the action of the splicing machinery, leading to a defective RNA molecule due to aberrant splicing; a mutation in the untranslated tail or polyadenylation signal of the gene can diminish the stability of the mRNA, causing a lower protein production.

Most mutations in the functional domain of the a gene cause loss-of-function. Most are rare and heterozygous. Although most inactivating mutations are recessive, a deletion of a single allele can also result in haploinsufficiency, a situation in which one normal allele is not sufficient to maintain a normal phenotype. Other heterozygous mutations can result in loss-of-function due to a dominant-negative effect, in which the affected allele impairs the function of the second normal allele.

In some instances, a mutation leads to a gain-of-function. These mutations are characterized by complete or incomplete dominant inheritance. In some genes, for example the parathyroid hormone (PTH) receptor and the calcium-sensing receptor, both loss-of-function and gain-of-function mutations have been found (see Chapter 20).

Although most disease-causing mutations can be detected, pathogenic mutations located in intronic sequences or in the

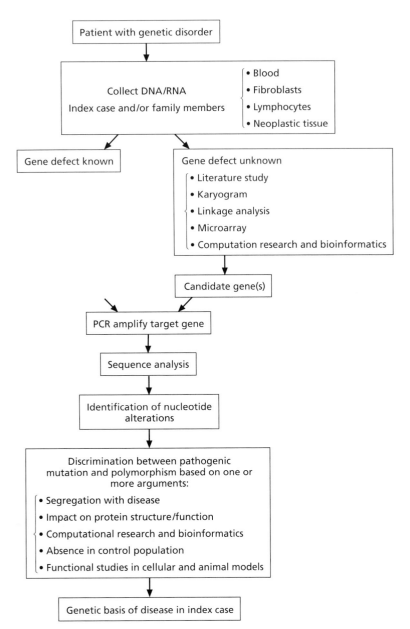

Figure 3.11 Flow diagram for the identification of disease-causing mutations by sequencing. See text for details.

promoter region of the gene that is involved in regulation of mRNA transcription, which are not amplified by the PCR, can be missed, as may microdeletions involving, for example, one of the two copies of an exon. In this situation, the normal allele is amplified and a false-negative score is obtained, so that the expression pattern of the mRNA or sequencing of the corresponding cDNA may be needed for the detection of the mutation. MLPA or multiplex amplifiable probe hybridization (MAPH) may be needed to detect these types of aberration [36].

Finally, epigenetic changes, such as imprinting and X-inactivation which involve methylation of DNA, can also be missed. They can change the expression of a particular gene, particularly when the gene is located in a genomic region subject

to epigenetic regulation such as chromosome region 11p15.5 encoding amongst others the IGF-2 gene [48].

Mutation detection in case of uncertainty about the gene involved

There are several ways to identify a gene responsible for a genetic endocrine disorder. One is to search the literature for candidate genes that can be screened for the occurrence of pathogenic deletions by FISH and MLPA or by direct sequencing. For example, the discovery of the etiology of the combined pituitary deficiency (GH, prolactin and TSH) in the Snell mouse (a mutation in the Pit-1 gene) led to the discovery of similar mutations in the human equivalent gene POU1F1 [49]. Later, the discovery of another transcription factor in pituitary ontogenesis, Prop-1 in the mouse, was followed by the detection of mutations in humans [50]. The resemblance of phenotypes observed in transgenic mice with human disease has led to a rapid increase in the elucidation of many genetic disorders of unknown etiology (see Chapter 6).

In other cases, finding a patient with an abnormal karyotype, caused, for example, by a translocation, can help in the identification of the gene involved. In such cases, it can be surmised that one of the breakpoints is located in the gene itself or in its close vicinity, which causes the disease. In such cases, the Human Genome Project will give information about the genes located in the neighborhood of the breakpoint. This strategy led, for example, to the discovery of the NSD-1 gene implicated in Sotos syndrome [45].

In the absence of more or less direct clues for a candidate gene, other techniques may be required to identify the responsible gene, such as "positional cloning," referring to the technique in which a gene is isolated on the basis of information about its chromosomal location. In the past, this was time-consuming and laborious but positional cloning has been simplified dramatically by the Human Genome Project and information on the chromosomal region involved in the disease can be derived from linkage analysis.

Linkage studies

Because most of the human genome does not code for protein, a large amount of sequence variation exists between individuals. These variations in DNA sequence, referred to as DNA polymorphisms, can be followed from one generation to the next and serve as genetic markers for linkage studies. Linkage means that the gene for the disease and the DNA marker are co-inherited. Polymorphic means that several variations (alleles) of the DNA marker occur in the population. Thus, if there is no candidate gene and if one or several large families with a disease are known, a genome-wide linkage study can be performed. In such an analysis, the location on the chromosome where the gene of interest is located is spotted by a linkage between the disease and an inherited polymorphic DNA marker situated on a known spot on a chromosome. If the mutated gene lies close to a polymorphic marker, there is a strong likelihood that the mutated gene joins the marker during the process of recombination in meiosis.

Linkage is expressed as a lod (logarithm of odds) score. High lod scores of +3 are generally accepted as supporting linkage and a score of −2 is consistent with the absence of linkage. Using a polymorphic marker set evenly distributed over all human chromosomes, it is possible to pinpoint the genomic region that is involved in the disease. The segregation in families of a polymorphic marker with disease can identify the chromosomal location of the disease-causing gene.

Restriction fragment length polymorphisms (RFLPs) were the first type of molecular markers used in linkage studies. Another useful type of DNA polymorphism consists of variable number of tandem repeats (VNTRs), composed of a variable number of

repetitions of a one-, two- or three-base sequence. Such polymorphisms, also known as simple sequence repeats (SSRs) or microsatellites, for example dinucleotide repeats such as CACACA, occur in many places in DNA. Polymorphic in this context means that the number of repetitive elements (repeats) in this marker (and thus its length) is highly variable within the population. The location of many dinucleotide repeats is known and the length can easily be analyzed by PCR.

In linkage analysis, RFLPs and SSRs are currently largely replaced by single nucleotide polymorphisms or SNPs. The human genome project has created large databases of genome-wide SNPs. It is estimated that 1 in every 600 base pairs in the human genome is a SNP. They are usually neutral. A fixed combination of alleles of several SNPs that are inherited together is called a haplotype. Technological development allows the simultaneous detection of 500 000 or more SNPs in a single experiment using high-throughput automated screening protocols.

A phenomenon called linkage disequilibrium is the basis for another strategy, which can afford a higher degree of resolution in mapping studies in some cases. This technique is not necessarily confined to large families but can be performed if material is available from large numbers of (apparently) unrelated patients with the disease.

Microarray

Microarray technology is a rapidly evolving approach to identify genes involved in disease processes. Microarrays (DNA chips) can be used for various purposes, such as the study of gene expression patterns (at the RNA level) in various tissues or cells, the diagnosis of gene mutations, SNP analysis or genome-wide searches for small deletions or amplifications. Microarrays are also used to develop genetic fingerprints of different types of malignancies.

On a chip or glass plate, a large number of single-stranded DNA sequences, representations of the coding sequences of genes or SNPs, are spotted. From the tissue or cells that one wishes to study, RNA is isolated. It is first transformed with reverse transcriptase to cDNA which is labeled with a fluorescent dye and hybridized on the array, where it binds to the complementary DNA sequences. When two samples are compared, two different fluorescent labels (red and green) are used. The intensity of fluorescence is measured for each spot and is a measure of the quantity of hybridized DNA on each spot and thus of the quantity of RNA in the original sample. One can also make a special array on which all possible mutations of one or more genes are represented. Hybridization with the patient sample shows which mutation is present.

In genetic research the application of bacterial artificial chromosome (BAC) and SNP microarrays is an important development. A BAC probe encodes a genomic DNA fragment of on average 200 000 bp. BAC DNA is used as probe in FISH. Microarray technology has allowed the generation of chips on which BACs covering the whole genome are spotted. This enables a genome-wide search for relatively small deletions or amplifications in a single experiment, which is in marked contrast to FISH analysis which allows evaluation of only a few probes. Even higher resolution can be reached with the high coverage SNP microarrays. The results of these arrays can be used in linkage analysis and linkage disequilibrium studies.

The quantitative nature of this technique makes it suited for the genome-wide detection of small deletions or amplifications. Microarray technology allows for the genetic evaluation of new patient groups in whom a genetic defect is expected but the absence of a family history or a candidate gene does not provide sufficient information to start more direct approaches in elucidating the genetic cause of the disease such as sequencing.

Conclusions

Endocrine tests, plasma hormone profiles and stimulation tests remain a vital part of pediatric endocrinology but DNA testing has become increasingly important and the spin-off from the Human Genome Project has led rapidly to further developments. The clinician who wants to use molecular tests for clinical and scientific purposes needs to keep pace with these developments.

References

1 Wit JM, Ranke MB, Kelnar CJH. ESPE classification of paediatric endocrine diagnoses. *Horm Res* 2007; **68** (Suppl 2): 1–120.

2 Kamp GA. *Growth hormone secretion, sensitivity and treatment in short children*. Leiden: Leiden University, 2000. Thesis.

3 Sackett DL, Straus SE, Richardon WS, Rosenberg W, Haynes RB. *Evidence-based Medicine: How to Practice and Teach EBM*, 2nd edn. Edinburgh: Churchill Livingstone, 2000.

4 Offringa M, Assendelft WJJ, Scholten RJPM. *Inleiding in Evidence-based Medicine*. Houten: Bohn Stafleu Van Loghum, 2000.

5 Hindmarsh PC, Brook CGD. Principles underlying endocrine tests. In: Brook CGD, Hindmarsh PC, eds. *Clinical Pediatric Endocrinology*, 4th edn. Oxford: Blackwell Science; 2001: 37–48.

6 Wheeler MJ. Hormone assays. In: Brook CGD, Hindmarsh PC, eds. *Clinical Pediatric Endocrinology*, 4th edn. Oxford: Blackwell Science, 2001: 27–36.

7 Elmlinger MW. Laboratory techniques, quality management and clinical validation of hormone measurement in endocrinology. In: Ranke MB, ed. *Diagnostics of Endocrine Function in Children and Adolescents*, 3rd edn. Basel: Karger, 2003: 1–29.

8 Chen JW, Ledet T, Orskov H, *et al*. A highly sensitive and specific assay for determination of IGF-1 bioactivity in human serum. *Am J Physiol Endocrinol Metab* 2003; **284**: E1149–E1155.

9 Hovens GC, Buiting AM, Karperien M, *et al*. A bioluminescence assay for thyrotropin receptor antibodies predicts serum thyroid hormone concentrations in patients with *de novo* Graves' disease. *Clin Endocrinol (Oxf)* 2006; **64**: 429–435.

10 Strasburger CJ, Wu Z, Pflaum CD, Dressendorfer RA. Immunofunctional assay of human growth hormone (hGH) in serum: a possible consensus for quantitative hGH measurement. *J Clin Endocrinol Metab* 1996; **81**: 2613–2620.

11 Miles LE, Hales CN. Labelled antibodies and immunological assay systems. *Nature* 1968; **219**: 186–189.

12 Honour JW, Brook CGD. Clinical indications for the use of urinary steroid profiles in neonates and children. *Ann Clin Biochem* 1997; **34**: 45–54.

13 Rosner W, Auchus RJ, Azziz R, Sluss PM, Raff H. Position statement. Utility, limitations and pitfalls in measuring testosterone: an Endocrine Society position statement. *J Clin Endocrinol Metab* 2007; **92**: 405–413.

14 Phillips DJ, Albertsson-Wikland K, Eriksson K, Wide L. Changes in the isoforms of luteinizing hormone and follicle-stimulating hormone during puberty in normal children. *J Clin Endocrinol Metab* 1997; **82**: 3103–3106.

15 Kohler G, Milstein C. Continuous cultures of fused cells secreting antibody of predefined specificity. *Nature* 1975; **256**: 495–497.

16 Ekins RP. Immunoassay design and optimisation. In: Price CP, Newman DJ, eds. *Principles and Practice of Immunoassay*, 2nd edn. London: Macmillan, 1997: 173–207.

17 Boyar R, Finkelstein J, Roffwarg H, Kapen S, Weitzman E, Hellman L. Synchronization of augmented luteinizing hormone secretion with sleep during puberty. *N Engl J Med* 1972; **287**: 582–586.

18 Apter D, Butzow TL, Laughlin GA, Yen SS. Gonadotropin-releasing hormone pulse generator activity during pubertal transition in girls: pulsatile and diurnal patterns of circulating gonadotropins. *J Clin Endocrinol Metab* 1993; **76**: 940–949.

19 Buckler JM. Plasma growth hormone response to exercise as diagnostic aid. *Arch Dis Child* 1973; **48**: 565–567.

20 Cole TJ, Green PJ. Smoothing reference centile curves: the LMS method and penalized likelihood. *Stat Med* 1992; **11**: 1305–1319.

21 Rikken B, van Doorn J, Ringeling A, Van den Brande JL, Massa G, Wit JM. Plasma concentrations of insulin-like growth factor (IGF)-I, IGF-II and IGF-binding protein-3 in the evaluation of childhood growth hormone deficiency. *Horm Res* 1998; **50**: 166–176.

22 Ricos C, Alvarez V, Cava F, *et al*. Current databases on biological variation: pros, cons and progress. *Scand J Clin Lab Invest* 1999; **59**: 491–500.

23 Albertsson-Wikland K, Rosberg S. Methods of evaluating spontaneous growth hormone secretion. In: Ranke MB, ed. *Diagnostics of Endocrine Function in Children and Adolescents*, 3rd edn. Basel: Karger, 2003: 129–159.

24 Clark RG, Jansson JO, Isaksson O, Robinson IC. Intravenous growth hormone: growth responses to patterned infusions in hypophysectomized rats. *J Endocrinol* 1985; **104**: 53–61.

25 Matthews DR, Hindmarsh PC. Hormone pulsatility. In: Brook CGD, Hindmarsh PC, eds. *Clinical Pediatric Endocrinology*, 4th edn. Oxford: Blackwell Science, 2001: 17–26.

26 Merriam GR, Wachter KW. Algorithms for the study of episodic hormone secretion. *Am J Physiol* 1982; **243**: E310–E318.

27 Veldhuis JD, Johnson ML. Cluster analysis: a simple, versatile and robust algorithm for endocrine pulse detection. *Am J Physiol* 1986; **250**: E486–E493.

28 Veldhuis JD, Carlson ML, Johnson ML. The pituitary gland secretes in bursts: appraising the nature of glandular secretory impulses by simultaneous multiple-parameter deconvolution of plasma hormone concentrations. *Proc Natl Acad Sci U S A* 1987; **84**: 7686–7690.

29 Pincus SM, Veldhuis JD, Rogol AD. Longitudinal changes in growth hormone secretory process irregularity assessed transpuber-

tally in healthy boys. *Am J Physiol Endocrinol Metab* 2000; **279**: E417–E424.

30 Albertsson-Wikland K, Rosberg S, Karlberg J, Groth T. Analysis of 24-hour growth hormone profiles in healthy boys and girls of normal stature: relation to puberty. *J Clin Endocrinol Metab* 1994; **78**: 1195–1201.

31 Saini S, Hindmarsh PC, Matthews DR *et al.* Reproducibility of 24-hour serum growth hormone profiles in man. *Clin Endocrinol* 1991; **34**: 455–462.

32 Spiliotis BE, August GP, Hung W, Sonis W, Mendelson W, Bercu BB. Growth hormone neurosecretory dysfunction: a treatable cause of short stature. *JAMA* 1984; **251**: 2223–2230.

33 Garibaldi LR, Picco P, Magier S, Chevli R, Aceto T Jr. Serum luteinizing hormone concentrations, as measured by a sensitive immunoradiometric assay, in children with normal, precocious or delayed pubertal development. *J Clin Endocrinol Metab* 1991; **72**: 888–898.

34 Bercu BB, Shulman D, Root AW, Spiliotis BE. Growth hormone (GH) provocative testing frequently does not reflect endogenous GH secretion *J Clin Endocrinol Metab* 1986; **63**: 709–716. [Published erratum appears in *J Clin Endocrinol Metab* 1987; **64**: 382.]

35 Rose SR, Ross JL, Uriarte M, Barnes KM, Cassorla FG, Cutler GB Jr. The advantage of measuring stimulated as compared with spontaneous growth hormone concentrations in the diagnosis of growth hormone deficiency. *N Engl J Med* 1988; **319**: 201–207.

36 White SJ, Vink GR, Kriek M, *et al.* Two-color multiplex ligation-dependent probe amplification: detecting genomic rearrangements in hereditary multiple exostoses. *Hum Mutat* 2004; **24**: 86–92.

37 New MI. Inborn errors of adrenal steroidogenesis. *Mol Cell Endocrinol* 2003; **211**: 75–83.

38 Pfaffle R. Diagnosis of endocrine disorders with molecular genetic methods. In: Ranke MB, ed. *Diagnostics of Endocrine Function in Children and Adolescents*, 3rd edn. Basel: Karger, 2003: 30–50.

39 Sanger F, Nicklen S, Coulson AR. DNA sequencing with chain-terminating inhibitors. *Proc Natl Acad Sci U S A* 1977; **74**: 5463–5467.

40 Orita M, Suzuki Y, Sekiya T, Hayashi K. Rapid and sensitive detection of point mutations and DNA polymorphisms using the polymerase chain reaction. *Genomics* 1989; **5**: 874–879.

41 Berg MA, Argente J, Chernausek S, *et al.* Diverse growth hormone receptor gene mutations in Laron syndrome. *Am J Hum Genet* 1993; **52**: 998–1005.

42 Lodish H, Berk A, Matsudaira P, *et al. Molecular Cell Biology*, 5th edn. New York: W.H. Freeman, 2003.

43 Abou-Samra AB, Juppner H, Force T, *et al.* Expression cloning of a common receptor for parathyroid hormone and parathyroid hormone-related peptide from rat osteoblast-like cells: a single receptor stimulates intracellular accumulation of both cAMP and inositol trisphosphates and increases intracellular free calcium. *Proc Natl Acad Sci U S A* 1992; **89**: 2732–2736.

44 Schipani E, Karga H, Karaplis AC, *et al.* Identical complementary deoxyribonucleic acids encode a human renal and bone parathyroid hormone (PTH)/PTH-related peptide receptor. *Endocrinology* 1993; **132**: 2157–2165.

45 Kurotaki N, Imaizumi K, Harada N, *et al.* Haploinsufficiency of NSD1 causes Sotos syndrome. *Nat Genet* 2002; **30**: 365–366.

46 Walenkamp MJE, de Muinck Keizer-Schrama SMPF, de Mos M, *et al.* Successful long-term growth hormone therapy in a girl with haploinsufficiency of the IGF-I receptor due to a terminal 15q26. 2- >qter deletion detected by multiplex ligation probe amplification. *J Clin Endocrinol Metab* 2008; **93**: 2421–2425.

47 Millar DS, Lewis MD, Horan M, *et al.* Novel mutations of the growth hormone 1 (GH1) gene disclosed by modulation of the clinical selection criteria for individuals with short stature. *Hum Mutat* 2003; **21**: 424–440.

48 Netchine I, Rossignol S, Dufourg MN, *et al.* 11p15 imprinting center region 1 loss of methylation is a common and specific cause of typical Russell–Silver syndrome: clinical scoring system and epigenetic–phenotypic correlations. *J Clin Endocrinol Metab* 2007; **92**: 3148–3154.

49 Pfaffle RW, DiMattia GE, Parks JS, *et al.* Mutation of the POU-specific domain of Pit-1 and hypopituitarism without pituitary hypoplasia. *Science* 1992; **257**: 1118–1121.

50 Wu W, Cogan JD, Pfaffle RW, *et al.* Mutations in PROP1 cause familial combined pituitary hormone deficiency. *Nat Genet* 1998; **18**: 147–149.

4 Congenital Disorders of the Hypothalamo-Pituitary-Somatotrope Axis

Ameeta Mehta[1], Evelien F. Gevers[2] & Mehul T. Dattani[3]

[1] BMJ Publishing Group and Developmental Endocrinology Research Group, UCL Institute of Child Health, London, UK
[2] MRC National Institute for Medical Research and Developmental Endocrinology Research Group, UCL Institute of Child Health, London, UK
[3] Developmental Endocrinology Research Group, UCL Institute of Child Health and Great Ormond Street Hospital for Children, London, UK

The pituitary gland is the central regulator of growth, reproduction and homeostasis. The gland lies within the sella turcica at the base of the brain to which it is attached by the pituitary stalk or infundibulum (Fig. 4.1). Its complex functions are mediated via hormone-signaling pathways that regulate finely balanced homeostatic control. These pathways coordinate complex signals from the brain and the hypothalamus to the adrenals, thyroid and gonads.

The mature gland consists of the adenohypophysis (anterior and intermediate lobes) and neurohypophysis (posterior lobe). The anterior pituitary consists of five different cell types, each defined by the hormone it produces: somatotropes [growth hormone (GH)], thyrotropes [thyrotropin or thyroid stimulating hormone (TSH)], corticotropes [corticotropin or adrenocorticotropic hormone (ACTH)], gonadotropes [follicle-stimulating hormone (FSH) and luteinizing hormone (LH)] and lactotropes (prolactin). GH secreted from pituitary somatotropes binds to its receptors and activates a signaling cascade that eventually leads to the production of insulin-like growth factor 1 (IGF-1), which then mediates the various growth-promoting actions of GH.

The intermediate lobe produces pro-opiomelanocortin (POMC), which is a precursor to melanocyte stimulating hormone (MSH), and endorphins, and this intermediate lobe involutes in the adult.

The posterior lobe consists of axons of neurons, the cell bodies of which reside in the hypothalamus, and secretes arginine vasopressin (AVP, also called antidiuretic hormone) and oxytocin.

The anterior pituitary develops from oral ectoderm while the posterior pituitary develops from neural ectoderm. Both lobes of the pituitary gland are histologically different as a result of embryological development and function almost as two separate glands.

The hypothalamus lies superior to the pituitary gland and the link between the two organs is critical for normal pituitary function. The hypothalamus virtually surrounds the third ventricle and has neural projections into the cerebral cortex and median eminence. Various stimulatory and inhibitory releasing hormones are secreted from hypothalamic nuclei and regulate the hypothalamo-pituitary-target gland axis (Table 4.1). They include GH-releasing hormone (GHRH), a 44-amino acid polypeptide which stimulates the release of GH; corticotropin-releasing hormone (CRH), a 41-amino acid polypeptide which stimulates the releases of ACTH; thyrotropin releasing hormone (TRH), a tripeptide that stimulates the release of TSH and prolactin; gonadotropin releasing hormone (GnRH), a decapeptide that stimulates the release of FSH and LH; somatostatin, a 14-amino acid peptide that inhibits the release of GH; and dopamine, a single amino acid derivative that inhibits the release of prolactin. Hormones secreted by the posterior lobe of the pituitary gland are synthesized in magnocellular neurons of the paraventricular and supraoptic nuclei within the hypothalamus.

The hypothalamus is supplied by blood from the circle of Willis and most venous blood drains into the vein of Galen. Blood from the superior hypophyseal arteries, which arise from the internal carotid arteries, flows through a capillary plexus in the median eminence to enter a sinusoidal network in the pituitary stalk. Blood passes from these sinusoids into a second capillary network plexus in the anterior pituitary. This venous portal system linking these two capillary networks is called the hypothalamo-pituitary portal system. The infundibulum or pituitary stalk carries the portal blood with delivery of hypothalamic hormones to the anterior pituitary as well as the neural tracts from magnocellular neurons of the paraventricular and supraoptic nuclei within the hypothalamus to the posterior pituitary. Any damage to the pituitary stalk can therefore result in anterior and posterior pituitary dysfunction.

Clinical features of hypopituitarism are variable, both in severity and in the number of hormone deficiencies. Onset of clinical features may be early in the neonatal period with a history of a stormy perinatal course. Isolated GH deficiency (IGHD) is by far

Brook's Clinical Pediatric Endocrinology, 6th edition. Edited by C. Brook, P. Clayton, R. Brown. © 2009 Blackwell Publishing, ISBN: 978-1-4051-8080-1.

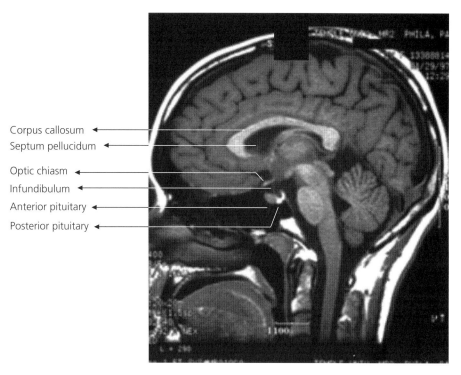

Corpus callosum
Septum pellucidum

Optic chiasm
Infundibulum
Anterior pituitary
Posterior pituitary

Figure 4.1 Magnetic resonance imaging of the brain illustrating neuroanatomical relations of the pituitary gland.

Table 4.1 Hormones secreted from the anterior lobe of the pituitary gland and their regulatory hormones.

Cell type	Hormone	Cell population (%)	Hypothalamic hormone	Hypothalamic nucleus of synthesis
Somatotrope	GH	40–50	GHRH (+) Somatostatin (–)	Arcuate, Anterior periventricular
Thyrotrope	TSH	3–5	TRH (+) Somatostatin (–)	Paraventricular, Anterior periventricular
Corticotrope	ACTH	15–20	CRH (+) AVP augments CRH	Paraventricular, Supraoptic
Gonadotrope	LH, FSH	10–15	GnRH (+)	Arcuate
Lactotrope	Prolactin	10–25	TRH (+) Dopamine (–)	Arcuate, Paraventricular

ACTH, adenocorticotropic hormone; AVP, arginine vasopressin; CRH, corticotropin releasing hormone; FSH, follicle stimulating hormone; GH, growth hormone; GHRH, growth hormone releasing hormone; GnRH, gonadotropin releasing hormone; LH, luteinizing hormone; TRH, thyrotropin releasing hormone; TSH, thyroid stimulating hormone.

the most common endocrinopathy, presenting later in infancy and childhood with growth failure. In many patients with hypopituitarism, the root of the problem lies within the hypothalamus rather than the pituitary. The evolution of additional hormone deficiencies with time is a well-recognized feature of hypopituitarism, and hence a complete evaluation of the hypothalamo-pituitary axis is indicated in any patient suspected of having one hormonal deficiency. These hormonal deficits can also be present as a component of a syndrome, with patients manifesting abnormalities in extra-pituitary structures, usually in structures sharing a common embryological origin, such as the eye and forebrain.

Hypothalamo-pituitary development

There has been an explosion in the understanding of the genetic basis of the development of hypothalamo-pituitary and midline forebrain structures over the past 25 years. Development of the pituitary gland has been extensively studied in the mouse. Although little is known about pituitary development in humans, it would appear to mirror that seen in the rodent; pituitary development is similar in all vertebrates (Fig. 4.2). The anterior and intermediate lobes of the pituitary gland are derived from oral ectoderm whilst the posterior pituitary is derived from neural ectoderm [1–3].

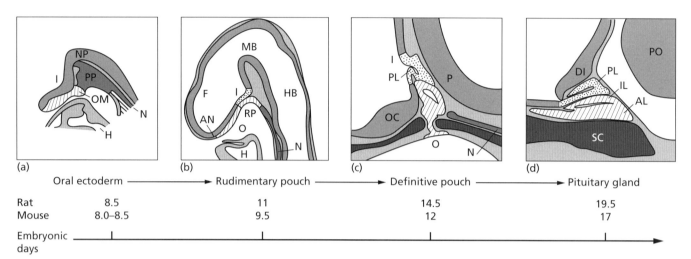

Figure 4.2 Rodent pituitary development. Four stages of pituitary development: (a) pituitary placode, (b) rudimentary pouch, (c) definitive pouch, (d) adult pituitary gland. AL, anterior lobe; AN, anterior neural pore; DI, diencephalon; F, forebrain; H, heart; HB, hindbrain; I, infundibulum; IL, intermediate lobe; MB, midbrain; N, notochord; NP, neural plate; O, oral cavity; OC, optic chiasm; OM, oral membrane; P, pontine flexure; PL, posterior lobe; PO, pons; PP, pituitary placode; RP, Rathke's pouch; SC, sphenoid cartilage. (From Sheng HZ, Westphal H. Early trends in pituitary organogenesis. *Trends Genet* 1999; **15**: 236–240 with permission.)

The development of the anterior pituitary occurs in four distinct stages, leading to the formation of a complicated secretory organ containing five different cell types secreting six different hormones.

1 *Formation of the pituitary placode from oral ectoderm.* Cell types of the pituitary gland are derived from the most anterior midline portion of the embryo in a region contiguous with the anterior neural ridge. The anterior neural ridge is displayed ventrally to form the oral epithelium which gives rise to the roof of the oral cavity. Onset of pituitary organogenesis coincides with a thickening (the pituitary placode) in the roof of the oral ectoderm at embryonic day (E) 8.5, corresponding to 4–6 weeks' gestation in humans.

2 *Formation of rudimentary Rathke's pouch.* Invagination of the oral ectoderm forms a rudimentary pouch and evagination of the ventral diencephalon forms the posterior pituitary. The pituitary placode makes contact with the floor of the ventral diencephalon. Apposition between the rudimentary Rathke's pouch and neural ectoderm of the diencephalon is critical to normal development and is maintained throughout early pituitary organogenesis.

3 *Formation of definitive Rathke's pouch.* The rudimentary Rathke's pouch deepens and folds on itself until it closes, forming a definitive pouch. The infundibulum or pituitary stalk is formed by evagination of the posterior part of the presumptive diencephalon.

4 *Formation of the adult pituitary gland.* The definitive pouch is completely detached from the oral cavity. Spatial and temporal differentiation of various cell types within the pituitary gland results in the development of individual hormone secreting cells in a sequential order.

Complex genetic interactions dictate normal pituitary development. A cascade of signaling molecules and transcription factors have a crucial role in organ commitment, cell proliferation, cell patterning and terminal differentiation and the final product is a culmination of this coordinated process (Fig. 4.3). Initially, cells within the primordium of the pituitary gland are competent to differentiate into all cell types. Following expression of the earliest markers of pituitary gland development [e.g. homeobox gene expressed in embryonic stem cells (*Hesx1*)], further signaling pathways are established from within the gland and ventral diencephalon that direct these cells towards terminal differentiation into mature hormone secreting cell types. Signaling molecules and transcription factors are expressed sequentially at critical periods of pituitary development and expression of many of these factors is subsequently attenuated (Fig. 4.4). Genes that are expressed early are implicated in organ commitment but are also implicated in repression and activation of downstream target genes that have specific roles in directing the cells towards a particular fate.

Spontaneous or artificially induced mutations in the mouse have led to significant insights into human pituitary disease, and identification of mutations associated with human pituitary disease have in turn been invaluable in defining the genetic cascade responsible for the development of this embryological tissue. Mutations involved specifically in human hypothalamo-pituitary disease are listed in Table 4.2.

Early developmental genes and transcription factors

A number of signaling molecules and transcription factors are implicated early in pituitary organogenesis and lineage differentiation. They are expressed sequentially at critical periods of pituitary development and the expression of many of these is then subsequently attenuated.

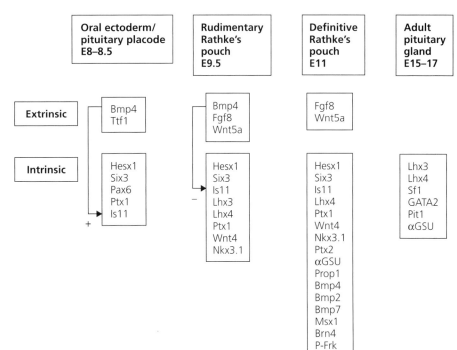

Oral ectoderm/ pituitary placode E8–8.5	Rudimentary Rathke's pouch E9.5	Definitive Rathke's pouch E11	Adult pituitary gland E15–17

Extrinsic

| Bmp4
Ttf1 | Bmp4
Fgf8
Wnt5a | Fgf8
Wnt5a | |

Intrinsic

| Hesx1
Six3
Pax6
Ptx1
Is11 | Hesx1
Six3
Is11
Lhx3
Lhx4
Ptx1
Wnt4
Nkx3.1 | Hesx1
Six3
Is11
Lhx4
Ptx1
Wnt4
Nkx3.1
Ptx2
αGSU
Prop1
Bmp4
Bmp2
Bmp7
Msx1
Brn4
P-Frk | Lhx3
Lhx4
Sf1
GATA2
Pit1
αGSU |

Figure 4.3 Transcription factors and signaling molecules involved in anterior pituitary development. (From Watkins-Chow DE, Camper SA. How many homeobox genes does it take to make a pituitary gland? *Trends Genet* 1998; **14**: 284–290.)

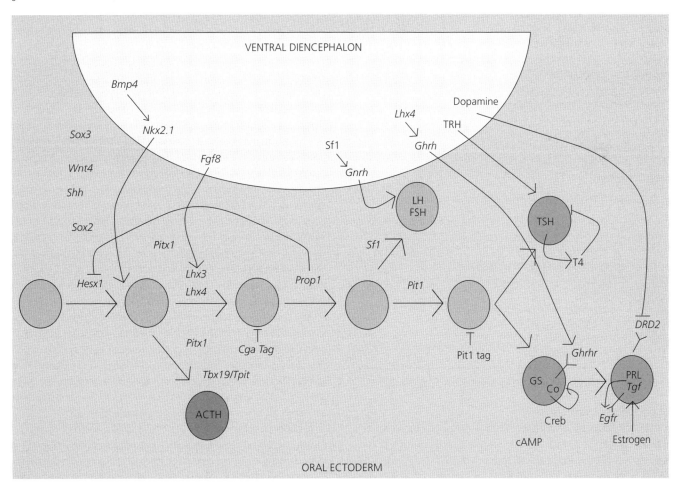

Figure 4.4 Schematic representation of the developmental cascade of genes implicated in human pituitary development with particular reference to pituitary cell differentiation.

Table 4.2 Genetic disorders of hypothalamo-pituitary development in humans.

Gene	Phenotype	Inheritance
Isolated hormone abnormalities		
GH1	Isolated GH deficiency	AR, AD
GHRHR	Isolated GH deficiency	AR
TSH β	Isolated TSH deficiency	AR
TRHR	Isolated TSH deficiency	AR
TPIT	Isolated ACTH deficiency	AR
GnRHR	Hypogonadotropic hypogonadism	AR
PC 1	ACTH deficiency, hypoglycemia, hypogonadotropic hypogonadism, obesity	AR
POMC	ACTH deficiency, obesity, red hair	AR
DAX1	Adrenal hypoplasia congenita and hypogonadotropic hypogonadism	XL
CRH	CRH deficiency	AR
KAL1	Kallman syndrome, renal agenesis, synkinesia	XL
FGFR1	Kallman syndrome, cleft lip and palate, facial dysmorphism	AD, AR
PROK2	Hypogonadotropic hypogonadism, anosmia	
PROKR2	Hypogonadotropic hypogonadism, anosmia	
Leptin	Hypogonadotropic hypogonadism, obesity	AR
Leptin-R	Hypogonadotropic hypogonadism, obesity	AR
GPR54	Hypogonadotropic hypogonadism	AR
FSH β	Primary amenorrhea, defective spermatogenesis	AR
LH β	Delayed puberty	AR
AVP-NPII	Diabetes insipidus	AR, AD
Combined pituitary hormone deficiency		
POU1F1	GH, TSH and prolactin deficiencies	AR, AD
PROP1	GH, TSH, LH, FSH, PRL and evolving ACTH deficiencies	AR
Specific syndrome		
HESX1	Septo-optic dysplasia	AR, AD
LHX3	GH, TSH, LH, FSH, PRL deficiencies, limited neck rotation	AR
LHX4	GH, TSH, ACTH deficiencies with cerebellar abnormalities	AD
SOX3	Hypopituitarism and mental retardation	XL
GLI2	Holoprosencephaly and multiple midline defects	AD
SOX2	Anophthalmia, hypopituitarism, learning difficulties, esophageal atresia	AD
GLI3	Pallister–Hall syndrome	AD
PITX2	Rieger syndrome	AD

R, receptor; AR, autosomal recessive; AD, autosomal dominant; XL, X-linked.

Morphogenetic signals

Extrinsic molecules within the ventral diencephalon and surrounding structures, such as bone morphogenetic proteins 2 and 4 (*Bmp2*, *-4*), fibroblast growth factor 8 (*Fgf8*), sonic hedgehog (*Shh*), wingless (*Wnt4*), thyroid transcription factor 1 (*Ttf1*; also called *Nkx2.1*), and molecules involved in Notch signaling have critical roles in early organogenesis [3,4]. Recent studies in the

mouse have shown that a close interaction between oral ectoderm and neural ectoderm is critical for initial development of the pituitary gland.

Rathke's pouch develops in a two-step process that requires at least two sequential inductive signals from the diencephalon. First, induction and formation of the rudimentary pouch is dependent upon *Bmp4*, and secondly, *Fgf8* activates two key regulatory genes, LIM homeobox 3 (*Lhx3*) and LIM homeobox 4 (*Lhx4*), that are essential for subsequent development of the rudimentary pouch into a definitive pouch. Both *Bmp4* and *Fgf8* are present only in the diencephalon and not in Rathke's pouch.

Murine mutations within the thyroid-specific enhancer binding protein (T*tf1*, also called *Nkx2.1*), expressed only in the presumptive ventral diencephalon, can cause severe defects in the development of not only the diencephalon but also the anterior pituitary gland. Conditional deletion of *Rbp-J*, which encodes the major mediator of the Notch pathway, leads to conversion of the late [pituitary specific transcription factor 1 (*Pit1*)] lineage into the early (corticotroph) lineage. Notch signaling is required for maintaining expression of *Prop1* (prophet of Pit1), which is required for generation of the *Pit1* lineage. Attenuation of Notch signaling is necessary for terminal differentiation in *Pit1* cells and maturation and proliferation of the GH-producing somatotroph [5]. There have been no reported mutations of these early morphogenetic signals in humans.

Hesx1

Homeobox gene expressed in embryonic stem cells (*Hesx1*) is one of the earliest markers of the pituitary primordium, suggesting that it has a critical role in early determination and differentiation of the pituitary gland. It is also called *Rpx* (Rathke's pouch homeobox) and is a member of the paired-like class of homeobox genes [6–9]. *Hesx1* is a transcriptional repressor, although its downstream targets are as yet unknown. A highly conserved region in the N-terminus of *Hesx1*, the engrailed homology domain, is crucial for its strong repressor function, and binds TLE1, a mammalian homolog of the *Drosophila* co-repressor Groucho. The homeodomain also interacts with the nuclear co-repressor NCoR1. The N-terminal domain-binding TLE permits cooperative binding of NCoR1, HDAC1 and Sin3A/B to the homeodomain, thereby making Hesx1 a strong repressor.

The gene is first expressed during mouse embryogenesis in a small patch of cells in the anterior midline visceral endoderm as gastrulation commences. *Hesx1* continues to be expressed in the developing anterior pituitary until E12, when it disappears in a spatiotemporal sequence that corresponds to progressive pituitary cell differentiation. Extinction of *Hesx1* is important for activation of other downstream genes such as *Prop1*.

It has been suggested that *Hesx1* and *Prop1* function as opposing transcription factors and that a careful temporal regulation of their expression is critical for normal pituitary development. Premature expression of *Prop1* can block pituitary organogenesis whereas prolonged expression of *Hesx1* can block *Prop1*-dependent activation. There is also evidence to suggest that *Prop1* activation is itself a prerequisite for extinction of *Hesx1*. *Lhx3* is also important for maintenance of *Hesx1* expression.

Targeted disruption of *Hesx1* in the mouse revealed a reduction in the prospective forebrain tissue, absence of developing optic vesicles, markedly decreased head size and severe microphthalmia reminiscent of the syndrome of septo-optic dysplasia (SOD) in humans. Other abnormalities included absence of the optic cups, the olfactory placodes and Rathke's pouch, reduced telencephalic vesicles, hypothalamic abnormalities and aberrant morphogenesis of Rathke's pouch. In 5% of null mutants, the phenotype was characterized by complete lack of the pituitary gland. In the majority of mutant mice, they were characterized by formation of multiple oral ectodermal invaginations and hence multiple pituitary glands.

Mutations in *HESX1* in humans were first reported in two siblings with SOD and subsequently other mutations have been shown to present with varying phenotypes characterized by IGHD, CPHD and SOD [8–13].

Pitx1 and *Pitx2*

Pituitary homeobox 1 (*Pitx1*) and pituitary homeobox 2 (*Pitx2*) are paired-like homeobox genes expressed in the fetal pituitary and in most cells of the adult pituitary gland. These genes have an important role in the development of Rathke's pouch and the anterior pituitary gland.

In the mouse, *Pitx1* is initially expressed in the first branchial arch mesenchyme at E9 and then throughout the oral epithelium lining the roof of the buccal cavity and in Rathke's pouch ectoderm. *Pitx1* expression continues throughout development in all regions of the anterior pituitary and overlaps with that of *Lhx3* and appears to be required for sustained expression of the latter. *Pitx1* is essential for sustained expression of alpha glycoprotein subunit unit (α-GSU), and for maintenance of cell-specific transcription in corticotropes and gonadotropes. A T-box factor, *Tpit*, present only in POMC expressing cells within the pituitary, is essential for initiating POMC cell differentiation and for activating POMC transcription synergistically with *Pitx1*. *Pitx1* also appears to modulate steroidogenic factor 1 (*sf1*) activity in gonadotropes, activation of the GH promoter and synergistic activation of the prolactin promoter with *Pit1*. Mice that are rendered deficient in *Pitx1* demonstrate abnormalities within the hind limb and palate. Gonadotropes and thyrotropes are reduced with an increase in the concentration of ACTH transcripts and peptide in corticotropes. In adults, *PITX1* is specifically expressed at higher concentrations in cells of the α-GSU lineage and a fraction of POMC-expressing cells. Most corticotropes in humans, however, do not express *PITX1*.

Pitx2 is first expressed in the mouse embryo in the oral epithelium and oral ectoderm. At E9.5 *Pitx2* is expressed in the developing Rathke's pouch in addition to mesenchyme near the optic eminence, basal plate of the central nervous system, forelimbs and domains of the abdominal cavity. It appears to be required for pituitary development shortly after formation of the committed pouch. It may be required for one or more anterior pituitary

cell types or may act in concert with other transcription factors. It is also expressed in lungs, kidney, testes and tongue. Additionally, *Pitx2* is implicated in left–right asymmetry because it is expressed in the lateral plate mesoderm and then continues to be expressed asymmetrically in several organs that are asymmetric with respect to left–right axis of the embryo. There are at least three isoforms of *Pitx2*. *Pitx2a* and *Pitx2b* are expressed in the adult pituitary in thyrotropes, gonadotropes, somatotropes and lactotropes but not corticotropes, where *Pitx1* is highly expressed. However, *Pitx2c* is expressed in all five cell lineages.

To date, no mutations have been described within *PITX1* in humans. Mutations in *PITX2* are associated with Rieger syndrome in humans [14].

Lhx3 and *Lhx4*

LIM homeobox 3 (*Lhx3*) and LIM homeobox 4 (*Lhx4*) belong to the LIM family of homeobox genes that are expressed early in Rathke's pouch. At least three different isoforms of *Lhx3* have been described in mammals, each with distinct expression patterns and transcriptional properties [15–17].

Lhx3 is detected in the developing nervous system. The *Lhx3a* isoform is first expressed at E8.5 in the mouse embryo while *Lhx3b* is first expressed at E9.5. Subsequently, *Lhx3* is expressed in the anterior and intermediate lobes of the pituitary gland, ventral hindbrain and spinal cord. Maintenance of *Lhx3* persists in the adult pituitary gland suggesting a maintenance function for one or more of the anterior pituitary cell types. *Lhx3* activates the α-GSU promoter and together with *Pit1* acts synergistically to activate the TSH-β and prolactin promoters and the *Pit1* enhancer. *Lhx3* is one of the earliest markers for cells that are destined to form the anterior and intermediate lobes and continued expression is essential for formation of gonadotropes, thyrotropes, somatotropes and lactotropes. In *Lhx3* null mutant mice, Rathke's pouch is initially formed but then fails to grow and *Hesx1* expression is switched off early. There is failure of expression of α-GSU, TSH-β, GH and Pit1 transcripts. Specification of the corticotrope cell lineage does occur, although there is failure of POMC cell proliferation, probably secondary to reduced T-Pit expression [18].

Lhx4 is a closely related gene that is expressed in specific areas of the brain and spinal cord. Like *Lhx3*, *Lhx4* is expressed throughout the invaginating pouch at E9.5. Subsequent expression at E12.5 is restricted to the future anterior lobe. Its expression is reduced by E15.5 [19]. Null mutants of *Lhx4* show formation of Rathke's pouch with expression of α-GSU, TSH-β, GH and Pit1 transcripts, demonstrating that various anterior pituitary cell lineages are specified although their numbers are reduced. *Lhx3*−/−, *Lhx4*−/− double mutant mice show a more severe phenotype than either single mutant with an early arrest of pituitary development, thereby suggesting that these two genes may act in a redundant manner during early pituitary development [20].

Human mutations in *LHX3* are associated with GH, TSH, prolactin and gonadotropin deficiencies with some patients demonstrating a neck phenotype characterized by limited neck rotation [21,22]. *LHX4* mutations in humans, reported in five pedigrees to date, resulted in variable hypopituitarism, more commonly GH, TSH and ACTH deficiencies with a hypoplastic sella and variable cerebellar hypoplasia [23–25].

Sox3

Sox3 is a member of the Sox [SRY-related high mobility group (HMG) box] family of transcription factors present in the mammalian sex determining gene, *SRY*, which were initially identified based on homology to the conserved binding motif of the HMG class [26,27]. Approximately 20 different Sox genes have been identified in mammals and variation in homology exhibited within the HMG box between different members allows them to be grouped into different subfamilies [28–30]. *Sox3* was among the first of the Sox genes to be cloned and, together with *Sox1* and *Sox2*, belongs to the Soxb1 subfamily exhibiting the highest degree of similarity to *SRY* [26,27,31]. Members of the Soxb1 subfamily of genes are expressed throughout the developing central nervous system and are some of the earliest neural markers that are believed to have a role in neuronal determination.

Sox3 is expressed in the earliest stages of development, with its main site of expression within the central nervous system, and has been strongly implicated in neurogenesis [32]. Subsequently, *Sox3* is expressed along the full length of the developing CNS, including the brain and spinal cord, in actively dividing undifferentiated neural progenitor cells where expression is maintained throughout development [33]. High concentrations of expression have also been noted in the ventral diencephalon, including the infundibulum and presumptive hypothalamus [34].

Targeted disruption of *Sox3* in mice results in mutants that have a variable and complex phenotype including craniofacial abnormalities, midline CNS defects, and a reduction in size and fertility [34,35]. *Sox3* mutant mice of both sexes are born with expected frequency showing no evidence for embryonic lethality, and approximately one-third of mutant mice are viable and fertile with no gross abnormalities. Heterozygous females are mosaic with respect to the mutation caused by X-inactivation and generally appear normal, although some display a mild craniofacial phenotype. However, approximately 43% of *Sox3* null mice do not survive to weaning, and the most severely affected mice exhibit profound growth insufficiency and general weakness with craniofacial defects including overgrowth and malalignment of the front teeth and abnormality of the shape of the pinna which was completely absent in some animals [34].

Rizzoti *et al.* [34] analyzed the pituitary gland and brain of *Sox3* mutant mice in detail, revealing the mutants to have a variable endocrine deficit, the extent of which was correlated with body weight. Pituitary concentrations of GH, LH, FSH and TSH were all lower in mutants compared to wild-type mice at 2 months of age. Histological analysis of the pituitary gland at this stage revealed a hypoplastic anterior lobe with the presence of an additional abnormal cleft disrupting the boundary between the anterior and intermediate lobes.

Further examination of *Sox3* mutant embryos revealed that Rathke's pouch displayed an abnormally expanded and bifurcated appearance in mutant embryos, which possibly results in the additional cleft observed at later stages of development and in the adult pituitary. *Sox3* is not expressed in Rathke's pouch; however, it is expressed at high concentrations in the ventral diencephalon including the infundibulum which provides necessary inductive signals for the formation of the anterior pituitary [4]. In *Sox3* mutants, the evagination of the infundibulum was less pronounced than observed in wild-type mice and the presumptive hypothalamus thinner and shorter [34]. This suggests that the hypopituitary phenotype observed in mutant mice arises as a secondary consequence of the absence of *Sox3* in the ventral diencephalon.

Duplications of Xq26-27 and mutations in *SOX3* have been implicated in variable hypopituitarism and mental retardation in humans [36–40].

Sox2

Sox2 is also a member of the Soxb1 subfamily. In the mouse, initial expression of *Sox2* is detected at E2.5 at the morula stage and then in the inner cell mass of the blastocyst at E3.5. Later expression of *Sox2*, following gastrulation, is restricted to the presumptive neuroectoderm and by E9.5 it is expressed throughout the brain, central nervous system, sensory placodes, branchial arches, gut endoderm, the esophagus and trachea [41,42]. Homozygous loss of *Sox2* results in peri-implantation lethality, whereas *Sox2* heterozygous mice appear relatively normal but show a reduction in size and male fertility [43]. Further studies that have resulted in the reduction of *SOX2* expression concentrations below 40%, compared to normal concentrations, result in anophthalmia in the affected mutants [44]. Given the observation of growth retardation and reduced fertility, Kelberman *et al.* [45] recently investigated the role of *Sox2* in murine pituitary development, showing that a proportion of heterozygous animals manifested a variable hypopituitary phenotype, with hypoplasia and abnormal morphology of the anterior pituitary gland with concomitant reduction in concentrations of GH, LH, ACTH and TSH.

Mutations in the gene have since been shown to be associated with hypopituitarism and severe eye abnormalities in humans [45].

Terminal cell differentiation

Terminal pituitary cell differentiation is a culmination of a complex interaction between extrinsic signaling molecules and transcription factors such as *Lhx3*, *Lhx4*, *Sox* genes, *GATA2*, *Isl1*, *Prop1* and *Pit1*. *GATA2* encodes a transcription factor that is important in the differentiation of gonadotropes and thyrotropes. Other transcription factors involved in the maturation of the gonadotrope lineage include *Sf*1 and *Dax*1 (dosage-sensitive sex reversal-adrenal hypoplasia congenita critical region on the X chromosome). *Pit1* and *Prop1* are best characterized in terms of function in both humans and mice.

Prop1

Prop1 (Prophet of *Pit1*) is a pituitary-specific paired-like homeodomain transcription factor first expressed in the dorsal portion of Rathke's pouch at E10–10.5 followed by maximal expression at E12 and subsequent extinction by E15.5 [46]. It is believed to be required for expression of *Pit1*, the critical lineage-determining transcription factor, because there is a failure of determination of *Pit1* lineages, lack of *Pit1* gene activation and absence of progression to mature cells in the Ames dwarf mice who harbor a homozygous missense mutation in the *Prop1* gene [47]. *Prop1* is also important in regulating the expression of *Hesx1*, the lineage-inhibiting transcription factor. Beta-catenin acts as a binary switch by interacting with *Prop1* to simultaneously activate expression of *Pit1* and to repress *Hesx1*, acting via TLE/Reptin/HDAC1 co-repressor complexes in the latter case [48].

Homozygous Ames dwarf mice exhibit severe proportional dwarfism, hypothyroidism and infertility and the emerging anterior pituitary gland is reduced in size by about 50% displaying an abnormal looping appearance. The adult Ames dwarf mouse exhibits GH, TSH and prolactin deficiency resulting from a severe reduction of somatotrope, lactotrope and caudomedial thyrotrope lineages. Additionally these mice have reduced gonadotropin expression correlating with low plasma LH and FSH concentrations. The size of the pituitary gland on magnetic resonance (MR) imaging is reduced considerably. Recent reports suggest that the *Prop1*-deficient fetal mouse pituitary retains mutant cells in the periluminal area of Rathke's pouch that fail to differentiate. The mutant pituitary then exhibits enhanced apoptosis and reduced proliferation [49]. At postnatal day 11, apoptosis-independent caspase-3 activation occurs in thyrotropes and somatotropes of normal but not *Prop1* and *Pit1* mutant pituitaries indicating a role for caspase-3 expression [50].

Humans with mutations in *PROP1* characteristically have GH, TSH, prolactin and gonadotropin deficiencies, suggesting a role for *PROP1* in gonadotrope differentiation in humans [51]. The phenotype also includes evolving ACTH deficiency in some patients.

Pit1

Pit1 (called *POU1F1* in humans) is a pituitary specific transcription factor belonging to the POU homeodomain family. It has also been called GH factor-1 as it was first identified as a regulator of *GH1* transcription. Apart from *GH1*, *Pit1* binding sites have also been identified in promoters of the prolactin and TSH-β genes. *Pit1* is expressed relatively late during pituitary development (E13.5 in the mouse) and its expression persists throughout life. Pit1 usually binds to multiple sites on target genes and dimerization of Pit1 on DNA seems to be important for high-affinity DNA binding and consequent transcriptional activation. Although Pit-1 is sufficient to activate the minimal elements in the *GH1* promoter necessary for cell-specific expression, it also requires other factors such as Zn-15, a zinc finger transcription factor, for synergistic activation of the *GH1* gene. *Pit1* is also essential for the development of somatotropes, lactotropes and thyrotropes in the anterior pituitary. Transcripts first appear in cells within the caudomedial region of the anterior pituitary at E14.5, followed by detection of the protein within somatotropes and lactotropes and subsequent expression of *GH1* and prolactin genes on E16 and E17 respectively. *Pit1* dependent thyrotropes arise on E15.5.

In the Snell dwarf mouse, a recessive point mutation results in absence of somatotropes, lactotropes and thyrotropes. A similar phenotype results in the Jackson dwarf mouse, which harbors a recessive null mutation of *Pit1*. Apart from its role in proliferation and maintenance of somatotropes, lactotropes and thyrotropes, Pit1 binding sites have also been found in promoter regions of the *GHRHR* and the *Pit1* gene itself. Data suggest that auto regulation of Pit1 is required to sustain *Pit1* gene expression once the Pit1 protein has reached a critical threshold [52,53].

Humans with mutations in *POU1F1* characteristically present with a pituitary phenotype characterized by GH, TSH and prolactin deficiencies [54].

Anterior pituitary hormones and their deficiencies

Growth hormone

Somatotropes account for 4–10% of the net weight of an adult pituitary gland. The human GH gene (*GH-N* or *GH1*) forms part of a cluster of five homologous genes along with human chorionic somatomammotropic hormone pseudogene 1 (*CSHP1*), human chorionic somatomammotropic hormone 1 (*CSH1*), *GH2* and human chorionic somatomammotropic hormone 2 (*CSH2*) located on the long arm of chromosome 17 (17q22-24) spanning 66.5 kilobases (kb). Its expression is regulated not only by a proximal promoter but also by a locus control region 15–32 kb upstream of the *GH-1* gene. The locus control region confers pituitary-specific, high level expression of human GH (hGH) [55]. The full-length transcript from the GH-N gene encodes a 191 amino-acid 22 kiloDalton (kDa) protein that contains two disulfide bridges and accounts for 85–90% of circulating GH. Alternative splicing of the mRNA transcript generates a 20 kDa form of GH that accounts for the remaining 10–15%. Within both the proximal promoter and the locus control region are located binding sites for the pituitary-specific transcription factor *Pit1*.

In the circulation, GH binds to two binding proteins (BP), high and low affinity GHBPs [56]. Little is known about low affinity GHBP, accounting for approximately 10–15% of GH binding, with a preference for binding to 20 kDa hGH. However, high affinity GHBP is a 61 kDa glycosylated protein that represents a soluble form of the extracellular domain of the GH receptor that can bind to both 20 and 22 kDa hGH, and thereby prolong the half-life of GH. *In vivo* studies that have co-administered GH and GHBP to hypophysectomized and GH deficient rats have demonstrated a potentiation of weight gain and bone growth, although similar studies have not as yet been performed in humans.

The half-life of hGH is short at less than 20 min. It binds to the GH receptor (GHR), which is present in a number of tissues. Binding of GH to the extracellular domain of the GHR results in receptor dimerization with phosphorylation of Janus (JAK) kinases as well as of the receptor itself. This induces phosphorylation of MAPK, STAT and PI3 kinase pathways. The end-result is activation of a number of genes that mediate the effects of GH. These include early response genes encoding transcription factors such as c-*jun*, c-*fos* and c-*myc* implicated in cell growth, proliferation and differentiation, and IGF-1 that mediates the growth-promoting effects of GH [57,58].

Action and regulation

Actions

GH is secreted in a pulsatile fashion under the control of the hypothalamus. Peak serum GH concentrations are achieved during sleep. GH secretion is also increased during emotional stress, exercise, hypoglycemia, protein meals and prolonged fasting. Pharmacological agents used to increase GH secretion include insulin, glucagon, clonidine, levodopa and propranolol. Apart from its actions on linear growth, GH is anabolic, lipolytic and diabetogenic. It increases calcium absorption and is believed to improve bone density. Administration of recombinant human GH (hGH) results in a reduction in body fat and an increase in muscle mass.

GH acts indirectly on bone growth by stimulating the synthesis of IGF-1, which is the main GH-dependent growth factor. IGF-1 is a single-chain polypeptide containing 70 amino acids. It shares considerable homology with insulin. It is synthesized in the liver and circulates bound to several binding glycoproteins. The principal binding protein is IGFBP3, the secretion of which is also regulated by GH. Measurement of IGF-1 correlates well with spontaneous GH secretion and is hence widely used in the diagnosis of GH deficiency. However, its concentration is altered in a number of other disease states such as hypothyroidism, malnutrition, poorly controlled diabetes and chronic disease.

Regulation

The secretion of GH is pulsatile with a predominant nocturnal component. Two hypothalamic hormones regulate pulsatility: GHRH, a 44 amino acid protein that stimulates GH secretion, and somatostatin, an inhibitory hormone containing 14 amino acids. The secretion of these hypothalamic hormones is further influenced by neurotransmitters and neuropeptides such as dopamine, catecholamines, histamine, serotonin, gamma aminobutyric acid and opiates. Both GH and growth factors such as IGF-1 and IGF-2 also negatively feedback on the hypothalamic regulators of GH secretion, whereas sex steroids such as testosterone and estrogen increase hGH secretion.

Recent use of synthetic GH releasing peptides has led to the identification of a GH secretagog receptor type 1a. The receptor is strongly expressed in the hypothalamus but specific binding sites for GH releasing peptides have also been identified in other regions of the CNS and peripheral endocrine and non-endocrine tissues in both humans and other organisms. The endogenous ligand for the GH secretagog receptor, ghrelin, has now been isolated from the stomach and is an octanoylated peptide consisting of 28 amino acids [59]. It is expressed predominantly in the stomach, but smaller amounts are also produced within the bowel, pancreas, kidney, the immune system, placenta, pituitary, testis, ovary and hypothalamus. Ghrelin leads not only to the secretion of GH, but also stimulates prolactin and ACTH secretion. Additionally, it influences endocrine pancreatic function and glucose metabolism, gonadal function, appetite and behavior. It also controls gastric motility and acid secretion, and has cardiovascular and antiproliferative effects. The role of endogenous ghrelin in normal growth during childhood remains unclear. Both ghrelin and GH releasing peptides release GH synergistically with GHRH but the efficacy of these compounds as growth-promoting agents is poor.

Isolated GH deficiency

Etiology and clinical features

Congenital GH deficiency encompasses a group of different etiological disorders. It may occur in isolation or associated with other anterior and posterior pituitary hormone deficiencies with or without extra-pituitary features such as optic nerve hypoplasia and midline forebrain defects. The condition may be sporadic or familial. The reported incidence is 1 in 3500 to 1 in 10 000 live births, with the majority of cases being idiopathic in origin. Familial cases account for 5–30% of cases and there are four well-described familial forms as shown in Table 4.3. Mutations within the genes encoding the transcription factors SOX3 and HESX1 can also cause IGHD.

IGHD type IA

Patients with IGHD type IA have a complete absence of GH and lack tolerance to exogenous GH treatment with production of hGH antibodies [60]. They present with early and profound growth failure. Serum GH concentrations are undetectable or extremely low on provocation testing. The condition is characterized by an initial response to exogenous hGH treatment, followed by development of antibodies to GH, resulting in a markedly decreased final height as an adult. The characteristic facial appearance of GH deficiency with mid-facial hypoplasia, delayed dentition and frontal bossing is well recognized. The disorder is inherited in an autosomal recessive manner and only a few cases have been reported to date. The majority of patients with type IA isolated GH deficiency have large deletions within the GH1 gene; those identified to date range from 6.7 to 45 kb [61]. However, microdeletions such as that of a single base pair at codon 10 leading to an altered reading frame with premature termination of translation and an ensuing truncated protein have also been described. Two further patients, a compound heterozygote with a 6.7 kb deletion and a 2 bp deletion in the third exon, and a patient who was homozygous for a missense mutation in the coding sequence leading to a premature stop codon also had a phenotype consistent with type IA IGHD. The exact prevalence

Table 4.3 Isolated growth hormone deficiency (GHD).

Inheritance	Type	Phenotype	Gene	Nature of mutations
Autosomal recessive	IA	Severe short stature, anti-GH antibodies on treatment	*GH-1*	Deletions, amino acid substitutions
	IB	Less severe short stature No anti-GH antibodies	*GH-1/GHRHR*	Splice site mutations, amino acid substitutions
Autosomal dominant	II	Less severe short stature No antibodies	*GH-1*	Splice site mutations
X-linked recessive	III	Short stature (GHD) with agammaglobulinemia	Not known	Not known

of this disorder is unclear. Sporadic cases may go unrecognized resulting in the possible low incidence of this disorder. A prevalence of 9–38% for *GH-1* deletions in markedly short [height ≤4 standard deviations (SD)] individuals has been suggested.

All reported families to date have been consanguineous. There is marked heterogeneity in the phenotype of these patients, in addition to considerable variability in antibody formation and response to hGH treatment, even within families with the same deletions. Patients with larger deletions (>7.6 kb) respond better to GH treatment compared with those with smaller deletions. Recombinant human IGF-1 (rhIGF1) has also been used, particularly in patients with a poor initial response to hGH treatment and formation of high antibody titers. With improvements in recombinant technology, purer forms of GH can now be produced which alleviate the problem of antibody formation to some extent.

IGHD type IB

IGHD type IB is also associated with a prenatal onset of GH deficiency, but is milder than IGHD type IA, with detectable concentrations of GH after provocation testing. The condition is inherited as an autosomal recessive trait. Children present with marked short stature and a poor growth velocity, and the condition is characteristically associated with a good response to exogenous hGH treatment with no formation of GH antibodies. IGHD type IB is a result of either homozygous splice site mutations within the *GH1* gene or mutations within the GHRH receptor (*GHRHR*). The human *GHRHR* gene consists of 13 exons spanning approximately 15 kb, and has been mapped to chromosome 7p15. It encodes a protein containing 423 amino acids. The receptor is a G-protein coupled receptor characterized by seven transmembrane domains with a high binding affinity for GHRH. Expression of *GHRHR* is upregulated by POU1F1. GHRHR is also required for proliferation of somatotropes and therefore has an important role in anterior pituitary development.

The first reported cases of *GHRHR* mutations were from the Indian subcontinent in two first cousins who were found to have a G > T substitution leading to a stop codon and a severely truncated protein lacking the membrane spanning domains with a consequent inability to bind to GHRH [62]. Since then, several patients with *GHRHR* mutations have been reported, including splice site mutations [63].

IGHD type II

This condition is inherited in an autosomal dominant manner. Patients present with short stature and respond well to exogenous hGH treatment with no formation of antibodies. IGHD type II is most commonly the result of splice site mutations in intron III (IVSIII) within the *GH1* gene. In addition, four missense mutations (R77C, R183H, P89L and V110F) have also been implicated in IGHD type II. The phenotype associated with these mutations is highly variable, particularly in association with the R183H mutation, with some individuals being of normal stature without any treatment [64]. More recently, mutations in an exon splice enhancer within exon 3 of the *GH1* gene have been associated with autosomal dominant GHD [65]. Splice site mutations lead to the production of two alternatively spliced GH molecules, 20 and 17.5 kDa hGH. The 17.5 kDa form of GH generated as a result of the skipping of exon 3 and subsequent loss of amino acids 32–71 has a dominant negative effect preventing secretion of normal wild-type 22 kDa GH with a consequent deleterious effect on pituitary somatotropes. In a murine model of this dominant negative mutation, there is evolution of the phenotype with later failure of prolactin, TSH and gonadotropin secretion [66].

Patients presenting with a splice site mutation within the first two base pairs of intervening sequence 3 (5′ IVS +1/+2 bp) leading to a skipping of exon 3 were found to be more likely to present at follow-up with other pituitary hormone deficiencies [67,68]. The development of multiple hormonal deficiencies is not age-dependent and there is a clear evidence of variability in the onset, severity and progression, even within the same family. A detailed analysis of different mutations identified in IGHD type II showed different mechanisms of secretory pathophysiology at a cellular level resulting in a different extent of co-localization and a differential effect on GH secretion. This might be caused by differences in folding or aggregation, processes that are necessary for sorting, packaging or secretion through the regulated secretory pathway [67].

The phenomenon of evolving CPHD could also be attributed to an invasion by activated macrophages leading to a significant bystander endocrine cell killing, which in time compromises cellular repletion of other cell lineages and ultimately to additional endocrine deficits, as observed in transgenic mice. Early treatment with rhGH in these patients may prevent the progressive dysfunction of the somatotropes and possibly other cell lines by suppressing the GHRH drive and hence production of the mutant 17.5 kDa protein, although this remains to be proven.

IGHD type III

This disorder is inherited in an X-linked recessive manner. In addition to GH deficiency, these patients may also manifest agammaglobulinemia. No abnormalities have been documented within the *GH-1* gene in these patients and the exact mechanism for the phenotype is unknown. Recently, a polyalanine expansion within SOX3, a transcription factor implicated in CNS development, has been described in a pedigree with X-linked mental retardation and GHD [40].

Thyrotropin or thyroid-stimulating hormone

TSH is a glycoprotein consisting of two non-covalently bound chains of amino acids (α and β) and is synthesized and stored within the thyrotropes of the anterior pituitary gland. The α chain consists of 92 amino acids and shares homology with other pituitary glycoproteins, FSH and LH. The gene encoding TSH α glycoprotein is located on chromosome 6q12-q21. The β chain contains 110 amino acids and is TSH-specific. The gene encoding the TSH β chain is located on chromosome 1p13.

Actions and regulation
Actions

The primary function of TSH is to stimulate the thyroid gland to secrete the thyroid hormones triiodothyronine (T3) and thyroxine (T4). Its actions include stimulation of the iodide pump on the cell membrane transporting iodide into the cell, stimulation of the synthesis of the thyroidal storage protein thyroglobulin, and stimulation and synthesis of T4 and T3 and their release from their complexes with thyroglobulin. TSH binds to its cell membrane receptor, which consists of seven transmembrane domains, four intracellular domains and a long extracellular sequence with six potential glycosylation sites. It is a G-protein coupled receptor that stimulates adenyl cyclase activity, activation of protein kinase A and subsequent phosphorylation.

Regulation

TSH secretion is pulsatile with peak concentrations at night. Its secretion is stimulated by hypothalamic TRH acting via its G-protein coupled receptor and inhibited by somatostatin and dopamine. The thyroid hormones negatively feedback both at the pituitary level on TSH secretion and at the hypothalamic level on TRH. Other factors impinging on TSH secretion include estrogen which increases the number of TRH receptors on the thyrotropes and a decrease in the ambient temperature acting as a potent stimulator of TSH.

Isolated TSH deficiency
Clinical features

Central hypothyroidism has a reported prevalence of 1 in 50 000 live births. Neonates can present with non-specific symptoms such as lethargy, poor feeding with failure to thrive, prolonged hyperbilirubinemia, and cold intolerance. Babies with central hypothyroidism may be born with a normal or above average birth weight and a birth length that is below average. Central hypothyroidism is generally milder than primary hypothyroidism, where a more severe phenotype characterized by coarse facies, constipation and severe mental retardation may be characteristic. Collu *et al.* [69] reported a patient with a TRH receptor mutation who presented only with short stature and delayed bone maturation. Although he had a subnormal intelligence quotient, this was possibly related to the low socio-economic status of the family because the IQ of unaffected sibs was similar.

Etiology

Isolated central hypothyroidism, characterized by insufficient TSH secretion resulting in low concentrations of thyroid hormones, is a very rare disorder. It may be sporadic, although familial cases have been reported with deficiencies of TSH and TRH. Dacou-Voutetakis *et al.* [70] first reported a homozygous nonsense mutation in exon 2 of the TSH β-subunit gene in three children affected by congenital TSH-deficient hypothyroidism within two related Greek families. Affected individuals showed symptoms of severe mental and growth retardation. This mutation gives rise to a truncated peptide including only the first 11 of 118 amino acids of the mature TSH β-subunit peptide. Collu *et al.* [69] were the first to report an inactivating mutation of the TRH receptor gene as a cause for isolated central hypothyroidism. The patient had complete absence of TSH and prolactin responses to TRH. Mutational analysis revealed that the patient was a compound heterozygote for two different mutations, having inherited a different mutated allele from each of the parents. The mutation resulted in a failure of TRH to bind the mutated TRH receptor with a consequent failure of TSH secretion.

Adrenocorticotropic hormone

ACTH is a 39 amino acid polypeptide with a short biological half-life of approximately 8 min. It is synthesized and stored within the corticotropes of the anterior pituitary that account for about 10% of the adenohypophysis. The initial precursor prohormone is POMC, located at chromosome 2p23.3 in humans. Post-translational processing of POMC is species-specific. The POMC gene spans approximately 12 kb and consists of three exons. Cleavage of the POMC precursor into biologically active peptides is a critical process. The main enzymes involved are prohormone convertases, particularly PC1 within the anterior pituitary corticotropes. PC1 cleaves POMC to generate N-POC and β lipotropin. N-POC is then cleaved to form pro-γ-melanocyte stimulating hormone, a joining peptide and ACTH. There is further evidence to suggest that another enzyme PC2 cleaves ACTH into αMSH and a corticotropin-like intermediate lobe peptide within the intermediate lobe and β lipotropin is cleaved into β endorphin and γ lipotropin. αMSH has an important role as an agonist for the melanocortin (MC) 1 receptor in causing pigment deposition in the hair follicle and as an agonist for the MC4 receptor in the hypothalamus where it controls appetite.

Actions and regulation

Actions

The primary function of ACTH is to stimulate the zona fasciculata and zona reticularis of the adrenal glands to produce glucocorticoids (mainly cortisol) and adrenal androgens. Like other peptide hormones, ACTH binds to its specific membrane receptor on the adrenocortical cells to increase the formation of cyclic AMP and activation of various protein kinases.

Regulation

The secretion of ACTH follows a circadian rhythm with peak concentrations in the early hours of the morning and low concentrations in the late evening. As a result, cortisol secretion is circadian with peak concentrations at around 0800 hours and a nadir at midnight. This rhythm can be disrupted by shifts in day–night patterns.

Hypothalamic CRH binds with high affinity to its specific cell membrane receptors on the corticotropes to increase transcription of the POMC gene and ACTH synthesis. CRH neurons are also found in other areas of the brain including the hypothalamus, brainstem and cerebral cortex. AVP acts synergistically with CRH to stimulate ACTH release from the corticotropes.

Various other neurotransmitters (serotonin, norepinephrine, neuropeptide Y, interleukins 1 and 6, tumor necrosis factor and leukemia inhibitory factor) are also involved in the regulation of ACTH secretion. Stressors such as surgical stress, infection, pain, acute illness, fever, hypoglycemia and other pathological states increase CRH secretion resulting in a profound increase in both ACTH and cortisol secretion. Exogenous glucocorticoids reverse this effect. The exact mechanism underlying the increased secretion of the steroid hormones is unclear, although it is thought to be mediated via interleukins.

Isolated ACTH deficiency

Clinical features

Isolated congenital ACTH deficiency is rare and is more commonly associated with other pituitary hormone deficiencies. The clinical features of isolated congenital ACTH deficiency are poorly defined and patients usually present in the neonatal period with non-specific symptoms such as poor feeding, failure to thrive and hypoglycemia. Signs of severe adrenal insufficiency include vascular collapse, shock and bradycardia. Serum aldosterone secretion is controlled by the renin-angiotensin system and hence abnormalities in salt excretion are unusual, although not unknown [71], in isolated ACTH deficiency. Females rely on adrenal androgens for the development of pubic and axillary hair and hence women with isolated ACTH deficiency will lack both.

Etiology

Only a few cases of isolated ACTH deficiency have been reported. Krude et al. [72] first described two patients with mutations in the POMC gene. The first patient was a compound heterozygote with one missense mutation leading to a frameshift at codon 144

and the other was a single nucleotide change leading to a premature stop codon. The second patient was homozygous for a point mutation in exon 2 leading to a start codon. Both patients presented with early-onset isolated ACTH deficiency and obesity with red hair resulting from the lack of αMSH production. Symptoms of hypoglycemia and cholestasis resolved with hydrocortisone supplementation. Both sets of heterozygous parents were asymptomatic.

Since the initial cases, there have been reports of a further three patients with POMC gene mutations, all presenting with isolated ACTH deficiency, red hair and obesity. A compound heterozygous mutation in the PC1 gene in a female patient with extreme early-onset obesity and ACTH deficiency was first described in 1997 [73]. In addition she had defective processing of other prohormones and presented with insulin dependent diabetes mellitus and hypogonadotropic hypogonadism [74]. More recently, a child with isolated ACTH deficiency, red hair and a severe enteropathy was found to harbor mutations within PC1 [75]. Several recessive mutations have been identified in TPIT, with a recessive mode of inheritance, resulting in severe ACTH deficiency, profound hypoglycemia associated with seizures in some cases and prolonged cholestatic jaundice in the neonatal period. Neonatal deaths have been reported in 25% of families with TPIT mutations in a large series, suggesting that isolated ACTH deficiency may be an underestimated cause of neonatal death [76].

Gonadotropins

The reproductive system is unique because of changes in the secretion of reproductive hormones taking place throughout life. The gonadotropins, FSH and LH, are glycoproteins composed of two subunits: α and β. The α-subunit is identical to the α-subunit of TSH (gene encoding the α-subunit is located on chromosome 6q12-q21) and the specific biological activity of both hormones resides in the β-subunit. The gene encoding the FSH β chain is found on chromosome 11p11.2 and that of the LH β chain is located on chromosome 19q13.2. The human chorionic gonadotropin β-subunit has similar biological activity to the LH β-subunit. LH secretion is pulsatile in both sexes but sexual dimorphism in physiological secretory patterns becomes evident with maturity of the hypothalamo-pituitary-gonadal axis. An increased nocturnal LH release is the first sign of the onset of puberty.

Actions and regulation

Actions

Both hormones bind to membrane receptors in their ovarian and testicular cells, activate the G-protein coupled complex and stimulate adenyl cyclase. FSH regulates gametogenesis in males and females while LH is thought to be primarily responsible for gonadal steroid secretion.

Regulation

Pulsatile release of hypothalamic GnRH regulates the secretion of the pituitary hormones LH and FSH which stimulate the testis and ovary at puberty to increase the gonadal steroid secretion and develop secondary sexual characteristics. There is a surge in gonadotropin and gonadal steroid secretion in the neonatal period with concentrations similar to those reached during puberty.

Following the first few months of life, the gonadotropin axis remains quiescent until puberty, when concentrations rise again. GnRH-synthesizing neuronal migration, from their first appearance in the embryonic medial olfactory placode to their final position in the mediobasal hypothalamus, is complete by around 19 weeks' gestation when pulsatile GnRH release is established. Several signaling factors such as anosmin-1 or KAL1 and FGFR1 are implicated in this migratory process. GnRH synthesis and release is also influenced by several neuroendocrine factors such as PC1 and leptin. Kiss-peptins are products of the *KiSS-1* gene, which bind to a G-protein coupled receptor known as GPR54. Although *KiSS-1* was initially discovered as a metastasis suppressor gene, recent evidence suggests that the kisspeptin/GPR54 system is a key regulator of the reproductive system, KiSS-1 neurons playing an important part in feedback regulation of gonadotropin secretion.

Recent studies have described a role for PROK2 and its receptor PROKR2 in the secretion of gonadotropins. Dopamine also appears to have a regulatory effect on gonadotropin secretion that is dose dependent. Estradiol and progesterone act via both the pituitary and hypothalamus to have a negative effect on gonadotropin secretion. However, if plasma estradiol concentrations are very high for a period greater than approximately 36 h in the absence of plasma progesterone, a positive feedback influence is exerted with an LH surge as seen in the mid-menstrual cycle in females. FSH secretion is also regulated by inhibin, a protein molecule secreted by the follicular granulosa cells in the female and Sertoli cells in the male.

Isolated gonadotropin deficiency
Clinical features
Hypogonadism may be caused by abnormalities within the hypothalamo-pituitary axis or within the gonad itself. Hypogonadotropic hypogonadism is particularly heterogeneous with a phenotype in males ranging from undescended testes at birth with absent pubertal development to normal puberty and infertility at the other extreme. It is four times more common in males than females with an incidence variably reported from 1 in 10 000 to 1 in 86 000 [77,78]. The most common presentation of isolated hypogonadotropic hypogonadism is at puberty with a lack of pubertal development, although the diagnosis is sometimes suspected at birth in patients who present with cryptorchidism and bilaterally undescended testes. The prevalence of abnormalities at birth is low suggesting that maternal human chorionic gonadotropin rather than fetal gonadotropins are responsible for testosterone secretion in the fetus.

The diagnosis of isolated hypogonadotropic hypogonadism at puberty is made with low concentrations of LH and FSH and a poor rise to stimulation with exogenous GnRH. Patients with constitutional delay in puberty (and growth) can present in a

similar manner and distinction between the two conditions is sometimes unclear. The condition is benign, more common in males and is a diagnosis of exclusion. Children with constitutional delay are generally short for chronological age although appropriate for skeletal age and progress to normal sexual maturation and function spontaneously, albeit at a later age. Because of the difficulty in distinction between the two conditions, it is sometimes necessary to treat the child with exogenous sex steroids in order to complete puberty at an appropriate age and revisit the diagnosis on completion of puberty.

Etiology
Hypogonadotropic hypogonadism may be isolated, as discussed below, or combined with other pituitary hormone deficiencies. Mutations in several transcription factors such as PROP1, LHX3, SOX2, SOX3 and HESX1 are associated with deficiencies of gonadotropic hormones [8,21,51]. The condition may be sporadic or familial inherited in an autosomal dominant, autosomal recessive or X-linked manner.

The association between isolated hypogonadotropic hypogonadism and anosmia (Kallman syndrome) was first reported by Maestre de San Juan. Kallman detailed the genetic basis to this disorder due to mutations in the *KAL-1* gene resulting in an X-linked inheritance. The anosmia results from agenesis of the olfactory bulbs, the development of which is closely linked to that of GnRH synthesizing neurons. Although these patients are capable of synthesizing and secreting a normal GnRH protein, the improper location of the GnRH neurons results in an inability of GnRH to reach the pituitary gland to stimulate the gonadotropins. Neuroimaging is often used in clinical practice to identify the abnormal olfactory bulbs in order to make the diagnosis. It is thought that approximately 75% of patients with Kallman syndrome demonstrate agenesis of the olfactory bulbs on neuroimaging [79]. Mutations in *KAL1* are responsible for the X-linked form of Kallman syndrome [80,81] and other features such as mirror movements, renal aplasia, high-arched palate, deafness and pes cavus are associated with the X-linked form of the disorder [81].

DAX-1 (dosage sensitive sex reversal, adrenal hypoplasia congenita critical region on the X chromosome) mutations in humans cause hypogonadotropic hypogonadism and adrenal hypoplasia congenita which can result in severe neonatal adrenal crisis. Most often, the hypogonadotropic hypogonadism presents at puberty [82]. The condition is inherited as an X-linked disorder due to inactivating mutations of *DAX1* gene. *DAX1* is a transcription factor that is expressed in several tissues and in the hypothalamus and pituitary. It closely interacts with SF1 (steroidogenic factor 1), another transcription factor that is critical for adrenal and gonadal development. Duplications of *DAX1* result in persistent Mullerian structures and XY sex reversal suggesting that the gene acts in a dosage sensitive manner. Females are phenotypically normal.

Inactivating mutations of the *GnRHR* were first reported in 1997 and since then seven different pedigrees have been described

[83]. There is a wide range of phenotypes described, from complete hypogonadism with undescended testes and presentation at birth, to those who present with mild pubertal delay [84]. Although mutations in *GnRHR* are rare, patients with milder phenotypes harboring mutations may not yet be identified. Recently, a homozygous missense mutation was identified within a novel gene, *GPR54*, in a highly consanguineous pedigree of patients with hypogonadotropic hypogonadism [85]. A second patient with isolated hypogonadotropic hypogonadism was found to be a compound heterozygote for two different mutations within the gene. Further pedigrees have been identified that harbor deletions within the gene. GPR54 is believed to be a regulator of GnRH secretion at the hypothalamic level. Mutations in *FGFR1*, *PROK2* and *PROKR2* have also been described in association with hypogonadotropic hypogonadism.

Mutations in *PC1* are associated with defective processing of prohormones and a mutation in *PC1* in a female patient has been reported with extreme early-onset obesity, ACTH deficiency, insulin dependent diabetes and hypogonadotropic hypogonadism [73].

Leptin is a secreted product of the adipocyte and acts as a satiety factor. Apart from its role in regulating nutrition, it appears to have an important role in several neuroendocrine functions by acting at a hypothalamic level. Mutations in leptin and its receptor are both associated with obesity, marked hyperphagia, metabolic abnormalities and hypogonadotropic hypogonadism [86,87]. Recently, treatment with leptin in a 12-year-old female patient with a frameshift mutation in the leptin gene has resulted in significant weight loss and normalization of nocturnal LH secretion [88].

Prolactin

Action, regulation and deficiency
Prolactin is a 199 amino acid protein with its gene located on chromosome 6p22.2-21.3. The principal functions of prolactin are growth and development of the breasts and initiation and maintenance of lactation in postpartum women. It also has some role in regulation of gonadal function by stimulating the generation of LH receptors in the gonads in both sexes. The mechanism of action of prolactin is similar to other protein molecules by stimulating the tyrosine kinase pathway and subsequent intracellular protein phosphorylation.

The release of prolactin is under the control of the hypothalamus with afferent impulses from sensory receptors, primarily around the nipples. The dominant hypothalamic influence is inhibitory and the principal inhibitory hormone is dopamine. Other molecules exerting an inhibitory role are norepinephrine, histamine and serotonin acting at either a hypothalamic or pituitary level. TRH, in addition to stimulating the release of TSH, is also the principal prolactin stimulatory hormone. Thyroxine and estrogen can modulate the number of TRH receptors in the lactotropes, thereby influencing prolactin release. Thyroxine, by negative feedback, decreases the number of TRH receptors while estrogens increase their availability.

The maternal pituitary is the main source of serum prolactin during pregnancy and the only known clinical effect of prolactin hyposecretion in adults is the failure of lactation in puerperal women. Prolactin deficiency may be combined with other anterior pituitary hormone deficiencies as seen in patients with *POU1F1* and *PROP1* mutations. Rarely it may occur as an isolated deficiency [89].

Posterior pituitary hormones

The neurohypophysis consists of the supraoptic and paraventricular hypothalamic nuclei containing the cell bodies of the magnocellular neurosecretory neurons that secrete vasopressin and oxytocin, the supraoptico-hypophyseal tract that includes the axons of these neurons, and the posterior pituitary where the axons terminate on capillaries of the inferior hypophyseal artery.

Arginine vasopressin
Vasopressin is a basic nanopeptide with a disulfide bridge between the cysteine residues at positions 1 and 6. Most mammals have the amino acid arginine at position 8. The vasopressin gene lies on chromosome 20p13, in tandem with the oxytocin gene and separated by 8 kb of DNA. The gene contains three exons and encodes a polypeptide precursor that consists of a 19 amino acid amino-terminal signal peptide, a 9 amino acid vasopressin peptide, a diamino acid linker, the 93 amino acid neurophysin peptide (NPII), a single amino acid linker, and a 39 amino acid carboxyl-terminal glycopeptide copeptin.

The preprohormone is synthesized in the magnocellular neuron cell body, following which the signal peptide is cleaved. The prohormone then folds and places AVP into a binding pocket of NPII, which protects AVP from proteolysis and promotes high-density packing in neurosecretory granules by oligomerization of AVP-NPII dimers. Following the formation of seven disulfide bonds within NPII and one within AVP, and the glycosylation of copeptin, the prohormone is packaged into neurosecretory granules and cleaved into the product peptides during axonal transport to the posterior pituitary. The mature hormone and NPII are then stored as a complex in secretory granules within the nerve terminals of the posterior pituitary. Stimulation of vasopressinergic neurons results in the opening of voltage-gated calcium channels in the nerve terminals, which through transient calcium influx results in fusion of the neurosecretory granules with the nerve terminal membrane and release of their contents into the circulation. The half-life of vasopressin is short, approximately 5–15 min.

Actions and regulation
Vasopressin acts via three G-protein coupled receptors: it achieves its pressor effects via V1 receptors, its main renal effects via V2 receptors (V2-R), and its action on corticotropes to secrete ACTH in synergy with CRH via V3 receptors. Activation of the V2-R

leads to a biphasic increase in the expression of the water channel protein aquaporin 2. This then allows reabsorption of water from the duct lumen along an osmotic gradient, with excretion of concentrated urine.

The main regulatory factors in determining vasopressin secretion are osmotic status, blood pressure and circulating volume. Neurotransmitters such as dopamine and norepinephrine are also thought to have a role in vasopressin secretion, as does angiotensin II.

Central diabetes insipidus

This is most commonly caused by lesions within the hypothalamo-pituitary axis such as germinoma, Langerhans cell histiocytosis and craniopharyngioma, post-traumatic head injury, post-surgery and secondary to inflammatory lesions such as sarcoidosis. Congenital causes of central diabetes insipidus (DI) are rare. Familial central DI is an autosomal dominant disorder of AVP secretion.

Patients present with polyuria and polydipsia, usually in the first 10 years of life. Overt hypertonic dehydration occurs only if the patient is unable to obtain water. Food consumption may be decreased leading to loss of weight and slow growth. During infancy, common clinical features include hyperthermia, vomiting, failure to thrive and constipation. Neonatal manifestations are uncommon, suggesting that the pathophysiology of familial central DI involves progressive postnatal degeneration of AVP-producing magnocellular neurons.

A number of mutations have been described in children with central DI in the AVP neurophysin gene. These include signal peptide mutations which decrease the ability of the signal peptidase to initiate removal of the signal peptide from the preprohormone [90]. A second group of mutations occurs within the AVP or amino-terminal domain of the NPII-coding sequence, and these interfere with the binding of AVP to NPII or in the folding of NPII [91]. A third group of mutations result in the synthesis of a truncated neurophysin molecule [92].

Recent studies have suggested that the mutations described to date may lead to abnormal folding and processing of the preprohormone. The mutant protein may then accumulate within the endoplasmic reticulum, where it then may kill the cells by interfering with the orderly processing of other essential proteins. Hence, heterozygous mutations within the AVP NII gene may result in the production of an abnormal preprohormone that cannot be processed properly and destroys AVP-processing neurons. A pedigree with autosomal recessive DI has also been described, with a homozygous mutation in exon 1 leading to partial loss of function.

Other causes include Wolfram syndrome, an autosomal recessive condition that includes DI, diabetes mellitus, optic atrophy and sensorineural deafness. *WFS1* is a novel gene on chromosome 4p16.1 encoding an 890 amino-acid glycoprotein (wolframin), predominantly localized in the endoplasmic reticulum. Mutations in *WFS1* underlie autosomal recessive Wolfram syndrome. Many mutations have been reported to date, over the

entire coding region, and are typically inactivating, suggesting that a loss of function causes the disease phenotype [93].

DI may also be a feature of midline disorders such as septo-optic dysplasia and holoprosencephaly.

Oxytocin

The oxytocin gene lies on chromosome 20p13 and consists of three exons, which, like vasopressin, encodes a polypeptide precursor with an amino-terminal signal peptide, the oxytocin peptide, neurophysin and a carboxy-terminal peptide. The human oxytocin promoter contains estrogen-response elements and interleukin-6 response elements. The significance of this is unclear. The half-life of oxytocin is short. Oxytocin binds to a G-protein coupled cell surface receptor on target cells to mediate a variety of physiological effects largely concerned with reproductive function, namely the regulation of lactation, parturition and reproductive behavior. In humans, women lacking posterior pituitary function can breast-feed normally, illustrating that oxytocin is not necessary for lactation in humans.

Combined pituitary hormone deficiency

Clinical features

Combined pituitary hormone deficiency (CPHD) is defined as a deficiency in two or more pituitary hormones. The condition varies considerably in severity. The signs and symptoms of hypopituitarism resulting from CPHD are essentially a combination of individual hormone abnormalities and may be non-specific in the early neonatal period becoming obvious with time. Occasionally the condition may be life-threatening, especially in patients with ACTH deficiency, and an early diagnosis is mandatory.

Neonatal presentation

The presentation of hypopituitarism in the neonatal period may be with symptoms of poor feeding, lethargy, apnea, jitteriness and poor weight gain. Hypoglycemia is present in the majority of patients with CPHD, probably because of ACTH deficiency, although it has also been reported in patients with IGHD. Measurement of capillary blood glucose is a routine practice in sick neonates and measurement of true blood glucose should be undertaken if the capillary glucose is less than 2.6 mmol/L. At the same time, blood should also be taken for measurement of random GH, cortisol, insulin, non-esterified fatty acids and ketone bodies. Low serum insulin in the presence of hypoglycemia will rule out hyperinsulinemia and low serum GH and cortisol concentrations should point towards a diagnosis of hypopituitarism. Patients with TSH deficiency may present with temperature instability and prolonged neonatal jaundice. Prolonged hyperbilirubinemia is, however, also a feature of hypopituitarism in patients without TSH deficiency. Conjugated hyperbilirubinemia is a marker of cortisol deficiency, and together with recurrent sepsis, apnea and seizures should prompt investigation for hypopituitarism. Measurement of serum cortisol concentration is therefore required. Although ACTH does not regulate the renin-angiotensin system, patients with hypopituitarism can present with hyponatremia but without hyperkalemia. Occasionally patients present with DI in the neonatal period, although this is much more common in patients with associated midline defects. A history of breech delivery or other instrumental delivery is more common in patients with hypopituitarism. Patients with gonadotropin deficiency, particularly LH, may present with undescended testes and a microphallus because growth of the penis is dependent upon normal secretion of LH and hence testosterone in the second and the third trimester.

Growth failure

Birth weight and birth length have been reported to be normal in patients with congenital hypopituitarism. However, there has been considerable controversy over the role of GH in the immediate postnatal period and in early infancy. Recent studies have shown evidence for severe growth failure in infants with congenital hypopituitarism [94,95]. Short stature is generally the primary complaint in patients with hypopituitarism who present later in infancy and childhood. Linear growth is dependent upon GH and thyroxine in childhood, and on sex steroids later during puberty.

The following features should warrant investigations for GH deficiency:

1 Severe short stature (height ≥3 SD below the mean for the population);
2 Height ≥2 SD below the mean for the population and a growth velocity over 1 year more than 1 SD below the mean, or a decrease in height >0.5 SD over 1 year in children >2 years of age;
3 Height SD ≥1.5 SD below the mid-parental height;
4 Height velocity ≥2 SD below the mean over 1 year or ≥1.5 SD over 2 years in the absence of short stature;
5 Other anterior pituitary hormone deficiencies;
6 Positive neonatal history in the presence of short stature or a reduced height velocity.
Bone maturation may be delayed for the chronological age.

Body habitus

Patients with GH deficiency have a characteristic facial appearance and body habitus. The head appears large with frontal bossing, a small nose, truncal obesity, immature facies, mid-facial hypoplasia and delayed dentition. Patients with GH deficiency have a reduced lean body mass and increased total body fat. Prolonged untreated hypopituitarism results in a considerable deficit in final height.

Development

Patients with untreated hypothyroidism under the age of 2 years can develop severe brain damage and global developmental delay. Prolonged undetected hypoglycemia can also result in profound central nervous system damage. DI associated with either severe hyponatremia (resulting from overtreatment) or hypernatremia (resulting from inadequate treatment or fluid deprivation) can also lead to brain damage.

Puberty

Male patients with hypogonadotropic hypogonadism may present with a microphallus and undescended testes. The diagnosis is less well-recognized in females at birth. Patients with hypogonadotropic hypogonadism can have a wide spectrum of abnormalities ranging from absent, delayed or arrested pubertal progress or infertility in later life. Additional GH deficiency will result in failure of the pubertal growth spurt.

Diabetes insipidus

Patients with panhypopituitarism can unusually present with DI. The symptoms are those of polyuria and polydipsia with weight loss. Cortisol is essential for the excretion of a water load and the diagnosis of DI may be masked in patients with both ACTH and AVP deficiency. Treatment with hydrocortisone will unmask DI with polyuria and polydipsia, and hence caution should be exercised in patients with multiple pituitary hormone abnormalities when they are commenced on glucocorticoid replacement treatment, with careful monitoring for DI. It is extremely unusual for DI to occur in patients without midline defects, such as septo-optic dysplasia and holoprosencephaly.

Visual problems

Patients with hypopituitarism and visual abnormalities should be reviewed by an ophthalmologist to rule out optic nerve hypoplasia and hence a diagnosis of septo-optic dysplasia. Neuroimaging is required to exclude this diagnosis.

Etiology

Idiopathic CPHD

Most patients with CPHD do not have a known underlying etiology and are classified as having idiopathic disease. The condition is highly variable with respect to clinical presentation. Even if hypopituitarism is not recognized in the immediate postnatal period, a careful history at the time of diagnosis may indicate the presence of perinatal symptoms.

Craft *et al.* [96] have suggested a causal relationship between gestational–perinatal complications and hypopituitarism with risk factors such as prematurity, gestational bleeding, complications of delivery, fetal distress or asphyxia. It is difficult to differentiate whether hypothalamo-pituitary defects are actually responsible for these perinatal complications or whether perinatal problems themselves lead to hypopituitarism. The discovery of pituitary transcription factors, mutations of which can lead to abnormalities of hypothalamo-pituitary morphology, suggests that the former may be the case at least in some patients. The fact that many males with hypopituitarism are born with genital abnormalities such as undescended testes and a micropenis also suggests that, in some cases at least, hypopituitarism is of prenatal onset.

Non-syndromic genetic CPHD

Mutations in PROP1

The human *PROP1* gene has been mapped to chromosome 5q and is a member of the paired-like homeobox gene family. The gene spans 3 kb and consists of three exons encoding a protein product of 226 amino acids. The DNA binding homeodomain consists of three alpha helical regions and most mutations reported to date affect this region.

Wu *et al.* [51] first reported mutations in *PROP1* in four unrelated pedigrees with an endocrine phenotype consistent with GH, TSH, prolactin, LH and FSH deficiencies. The first family harbored a homozygous mutation (R120C) in the paired like homeodomain. The second and third pedigrees were found to have what is now believed to be a mutational "hot spot" within the *PROP1* gene, a 2 bp deletion (delA301, G302, also known as 296del GA). This mutation involves a 2 bp GA or AG deletion among three tandem GA repeats (296-GAGAGAG-302) within exon 2 resulting in a frameshift with a stop codon at codon 109, thereby leading to a truncated protein (S109X) that contains the N-terminus and only the first helix of the homeodomain, thereby disrupting both DNA-binding and transcriptional activation. The patient in the fourth pedigree was a compound heterozygote (delA301, G302/F117I). To date, 22 distinct mutations have been identified in over 170 patients (Fig. 4.5), suggesting that mutations in *PROP1* are the most common cause of CPHD, in approximately 50% of familial cases [97,98].

The incidence in sporadic cases is much lower [98,99]. Affected individuals exhibit recessive inheritance. The most common *PROP1* mutation (50–72%) detected in multiple unrelated families is the 2 bp deletion within exon 2 resulting in a frameshift at codon 109 (see above) [51,97,98,100]. This probably represents a mutational hot spot [98] and along with the 150delA mutation accounts for approximately 97% of all mutations in *PROP1*.

The timing of initiation and severity of hormonal deficiencies in patients with mutations in *PROP1* is highly variable. Although most patients present with early-onset GH deficiency, normal growth in early childhood and normal final height in an untreated patient with a *PROP1* mutation have been reported [101]. The normal final height was achieved at the expense of considerable weight gain at the time of puberty. As observed in patients with *POU1F1* mutations, the TSH deficiency in these patients is highly variable and may not be present from birth. The spectrum of gonadotropin deficiency can range from presentation with a microphallus and undescended testes, hypogonadism with lack of puberty, to spontaneous pubertal development with subsequent arrest, and infertility [47].

The exact mechanism underlying this "acquired" deficiency is unclear, although it suggests that Prop1 is not required for gonadotrope determination but is required for differentiation. Individuals with mutations in *PROP1* exhibit normal ACTH and hence cortisol concentrations in early life but often demonstrate an evolving cortisol deficiency associated with increasing age [100,102–105], although it has also been described in a 7-year-old patient [105]. The underlying mechanism for cortisol deficiency is unknown, especially as *PROP1* is not expressed in corticotropes, although it appears to be required for maintenance of the corticotrope population. Various hypotheses have been postulated such as a gradual attrition of corticotropes or an expanding pituitary and its subsequent involution [102], although there appears to be no correlation between involution of the pituitary gland and development of ACTH deficiency.

Pituitary morphology in patients with mutations in *PROP1* is variable. Most individual reports have documented a normal pituitary stalk and posterior lobe, with a small or normal anterior pituitary on MR scanning. However, in some cases, an enlarged anterior pituitary has also been reported [51,100,106]. Longitudinal analyses of anterior pituitary size have revealed that a significant number of patients demonstrate pituitary enlargement in early childhood, which can wax and wane in size, with subsequent involution in older patients (Fig. 4.6) [99,104,107]. The pituitary enlargement consists of a mass lesion interposed between the anterior and posterior lobes, possibly originating from the intermediate lobe [107]. To date, the underlying mechanism leading to pituitary gland enlargement remains unknown. The only biopsy report of the "tumor" was non-specific with presence of amorphous material, no signs of apoptosis and no recognizable cells. Prolonged expression of *HESX1* or *LHX3* and hence of undifferentiated precursor cells that remain viable for a longer

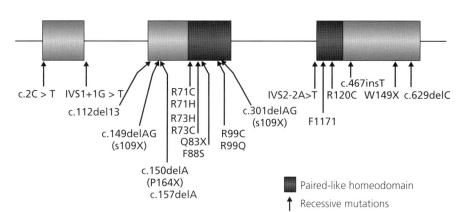

Figure 4.5 Human mutations in *PROP1* causing combined pituitary hormone deficiency. All mutations are inherited recessively.

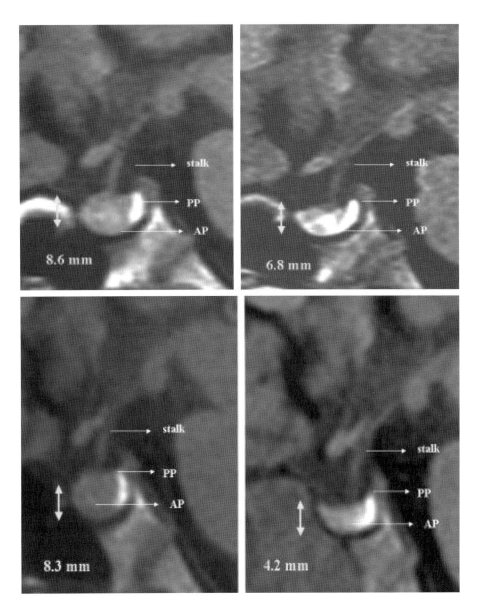

Figure 4.6 Magnetic resonance imaging of a 9-year-old boy with a 13 base pair deletion in PROP1 showing: (a) an enlarged sella turcica with a markedly enlarged anterior pituitary (AP, 8.6 mm), with enhancing lesions suggestive of possible haemorrhage at initial presentation; (b) an anterior pituitary size of 6.8 mm 4 months later; (c) an anterior pituitary size of 8.3 mm 12 months later; (d) an anterior pituitary size of 4.2 mm 21 months later. PP, posterior pituitary.

time have been implicated [46]. A recent report suggesting that *Prop1*-deficient fetal mouse pituitary retains mutant cells in the periluminal area of Rathke's pouch that fail to differentiate and exhibit enhanced apoptosis and reduced proliferation may be a possible explanation [49].

Mutations in POU1F1

The human *POU1F1* gene has been localized to chromosome 3p11 and consists of six exons spanning 17 kb. It encodes a 291 amino acid protein with a molecular mass of 33 kD. The protein has three functional domains: a transactivation domain, a POU specific domain and a POU homeodomain. The POU specific and POU homeodomains are both critical for high affinity DNA-binding on GH and prolactin promoters.

The first mutation within *POU1F1* was identified by Tatsumi *et al.* [54] in a child with GH, prolactin and profound TSH defi-

ciency. The patient was homozygous for a nonsense mutation in *POU1F1* resulting in a severely truncated protein of 171 amino acids, lacking half of the POU-specific domain and all of the POU-homeodomain. Such a protein would be incapable of binding to GH and PRL promoters and thus unable to activate the transcription of these genes. The inheritance is both as an autosomal dominant and recessive, the former associated with a dominant negative effect whereby the mutant protein interferes with the function of the normal protein. More recently, a patient with GH deficiency, normal basal serum prolactin but lack of response to stimulation with TRH and evolving secondary hypothyroidism has been identified with a novel mutation (K216E) that can bind to DNA and activate transcription, but that does not support retinoic acid induction of the *POU1F1* gene distal enhancer either alone or in combination with wild-type *POU1F1* [108]. Hence functional analysis of many of these mutations suggests that some mutations disrupt DNA binding whereas others disrupt transcriptional activation or other properties such as autoregulation.

The spectrum of hormone deficiency can also vary in patients with *POU1F1* mutations. GH deficiency generally presents early in life, along with prolactin deficiency. However, TSH deficiency can be variable with presentation later in childhood [109,110] or preserved [111]. A total of 27 mutations within *POU1F1* have been described (22 recessive, five dominant) in over 60 patients, all with a broadly similar phenotype of GH, TSH and prolactin deficiency (Fig. 4.7). Although the majority of mutations within *POU1F1* are recessive, the heterozygous point mutation R271W appears to be a "hot spot" for mutations within *POU1F1* [112], and has been identified in several unrelated patients from different ethnic backgrounds [113–119].

MR imaging demonstrates a small or normal anterior pituitary with no other extra-pituitary abnormalities. Abnormalities within midline structures are not associated with *POU1F1* mutations. Deficiency of GH, prolactin and TSH is more profound in patients harboring mutations in *POU1F1* than in patients with *PROP1* mutations. Table 4.4 compares the phenotype in patients with hypopituitarism as a result of mutations in *PROP1*, *POU1F1* and *LHX3*.

Syndromic CPHD
Septo-optic dysplasia

Septo-optic dysplasia (SOD) is a rare congenital heterogeneous anomaly with a prevalence ranging from 6.3 to 10.9 per 100000 [120,121]. The condition is defined by the presence of any two of three features: midline forebrain defects, optic nerve hypoplasia (ONH) and hypopituitarism. The first reported case of ONH associated with absence of the septum pellucidum was in a 7-month-old infant with congenital blindness, absent pupillary reflexes and normal development, more than 50 years ago. Prior to that, ONH had only been described as a rare and isolated anomaly for almost a century. De Morsier, in 1956, described the postmortem findings of ONH and agenesis of the septum pellucidum and coined the term "septo-optic dysplasia", also known as De Morsier syndrome. Approximately 30% of patients with SOD manifest the complete clinical triad, 62% of patients have some degree of hypopituitarism, and 60% have an absent septum pellucidum [122,123]. The condition is equally prevalent in males and females.

ONH may be unilateral or bilateral and may be the first presenting feature, with the later onset of endocrine dysfunction. Bilateral ONH is more common (88% compared with 12% unilateral cases). Additionally, there appears to be little correlation between the size of the optic nerve and its visual function. Neuroradiological abnormalities are present in up to 75–80% of patients with ONH [124,125]. Pituitary hypoplasia may manifest as endocrine deficits varying from isolated GH deficiency to panhypopituitarism. There has been some suggestion that abnormalities of the septum pellucidum and hypothalamo-pituitary axis on neuroimaging can predict the severity of endocrine dysfunction [126]. A decrease in growth rate resulting from GH deficiency is the most common feature, with hypoglycemia and polyuria and polydipsia being less common. Either sexual precocity or failure to develop in puberty may occur. Abnormal hypothalamic neuroanatomy or function and DI may be a feature. The

Table 4.4 Clinical features of hypopituitarism due to mutations in *POU1F1*, *PROP1* and *LHX3* causing combined pituitary hormone deficiency (CPHD) in humans.

Phenotype	*PROP1*	*POU1F1*	*LHX3*
Presentation	Delayed	Congenital	Congenital
GH	Deficient	Deficient	Deficient
TSH	Deficient	Deficient	Deficient
Prolactin	Deficient	Deficient	Deficient
LH, FSH	Deficient	Normal	Deficient
ACTH	May evolve	Normal	Normal
Pituitary size	S, N, E	S, N	S, N, E
Non-pituitary phenotype	Nil	Nil	Short cervical spine

E, enlarged; N, normal; S, small.

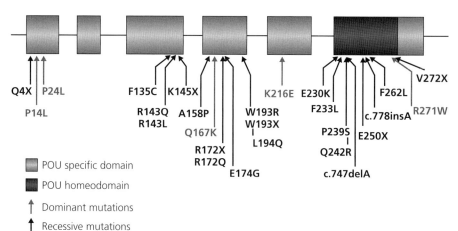

POU specific domain
POU homeodomain
↑ Dominant mutations
↑ Recessive mutations

Q4X P24L
P14L
F135C K145X
R143Q A158P
R143L
Q167K
R172X
R172Q
E174G
K216E E230K
F233L
W193R
W193X
L194Q
P239S
Q242R
c.747delA
F262L
c.778insA R271W
E250X
V272X

Figure 4.7 The reported *POU1F1* mutations to date.

endocrinopathy may be evolving with a progressive loss of endocrine function over time. The most common endocrinopathy is GH deficiency followed by TSH and ACTH deficiency. Gonadotropin secretion may be retained in the face of other pituitary hormone deficiencies [127]. Commencement of GH treatment in SOD children with GH deficiency may be associated with accelerated pubertal maturation.

Neurological deficit is common, but not invariably so, and in one study, was documented in 15 of 24 children with a severe degree of optic nerve hypoplasia. The deficit ranged from global retardation to focal deficits such as epilepsy or hemiparesis. Other neuroanatomical abnormalities include cavum septum pellucidum, cerebellar hypoplasia, schizencephaly and aplasia of the fornix. An association between SOD and other congenital anomalies such as digital abnormalities has been reported [128–130].

Both genetic and environmental factors have been implicated in the etiology of the condition [131,132]. Environmental agents such as viral infections, vascular or degenerative changes and exposure to alcohol or drugs have been implicated in the etiology of SOD. The condition presents more commonly in children born to younger mothers and clusters in geographical areas with a high frequency of teenage pregnancies [121,133,134]. Because forebrain and pituitary development occurs as early as 3–6 weeks' gestation in the human embryo, and is closely linked, any insult at this critical stage of development could account for the features of SOD.

In the light of the phenotype demonstrated in *Hesx1* null mutant mice, the human homolog of the gene was screened for mutations in patients with SOD. *HESX1* maps to chromosome 3p21.1-3p21.2, and its coding region spans 1.7 kb with a highly conserved genomic organization consisting of four coding exons. A homozygous missense mutation (Arg160Cys) was found in the homeobox of *HESX1* in two siblings within a highly consanguineous family in which two affected siblings presented with ONH, absence of the corpus callosum, and hypoplasia of the anterior pituitary gland with panhypopituitarism [8]. The parents were heterozygous for the mutation and phenotypically normal. Screening of extended members of the family revealed a further nine phenotypically normal heterozygotes within this highly consanguineous pedigree, consistent with an autosomal recessive inheritance. The mutation led to a complete loss of DNA-binding, and the mutation unusually was associated with an *in vitro* dominant negative effect even though heterozygotes for the mutation did not manifest a phenotype. Haplotype analysis using markers which closely flanked *HESX1* revealed that such heterozygous *HESX1* mutations are associated with a dominant inheritance that is incompletely penetrant, although the insertion (Table 4.5) was a *de novo* mutation.

The phenotypes associated with heterozygous mutations are, on the whole, milder, classically characterized by isolated GHD with an ectopic/undescended posterior pituitary. However, the overall frequency of *HESX1* mutations in SOD has been low,

Table 4.5 Reported mutations in *HESX1*.

Mutation	Inheritance	Endocrine phenotype	Neuroradiological findings	Reference
Q6H	Dominant	GH, TSH, LH, FSH deficiency	AP hypoplasia, ectopic PP	[9]
I26T	Recessive	GH, LH, FSH deficiency; evolving ACTH, TSH deficiency	AP hypoplasia, ectopic PP, normal ON	[10]
c.306–307insAG	Dominant	GH, LH, FSH deficiency; hypothyroidism	AP hypoplasia, ON hypoplasia	[13]
Q117P	Dominant	GH, TSH, ACTH, LH, FSH deficiency	AP hypoplasia, ectopic PP	[345]
c.357+2T > C	Recessive	GH, TSH, ACTH, PRL deficiency	AP aplasia, normal PP, normal ON	[346]
Alu insertion (exon 3)	Recessive	Panhypopituitarism	AP aplasia, hypoplastic sella, normal PP and infundibulum	[347]
E149K	Dominant	GH deficiency	AP hypoplasia, ectopic PP, infundibular hypoplasia	[134]
c.449–450delCA	Recessive	GH, TSH, ACTH deficiency	AP aplasia, normal PP, normal ON, thin CC, hydrocephalus	[346]
R160C	Recessive	GH, TSH, ACTH, LH, FSH deficiency	AP hypoplasia, ectopic PP, ON hypoplasia, ACC	[8]
S170L	Dominant	GH deficiency	Normal AP, ON hypoplasia, ectopic PP, partial ACC	[9]
K176T	Dominant	GH deficiency, evolving ACTH, TSH deficiency	Ectopic PP	[345]
g.1684delG	Dominant	GH deficiency	AP hypoplasia, ON hypoplasia, ACC, absent PP bright spot	[12]
T181A	Dominant	GH deficiency	AP hypoplasia, normal ON, absent PP bright spot	[9]

AP, anterior pituitary; CC, corpus callosum; ON, optic nerve; PP, posterior pituitary; SP septum pellucidum.

suggesting that mutations in other known or unknown genes may contribute to this complex disorder (Table 4.5).

Hypopituitarism and neck abnormalities

LHX3 maps to human chromosome 9q34. *LHX3* mutations are a rare cause of CPHD including deficiencies for GH, prolactin, TSH, and LH/FSH in all patients. To date, homozygous mutations in *LHX3* [a missense mutation (Y116C) in the LIM2 domain, a novel, single base pair deletion in exon 2, deletion of the entire gene (del/del), mutations causing truncated proteins (E173ter, W224ter), and a mutation causing a substitution in the homeodomain (A210V)] have currently been identified in 12 patients from seven unrelated consanguineous families [21,22,135]. The mutations are associated with diminished DNA binding and pituitary gene activation, consistent with observed hormone deficiencies.

Whereas most patients have severe hormone deficiencies manifesting after birth, milder forms have been observed. The lack of limited neck rotation, initially thought to be a universal feature of patients with *LHX3* mutations, extends the known molecular defects and range of phenotypes found in LHX3-associated diseases [22]. Hypopituitarism was additionally associated in all patients, apart from those with W224ter mutations, with a short rigid cervical spine with limited head rotation and trunk movement. Pituitary morphology on MR scanning was variable in these patients, as with mutations in *PROP1*, ranging from a small to a markedly enlarged anterior pituitary not evident in a previous MR scan, to a recent report of a hypointense lesion with a "microadenoma" [135].

Hypopituitarism with cerebellar abnormalities

The human *LHX4* gene extends over 45 kb on chromosome 1q25. Mutations within *LHX4* have been reported in seven patients to date with variable hypopituitarism and MR abnormalities. Mutational analysis of the first reported patient, with CPHD (GH, TSH and ACTH deficiency), revealed a heterozygous intronic mutation in *LHX4* [24]. MR imaging revealed anterior pituitary hypoplasia, an undescended posterior pituitary, an absent pituitary stalk, a poorly formed sella and pointed cerebellar tonsils. The second patient presented with a similar phenotype but also had additional prolactin, LH and FSH deficiencies, Chiari malformation and respiratory distress syndrome and was found to have a heterozygous missense mutation (P366T) in exon 6, which was present in the LIM4 specific domain [25].

More recently, Pfaeffle *et al.* [23] have reported three novel heterozygous mutations (A120P, L190R, R84C) in three unrelated families. All patients had evidence of variable hypopituitarism between and within families and a hypoplastic anterior pituitary on neuroimaging. However, an undescended posterior pituitary was not observed in patients of the first family, two of whom demonstrated pituitary cysts. Mutations in *LHX4* are rare and the resultant phenotype in patients with mutations suggests that *LHX4* tightly coordinates brain development and skull shape. Haploinsufficiency of *LHX4* results in defective regulation of

POU1F1 and downstream activation of *GH1* expression, providing a mechanism at the molecular level in patients with mutations in *LHX4* [136]. However, ACTH deficiency observed in these patients cannot be explained by this mechanism suggesting that other *LHX4*-dependent pathways may exist independent of *POU1F1* in the developing pituitary gland.

Rieger syndrome

Mutations within *PITX2* or *RIEG* are associated with Rieger syndrome in humans. Rieger syndrome is an autosomal dominant condition with variable manifestations including anomalies of the anterior chamber of the eye, dental hypoplasia, a protuberant umbilicus, mental retardation and pituitary abnormalities. All mutations identified within *PITX2* to date are heterozygous, affecting the homeodomain of the gene, although none of the patients with these mutations presented with pituitary hormone deficiencies [1].

Hypopituitarism with mental retardation

A number of pedigrees have been described with X-linked hypopituitarism involving duplications of Xq26-q27 [36,37,39], with the smallest described to date being approximately 690 kb [38]. The phenotype is that of variable mental retardation and hypopituitarism associated with anterior pituitary hypoplasia, infundibular hypoplasia and an ectopic posterior pituitary, with variable abnormalities of the corpus callosum. All duplications encompass the *SOX3* gene (OMIM 313430). SOX3 is encoded by a single exon producing a transcript with a coding region of approximately 1.3 kb, mapping to chromosome Xq27. The SOX3 protein consists of a short 66 amino acid N-terminal domain of unknown function, the 79 amino acid DNA binding HMG domain and a longer C-terminal domain, containing four polyalanine stretches, shown to be involved in transcriptional activation [27,137]. Further implication of *SOX3* in hypopituitarism comes from identification of patients with hypopituitarism and an expansion of a polyalanine tract within the gene [38,40]. Mutations in the gene are associated with both panhypopituitarism and IGHD. A proportion of *Sox3* null mice also exhibit pituitary and hypothalamic defects, in addition to craniofacial abnormalities, reduced size and fertility and defects of CNS midline structures. This suggests that *Sox3/SOX3* dosage is critical for normal hypothalamic-pituitary development as over-dosage (patients presenting with Xq27 duplications) and under-dosage (the phenotype of *Sox3* null mice as well as patients with loss of function polyalanine expansions) of Sox3 are both associated with infundibular hypoplasia and variable hypopituitarism [38,40].

Hypopituitarism and severe eye defects

Like its murine counterpart, the human *SOX2* gene (OMIM 184429) is composed of a single exon encoding a 317 amino acid protein containing an N-terminal domain of unknown function, a DNA binding HMG domain and a C-terminal transcriptional activation domain. Twelve heterozygous *de novo* mutations in

SOX2 were previously reported in 14 human patients associated with bilateral anophthalmia or severe microphthalmia with additional abnormalities including developmental delay, learning difficulties, esophageal atresia and genital abnormalities [42,138–141]. All of these mutations occured *de novo* and included five nonsense, four frameshift, one deletion and two missense mutations. We have subsequently reported six patients harboring *de novo* heterozygous mutations in *SOX2* resulting in loss-of-function of the mutant protein, four of which were previously unreported (c.60insG, c.387delC, Y160X and c.479delA).

Clinical evaluation revealed that in addition to anophthalmia or microphthalmia, *SOX2* mutations were also associated with anterior pituitary hypoplasia and hypogonadotropic hypogonadism, which resulted in the absence of puberty in all six patients and genital abnormalities in males. All affected individuals exhibited learning difficulties with other variable manifestations including hippocampal abnormalities, defects of the corpus callosum, esophageal atresia and sensorineural hearing loss [45]. The mutations were associated with significant loss-of-function which included loss of DNA binding, nuclear localization, and transcriptional activation, suggesting these phenotypes arise as a result of haploinsufficiency of *SOX2* in development.

More recently, Sato *et al.* [142] have reported an additional patient with a missense mutation in the HMG domain (L75Q) resulting in decreased DNA binding affinity of the mutant protein. The affected individual manifested unilateral right-sided anophthalmia and isolated hypogonadotropic hypogonadism, with a normal anterior pituitary and normal mental development, further supporting a critical role for SOX2 in the regulation of correct gonadotropin production in addition to eye development [142]. SOX2 has also been shown to interact with β-catenin, and can therefore interact with the Wnt signaling pathway [143].

Holoprosencephaly

Abnormal cleavage of the forebrain leads to holoprosencephaly (HPE). Three types have been identified: alobar, semilobar and lobar. The condition is also associated with other anomalies such as nasal and ocular defects, abnormalities of the olfactory nerves and bulbs, corpus callosum, hypothalamus and pituitary gland. Phenotypes can be highly variable and the pituitary abnormality most commonly associated with HPE is DI, although anterior pituitary hormone deficiencies may be associated with the condition.

Major advances have recently been made in understanding the etiology of this condition. At least 12 chromosomal regions on 11 chromosomes contain genes implicated in HPE. Autosomal recessive and dominant forms of the condition have been described. Mutations in various genes such as *SHH*, *ZIC2*, *TG1F* and *SIX3* have now been implicated in this condition. Three *GLI* genes have been implicated in the mediation of SHH signals. Heterozygous mutations within *GLI2* were identified in seven of 390 patients with HPE [144]. The phenotype and penetrance was variable, with the parent carrying a mutation but showing no

obvious phenotype in some cases. In all affected patients, pituitary gland function was abnormal, accompanied by variable craniofacial abnormalities. Other features included post-axial polydactyly, single nares, single central incisor and partial agenesis of the corpus callosum.

Miscellaneous conditions

A number of conditions are associated with variable hypopituitarism. These include Pallister–Hall syndrome, Fanconi anemia, solitary single central incisor, cleft lip and palate and ectrodactyly-ectodermal dysplasia-clefting syndrome.

Investigation and treatment of hypopituitarism

Investigations for hypopituitarism

The diagnosis of hypopituitarism is based upon a combination of provocative testing of the hypothalamo-pituitary axis, measurement of IGF-1 and IGFBP3, neuroradiology, and the clinical phenotype [145]. Normal secretion of a hormone is dependent upon the presence of an intact hypothalamo-pituitary-target gland axis. The axis can be stimulated to test for hormone deficiency and can be suppressed to test for hormonal excess and this forms the basis for several pituitary stimulation tests. Children with congenital abnormalities of the hypothalamo-pituitary axis are at risk of serious morbidity from hypoglycemia, adrenal crisis, delayed mental development and even mortality. The diagnosis of CPHD may be evident in the newborn period when the infant presents with hypoglycemia, or prolonged neonatal hyperbilirubinemia. Additionally, males may present with undescended testes and a microphallus. The diagnosis is often clear on assessing basal thyroid function, with a low concentration of free thyroxine (FT4) and a concomitant low concentration of TSH. The random cortisol is low, and a 24-h plasma cortisol may confirm low concentrations of cortisol throughout the day. The concentration of the GH-dependent factors IGF-1 and IGFBP3 is also useful, although in isolation the sensitivity and specificity of the test is poor. Growth hormone provocation tests are contraindicated in children less than 1 year of age.

In the older child, the diagnosis of CPHD is based upon the documentation of a low growth velocity in conjunction with GHD on provocative testing. TSH deficiency is characterized by a low TSH in conjunction with a low thyroxine concentration. A routine TRH test is not mandatory to establish the diagnosis of central hypothyroidism in children with CPHD [146], although recent studies have suggested that the test might be more useful in infants [147]. Basal serum prolactin concentrations of <500 mU/L are usually indicative of prolactin deficiency and may be confirmed by a suboptimal response to TRH. Gonadotropin deficiency is confirmed by a poor response to GnRH, although the latter is dependent upon the age at which the test is performed. ACTH deficiency can be diagnosed as a poor cortisol response to provocation with either hypoglycemia or exogenous ACTH (synacthen). In some patients, 24-h plasma cortisol sampling may prove necessary as it provides a better marker of endogenous physiological cortisol secretion as opposed to the measure of cortisol reserve [148]. In males, stimulation of testes with human chorionic gonadotropin can be used in the diagnosis of hypogonadotropic hypogonadism, when the testes often show a very poor testosterone response to human chorionic gonadotropin.

MR imaging of the brain is extremely useful in detecting abnormalities of forebrain and pituitary development, and in assessing the size of the optic chiasm and optic nerves [126,149]. The size of the anterior pituitary gland is highly variable, as it can be normal, hypoplastic or enlarged. The posterior gland may be eutopic or ectopic. Midline defects of the forebrain may also be present.

The role of genetics remains to be established and is only offered on a research basis at present. Appropriate mutational screening is an important adjunct to assessment and management of the patient as it not only provides a better understanding of the pathophysiological process but it can also help in management of the patient as observed in those with IGHD type II and those with mutations in *PROP1*. Mutations within *PROP1* or *HESX1* can alert one to the possibility of evolving cortisol deficiency. Additionally, the detection of a mutation within one of the pituitary transcription factors in a patient with an enlarged pituitary will circumvent the need for surgery. Detection of mutations can also lead to early diagnosis, and hence reduce the morbidity that is associated with a late diagnosis.

There is at present no need for prenatal diagnosis because the condition is eminently treatable. Given the variable penetrance of many of the dominant mutations, prenatal diagnosis should certainly not be offered until our understanding of the genetic basis to many of these conditions is significantly advanced. However, the concentrations of cortisol and thyroxine should be checked postnatally in order to diagnose the condition as quickly as possible and thereby institute treatment rapidly with a view to preventing brain damage that might ensue if the child has undiagnosed hypothyroidism or hypoglycemia.

Management of hypopituitarism

The mainstay of treatment is replacement therapy with the appropriate hormones. Thyroxine should be commenced if the free or total thyroxine concentration is low, ensuring that the cortisol secretion is normal or that hydrocortisone treatment is commenced if required prior to thyroxine treatment. Growth should be carefully monitored, and if the growth velocity is poor and GHD confirmed on provocative testing, then treatment with recombinant hGH (rhGH) should be commenced. rhGH should be continued until linear growth ceases, although there is now a case for the use of GH treatment in young adults with GHD given the possible metabolic effects on fat, lean body mass and bone mineral density. Sex steroids in the form of estrogen or testosterone should be commenced at the time of puberty if gonadotropin deficiency is confirmed. Hydrocortisone should be commenced if cortisol secretion is impaired. If a mutation within *PROP1* is

documented and the cortisol secretion is normal, cortisol secretion should be assessed at regular intervals because it may become impaired at a later date. If a pituitary mass is present, serial MR imaging scans are indicated in order to monitor the size of the mass.

In patients with SOD, adequate ophthalmological, neurological and social support should be offered to the patients and their families, given the visual disability that is a part of the condition.

It is important to remember that these conditions can evolve and so regular monitoring of thyroxine concentrations as well as cortisol concentrations is recommended, on or off treatment.

Growth hormone receptor and downstream signaling

Cellular actions of GH occur through the binding of GH to its single membrane passing receptor (GHR). Only one GHR has been described and probably most, if not all, actions of GH occur through binding to this receptor. After binding of GH to its receptor, intracellular signaling cascades are activated, resulting in the transcriptional activation of target genes. Aberrations in this process result in GH insensitivity (GHI) and are discussed below.

Biology of GH and IGF-1 signaling
Growth hormone receptor
The GHR is a member of the type I class of cytokine receptor family that also includes single transmembrane receptors for prolactin, leptin, erythropoietin, thrombopoietin, leukemia inhibitory factor (LIF) and several interleukins and colony-stimulating factors. Members share 15–20% homology in the cytokine homolog domain, which is located in the extracellular part of the receptor and is involved in ligand binding. Based on structural and sequence homology, the family can be subdivided into five groups [150,151]. GHR belongs to group 1 together with receptors for prolactin, erythropoietin and thrombopoietin. All of these receptors form homodimers and contain conserved Box1 and Box2 domains and signal through JAK2 and Stat5 (signal transducer and activator of transcription). Members of other groups of the cytokine receptor family also signal through JAKs and Stats but not necessarily JAK2 and Stat5.

The *GHR* gene is located on human chromosome 5p13.1-p12, and spans approx 87 kb in the human genome. In most species, *GHR* contains several alternative promoters positioned in clusters up to 40 kb upstream of exon 2, which are expressed in a tissue-specific fashion [152–155], allowing for tissue-specific regulation of GHR expression.

Apart from the main 4.6 Kb GHR transcript, there are several GHR isoforms varying in size and sequence, arising from alternative processing of the primary transcript, for example GHR 1-277 and GHR 1-279 that lack most of the intracellular domain. Two genomic *GHR* isoforms that exist only in humans have arisen from ancestral homologous recombination. They differ in the retention or deletion of exon 3 [152]. The functional differences between these two isoforms have been the subject of much recent research and are discussed below.

The *GHR* gene encodes for the GHR proreceptor. After cleavage of an 18 amino acid signaling peptide, the mature receptor has a 246 amino acid extracellular domain, 24 amino acid transmembrane domain and a 350 amino acid intracellular domain. The extracellular domain contains a distal part involved in GH binding and a more proximal part involved in GHR dimerization (Fig. 4.8) [156,157]. The intracellular domain contains a proline-rich Box1 which is associated with JAK2 binding. Tyrosine residues in the intracellular domain of GHR have a key role in signaling. Just distal to Box2 is a small domain, the UbE motif, which is necessary for ubiquitination and internalization of GHR.

GHR is expressed on the cell plasma membrane but is constitutively internalized, both by clathrin coated pits and caveolae. GHRs are transported to the endosomes from where they can be recycled to the plasma membrane or targeted for degradation. Degradation occurs in the proteasome, an enzyme complex that degrades ubiquitinated proteins. Ubiquitination of GHR, i.e. addition of ubiquitin groups, increases after GH binding to GHR, and is dependent on the UbE motif [158]. Internalization is important for the regulation and termination of signaling.

Growth hormone binding protein

The main GH binding protein (GHBP) is the soluble extracellular domain of the GHR and has an identical affinity for GH as GHR [159]. It binds to GH and increases its half-life in the circulation and may serve a function in the transportation of GH to target tissues and subsequent binding to the receptor. Although in rodents GHBP arises through alternative splicing, human GHBP arises from proteolytic cleavage of the cell membrane anchored GHR, for example by TNF α converting enzyme (TACE) [160]. GHBP is, like GHR, present in many tissues, but GHBP in the circulation is mostly derived from the liver. Although GHR and GHBP are regulated by and are very sensitive to GH, and GHR and GHBP often change in parallel [161–163], measurement of plasma GHBP has not been shown to reflect GHR and GH responsiveness [164]. The absence of GHBP in the circulation may suggest an abnormality of the GHR and support a diagnosis of GHI but *GHR* mutations do not necessarily affect GHBP concentrations, and GHBP may even be high [165]. Liver dysfunction also impairs GHBP production [166].

GH signal transduction
Initiation of signaling by GH
GHR, like its family group member EPO-R, is preformed as a dimer and is transported in a non-ligand bound state to the cell surface [157]. GH then binds in a sequential manner to the GHR dimer where the first GHR binds to the stronger site 1 of the GH molecule followed by the second GHR binding to the weaker site 2. Binding of GH results in a conformational change whereby

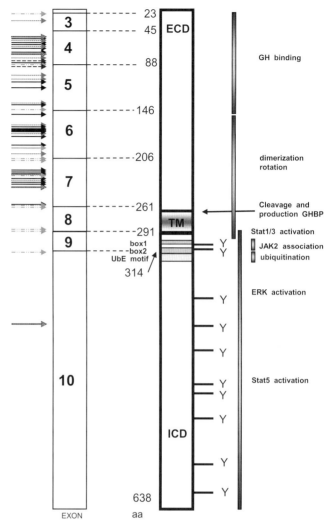

Figure 4.8 Schematic representation of the mature growth hormone (GH) receptor (middle), associated domain functions (right side) and corresponding coding regions in *GHR* (left side). Homozygous recessive and heterozygous dominant negative mutations are indicated with arrows. aa, amino acid number counted from aa 1 as the start of the 18 aa signal peptide, which is not shown in the figure; ECD, extracellular domain; GHBP, GH binding protein; ICD, intracellular domain; JAK2, Janus kinase 2; STAT, signal transducer and activator of transcription; TM, transmembrane domain; UbE, ubiquitination domain. Arrows depict gene defects: ⟶ nonsense mutation, ┈┈▸ missense mutation, ─·─·▸ splice site mutation, ─ ─ ─▸ large deletion, ⟹ small deletion with premature termination codon.

rotation of the GHRs results in repositioning of the intracellular domains and of Box1-associated JAK2 molecules. As a result, JAK2 is autophosphorylated and activated which in turn leads to cross-phosphorylation of distal tyrosine residues of GHR which enables SH2 (*Src* homology 2) domain molecules to dock to these sites [167,168]. Stat5a and Stat5b molecules contain SH2 domains and bind to these phosphorylated tyrosine sites and then they in turn become phosphorylated. Phosphorylated Stat5 molecules (homo- and hetero-) dimerize and translocate to the nucleus where they bind DNA, as dimers or as tetramers, and activate target genes (Fig. 4.9) [169].

Signal transducer and activator of transcription 5

The Stat family consists of Stats 1–4, Stat5a, Stat5b and Stat6. *STAT5A* and *STAT5B* genes are located on chromosome 17q11.2 and have originated from gene duplication, and encode for the 787 amino acid proteins Stat5a and Stat5b that are 95% homologous. Stat5 has, like all Stats, an N-terminal coiled-coil domain, which provides a hydrophilic interface for protein binding, a DNA binding domain, a linker domain, a SH2 domain necessary for the binding of docking sites and for dimerization, and a transcriptional activation domain (Fig. 4.10) [170]. The transcriptional activation domain contains the tyrosine residue 699 available for phosphorylation, and both the DNA binding domain and the N-terminal domain are crucial for stable Stat–DNA interaction.

Both Stat5a and Stat5b can be activated by GH, and they have both overlapping and distinct functions [171–176]. Gene inactivation mouse models have shown that deletion of *Stat5b*, but not of other Stat genes, even though GH also activates Stat1 and Stat3,

affects growth, and that Stat5b is of greater importance for stimulation of growth than Stat5a [170,171,177–179]. *Stat5b* null mice have severe postnatal growth retardation especially in males, although this is not as severe as in *Ghr* null mice. They have increased GH secretion, reduced hepatic IGF-1, IGFBP3 and acid labile subunit (ALS) expression, and increased obesity (177). *Stat5a* null mice have normal growth but impaired mammary gland formation and lactogenesis, reflecting impaired signaling of prolactin [172]. *Stat5a/b* double null mice are more severely affected than the single null mice, and display more severe growth retardation, although *Ghr* null mice are still more severely affected [180,181]. *Stat5a/b* double null mice also have a severe combined immunodeficiency, with reduced CD8 T-cell number and a failure of hematopoietic stem cells to develop lymphoid lineages [182]. Transgenic Stat5 expression results in expansion of CD8 cells and lymphomagenesis [183] and also in increased proliferation and differentiation in mammary cells [184], suggesting a critical role for Stat5 in cell proliferation, particularly in immune cells.

Stat5b is phosphorylated upon stimulation by a pulse of GH, and after this rapid activation becomes temporarily refractive to

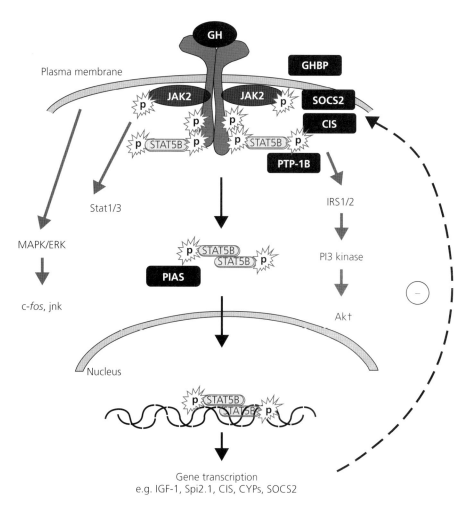

Figure 4.9 Schematic representation of main GH signaling pathways. Black boxes represent proteins involved in negative feedback of GH signaling. CIS, cytokine inducible SH2 containing protein 1; CYP, cytochrome P450 enzyme; GH, growth hormone; GHBP, growth hormone binding protein; IGF-1, insulin-like growth factor 1; IRS1/2, insulin receptor substrate 1/2; JAK2, Janus kinase 2; MAPK/ERK, mitogen activated protein kinase/extracellular signal-regulated kinases; P, phosphor; PI3 kinase, phosphoinositide-3 kinase; PIAS, protein inhibitors of activated STATs; PTP-1B, protein tyrosine phosphatase B1; SOCS2, suppressor of cytokine signaling 2; STAT, signal transducer and activator of transcription.

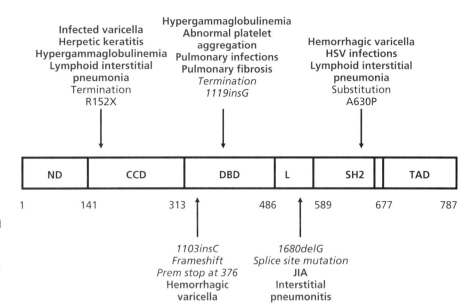

Figure 4.10 Localization of *STAT5B* mutations and their resulting immune phenotype. CCD, coiled-coil domain; DBD, DNA binding domain; L, linker domain; ND, N-terminal domain; SH2, *Svc* homology 2-containing domain; TAD, transactivation domain. Base pair insertions and deletions are in italics.

further or continuous stimulation [185,186]. GH secretion is more continuous in females, and indeed, in female rodents, Stat5b is phosphorylated to a lesser extent although phosphorylation still occurs. This gender-specific signaling has an important role in the regulation of gender-specific proteins, especially CYP450 enzymes [187,188] which have a role in hepatic metabolism of steroids and foreign compounds. The *Stat5b* null male mice are resistant to GH pulses [189] and their hepatic male-specific genes are decreased to female concentrations while female predominant genes are expressed at higher concentrations than in WT males. Hepatic nucleic factors (HNFs), especially HNF3, 4α and 6, interact with Stat5b to induce these Stat5b-dependent gender-specific gene expression patterns [176,188,190].

Stat5 response elements

Phosphorylated Stat5a and Stat5b bind Stat5 response elements (Stat5 RE) as dimers or tetramers but their binding is enhanced by the interaction of co-activators binding to adjacent DNA binding sites, like the γ-interferon activated sequence (GAS) motif [169], the glucocorticoid receptor (GR) response element [191], C/EBP and HNFs [188]. Inactivation of the GR binding site also results in reduced GH signaling, severe growth delay and reduced expression of GH-dependent genes in mice [191]. Stat5 RE have been located in the second and third intron of the human *IGF-1* gene and 73 kb upstream of the initiation site, although the effectiveness of the distant site is much less [192,193]. Besides *IGF-1*, *Spi2.1*, *CIS*, *SOCS2*, *HNF6* and several genes for CYP450 enzymes contain functional Stat5 RE [188,194–196]. *IGFBP3* and *ALS* are also direct GH target genes dependent on Stat5b but it is still unclear whether each gene is a direct target for Stat5b [197]. More genes with functional Stat5 binding sites are being identified now, including genes involved in lactogenesis [whey acid protein (*WAP*), *beta-casein*] [198] and immune function (*IL-2β*, *PIM1*, *IFN-γ*) [199].

Negative regulation of signaling

Activation of JAK-STAT signaling occurs rapidly, within minutes after GH stimulation, but is transient because of the tight control of the termination of signaling. This negative regulation of signaling occurs at several levels: GHR internalization, suppressors of cytokine signaling (SOCS), protein tyrosine phosphatases (PTPs) and protein inhibitors of activated Stats (PIAS).

The SOCS family of proteins comprises cytokine inducible-Src homology 2 protein (CIS) and SOCS 1–7. GH, PRL and many other cytokines can induce CIS, SOCS1, -2 and -3. SOCS family proteins inhibit JAK-STAT signaling by inhibiting JAK proteins, binding positive regulators of signaling or docking sites, and promoting GHR ubiquitination. The role of the several family members has become clearer from phenotypes associated with their overexpression. Mice overexpressing CIS have mild growth retardation and have also altered T-cell function and impaired mammary gland development, whereas *Socs2* null mice show gigantism similar to bovine GH overexpressing mice (30–40% overgrowth), are hyperresponsive to GH and have increased extrahepatic IGF-1 production. Stat5 signaling is indeed prolonged in hepatocytes of these mice and cross-breeding with *Stat5b* null mice showed that Stat5b is necessary for the gigantism [200].

PTPs dephosphorylate activated phosphorylated proteins in cytokine signaling pathways but also insulin signaling pathways. Several PTPs, like PTP-1, PTP-H1 and PTP-B1 and TC-PTP attenuate GH signaling, and PTP-1B is involved in fasting induced GH insensitivity [201–203]. PTPN11 mainly functions in RAS-

MAPK signaling, and abnormalities result not only in Noonan syndrome but also in associated mild GH resistance [204].

Other signaling pathways

Apart from activating Stat5a and Stat5b, GH is also able to activate Stat1 and Stat3 and to activate the MAPK-ERK pathway, PI3 kinase pathway and phospholipase C/DAG/PKC/Ca^{2+} pathway (Fig. 4.9) [205]. However, of these signaling pathways, Stat5b signaling is the most important for the regulation of growth. The role of other pathways has not been fully elucidated, although "knock-in" mice models with various truncated GHRs start to give us some insight [206].

IGF-1, its binding proteins and the acid-labile subunit

IGF-1 and IGF binding protein 3 (IGFBP3) are the main end products of the interaction of GH with its receptor. IGF-1 is a major regulator of growth and promotes proliferation, differentiation and cell survival. In addition, it promotes metabolic actions necessary for growth, such as protein synthesis, calcium accretion and fatty acid and glucose transport [207,208]. IGF-1 is of major importance for intrauterine growth but GH is not a main regulator of fetal IGF-1 production and growth, and fetal IGF-1 is more dependent on maternal feeding and metabolism [209,210]. In accordance, there is a strong relation between birth weight and umbilical cord IGF-1 concentrations [211,212], whereas children with severe GH deficiency, *GH1* gene deletion or GH insensitivity have only marginally reduced birth weights and lengths [94,213,214].

Mice with a targeted deletion of *Igf1* have severe prenatal (40% reduction in birth weight) and postnatal growth deficiency, sensorineural hearing loss and many die shortly after birth [215–217]. Hemizygous mice are mildly affected [218]. Interestingly, *Igf1* haploinsufficiency is also found in dogs and is a major determinant of their size [219].

The *IGF-1* gene is located on chromosome 12q22-24.1. Alternative processing of the gene results in several IGF-1 mRNAs and precursor proteins and allows for complex tissue specific regulation of IGF-1 expression but does not affect the structure of the main mature 70 amino acid IGF-1 peptide. IGF-1 circulates as a 150 kD ternary complex, bound to IGFBP3 and ALS. ALS is an 85 kDa glycoprotein almost exclusively produced in the liver, and its production is, like IGFBP3, stimulated directly by GH. ALS stabilizes the ternary complex, increases its size and therefore extends its half-life to approximately 15 hours, whereas free IGF-1 has a half-life in the order of minutes [220]. Of the six IGFBPs secreted into the circulation, only IGFBP3 and IGFBP5 are GH-induced, and only these two IGFBPs bind ALS [221]. Since GH can induce all three building blocks of the ternary complex, it can be maintained in a stable complex. At least 80% of IGF-1 in the serum is bound in the ternary complex with ALS and IGFBP3 or IGFBP5 [222]. IGFBP1 is regulated by insulin, and increases free IGF-1 after a meal. IGFBP2 is the most abundant IGFBP in the circulation and concentrations can increase further in chronic disease.

The major source of circulating IGF-1 is the liver and IGF-1 concentrations correlate with hepatic function [223]. In the postnatal period, GH is the main regulator of IGF-1 production and indeed the degree of postnatal growth failure due to genetic IGF-1 deficiency and GH deficiency are similar [224]. Nutritional and immunological status is of major importance for IGF-1 production. Malnutrition and fasting result in a rapid decrease in hepatic IGF-1 production and this is partly due to reduced GH sensitivity [201,225], whereas IGF-1 concentrations are often high in obesity [226]. Increased activity of the immune system in systemic inflammatory disease such as Crohn disease or juvenile arthritis suppresses IGF-1 production [227]. Children with renal dysfunction also have low IGF-1 concentrations and bioavailability [228,229]. Thyroid hormone, androgens and low dose estrogen stimulate IGF-1 production [230]. GH is also the major regulator of IGFBP3, but glucocorticoids, parathyroid hormone, and estrogens also affect IGFBP3 production.

Type I IGF-1 receptor

The *IGF-1R* gene is located on human chromosome 15q26.3. The type I IGF-1 receptor (IGF-1R) protein consists of transmembrane α and β subunits that are synthesized as preproglycoproteins. The mature protein is organized in a heterotetrameric fashion (α2β2). The α chain is involved in ligand binding, whereas the β chain contains a tyrosine kinase domain. IGF-1 binding results in phosphorylation of intracellular tyrosine residues of the receptor, facilitating binding of signaling molecules. Insulin receptor substrates and Shc proteins become activated and transmit signals through the Ras/Raf/MAPK pathway and the PI3K/Akt pathway, resulting in cell proliferation and cell survival [208]. IGF-1 acts primarily through IGF-1R, but can bind with lower affinity to the highly homologous insulin receptor, and to IGF-1R/IR heterodimers. Vice versa, insulin is able to signal through the IGF-1R [207,231]. Signs of such alternative signaling can become apparent in pathological IGF-1 or insulin signaling.

Deletion of *IGF-1r* in mice results in severe prenatal growth retardation and respiratory failure at birth invariably resulting in death, and the growth failure is more severe than in *Igf-1* null mutants (45% vs. 60% of normal birth weight) [215]. Mice carrying one *Igf-1r* allele have only a mild growth defect (85% of normal) [232]. Interestingly, they also show increased longevity which is not due to altered energy metabolism [233].

Peripheral target tissues

The growth plate is the final target organ for GH and IGF-1 to promote longitudinal growth. However, the growth plate is also a target for other growth factors and abnormalities in their expression or signaling can cause as severe a growth deficiency as GH/IGF-1 pathology, for example in anomalous PTH-R signaling (Jansen metaphyseal and Blomstrand chondrodysplasia), FGFR3 signaling (achondroplasia, hypochondroplasia), NPR2 (natriuretic peptide receptor 2) signaling (acromesomelic dysplasia, Maroteaux type) and SHOX insufficiency (Turner syndrome, Leri–Weil dyschondrostosis, Langer mesomelic dysplasia).

The hierarchical organization of the growth plate is of value for the unraveling of hormone action. It contains a zone of immature resting chondrocytes, a zone of proliferating cells and a zone of fully differentiated chondrocytes that produce extracellular matrix and hypertrophy, which results in growth. The perichondrium surrounding the growth plate contains undifferentiated mesenchymal cells, which can differentiate into chondrocytes. In rodents, GHRs are most pronounced in the resting cells and the prehypertropic chondrocytes [234], whereas IGF-1R is present in proliferating chondrocytes [235]. Low amounts of IGF-1 are present in proliferating cells [236]. Both GH and IGF-1 are able to affect growth plate chondrocytes [237] but discussion continues about the physiological impact of their endocrine and paracrine/autocrine actions.

There is now support from many studies for differential roles for IGF-1 and GH in longitudinal growth. Although IGF-1 is of great importance for normal intrauterine and postnatal growth, the role of hepatic generated and circulating IGF-1 in the regulation of growth may be of less importance than previously thought [238], because mice lacking hepatic IGF-1 production and mice lacking ALS production, which results in extremely rapid clearance of IGF-1, are of near-normal size [239–241], GH affects cell cycle times of resting cells in the growth plate, and GH can induce Stat5 phosphorylation and IGF-1 production in chondrocytes *in vitro* and *in vivo* [242–244]. Additionally, mice overexpressing bovine GH (bGH) show gigantism [245], in contrast to mice overexpressing IGF-1 [246]. IGF-1 is able to stimulate growth in severely growth retarded children and rodents [165,247], but systemic treatment fails to normalize bone length in *Ghr* null mice [248] and double *Ghr/Igf-1* null mice are more severely affected than the single null mice [249]. However, complete absence of circulating IGF-1 does have a small effect on growth [250]. These studies suggest that the direct effects of GH and the local production of IGF-1 are at least as important as their endocrine effects.

Clinical aspects of growth hormone insensitivity

The clinical entity of dwarfism, high circulating GH and insensitivity to GH has been named Laron dwarfism, Laron syndrome, GH insensitivity or GHR deficiency. The label "GH insensitivity" captures the spectrum of consequences of *GHR* defects best. Classic GH insensitivity (GHI) is a fully penetrant autosomal recessive disease caused by mutations in *GHR*. Other causes for GHI are given in Table 4.6.

Abnormalities of GH

Mutations in *GH1* can lead to IGHD, but they can also result in production and secretion of bioactive GH that is unable to activate GH signaling pathways. Patients with bioactive GH present with short stature, normal or increased GH concentrations, and low IGF-1 concentrations, suggestive of GHI. However, in contrast to classic GHI, they are able to produce IGF-1 in an IGF generation test and respond well to rhGH treatment, so that, strictly speaking, they are not GH insensitive.

Table 4.6 Classification of growth hormone (GH) insensitivity.

1 Congenital GH insensitivity

GH axis
(a) Bioinactive GH
(b) *GHR* defects:
  i. Extracellular
  ii. Transmembrane
  iii. Intracellular
(c) GH-signal transduction defects
  i. *STAT5B* defects
  ii. *PTPN11* defects

IGF-1 axis
(a) *IGF-1* defects
(b) *IGF-1R* defects
  i. *IGF-1R* gene mutation
  ii. *IGF-1R* haploinsufficiency
(c) *IGFALS* defects

2 Acquired GH insensitivity
  i. GH autoantibodies
  ii. Malnutrition
  iii. Liver disease
  iv. Uncontrolled diabetes
  v. Catabolic states (intensive care, postoperatively)
  vi. Chronic inflammation (inflammatory bowel disease, arthritis)
  vii. Other

The first patient with bioactive GH was described by Kowarski *et al.* [251], and therefore this clinical entity is also referred to as "Kowarski syndrome". A few patients were described in the 1980s, based on their clinical and biochemical phenotype. More recently, several *GH1* gene mutations have been described that would result in bioactive GH, but the reduction in GH bioactivity and the relation with the phenotype has been difficult to establish in some cases [252–254]. Of note, one heterozygous mutation (I179M) results in a mutant GH that would selectively affect ERK, but not Stat5, signaling; however, the pathophysiological impact is unclear because the genotype does not co-segregate with the phenotype [255]. Another homozygous mutation (C53S) results in the absence of the disulfide bridge linking C53 and C165 in the GH protein, which reduces the capacity to bind GHR and activate JAK2-Stat5 signaling [256]. The patient presented with short stature (−3.6 SD), moderately increased GH secretion, decreased IGF-1 concentration (−3.4 SD), and a normal GHBP concentration, with a good response to rhGH treatment. The mutant GH protein was detected in some GH assays, but not in others, emphasizing that this disorder and IGHD resulting from *GH1* mutations lie within the same diagnostic spectrum.

Abnormalities of *GHR*

In 1966, Laron *et al.* [257] described the clinical phenotype of the "Laron dwarf" and in 1989, 2 years after the cloning of *GHR*, the first GHR defect in "Laron syndrome" was described [258].

Classic GH insensitivity (GHI) is a fully penetrant autosomal recessive disease and many patients belong to consanguineous or inbred families. Most mutations affect the extracellular domain of the GHR, and interfere with GH binding or GHR production/ trafficking [259]. To date, approximately 250 patients have been described worldwide with 60 different mutations. Most common mutations are nonsense and missense mutations, but splice site mutations, and gross and small deletions also occur; most mutations are in exons 4, 5, 6 and 7 (Fig. 4.8) [165]. The largest isolated cohorts are in the Mediterranean, Israel and Ecuador. Members of the Ecuadorian cohort all have the same mutation in exon 6 (E180) that leads to the creation of a novel splice site, resulting in a protein lacking amino acids 181–188 [214].

Mutations affecting the extracellular domain – classic GHI

Birthweight in GHI is usually in the normal range, although birth length may be slightly reduced (42–46 cm), similar to babies born with a deletion of *GH1*. Postnatal growth fails immediately after birth and the growth deficit increases with age. Growth charts for GHI exist [260], and the mean adult height of untreated women is 123 cm (range 105–140 cm) and that of untreated men is 139 cm (range 116–142 cm) in the Israeli cohort and somewhat less in the Ecuadorian cohort. Individual heights range between −4 and −10 SD, and there is no genotype–phenotype correlation [261]. Young children resemble those with severe isolated GH deficiency and are short and obese, have frontal bossing, a saddle nose, mid-facial hypoplasia, thin sparse hair, acromicria, a high-pitched voice and microphallus. Head circumference is in the low normal range, proportional to the growth deficit, in contrast to *IGF-1* and *IGF-1R* gene mutations [224,262]. Teething is often delayed and motor development may be slightly delayed. Children often have recurrent hypoglycemia. Puberty is slightly delayed, especially in boys, and menarche in girls is between 13 and 15 years; however, fertility is normal. Lean body mass, muscle mass and muscle strength are reduced. Because of the reduced muscle and bone mass, body mass index (BMI) does not accurately reflect degree of adiposity, which can be as high as 50% fat. Bones are thin, but bone density is normal for the bone size. The skin is thin and sweating is reduced. Intellect is generally normal [214,259,263–265]. The height of heterozygous carriers is in the lower normal range but not statistically different from non-carriers [266].

Spontaneous GH secretion is increased, with increased trough and peak concentrations, and an increased response to stimulation but a normal pulsatile pattern and a normal suppression by exogenous IGF-1 [214,259]. Pituitary size is normal, but prolactin concentrations can be occasionally increased [267]. GHBP is typically low or low normal in patients with extracellular domain mutations. Circulating IGF-1 concentrations are variable, and range from just below normal to undetectable concentrations, but IGFBP3 and ALS concentrations are extremely low. Despite the low concentrations, height correlates with IGFBP3 SD [261,268]. Concentrations of IGFBP1 and IGFBP2 are increased. Serum lipid and insulin concentrations are relatively high and insulin insensitivity increases with advancing age and increasing obesity [214]. Table 4.7 summarizes these clinical features of GHI.

Hemoglobin, hematocrit and red blood cell count may be subnormal, in line with a role for GH and IGF-1 in erythropoiesis [269,270]. GHI is not associated with altered immune function, neither in humans nor in animal models [180]. Although GH and IGF-1 can stimulate the immune system [271], they are not obligatory for normal immune function [272].

GHI with normal GHBP concentrations, often called atypical GHI, is associated with lack of facial abnormalities; most of these patients do not have confirmed *GHR* mutations and may have defects further downstream [165]. Unusually, two mutations in the extracellular domain have been described in patients who have normal GHBP concentrations and normal facial appearance; one is a mutation in the extracellular domain (exon 6, D152H) that only results in a mild decrease of GH binding, but prevents dimerization [273], and the other is a homozygous mutation in intron 6 that results in an active splice site and the formation of a pseudoexon between exons 6 and 7, adding 36 amino acid in frame in the extracellular domain. This unusual mutation results in abnormal cellular trafficking of GHR and reduced number of GHRs on the plasma membrane [274,275].

Mutations affecting the transmembrane domain

Only two mutations have been described that affect the transmembrane region of the GHR protein: a homozygous mutation in the splice acceptor site (G > T 785-1) of intron 7 and one in the splice donor site (G > C 875+1) of intron 8, both resulting in the skipping of exon 8 which encodes for the transmembrane domain [276,277]. Patients have severe growth deficiency (−5.1 to −5.4 SD) and high concentrations of GHBP as a result of the failure of the receptor to anchor in the plasma membrane.

Table 4.7 Hallmarks of growth hormone insensitivity (GHI) due to extracellular domain mutations in *GHR*.

Autosomal recessive; heterozygous parents of low-normal height
Normal birth weight with slightly reduced birth length
Occasional to frequent hypoglycemia
Severe postnatal growth deficiency (height −4 to −10 SD)
Facial dysmorphism
Truncal obesity
Mild delay in puberty
Increased GH secretion with occasionally increased prolactin secretion
Low GHBP concentrations (exceptionally normal GHBP concentrations)
Low-normal to undetectable IGF-1 concentrations
Low IGFBP3 concentrations
No or poor response in IGF generation test
Normal intellectual capacity
Insulin insensitivity developing with age and obesity

GHBP, growth hormone binding protein; IGF, insulin-like growth factor.

Mutations affecting the intracellular domain

A few children with GHI have mutations affecting the intracellular domain of GHR. A dominant negative heterozygous mutation in the splice acceptor site of intron 8 (G > C 876-1) or the splice donor site of intron 9 (G > A 945+1) results in skipping of exon 9 and a severe truncation of the intracellular domain to 7 amino acids [278,279]. GHR internalization, which normally occurs after GH binding, is blocked while dimer formation with wild-type receptors still occurs, so that non-signaling truncated receptor dimers outnumber wild-type receptors on the plasma membrane, thereby having a dominant negative effect. GHBP concentrations are extremely high because of the defective GHR internalization, but height is only mildly affected (−3.0 to −3.5 SD), possibly because of residual signaling through wild-type GHR dimers.

A homozygous deletion in exon 10 results in a premature stop codon and truncation after Box1 of the GHR preventing Stat5 signaling, but not other signaling, and results in severe short stature (−6 to −8.7 SD) and an extremely low concentration of IGFBP3 but normal GHBP concentration [280].

GHR abnormalities and idiopathic short stature

The group of children with idiopathic short stature (ISS) is by nature heterogeneous and abnormalities of the GH-GHR-signal transduction pathways may underlie the clinical phenotype in a subgroup of these patients. Heterozygous *GHR* mutations have been identified in approximately 5% of patients with ISS [281,282], but data supporting the causal relation between the mutation and the phenotype of short stature are lacking; additionally, the height of heterozygous parents of patients with classic GHI is in the normal range [266]. It is likely that mutations of components of the signaling transduction pathways downstream of GHR and IGF-1R will be identified in the future. Mutations in *SHOX* have been described in ISS [283] and mutations in other genes involved in skeletal development may account for a further small cohort of patients with ISS. For example, C-type natriuretic peptide (CNP) is expressed in growth plate chondrocytes and stimulates matrix production and chondrocyte differentiation. Null mice for *Cnp* or its receptor natriuretic peptide receptor B (*Npr2*) are dwarfed and human homozygous loss-of-function mutations cause acromesomelic dysplasia, Maroteaux type. Heterozygous carriers are normally proportioned but have mild short stature [284–286]. As a group, children with ISS often have IGF-1 concentrations in the low normal range, although IGFBP3 concentrations are usually normal, in contrast to patients with severe GHD and GHI [287,288].

Exon 3 deleted GHR

Several GHR isoforms exist in humans, and expression of an alternative GHR transcript that lacks exon 3 (*GHRd3*) and encodes a protein that lacks 22 amino acid in the extracellular domain has recently been related to an increased response to GH treatment as compared with the full-length GHR (*GHRfl*), both *in vivo* and *in vitro* [289]. The occurrence of the *GHRd3* poly-

morphism is the result of ancestral homologous recombination of elements flanking exon 3. Approximately 25% of the *GHR* alleles are *GHRd3* and 75% are *GHRfl* in European populations [290]. Exon 3 deletion does not affect GH binding [291], and the molecular mechanism for the increased response to GH is still lacking. There is no relation with adult height in the normal population [292], but an initial retrospective analysis performed in a cohort of GH-treated small for gestational age (SGA) and ISS children showed a twofold increase in height velocity response to GH treatment in patients with the *GHRd3/d3* genotype compared with the *GHRfl/fl* genotype. Subsequent retrospective studies have been conflicting [292–295]. In a recent large retrospective study of 181 patients with IGHD, patients with the *d3/d3* genotype had an increased height velocity during the first 2 years of GH treatment but not in the subsequent 2 years, and there was no difference in final height between the genotypes in the 95 patients who had reached final height [296]. The clinical impact of this genotype variation in the several causes of short stature is therefore still unclear and it remains to be seen whether *GHR* genotype could or should be used as a pharmacogenomic marker to optimize individual GH treatment in the future.

Abnormalities of *STAT5B*

The first *STAT5B* mutation was described in a patient with the clinical phenotype of GHI: severe short stature, facial dysmorphism, extremely low IGF-1, IGFBP3 and ALS concentrations and no response to rhGH. The normal GHBP concentration and the presence of lymphoid interstitial pneumonia and frequent severe infections such as hemorrhagic varicella and herpes zoster suggested that this condition was distinct from classic GHI. Mutation analysis revealed a homozygous mutation in the SH2 domain of Stat5b, which prevents the mutant Stat5b from being phosphorylated [297]. Four more mutations have been described [298–301], in several domains of Stat5b (Fig. 4.10), and, in contrast to the phenotype of Stat5b null mice, both genders seem similarly affected.

All patients have a similar endocrine phenotype of normal or low-normal birth weight, severe postnatal growth deficiency, normal head circumference, delayed puberty and a biochemical profile consistent with severe GHI, including increased prolactin secretion, but the immune phenotype varies (Table 4.8). Most patients have had severe infections that require T-cell mediated immunity; lymphoid interstitial pneumonitis, juvenile idiopathic arthritis and hypergammaglobulinemia are variably present, without a clear genotype–phenotype relation. Response of Stat1 and Stat3 activation to GH is exaggerated. The heights of patients with *GHR* mutations and those with *Stat5b* mutations are of similar magnitude, suggesting that most of the growth-promoting effect of GH is Stat5-dependent, and this is in line with the much milder growth deficiency in a patient with diminished ERK signaling [255] and with mice models of altered GHR signaling [206]. Heterozygous carriers are of normal stature and have normal immune function.

Table 4.8 Clinical and biochemical features of growth hormone insensitivity (GHI) due to mutations of *STATB*, *IGFALS*, *IGF-1* and *IGF-1R*.

Gene defect	STAT5B	IGFALS	IGF-1	IGF-1R
Mode of inheritance	AR	AR	AR	AD
Number of patients described	6	6	2	5 (+mothers)
IUG				
Birth weight	−0.7 to −2.5 SD	↔	−3.9 SD	−1.5 to −3.5 SD
Birth length	−0.4 to 0 SD	↔	−4.3 to −5.4 SD	−1.0 to −5.8 SD
Birth HC	NA	NA	−4.9 SD	−4.6 to −5.6 SD
Neonatal problems	−	−	Hypoglycemia, NG feeding (1)	−
Auxology				
Height	−5.6 to −9.9 SD	−1 to −3.1 SD	−6.9 to −8.5 SD	−2.6 to −5.0 SD
Head circumference	−1.4 SD	−0.6 to −1.8 SD	−8.0 SD	NA
Pubertal development	Delayed	Normal–delayed	Delayed	↔
BMI	NA/mild increase	↔	−1.9 to −2.0 SD	↔
Parents' height	−0.8 to −2.8 SD (HZ)	−2.2 to +0.6 SD (HZ)	−2.4 to +0.3 SD (HZ)	−1.6 to −4.0 SD (HZ) −2.2 to +0.5 SD(NML)
Related problems	Lymphoid interstitial pneumonia (3–4), Immune deficiency (3), Hypergammaglobulinemia (2) Abnormal thrombocyte aggregation (1) JIA (1)	Mild speech disorder (1)	Sensorineural deafness Cataract (1) Shallow anterior chambers (1) Restricted movement of elbows (1)	Mild delay in motor (3) and speech (1) development Delayed tooth eruption (1)
Dysmorphisms	Prominent forehead Saddle nose High-pitched voice	Mild micrognathia Tooth irregularities (1)	Microcephaly Micrognathia Bilat. ptosis (1) Bilat. clinodactyly (1) Myopia (1)	Microcephaly (5) Triangular face (2)
Mental retardation	No	Mild (1)	Severe	Mild (2)
Investigations				
GH stimulation test	⇑	⇑	⇑	↔/↑
Spont GH secretion	↑	↑	⇑	↔/↑
Prolactin	⇑	↔/NA	↔/NA	↔/NA
GHBP	↔	↔/↑	↔	NA
IGF-1	Undetectable/very low	−4.5 to −10 SD	Undetectable/+7 SD	↔/⇑
IGF-2	⇓	−3.5 SD	↔	↔
IGFBP3	Undetectable/very low	−4 to −10 SD	↔	↔/↑
IGF-1/BP3 generation	No response	No response	No response	NA/⇑
ALS	Undetectable/very low	Undetectable	↔/⇑	NA/⇑
Insulin-sensitivity	NA/↔	↓	⇓ (1)	NA
Bone age	NA/ severe delay	Mild delay	Mild delay	Mild delay
Bone density	NA	↔	−4.4 to −4.8 SD	↔ (1)
MRI brain	NA/normal	Normal	Slightly enlarged lateral ventricles	NA/normal

Number of affected patients in brackets, if not all patients are affected. AD, autosomal dominant; AR, autosomal recessive; HZ, heterozygous; IUG, intrauterine growth; JIA, juvenile idiopathic arthritis; NG, nasogastric; NML, normal; − absent, ↔ normal, ↑ mildly increased, ⇑ increased, ↓ mildly decreased, ⇓ decreased.

SINGLETON HOS...
STAFF LIBRARY

The immune function of two patients, who both had signs of interstitial pneumonitis and hypergammaglobulinemia, was further examined. T-cell lymphopenia with normal CD4+/CD8+ ratios was noted, but with a very low number of NK (natural killer) cells and CD4+ and CD25+ T cells, and an impaired proliferation response to interleukin 2 (IL-2). Despite the lymphopenia, T cells show hyperactivation [301,302]. IL-2 also uses Stat5b, like GH, for its signaling, and indeed the immune phenotype of Stat5b null mice and mice lacking Il2 or its receptor, that includes autoimmunity and lymphoid cell hyperplasia, are very similar [303]. Regulatory T cells are involved in suppression of immunity and prevention of autoimmunity [304] and the lymphoid interstitial pneumonitis and JIA of Stat5b deficient patients could be the result of these immunological abnormalities.

Abnormalities of PTPN11 – Noonan syndrome

Noonan syndrome is caused by abnormalities within signaling pathways associated with GH signaling. Cardinal features include cardiac abnormalities (pulmonary stenosis and hypertropic cardiomyopathy), broad or webbed neck, chest deformities, short stature and facial dysmorphism (triangular face, hypertelorism, low set ears and ptosis). Other variable features include bleeding diathesis, cryptorchidism and delay of puberty.

Mutations in PTPN11 (protein tyrosine phosphatase N11), SOS1 and KRAS have been identified in patients with Noonan syndrome in frequencies of approximately 50%, 10% and less than 5% of the cases [305–307]. PTPN11 encodes the protein SHP2 (SRC homology domain 2 containing protein tyrosyl phosphatase 2), which is widely expressed in both embryological and adult tissues and is involved in the regulation of signal transduction. Activating mutations of PTPN11 result in overactive SHP2, which enhances RAS/MAPK signaling, and this in turn underlies many of the features of Noonan syndrome. However, SHP2 is also involved in GH signaling and normally binds to the GHR and inhibits GH signaling [308]. Indeed, overactive SHP2 blocks GH-JAK-STAT5 signaling through binding to tyrosyl phosphorylation sites of the GH receptor. Patients with a PTPN11 mutation are mildly GH insensitive and slightly shorter than suggested by their target height [204,309]. Their IGF-1 and ALS concentrations are relatively low, whereas their IGFBP3 concentrations are normal. GH treatment increases height velocity in the short term, but less so in Noonan patients with PTPN11 mutations than in those without [309,310]. Activating PTPN11 mutations are also associated with leukemia and other neoplasms but these mutations usually result in greater SHP2 activity than those found in Noonan syndrome [311].

Abnormalities of IGF-1

The first IGF-1 gene defect was described in 1996 [224]. A homozygous splice site mutation resulted in a deletion of exon 4 and 5 of the IGF-1 gene and in a premature stop codon, which led to a reduction of the IGF-1 peptide from 70 amino acids to 25 amino acids. The patient was born with severe proportional intrauterine growth retardation (IUGR) [birth weight 1.4 kg (−3.9 SD), birth length 37 cm (−5.4 SD) and head circumference 27 cm (−4.9 SD) at a gestational age of 37 weeks] and had feeding problems in the neonatal period but only mild hypoglycemia and jaundice (Table 4.8). He had severe postnatal growth failure and his height and weight were −6.8 SD and −6.5 SD, respectively at the age of 15 years, but his fat mass was relatively normal. He had severe microcephaly and mental retardation as well as sensorineural deafness. He was mildly dysmorphic (bilateral ptosis, micrognathia, low hairline, bilateral clinodactyly, one-sided single palmar crease) and his puberty was slightly delayed at the age of 15. His spontaneous GH secretion was increased, whereas the IGF-1 was undetectable. IGFBP3 was normal, as was ALS, but IGF-2 was mildly elevated. An IGF-1 generation test did not increase IGF-1. Bone age was delayed and there was a mild degree of hyperinsulinism. The parents were heterozygous for the same defect and had heights and IGF-1 concentrations in the low normal range. The patient was treated with GH, but failed to respond.

A second patient was described 10 years later [312]. This patient had a homozygous missense mutation resulting in a V44M alteration. The altered protein had a 90-fold reduced affinity for IGF-1R [313]. The clinical picture of IUGR, severe short stature, microcephaly, micrognathia, deafness and severe mental retardation, is very similar to that of the earlier described patient. A homozygous mutation in the polyadenylation signal has also been described in a patient with a phenotype similar to the cases above [314], but subsequent studies suggest that this is a polymorphic variant [315].

IGF-1 gene abnormalities have been speculated to underlie the growth phenotype in children born SGA failing to show catch-up growth. Associations with polymorphism in non-coding regions have been suggested [316,317] but no functional mutations or polymorphisms in the IGF-1 coding region have been identified [315].

Abnormalities of IGFALS

A total of six families with gene abnormalities of IGFALS all resulting in severe ALS deficiency have been described (Table 4.8) [318–321]. Patients with homozygous mutations have undetectable ALS by ELISA and Western ligand and immunoblotting and extremely low IGF-1 and IGFBP3 serum concentrations. All have only a very mild growth deficiency (height −1.2 to −3.1 SD) with no clear prenatal growth deficiency, but a delay in pubertal development. Insulin sensitivity is markedly reduced with insulin concentrations reaching values in the low hundreds (μIU/mL) during an oral glucose tolerance test.

ALS was also undetectable in three affected siblings with compound heterozygous mutations. These patients had a milder growth phenotype (height −0.5 to −1.0 SD) but also had pubertal delay and insulin insensitivity. The mild growth deficiency seen in these patients with ALS deficiency is in line with the phenotype of the Igfals null mice [241]. Some patients had an increased GH secretion which could support maintenance of a normal plasma concentration of free IGF-1 and could also contribute to the reduced insulin sensitivity although altered IGF-1 bioavailibility is the main contributor to altered glucose sensing [318].

Abnormalities of *IGF-1R*

In 2003, *IGF-1R* mutations were described for the first time in patients selected from a population of patients with IUGR without catch-up growth or with short stature and increased IGF-1 concentrations [322]. The first patient was found to have a compound heterozygous mutation but all of the other four described mutations are heterozygous mutations [262,323–325]. All but one result in reduced IGF-1R signaling, although the primary defects affect ligand binding, dimerization or tyrosine kinase activity of the IGF-1R. Affected patients are characterized by IUGR (approximately −3 SD) with reduced birth length, microcephaly and short stature (Table 4.8). Typically, there is no catch-up growth and postnatal growth is parallel to the lowest centile. Some patients have dysmorphic features. Despite the IUGR, there is no hypoglycemia, in contrast to *GHR* mutations. In contrast to IGF-1 deficiency, there is no severe mental retardation, although mild retardation has been reported in two patients. Pubertal progression and fertility is normal. IGF-1 concentrations can be normal or mildly to severely elevated whereas IGFBP3 is normal in most cases. GH secretion may be increased, although prolactin concentrations are normal. Bone age seems less delayed than in typical isolated GHD or GHI.

The five mutations were identified in different regions of the *IGF-1R* gene and resulted in severe truncation, abnormal cleavage to the mature receptor, reduced ligand binding or reduced signaling. The effect on growth was variable, the cleavage site mutation affecting growth the least (height −2 SD) and the ligand binding domain mutation affecting growth the most (height −5 SD).

The relative high number of mutations found since 2003 suggest that heterozygous *IGF-1R* mutations may not be uncommon, although they still only explain approximately 2% of the short stature in populations selected for IUGR and abnormal growth [322]. A few patients with heterozygous terminal deletions of the long arm of chromosome 15 (15q26.2-qter) and one of a ring chromosome 15 have been described [326,327], resulting in IGF-1R haploinsufficiency. These patients have IUGR and short stature of varying severity. Conversely, trisomy 15q26-qter results in a high birth weight, mild postnatal overgrowth and macrocephaly although other genes apart from *IGF-1R* could be involved in this phenotype [328].

Treatment with rhGH has been shown to improve short-term growth in some of the patients with *IGF-1R* mutations [322].

Abnormalities of *IGF-2*

Although abnormalities of *IGF-2* do not result in GHI, we mention IGF-2 for completion. The *IGF-2* gene is located on chromosome 11p15 in a 1 Mb cluster of genes implicated in growth regulation, many of which are imprinted. Besides the paternally imprinted IGF-2 gene, this cluster includes H19, a maternally expressed growth suppressor gene, p57KIP2, a mostly maternally expressed growth suppressor gene and LIT1, which is

paternally expressed and methylates upstream targets. Epigenetic defects that result in loss of paternal methylation and silencing of IGF-2 may underlie up to 50% of the patients with Russell–Silver syndrome [329]. Disturbances in the imprinting and methylation of this region that give rise to an increased expression of paternal growth promoting genes and decreased expression of maternally expressed growth suppressing genes can result in Beckwith–Wiedemann syndrome.

Investigation of GHI

Basal investigations

Initial investigation of suspected GHI should at least include a GH stimulation test, IGF-1 and IGFBP3 concentration, inflammation markers, bone age and chromosome analysis. A skeletal survey may be performed to exclude chondrodysplasia. If assays are available, assessment of GHBP, ALS and IGFBP1 and IGFBP2 concentrations is useful. An overnight GH profile will give more information on GH secretion but only needs to be performed in cases of diagnostic difficulty. IGF-1 and IGFBP3 concentrations are measured by immunoassay, but assays require dissociation of IGF-1 and IGFBPs and extraction of IGFBPs to prevent interference in IGF-1 measurements. Most current assays block IGFBP binding sites by addition of IGF-2, and therefore the antibody for IGF-1 needs to be of high specificity. Total IGF-1 is measured and measurement of free IGF-1 is more complex and not generally used in clinical laboratories. Because of the use of different antibodies and different methods, comparability of values obtained with different assays is of limited value. Age- and gender-specific normative data are normally available from the commercial supplier and should be used because IGF-1 and IGFBP3 can still increase during puberty in GHI. Another pitfall is that proteolyzed IGFBP3 may still be functionally active but may not be recognized by the antibody used in the assay [330]. IGFBP3 concentration may be a better indicator of GH action than IGF-1. IGFBP3 concentrations are generally low in GHD and GHI, whereas concentrations are generally normal in ISS and chronic disease [287,288]. Both IGF-1 and IGFBP3 assays lack the sensitivity to diagnose GHD or GHI [331] but assessment of the combination of IGF-1 and IGFBP3 (and ALS if available) may provide useful information.

IGF generation tests

Criteria to further investigate GHI and perform an IGF generation test are as follows:

1 Proportional short stature with a height below the parental target height and a height < −2.5 SD;

2 Low serum IGF-1 and/or IGFBP3 concentration (<−2 SD for age);

3 Increased or normal GH response on a GH stimulation test.

However, these criteria have their pitfalls, because IGF is also regulated by factors other than GH. The IGF-1 generation test has a low sensitivity and specificity [332], although with improving assays and standardization of protocols, it can still provide useful information and is currently the only test available to assess

GH sensitivity. It is not usually difficult to recognize severe GHI, but reduced GH sensitivity may be more difficult to establish. Many different protocols for IGF-1 generation have been used. The most frequently used protocol uses GH treatment in a dose of 0.033 mg/kg/day given by subcutaneous injections in the evening for 4 consecutive days. Blood is taken before the first GH injection and again after the last GH dose, for measurement of IGF-1 and IGFBP3. There are no good normative data because a wide range of responsiveness exists in the normal population but usually an increase in IGF-1 and IGFBP3 by at least 20% or twice the coefficient of variation of the assay is regarded as normal [287,333], although IGF-1 usually shows a greater response than IGFBP3 [288]. In (partial) GHI, the IGF-1 and IGFBP3 concentrations remain low for age while in children with bioinactive GH and neurosecretory dysfunction, there is a normal IGF-1 and IGFBP3 response to exogenous GH. In the heterogeneous group of ISS, IGF-1 generation is also within the normal limits [287].

Alternatively, a low dose IGF-1 generation test has recently been suggested (0.011 mg/kg/day) to assess mild GHI [287]. A combination of a low and a high dose IGF-1 generation test (0.025 and 0.050 mg/kg for 8 days) may increase sensitivity and specificity [288,334]. A trial of GH treatment for 4–6 months with assessment of height velocity, IGF-1 and IGFBP3 may also give valuable information. At this stage, when the IGF generation test does not provide a clear-cut result, 20 min sampling for overnight GH profile could also be undertaken.

Treatment in GH insensitivity

Before the production of recombinant human IGF-1, there was no treatment available for GHI. When recombinant human IGF-1 became available in the 1990s, trials with IGF-1 treatment were performed in specialized centers. Apart from proven *GHR* mutations, treatment groups also included patients with a GHI phenotype and abnormal IGF-1 generation test but without proven mutation in *GHR* and GHD patients that had developed GH antibodies. All studies were uncontrolled, apart from one in Ecuador that was placebo-controlled and blinded [335]. Most studies used twice daily subcutaneous IGF-1 injections in a dose of 40–120 μg/kg, and most studies showed an increase in height velocity (HV) from approximately 3–4 cm/year to 8–9 cm/year in the first year and 5.5–7 cm/year in the second year of treatment with a corresponding increase in height SD of approximately 1–1.5 SD. The response decreased in the subsequent years although HV remained above the baseline HV [335–337]. Long-term results for the US study showed that HV remained around 4.5–5 cm/year for at least 8 years. Six patients who had reached near final height had gained more than 10 cm over predicted height, and measured 112–164 cm [338].

Because of concerns of hypoglycemia, a small, double blind, placebo controlled study was performed which showed that on placebo injections, 2.6% of the glucose measurements were below the hypoglycemia threshold (<50 mg/dL) whereas 5.5% were during rhIGF-1 treatment, although this difference was not statistically significant. To reduce the risk of hypoglycemia, rhIGF-1

has to be administered within 30 min of a meal. Other side effects include lipohypertrophy at the injection site, hyperstimulation of lymphoid tissue and benign intracranial hypertension that responds to temporary cessation of treatment. In the trials, coarsening of facial features was noted in many patients, especially during puberty. Cholesterol and free fatty acids increased slightly over the years, but percentage body fat remained stable in the long term. There are four conditions for which rhIGF-1 is the only specific growth therapy currently available: GHI due to GHR *gene* mutation, *Stat5b* gene mutations, *IGF-1* gene mutation and GH inactivating antibodies [339]. The usual dose is 40 μg/kg twice daily but can be increased to 80–120 μg/kg. Besides mecasermin (rhIGF-1), mecasermin rifanbate, an equimolar complex of IGF-1 and IGFBP3, is commercially available although it is not currently marketed for the indications above. Because of its extended half-life [340], treatment with mecasermin rifanbate is only once daily but doses are higher, starting with 0.5 mg/kg and increasing to 1.0–2.0 mg/kg, providing 200–400 μg/kg rhIGF-1 to obtain pharmacological effects [341]. In contrast to rhGH treatment in GH deficiency, rhIGF-1 treatment only partially restores the growth defect, most likely due to suboptimal delivery, in space and time, of IGF-1 to target cells. As expected [342], and as observed in leprechaunism and diabetes, IGF-1 treatment also very effectively improves the insulin insensitivity in IGF-1 deficiency [343]. Lastly, IGFBP displacers, i.e. IGF analogs that bind IGFBPs but not IGF-1R and therefore "displace" IGF-1 from IGFBPs, have been used in animal studies and shown to increase free IGF-1 and to improve growth in hypophysectomized rats [344].

References

1 Cohen LE, Radovick S. Molecular basis of combined pituitary hormone deficiencies. *Endocr Rev* 2002; **23**: 431–442.

2 Dattani MT, Robinson IC. The molecular basis for developmental disorders of the pituitary gland in man. *Clin Genet* 2000; **57**: 337–346.

3 Dasen JS, Rosenfeld MG. Signaling and transcriptional mechanisms in pituitary development. *Annu Rev Neurosci* 2001; **24**: 327–355.

4 Rizzoti K, Lovell-Badge R. Early development of the pituitary gland: induction and shaping of Rathke's pouch. *Rev Endocr Metab Disord* 2005; **6**: 161–172.

5 Zhu X, Zhang J, Tollkuhn J, Ohsawa R, Bresnick EH, Guillemot F, et al. Sustained Notch signaling in progenitors is required for sequential emergence of distinct cell lineages during organogenesis. *Genes Dev* 2006; **20**: 2739–2753.

6 Thomas PQ, Johnson BV, Rathjen J, Rathjen PD. Sequence, genomic organization, and expression of the novel homeobox gene Hesx1. *J Biol Chem* 1995; **270**: 3869–3875.

7 Hermesz E, Mackem S, Mahon KA. Rpx: a novel anterior-restricted homeobox gene progressively activated in the prechordal plate, anterior neural plate and Rathke's pouch of the mouse embryo. *Development* 1996; **122**: 41–52.

8 Dattani MT, Martinez-Barbera JP, Thomas PQ, Brickman JM, Gupta R, Martensson IL, et al. Mutations in the homeobox gene

HESX1/Hesx1 associated with septo-optic dysplasia in human and mouse. *Nat Genet* 1998; **19**: 125–133.

9 Thomas PQ, Dattani MT, Brickman JM, McNay D, Warne G, Zacharin M, et al. Heterozygous HESX1 mutations associated with isolated congenital pituitary hypoplasia and septo-optic dysplasia. *Hum Mol Genet* 2001; **10**: 39–45.

10 Carvalho LR, Woods KS, Mendonca BB, Marcal N, Zamparini AL, Stifani S, et al. A homozygous mutation in HESX1 is associated with evolving hypopituitarism due to impaired repressor-corepressor interaction. *J Clin Invest* 2003; **112**: 1192–1201.

11 Brickman JM, Clements M, Tyrell R, McNay D, Woods K, Warner J, et al. Molecular effects of novel mutations in Hesx1/HESX1 associated with human pituitary disorders. *Development* 2001; **128**: 5189–5199.

12 Cohen RN, Cohen LE, Botero D, Yu C, Sagar A, Jurkiewicz M, et al. Enhanced repression by HESX1 as a cause of hypopituitarism and septooptic dysplasia. *J Clin Endocrinol Metab* 2003; **88**: 4832–4839.

13 Tajima T, Hattorri T, Nakajima T, Okuhara K, Sato K, Abe S, et al. Sporadic heterozygous frameshift mutation of HESX1 causing pituitary and optic nerve hypoplasia and combined pituitary hormone deficiency in a Japanese patient. *J Clin Endocrinol Metab* 2003; **88**: 45–50.

14 Semina EV, Reiter R, Leysens NJ, Alward WL, Small KW, Datson NA, et al. Cloning and characterization of a novel bicoid-related homeobox transcription factor gene, RIEG, involved in Rieger syndrome. *Nat Genet* 1996; **14**: 392–399.

15 Schmitt S, Biason-Lauber A, Betts D, Schoenle EJ. Genomic structure, chromosomal localization, and expression pattern of the human LIM-homeobox3 (LHX 3) gene. *Biochem Biophys Res Commun* 2000; **274**: 49–56.

16 Zhadanov AB, Bertuzzi S, Taira M, Dawid IB, Westphal H. Expression pattern of the murine LIM class homeobox gene Lhx3 in subsets of neural and neuroendocrine tissues. *Dev Dyn* 1995; **202**: 354–364.

17 Bach I, Rhodes SJ, Pearse RV, Heinzel T, Gloss B, Scully KM, et al. P-Lim, a LIM homeodomain factor, is expressed during pituitary organ and cell commitment and synergizes with Pit-1. *Proc Natl Acad Sci U S A* 1995; **92**: 2720–2724.

18 Ellsworth BS, Butts DL, Camper SA. Mechanisms underlying pituitary hypoplasia and failed cell specification in Lhx3-deficient mice. *Dev Biol* 2008; **313**: 118–129.

19 Sheng HZ, Moriyama K, Yamashita T, Li H, Potter SS, Mahon KA, et al. Multistep control of pituitary organogenesis. *Science* 1997; **278**: 1809–1812.

20 Sobrier ML, Attie-Bitach T, Netchine I, Encha-Razavi F, Vekemans M, Amselem S. Pathophysiology of syndromic combined pituitary hormone deficiency due to a LHX3 defect in light of LHX3 and LHX4 expression during early human development. *Gene Expr Patterns* 2004; **5**: 279–284.

21 Netchine I, Sobrier ML, Krude H, Schnabel D, Maghnie M, Marcos E, et al. Mutations in LHX3 result in a new syndrome revealed by combined pituitary hormone deficiency. *Nat Genet* 2000; **25**: 182–186.

22 Pfaeffle RW, Savage JJ, Hunter CS, Palme C, Ahlmann M, Kumar P, et al. Four novel mutations of the LHX3 gene cause combined pituitary hormone deficiencies with or without limited neck rotation. *J Clin Endocrinol Metab* 2007; **92**: 1909–1919.

23 Pfaeffle RW, Hunter CS, Savage JJ, Duran-Prado M, Mullen RD, Neeb ZP, et al. Three novel missense mutations within the LHX4 gene are associated with variable pituitary hormone deficiencies. *J Clin Endocrinol Metab* 2008; **93**: 1062–1071.

24 Machinis K, Pantel J, Netchine I, Leger J, Camand OJ, Sobrier ML, et al. Syndromic short stature in patients with a germline mutation in the LIM homeobox LHX4. *Am J Hum Genet* 2001; **69**: 961–968.

25 Tajima T, Hattori T, Nakajima T, Okuhara K, Tsubaki J, Fujieda K. A novel missense mutation (P366T) of the LHX4 gene causes severe combined pituitary hormone deficiency with pituitary hypoplasia, ectopic posterior lobe and a poorly developed sella turcica. *Endocr J* 2007; **54**: 637–641.

26 Gubbay J, Collignon J, Koopman P, Capel B, Economou A, Munsterberg A, et al. A gene mapping to the sex-determining region of the mouse Y chromosome is a member of a novel family of embryonically expressed genes. *Nature* 1990; **346**: 245–250.

27 Stevanovic M, Lovell-Badge R, Collignon J, Goodfellow PN. SOX3 is an X-linked gene related to SRY. *Hum Mol Genet* 1993; **2**: 2013–2018.

28 Pevny LH, Lovell-Badge R. Sox genes find their feet. *Curr Opin Genet Dev* 1997; **7**: 338–344.

29 Wegner M. From head to toes: the multiple facets of Sox proteins. *Nucleic Acids Res* 1999; **27**: 1409–1420.

30 Bowles J, Schepers G, Koopman P. Phylogeny of the SOX family of developmental transcription factors based on sequence and structural indicators. *Dev Biol* 2000; **227**: 239–255.

31 Stevanovic M, Zuffardi O, Collignon J, Lovell-Badge R, Goodfellow P. The cDNA sequence and chromosomal location of the human SOX2 gene. *Mamm Genome* 1994; **5**: 640–642.

32 Pevny L, Placzek M. SOX genes and neural progenitor identity. *Curr Opin Neurobiol* 2005; **15**: 7–13.

33 Bylund M, Andersson E, Novitch BG, Muhr J. Vertebrate neurogenesis is counteracted by Sox1-3 activity. *Nat Neurosci* 2003; **6**: 1162–1168.

34 Rizzoti K, Brunelli S, Carmignac D, Thomas PQ, Robinson IC, Lovell-Badge R. SOX3 is required during the formation of the hypothalamo-pituitary axis. *Nat Genet* 2004; **36**: 247–255.

35 Weiss J, Meeks JJ, Hurley L, Raverot G, Frassetto A, Jameson JL. Sox3 is required for gonadal function, but not sex determination, in males and females. *Mol Cell Biol* 2003; **23**: 8084–8091.

36 Hamel BC, Smits AP, Otten BJ, van den HB, Ropers HH, Mariman EC. Familial X-linked mental retardation and isolated growth hormone deficiency: clinical and molecular findings. *Am J Med Genet* 1996; **64**: 35–41.

37 Hol FA, Schepens MT, van Beersum SE, Redolfi E, Affer M, Vezzoni P, et al. Identification and characterization of an Xq26-q27 duplication in a family with spina bifida and panhypopituitarism suggests the involvement of two distinct genes. *Genomics* 2000; **69**: 174–181.

38 Woods KS, Cundall M, Turton J, Rizotti K, Mehta A, Palmer R, et al. Over- and underdosage of SOX3 is associated with infundibular hypoplasia and hypopituitarism. *Am J Hum Genet* 2005; **76**: 833–849.

39 Solomon NM, Nouri S, Warne GL, Lagerstrom-Fermer M, Forrest SM, Thomas PQ. Increased gene dosage at Xq26-q27 is associated with X-linked hypopituitarism. *Genomics* 2002; **79**: 553–559.

40 Laumonnier F, Ronce N, Hamel BC, Thomas P, Lespinasse J, Raynaud M, et al. Transcription factor SOX3 is involved in X-linked

mental retardation with growth hormone deficiency. *Am J Hum Genet* 2002; **71**: 1450–1455.

41 Wood HB, Episkopou V. Comparative expression of the mouse Sox1, Sox2 and Sox3 genes from pre-gastrulation to early somite stages. *Mech Dev* 1999; **86**: 197–201.

42 Williamson KA, Hever AM, Rainger J, Rogers RC, Magee A, Fiedler Z, *et al*. Mutations in SOX2 cause anophthalmia-esophageal-genital (AEG) syndrome. *Hum Mol Genet* 2006; **15**: 1413–1422.

43 Avilion AA, Nicolis SK, Pevny LH, Perez L, Vivian N, Lovell-Badge R. Multipotent cell lineages in early mouse development depend on SOX2 function. *Genes Dev* 2003; **17**: 126–140.

44 Taranova OV, Magness ST, Fagan BM, Wu Y, Surzenko N, Hutton SR, *et al*. SOX2 is a dose-dependent regulator of retinal neural progenitor competence. *Genes Dev* 2006; **20**: 1187–1202.

45 Kelberman D, Rizzoti K, Avilion A, Bitner-Glindzicz M, Cianfarani S, Collins J, *et al*. Mutations within Sox2/SOX2 are associated with abnormalities in the hypothalamo-pituitary-gonadal axis in mice and humans. *J Clin Invest* 2006; **116**: 2442–2455.

46 Sornson MW, Wu W, Dasen JS, Flynn SE, Norman DJ, O'Connell SM, *et al*. Pituitary lineage determination by the Prophet of Pit-1 homeodomain factor defective in Ames dwarfism. *Nature* 1996; **384**: 327–333.

47 Parks JS, Brown MR, Hurley DL, Phelps CJ, Wajnrajch MP. Heritable disorders of pituitary development. *J Clin Endocrinol Metab* 1999; **84**: 4362–4370.

48 Olson LE, Tollkuhn J, Scafoglio C, Krones A, Zhang J, Ohgi KA, *et al*. Homeodomain-mediated beta-catenin-dependent switching events dictate cell-lineage determination. *Cell* 2006; **125**: 593–605.

49 Ward RD, Raetzman LT, Suh H, Stone BM, Nasonkin IO, Camper SA. Role of PROP1 in pituitary gland growth. *Mol Endocrinol* 2005; **19**: 698–710.

50 Ward RD, Stone BM, Raetzman LT, Camper SA. Cell proliferation and vascularization in mouse models of pituitary hormone deficiency. *Mol Endocrinol* 2006; **20**: 1378–1390.

51 Wu W, Cogan JD, Pfaffle RW, Dasen JS, Frisch H, O'Connell SM, *et al*. Mutations in PROP1 cause familial combined pituitary hormone deficiency. *Nat Genet* 1998; **18**: 147–149.

52 Li S, Crenshaw EB, III, Rawson EJ, Simmons DM, Swanson LW, Rosenfeld MG. Dwarf locus mutants lacking three pituitary cell types result from mutations in the POU-domain gene pit-1. *Nature* 1990; **347**: 528–533.

53 Andersen B, Rosenfeld MG. POU domain factors in the neuroendocrine system: lessons from developmental biology provide insights into human disease. *Endocr Rev* 2001; **22**: 2–35.

54 Tatsumi K, Miyai K, Notomi T, Kaibe K, Amino N, Mizuno Y, *et al*. Cretinism with combined hormone deficiency caused by a mutation in the PIT1 gene. *Nat Genet* 1992; **1**: 56–58.

55 Bennani-Baiti IM, Asa SL, Song D, Iratni R, Liebhaber SA, Cooke NE. DNase I-hypersensitive sites I and II of the human growth hormone locus control region are a major developmental activator of somatotrope gene expression. *Proc Natl Acad Sci U S A* 1998; **95**: 10655–10660.

56 Baumann G. Genetic characterization of growth hormone deficiency and resistance: implications for treatment with recombinant growth hormone. *Am J Pharmacogenomics* 2002; **2**: 93–111.

57 Carter-Su C, King AP, Argetsinger LS, Smit LS, Vanderkuur J, Campbell GS. Signalling pathway of GH. *Endocr J* 1996; **43** (Suppl): S65–S70.

58 Smit LS, Meyer DJ, Billestrup N, Norstedt G, Schwartz J, Carter-Su C. The role of the growth hormone (GH) receptor and JAK1 and JAK2 kinases in the activation of Stats 1, 3, and 5 by GH. *Mol Endocrinol* 1996; **10**: 519–533.

59 Kojima M, Hosoda H, Date Y, Nakazato M, Matsuo H, Kangawa K. Ghrelin is a growth-hormone-releasing acylated peptide from stomach. *Nature* 1999; **402**: 656–660.

60 Illig R. Growth hormone antibodies in patients treated with different preparations of human growth hormone (HGH). *J Clin Endocrinol Metab* 1970; **31**: 679–688.

61 Phillips JA III, Hjelle BL, Seeburg PH, Zachmann M. Molecular basis for familial isolated growth hormone deficiency. *Proc Natl Acad Sci U S A* 1981; **78**: 6372–6375.

62 Wajnrajch MP, Gertner JM, Harbison MD, Chua SC Jr, Leibel RL. Nonsense mutation in the human growth hormone-releasing hormone receptor causes growth failure analogous to the little (lit) mouse. *Nat Genet* 1996; **12**: 88–90.

63 Carakushansky M, Whatmore AJ, Clayton PE, Shalet SM, Gleeson HK, Price DA, *et al*. A new missense mutation in the growth hormone-releasing hormone receptor gene in familial isolated GH deficiency. *Eur J Endocrinol* 2003; **148**: 25–30.

64 Hess O, Hujeirat Y, Wajnrajch MP, Allon-Shalev S, Zadik Z, Lavi I, *et al*. Variable phenotypes in familial isolated growth hormone deficiency caused by a G6664A mutation in the GH-1 gene. *J Clin Endocrinol Metab* 2007; **92**: 4387–4393.

65 Moseley CT, Mullis PE, Prince MA, Phillips JA III. An exon splice enhancer mutation causes autosomal dominant GH deficiency. *J Clin Endocrinol Metab* 2002; **87**: 847–852.

66 McGuinness L, Magoulas C, Sesay AK, Mathers K, Carmignac D, Manneville JB, *et al*. Autosomal dominant growth hormone deficiency disrupts secretory vesicles in vitro and in vivo in transgenic mice. *Endocrinology* 2003; **144**: 720–731.

67 Salemi S, Yousefi S, Baltensperger K, Robinson IC, Eble A, Simon D, *et al*. Variability of isolated autosomal dominant GH deficiency (IGHD II): impact of the P89L GH mutation on clinical follow-up and GH secretion. *Eur J Endocrinol* 2005; **153**: 791–802.

68 Turton JP, Buchanan CR, Robinson IC, Aylwin SJ, Dattani MT. Evolution of gonadotropin deficiency in a patient with type II autosomal dominant GH deficiency. *Eur J Endocrinol* 2006; **155**: 793–799.

69 Collu R, Tang J, Castagne J, Lagace G, Masson N, Huot C, *et al*. A novel mechanism for isolated central hypothyroidism: inactivating mutations in the thyrotropin-releasing hormone receptor gene. *J Clin Endocrinol Metab* 1997; **82**: 1561–1565.

70 Dacou-Voutetakis C, Feltquate DM, Drakopoulou M, Kourides IA, Dracopoli NC. Familial hypothyroidism caused by a nonsense mutation in the thyroid-stimulating hormone beta-subunit gene. *Am J Hum Genet* 1990; **46**: 988–993.

71 Lin L, Hindmarsh PC, Metherell LA, Alzyoud M, Al Ali M, Brain CE, *et al*. Severe loss-of-function mutations in the adrenocorticotropin receptor (ACTHR, MC2R) can be found in patients diagnosed with salt-losing adrenal hypoplasia. *Clin Endocrinol (Oxf)* 2007; **66**: 205–210.

72 Krude H, Biebermann H, Luck W, Horn R, Brabant G, Gruters A. Severe early-onset obesity, adrenal insufficiency and red hair pigmentation caused by POMC mutations in humans. *Nat Genet* 1998; **19**: 155–157.

73 Jackson RS, Creemers JW, Ohagi S, Raffin-Sanson ML, Sanders L, Montague CT, et al. Obesity and impaired prohormone processing associated with mutations in the human prohormone convertase 1 gene. *Nat Genet* 1997; **16**: 303–306.

74 O'Rahilly S, Gray H, Humphreys PJ, Krook A, Polonsky KS, White A, et al. Brief report: impaired processing of prohormones associated with abnormalities of glucose homeostasis and adrenal function. *N Engl J Med* 1995; **333**: 1386–1390.

75 Jackson RS, Creemers JW, Farooqi IS, Raffin-Sanson ML, Varro A, Dockray GJ, et al. Small-intestinal dysfunction accompanies the complex endocrinopathy of human proprotein convertase 1 deficiency. *J Clin Invest* 2003; **112**: 1550–1560.

76 Lamolet B, Pulichino AM, Lamonerie T, Gauthier Y, Brue T, Enjalbert A, et al. A pituitary cell-restricted T box factor, Tpit, activates POMC transcription in cooperation with Pitx homeoproteins. *Cell* 2001; **104**: 849–859.

77 Fromantin M, Gineste J, Didier A, Rouvier J. [Impuberism and hypogonadism at induction into military service. Statistical study]. *Probl Actuels Endocrinol Nutr* 1973; **16**: 179–199.

78 Filippi G. Klinefelter's syndrome in Sardinia. Clinical report of 265 hypogonadic males detected at the time of military check-up. *Clin Genet* 1986; **30**: 276–284.

79 Quinton R, Duke VM, de Zoysa PA, Platts AD, Valentine A, Kendall B, et al. The neuroradiology of Kallmann's syndrome: a genotypic and phenotypic analysis. *J Clin Endocrinol Metab* 1996; **81**: 3010–3017.

80 Bick D, Franco B, Sherins RJ, Heye B, Pike L, Crawford J, et al. Brief report: intragenic deletion of the KALIG-1 gene in Kallmann's syndrome. *N Engl J Med* 1992; **326**: 1752–1755.

81 Hardelin JP, Levilliers J, Blanchard S, Carel JC, Leutenegger M, Pinard-Bertelletto JP, et al. Heterogeneity in the mutations responsible for X chromosome-linked Kallmann syndrome. *Hum Mol Genet* 1993; **2**: 373–377.

82 Tabarin A, Achermann JC, Recan D, Bex V, Bertagna X, Christin-Maitre S, et al. A novel mutation in DAX1 causes delayed-onset adrenal insufficiency and incomplete hypogonadotropic hypogonadism. *J Clin Invest* 2000; **105**: 321–328.

83 de Roux N, Young J, Misrahi M, Genet R, Chanson P, Schaison G, et al. A family with hypogonadotropic hypogonadism and mutations in the gonadotropin-releasing hormone receptor. *N Engl J Med* 1997; **337**: 1597–1602.

84 Lin L, Ercan O, Raza J, Burren CP, Creighton SM, Auchus RJ, et al. Variable phenotypes associated with aromatase (CYP19) insufficiency in humans. *J Clin Endocrinol Metab* 2007; **92**: 982–990.

85 de Roux N, Genin E, Carel JC, Matsuda F, Chaussain JL, Milgrom E. Hypogonadotropic hypogonadism due to loss of function of the KiSS1-derived peptide receptor GPR54. *Proc Natl Acad Sci U S A* 2003; **100**: 10972–10976.

86 Montague CT, Farooqi IS, Whitehead JP, Soos MA, Rau H, Wareham NJ, et al. Congenital leptin deficiency is associated with severe early-onset obesity in humans. *Nature* 1997; **387**: 903–908.

87 Farooqi IS, Wangensteen T, Collins S, Kimber W, Matarese G, Keogh JM, et al. Clinical and molecular genetic spectrum of congenital deficiency of the leptin receptor. *N Engl J Med* 2007; **356**: 237–247.

88 Farooqi IS, Jebb SA, Langmack G, Lawrence E, Cheetham CH, Prentice AM, et al. Effects of recombinant leptin therapy in a child with congenital leptin deficiency. *N Engl J Med* 1999; **341**: 879–884.

89 Kauppila A, Chatelain P, Kirkinen P, Kivinen S, Ruokonen A. Isolated prolactin deficiency in a woman with puerperal alactogenesis. *J Clin Endocrinol Metab* 1987; **64**: 309–312.

90 Ito M, Oiso Y, Murase T, Kondo K, Saito H, Chinzei T, et al. Possible involvement of inefficient cleavage of preprovasopressin by signal peptidase as a cause for familial central diabetes insipidus. *J Clin Invest* 1993; **91**: 2565–2571.

91 Bahnsen U, Oosting P, Swaab DF, Nahke P, Richter D, Schmale H. A missense mutation in the vasopressin-neurophysin precursor gene cosegregates with human autosomal dominant neurohypophyseal diabetes insipidus. *EMBO J* 1992; **11**: 19–23.

92 Nagasaki H, Ito M, Yuasa H, Saito H, Fukase M, Hamada K, et al. Two novel mutations in the coding region for neurophysin-II associated with familial central diabetes insipidus. *J Clin Endocrinol Metab* 1995; **80**: 1352–1356.

93 Cryns K, Sivakumaran TA, van den Ouweland JM, Pennings RJ, Cremers CW, Flothmann K, et al. Mutational spectrum of the WFS1 gene in Wolfram syndrome, nonsyndromic hearing impairment, diabetes mellitus, and psychiatric disease. *Hum Mutat* 2003; **22**: 275–287.

94 Mehta A, Hindmarsh PC, Stanhope RG, Turton JP, Cole TJ, Preece MA, et al. The role of growth hormone in determining birth size and early postnatal growth, using congenital growth hormone deficiency (GHD) as a model. *Clin Endocrinol (Oxf)* 2005; **63**: 223–231.

95 Pena-Almazan S, Buchlis J, Miller S, Shine B, MacGillivray M. Linear growth characteristics of congenitally GH-deficient infants from birth to one year of age. *J Clin Endocrinol Metab* 2001; **86**: 5691–5694.

96 Craft WH, Underwoood LE, Van Wyk JJ. High incidence of perinatal insult in children with idiopathic hypopituitarism. *J Pediatr* 1980; **96**(3 Pt 1): 397–402.

97 Deladoey J, Fluck C, Buyukgebiz A, Kuhlmann BV, Eble A, Hindmarsh PC, et al. "Hot spot" in the PROP1 gene responsible for combined pituitary hormone deficiency. *J Clin Endocrinol Metab* 1999; **84**: 1645–1650.

98 Cogan JD, Wu W, Phillips JA, III, Arnhold IJ, Agapito A, Fofanova OV, et al. The PROP1 2-base pair deletion is a common cause of combined pituitary hormone deficiency. *J Clin Endocrinol Metab* 1998; **83**: 3346–3349.

99 Turton JP, Mehta A, Raza J, Woods KS, Tiulpakov A, Cassar J, et al. Mutations within the transcription factor PROP1 are rare in a cohort of patients with sporadic combined pituitary hormone deficiency (CPHD). *Clin Endocrinol (Oxf)* 2005; **63**: 10–18.

100 Mendonca BB, Osorio MG, Latronico AC, Estefan V, Lo LS, Arnhold IJ. Longitudinal hormonal and pituitary imaging changes in two females with combined pituitary hormone deficiency due to deletion of A301,G302 in the PROP1 gene. *J Clin Endocrinol Metab* 1999; **84**: 942–945.

101 Arroyo A, Pernasetti F, Vasilyev VV, Amato P, Yen SS, Mellon PL. A unique case of combined pituitary hormone deficiency caused by a PROP1 gene mutation (R120C) associated with normal height and absent puberty. *Clin Endocrinol (Oxf)* 2002; **57**: 283–291.

102 Asteria C, Oliveira JH, Abucham J, Beck-Peccoz P. Central hypocortisolism as part of combined pituitary hormone deficiency due to mutations of PROP-1 gene. *Eur J Endocrinol* 2000; **143**: 347–352.

103 Pernasetti F, Toledo SP, Vasilyev VV, Hayashida CY, Cogan JD, Ferrari C, et al. Impaired adrenocorticotropin-adrenal axis in com-

bined pituitary hormone deficiency caused by a two-base pair deletion (301-302delAG) in the prophet of Pit-1 gene. *J Clin Endocrinol Metab* 2000; **85**: 390–397.

104 Riepe FG, Partsch CJ, Blankenstein O, Monig H, Pfaffle RW, Sippell WG. Longitudinal imaging reveals pituitary enlargement preceding hypoplasia in two brothers with combined pituitary hormone deficiency attributable to PROP1 mutation. *J Clin Endocrinol Metab* 2001; **86**: 4353–4357.

105 Agarwal G, Bhatia V, Cook S, Thomas PQ. Adrenocorticotropin deficiency in combined pituitary hormone deficiency patients homozygous for a novel PROP1 deletion. *J Clin Endocrinol Metab* 2000; **85**: 4556–4561.

106 Vallette-Kasic S, Barlier A, Teinturier C, Diaz A, Manavela M, Berthezene F, *et al.* PROP1 gene screening in patients with multiple pituitary hormone deficiency reveals two sites of hypermutability and a high incidence of corticotroph deficiency. *J Clin Endocrinol Metab* 2001; **86**: 4529–4535.

107 Voutetakis A, Argyropoulou M, Sertedaki A, Livadas S, Xekouki P, Maniati-Christidi M, *et al.* Pituitary magnetic resonance imaging in 15 patients with Prop1 gene mutations: pituitary enlargement may originate from the intermediate lobe. *J Clin Endocrinol Metab* 2004; **89**: 2200–2206.

108 Cohen LE, Zanger K, Brue T, Wondisford FE, Radovick S. Defective retinoic acid regulation of the Pit-1 gene enhancer: a novel mechanism of combined pituitary hormone deficiency. *Mol Endocrinol* 1999; **13**: 476–484.

109 Pfaffle RW, DiMattia GE, Parks JS, Brown MR, Wit JM, Jansen M, *et al.* Mutation of the POU-specific domain of Pit-1 and hypopituitarism without pituitary hypoplasia. *Science* 1992; **257**: 1118–1121.

110 Pfaffle RW, Martinez R, Kim C, Frisch H, Lebl J, Otten B, *et al.* GH and TSH deficiency. *Exp Clin Endocrinol Diabetes* 1997; **105** (Suppl 4): 1–5.

111 Turton JP, Reynaud R, Mehta A, Torpiano J, Saveanu A, Woods KS, *et al.* Novel mutations within the POU1F1 gene associated with variable combined pituitary hormone deficiency (CPHD). *J Clin Endocrinol Metab* 2005; **90**: 4762–4770.

112 Cohen LE, Wondisford FE, Salvatoni A, Maghnie M, Brucker-Davis F, Weintraub BD, *et al.* A "hot spot" in the Pit-1 gene responsible for combined pituitary hormone deficiency: clinical and molecular correlates. *J Clin Endocrinol Metab* 1995; **80**: 679–684.

113 Ohta K, Nobukuni Y, Mitsubuchi H, Fujimoto S, Matsuo N, Inagaki H, *et al.* Mutations in the Pit-1 gene in children with combined pituitary hormone deficiency. *Biochem Biophys Res Commun* 1992; **189**: 851–855.

114 Radovick S, Nations M, Du Y, Berg LA, Weintraub BD, Wondisford FE. A mutation in the POU-homeodomain of Pit-1 responsible for combined pituitary hormone deficiency. *Science* 1992; **257**: 1115–1118.

115 Okamoto N, Wada Y, Ida S, Koga R, Ozono K, Chiyo H, *et al.* Monoallelic expression of normal mRNA in the PIT1 mutation heterozygotes with normal phenotype and biallelic expression in the abnormal phenotype. *Hum Mol Genet* 1994; **3**: 1565–1568.

116 Holl RW, Pfaffle R, Kim C, Sorgo W, Teller WM, Heimann G. Combined pituitary deficiencies of growth hormone, thyroid stimulating hormone and prolactin due to Pit-1 gene mutation: a case report. *Eur J Pediatr* 1997; **156**: 835–837.

117 Aarskog D, Eiken HG, Bjerknes R, Myking OL. Pituitary dwarfism in the R271W Pit-1 gene mutation. *Eur J Pediatr* 1997; **156**: 829–834.

118 Rodrigues Martineli AM, Braga M, De Lacerda L, Raskin S, Graf H. Description of a Brazilian patient bearing the R271W Pit-1 gene mutation. *Thyroid* 1998; **8**: 299–304.

119 Ward L, Chavez M, Huot C, Lecocq P, Collu R, Decarie JC, *et al.* Severe congenital hypopituitarism with low prolactin concentrations and age-dependent anterior pituitary hypoplasia: a clue to a PIT-1 mutation. *J Pediatr* 1998; **132**: 1036–1038.

120 Tornqvist K, Ericsson A, Kallen B. Optic nerve hypoplasia: risk factors and epidemiology. *Acta Ophthalmol Scand* 2002; **80**: 300–304.

121 Patel L, McNally RJ, Harrison E, Lloyd IC, Clayton PE. Geographical distribution of optic nerve hypoplasia and septo-optic dysplasia in Northwest England. *J Pediatr* 2006; **148**: 85–88.

122 Arslanian SA, Rothfus WE, Foley TP Jr, Becker DJ. Hormonal, metabolic, and neuroradiologic abnormalities associated with septo-optic dysplasia. *Acta Endocrinol (Copenh)* 1984; **107**: 282–288.

123 Morishima A, Aranoff GS. Syndrome of septo-optic-pituitary dysplasia: the clinical spectrum. *Brain Dev* 1986; **8**: 233–239.

124 Brodsky MC, Glasier CM. Optic nerve hypoplasia. Clinical significance of associated central nervous system abnormalities on magnetic resonance imaging. *Arch Ophthalmol* 1993; **111**: 66–74.

125 Zeki SM, Hollman AS, Dutton GN. Neuroradiological features of patients with optic nerve hypoplasia. *J Pediatr Ophthalmol Strabismus* 1992; **29**: 107–112.

126 Birkebaek NH, Patel L, Wright NB, Grigg JR, Sinha S, Hall CM, *et al.* Endocrine status in patients with optic nerve hypoplasia: relationship to midline central nervous system abnormalities and appearance of the hypothalamic-pituitary axis on magnetic resonance imaging. *J Clin Endocrinol Metab* 2003; **88**: 5281–5286.

127 Nanduri VR, Stanhope R. Why is the retention of gonadotrophin secretion common in children with panhypopituitarism due to septo-optic dysplasia? *Eur J Endocrinol* 1999; **140**: 48–50.

128 Pagon RA, Stephan MJ. Septo-optic dysplasia with digital anomalies. *J Pediatr* 1984; **105**: 966–968.

129 Orrico A, Galli L, Zappella M, Monti L, Vatti GP, Venturi C, *et al.* Septo-optic dysplasia with digital anomalies associated with maternal multidrug abuse during pregnancy. *Eur J Neurol* 2002; **9**: 679–682.

130 Harrison IM, Brosnahan D, Phelan E, Fitzgerald RJ, Reardon W. Septo-optic dysplasia with digital anomalies: a recurrent pattern syndrome. *Am J Med Genet A* 2004; **131**: 82–85.

131 Rainbow LA, Rees SA, Shaikh MG, Shaw NJ, Cole T, Barrett TG, *et al.* Mutation analysis of POUF-1, PROP-1 and HESX-1 show low frequency of mutations in children with sporadic forms of combined pituitary hormone deficiency and septo-optic dysplasia. *Clin Endocrinol (Oxf)* 2005; **62**: 163–168.

132 Wales JK, Quarrell OW. Evidence for possible Mendelian inheritance of septo-optic dysplasia. *Acta Paediatr* 1996; **85**: 391–392.

133 Murray PG, Paterson WF, Donaldson MD. Maternal age in patients with septo-optic dysplasia. *J Pediatr Endocrinol Metab* 2005; **18**: 471–476.

134 McNay DE, Turton JP, Kelberman D, Woods KS, Brauner R, Papadimitriou A, *et al.* HESX1 mutations are an uncommon cause of septooptic dysplasia and hypopituitarism. *J Clin Endocrinol Metab* 2007; **92**: 691–697.

135 Bhangoo AP, Hunter CS, Savage JJ, Anhalt H, Pavlakis S, Walvoord EC, et al. Clinical case seminar: a novel LHX3 mutation presenting as combined pituitary hormonal deficiency. J Clin Endocrinol Metab 2006; 91: 747–753.

136 Machinis K, Amselem S. Functional relationship between LHX4 and POU1F1 in light of the LHX4 mutation identified in patients with pituitary defects. J Clin Endocrinol Metab 2005; 90: 5456–5462.

137 Kamachi Y, Uchikawa M, Collignon J, Lovell-Badge R, Kondoh H. Involvement of Sox1, 2 and 3 in the early and subsequent molecular events of lens induction. Development 1998; 125: 2521–2532.

138 Fantes J, Ragge NK, Lynch SA, McGill NI, Collin JR, Howard-Peebles PN, et al. Mutations in SOX2 cause anophthalmia. Nat Genet 2003; 33: 461–463.

139 Ragge NK, Lorenz B, Schneider A, Bushby K, de Sanctis L, de Sanctis U, et al. SOX2 anophthalmia syndrome. Am J Med Genet A 2005; 135: 1–7.

140 Hagstrom SA, Pauer GJ, Reid J, Simpson E, Crowe S, Maumenee IH, et al. SOX2 mutation causes anophthalmia, hearing loss, and brain anomalies. Am J Med Genet A 2005; 138: 95–98.

141 Zenteno JC, Gascon-Guzman G, Tovilla-Canales JL. Bilateral anophthalmia and brain malformations caused by a 20-bp deletion in the SOX2 gene. Clin Genet 2005; 68: 564–566.

142 Sato N, Kamachi Y, Kondoh H, Shima Y, Morohashi K, Horikawa R, et al. Hypogonadotropic hypogonadism in an adult female with a heterozygous hypomorphic mutation of SOX2. Eur J Endocrinol 2007; 156: 167–171.

143 Kelberman D, de Castro SC, Huang S, Crolla JA, Palmer R, Gregory JW, et al. SOX2 plays a critical role in the pituitary, forebrain and eye during human embryonic development. J Clin Endocrinol Metab 2008; 93: 1865–1873.

144 Roessler E, Du YZ, Mullor JL, Casas E, Allen WP, Gillessen-Kaesbach G, et al. Loss-of-function mutations in the human GLI2 gene are associated with pituitary anomalies and holoprosencephaly-like features. Proc Natl Acad Sci U S A 2003; 100: 13424–13429.

145 Tillmann V, Tang VW, Price DA, Hughes DG, Wright NB, Clayton PE. Magnetic resonance imaging of the hypothalamic-pituitary axis in the diagnosis of growth hormone deficiency. J Pediatr Endocrinol Metab 2000; 13: 1577–1583.

146 Mehta A, Hindmarsh PC, Stanhope RG, Brain CE, Preece MA, Dattani MT. Is the thyrotropin-releasing hormone test necessary in the diagnosis of central hypothyroidism in children. J Clin Endocrinol Metab 2003; 88: 5696–5703.

147 van Tijn DA, de Vijlder JJ, Vulsma T. Role of the thyrotropin-releasing hormone stimulation test in diagnosis of congenital central hypothyroidism in infants. J Clin Endocrinol Metab 2008; 93: 410–419.

148 Mehta A, Hindmarsh PC, Dattani MT. An update on the biochemical diagnosis of congenital ACTH insufficiency. Clin Endocrinol (Oxf) 2005; 62: 307–314.

149 Birkebaek NH, Patel L, Wright NB, Grigg JR, Sinha S, Hall CM, et al. Optic nerve size evaluated by magnetic resonance imaging in children with optic nerve hypoplasia, multiple pituitary hormone deficiency, isolated growth hormone deficiency, and idiopathic short stature. J Pediatr 2004; 145: 536–541.

150 Boulay JL, O'Shea JJ, Paul WE. Molecular phylogeny within type I cytokines and their cognate receptors. Immunity 2003; 19: 159–163.

151 Liongue C, Ward AC. Evolution of Class I cytokine receptors. BMC Evol Biol 2007; 7: 120.

152 Edens A, Talamantes F. Alternative processing of growth hormone receptor transcripts. Endocr Rev 1998; 19: 559–582.

153 Wei Y, Rhani Z, Goodyer CG. Characterization of growth hormone receptor messenger ribonucleic acid variants in human adipocytes. J Clin Endocrinol Metab 2006; 91: 1901–1908.

154 Rivers CA, Norman MR. The human growth hormone receptor gene: characterisation of the liver-specific promoter. Mol Cell Endocrinol 2000; 160: 51–59.

155 Gates GC, Rhani Z, Zheng H. Expression of the hepatic specific V1 messenger ribonucleic acid of the human growth hormone receptor gene is regulated by hepatic nuclear factor (HNF)-4α2 and HNF-4 α 8. Mol Endocrinol 2008; 22: 485–500.

156 Behncken SN, Waters MJ. Molecular recognition events involved in the activation of the growth hormone receptor by growth hormone. J Mol Recognit 1999; 12: 355–362.

157 Brown RJ, Adams JJ, Pelekanos RA, Wan Y, McKinstry WJ, Palethorpe K, et al. Model for growth hormone receptor activation based on subunit rotation within a receptor dimer. Nat Struct Mol Biol 2005; 12: 814–821.

158 Strous GJ, dos Santos CA, Gent J, Govers R, Sachse M, Schantl J, et al. Ubiquitin system-dependent regulation of growth hormone receptor signal transduction. Curr Top Microbiol Immunol 2004; 286: 81–118.

159 Leung DW, Spencer SA, Cachianes G, Hammonds RG, Collins C, Henzel WJ, et al. Growth hormone receptor and serum binding protein: purification, cloning and expression. Nature 1987; 330: 537–543.

160 Zhang Y, Jiang J, Black RA, Baumann G, Frank SJ. Tumor necrosis factor-alpha converting enzyme (TACE) is a growth hormone binding protein (GHBP) sheddase: the metalloprotease TACE/ADAM-17 is critical for (PMA-induced) GH receptor proteolysis and GHBP generation. Endocrinology 2000; 141: 4342–4348.

161 Carmignac DF, Gabrielsson BG, Robinson IC. Growth hormone binding protein in the rat: effects of gonadal steroids. Endocrinology 1993; 133: 2445–2452.

162 Gevers EF, Wit JM, Robinson IC. Growth, growth hormone (GH)-binding protein, and GH receptors are differentially regulated by peak and trough components of the GH secretory pattern in the rat. Endocrinology 1996; 137: 1013–1018.

163 Baumann G. Growth hormone binding protein: the soluble growth hormone receptor. Minerva Endocrinol 2002; 27: 265–276.

164 Amit T, Youdim MB, Hochberg Z. Clinical review 112: does serum growth hormone (GH) binding protein reflect human GH receptor function? J Clin Endocrinol Metab 2000; 85: 927–932.

165 Savage MO, Attie KM, David A, Metherell LA, Clark AJ, Camacho-Hubner C. Endocrine assessment, molecular characterization and treatment of growth hormone insensitivity disorders. Nat Clin Pract Endocrinol Metab 2006; 2: 395–407.

166 Donaghy AJ, Delhanty PJ, Ho KK, Williams R, Baxter RC. Regulation of the growth hormone receptor/binding protein, insulin-like growth factor ternary complex system in human cirrhosis. J Hepatol 2002; 36: 751–758.

167 Sotiropoulos A, Perrot-Applanat M, Dinerstein H, Pallier A, Postel-Vinay MC, Finidori J, et al. Distinct cytoplasmic regions of the growth hormone receptor are required for activation of JAK2,

mitogen-activated protein kinase, and transcription. *Endocrinology* 1994; **135**: 1292–1298.

168 Frank SJ, Gilliland G, Kraft AS, Arnold CS. Interaction of the growth hormone receptor cytoplasmic domain with the JAK2 tyrosine kinase. *Endocrinology* 1994; **135**: 2228–2239.

169 Soldaini E, John S, Moro S, Bollenbacher J, Schindler U, Leonard WJ. DNA binding site selection of dimeric and tetrameric Stat5 proteins reveals a large repertoire of divergent tetrameric Stat5a binding sites. *Mol Cell Biol* 2000; **20**: 389–401.

170 Levy DE, Darnell JE Jr. Stats: transcriptional control and biological impact. *Nat Rev Mol Cell Biol* 2002; **3**: 651–662.

171 Teglund S, McKay C, Schuetz E, van Deursen JM, Stravopodis D, Wang D, *et al*. Stat5a and Stat5b proteins have essential and nonessential, or redundant, roles in cytokine responses. *Cell* 1998; **93**: 841–850.

172 Liu X, Robinson GW, Wagner KU, Garrett L, Wynshaw-Boris A, Hennighausen L. Stat5a is mandatory for adult mammary gland development and lactogenesis. *Genes Dev* 1997; **11**: 179–186.

173 Choi HK, Waxman DJ. Growth hormone, but not prolactin, maintains, low-level activation of STAT5a and STAT5b in female rat liver. *Endocrinology* 1999; **140**: 5126–5135.

174 Gallego MI, Binart N, Robinson GW, Okagaki R, Coschigano KT, Perry J, *et al*. Prolactin, growth hormone, and epidermal growth factor activate Stat5 in different compartments of mammary tissue and exert different and overlapping developmental effects. *Dev Biol* 2001; **229**: 163–175.

175 Holloway MG, Cui Y, Laz EV, Hosui A, Hennighausen L, Waxman DJ. Loss of sexually dimorphic liver gene expression upon hepatocyte-specific deletion of Stat5a-Stat5b locus. *Endocrinology* 2007; **148**: 1977–1986.

176 Clodfelter KH, Miles GD, Wauthier V, Holloway MG, Zhang X, Hodor P, *et al*. Role of STAT5a in regulation of sex-specific gene expression in female but not male mouse liver revealed by microarray analysis. *Physiol Genomics* 2007; **31**: 63–74.

177 Udy GB, Towers RP, Snell RG, Wilkins RJ, Park SH, Ram PA, *et al*. Requirement of STAT5b for sexual dimorphism of body growth rates and liver gene expression. *Proc Natl Acad Sci U S A* 1997; **94**: 7239–7244.

178 Dupuis S, Dargemont C, Fieschi C, Thomassin N, Rosenzweig S, Harris J, *et al*. Impairment of mycobacterial but not viral immunity by a germline human STAT1 mutation. *Science* 2001; **293**: 300–303.

179 Minegishi Y, Saito M, Tsuchiya S, Tsuge I, Takada H, Hara T, *et al*. Dominant-negative mutations in the DNA-binding domain of STAT3 cause hyper-IgE syndrome. *Nature* 2007; **448**: 1058–1062.

180 Zhou Y, Xu BC, Maheshwari HG, He L, Reed M, Lozykowski M, *et al*. A mammalian model for Laron syndrome produced by targeted disruption of the mouse growth hormone receptor/binding protein gene (the Laron mouse). *Proc Natl Acad Sci U S A* 1997; **94**: 13215–13220.

181 Coschigano KT, Clemmons D, Bellush LL, Kopchick JJ. Assessment of growth parameters and life span of GHR/BP gene-disrupted mice. *Endocrinology* 2000; **141**: 2608–2613.

182 Yao Z, Cui Y, Watford WT, Bream JH, Yamaoka K, Hissong BD, *et al*. Stat5a/b are essential for normal lymphoid development and differentiation. *Proc Natl Acad Sci U S A* 2006; **103**: 1000–1005.

183 Kelly J, Spolski R, Imada K, Bollenbacher J, Lee S, Leonard WJ. A role for Stat5 in CD8+ T cell homeostasis. *J Immunol* 2003; **170**: 210–217.

184 Iavnilovitch E, Groner B, Barash I. Overexpression and forced activation of stat5 in mammary gland of transgenic mice promotes cellular proliferation, enhances differentiation, and delays postlactational apoptosis. *Mol Cancer Res* 2002; **1**: 32–47.

185 Gebert CA, Park SH, Waxman DJ. Down-regulation of liver JAK2-STAT5b signaling by the female plasma pattern of continuous growth hormone stimulation. *Mol Endocrinol* 1999; **13**: 213–227.

186 Gebert CA, Park SH, Waxman DJ. Termination of growth hormone pulse-induced STAT5b signaling. *Mol Endocrinol* 1999; **13**: 38–56.

187 Ahluwalia A, Clodfelter KH, Waxman DJ. Sexual dimorphism of rat liver gene expression: regulatory role of growth hormone revealed by deoxyribonucleic Acid microarray analysis. *Mol Endocrinol* 2004; **18**: 747–760.

188 Waxman DJ, O'Connor C. Growth hormone regulation of sex-dependent liver gene expression. *Mol Endocrinol* 2006; **20**: 2613–2629.

189 Davey HW, Park SH, Grattan DR, McLachlan MJ, Waxman DJ. STAT5b-deficient mice are growth hormone pulse-resistant: role of STAT5b in sex-specific liver P450 expression. *J Biol Chem* 1999; **274**: 35331–35336.

190 Clodfelter KH, Holloway MG, Hodor P, Park SH, Ray WJ, Waxman DJ. Sex-dependent liver gene expression is extensive and largely dependent upon signal transducer and activator of transcription 5b (STAT5b): STAT5b-dependent activation of male genes and repression of female genes revealed by microarray analysis. *Mol Endocrinol* 2006; **20**: 1333–1351.

191 Tronche F, Opherk C, Moriggl R, Kellendonk C, Reimann A, Schwake L, *et al*. Glucocorticoid receptor function in hepatocytes is essential to promote postnatal body growth. *Genes Dev* 2004; **18**: 492–497.

192 Eleswarapu S, Gu Z, Jiang H. Growth hormone regulation of IGF-1 gene expression may be mediated by multiple distal STAT5 binding sites. *Endocrinology* 2008; **149**: 2230–2240.

193 Chia DJ, Ono M, Woelfle J, Schlesinger-Massart M, Jiang H, Rotwein P. Characterization of distinct Stat5b binding sites that mediate growth hormone-stimulated IGF-1 gene transcription. *J Biol Chem* 2006; **281**: 3190–3197.

194 Vidal OM, Merino R, Rico-Bautista E, Fernandez-Perez L, Chia DJ, Woelfle J, *et al*. In vivo transcript profiling and phylogenetic analysis identifies suppressor of cytokine signaling 2 as a direct signal transducer and activator of transcription 5b target in liver. *Mol Endocrinol* 2007; **21**: 293–311.

195 Matsumoto A, Masuhara M, Mitsui K, Yokouchi M, Ohtsubo M, Misawa H, *et al*. CIS, a cytokine inducible SH2 protein, is a target of the JAK-STAT5 pathway and modulates STAT5 activation. *Blood* 1997; **89**: 3148–3154.

196 Wood TJ, Sliva D, Lobie PE, Goullieux F, Mui AL, Groner B, *et al*. Specificity of transcription enhancement via the STAT responsive element in the serine protease inhibitor 2.1 promoter. *Mol Cell Endocrinol* 1997; **130**: 69–81.

197 Woelfle J, Rotwein P. In vivo regulation of growth hormone-stimulated gene transcription by STAT5b. *Am J Physiol Endocrinol Metab* 2004; **286**: E393–E401.

198 Mukhopadhyay SS, Wyszomierski SL, Gronostajski RM, Rosen JM. Differential interactions of specific nuclear factor I isoforms with

the glucocorticoid receptor and STAT5 in the cooperative regulation of WAP gene transcription. *Mol Cell Biol* 2001; **21**: 6859–6869.

199 Kim HP, Imbert J, Leonard WJ. Both integrated and differential regulation of components of the IL-2/IL-2 receptor system. *Cytokine Growth Factor Rev* 2006; **17**: 349–366.

200 Greenhalgh CJ, Rico-Bautista E, Lorentzon M, Thaus AL, Morgan PO, Willson TA, et al. SOCS2 negatively regulates growth hormone action *in vitro* and *in vivo*. *J Clin Invest* 2005; **115**: 397–406.

201 Gu F, Dube N, Kim JW, Cheng A, Ibarra-Sanchez MJ, Tremblay ML, et al. Protein tyrosine phosphatase 1B attenuates growth hormone-mediated JAK2-STAT signaling. *Mol Cell Biol* 2003; **23**: 3753–3762.

202 Ram PA, Waxman DJ. Interaction of growth hormone-activated STATs with SH2-containing phosphotyrosine phosphatase SHP-1 and nuclear JAK2 tyrosine kinase. *J Biol Chem* 1997; **272**: 17694–17702.

203 Pasquali C, Curchod ML, Walchli S, Espanel X, Guerrier M, Arigoni F, et al. Identification of protein tyrosine phosphatases with specificity for the ligand-activated growth hormone receptor. *Mol Endocrinol* 2003; **17**: 2228–2239.

204 Binder G, Neuer K, Ranke MB, Wittekindt NE. PTPN11 mutations are associated with mild growth hormone resistance in individuals with Noonan syndrome. *J Clin Endocrinol Metab* 2005; **90**: 5377–5381.

205 Lanning NJ, Carter-Su C. Recent advances in growth hormone signaling. *Rev Endocr Metab Disord* 2006; **7**: 225–235.

206 Rowland JE, Lichanska AM, Kerr LM, White M, d'Aniello EM, Maher SL, et al. *In vivo* analysis of growth hormone receptor signaling domains and their associated transcripts. *Mol Cell Biol* 2005; **25**: 66–77.

207 LeRoith D, Yakar S. Mechanisms of disease: metabolic effects of growth hormone and insulin-like growth factor 1. *Nat Clin Pract Endocrinol Metab* 2007; **3**: 302–310.

208 Samani AA, Yakar S, LeRoith D, Brodt P. The role of the IGF system in cancer growth and metastasis: overview and recent insights. *Endocr Rev* 2007; **28**: 20–47.

209 Luther J, Aitken R, Milne J, Matsuzaki M, Reynolds L, Redmer D, et al. Maternal and fetal growth, body composition, endocrinology, and metabolic status in undernourished adolescent sheep. *Biol Reprod* 2007; **77**: 343–350.

210 Randhawa R, Cohen P. The role of the insulin-like growth factor system in prenatal growth. *Mol Genet Metab* 2005; **86**: 84–90.

211 Davidson S, Hod M, Merlob P, Shtaif B. Leptin, insulin, insulin-like growth factors and their binding proteins in cord serum: insight into fetal growth and discordancy. *Clin Endocrinol (Oxf)* 2006; **65**: 586–592.

212 Geary MP, Pringle PJ, Rodeck CH, Kingdom JC, Hindmarsh PC. Sexual dimorphism in the growth hormone and insulin-like growth factor axis at birth. *J Clin Endocrinol Metab* 2003; **88**: 3708–3714.

213 Gluckman PD, Gunn AJ, Wray A, Cutfield WS, Chatelain PG, Guilbaud O, et al. Congenital idiopathic growth hormone deficiency associated with prenatal and early postnatal growth failure. The International Board of the Kabi Pharmacia International Growth Study. *J Pediatr* 1992; **121**: 920–923.

214 Rosenbloom AL, Guevara-Aguirre J, Rosenfeld RG, Francke U. Growth hormone receptor deficiency in Ecuador. *J Clin Endocrinol Metab* 1999; **84**: 4436–4443.

215 Liu JP, Baker J, Perkins AS, Robertson EJ, Efstratiadis A. Mice carrying null mutations of the genes encoding insulin-like growth factor 1 (Igf-1) and type 1 IGF receptor (Igf1r). *Cell* 1993; **75**: 59–72.

216 Baker J, Liu JP, Robertson EJ, Efstratiadis A. Role of insulin-like growth factors in embryonic and postnatal growth. *Cell* 1993; **75**: 73–82.

217 Cediel R, Riquelme R, Contreras J, Diaz A, Varela-Nieto I. Sensorineural hearing loss in insulin-like growth factor I-null mice: a new model of human deafness. *Eur J Neurosci* 2006; **23**: 587–590.

218 Mohan S, Baylink DJ. Impaired skeletal growth in mice with haploinsufficiency of IGF-1: genetic evidence that differences in IGF-1 expression could contribute to peak bone mineral density differences. *J Endocrinol* 2005; **185**: 415–420.

219 Sutter NB, Bustamante CD, Chase K, Gray MM, Zhao K, Zhu L, et al. A single IGF1 allele is a major determinant of small size in dogs. *Science* 2007; **316**: 112–115.

220 Clemmons DR. Role of insulin-like growth factor binding proteins in controlling IGF actions. *Mol Cell Endocrinol* 1998; **140**: 19–24.

221 Twigg SM, Baxter RC. Insulin-like growth factor (IGF)-binding protein 5 forms an alternative ternary complex with IGFs and the acid-labile subunit. *J Biol Chem* 1998; **273**: 6074–6079.

222 Boisclair YR, Rhoads RP, Ueki I, Wang J, Ooi GT. The acid-labile subunit (ALS) of the 150 kDa IGF-binding protein complex: an important but forgotten component of the circulating IGF system. *J Endocrinol* 2001; **170**: 63–70.

223 Holt RI, Jones JS, Stone NM, Baker AJ, Miell JP. Sequential changes in insulin-like growth factor I (IGF-I) and IGF-binding proteins in children with end-stage liver disease before and after successful orthotopic liver transplantation. *J Clin Endocrinol Metab* 1996; **81**: 160–168.

224 Woods KA, Camacho-Hubner C, Savage MO, Clark AJ. Intrauterine growth retardation and postnatal growth failure associated with deletion of the insulin-like growth factor I gene. *N Engl J Med* 1996; **335**: 1363–1367.

225 Beauloye V, Willems B, de C, V, Frank SJ, Edery M, Thissen JP. Impairment of liver GH receptor signaling by fasting. *Endocrinology* 2002; **143**: 792–800.

226 Gleeson HK, Lissett CA, Shalet SM. Insulin-like growth factor-I response to a single bolus of growth hormone is increased in obesity. *J Clin Endocrinol Metab* 2005; **90**: 1061–1067.

227 Bergad PL, Schwarzenberg SJ, Humbert JT, Morrison M, Amarasinghe S, Towle HC, et al. Inhibition of growth hormone action in models of inflammation. *Am J Physiol Cell Physiol* 2000; **279**: C1906–C1917.

228 Tonshoff B, Kiepe D, Ciarmatori S. Growth hormone/insulin-like growth factor system in children with chronic renal failure. *Pediatr Nephrol* 2005; **20**: 279–289.

229 Mahesh S, Kaskel F. Growth hormone axis in chronic kidney disease. *Pediatr Nephrol* 2008; **23**: 41–48.

230 Clemmons DR. Clinical utility of measurements of insulin-like growth factor 1. *Nat Clin Pract Endocrinol Metab* 2006; **2**: 436–446.

231 Denley A, Carroll JM, Brierley GV, Cosgrove L, Wallace J, Forbes B, et al. Differential activation of insulin receptor substrates 1 and 2 by insulin-like growth factor-activated insulin receptors. *Mol Cell Biol* 2007; **27**: 3569–3577.

232 Kido Y, Nakae J, Hribal ML, Xuan S, Efstratiadis A, Accili D. Effects of mutations in the insulin-like growth factor signaling system on embryonic pancreas development and beta-cell compensation to insulin resistance. *J Biol Chem* 2002; **277**: 36740–36747.

233 Holzenberger M, Dupont J, Ducos B, Leneuve P, Geloen A, Even PC, *et al*. IGF-1 receptor regulates lifespan and resistance to oxidative stress in mice. *Nature* 2003; **421**: 182–187.

234 Gevers EF, van der Eerden BC, Karperien M, Raap AK, Robinson IC, Wit JM. Localization and regulation of the growth hormone receptor and growth hormone-binding protein in the rat growth plate. *J Bone Miner Res* 2002; **17**: 1408–1419.

235 Wang E, Wang J, Chin E, Zhou J, Bondy CA. Cellular patterns of insulin-like growth factor system gene expression in murine chondrogenesis and osteogenesis. *Endocrinology* 1995; **136**: 2741–2751.

236 Lazowski DA, Fraher LJ, Hodsman A, Steer B, Modrowski D, Han VK. Regional variation of insulin-like growth factor-I gene expression in mature rat bone and cartilage. *Bone* 1994; **15**: 563–576.

237 Hunziker EB, Wagner J, Zapf J. Differential effects of insulin-like growth factor I and growth hormone on developmental stages of rat growth plate chondrocytes *in vivo*. *J Clin Invest* 1994; **93**: 1078–1086.

238 Kaplan SA, Cohen P. The somatomedin hypothesis 2007: 50 years later. *J Clin Endocrinol Metab* 2007; **92**: 4529–4535.

239 Sjogren K, Liu JL, Blad K, Skrtic S, Vidal O, Wallenius V, *et al*. Liver-derived insulin-like growth factor I (IGF-I) is the principal source of IGF-I in blood but is not required for postnatal body growth in mice. *Proc Natl Acad Sci U S A* 1999; **96**: 7088–7092.

240 Liu JL, Yakar S, LeRoith D. Mice deficient in liver production of insulin-like growth factor I display sexual dimorphism in growth hormone-stimulated postnatal growth. *Endocrinology* 2000; **141**: 4436–4441.

241 Ueki I, Ooi GT, Tremblay ML, Hurst KR, Bach LA, Boisclair YR. Inactivation of the acid labile subunit gene in mice results in mild retardation of postnatal growth despite profound disruptions in the circulating insulin-like growth factor system. *Proc Natl Acad Sci U S A* 2000; **97**: 6868–6873.

242 Gevers EF, Milne J, Robinson IC, Loveridge N. Single cell enzyme activity and proliferation in the growth plate: effects of growth hormone. *J Bone Miner Res* 1996; **11**: 1103–1111.

243 Reinecke M, Schmid AC, Heyberger-Meyer B, Hunziker EB, Zapf J. Effect of growth hormone and insulin-like growth factor I (IGF-I) on the expression of IGF-I messenger ribonucleic acid and peptide in rat tibial growth plate and articular chondrocytes *in vivo*. *Endocrinology* 2000; **141**: 2847–2853.

244 Gevers EF, Robinson IC. GH and Stat5 signaling *in vivo*: insulin attenuates GH-resistance induced by fasting. Proceedings of the 89th Annual Meeting of The Endocrine Society, Toronto. 2007: 2–388.

245 Palmiter RD, Brinster RL, Hammer RE, Trumbauer ME, Rosenfeld MG, Birnberg NC, *et al*. Dramatic growth of mice that develop from eggs microinjected with metallothionein-growth hormone fusion genes. *Nature* 1982; **300**: 611–615.

246 Mathews LS, Hammer RE, Behringer RR, D'Ercole AJ, Bell GI, Brinster RL, *et al*. Growth enhancement of transgenic mice expressing human insulin-like growth factor I. *Endocrinology* 1988; **123**: 2827–2833.

247 Liao L, Dearth RK, Zhou S, Britton OL, Lee AV, Xu J. Liver-specific overexpression of the insulin-like growth factor-I enhances somatic growth and partially prevents the effects of growth hormone deficiency. *Endocrinology* 2006; **147**: 3877–3888.

248 Sims NA, Clement-Lacroix P, Da Ponte F, Bouali Y, Binart N, Moriggl R, *et al*. Bone homeostasis in growth hormone receptor-null mice is restored by IGF-I but independent of Stat5. *J Clin Invest* 2000; **106**: 1095–1103.

249 Lupu F, Terwilliger JD, Lee K, Segre GV, Efstratiadis A. Roles of growth hormone and insulin-like growth factor 1 in mouse postnatal growth. *Dev Biol* 2001; **229**: 141–162.

250 Yakar S, Rosen CJ, Beamer WG, Ackert-Bicknell CL, Wu Y, Liu JL, *et al*. Circulating concentrations of IGF-1 directly regulate bone growth and density. *J Clin Invest* 2002; **110**: 771–781.

251 Kowarski AA, Schneider J, Ben Galim E, Weldon VV, Daughaday WH. Growth failure with normal serum RIA-GH and low somatomedin activity: somatomedin restoration and growth acceleration after exogenous GH. *J Clin Endocrinol Metab* 1978; **47**: 461–464.

252 Takahashi Y, Kaji H, Okimura Y, Goji K, Abe H, Chihara K. Brief report: short stature caused by a mutant growth hormone. *N Engl J Med* 1996; **334**: 432–436.

253 Millar DS, Lewis MD, Horan M, Newsway V, Easter TE, Gregory JW, *et al*. Novel mutations of the growth hormone 1 (GH1) gene disclosed by modulation of the clinical selection criteria for individuals with short stature. H*um Mutat* 2003; **21**: 424–440.

254 Petkovic V, Thevis M, Lochmatter D, Besson A, Eble A, Fluck CE, *et al*. GH mutant (R77C) in a pedigree presenting with the delay of growth and pubertal development: structural analysis of the mutant and evaluation of the biological activity. *Eur J Endocrinol* 2007; **157** (Suppl 1): S67–S74.

255 Lewis MD, Horan M, Millar DS, Newsway V, Easter TE, Fryklund L, *et al*. A novel dysfunctional growth hormone variant (Ile179Met) exhibits a decreased ability to activate the extracellular signal-regulated kinase pathway. *J Clin Endocrinol Metab* 2004; **89**: 1068–1075.

256 Besson A, Salemi S, Deladoey J, Vuissoz JM, Eble A, Bidlingmaier M, *et al*. Short stature caused by a biologically inactive mutant growth hormone (GH-C53S). *J Clin Endocrinol Metab* 2005; **90**: 2493–2499.

257 Laron Z, Pertzelan A, Mannheimer S. Genetic pituitary dwarfism with high serum concentration of growth hormone: a new inborn error of metabolism? *Isr J Med Sci* 1966; **2**: 152–155.

258 Godowski PJ, Leung DW, Meacham LR, Galgani JP, Hellmiss R, Keret R, *et al*. Characterization of the human growth hormone receptor gene and demonstration of a partial gene deletion in two patients with Laron-type dwarfism. *Proc Natl Acad Sci U S A* 1989; **86**: 8083–8087.

259 Laron Z. Laron syndrome (primary growth hormone resistance or insensitivity): the personal experience 1958–2003. *J Clin Endocrinol Metab* 2004; **89**: 1031–1044.

260 Laron Z, Lilos P, Klinger B. Growth curves for Laron syndrome. *Arch Dis Child* 1993; **68**: 768–770.

261 Woods KA, Dastot F, Preece MA, Clark AJ, Postel-Vinay MC, Chatelain PG, *et al*. Phenotype: genotype relationships in growth hormone insensitivity syndrome. *J Clin Endocrinol Metab* 1997; **82**: 3529–3535.

262 Walenkamp MJ, van der Kamp HJ, Pereira AM, Kant SG, van Duyvenvoorde HA, Kruithof MF, *et al*. A variable degree of intrauterine and postnatal growth retardation in a family with a missense mutation in the insulin-like growth factor I receptor. *J Clin Endocrinol Metab* 2006; **91**: 3062–3070.

263 Laron Z, Ginsberg S, Lilos P, Arbiv M, Vaisman N. Body composition in untreated adult patients with Laron syndrome (primary GH insensitivity). *Clin Endocrinol (Oxf)* 2006; **65**: 114–117.

264 Kranzler JH, Rosenbloom AL, Martinez V, Guevara-Aguirre J. Normal intelligence with severe insulin-like growth factor I deficiency due to growth hormone receptor deficiency: a controlled study in a genetically homogeneous population. *J Clin Endocrinol Metab* 1998; **83**: 1953–1958.

265 Bachrach LK, Marcus R, Ott SM, Rosenbloom AL, Vasconez O, Martinez V, *et al*. Bone mineral, histomorphometry, and body composition in adults with growth hormone receptor deficiency. *J Bone Miner Res* 1998; **13**: 415–421.

266 Rosenbloom AL, Guevara-Aguirre J, Berg MA, Francke U. Stature in Ecuadorians heterozygous for growth hormone receptor gene E180 splice mutation does not differ from that of homozygous normal relatives. *J Clin Endocrinol Metab* 1998; **83**: 2373–2375.

267 Silbergeld A, Klinger B, Schwartz H, Laron Z. Serum prolactin in patients with Laron-type dwarfism: effect of insulin-like growth factor I. *Horm Res* 1992; **37**: 160–164.

268 Burren CP, Woods KA, Rose SJ, Tauber M, Price DA, Heinrich U, *et al*. Clinical and endocrine characteristics in atypical and classical growth hormone insensitivity syndrome. *Horm Res* 2001; **55**: 125–130.

269 Sivan B, Lilos P, Laron Z. Effects of insulin-like growth factor-I deficiency and replacement therapy on the hematopoietic system in patients with Laron syndrome (primary growth hormone insensitivity). *J Pediatr Endocrinol Metab* 2003; **16**: 509–520.

270 Christ ER, Cummings MH, Westwood NB, Sawyer BM, Pearson TC, Sonksen PH, *et al*. The importance of growth hormone in the regulation of erythropoiesis, red cell mass, and plasma volume in adults with growth hormone deficiency. *J Clin Endocrinol Metab* 1997; **82**: 2985–2990.

271 Jeay S, Sonenshein GE, Postel-Vinay MC, Kelly PA, Baixeras E. Growth hormone can act as a cytokine controlling survival and proliferation of immune cells: new insights into signaling pathways. *Mol Cell Endocrinol* 2002; **188**: 1–7.

272 Dorshkind K, Horseman ND. The roles of prolactin, growth hormone, insulin-like growth factor-I, and thyroid hormones in lymphocyte development and function: insights from genetic models of hormone and hormone receptor deficiency. *Endocr Rev* 2000; **21**: 292–312.

273 Duquesnoy P, Sobrier ML, Duriez B, Dastot F, Buchanan CR, Savage MO, *et al*. A single amino acid substitution in the exoplasmic domain of the human growth hormone (GH) receptor confers familial GH resistance (Laron syndrome) with positive GH-binding activity by abolishing receptor homodimerization. *EMBO J* 1994; **13**: 1386–1395.

274 Metherell LA, Akker SA, Munroe PB, Rose SJ, Caulfield M, Savage MO, *et al*. Pseudoexon activation as a novel mechanism for disease resulting in atypical growth-hormone insensitivity. *Am J Hum Genet* 2001; **69**: 641–646.

275 David A, Camacho-Hubner C, Bhangoo A, Rose SJ, Miraki-Moud F, Akker SA, *et al*. An intronic growth hormone receptor mutation causing activation of a pseudoexon is associated with a broad spectrum of growth hormone insensitivity phenotypes. *J Clin Endocrinol Metab* 2007; **92**: 655–659.

276 Woods KA, Fraser NC, Postel-Vinay MC, Savage MO, Clark AJ. A homozygous splice site mutation affecting the intracellular domain of the growth hormone (GH) receptor resulting in Laron syndrome with elevated GH-binding protein. *J Clin Endocrinol Metab* 1996; **81**: 1686–1690.

277 Silbergeld A, Dastot F, Klinger B, Kanety H, Eshet R, Amselem S, *et al*. Intronic mutation in the growth hormone (GH) receptor gene from a girl with Laron syndrome and extremely high serum GH binding protein: extended phenotypic study in a very large pedigree. *J Pediatr Endocrinol Metab* 1997; **10**: 265–274.

278 Ayling RM, Ross R, Towner P, Von Laue S, Finidori J, Moutoussamy S, *et al*. A dominant-negative mutation of the growth hormone receptor causes familial short stature. *Nat Genet* 1997; **16**: 13–14.

279 Iida K, Takahashi Y, Kaji H, Nose O, Okimura Y, Abe H, *et al*. Growth hormone (GH) insensitivity syndrome with high serum GH-binding protein concentrations caused by a heterozygous splice site mutation of the GH receptor gene producing a lack of intracellular domain. *J Clin Endocrinol Metab* 1998; **83**: 531–537.

280 Milward A, Metherell L, Maamra M, Barahona MJ, Wilkinson IR, Camacho-Hubner C, *et al*. Growth hormone (GH) insensitivity syndrome due to a GH receptor truncated after Box1, resulting in isolated failure of STAT 5 signal transduction. *J Clin Endocrinol Metab* 2004; **89**: 1259–1266.

281 Goddard AD, Covello R, Luoh SM, Clackson T, Attie KM, Gesundheit N, *et al*. Mutations of the growth hormone receptor in children with idiopathic short stature. The Growth Hormone Insensitivity Study Group. *N Engl J Med* 1995; **333**: 1093–1098.

282 Goddard AD, Dowd P, Chernausek S, Geffner M, Gertner J, Hintz R, *et al*. Partial growth-hormone insensitivity: the role of growth-hormone receptor mutations in idiopathic short stature. *J Pediatr* 1997; **131**: S51–S55.

283 Jorge AA, Souza SC, Nishi MY, Billerbeck AE, Liborio DC, Kim CA, *et al*. SHOX mutations in idiopathic short stature and Leri-Weill dyschondrosteosis: frequency and phenotypic variability. *Clin Endocrinol (Oxf)* 2007; **66**: 130–135.

284 Chusho H, Tamura N, Ogawa Y, Yasoda A, Suda M, Miyazawa T, *et al*. Dwarfism and early death in mice lacking C-type natriuretic peptide. *Proc Natl Acad Sci U S A* 2001; **98**: 4016–4021.

285 Bartels CF, Bukulmez H, Padayatti P, Rhee DK, Ravenswaaij-Arts C, Pauli RM, *et al*. Mutations in the transmembrane natriuretic peptide receptor NPR-B impair skeletal growth and cause acromesomelic dysplasia, type Maroteaux. *Am J Hum Genet* 2004; **75**: 27–34.

286 Olney RC, Bukulmez H, Bartels CF, Prickett TC, Espiner EA, Potter LR, *et al*. Heterozygous mutations in natriuretic peptide receptor-B (NPR2) are associated with short stature. *J Clin Endocrinol Metab* 2006; **91**: 1229–1232.

287 Blair JC, Camacho-Hubner C, Miraki MF, Rosberg S, Burren C, Lim S, *et al*. Standard and low-dose IGF-I generation tests and spontaneous growth hormone secretion in children with idiopathic short stature. *Clin Endocrinol (Oxf)* 2004; **60**: 163–168.

288 Buckway CK, Selva KA, Pratt KL, Tjoeng E, Guevara-Aguirre J, Rosenfeld RG. Insulin-like growth factor binding protein-3 generation as a measure of GH sensitivity. *J Clin Endocrinol Metab* 2002; **87**: 4754–4765.

289 Dos SC, Essioux L, Teinturier C, Tauber M, Goffin V, Bougneres P. A common polymorphism of the growth hormone receptor is associated with increased responsiveness to growth hormone. *Nat Genet* 2004; **36**: 720–724.

290 Pantel J, Machinis K, Sobrier ML, Duquesnoy P, Goossens M, Amselem S. Species-specific alternative splice mimicry at the growth

hormone receptor locus revealed by the lineage of retroelements during primate evolution. *J Biol Chem* 2000; **275**: 18664–18669.

291 Sobrier ML, Duquesnoy P, Duriez B, Amselem S, Goossens M. Expression and binding properties of two isoforms of the human growth hormone receptor. *FEBS Lett* 1993; **319**: 16–20.

292 Lettre G, Butler JL, Ardlie KG, Hirschhorn JN. Common genetic variation in eight genes of the GH/IGF1 axis does not contribute to adult height variation. *Hum Genet* 2007; **122**: 129–139.

293 Carrascosa A, Audi L, Fernandez-Cancio M, Esteban C, Andaluz P, Vilaro E, et al. The exon 3-deleted/full-length growth hormone receptor polymorphism did not influence growth response to growth hormone therapy over 2 years in prepubertal short children born at term with adequate weight and length for gestational age. *J Clin Endocrinol Metab* 2008; **93**: 764–770.

294 Binder G, Baur F, Schweizer R, Ranke MB. The d3-growth hormone (GH) receptor polymorphism is associated with increased responsiveness to GH in Turner syndrome and short small-for-gestational-age children. *J Clin Endocrinol Metab* 2006; **91**: 659–664.

295 Schreiner F, Stutte S, Bartmann P, Gohlke B, Woelfle J. Association of the growth hormone receptor d3-variant and catch-up growth of preterm infants with birth weight of less than 1500 grams. *J Clin Endocrinol Metab* 2007; **92**: 4489–4493.

296 Raz B, Janner M, Petkovic V, Lochmatter D, Eble A, Dattani MT, et al. Influence of growth hormone receptor d3 and full-length isoforms on growth hormone response and final height in patients with severe growth hormone deficiency. *J Clin Endocrinol Metab* 2008; **93**: 974–980.

297 Kofoed EM, Hwa V, Little B, Woods KA, Buckway CK, Tsubaki J, et al. Growth hormone insensitivity associated with a STAT5b mutation. *N Engl J Med* 2003; **349**: 1139–1147.

298 Hwa V, Little B, Adiyaman P, Kofoed EM, Pratt KL, Ocal G, et al. Severe growth hormone insensitivity resulting from total absence of signal transducer and activator of transcription 5b. *J Clin Endocrinol Metab* 2005; **90**: 4260–4266.

299 Vidarsdottir S, Walenkamp MJ, Pereira AM, Karperien M, van Doorn J, van Duyvenvoorde HA, et al. Clinical and biochemical characteristics of a male patient with a novel homozygous STAT5b mutation. *J Clin Endocrinol Metab* 2006; **91**: 3482–3485.

300 Hwa V, Camacho-Hubner C, Little BM, David A, Metherell LA, El Khatib N, et al. Growth hormone insensitivity and severe short stature in siblings: a novel mutation at the exon 13-intron 13 junction of the STAT5b gene. *Horm Res* 2007; **68**: 218–224.

301 Bernasconi A, Marino R, Ribas A, Rossi J, Ciaccio M, Oleastro M, et al. Characterization of immunodeficiency in a patient with growth hormone insensitivity secondary to a novel STAT5b gene mutation. *Pediatrics* 2006; **118**: e1584–e1592.

302 Cohen AC, Nadeau KC, Tu W, Hwa V, Dionis K, Bezrodnik L, et al. Cutting edge: Decreased accumulation and regulatory function of CD4+ CD25(high) T cells in human STAT5b deficiency. *J Immunol* 2006; **177**: 2770–2774.

303 Snow JW, Abraham N, Ma MC, Herndier BG, Pastuszak AW, Goldsmith MA. Loss of tolerance and autoimmunity affecting multiple organs in STAT5A/5B-deficient mice. *J Immunol* 2003; **171**: 5042–5050.

304 Antov A, Yang L, Vig M, Baltimore D, Van Parijs L. Essential role for STAT5 signaling in CD25$^+$CD4$^+$ regulatory T cell homeostasis and the maintenance of self-tolerance. *J Immunol* 2003; **171**: 3435–3441.

305 Tartaglia M, Pennacchio LA, Zhao C, Yadav KK, Fodale V, Sarkozy A, et al. Gain-of-function SOS1 mutations cause a distinctive form of Noonan syndrome. *Nat Genet* 2007; **39**: 75–79.

306 Tartaglia M, Mehler EL, Goldberg R, Zampino G, Brunner HG, Kremer H, et al. Mutations in PTPN11, encoding the protein tyrosine phosphatase SHP-2, cause Noonan syndrome. *Nat Genet* 2001; **29**: 465–468.

307 Roberts AE, Araki T, Swanson KD, Montgomery KT, Schiripo TA, Joshi VA, et al. Germline gain-of-function mutations in SOS1 cause Noonan syndrome. *Nat Genet* 2007; **39**: 70–74.

308 Stofega MR, Herrington J, Billestrup N, Carter-Su C. Mutation of the SHP-2 binding site in growth hormone (GH) receptor prolongs GH-promoted tyrosyl phosphorylation of GH receptor, JAK2, and STAT5B. *Mol Endocrinol* 2000; **14**: 1338–1350.

309 Limal JM, Parfait B, Cabrol S, Bonnet D, Leheup B, Lyonnet S, et al. Noonan syndrome: relationships between genotype, growth, and growth factors. *J Clin Endocrinol Metab* 2006; **91**: 300–306.

310 Ferreira LV, Souza SA, Arnhold IJ, Mendonca BB, Jorge AA. PTPN11 (protein tyrosine phosphatase, nonreceptor type 11) mutations and response to growth hormone therapy in children with Noonan syndrome. *J Clin Endocrinol Metab* 2005; **90**: 5156–5160.

311 Tartaglia M, Gelb BD. Noonan syndrome and related disorders: genetics and pathogenesis. *Annu Rev Genomics Hum Genet* 2005; **6**: 45–68.

312 Walenkamp MJ, Karperien M, Pereira AM, Hilhorst-Hofstee Y, van Doorn J, Chen JW, et al. Homozygous and heterozygous expression of a novel insulin-like growth factor-I mutation. *J Clin Endocrinol Metab* 2005; **90**: 2855–2864.

313 Denley A, Wang CC, McNeil KA, Walenkamp MJ, van Duyvenvoorde H, Wit JM, et al. Structural and functional characteristics of the Val44Met insulin-like growth factor I missense mutation: correlation with effects on growth and development. *Mol Endocrinol* 2005; **19**: 711–721.

314 Bonapace G, Concolino D, Formicola S, Strisciuglio P. A novel mutation in a patient with insulin-like growth factor 1 (IGF1) deficiency. *J Med Genet* 2003; **40**: 913–917.

315 Coutinho DC, Coletta RR, Costa EM, Pachi PR, Boguszewski MC, Damiani D, et al. Polymorphisms identified in the upstream core polyadenylation signal of IGF1 gene exon 6 do not cause pre- and postnatal growth impairment. *J Clin Endocrinol Metab* 2007; **92**: 4889–4892.

316 Arends N, Johnston L, Hokken-Koelega A, van Duijn C, de Ridder M, Savage M, et al. Polymorphism in the IGF-I gene: clinical relevance for short children born small for gestational age (SGA). *J Clin Endocrinol Metab* 2002; **87**: 2720.

317 Johnston LB, Dahlgren J, Leger J, Gelander L, Savage MO, Czernichow P, et al. Association between insulin-like growth factor I (IGF-I) polymorphisms, circulating IGF-I, and pre- and postnatal growth in two European small for gestational age populations. *J Clin Endocrinol Metab* 2003; **88**: 4805–4810.

318 Domene HM, Bengolea SV, Martinez AS, Ropelato MG, Pennisi P, Scaglia P, et al. Deficiency of the circulating insulin-like growth factor system associated with inactivation of the acid-labile subunit gene. *N Engl J Med* 2004; **350**: 570–577.

319 Domene HM, Scaglia PA, Lteif A, Mahmud FH, Kirmani S, Frystyk J, et al. Phenotypic effects of null and haploinsufficiency of acid-labile subunit in a family with two novel IGFALS gene mutations. *J Clin Endocrinol Metab* 2007; **92**: 4444–4450.

320 Hwa V, Haeusler G, Pratt KL, Little BM, Frisch H, Koller D, et al. Total absence of functional acid labile subunit, resulting in severe insulin-like growth factor deficiency and moderate growth failure. *J Clin Endocrinol Metab* 2006; **91**: 1826–1831.

321 Heath KE, Argente J, Barrios V, Pozo J, Diaz-Gonzalez F, Martos-Moreno GA, et al. Primary acid-labile subunit deficiency due to recessive IGFALS mutations results in postnatal growth deficit associated with low circulating IGF-I and IGFBP-3 concentrations, and hyperinsulinemia. *J Clin Endocrinol Metab* 2008; **93**: 1616–1624.

322 Abuzzahab MJ, Schneider A, Goddard A, Grigorescu F, Lautier C, Keller E, et al. IGF-I receptor mutations resulting in intrauterine and postnatal growth retardation. *N Engl J Med* 2003; **349**: 2211–2222.

323 Raile K, Klammt J, Schneider A, Keller A, Laue S, Smith R, et al. Clinical and functional characteristics of the human Arg59Ter insulin-like growth factor i receptor (IGF1R) mutation: implications for a gene dosage effect of the human IGF1R. *J Clin Endocrinol Metab* 2006; **91**: 2264–2271.

324 Kawashima Y, Kanzaki S, Yang F, Kinoshita T, Hanaki K, Nagaishi J, et al. Mutation at cleavage site of insulin-like growth factor receptor in a short-stature child born with intrauterine growth retardation. *J Clin Endocrinol Metab* 2005; **90**: 4679–4687.

325 Inagaki K, Tiulpakov A, Rubtsov P, Sverdlova P, Peterkova V, Yakar S, et al. A familial insulin-like growth factor-I receptor mutant leads to short stature: clinical and biochemical characterization. *J Clin Endocrinol Metab* 2007; **92**: 1542–1548.

326 Peoples R, Milatovich A, Francke U. Hemizygosity at the insulin-like growth factor I receptor (IGF1R) locus and growth failure in the ring chromosome 15 syndrome. *Cytogenet Cell Genet* 1995; **70**: 228–234.

327 Rujirabanjerd S, Suwannarat W, Sripo T, Dissaneevate P, Permsirivanich W, Limprasert P. De novo subtelomeric deletion of 15q associated with satellite translocation in a child with developmental delay and severe growth retardation. *Am J Med Genet A* 2007; **143**: 271–276.

328 Okubo Y, Siddle K, Firth H, O'Rahilly S, Wilson LC, Willatt L, et al. Cell proliferation activities on skin fibroblasts from a short child with absence of one copy of the type 1 insulin-like growth factor receptor (IGF1R) gene and a tall child with three copies of the IGF1R gene. *J Clin Endocrinol Metab* 2003; **88**: 5981–5988.

329 Gicquel C, Rossignol S, Cabrol S, Houang M, Steunou V, Barbu V, et al. Epimutation of the telomeric imprinting center region on chromosome 11p15 in Silver–Russell syndrome. *Nat Genet* 2005; **37**: 1003–1007.

330 Clemmons DR. Value of insulin-like growth factor system markers in the assessment of growth hormone status. *Endocrinol Metab Clin North Am* 2007; **36**: 109–129.

331 Cianfarani S, Liguori A, Boemi S, Maghnie M, Iughetti L, Wasniewska M, et al. Inaccuracy of insulin-like growth factor (IGF) binding protein (IGFBP)-3 assessment in the diagnosis of growth hormone (GH) deficiency from childhood to young adulthood: association to low GH dependency of IGF-II and presence of circulating IGFBP-3 18-kilodalton fragment. *J Clin Endocrinol Metab* 2005; **90**: 6028–6034.

332 Jorge AA, Souza SC, Arnhold IJ, Mendonca BB. Poor reproducibility of IGF-I and IGF binding protein-3 generation test in children with short stature and normal coding region of the GH receptor gene. *J Clin Endocrinol Metab* 2002; **87**: 469–472.

333 Savage MO, Blum WF, Ranke MB, Postel-Vinay MC, Cotterill AM, Hall K, et al. Clinical features and endocrine status in patients with growth hormone insensitivity (Laron syndrome). *J Clin Endocrinol Metab* 1993; **77**: 1465–1471.

334 Rosenfeld RG, Buckway C, Selva K, Pratt KL, Guevara-Aguirre J. Insulin-like growth factor (IGF) parameters and tools for efficacy: the IGF-I generation test in children. *Horm Res* 2004; **62** (Suppl 1): 37–43.

335 Guevara-Aguirre J, Rosenbloom AL, Vasconez O, Martinez V, Gargosky SE, Allen L, et al. Two-year treatment of growth hormone (GH) receptor deficiency with recombinant insulin-like growth factor I in 22 children: comparison of two dosage concentrations and to GH-treated GH deficiency. *J Clin Endocrinol Metab* 1997; **82**: 629–633.

336 Backeljauw PF, Underwood LE. Therapy for 6.5–7.5 years with recombinant insulin-like growth factor I in children with growth hormone insensitivity syndrome: a clinical research center study. *J Clin Endocrinol Metab* 2001; **86**: 1504–1510.

337 Ranke MB, Savage MO, Chatelain PG, Preece MA, Rosenfeld RG, Wilton P. Long-term treatment of growth hormone insensitivity syndrome with IGF-I. Results of the European Multicentre Study. The Working Group on Growth Hormone Insensitivity Syndromes. *Horm Res* 1999; **51**: 128–134.

338 Chernausek SD, Backelauw PF, Frane J, Kuntze J, Underwood LE. Long-term treatment with recombinant insulin-like growth factor (IGF)-I in children with severe IGF-I deficiency due to growth hormone insensitivity. *J Clin Endocrinol Metab* 2007; **92**: 902–910.

339 Collett-Solberg PF, Misra M. The role of recombinant human insulin-like growth factor-I in treating children with short stature. *J Clin Endocrinol Metab* 2008; **93**: 10–18.

340 Camacho-Hubner C, Rose S, Preece MA, Sleevi M, Storr HL, Miraki-Moud F, et al. Pharmacokinetic studies of recombinant human insulin-like growth factor I (rhIGF-I)/rhIGF-binding protein-3 complex administered to patients with growth hormone insensitivity syndrome. *J Clin Endocrinol Metab* 2006; **91**: 1246–1253.

341 Camacho-Hubner C, Underwood LE, Yordam N, Yuksel B, Smith AV, Attie KM, et al. Once daily rhIGF-1/rhIGFBP-3 treatment improves growth in children with severe primary IGF-1 deficiency: results of a multicenter clinical trial. Proceedings of the 88th Annual Meeting of The Endocrine Society, Boston, OR, 40–1: 2006.

342 Clemmons DR. Involvement of insulin-like growth factor-I in the control of glucose homeostasis. *Curr Opin Pharmacol* 2006; **6**: 620–625.

343 Woods KA, Camacho-Hubner C, Bergman RN, Barter D, Clark AJ, Savage MO. Effects of insulin-like growth factor I (IGF-I) therapy on body composition and insulin resistance in IGF-I gene deletion. *J Clin Endocrinol Metab* 2000; **85**: 1407–1411.

344 Lowman HB, Chen YM, Skelton NJ, Mortensen DL, Tomlinson EE, Sadick MD, et al. Molecular mimics of insulin-like growth factor 1 (IGF-1) for inhibiting IGF-1: IGF-binding protein interactions. *Biochemistry* 1998; **37**: 8870–8878.

345 Coya R, Vela A, Perez dN, Rica I, Castano L, Busturia MA, et al. Panhypopituitarism: genetic versus acquired etiological factors. *J Pediatr Endocrinol Metab* 2007; **20**: 27–36.

346 Sobrier ML, Maghnie M, Vie-Luton MP, Secco A, Di Iorgi N, Lorini R, *et al.* Novel HESX1 mutations associated with a life-threatening neonatal phenotype, pituitary aplasia, but normally located posterior pituitary and no optic nerve abnormalities. *J Clin Endocrinol Metab* 2006; **91**: 4528–4536.

347 Sobrier ML, Netchine I, Heinrichs C, Thibaud N, Vie-Luton MP, Van Vliet G, *et al.* Alu-element insertion in the homeodomain of HESX1 and aplasia of the anterior pituitary. *Hum Mutat* 2005; **25**: 503.

5 Acquired Disorders of the Hypothalamo-Pituitary Axis

Kyriaki S. Alatzoglou[1] & Mehul T. Dattani[2]

[1] Developmental Endocrinology Research Group, UCL Institute of Child Health, London, UK
[2] Developmental Endocrinology Research Group, UCL Institute of Child Health and Great Ormond Street Hospital for Children, London, UK

The pituitary gland and hypothalamus are central regulators of growth, metabolism and development. Hypopituitarism is the deficiency of one or more pituitary hormones and has a prevalence of 45 cases per million and an annual incidence of about 4 cases per 100 000 [1]. The fine balance of the hypothalamo-pituitary axis can be affected by a variety of pathological conditions that lead to hormone deficiencies or dysregulation [2]. These include tumors affecting the hypothalamo-pituitary area, damage secondary to trauma, surgery, irradiation, infection, autoimmune processes, infiltration by granulomatous disease or iron overload states and vascular causes (Table 5.1).

CNS tumors

Tumors in the hypothalamo-pituitary area may cause endocrine disturbance either directly, or secondary to treatment (surgery, radiotherapy). Clinically evident endocrine effects are caused by hormone hypersecretion from the mass or, more commonly, from pituitary hormone deficiencies. These are the result of direct pressure of the expanding mass on the anterior pituitary cells and, in case of hypothalamic and stalk involvement, secondary to reduced synthesis and transport of hypothalamic releasing hormones. Furthermore, hypothalamic involvement leads to important non-endocrine sequelae such as temperature dysregulation, hyperphagia, obesity and sleep disorders that affect the quality of life of survivors.

Growth hormone (GH) secreting cells are especially vulnerable to pressure effects and radiation injury. As a result, GH deficiency and growth failure are early endocrine manifestations, followed by gonadotropin and thyroid stimulating hormone deficiency. Because of the proximity of the sellar area to vital structures (ventricles, optic nerves and chiasm), pituitary tumors in chil-

dren often present with signs and symptoms of increased intracranial pressure or visual disturbances [3]. Tumors that affect the pituitary area can be benign or malignant, cystic or solid. Rarely they are secondary to metastases from distant organs in children. Tumors of the sellar area are summarized in Table 5.2.

Craniopharyngioma

Epidemiology and histology

Craniopharyngiomas are rare epithelial tumors of embryonal origin, derived from remnants of Rathke's pouch [4]. In children they represent 5–15% of intracranial tumors and are the most common neoplasm of the hypothalamo-pituitary area, accounting for approximately 80% of tumors in this location [5,6]. Their incidence is 1.3 per million per year and about one-quarter affect children younger than 14 years [7]. In the UK, there are 15 new cases per year in children under 15 years of age [8]. There is a bimodal peak in incidence, the first between 5 and 14 years and the second in adults older than 50 years. However, they can be diagnosed at any age and have even been reported in the neonatal period [9–11].

At presentation, most craniopharyngiomas have a combined intrasellar and suprasellar location (74.2%) and almost half have hypothalamic involvement (51.6%). A smaller percentage is exclusively suprasellar (22.6%) or confined within the sella turcica (6–3%). Almost one-third invade the floor of the third ventricle and may cause obstructive hydrocephalus [12,13]. Craniopharyngiomas in children are predominantly cystic (56.7%), multicystic (16.7%), predominantly solid (13.3%), purely solid (10%) or purely cystic (3.3%). The cystic fluid is viscous and rich in cholesterol and the incidence of calcification is much higher in children (83.3%) than adults [14].

There are two main histological types: the adamantinomatous type, which consists of epithelial neoplastic cells that resemble those found in lesions of the jaw (the more common) and the papillary type found almost exclusively in adults. Although

Brook's Clinical Pediatric Endocrinology, 6th edition. Edited by C. Brook, P. Clayton, R. Brown. © 2009 Blackwell Publishing, ISBN: 978-1-4051-8080-1.

Table 5.1 Causes of acquired hypopituitarism.

I. Tumors in/around pituitary area

1 *Solid or mixed lesions*
Craniopharygioma
Germinoma
Optic glioma
Dysgerminoma
Ependymoma
Pituitary adenoma
Meningioma
Chordoma

2 *Cystic lesions*
Rathke's cleft cyst
Arachnoid cyst
Dermoid cyst

3 *Metastatic tumors* (rare)
i.e. Childhood Hodgkin and nasopharyngeal carcinoma

II. Radiotherapy

1 Radiotherapy for CNS tumors (locally and for tumors located distally)
2 CNS irradiation for hematologic malignancies and bone marrow transplant

III. Brain trauma

1 Traumatic brain injury (e.g. road traffic accident, child abuse, accidental)
2 Post neurosurgery
3 Subarachnoid hemorrhage (pituitary apoplexy, vascular causes)

IV. Inflammation/infection

1 Meningitis, encephalitis
2 Pituitary abscess
3 Sarcoidosis
4 Tuberculosis
5 Auto-immune processes: i.e. autoimmune lymphocytic hypophysitis

V. Infiltration

1 Langerhans cell histiocytosis
2 Iron overload: hemochromatosis, thalassemia and diseases requiring chronic transfusions

VI. Psychosocial deprivation

Table 5.2 Tumors involving the hypothalamo-pituitary area.

Craniopharyngioma
Pituitary adenoma
Optic tract glioma
Pilocytic astrocytoma
Ependymoma
Germinoma
Hamartoma
Meningioma
Rathke's cleft cyst
Dermoid/epidermoid cyst
Arachnoid cyst
Langerhans cell histiocytosis

---

craniopharyngiomas are histologically benign, they can extend from their initial site, develop papillae and invade surrounding tissues including the hypothalamus and optic chiasm. This attachment makes their complete excision difficult, if not impossible, and contributes to tumor recurrence and morbidity.

Genetics

Craniopharyngiomas are sporadic but there have been rare case reports of affected family members suggesting recessive inheritance [15,16]. Genetic studies aim to elucidate their origin and pathogenesis and to identify markers that can predict the behavior of the tumor. The genetic basis of these tumors is unclear. Multiple chromosomal abnormalities, including deletions and translocations, have been reported in a few cases [17,18] but subsequent studies did not yield consistent results [19].

Only a small subset of craniopharyngiomas (two of eight tumors examined) are monoclonal, deriving from a single progenitor cell [20]. Further study of tumors with monoclonal characteristics using comparative genomic hybridization (CGH), showed no genetic abnormality in 30%, whereas 67% (6 of 9) exhibited at least one change. The most common genetic abnormality was an increase in the DNA copy number with different areas being involved (i.e. 1p32-tel, 9q22-tel, 12q22-tel, 22q12-tel) [21]. However, a recent study of 11 pediatric adamantinomatous craniopharyngiomas using CGH showed no alteration in the DNA copy number, suggesting that the acquisition of chromosomal imbalances is a rare event and probably does not have a role on the etiology of childhood craniopharyngiomas [22]. A possible explanation for these conflicting results may be that most studies do not discriminate between early and late onset forms of the disease.

Candidate genes for the pathogenesis of craniopharyngiomas include *patched (PTCH)* and potential oncogenes such as those coding for the alpha subunits of the stimulatory (*Gsa*) or inhibitory (*Gi2a*) GTP-binding protein. So far mutations have been identified in neither them [20] nor in the tumor suppression gene *p53* [23]. There is evidence, however, that the activation of β-catenin may have a role in the pathogenesis of adamantinomatous craniopharyngiomas. β-Catenin is a cytoplasmic protein important for cell–cell adhesion and association with cadherins. It is also a downstream component of the *Wnt* signaling pathway that regulates many developmental processes such as cell proliferation, axis orientation and organ development. Sekine *et al.* [24] found mutations in β-catenin in all adamantinomatous craniopharyngiomas they examined. Although further studies confirmed that it is the adamantinomatous, and not papillary, craniopharyngiomas that have heterozygous missense mutations in β-catenin, the reported rate was lower (16%, 7 of the 43 examined) [25].

Presentation

At presentation most children (up to 75%) have symptoms related to increased intracranial pressure, including headache, vomiting and visual disturbances (Table 5.3) [26]. Compared with adults, the incidence of headache, nausea or vomiting and hydrocephalus are significantly higher in children [13].

Seventy to 80% of children have evidence of endocrine deficiencies at presentation (Table 5.4) and growth failure is observed in 32–52%. Low concentrations of IGF-1 have been reported in 80% of children at time of diagnosis [26–28]. GH deficiency is the most common hormone deficiency, documented in 75–100% of those tested before treatment, followed by adenocrticotropic hormone (ACTH; 20–70%) and thyroid stimulating hormone (TSH; 3–30%) deficiencies [13,26,29,30]. Compression of the pituitary stalk or damage of hypothalamic dopaminergic neurons results in elevated prolactin (PRL) concentrations in 8–20% of children at diagnosis.

Table 5.3 Symptoms at presentation in 41 cases of childhood craniopharyngiomas. (After Karavitaki *et al.* [13].)

Symptom	Percentage (%)
Headache	78
Nausea/vomiting	54
Visual field defects	46
Decreased visual acuity	39
Growth failure	32
Papilloedema	29
Cranial nerve palsies	27
Anorexia/weight loss	20
Poor energy	22
Lethargy	17
Polyuria/polydipsia	15
Cognitive impairment	10
Change in behavior	10
Decrease consciousness/coma	10
Optic atrophy	5
Hyperphagia/excessive weight gain	5
Ataxia/unsteadiness	7
Hemiparesis	7
Blindness	3

Table 5.4 Incidence of pituitary hormone deficiencies and hyperprolactinemia in children with craniopharyngioma at diagnosis. Data are presented as percentage of patients tested for the defect.

Study	GHD	ACTHD	TSHD	GnD	PRL	DI
Karavitaki *et al.* [13]	100%	68%	25%	–	–	22%
deVries *et al.* [26]	85%	71%	2.7%	–	8%	52%
Bin-Abbas *et al.* [28]	–	19%	25%	–	–	32%
Honegger *et al.* [30]	74%	27%	20%	91%	17%	10%
DeVile *et al.* [31]	87%	32%	32%	50%	32%	29%
Sklar *et al.* [27]	75%	25%	25%	40%	20%	–

ACTHD, adenocorticotropic hormone deficiency; DI, diabetes insipidus; GHD, growth hormone deficiency; GnD, gonadotropin deficiency; PRL, prolactin; TSHD, thyroid stimulating hormone deficiency.

The incidence of diabetes insipidus (DI) at presentation varies between 10 and 29% of patients, depending on the study [31]. However, in a recent study almost half of patients had DI at presentation. The authors suggested that the incidence of DI is either underestimated or may be masked by the simultaneous presence of ACTH deficiency [26].

In adolescents, craniopharyngiomas present with delayed puberty or pubertal arrest: in a series of 56 patients, all adolescents complained of delayed puberty [26]. This is consistent with the finding that hypogonadism is one of the most frequent presenting complaints in adults [4]. Rare presentations include precious puberty [32] and the syndrome of inappropriate antidiuretic hormone secretion (SIADH) [33].

Compared with adults, there is no significant difference in the incidence of GH, ACTH and TSH deficiency or DI in children. In contrast to what is observed in other pituitary tumors, such as adenomas, the treatment of craniopharyngioma does not reverse the pre-existing pituitary deficiencies [4].

Magnetic resonance imaging findings

Craniopharyngiomas appear as mass lesions in the sellar and/or suprasellar area which may extend to the hypothalamus and invade the third ventricle. Adamantinomatous craniopharyngiomas are predominantly cystic and the cystic portion of the lesion appears hyperintense in T1 and T2 images. The solid part of the tumor shows areas of high and low signal intensity that represent areas of calcification and hemosiderin deposits [34]. In the majority of cases (58–76%) the size of craniopharyngiomas, as estimated by magnetic resonance imaging (MRI) or computed tomography (CT), has been reported to be 2–4 cm, while it is smaller than 2 cm in 4–28% of cases and more than 4 cm in 14–20% [6,14,35]. The imaging characteristics of craniopharyngiomas may provide clues for the differential diagnosis from other mass lesions in the area (Figs 5.1–5.3).

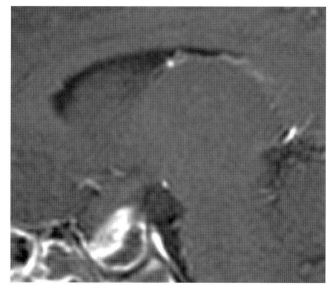

Figure 5.1 Craniopharyngioma. Enhancing solid mass with cystic component occupying the sella turcica.

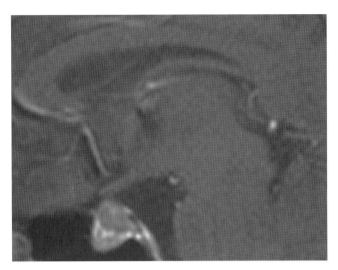

Figure 5.2 Pituitary adenoma. Mass that involves the pituitary gland, with parasellar extension.

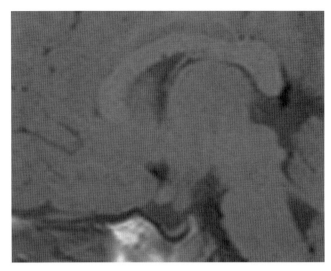

Figure 5.3 Langerhans cell histiocytosis. Thickened pituitary stalk, absence of the bright spot of posterior pituitary and anterior pituitary hypoplasia.

Treatment and outcome

Management is complex, controversial and best achieved by a multidisciplinary approach in specialized centers (Fig. 5.4). Aims of treatment are to relieve acute signs and symptoms of compression (raised intracranial pressure, threatening visual failure), to preserve hypothalamic function, thus reducing later morbidity and mortality, and to provide long-term control and prevent recurrence [36–38].

The extent of surgical resection is probably the most important factor influencing recurrence of craniopharyngioma [39]. In patients who had surgery only, the 10-year recurrence-free survival rate after total removal was 83%, after subtotal removal 50.5% and after partial removal 15.6%. Tumors usually recur in the first 5 years and relatively rarely thereafter [14], although, even after complete resection confirmed radiologically, relapses can occur in 15–25% of patients [14,39]. In older series, when patients were treated with radical and repeated surgical resections, mortality was high (25–50%) and hypothalamic, visual and cognitive morbidity occurred in the vast majority (75%), especially in craniopharyngiomas with suprasellar or retro-chiasmatic extension [12].

Guidelines for the multidisciplinary management of children with craniopharyngioma have been published [8,36,37] and patients can be categorized in two risk groups with respect to management and prognosis. The good risk group includes older children with small tumors (2–4 cm) and no hypothalamic syndrome or hydrocephalus, while younger children with larger tumors (>2–4 cm) and hypothalamic syndrome or hydrocephalus have a poor risk. Complete radical resection, with or without adjuvant radiotherapy, is suggested for the good risk group, while limited surgery and immediate or delayed radiotherapy is the treatment of choice for the poor risk group [37,40].

Although clinical characteristics of the tumor have been shown to be prognostic for relapse (i.e. size and location) [41], there are still no identified biochemical factors to predict the behavior of

the tumor and recurrence risk. Studies have focused on factors responsible for the vascularization of the tumor and expression of molecules that mediate adhesiveness to surrounding tissues. Study of the expression of vascular endothelial growth factor (VEGF) and the microvascular density (MVD) of craniopharyngiomas have shown that VEGF expression and MVD were higher in the adamantinomatous than papillary type. This agrees with the observation that the former have a tendency to infiltrate and relapse but there was no significant difference in the expression pattern between patients who had recurrence and those who remained recurrence free [42].

The tendency of craniopharyngiomas to adhere to surrounding tissues may be regulated by the expression of integrins and galectins, which are members of the lectin family and modulate the function of integrins. Adamantinomatous craniopharyngiomas express integrin subunits (i.e. a2,a5,b1,b5), while optic chiasm and pituitary stalk express vibronectin, thrombospondin and forms of collagen. The interaction between these molecules may explain the adhesiveness to these tissues. This interaction is likely to be more complex and correlations with clinical characteristics are yet to be made [43].

Pituitary adenomas

Pituitary adenomas represent less than 3% of supratentorial tumors in childhood and about 3.5–6% of all surgically treated pediatric pituitary tumors. In most cases they are hormonally active, arising from any of the five cell types of the anterior pituitary, and may produce prolactin (prolactinomas, 52%), ACTH leading to Cushing disease (corticotropinomas 33.3%), GH (somatotropinomas 8%) or, more rarely, TSH (thyrotropinomas). Non-functioning pituitary adenomas are rare in children (2.7%) compared to adults where they represent almost 20% of pituitary adenomas. While the majority of childhood pituitary adenomas are prolactinomas pre-

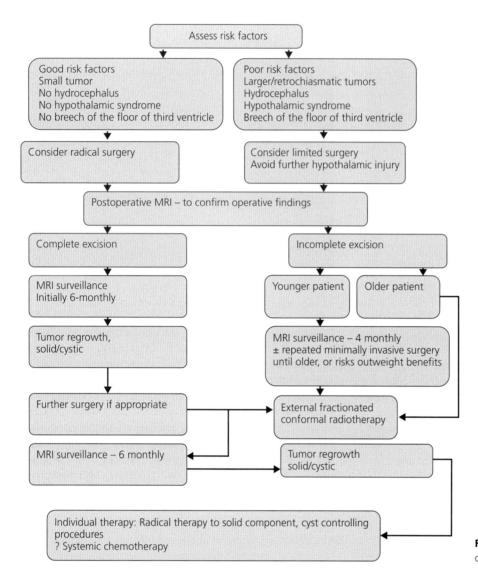

Figure 5.4 Recommended management plan for a child with craniopharyngioma. (After Spoudeas [8].)

senting in adolescence, corticotropinomas are the most common tumors in prepubertal children [44,45].

Pituitary adenomas occur in isolation or may be part of a genetic syndrome such as multiple endocrine neoplasia type 1 (MEN1), McCune–Albright syndrome or Carney complex [46]. Their pathogenesis is not clear but there is increasing evidence that dysregulation in hormone receptor signaling, changes in molecules that regulate cell cycle or are important for adhesion to extracellular matrix, as well as changes in growth factors may be implicated [47].

Their clinical presentation results from pituitary hormone hypersecretion or deficiencies, disruption of growth and sexual maturation, and pressure effects. On MRI, pituitary adenomas show slow uptake of gadolinium and appear as hypo-enhancing lesions that may displace the pituitary stalk [34].

Prolactinomas

Prolactinomas are the most common pituitary adenoma. The majority are microprolactinomas and present in children older than 12 years with a female preponderance (female to male ratio 4.5:1) [44]. Macroadenomas are more frequent at diagnosis in boys than in girls, although this difference does not appear to be significant (76.2% vs 48.3%; $P = 0.09$) [48]. In prepubertal children, prolactinomas present with headache, visual disturbance and growth failure. Around puberty the main symptoms arise from the suppression of gonadotropin secretion, either as a result of hyperprolactinemia, or secondary to local compression. Females present with amenorrhea or menstrual irregularities, pubertal arrest and galactorrhea. In a series reported by Cannavo et al. [49], the incidence of galactorrhea was as high as 91%. Adolescent males present with symptoms related to mass effect, such as headache and visual impairment, as well as pubertal arrest and growth failure. Almost one-third of patients with prolactinomas have additional pituitary hormone deficiencies. Associated hormone deficiencies are rare in microprolactinomas (4.7%), whereas they are common in patients with macroprolactinomas and extrasellar extension (77.8%) [48,49].

For the diagnosis of prolactinoma, it is important to obtain both radiological (MRI) and biochemical evidence of sustained hyperprolactinemia. In children, as in adults, serum prolactin usually parallels the tumor size and patients with prolactin concentration exceeding 2–3000 mU/L are likely to have a prolactinoma. However, moderate elevation of PRL concentration may be the result of pituitary stalk compression by another tumor, rather than a prolactinoma per se. Therefore, the differential diagnosis should include secondary hyperprolactinemia resulting from impaired hypothalamic production of dopamine or stalk compression (e.g. sellar and parasellar masses, granulomatous infiltration, head trauma), medication (i.e. phenothiazines, metoclopramide) and the presence of macroprolactin [50,51].

Unless there are complications requiring surgical decompression (visual loss, hydrocephalus), the treatment of choice is pharmacological with dopamine agonists. Bromocriptine at a dose ranging from 2.5 to 20 mg/day orally achieves normalization of prolactin concentrations in 38.5% of patients but side effects, including gastrointestinal disturbance and postural hypotension, often lead to poor compliance. Cabergoline, at doses ranging from 0.5 to 3.5 mg/week, is effective in adolescent patients with large tumors and appears to be better tolerated than bromocriptine [52] but there are studies reporting clinically significant mitral valve regurgitation in patients on long-term cabergoline [53]. This effect seems to be dose dependent and has been observed in adult patients treated for Parkinson's disease with higher dosing regimens than the ones used for the treatment of prolactinomas. Irrespective of the type of treatment, the reduction of tumor size, by dopamine agonists or surgery, may result in restoration of normal pituitary function [54].

Corticotropinomas

Corticotropinomas are the most common pituitary adenomas in prepubertal children, representing up to 54.8% of pituitary adenomas in those under 11 years of age [44]. Cushing disease caused by an ACTH-secreting pituitary adenoma is the most common cause of Cushing syndrome in children over 5 years of age [55]. Corticotropinomas are usually microadenomas, with a diameter less than 5 mm, while macroadenomas are rare and have been described as an early manifestation of MEN1 [56].

Children present clinically with rapid weight gain and characteristic changes in facial appearance (100%), striae (53–64%), hypertension (32–47%), emotional liability (53%) and fatigue (59–64%), while muscle weakness and easy bruising are rare [55,57]. Other features include virilization and pseudoprecocious puberty [58]. Psychological changes observed include compulsive behavior and overachievement at school, which differ from the depression and memory and sleep problems observed in adults [45]. The growth pattern is characterized by short stature (height less than −2 SD in 40%), with a discrepancy between height SD and body mass index (BMI) SD [55].

Diagnostic investigations include endocrine and radiological investigations as well as bilateral inferior petrosal sinus sampling (BIPSS) [59,60]. BIPSS leads to successful localization of the microadenoma in 58–74% of patients [57,61]. The treatment of choice is transphenoidal excision and the cure rate ranges between 45% and 78% depending on series, while almost 40% require postoperative radiotherapy to achieve remission [62–64]. Postoperative complications include growth hormone deficiency (36%), transient DI (12%), panhypopituitarism (4%) and transient cerebrospinal fluid rhinorrhea (4%) [57].

Optic gliomas

Tumors of the optic pathway represent 4–6% of all pediatric intracranial tumors and the most common are optic gliomas (65%). Most are low-grade lesions with favorable prognosis if treated optimally [65]. Gliomas confined to the optic nerve have a predilection for females (60–70%) and are associated with neurofibromatosis type 1 (NF-1) in more than half of cases, while 38% are sporadic. Children with sporadic gliomas are more likely to manifest increased intracranial pressure, decreased visual activity and endocrine complications [66]. The most frequent symptoms at presentation are visual defects (diminished vision, optic atrophy, strabismus, nystagmus, proptosis), ataxia and precocious puberty [67].

Because of their close anatomic relation to the hypothalamus and pituitary, dysregulation of the hypothalamo-pituitary axis is common and brought about either by the tumor itself or secondary to treatment. Premature sexual maturation (PSM) is a frequently presenting symptom, while the most common defect post cranial irradiation is growth hormone deficiency (GHD) [68]. In a study of 100 patients with precocious puberty caused by central lesions, 45 had been diagnosed with optic glioma or astrocytoma. All patients treated for optic glioma had hypothalamo-pituitary deficiencies, including GHD (100%), thyrotropin deficiency (71.4%), ACTH deficiency (12.5%) and gonadotropin deficiency (34.3%) [69]. Because this study was designed to investigate patients who presented with central precocious puberty, with respect to its etiology, the high incidence of endocrine abnormalities may be a result of selection bias.

In another series of 68 children treated for optic glioma the incidence of endocrine dysfunction was 42.6% and GHD occurred in 38%. Hypogonadotropic hypogonadism was diagnosed in 36% (9 of 25 teenage patients), hypothyroidism in 20.5%, PSM in 19.6% of the age-specific population, and hypoadrenalism and DI each in 11.8%. All patients with ACTH deficiency also had GHD and hypothyroidism [70]. In the same study GHD and hypogonadism were significantly correlated with radiotherapy and there was also significant association between tumor resection and hypoadrenalism, hypothyroidism and DI.

Cystic lesions

Cystic lesions in the pituitary area include Rathke's cleft cysts, arachnoidal cysts, cystic adenomas and craniopharyngiomas.

Rathke's cleft cysts are benign remnants of Rathke's pouch. They are usually small (less than 5 mm), asymptomatic and found in almost 20% of routine autopsies [71]. They consist of well-differentiated columnar or cuboidal epithelial cells and the content of the cyst varies. Rathke's cleft cysts can grow and become symptomatic, especially if they have suprasellar extension. Symptoms include headache, visual defects and pituitary dysfunction ranging from increased prolactin to pituitary hormone deficiencies [72]. Differential diagnosis from other cystic lesions in the area is not always easy, because the cyst fluid shows variable signal intensities on MRI and can appear as hypo- or hyperdense. Almost 50% of Rathke's cleft cysts show rim enhancement. Treatment should include both fluid drainage and cyst wall removal in order to avoid relapses [73] and recurrence is rare (2 of 14 patients in one series).

Arachnoid cysts consist of a collection of cerebrospinal fluid (CSF)-like fluid surrounded by a wall made of arachnoid structures. They are mainly suprasellar, with only rare cases being intrasellar [74]. Suprasellar cysts are usually diagnosed following non-endocrine symptoms such as neurological deficits, macrocephaly and visual symptoms, as was demonstrated in a study of 30 patients (mean age at diagnosis 4.3 ± 1 year) [75]. Because of the proximity of the lesion to the hypothalamo-pituitary area, arachnoid cysts may cause central precocious puberty, amenorrhea and hyperprolactinemia in addition to thyrotropin, ACTH or GH deficiency and almost one-third of patients develop precocious puberty. Precocious puberty may be followed by pubertal arrest, a sequence that may be the result of hypothalamo-pituitary dysfunction [75].

A study of 100 patients with precocious puberty caused by CNS lesions showed that 10% of cases were due to suprasellar arachnoid cysts and 60% of patients with arachnoid cysts were also GH deficient [69]. When it comes to treatment, the use of endoscopic exploration during transphenoid surgery offers advantages for the management of cystic pituitary lesions [76].

Traumatic brain injury

Traumatic brain injury has been recognized as a cause of acquired hypopituitarism in a number of adult studies. Data on pediatric patients are sporadic but there is a growing awareness that hypopituitarism is under-diagnosed with possible negative effects on growth and development [77]. These effects may be significant considering the scale of the problem: in the UK, 180 children per 100 000 population per year sustain a head injury, with 5.6 per 100 000 requiring intensive care of whom almost one-third undergo neurosurgery. The incidence of traumatic brain injury peaks in adolescence and early adulthood, with rates approaching 250 per 100 000 [78,79].

Although the pituitary gland is protected within the sella turcica, the rich vascular network of the hypothalamus and pituitary and the structure of the pituitary stalk make it vulnerable to the effects of trauma (Table 5.5). The pathophysiology of hypopituitarism related to trauma is not clearly defined but it is

Table 5.5 Mechanisms of pituitary damage in traumatic brain injury.

I. Ischemia and infarction
Vascular rupture
Vascular compression secondary to edema/increased intracranial pressure
Hypovolemia/hypotension
Hypoxia
Vasospasm

II. Direct trauma to:
Anterior pituitary
Hypothalamic nuclei
Stalk transection
Basal skull trauma

thought that it is the result of direct trauma or of vascular injury resulting in ischemia and infarction [80,81]. This is supported by the anatomical findings of autopsies following head trauma, which include anterior lobe necrosis, pituitary fibrosis, hemorrhage, infarction or necrosis of the pituitary stalk [82].

It is of note that the peripheral layer of anterior pituitary cells, under the capsule, receive arterial blood from the capsule and not from the system of portal veins and this may explain why these cells and those in a small area adjacent to the posterior lobe are the only surviving cells in cases of pure anterior lobe necrosis [83]. Somatotrope cells are located in the wings of the pituitary gland, their vascular supply comes from portal vessels and they are vulnerable to the disruption of blood supply after head injury. However, ACTH and TSH secreting cells are located in the medial portion of the pituitary and receive blood supply from portal vessels and the anterior pituitary artery. This may explain why GHD is the most common deficiency seen after trauma [84].

Hormone deficiencies may be identified in the first days to weeks post trauma (acute phase) or may develop over time (late effect). Because there is overlap between the symptoms and signs of hypopituitarism and those of neuropsychological sequelae, it is possible that late-evolving or partial deficiencies can remain undiagnosed for long periods. It is not surprising, therefore, that in different studies the time to diagnosis ranges from 1 to 40 years [83,85–88].

Acute phase

In the acute phase, alterations in endocrine function may reflect an adaptive response to acute illness. The clinically significant alterations involve mainly the regulation of fluid and electrolyte balance (DI, SIADH, cerebral salt wasting) and the hypothalamo-pituitary-adrenal axis. Most of the pituitary hormone changes observed in the acute phase are transient and their development cannot predict the development of permanent hypopituitarism [88]. It has been suggested recently that trauma severity may be the only predictor of permanent hypopituitarism [89], although not all studies have arrived at this conclusion.

It would appear that the majority of patients show a degree of pituitary hormone dysfunction in the first days after brain trauma (53–76%) but there is wide variation in the reported hormone responses, which reflects differences in patient selection and time of testing [90]. All anterior pituitary hormones can be affected [82].

In a study of 50 adult patients evaluated at a median of 12 days after injury, almost all (80%) had evidence of hypogonadism and there was positive correlation between serum testosterone concentration and Glasgow Coma Scale (GCS) scores upon admission [87]. This is a high percentage compared to studies that have shown evidence of hypogonadotropic hypogonadism in only 24–67% of patients in the acute setting [89,90]. It is not clear if this acute decline in the function of gonadotropes is the result of direct injury and hypoxia or if it represents an adaptive mechanism at the time of illness to downregulate the synthesis of anabolic steroids and conserve metabolic substrates for vital organs.

In the first days after injury, almost 50% of patients have hyperprolactinemia, 18% show subnormal GH response and 16% have abnormal cortisol response to provocation, while TSH deficiency is evident in 2% [91]. The diagnosis of ACTH and subsequent glucocorticoid deficiency in the acute phase is difficult. At the time of critical illness there is activation of the hypothalamo-pituitary-adrenal axis, lowering of corticosteroid binding globulin, increased free cortisol and increased tissue sensitivity to glucocorticoids [92]. Therefore, the available normal values do not represent an appropriate response to acute stress and dynamic testing is usually contraindicated in the acute setting. Acute glucocorticoid insufficiency may be life-threatening but it seems that there is no reliable factor to predict the development of ACTH deficiency in patients with traumatic brain injury. There is no difference in GCS, CT scan appearance or presence of other pituitary hormone deficiencies between ACTH deficient and ACTH sufficient patients but ACTH deficient patients tend to have lower basal serum cortisol concentration [82]. A high index of suspicion is required for early diagnosis and treatment.

A well-recognized and potentially hazardous complication of the acute phase is DI. Its incidence varies between 2.9% and 26% depending on the series and criteria used for diagnosis [93,94].

The variation in the reported incidence may also be because its diagnosis may be missed in cases of partial DI or if there is concomitant ACTH deficiency. In a recent prospective study of 50 patients, Agha et al. [94] diagnosed DI and partial DI in 26% of patients in the acute phase, an incidence that is higher than in previously reported series. The incidence of acute DI was associated with more severe head injury and there were no new cases after the acute phase. The majority of patients recovered after 6 months (69%): only 6% had permanent DI 12 months after the injury [94].

Permanent endocrine sequelae

Pituitary hormone deficiencies present in the acute phase are usually transient but may persist, appear or evolve over time (Table 5.6). In adults, the incidence of permanent hypopituitarism ranges between 23% and 69%, depending on the study. The growth hormone axis is most frequently affected (10–33%), followed by the gonadal (8–23%), adrenal (5–23%) and thyroid (2–22%) axes. The prevalence of permanent DI varies between 0 and 6% [85,94–96].

There are sporadic reports of hypopituitarism following traumatic brain injury in children but prospective studies are in progress (Table 5.6). The incidence of hypopituitarism is reported to range from 10% to 60% and although this is lower in children than adults, it is not uncommon [97–99]. In general, the long-term outcome of brain injury seems to be more favorable in children but recent studies have shown that the problem was probably underestimated. More than half of children (67%) who sustain head injury before the age of 2 years have mild disability at a 2-year follow-up and less than half (45%) function at a level appropriate for age [100]. Furthermore, in a prospective study of 330 children with moderate or severe head injury, 40% had measurable impairment in health related quality of life [101]. The extent to which endocrine dysfunction contributes to these outcomes has yet to be defined.

GHD appears to be the main endocrine manifestation, followed by gonadotropin deficiency. GHD can present as growth failure, while delayed or arrested puberty and secondary amenorrhea may present in adolescents and in patients in the transition phase. Hypopituitarism may contribute to the lack of energy,

Table 5.6 Incidence of late hypopituitarism following traumatic brain injury (TBI).

Study	n	Age	Interval TBI/diagnosis	AP dysfunction (%)	GH (%)	ACTH (%)	Gonadal (%)	Thyroid (%)	DI (%)
Kelly et al. [84]	22	Adult	3 months–23 years	36	18	4.5	22	4.5	
Lieberman et al. [85]	70	18–58	1 month–23 years	68	15	7	–	22	–
Agha et al. [87]	102	15–65	6–36 months	28.4	10.7	12.7	11.8	1	
Leal-Cerro et al. [95]	170	29.2 ± 1.1	12 months–5 years	25	5.8	6.4	17	5.8	
Aimaretti et al. [96]	70	39.3 ± 2.4	3 and 12 months	22.7	20	7.1	11.4	5.7	2.8
Tanriverdi et al. [88]	52	Adult	12 months	51	33	19	8	6	
Klose et al. [89]	46	19–63	0–12 days & 3, 6 and 12 months	10.5 (4% isolated)	10.5	6.5	2	2	2

fatigability and reduced bone mineral density that can be seen after severe head trauma [102]. In a number of case reports, central precocious puberty has been described in association with head injury presenting 0.4–1.6 years after the event [103].

In 23 patients aged 16–25 years followed up at 3 years after the event, hypopituitarism was present in 35% and the most common finding was an isolated pituitary hormone deficiency in 21.7%, followed by panhypopituitarism in 8.6%, and multiple hormone deficiencies in 4.3%. Retesting these patients at 1 year showed that hypopituitarism remained in 30% and GH and gonadotropin deficiencies were the main abnormalities [97]. Of 48 pediatric patients studied after moderate to severe head trauma and evaluated prospectively (n = 26) or retrospectively (n = 22), there was evidence of hypothalamo-pituitary dysfunction at 6 months to 7 years in five (10.4%). Two patients had isolated GHD, one ACTH deficiency, one gonadotropin deficiency and one combined GH/ACTH/TSH and gonadotropin deficiency. The only case of reported DI was transient [98].

In contrast to the above mentioned studies, Niederland *et al.* [99] reported that 61% of children with history of traumatic brain injury had pituitary dysfunction almost 3 years after head trauma and 42% (11 of 26) had GHD. Although complete auxological data were missing, it seemed that this subgroup did not show any slowing of the growth rate prior to diagnosis compared with children who had sufficient GH response. Basal cortisol concentration was suboptimal in 34% (9/26), 12% had an inappropriate TSH response to TRH stimulation and one patient had an increased PRL concentration [99].

Patients with hypopituitarism after head injury may have no clinical signs and symptoms suggestive of this disorder and prompt diagnosis requires a high degree of suspicion [104]. A consensus guideline on screening suggests that all patients who had traumatic brain injury, regardless of its severity, should undergo baseline endocrine evaluation 3 and 12 months after the event or discharge from ITU [105]. For children and adolescents, an algorithm for endocrine assessment and follow-up has also been suggested [77].

Infiltrative and inflammatory disorders

Hypophysitis

Hypophysitis is an inflammation of the pituitary gland that can be either primary or secondary to infection, systemic disease or irritation from adjacent lesions (Table 5.7). This inflammatory process mimics tumors of the pituitary area clinically and radiologically [106]. There are three histological types of primary hypophysitis: lymphocytic, granulomatous and xanthomatous.

Lymphocytic hypophysitis is the most common, involving the anterior pituitary and sometimes infiltrating the infundibulum and posterior lobe. Lymphocytic hypophysitis occurs mainly in young women and is associated with pregnancy or the presence of autoimmune diseases, including Hashimoto thyroiditis, Graves disease, type 1 diabetes and systemic lupus erythematosus (SLE)

Table 5.7 Main causes of hypophysitis.

I. Primary hypophysitis
Lymphocytic
Granulomatous
Xanthomatous

II. Secondary hypophysitis
Local lesions
Germinomas
Craniopharyngiomas
Pituitary adenomas

Systemic disease
Sarcoidosis
Wegener granulomatosis
Langerhans cell histiocytosis
Tuberculosis

[107]. In all histological types of hypophysitis, the underlying mechanism involves T-cell toxicity mediated by CD8+ T cells [108].

Primary hypophysitis can present with symptoms and signs of increased intracranial pressure, pressure on adjacent structures (i.e. headaches, visual disturbances, cranial nerve palsies) and pituitary hormone deficiencies. Data from adult studies show that the majority of patients (94%) have evidence of at least one pituitary hormone deficiency, the most common being gonadotropin deficiency (82%), followed by TSH (77%), ACTH (71%) and GH (62%) deficiencies. Hyperprolactinemia has been documented in 21% and posterior pituitary dysfunction and DI in 45% of cases. It would appear that the most severe endocrine deficiencies are observed in the granulomatous type. In these cases MRI scanning reveals enlargement of the pituitary gland with thickening of the stalk, and about 60% show suprasellar extension [109].

There are case reports of hypophysitis in children and adolescents and in most cases diagnosis has been made only after biopsy and histologic examination. In many cases, hypophysitis presented with DI and hypopituitarism and preceded the diagnosis of an intracranial tumor, such as germinoma [110–112]. In other reports, it presented with DI and hypogonadotropic hypogonadism [113] or in association with common variable immunodeficiency [114]. Once the diagnosis is established, management is generally conservative, unless there are signs of increased intracranial pressure or optic nerve compression [107].

Langerhans cell histiocytosis

Langerhans cell histiocytosis (LCH) is characterized by clonal proliferation and accumulation of abnormal dendritic cells which can affect either a single site or many systems causing multiorgan dysfunction [115]. In children, the median age of diagnosis ranges between 1.8 and 3.4 years [116,117].

LCH infiltrates the hypothalamo-pituitary area in 15–35% of patients with subsequent development of at least one pituitary

Table 5.8 Incidence of endocrine dysfunction in 145 patients with pituitary involvement. (After Donadieu *et al.* [121].)

Endocrinopathy	Number (%)	Median age at diagnosis (range)
Diabetes insipidus	141 (97%)	3.9 (1–33)
Growth hormone deficiency	61 (42%)	7.7 (2.5–19)
Central hypothyroidism	23 (16%)	9.7 (2.5–19)
Gonadotropin deficiency	17 (12%)	16 (13–35)
Corticotropin deficiency	10 (7%)	11.7 (2.5–17.8)
Panhypopituitarism	9 (6%)	

hormone deficiency (Table 5.8) [118–120]. In a study of 589 pediatric patients with LCH, 145 (25%) had pituitary dysfunction. In 60, pituitary involvement was present at the time of diagnosis and in 20 of them it was the first manifestation of the disease. Patients at high risk of pituitary involvement seem to be those with multisystem disease involving skull, facial bones, mastoid, sinuses and mucous membranes (i.e. gums, ear, nose and throat region). Compared with patients without pituitary involvement, patients with pituitary involvement have a higher rate of relapse (10% at 5 years versus 4.8% at 5 years), and a higher incidence of neurodegenerative LCH [121].

DI is the most frequently reported permanent consequence of LCH [122] and the most common endocrinopathy; almost all patients with pituitary involvement have DI that presents early in the course of the disease, within the first 3–5 years, and occasionally may precede the diagnosis [123]. Children with LCH and DI may also have anterior pituitary hormone deficiencies, with most deficits developing in the 6 years after the diagnosis of DI [124].

The second most common endocrinopathy is GHD, which occurs in 14% of patients with LCH and in more than 40% of patients who have pituitary involvement [119,120]. In the majority, GHD is associated with DI, with a median interval of 2.9–3.5 years between the diagnosis of DI and development of GHD [124,125]. Isolated GHD or the association of GHD with other anterior pituitary hormone deficiencies occurs less commonly.

Pituitary MRI findings in patients with LCH include thickening of the pituitary stalk, suggestive of the infiltrative process, enhancing changes in the pituitary gland and hypothalamus and absence of the bright signal of the posterior pituitary in T1-weighted images, caused by the loss of the phospholipid rich ADH secretory granules [34]. The latter is an invariable feature of patients who develop DI [126,127].

Although 75% show a thickened pituitary stalk at the time of diagnosis of DI, only 24% have persistent stalk thickening after 5 years. These changes are variable and do not correlate with treatment or with clinical recovery because DI persists in all cases [128].

The role of MRI in predicting the development of anterior hormone deficiencies is uncertain. It has been reported that patients who become growth hormone deficient are more likely to have a smaller anterior pituitary, while the size of the stalk and posterior pituitary are not significantly different [125]. This is consistent with the observation that the progressive reduction in anterior pituitary size in patients with LCH may be the consequence of vascular damage [129]. In other reports, however, the occurrence of anterior pituitary hormone deficiencies is linked to a thickening of the stalk at diagnosis [128] or there is no correlation between the size of pituitary gland and the development of endocrinopathies [120].

Long-term follow-up of patients with LCH has shown that established hormone deficiencies cannot be reversed by treatment [127] but isolated case reports have suggested that the purine analog 2-chlorodeoxyadenosine (2-CDA) may reverse established DI [130]. Subsequent studies of this form of therapy, used in refractory cases of LCH involving the CNS, showed that 2-CDA may result in partial or complete radiolological improvement of the mass lesion but the endocrine consequences of the disease, including DI and panhypopituitarism, do not reverse [131]. Patients treated with the JLSG-96 protocol who have been followed up for 5 years developed DI with an incidence of 3.1–8.9%, depending on the extension of the disease (single system multisite, versus multisystem) [132].

Pituitary dysfunction in LCH is thought to occur secondary to the infiltration of the hypothalamo-pituitary area by the disease. However, there is evidence that inflammatory factors are implicated in pathogenesis. An intriguing finding is that circulating antibodies to vasopressin have been detected in 4 of 6 patients with DI resulting from LCH (66%) and 9 of 12 patients with idiopathic DI (75%) [133]. Although this is suggestive of an autoimmune mechanism, their role in the development of DI in cases of LCH is not clear and their presence cannot be used reliably in the differential diagnosis of central DI.

Radiotherapy used for the treatment of LCH is within the dose range of 10–15 Gy, which is known to be unlikely to cause growth hormone insufficiency (GHI). However, in a recent study, radiotherapy has been associated with an increased risk of GHD, despite the fact that the dose was less than 15 Gy [125], a finding that may reflect the severity and extent of the disease rather than the direct effect of radiotherapy. The extent of the disease may in turn be determined by the increased expression of pro-inflammatory agents such as matrix metalloproteases (MMP12), as there are a number of studies showing that dysregulation of cytokines and chemokines is implicated in the pathogenesis of LCH and may have a role in the development of extensive multisystem LCH [134,135]. The role of inflammatory factors in the clinical manifestations of LCH is also underlined by the single case report of precocious puberty in association with LCH, in a girl who did not have radiotherapy as part of LCH treatment. Although it is difficult to establish that this association did not occur by chance, there is the hypothesis that the increased amount of cytokines produced by the LCH lesion may cause neurosecretory dysfunction and damage the gonadotropin releasing hormone pulse generator [136].

Sarcoid

Sarcoid is a multisystem granulomatous disease of unknown aetiology that clinically affects the central nervous system in 5–10% of cases [137]. The effects on the hypothalamo-pituitary axis are the result of infiltration by granulomatous tissue; on MRI the lesion may infiltrate the hypothalamus and pituitary. It enhances with gadolinium and there is thickening of the pituitary stalk. The most frequently reported endocrine abnormality is DI in 25–50% of patients with neurosarcoidosis [138,139]. This is followed by hyperprolactinemia, although anterior pituitary dysfunction with hypogonadism has also been reported [140]. Sarcoidosis of the nervous system has a poor prognosis but long-term remissions have been reported with high-dose intravenous pulsed methylprednisolone therapy. Hormonal defects of less than 1 year duration may respond to steroid treatment but longer standing deficits usually persist [141].

CNS infection

Hypothalamo-pituitary dysfunction has been reported after meningitis or encephalitis, with most cases being reported as isolated case reports. Despite the bias in the selection of cases, one can assume that the incidence of endocrine deficiencies depends on the virulence of the infectious organism, the severity and localization of the disease and the immune status of the host. In a recent study of 19 adult patients who have been investigated 10–56 months following CNS infection, 21% had ACTH deficiency and 11% had gonadotropin deficiency, while there was no GHD or DI reported [142]. Hypopituitarism has been reported following infection by a variety of agents (Table 5.9) [143–150].

Tuberculosis

Tuberculous meningitis has long been recognized as a cause of hypopituitarism but the incidence is difficult to establish because of selection bias and small-scale studies. In 49 patients who had tuberculous meningitis in childhood, 20% had abnormal hypothalamo-pituitary function observed over a mean interval of 18.5 ± 8.5 years from the initial insult. Among patients with hypopituitarism, GH was the most commonly affected hormone, either in isolation (30%) or in combination with gonadotropin deficiency (40%). Isolated hypogonadotropic hypogonadism was observed in 20% and ACTH deficiency and hyperprolactinemia each in 10%. Half of patients with documented hypopituitarism had normal MRI, while other findings included pituitary atrophy (2/10), increased enhancement in the suprasellar area (1/10) or ventricular dilatation (1/10) [151].

Another consequence of systemic tuberculosis (TB) infection is the development of pituitary tuberculomas. Despite the global incidence of TB, intracranial tuberculomas account for only 0.15–4% of space occupying lesions, occurring mainly in developing countries and in patients belonging to high-risk groups. Pituitary involvement in these cases may be secondary to hematogenous spread, tuberculous meningitis or direct extension from

Table 5.9 Hypopituitarism following CNS infection.

I. Bacterial meningitis/encephalitis
Group B streptococcus
Haemophilus influenzae
Streptococcus pneumonia

II. *Mycobacterium tuberculosis*

III. Spirochetes: *Borrelia burgdorferi*

IV. Protozoan/fungal infections
Trypanosoma cruzi
Cryptococcus
Cysticercosis
Aspergillosis

IV. Viral menigoencephalitis
Congenital CMV
Coxsackie virus
Herpes simplex virus
Enterovirus
Varicella

V. Meningitis/encephalitis of unknown cause

CMV, cytomegalovirus.

sinus tuberculosis [152]. There are isolated reports of hypothalamic tuberculomas, where it is thought that damage to the hypothalamus may be caused by infarction or chronic scarring and calcification [153].

The diagnosis of pituitary tuberculoma requires a high index of suspicion, because less than one-third of patients have evidence of previous or concurrent TB infection [154,155]. On MRI tuberculoma appears as an enhancing mass with suprasellar extension and compression of the optic chiasm. Although in almost all cases there is thickening of the pituitary stalk, this sign is not specific and there are no robust radiological data to differentiate tuberculomas from other granulomatous pituitary lesions such as sarcoid, syphilis, histiocytosis or Wegener granulomatosis and the diagnosis requires exclusion of these causes [156]. Furthermore, the majority of lesions are negative for acid-fast bacilli and diagnosis has been based on the histological finding of a chronic granulomatous inflammatory process and the subsequent response to antituberculous therapy [154,157].

At presentation, the symptoms and signs of pituitary tuberculomas may be insidious and of variable duration ranging from 15 days to 2 years. Persistent headache is present in all patients, followed by visual field defects (64%) and cranial nerve palsies (22%). In patients with pituitary tuberculomas the incidence of hypopituitarism has been reported at 22–60%, while diabetes insipidus may occur in 10%. However, it is possible that the higher incidence is a result of selection bias. The most frequent anterior pituitary hormone disturbances are ACTH and TSH deficiency, gonadotropin deficiency and hyperprolactinemia [155]. In rare cases, pituitary tuberculomas present acutely with clinical and laboratory evidence of acute meningitis, anterior pituitary dysfunction with low cortisol and thyroxin and DI. MRI in these cases has revealed a mass in the suprasellar region with solid and cystic components and thickening of the pituitary stalk, while on biopsy the lesion was positive for acid-fast bacilli [152].

Thalassemia

The majority of complications of thalassemia are the consequence of the toxic effects of iron which is deposited in organs of the reticulo-endothelial system, the heart and all target organs of the endocrine system, including the pituitary [158].

The anterior pituitary is very sensitive to iron overload resulting in defective GH secretion, reduced responsiveness of GH to growth hormone releasing hormone (GHRH) and hypogonadotropic hypogonadism. The gonadotroph cells seem to be particularly vulnerable, which may be related to the way that iron is transported in cells. Extracellular iron is bound to transferrin (Tf) and enters cells by endocytosis through transferrin receptors (TfR). Initial histological studies in patients with hemochromatosis have shown that although non-heme bound iron is deposited in all five cell types of the anterior pituitary, its deposition is more pronounced in the gonadotropes [159]. Subsequent studies in rat anterior pituitaries demonstrated that transferrin receptors are expressed only in somatotropes and gonadotropes [160].

Gonadotropin secreting cells from human pituitary adenomas selectively stain immunopositive for the expression of TfR, an observation that suggests that these cells have a special requirement for iron compared to other cell types, and are therefore susceptible to damage in iron overload syndromes [161]. The above results were not reproduced in a study that examined the expression of TfR in specimens from 50 human pituitaries and 42 samples from pituitary adenomas. Immunoreactivity for TfR was present in most cells from the specimens from normal anterior pituitaries as well as in all types of adenomas, and was not restricted to gonadotropinomas. Furthermore, iron loaded gonadotropes did not stain immunopositive for TfR. This may reflect either the downregulation of the expression of the receptor in iron loaded cells, or the fact that pituitary cells may have additional mechanisms to acquire iron [162].

Failure of pubertal development and growth impairment are the most prominent endocrine complications and may occur despite early initiation of chelation. It is estimated that 56% of thalassemic patients have at least one endocrinopathy; almost half have hypogonadism (40–59%) and 33–36% manifest growth failure [163–165].

Children with thalassemia usually maintain their growth rate in childhood with growth failure manifesting at puberty, leading to disproportionate short stature and truncal shortening [166]. This was demonstrated in a study of 238 well-treated thalassemic children whose growth deficit was minimal at the age of 2 years,

became accentuated with time and showed no notable pubertal growth spurt in adolescence [167]. The incidence of short stature is almost 30%, with no difference between males and females [168].

Many factors contribute to the growth deficit observed in thalassemia [169]. It may be the result of chronic anemia and tissue hypoxia, although this effect is expected to be diminished in an era of hypertransfusion regimens and bone marrow transplantation. Delayed puberty and hypothyroidism can also contribute to suboptimal growth and these endocrine deficiencies should be detected and treated.

Iron overload and toxicity from free radical damage adversely affects growth, as has long been observed in poorly chelated patients but overchelation as well as poor chelation can lead to growth retardation, because of the toxic effects of desferrioxamine (DFO) on spinal cartilage. This is consistent with the observation that patients who start high dose chelation early in life show metaphyseal changes and platyspondyly. This effect may be a result of inhibition of DNA synthesis and fibroblast proliferation as well as chelation of trace elements [170]. Three to 35% of patients have been reported to present with bony lesions typical of DFO overtreatment, depending on the population studied [171,172].

In order to maximize growth in thalassemia, careful dosage of DFO is required, avoiding either inadequate or excessive dosing regimens. It has been suggested that chelation should start after 3 years of age, with a maximum dose of DFO of 35 mg/kg/day in children under 5 years and up to 40 mg/kg/day until growth is complete, with careful monitoring of height velocity and sitting and standing height twice yearly in order to adjust the dosage as necessary [173].

The investigation of the GH axis and its contribution to the growth deficit observed in thalassemic patients has yielded variable results. Studies have reported normal reserve of GH, GHD or a relative resistance to the action of GH. These variations may be because of the heterogeneity of the populations studied with respect to their pubertal status, type of GH provocation test and whether it was primed or not, the severity of disease, the genotype, transfusion regimens and chelating therapy (i.e. dose, duration, compliance).

Of 32 patients with thalassemia studied between the ages of 3 and 26 years, 14 of whom were prepubertal, 13 (40%) had short stature and they were tested with at least one GH provocation test. Ten had normal GH on provocation and three had GHD but, on overnight profile, those who had been considered GH sufficient showed a reduced maximum peak and reduced mean GH concentration, indicating that the patients were probably GH insufficient, possibly as a result of neuroendocrine dysfunction rather than direct pituitary damage. In the same study, the concentration of IGF-1 was reduced in children with short stature and in those with normal stature but with a low growth velocity. However, all patients had an appropriate response to an IGF-1 generation test, thereby excluding insensitivity to GH action [174].

A subsequent study of 28 thalassemic children and adolescents showed that 45% of short children were GH deficient, with a peak GH ≤20 mU/L in response to two GH provocation tests (insulin and clonidine), while 55% had sufficient GH secretion. As there was no difference in growth between the two groups, the impairment of GH secretion could not be considered as the main cause of height deficit in these patients. Furthermore, eight patients with GHD also had an IGF-1 generation test and five of them (63%) demonstrated an IGF-1 increase less than 50%, a finding that was interpreted as a degree of GH insensitivity and is in contrast with the previously mentioned results [175].

The follow-up of 39 patients for a mean duration of 16 years demonstrated that, although growth retardation occurs in almost one-third of patients with 36% having a final height ≤2 SD, GHD is rare (diagnosed in 1 of 15 tested). In addition, there was no association between the short final height and the age at diagnosis, the presence of hypogonadism, hypothyroidism or non-endocrine complications. However, mean serum ferritin over the study period was significantly higher in patients with short stature than those with final height ≥2 SD. This difference was significant only for the prepubertal years; a mean ferritin concentration of more than 3000 ng/mL before puberty was found to be a predictor for final short stature [176].

Retesting of 16 adult thalassemic patients who had been diagnosed as GHD in childhood and treated with rhGH showed that most had sufficient GH secretion, while 19% had a GH peak less than 10 ng/mL [177]. However, the evaluation of GH secretion in 94 adult patients with thalassemia, who had not previously been tested, showed that the incidence of GHD is not rare and probably increases over time. Severe GHD was diagnosed in 22.3% of patients, while a further 19% had partial GHD. Low IGF-1 concentrations (less than −1.8 SD) were observed in 95% of patients with severe GHD, 94% of those with partial GHD and 80% of patients with normal GH reserve. The finding of low IGF-1 with normal GH was probably due to reduced IGF-1 synthesis in the liver secondary to hepatic hemosiderosis. The authors did not observe any correlation between ferritin concentration and the status of GH secretion [178]. However, a single ferritin concentration around the time of the study does not reflect the exposure to iron overload through childhood, and in this case it would have been interesting to have data correlating the endocrine abnormalities to the degree of iron deposition in the liver and the pituitary.

Hypogonadotropic hypogonadism resulting from iron toxicity on gonadotrope cells is the most common endocrine complication, although primary gonadal failure may also occur. It manifests as pubertal delay, growth failure, primary or secondary amenorrhea and infertility. The damaging role of iron overload on gonadotrope cell function has been demonstrated by an early study showing that initiation of chelation therapy before the age of 10 years resulted in normal sexual maturation in the majority of patients (90%), compared to 38% of those who started chelation after the age of 10 years [179]. However, the mean ferritin concentration in this study was rather low (1562 ± 445 ng/mL),

which may explain why these very encouraging results have not been reproduced in subsequent studies. In a study of 1861 patients, 51% of boys and 47% of girls over 15 years of age had pubertal failure [165]. The results of the study by Shalitin et al. [176] were comparable, as the authors showed that despite early treatment with DFO (mean age 4.9 years), 59% of patients had hypogonadism. Mean serum ferritin was significantly higher in patients with hypogonadism and a mean concentration of 2500 ng/mL during the prepubertal years has been defined as the cutoff for the development of hypogonadism [176].

Consistent with these findings are results from MRI that have been used to monitor pituitary iron deposition using the signal intensity ratio (SIR) and T2 relaxation rate [180]. Thalassemic patients with hypogonadotropic hypogonadism have more pronounced pituitary iron deposition and reduced pituitary height than thalassemic patients without pituitary dysfunction [181]. This may be the result of cell destruction and irreversible damage from the toxic effect of iron on gonadotropes. The extent of iron deposition in the pituitary, however, cannot be predicted by the degree of hemosiderosis in the liver and this observation probably reflects the fact that different organs have different iron kinetics [182].

Psychosocial deprivation

An extreme form of failure to thrive is observed in children who live under stressful social circumstances or have been subjected to abuse and neglect. They present with short stature and a characteristic behavioral pattern that includes hyperphagia, bizarre eating habits that mimic organic compulsive eating disorders, vomiting and polydipsia [183]. On overnight profile, GH secretion in these children shows a spectrum of abnormalities that involve the basal values, pulse frequency and pulse amplitude. A characteristic of this condition, however, is that GH insufficiency is reversible after 3 weeks in hospital, after removal from the stressful environment [184].

References

1 Regal M, Paramo C, Sierra SM, Garcia-Mayor RV. Prevalence and incidence of hypopituitarism in an adult Caucasian population in northwestern Spain. *Clin Endocrinol (Oxf)* 2001; **55**: 735–740.

2 Schneider HJ, Aimaretti G, Kreitschmann-Andermahr I, Stalla GK, Ghigo E. Hypopituitarism. *Lancet* 2007; **369**: 1461–1470.

3 Jagannathan J, Dumont AS, Jane JA Jr. Diagnosis and management of pediatric sellar lesions. *Front Horm Res* 2006; **34**: 83–104.

4 Karavitaki N, Cudlip S, Adams CB, Wass JA. Craniopharyngiomas. *Endocr Rev* 2006; **27**: 371–397.

5 Kaatsch P, Rickert CH, Kuhl J, Schuz J, Michaelis J. Population-based epidemiologic data on brain tumors in German children. *Cancer* 2001; **92**: 3155–3164.

6 May JA, Krieger MD, Bowen I, Geffner ME. Craniopharyngioma in childhood. *Adv Pediatr* 2006; **53**: 183–209.

7 Bunin GR, Surawicz TS, Witman PA, Preston-Martin S, Davis F, Bruner JM. The descriptive epidemiology of craniopharyngioma. *J Neurosurg* 1998; **89**: 547–551.

8 Spoudeas HA, ed. *Paediatric Endocrine Tumours: A Multi-Disciplinary Statement of Best Practice from a Working Group Convened Under the Auspices of the BSPED and UKCCSG (Rare Tumour Working Groups).* 2005: 16–46.

9 Arai T, Ohno K, Takada Y, Aoyagi M, Hirakawa K. Neonatal craniopharyngioma and inference of tumor inception time: case report and review of the literature. *Surg Neurol* 2003; **60**: 254–259.

10 Muller-Scholden J, Lehrnbecher T, Muller HL, et al. Radical surgery in a neonate with craniopharyngioma: report of a case. *Pediatr Neurosurg* 2000; **33**: 265–269.

11 Wellons JC III, Tubbs RS. Staged surgical treatment of a giant neonatal craniopharyngioma: case illustration. *J Neurosurg* 2006; **105** (Suppl): 76.

12 Muller HL, Gebhardt U, Etavard-Gorris N, et al. Prognosis and sequela in patients with childhood craniopharyngioma: results of HIT-ENDO and update on KRANIOPHARYNGEOM 2000. *Klin Padiatr* 2004; **216**: 343–348.

13 Karavitaki N, Brufani C, Warner JT, et al. Craniopharyngiomas in children and adults: systematic analysis of 121 cases with long-term follow-up. *Clin Endocrinol (Oxf)* 2005; **62**: 397–409.

14 Fahlbusch R, Honegger J, Paulus W, Huk W, Buchfelder M. Surgical treatment of craniopharyngiomas: experience with 168 patients. *J Neurosurg* 1999; **90**: 237–250.

15 Boch AL, van ER, Kujas M. Craniopharyngiomas in two consanguineous siblings: case report. *Neurosurgery* 1997; **41**: 1185–1187.

16 Green AL, Yeh JS, Dias PS. Craniopharyngioma in a mother and daughter. *Acta Neurochir (Wien)* 2002; **144**: 403–404.

17 Gorski GK, McMorrow LE, Donaldson MH, Freed M. Multiple chromosomal abnormalities in a case of craniopharyngioma. *Cancer Genet Cytogenet* 1992; **60**: 212–213.

18 Karnes PS, Tran TN, Cui MY, et al. Cytogenetic analysis of 39 pediatric central nervous system tumors. *Cancer Genet Cytogenet* 1992; **59**: 12–19.

19 Rickert CH, Paulus W. Lack of chromosomal imbalances in adamantinomatous and papillary craniopharyngiomas. *J Neurol Neurosurg Psychiatry* 2003; **74**: 260–261.

20 Sarubi JC, Bei H, Adams EF, et al. Clonal composition of human adamantinomatous craniopharyngiomas and somatic mutation analyses of the patched (PTCH), Gsalpha and Gi2alpha genes. *Neurosci Lett* 2001; **310**: 5–8.

21 Rienstein S, Adams EF, Pilzer D, Goldring AA, Goldman B, Friedman E. Comparative genomic hybridization analysis of craniopharyngiomas. *J Neurosurg* 2003; **98**: 162–164.

22 Yoshimoto M, de T, Sr., da Silva NS, et al. Comparative genomic hybridization analysis of pediatric adamantinomatous craniopharyngiomas and a review of the literature. *J Neurosurg* 2004; **101** (Suppl): 85–90.

23 Nozaki M, Tada M, Matsumoto R, Sawamura Y, Abe H, Iggo RD. Rare occurrence of inactivating p53 gene mutations in primary non-astrocytic tumors of the central nervous system: reappraisal by yeast functional assay. *Acta Neuropathol* 1998; **95**: 291–296.

24 Sekine S, Shibata T, Kokubu A, et al. Craniopharyngiomas of adamantinomatous type harbor beta-catenin gene mutations. *Am J Pathol* 2002; **161**: 1997–2001.

25 Oikonomou E, Barreto DC, Soares B, De ML, Buchfelder M, Adams EF. Beta-catenin mutations in craniopharyngiomas and pituitary adenomas. *J Neurooncol* 2005; **73**: 205–209.

26 deVries L, Lazar L, Phillip M. Craniopharyngioma: presentation and endocrine sequelae in 36 children. *J Pediatr Endocrinol Metab* 2003; **16**: 703–710.

27 Sklar CA. Craniopharyngioma: endocrine abnormalities at presentation. *Pediatr Neurosurg* 1994; **21** (Suppl 1): 18–20.

28 Bin-Abbas B, Mawlawi H, Sakati N, Khafaja Y, Chaudhary MA, Al-Ashwal A. Endocrine sequelae of childhood craniopharyngioma. *J Pediatr Endocrinol Metab* 2001; **14**: 869–874.

29 Muller HL, Emser A, Faldum A, et al. Longitudinal study on growth and body mass index before and after diagnosis of childhood craniopharyngioma. *J Clin Endocrinol Metab* 2004; **89**: 3298–3305.

30 Honegger J, Buchfelder M, Fahlbusch R. Surgical treatment of craniopharyngiomas: endocrinological results. *J Neurosurg* 1999; **90**: 251–257.

31 DeVile CJ, Grant DB, Hayward RD, Stanhope R. Growth and endocrine sequelae of craniopharyngioma. *Arch Dis Child* 1996; **75**: 108–114.

32 de VL, Weintrob N, Phillip M. Craniopharyngioma presenting as precocious puberty and accelerated growth. *Clin Pediatr (Phila)* 2003; **42**: 181–184.

33 Gonzales-Portillo G, Tomita T. The syndrome of inappropriate secretion of antidiuretic hormone: an unusual presentation for childhood craniopharyngioma – report of three cases. *Neurosurgery* 1998; **42**: 917–921.

34 Argyropoulou MI, Kiortsis DN. MRI of the hypothalamic-pituitary axis in children. *Pediatr Radiol* 2005; **35**: 1045–1055.

35 Molla E, Marti-Bonmati L, Revert A, et al. Craniopharyngiomas: identification of different semiological patterns with MRI. *Eur Radiol* 2002; **12**: 1829–1836.

36 Muller HL, Albanese A, Calaminus G, et al. Consensus and perspectives on treatment strategies in childhood craniopharyngioma: results of a meeting of the Craniopharyngioma Study Group (SIOP), Genova, 2004. *J Pediatr Endocrinol Metab* 2006; **19** (Suppl 1): 453–454.

37 Spoudeas HA, Saran F, Pizer B. A multimodality approach to the treatment of craniopharyngiomas avoiding hypothalamic morbidity: a UK perspective. *J Pediatr Endocrinol Metab* 2006; **19** (Suppl 1): 447–451.

38 Garre ML, Cama A. Craniopharyngioma: modern concepts in pathogenesis and treatment. *Curr Opin Pediatr* 2007; **19**: 471–479.

39 Lena G, Paz PA, Scavarda D, Giusiano B. Craniopharyngioma in children: Marseille experience. *Childs Nerv Syst* 2005; **21**: 778–784.

40 Scarzello G, Buzzaccarini MS, Perilongo G, et al. Acute and late morbidity after limited resection and focal radiation therapy in craniopharyngiomas. *J Pediatr Endocrinol Metab* 2006; **19** (Suppl 1): 399–405.

41 Meuric S, Brauner R, Trivin C, Souberbielle JC, Zerah M, Sainte-Rose C. Influence of tumor location on the presentation and evolution of craniopharyngiomas. *J Neurosurg* 2005; **103** (Suppl): 421–426.

42 Xu J, Zhang S, You C, Wang X, Zhou Q. Microvascular density and vascular endothelial growth factor have little correlation with prognosis of craniopharyngioma. *Surg Neurol* 2006; **66** (Suppl 1): S30–S34.

43 Lefranc F, Mijatovic T, Decaestecker C, *et al.* Monitoring the expression profiles of integrins and adhesion/growth-regulatory galectins in adamantinomatous craniopharyngiomas: their ability to regulate tumor adhesiveness to surrounding tissue and their contribution to prognosis. *Neurosurgery* 2005; **56**: 763–776.

44 Kunwar S, Wilson CB. Pediatric pituitary adenomas. *J Clin Endocrinol Metab* 1999; **84**: 4385–4389.

45 Lafferty AR, Chrousos GP. Pituitary tumors in children and adolescents. *J Clin Endocrinol Metab* 1999; **84**: 4317–4323.

46 Beckers A, Daly AF. The clinical, pathological, and genetic features of familial isolated pituitary adenomas. *Eur J Endocrinol* 2007; **157**: 371–382.

47 Ezzat S, Asa SL. Mechanisms of disease: the pathogenesis of pituitary tumors. *Nat Clin Pract Endocrinol Metab* 2006; **2**: 220–230.

48 Colao A, Loche S, Cappa M, *et al.* Prolactinomas in children and adolescents: clinical presentation and long-term follow-up. *J Clin Endocrinol Metab* 1998; **83**: 2777–2780.

49 Cannavo S, Venturino M, Curto L, *et al.* Clinical presentation and outcome of pituitary adenomas in teenagers. *Clin Endocrinol (Oxf)* 2003; **58**: 519–527.

50 Casanueva FF, Molitch ME, Schlechte JA, *et al.* Guidelines of the Pituitary Society for the diagnosis and management of prolactinomas. *Clin Endocrinol (Oxf)* 2006; **65**: 265–273.

51 Melmed S. Update in pituitary disease. *J Clin Endocrinol Metab* 2008; **93**: 331–338.

52 Gillam MP, Molitch ME, Lombardi G, Colao A. Advances in the treatment of prolactinomas. *Endocr Rev* 2006; **27**: 485–534.

53 Zanettini R, Antonini A, Gatto G, Gentile R, Tesei S, Pezzoli G. Valvular heart disease and the use of dopamine agonists for Parkinson's disease. *N Engl J Med* 2007; **356**: 39–46.

54 Colao A, Vitale G, Cappabianca P, *et al.* Outcome of cabergoline treatment in men with prolactinoma: effects of a 24-month treatment on prolactin levels, tumor mass, recovery of pituitary function, and semen analysis. *J Clin Endocrinol Metab* 2004; **89**: 1704–1711.

55 Savage MO, Storr HL, Chan LF, Grossman AB. Diagnosis and treatment of pediatric Cushing's disease. *Pituitary* 2007; **10**: 657–671.

56 Stratakis CA, Schussheim DH, Freedman SM, *et al.* Pituitary macroadenoma in a 5-year-old: an early expression of multiple endocrine neoplasia type 1. *J Clin Endocrinol Metab* 2000; **85**: 4776–4780.

57 Joshi SM, Hewitt RJ, Storr HL, *et al.* Cushing's disease in children and adolescents: 20 years of experience in a single neurosurgical center. *Neurosurgery* 2005; **57**: 281–285.

58 Magiakou MA, Chrousos GP. Cushing's syndrome in children and adolescents: current diagnostic and therapeutic strategies. *J Endocrinol Invest* 2002; **25**: 181–194.

59 Storr HL, Chan LF, Grossman AB, Savage MO. Paediatric Cushing's syndrome: epidemiology, investigation and therapeutic advances. *Trends Endocrinol Metab* 2007; **18**: 167–174.

60 Arnaldi G, Angeli A, Atkinson AB, *et al.* Diagnosis and complications of Cushing's syndrome: a consensus statement. *J Clin Endocrinol Metab* 2003; **88**: 5593–5602.

61 Batista D, Gennari M, Riar J, *et al.* An assessment of petrosal sinus sampling for localization of pituitary microadenomas in children with Cushing disease. *J Clin Endocrinol Metab* 2006; **91**: 221–224.

62 Storr HL, Afshar F, Matson M, *et al.* Factors influencing cure by transsphenoidal selective adenomectomy in paediatric Cushing's disease. *Eur J Endocrinol* 2005; **152**: 825–833.

63 Devoe DJ, Miller WL, Conte FA, *et al.* Long-term outcome in children and adolescents after transsphenoidal surgery for Cushing's disease. *J Clin Endocrinol Metab* 1997; **82**: 3196–3202.

64 Atkinson AB, Kennedy A, Wiggam MI, McCance DR, Sheridan B. Long-term remission rates after pituitary surgery for Cushing's disease: the need for long-term surveillance. *Clin Endocrinol (Oxf)* 2005; **63**: 549–559.

65 Walker D. Recent advances in optic nerve glioma with a focus on the young patient. *Curr Opin Neurol* 2003; **16**: 657–664.

66 Czyzyk E, Jozwiak S, Roszkowski M, Schwartz RA. Optic pathway gliomas in children with and without neurofibromatosis 1. *J Child Neurol* 2003; **18**: 471–478.

67 Jahraus CD, Tarbell NJ. Optic pathway gliomas. *Pediatr Blood Cancer* 2006; **46**: 586–596.

68 Adan L, Trivin C, Sainte-Rose C, Zucker JM, Hartmann O, Brauner R. GH deficiency caused by cranial irradiation during childhood: factors and markers in young adults. *J Clin Endocrinol Metab* 2001; **86**: 5245–5251.

69 Trivin C, Couto-Silva AC, Sainte-Rose C, *et al.* Presentation and evolution of organic central precocious puberty according to the type of CNS lesion. *Clin Endocrinol (Oxf)* 2006; **65**: 239–245.

70 Collet-Solberg PF, Sernyak H, Satin-Smith M, *et al.* Endocrine outcome in long-term survivors of low-grade hypothalamic/chiasmatic glioma. *Clin Endocrinol (Oxf)* 1997; **47**: 79–85.

71 el-Mahdy W, Powell M. Transsphenoidal management of 28 symptomatic Rathke's cleft cysts, with special reference to visual and hormonal recovery. *Neurosurgery* 1998; **42**: 7–16.

72 Isono M, Kamida T, Kobayashi H, Shimomura T, Matsuyama J. Clinical features of symptomatic Rathke's cleft cyst. *Clin Neurol Neurosurg* 2001; **103**: 96–100.

73 Billeci D, Marton E, Tripodi M, Orvieto E, Longatti P. Symptomatic Rathke's cleft cysts: a radiological, surgical and pathological review. *Pituitary* 2004; 7: 131–137.

74 Dubuisson AS, Stevenaert A, Martin DH, Flandroy PP. Intrasellar arachnoid cysts. *Neurosurgery* 2007; **61**: 505–513.

75 Adan L, Bussieres L, Dinand V, Zerah M, Pierre-Kahn A, Brauner R. Growth, puberty and hypothalamic-pituitary function in children with suprasellar arachnoid cyst. *Eur J Pediatr* 2000; **159**: 348–355.

76 Cavallo LM, Prevedello D, Esposito F, *et al.* The role of the endoscope in the transsphenoidal management of cystic lesions of the sellar region. *Neurosurg Rev* 2008; **31**: 55–64.

77 Acerini CL, Tasker RC. Traumatic brain injury induced hypothalamic-pituitary dysfunction: a paediatric perspective. *Pituitary* 2007; **10**: 373–380.

78 Parslow RC, Morris KP, Tasker RC, Forsyth RJ, Hawley CA. Epidemiology of traumatic brain injury in children receiving intensive care in the UK. *Arch Dis Child* 2005; **90**: 1182–1187.

79 Tasker RC, Morris KP, Forsyth RJ, Hawley CA, Parslow RC. Severe head injury in children: emergency access to neurosurgery in the United Kingdom. *Emerg Med J* 2006; **23**: 519–522.

80 Oertel M, Boscardin WJ, Obrist WD, *et al.* Posttraumatic vasospasm: the epidemiology, severity, and time course of an underestimated phenomenon: a prospective study performed in 299 patients. *J Neurosurg* 2005; **103**: 812–824.

81 Urban RJ. Hypopituitarism after acute brain injury. *Growth Horm IGF Res* 2006; **16** (Suppl A): S25–S29.

82 Agha A, Thompson CJ. Anterior pituitary dysfunction following traumatic brain injury (TBI). *Clin Endocrinol (Oxf)* 2006; **64**: 481–488.

83 Benvenga S, Campenni A, Ruggeri RM, Trimarchi F. Clinical review 113: Hypopituitarism secondary to head trauma. *J Clin Endocrinol Metab* 2000; **85**: 1353–1361.

84 Kelly DF, Gonzalo IT, Cohan P, Berman N, Swerdloff R, Wang C. Hypopituitarism following traumatic brain injury and aneurysmal subarachnoid hemorrhage: a preliminary report. *J Neurosurg* 2000; **93**: 743–752.

85 Lieberman SA, Oberoi AL, Gilkison CR, Masel BE, Urban RJ. Prevalence of neuroendocrine dysfunction in patients recovering from traumatic brain injury. *J Clin Endocrinol Metab* 2001; **86**: 2752–2756.

86 Bondanelli M, De ML, Ambrosio MR, et al. Occurrence of pituitary dysfunction following traumatic brain injury. *J Neurotrauma* 2004; **21**: 685–696.

87 Agha A, Rogers B, Sherlock M, et al. Anterior pituitary dysfunction in survivors of traumatic brain injury. *J Clin Endocrinol Metab* 2004; **89**: 4929–4936.

88 Tanriverdi F, Senyurek H, Unluhizarci K, Selcuklu A, Casanueva FF, Kelestimur F. High risk of hypopituitarism after traumatic brain injury: a prospective investigation of anterior pituitary function in the acute phase and 12 months after trauma. *J Clin Endocrinol Metab* 2006; **91**: 2105–2111.

89 Klose M, Juul A, Struck J, Morgenthaler NG, Kosteljanetz M, Feldt-Rasmussen U. Acute and long-term pituitary insufficiency in traumatic brain injury: a prospective single-centre study. *Clin Endocrinol (Oxf)* 2007; **67**: 598–606.

90 Dimopoulou I, Tsagarakis S, Theodorakopoulou M, et al. Endocrine abnormalities in critical care patients with moderate-to-severe head trauma: incidence, pattern and predisposing factors. *Intensive Care Med* 2004; **30**: 1051–1057.

91 Agha A, Rogers B, Mylotte D, et al. Neuroendocrine dysfunction in the acute phase of traumatic brain injury. *Clin Endocrinol (Oxf)* 2004; **60**: 584–591.

92 Cooper MS, Stewart PM. Corticosteroid insufficiency in acutely ill patients. *N Engl J Med* 2003; **348**: 727–734.

93 Boughey JC, Yost MJ, Bynoe RP. Diabetes insipidus in the head-injured patient. *Am Surg* 2004; **70**: 500–503.

94 Agha A, Sherlock M, Phillips J, Tormey W, Thompson CJ. The natural history of post-traumatic neurohypophysial dysfunction. *Eur J Endocrinol* 2005; **152**: 371–377.

95 Leal-Cerro A, Flores JM, Rincon M, et al. Prevalence of hypopituitarism and growth hormone deficiency in adults long-term after severe traumatic brain injury. *Clin Endocrinol (Oxf)* 2005; **62**: 525–532.

96 Aimaretti G, Ambrosio MR, Di SC, et al. Residual pituitary function after brain injury-induced hypopituitarism: a prospective 12-month study. *J Clin Endocrinol Metab* 2005; **90**: 6085–6092.

97 Aimaretti G, Ambrosio MR, Di SC, et al. Hypopituitarism induced by traumatic brain injury in the transition phase. *J Endocrinol Invest* 2005; **28**: 984–989.

98 Einaudi S, Matarazzo P, Peretta P, et al. Hypothalamo-hypophysial dysfunction after traumatic brain injury in children and adoles-cents: a preliminary retrospective and prospective study. *J Pediatr Endocrinol Metab* 2006; **19**: 691–703.

99 Niederland T, Makovi H, Gal V, Andreka B, Abraham CS, Kovacs J. Abnormalities of pituitary function after traumatic brain injury in children. *J Neurotrauma* 2007; **24**: 119–127.

100 Keenan HT, Hooper SR, Wetherington CE, Nocera M, Runyan DK. Neurodevelopmental consequences of early traumatic brain injury in 3-year-old children. *Pediatrics* 2007; **119**: e616–e623.

101 McCarthy ML, MacKenzie EJ, Durbin DR, et al. Health-related quality of life during the first year after traumatic brain injury. *Arch Pediatr Adolesc Med* 2006; **160**: 252–260.

102 Acerini CL, Tasker RC, Bellone S, Bona G, Thompson CJ, Savage MO. Hypopituitarism in childhood and adolescence following traumatic brain injury: the case for prospective endocrine investigation. *Eur J Endocrinol* 2006; **155**: 663–669.

103 Einaudi S, Bondone C. The effects of head trauma on hypothalamic-pituitary function in children and adolescents. *Curr Opin Pediatr* 2007; **19**: 465–470.

104 Casanueva FF, Ghigo E, Polak M, Savage MO. The importance of investigation of pituitary function in children and adolescents following traumatic brain injury. *J Endocrinol Invest* 2006; **29**: 764–766.

105 Ghigo E, Masel B, Aimaretti G, et al. Consensus guidelines on screening for hypopituitarism following traumatic brain injury. *Brain Inj* 2005; **19**: 711–724.

106 Cheung CC, Ezzat S, Smyth HS, Asa SL. The spectrum and significance of primary hypophysitis. *J Clin Endocrinol Metab* 2001; **86**: 1048–1053.

107 Caturegli P, Newschaffer C, Olivi A, Pomper MG, Burger PC, Rose NR. Autoimmune hypophysitis. *Endocr Rev* 2005; **26**: 599–614.

108 Gutenberg A, Buslei R, Fahlbusch R, Buchfelder M, Bruck W. Immunopathology of primary hypophysitis: implications for pathogenesis. *Am J Surg Pathol* 2005; **29**: 329–338.

109 Gutenberg A, Hans V, Puchner MJ, et al. Primary hypophysitis: clinical-pathological correlations. *Eur J Endocrinol* 2006; **155**: 101–107.

110 Mikami-Terao Y, Akiyama M, Yanagisawa T, et al. Lymphocytic hypophysitis with central diabetes insipidus and subsequent hypopituitarism masking a suprasellar germinoma in a 13-year-old girl. *Childs Nerv Syst* 2006; **22**: 1338–1343.

111 Fehn M, Bettendorf M, Ludecke DK, Sommer C, Saeger W. Lymphocytic hypophysitis masking a suprasellar germinoma in a 12-year-old girl: a case report. *Pituitary* 1999; **1**: 303–307.

112 Bettendorf M, Fehn M, Grulich-Henn J, et al. Lymphocytic hypophysitis with central diabetes insipidus and consequent panhypopituitarism preceding a multifocal, intracranial germinoma in a prepubertal girl. *Eur J Pediatr* 1999; **158**: 288–292.

113 Cemeroglu AP, Blaivas M, Muraszko KM, Robertson PL, Vazquez DM. Lymphocytic hypophysitis presenting with diabetes insipidus in a 14-year-old girl: case report and review of the literature. *Eur J Pediatr* 1997; **156**: 684–688.

114 Younes JS, Secord EA. Panhypopituitarism in a child with common variable immunodeficiency. *Ann Allergy Asthma Immunol* 2002; **89**: 322–325.

115 de Graaf JH, Egeler RM. New insights into the pathogenesis of Langerhans cell histiocytosis. *Curr Opin Pediatr* 1997; **9**: 46–50.

116 Bhatia S, Nesbit ME Jr, Egeler RM, Buckley JD, Mertens A, Robison LL. Epidemiologic study of Langerhans cell histiocytosis in children. *J Pediatr* 1997; **130**: 774–784.

117 Howarth DM, Gilchrist GS, Mullan BP, Wiseman GA, Edmonson JH, Schomberg PJ. Langerhans cell histiocytosis: diagnosis, natural history, management, and outcome. *Cancer* 1999; **85**: 2278–2290.

118 Bernstrand C, Sandstedt B, Ahstrom L, Henter JI. Long-term follow-up of Langerhans cell histiocytosis: 39 years' experience at a single centre. *Acta Paediatr* 2005; **94**: 1073–1084.

119 Amato MC, Elias LL, Elias J, *et al*. Endocrine disorders in pediatric-onset Langerhans cell histiocytosis. *Horm Metab Res* 2006; **38**: 746–751.

120 Nanduri VR, Bareille P, Pritchard J, Stanhope R. Growth and endocrine disorders in multisystem Langerhans' cell histiocytosis. *Clin Endocrinol (Oxf)* 2000; **53**: 509–515.

121 Donadieu J, Rolon MA, Thomas C, *et al*. Endocrine involvement in pediatric-onset Langerhans' cell histiocytosis: a population-based study. *J Pediatr* 2004; **144**: 344–350.

122 Haupt R, Nanduri V, Calevo MG, *et al*. Permanent consequences in Langerhans cell histiocytosis patients: a pilot study from the Histiocyte Society-Late Effects Study Group. *Pediatr Blood Cancer* 2004; **42**: 438–444.

123 Prosch H, Grois N, Prayer D, *et al*. Central diabetes insipidus as presenting symptom of Langerhans cell histiocytosis. *Pediatr Blood Cancer* 2004; **43**: 594–599.

124 Maghnie M, Cosi G, Genovese E, *et al*. Central diabetes insipidus in children and young adults. *N Engl J Med* 2000; **343**: 998–1007.

125 Donadieu J, Rolon MA, Pion I, *et al*. Incidence of growth hormone deficiency in pediatric-onset Langerhans cell histiocytosis: efficacy and safety of growth hormone treatment. *J Clin Endocrinol Metab* 2004; **89**: 604–609.

126 Maghnie M, Arico M, Villa A, Genovese E, Beluffi G, Severi F. MR of the hypothalamic-pituitary axis in Langerhans cell histiocytosis. *AJNR Am J Neuroradiol* 1992; **13**: 1365–1371.

127 Kaltsas GA, Powles TB, Evanson J, *et al*. Hypothalamo-pituitary abnormalities in adult patients with Langerhans cell histiocytosis: clinical, endocrinological, and radiological features and response to treatment. *J Clin Endocrinol Metab* 2000; **85**: 1370–1376.

128 Grois N, Prayer D, Prosch H, Minkov M, Potschger U, Gadner H. Course and clinical impact of magnetic resonance imaging findings in diabetes insipidus associated with Langerhans cell histiocytosis. *Pediatr Blood Cancer* 2004; **43**: 59–65.

129 Maghnie M, Genovese E, Arico M, *et al*. Evolving pituitary hormone deficiency is associated with pituitary vasculopathy: dynamic MR study in children with hypopituitarism, diabetes insipidus, and Langerhans cell histiocytosis. *Radiology* 1994; **193**: 493–499.

130 Ottaviano F, Finlay JL. Diabetes insipidus and Langerhans cell histiocytosis: a case report of reversibility with 2-chlorodeoxyadenosine. *J Pediatr Hematol Oncol* 2003; **25**: 575–577.

131 Dhall G, Finlay JL, Dunkel IJ, *et al*. Analysis of outcome for patients with mass lesions of the central nervous system due to Langerhans cell histiocytosis treated with 2-chlorodeoxyadenosine. *Pediatr Blood Cancer* 2008; **50**: 72–79.

132 Morimoto A, Ikushima S, Kinugawa N, *et al*. Improved outcome in the treatment of pediatric multifocal Langerhans cell histiocytosis: results from the Japan Langerhans Cell Histiocytosis Study Group-96 protocol study. *Cancer* 2006; **107**: 613–619.

133 Maghnie M, Ghirardello S, De BA, *et al*. Idiopathic central diabetes insipidus in children and young adults is commonly associated with vasopressin-cell antibodies and markers of autoimmunity. *Clin Endocrinol (Oxf)* 2006; **65**: 470–478.

134 Rust R, Kluiver J, Visser L, *et al*. Gene expression analysis of dendritic/Langerhans cells and Langerhans cell histiocytosis. *J Pathol* 2006; **209**: 474–483.

135 De FP, Badulli C, Cuccia M, *et al*. Specific polymorphisms of cytokine genes are associated with different risks to develop single-system or multi-system childhood Langerhans cell histiocytosis. *Br J Haematol* 2006; **132**: 784–787.

136 Municchi G, Marconcini S, D'Ambrosio A, Berardi R, Acquaviva A. Central precocious puberty in multisystem Langerhans cell histiocytosis: a case report. *Pediatr Hematol Oncol* 2002; **19**: 273–278.

137 Iannuzzi MC, Rybicki BA, Teirstein AS. Sarcoidosis. *N Engl J Med* 2007; **357**: 2153–2165.

138 Bihan H, Christozova V, Dumas JL, *et al*. Sarcoidosis: clinical, hormonal, and magnetic resonance imaging (MRI) manifestations of hypothalamic-pituitary disease in 9 patients and review of the literature. *Medicine (Baltimore)* 2007; **86**: 259–268.

139 Takano K. Sarcoidosis of the hypothalamus and pituitary. *Intern Med* 2004; **43**: 894–895.

140 Murialdo G, Tamagno G. Endocrine aspects of neurosarcoidosis. *J Endocrinol Invest* 2002; **25**: 650–662.

141 Molina A, Mana J, Villabona C, Fernandez-Castaner M, Soler J. Hypothalamic-pituitary sarcoidosis with hypopituitarism: long-term remission with methylprednisolone pulse therapy. *Pituitary* 2002; **5**: 33–36.

142 Schaefer S, Boegershausen N, Meyer S, Ivan D, Schepelmann K, Kann PH. Hypothalamic-pituitary insufficiency following infectious diseases of the central nervous system. *Eur J Endocrinol* 2008; **158**: 3–9.

143 Franco-Paredes C, Evans J, Jurado R. Diabetes insipidus due to *Streptococcus pneumoniae* meningitis. *Arch Intern Med* 2001; **161**: 1114–1115.

144 Marcus BJ, Collins KA. Childhood panhypopituitarism presenting as child abuse: a case report and review of the literature. *Am J Forensic Med Pathol* 2004; **25**: 265–269.

145 Carrera MJ, Salar A, Pascual J, Mir M, Chillaron JJ, Cano JF. Hypopituitarism associated with mycotic aneurysm of the cavernous carotid artery in a renal transplant recipient. *Nephrol Dial Transplant* 2006; **21**: 3299–3300.

146 Choi HJ, Cornford M, Wang L, Sun J, Friedman TC. Acute Chagas' disease presenting with a suprasellar mass and panhypopituitarism. *Pituitary* 2004; **7**: 111–114.

147 Pinzer T, Reiss M, Bourquain H, Krishnan KG, Schackert G. Primary aspergillosis of the sphenoid sinus with pituitary invasion: a rare differential diagnosis of sellar lesions. *Acta Neurochir (Wien)* 2006; **148**: 1085–1090.

148 Mena W, Royal S, Pass RF, Whitley RJ, Philips JB III. Diabetes insipidus associated with symptomatic congenital cytomegalovirus infection. *J Pediatr* 1993; **122**: 911–913.

149 Lee YJ, Yang D, Shyur SD, Chiu NC. Neurogenic diabetes insipidus in a child with fatal Coxsackie virus B1 encephalitis. *J Pediatr Endocrinol Metab* 1995; **8**: 301–304.

150 Vesely DL, Mastrandrea P, Samson C, Argyelan G, Charvit S. Postherpes encephalitic anterior pituitary insufficiency with hypothermia and hypotension. *Am J Med Sci* 2000; **320**: 273–277.

151 Lam KS, Sham MM, Tam SC, Ng MM, Ma HT. Hypopituitarism after tuberculous meningitis in childhood. *Ann Intern Med* 1993; **118**: 701–706.

152 Dutta P, Bhansali A, Singh P, Bhat MH. Suprasellar tubercular abscess presenting as panhypopituitarism: a common lesion in an uncommon site with a brief review of literature. *Pituitary* 2006; **9**: 73–77.

153 Indira B, Panigrahi MK, Vajramani G, Shankar SK, Santosh V, Das BS. Tuberculoma of the hypothalamic region as a rare case of hypopituitarism: a case report. *Surg Neurol* 1996; **45**: 347–350.

154 Paramo C, de la FJ, Nodar A, Miramontes S, Quintela JL, Garcia-Mayor RV. Intrasellar tuberculoma: a difficult diagnosis. *Infection* 2002; **30**: 35–37.

155 Sharma MC, Arora R, Mahapatra AK, Sarat-Chandra P, Gaikwad SB, Sarkar C. Intrasellar tuberculoma: an enigmatic pituitary infection: a series of 18 cases. *Clin Neurol Neurosurg* 2000; **102**: 72–77.

156 Unlu E, Puyan FO, Bilgi S, Kemal HM. Granulomatous hypophysitis: presentation and MRI appearance. *J Clin Neurosci* 2006; **13**: 1062–1066.

157 Domingues FS, de Souza JM, Chagas H, Chimelli L, Vaisman M. Pituitary tuberculoma: an unusual lesion of sellar region. *Pituitary* 2002; **5**: 149–153.

158 Rund D, Rachmilewitz E. Beta-thalassemia. *N Engl J Med* 2005; **353**: 1135–1146.

159 Oerter KE, Kamp GA, Munson PJ, Nienhuis AW, Cassorla FG, Manasco PK. Multiple hormone deficiencies in children with hemochromatosis. *J Clin Endocrinol Metab* 1993; **76**: 357–361.

160 Tilemans D, Vijver VV, Verhoeven G, Denef C. Production of transferrin-like immunoreactivity by rat anterior pituitary and intermediate lobe. *J Histochem Cytochem* 1995; **43**: 657–664.

161 Atkin SL, Burnett HE, Green VL, White MC, Lombard M. Expression of the transferrin receptor in human anterior pituitary adenomas is confined to gonadotrophinomas. *Clin Endocrinol (Oxf)* 1996; **44**: 467–471.

162 Tampanaru-Sarmesiu A, Stefaneanu L, Thapar K, Kontogeorgos G, Sumi T, Kovacs K. Transferrin and transferrin receptor in human hypophysis and pituitary adenomas. *Am J Pathol* 1998; **152**: 413–422.

163 Fung EB, Harmatz PR, Lee PD, *et al.* Increased prevalence of iron-overload associated endocrinopathy in thalassaemia versus sickle-cell disease. *Br J Haematol* 2006; **135**: 574–582.

164 Borgna-Pignatti C, Cappellini MD, De SP, *et al.* Survival and complications in thalassemia. *Ann N Y Acad Sci* 2005; **1054**: 40–47.

165 Multicentre study on prevalence of endocrine complications in thalassaemia major. Italian Working Group on Endocrine Complications in Non-endocrine Diseases. *Clin Endocrinol (Oxf)* 1995; **42**: 581–586.

166 Skordis N. The growing child with thalassaemia. *J Pediatr Endocrinol Metab* 2006; **19**: 467–469.

167 DeSanctis V, Roos M, Gasser T, Fortini M, Raiola G, Galati MC. Impact of long-term iron chelation therapy on growth and endocrine functions in thalassaemia. *J Pediatr Endocrinol Metab* 2006; **19**: 471–480.

168 DeSanctis V, Eleftheriou A, Malaventura C. Prevalence of endocrine complications and short stature in patients with thalassaemia major: a multicenter study by the Thalassaemia International Federation (TIF). *Pediatr Endocrinol Rev* 2004; **2** (Suppl 2): 249–255.

169 Raiola G, Galati MC, De SV, *et al.* Growth and puberty in thalassemia major. *J Pediatr Endocrinol Metab* 2003; **16** (Suppl 2): 259–266.

170 DeSanctis V, Katz M, Vullo C, Bagni B, Ughi M, Wonke B. Effect of different treatment regimes on linear growth and final height in beta-thalassaemia major. *Clin Endocrinol (Oxf)* 1994; **40**: 791–798.

171 Chan YL, Li CK, Pang LM, Chik KW. Desferrioxamine-induced long bone changes in thalassaemic patients: radiographic features, prevalence and relations with growth. *Clin Radiol* 2000; **55**: 610–614.

172 DeSanctis V, Stea S, Savarino L, *et al.* Osteochondrodystrophic lesions in chelated thalassemic patients: an histological analysis. *Calcif Tissue Int* 2000; **67**: 134–140.

173 Porter JB, Davis BA. Monitoring chelation therapy to achieve optimal outcome in the treatment of thalassaemia. *Best Pract Res Clin Haematol* 2002; **15**: 329–368.

174 Roth C, Pekrun A, Bartz M, *et al.* Short stature and failure of pubertal development in thalassaemia major: evidence for hypothalamic neurosecretory dysfunction of growth hormone secretion and defective pituitary gonadotropin secretion. *Eur J Pediatr* 1997; **156**: 777–783.

175 Cavallo L, Gurrado R, Gallo F, Zacchino C, De MD, Tato L. Growth deficiency in polytransfused beta-thalassaemia patients is not growth hormone dependent. *Clin Endocrinol (Oxf)* 1997; **46**: 701–706.

176 Shalitin S, Carmi D, Weintrob N, *et al.* Serum ferritin level as a predictor of impaired growth and puberty in thalassemia major patients. *Eur J Haematol* 2005; **74**: 93–100.

177 La Rosa C, De Sanctis V, Mangiagli A, *et al.* Growth hormone secretion in adult patients with thalassaemia. *Clin Endocrinol (Oxf)* 2005; **62**: 667–671.

178 Scacchi M, Danesi L, Cattaneo A, *et al.* Growth hormone deficiency (GHD) in adult thalassaemic patients. *Clin Endocrinol (Oxf)* 2007; **67**: 790–795.

179 Bronspiegel-Weintrob N, Olivieri NF, Tyler B, Andrews DF, Freedman MH, Holland FJ. Effect of age at the start of iron chelation therapy on gonadal function in beta-thalassemia major. *N Engl J Med* 1990; **323**: 713–719.

180 Argyropoulou MI, Kiortsis DN, Astrakas L, Metafratzi Z, Chalissos N, Efremidis SC. Liver, bone marrow, pancreas and pituitary gland iron overload in young and adult thalassemic patients: a T2 relaxometry study. *Eur Radiol* 2007; **17**: 3025–3030.

181 Argyropoulou MI, Kiortsis DN, Metafratzi Z, Bitsis S, Tsatoulis A, Efremidis SC. Pituitary gland height evaluated by MR in patients with beta-thalassaemia major: a marker of pituitary gland function. *Neuroradiology* 2001; **43**: 1056–1058.

182 Argyropoulou MI, Kiortsis DN, Efremidis SC. MRI of the liver and the pituitary gland in patients with beta-thalassaemia major: does hepatic siderosis predict pituitary iron deposition? *Eur Radiol* 2003; **13**: 12–16.

183 Skuse D, Albanese A, Stanhope R, Gilmour J, Voss L. A new stress-related syndrome of growth failure and hyperphagia in children, associated with reversibility of growth-hormone insufficiency. *Lancet* 1996; **348**: 353–358.

184 Albanese A, Hamill G, Jones J, Skuse D, Matthews DR, Stanhope R. Reversibility of physiological growth hormone secretion in children with psychosocial dwarfism. *Clin Endocrinol (Oxf)* 1994; **40**: 687–692.

6 Evaluation of Growth Disorders

Jerry K. Wales

Academic Unit of Child Health, Sheffield Children's Hospital, Sheffield, UK

Growth assessment requires an understanding of the physiology of growth. One of the most important aspects is accurate measurement and correct use of comparative standards. A structured approach to the clinical assessment of a child presenting with a growth disorder allows for a diagnostic framework from which specific clues can be spotted and further addressed. Short and tall stature will be dealt with separately along the lines of the current classification proposed by European Society for Pediatric Endocrinology (ESPE) [1] with attention to presentations in early and later childhood and, if appropriate, in young adult life.

Physiology of growth

Childhood growth is the product of a complex interaction of nutrient supply (over and above that required for basic metabolism) and hormones acting on the growth plates, with surplus energy being converted to muscle or deposited as fat. The process is easily disrupted and can serve as a marker for pathologies in any system and in the social environment.

There are four recognizable human growth phases, fetal, infantile, childhood and pubertal, each with different predominating control mechanisms [2,3].

Fetal growth peaks at 10 cm/month at the end of the second trimester with maximum weight gain in the third trimester [4]. Nutrient supply via the placenta is the main growth rate-limiting step but the placenta is also an active endocrine organ, producing growth factors such as growth hormone variant, human placental lactogen and organ-specific hormones such as corticotropin-releasing hormone (CRH), hepatic and epidermal growth factors (the latter acting on the adrenal).

The placenta in early pregnancy allows a small amount of thyroxine to pass to the fetus which has important effects on brain development; thereafter it is relatively impermeable to thyroxine

and deactivates fetal thyroid hormone. It acts as a barrier to two-way fetal and maternal steroid production, as well as producing placental steroids. The fetal pancreas releases insulin in response to nutrient supply and this has direct growth-promoting effects. Additionally, the fetus manufactures insulin-like growth factors (IGF), of which IGF-2 predominates and modulates the growth factor actions with specific binding proteins [5].

Placental failure or damage results in a growth-restricted infant, which may be symmetrical if occurring early in pregnancy (weight, length and head circumference all affected) or asymmetrical (mostly weight affected) from later problems. Congenital viral infections or genetic abnormalities tend to produce symmetrical growth restriction. Premature birth may result in suboptimal growth at a critical phase and, although later catch-up growth is usual, there may be late metabolic consequences [6].

Infantile growth is an extension of the fetal growth phase before growth becomes hormone dependent. Early growth in height and weight requires adequate nutrition but also normal thyroid function and bone metabolism. The hypothalamo-pituitary axis (HPA) becomes increasingly active and infants with growth hormone deficiency are shorter than may be expected even during the first year [7].

Childhood growth requires growth hormone (GH) action on epiphyseal cartilage cells to produce IGF-1, the major postnatal growth factor that stimulates cell division and growth. GH is secreted in an intermittent, pulsatile pattern largely due to the reciprocal interactions of GH releasing hormone (GHRH) and somatostatin (SS) or somatotrophin release inhibiting factor (SRIF) [8]. Withdrawal of SS appears to be the most important factor in determining the time of a GH pulse. Ghrelin, a 28 amino acid peptide secreted from the upper gastrointestinal tract, acts with GHRH to promote GH release and is also orexigenic thus linking food intake and growth promotion [9].

Growth hormone is a single-chain amino acid polypeptide (191AA) produced by the anterior pituitary (Fig. 6.1). Alternative splicing of the GH gene on the long arm of chromosome 17 produces other active shorter circulating variants. GH circulates in association with soluble extracellular receptor GH binding protein

Brook's Clinical Pediatric Endocrinology, 6th edition. Edited by C. Brook, P. Clayton, R. Brown. © 2009 Blackwell Publishing, ISBN: 978-1-4051-8080-1.

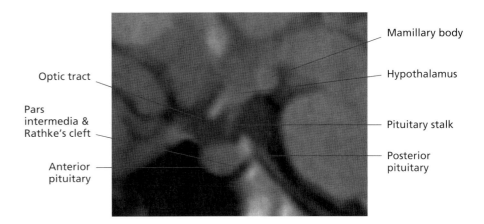

Optic tract

Pars
intermedia &
Rathke's cleft

Anterior
pituitary

Mamillary body

Hypothalamus

Pituitary stalk

Posterior
pituitary

Figure 6.1 Normal pituitary.

(GHBP) which causes dimerization of the GH receptor at the cell membrane. Activated receptors clump together in pits on the cell surface and are then internalized. There is then activation of intracellular signaling leading to production of IGF-1.

The GH receptor does not have intrinsic tyrosine kinase activity but activates a signaling peptide, JAK2, leading to autophosphorylation and the initiation of a phosphorylation cascade. A number of downstream pathways [mitogen activated protein kinase (MAPK), signal transducers and activators of transcription (STAT) and phosphatidylinositol 3-kinase (PI3-K)] result in GH signal transduction and the activation of the *IGF-1* gene. IGF-1 is a single-chain polypeptide hormone with structural homology to insulin that is present in the circulation at concentrations approximately 1000-fold that of insulin. IGF-1 production from the liver results in the measurable circulating IGF-1. Local production of IGF-1 at the growth plate acts on the IGF-1 receptor (which can also bind insulin) and causes cell division and maturation leading to bone lengthening [10].

The actions of IGF-1 are modulated by several binding proteins (IGFBPs), which prevent the high concentrations of IGF-1 causing hypoglycemia. IGFBPs act as co-transporters of IGF-1 out of the circulation and prevent rapid breakdown of the peptide. IGFBP3 is the most important, a GH-dependent binding protein that forms a ternary complex with IGF-1 and another protein, acid labile subunit (ALS), in the circulation. IGF binding proteins are modulated by immune peptides such as cytokines, reducing the availability of IGF-1 in states of inflammation or starvation [11].

Energy remaining for growth is what is left after the subtraction of the energy required to maintain basal metabolic rate, daily activity and diet-induced thermogenesis from the total energy intake. Because this is a small proportion (about 10%) of the total, quite severe energy restriction is required postnatally to disrupt growth. For bone lengthening to occur the growth plate must be normal and thyroxine, vitamin D and calcium are needed for normal epiphyseal cell division and differentiation. The growth promoting actions of GH thus require adequate nutrition, normal endocrine function and a normal skeleton.

Growth hormone, IGF-1 and neurotransmitters control GH release, which can thereby be modulated by input from higher centers [8]: for instance, severe psychosocial deprivation can produce marked growth restriction and reversible complete growth hormone deficiency (GHD) [12].

At puberty the pulsatility of GH secretion increases two- to threefold following which the secretion of GH falls toward prepubertal values and then declines further from middle age ("the somatopause"). The production of testosterone and estrogen from the gonads boosts growth of the spine in particular – hence the long-legged body habitus of a hypogonadotropic individual with normal GH production (such as untreated Klinefelter syndrome). Estrogen in both sexes (produced in the male by peripheral aromatization of testosterone) matures the epiphyses towards eventual bony fusion after which growth ceases.

Adult size is determined by the size of both parents but the mechanisms underlying the programing of adult stature are obscure. At 2 years of age a child should occupy a height centile determined equally by the sizes of both parents but before then a considerable amount of "channel-crossing" on the centile charts may occur. Catch-down growth is an adjustment from intrauterine factors that produce increased fetal growth, usually hyperinsulinemia. About two-thirds of intrauterine growth restricted (IUGR) babies show catch-up growth and cross centile channels after removal of any adverse intrauterine factors producing nutritional restraint. Most of this catch-up starts soon after birth and is completed by 18 months to 2 years [13].

With improved nutrition, especially protein and total calorie intake, there is a generational secular trend towards increasing height, weight and earlier sexual maturation. This is most obvious in societies where there has been a major change in socioeconomic status (e.g. Japan after the World War II or East Germany after reunification). In countries with a high standard of living, there has been a slowing of this trend and it is possible that there is a "maximum optimal final population height" for humans [14].

Anthropometry

The accurate assessment of a growth disorder must start with appropriate measurements taken by a trained observer using well-calibrated and maintained equipment [15]. All too often the task is delegated to someone who produces misleading information from measurement and unrecognized equipment error. Different measurements assess different body compartments (Fig. 6.2).

Length

Convention (and hence the comparative standards) dictates that under the age of 2 years supine length is measured. It may also be necessary in older children with neuromuscular problems. Two people are needed, one to hold the head against an immovable vertical plate board with the face horizontal and a second to extend the hips and knees to bring the soles of the feet down along a movable footboard: length is recorded to the nearest completed millimeter.

Height should be measured with the patient in bare feet with the heels in the same upright plane as the back of the head, often against a vertical wall. The subject should be relaxed and not standing tensely; the face should be maintained with the outer canthus and upper ear horizontal. Gentle upward traction on the mastoid processes by the measurer straightens the spine and the reading is made to the nearest completed millimeter at the end of a breath.

When repeated observations of height are taken to measure growth velocity, they should be performed at approximately the same time of day to avoid errors resulting from spinal compression and preferably by the same observer, especially if taken at intervals of less than 1 year. Morning height is 8 mm more than the afternoon value, representing about 15% of the yearly growth of a prepubertal child. Inter-observer errors are considerably greater than intra-observer errors. Short stature is defined as a height more than −2 SD (2.3%) below the mean.

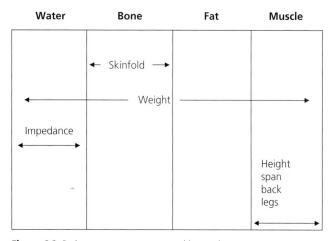

Figure 6.2 Body compartments as assessed by auxology.

Weight

Infants must be weighed naked and children in minimal clothing. Wet diapers can add up to as much as 10% of the baby's apparent weight and sports shoes, T-shirt and denims are equivalent to about 9 months of mid-childhood growth.

Body proportions and head size

Measurement of the length of the back can establish relative body proportions. This is very important in diagnostic assessment. In infancy the same technique and equipment used to measure length are used but the legs are lifted vertically and the footboard brought into contact with the buttocks. After 2 years, sitting height in an ambulant child is measured by placing a seat of known height with a horizontal top under the height measuring device or using a sitting height stadiometer. Leg length is then estimated by subtracting sitting height (equivalent to back + head length) from standing height. Upper/lower segment charts then allow comparison of body segments.

Arm span, estimated by measuring the fingertip-to-fingertip distance with the arms held horizontally, is an approximate surrogate for height (span = height ± 3.5 cm) in the patient unable to stand or with severe spinal deformity. It may bear an abnormal relationship to height in some skeletal dysplasias or Marfan syndrome.

Head circumference may also be disproportionately large or small in some growth disorders and can provide further diagnostic clues. It should be measured using a non-stretchable paper or metal tape, usually as the mean of three estimations to establish the maximum occipito-frontal circumference (OFC).

Body composition and adiposity

Body mass index [BMI; weight (kg)/height (m)^2] allows a crude estimate of adiposity in comparison to age-related standards. In practice it is not difficult to differentiate the muscular from the fat child. Skinfold measurements allow for estimation of fat distribution on the limbs, trunk and abdomen which can be occasionally useful in diagnosis. They are of most value when used serially to establish response to treatment or to note the characteristic changes of increasing truncal adiposity compared to the limbs in early puberty in boys. The same design of calipers is needed that were used to construct the comparative standards being used. Triceps and subscapular skinfolds are most commonly used but the addition of biceps and suprailiac skinfolds allows the values to be used in formulae that estimate total body fat mass.

Bioelectrical impedance devices are increasingly incorporated into weighing scales and measure the conductance of a tiny charge through body water. This allows estimation of lean body mass by software using published regression equations for different clinical situations. The estimate is very dependent on factors such as ambient temperature, time since a meal or bladder voiding and should be interpreted with caution.

Crude estimates of undernutrition can be made using mid-upper-arm circumference (MUAC; measured at a point half way between elbow and shoulder) using a flexible non-stretch tape measure, and waist and hip circumferences as a measure of overnutrition. Waist circumference is usually measured between the lower ribs and the ischial ridge at the level of the umbilicus at the end of a normal expiration. Other definitions have been described such as the point at which lateral bending produces a skin crease. Hip circumference is usually measured at the level of both greater trochanters. The waist:hip or waist:height ratio may then be calculated as an estimate of body shape. It is again important that the measurer establishes which of several measurement techniques and body landmarks is applicable to the comparative standards being used.

Other measurements

It is sometimes helpful to assess other body sizes and their relationships directly. Standard centile charts exist for almost every possible anthropometric variable and have been published as a compendium for use in dysmorphology.

In short-limbed conditions and if hemihypertrophy is suspected, direct measurement of limb segments using a specially designed anthropometer or a metal builder's tape measure may be useful.

Bone age or skeletal maturity

Most methods assess the degree of development of the large number of bones available on a radiograph of the left hand and wrist [15]. The individual ossification centers may be "aged" in comparison to a standard atlas (e.g. Gruelich and Pyle method) or by assigning a score to 20 of the individual bones [e.g. the Tanner–Whitehouse 2 or 3 (TW2 or TW3) methods]. Computerized assessment of digital radiographs may become routine but has not yet been perfected. Accurate estimation of bone age may be difficult or impossible in some skeletal dysplasias or after high-dose steroid treatment.

Equations that use height (± recent height velocity) combined with a "bone maturity score" allow a predicted adult height to be estimated with a range of error of ±2 SD. Because the methodology was described for normal children, the validity of such prediction for children with pathology is doubtful, especially if bone age is advanced. If bone age is estimated at the same time as a measurement, height can be plotted for the bone age of a child as well as for the chronological age to give a visual representation of height remaining (Fig. 6.3). Bone age advances at a more rapid pace than chronological age (up to 2.5 years per year) during puberty, which can lead to an over-optimistic prediction of final height and indicates the need for control groups to be used in all situations where response to a growth promoting treatment is being assessed.

Definition of normal

Growth charts

Cross-sectional standards for height, weight, BMI and head circumference are available for many populations and should be updated regularly to take secular changes into account. There are also many disease-specific charts available once a diagnosis has been reached (Table 6.1).

A common layout is to use the 0.4th, 2nd, 9th, 25th and 50th centile approximating to two-thirds of one standard deviation per major interval with corresponding values above the mean to give nine centile lines. This design means that only 1/250 children would fall below the 0.4th or above the 99.6th centile in a normal population, which may form the basis for a referral protocol from height screening programs [16].

By 2 years of age, the correlation between the current height of the child and mid-parental height is about 0.75; at final height it is about 0.8 in a normal child. Whatever chart is used, it is possible rapidly to estimate the expected genetic potential of the subject by plotting the centile value of each parent on the right-hand y-axis and drawing the mid-parental centile. Many equations have been used to estimate genetic height potential. On the current UK charts (Fig. 6.3) the calculation is shown as:

Target height for a boy: (father's height + mother's height)/2 = A

A + 7 = mid-parental height, range ± 10 cm

Target height for a girl: (mother's height + father's height)/2 = A

A − 7 = mid-parental height, range ± 8.5 cm

An alternative method is to plot on or calculate the centile position of the parents from the adult y-axis. Here the mid-parental centile position can be calculated on the y-axis of any chart and a centile range of the equivalent adult span of ±10 cm (male) or 8.5 cm (female) used as the target range. If the economic situation of the child is much better than that of the parents in their youth, one can add 4.5 cm to the estimated genetic height potential to allow for secular trends in height.

Height velocity

Change of height with time is more important than absolute height at a point and can be made visually by assessing deviation upwards or downwards through the centile lines or by calculating a height velocity. Height velocity standards constructed from longitudinal observations made at 12-monthly intervals on relatively small populations are available. Caution should be used if clinical inferences are to be drawn from measurements taken over shorter intervals. Height velocity is calculated by the formula:

Ht 2 – Ht 1 / interval in years

Height centile lines diverge with age because tall children must grow slightly faster than short ones but growth is episodic not linear, so, unlike height, height velocity varies around a centile rather than following a channel. A tall child with a height on the 91st centile will have velocities on either side of the 75th height velocity centile and a shorter child on the 9th centile will oscillate around the 25th velocity centile. Hence "normal" height velocity

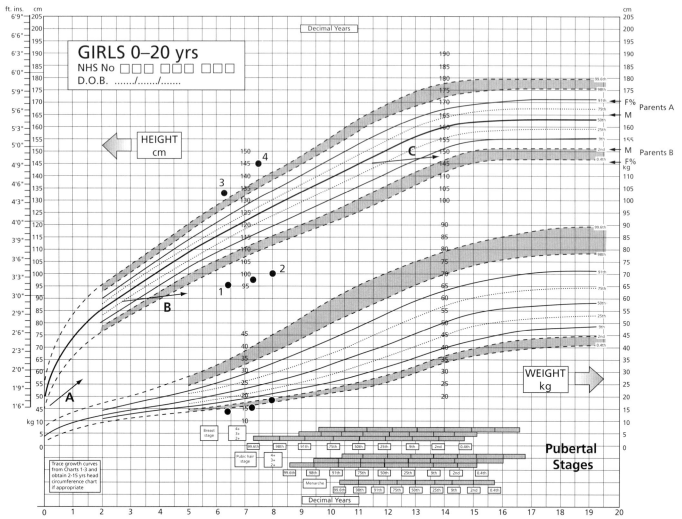

Figure 6.3 Growth chart. Line A, Failure of the fetal/infantile component of growth: SGA, placental and maternal ill-health, intrauterine infection, genetic syndromes, primordial nanism, some dysplasias [measure occipito-frontal circumference (OFC) and body segments]. Line B, Failure of the childhood component of growth: GHD, hypothyroidism, psychosocial deprivation, severe malnutrition, some dysplasias (measure OFC and segments). Line C, Failure of the pubertal component of growth: constitutional delayed puberty, hypogonadism, hypochondroplasia. At point 1 the girl is at the bottom end of her genetic range for parents B, but abnormally short for parents A. Subsequent growth rate is poor and worse for height than weight indicating a high chance of an endocrine abnormality causing the short stature. At point 3 the girl is at the top end of her genetic range for parents A, but abnormally tall for parents B. By point 4 her growth rate is abnormal indicating an acquired cause of tall stature (e.g. thyrotoxicosis, early sex hormone exposure, gigantism).

may be thought of as oscillating 25–75% except for children with delayed puberty, when the exaggerated prepubertal nadir of growth produces values less than 4 cm/year and below the 25th centile. The theoretical chance of annual growth velocities in a normal child being below the 25th centile over 2 years would be 0.25 × 0.25 or 6.25%.

On average, growth is slower in winter than summer and, if monitored longitudinally in a normal child, can show relatively fixed periods of mild acceleration (e.g. the "preschool growth spurt") or deceleration (e.g. the prepubertal nadir") [17].

Standard deviation scores

Any normally distributed measurement for which population standards exist may be expressed as a standard deviation score (SD or Z score), which allows for comparison of children within the reference population of different ages and sex:

$$SD \text{ (Z score)} = x - \bar{x}/SD,$$

where x is the measured value; $\bar{x}$ the mean and SD the standard deviation for a given population. In a characteristic normally

Table 6.1 Some syndromes with specific growth charts.

Turner	Height, height velocity, weight
Trisomy 21	Height, weight, OFC
Noonan	Height
Prader–Willi	Height, weight, OFC, hand and foot length
Russell–Silver	Height
Cornelia de Lange	Height, weight, OFC
Laron	Height
Achondroplasia	Height, OFC, segments
Hypochondroplasia	Height and segments
Pseudoachondroplasia	Height
Spondyloepiphyseal dysplasia	Height
Diastropic dysplasia	Height
Cartilage-hair hypoplasia	Height
Marfan syndrome	Height

OFC, occipito-frontal circumference.

distributed population, the SD has a mean of 0 and a SD of 1, −1 to +1 including 68.26% and −2 to +2 95.44% of the population, respectively. Only 0.13% of a population has a SD of more or less than 3.

How to use a growth chart

First plot simple height and weight and compare the individual with the population. Always use a simple dot rather than crosses or circles that can obscure data and do not joining successive points with a line. What is the relationship of the subject's weight to height? Are they relatively heavier than short; tall and thin; tall and heavy, etc. – all of which patterns may increase the likelihood of pathology. Plot height for bone age (if available) and stage of puberty (given on many centile charts; Fig. 6.3). Compare the subject's centile position to that of their parent(s) and sibling(s).

It is usually possible to assess visually if the subject is likely to achieve his/her predicted adult height, given the degree of bone or sexual maturation. A bone age-based height prediction can be used if the skeleton is normal.

Plot sitting height and leg length to assess disproportion and compare the head circumference to height (and parental head size) to assess possible macrocephaly or microcephaly as part of documentation of dysmorphology.

At subsequent visits or, where prior information exists, height velocity can be estimated visually on the cross-sectional chart or plotted on a longitudinal chart. Because of the sex hormone-augmented growth of the back and increased secretion of growth hormone, the pubertal height spurt is dependent on the timing of gonadal steroid production. This is variable, with some individuals maturing early or later than their contemporaries, often with a family pattern that is obtainable from the history. It is important to take into account this "tempo" of maturation when assessing growth around puberty. Figure 6.3 shows some examples of the use of the growth chart in practice.

Structured clinical assessment

History
The general points to be noted in the assessment of any child with a growth disorder are shown in Table 6.2.

Examination
A systematic approach to the general examination of a child with a growth disorder starts at the periphery, moves to the arms and to the head and neck before the body, skin and parents (Table 6.3).

Short stature

The ESPE classification system of growth disorders has been used to base the structure of the following section, which will also be structured to differentiate early presenting from late presenting growth disorders, where possible [1]. Short stature may be categorized as:

(a) *Primary growth failure*
Clinically defined syndromes with chromosomal abnormalities
Clinically defined syndromes without known chromosomal abnormalities
Intrauterine growth retardation with failure to demonstrate catch-up
Skeletal dysplasias
Disorders of calcium and phosphate, metabolic disorders and primary disorders of bone.
(b) *Secondary growth failure*
Disorders in specific systems
Endocrine disorders, including:
    Growth hormone deficiency (congenital/acquired)
    Growth hormone insensitivity
Iatrogenic short stature
Psychosocial short stature.
(c) *Constitutional short stature*
Idiopathic familial short stature
Constitutional short stature with pubertal delay
Non-familial short stature with or without pubertal delay.

Epidemiology
Organic pathology causing short stature is rare. In a study of 114 000 children measured once or serially (80 000) for 2 years the frequencies of growth abnormalities outside those already known in the growth clinic were examined [18]. Of 1200 identified initially as <−2 SD below the mean, most were in the normal centile range and growing at a normal rate on remeasurement. Of the 555 children with heights <3rd centile and growing poorly, familial short stature and constitutional delay in growth accounted for 75% and 10% had a systemic illness. Only 5% had an endocrine disorder. Thirty-three had GH deficiency, although half of these were already diagnosed. Six girls had undiagnosed Turner

Table 6.2 Points to note in the history of a child presenting with a growth disorder.

Presenting complaint	Parents and child (this may be different and different again from professional concern)
How long have they been worried?	
Specific symptoms	In any system that may indicate chronic illness
Details of the pregnancy, gestational age, mode of delivery, neonatal ill health, birth measurements	Maternal ill health, prescription medication or drug/alcohol use
Neonatal problems	e.g. hypoglycemia (congenital hypopituitarism), jaundice (congenital hypothyroidism or hypopituitarism), floppiness and feeding difficulty (Prader–Willi syndrome), puffy hands and feet, coarctation (Turner syndrome)
Current growth rate, past medical records, home measurements	Is the child growing out of their clothes and shoes before they wear out? Any recent change in weight pattern?
Family history	Parental and sibling heights, (preferably measured), maternal menarche, delayed or early shaving/growth in father, marked short/tall stature, consanguinity In particular any endocrine disorders, endocrine malignancy and autoimmunity, early heart disease or eye problems
Social details	Home Sport, career aspirations Teasing/bullying at school
Developmental or educational concentration, behavior	
Medication	Any regular treatment (including topical and inhaled steroid preparations, substance abuse, methylphenidate)
Past medical events	Even "trivial" procedures; e.g. herniae, undescended testes
Diet	
Any symptoms suggestive of early sexual development	Moody, sweaty, body odor, spots, PV discharge, hair, breast, penis growth

syndrome. The incidence of GHD (defined as a peak response to stimulation of <10 ng/dL in this study) was 1 in 3500.

In another study, 180 of 14 000 children at school entry were found to have heights below the 3rd centile, the majority with familial short stature; 32/180 had organic disease, already recognized in 25. Only 1 in 3500 of the total population had an unrecognized remediable cause of short stature [19].

Primary growth failure

Primary growth failure is divided into those with or without clinical syndromes with chromosomal abnormalities. To some extent, this is artificial because many conditions that had no previously known chromosomal abnormality have been found increasingly to have abnormalities such as subtle deletions. Numeric abnormalities, especially Turner syndrome, are important, usually resulting in well-defined abnormalities accompanied by short stature.

Clinically defined syndromes with numeric chromosomal abnormalities

Conditions in this category include Turner syndrome (45XO and variants), Down syndrome (trisomy 21), Edward syndrome (trisomy 18), Patau syndrome (trisomy 13) and triploidy. Only Turner syndrome presents primarily as a growth disorder because the other conditions usually have such severe associated abnormalities, including neurodevelopmental delay, that they present early in life.

Turner syndrome and SHOX insufficiency

Turner syndrome can present antenatally, in the neonate, in infancy, at puberty or in adulthood.

First described by Ullrich in 1930 and Turner 8 years later [20,21], this is the most common female sex chromosome abnormality. Most affected fetuses abort spontaneously early in pregnancy but enough survive to give a prevalence rate of approximately 1 in 2500 live female births. Presumably fetuses with the least severe chromosomal abnormality and highest tissue mosaicism are the ones that survive to term.

In approximately 50% of cases, the entire X chromosome is missing in peripheral blood lymphocytes but there are several other possible karyotypic abnormalities that produce the syndrome and frequently tissue mosaicism. Partial absence of the second X chromosome, inversions and ring chromosomes may all be present in this syndrome, with a frequency given in Table 6.4 [22]. The presence of Y chromosomal material may be associated with the later development of gonadoblastoma and must be excluded early. In some individuals, the mosaicism may be such that the blood karyotype is entirely 46XX but the features of

Table 6.3 Points to note in the examination of a child presenting with a growth disorder.

General observation	Activity, demeanor and interaction
Hands	Dermatoglyphics
	Joint mobility
	Long or short fingers/abnormal thumb
	Abnormal/extra digits
	Clubbing. Nail size/shape
	Pigmentation, abnormal color
Wrist	Rickets
Arms	Span
	Abnormal bones; fusion with limited rotation; angulation
Neck	Webbing; extra skin; low hairline
	Goitre tremor, exophthalmos or other signs of thyrotoxicosis
Hair	Pattern, whorls, hair loss, texture
Head and eyes	Skull shape
Any midline defects are of particular importance	e.g. Hypertelorism or hypotelorism, epicanthic folds; ptosis; blepharophimosis, microphthalmia and exophthalmos
	Abnormal retinae and discs, visual field deficit, appearance and the position of the lens
Mouth and palate	Tooth eruption, abnormality of enamel and teeth
	Tongue and lips (neuromas in MEN2b)
Ears	Position and shape
Central nervous system	Developmental level
Chest	Shape, lung abnormality
Breast tissue	Puberty, structural abnormalities
Spine abnormality	Scoliosis, kyphosis, lordosis
Cardiovascular system	Blood pressure, heart abnormality
Abdomen	Organomegaly, masses, herniae
Genitalia	Stage puberty
	Structural abnormalities – hypogonadism, cryptorchidism
Body shape	Muscle and fat distribution
	Asymmetry
Skin	Birthmarks, naevi, pigmentation, fragility, pigmented scars
	Hirsutism
Parents	Size, proportions, dysmorphic features, development

MEN2b, multiple endocrine neoplasia type 2b.

Table 6.4 Recognized chromosomal abnormalities in Turner syndrome.

45X	40%
45X/46 Xi(Xq)	10% (mosaic isochromosome long arm)
46Xi (Xq)	6% (isochromosome long arm)
45X, 46Xr (X)	5% (ring)
45X, 46XX	12% (mosaic)
45X, 46XY	4% (gonadoblastoma risk 20–30%)
45X, 46Xi (Yp)	2.5% (gonadoblastoma risk 20–30%)
Other including: 45X/47XXX, 45X/46XX/47XXX Tissue, not blood	18%

Turner syndrome are present. In such cases, it may be useful to examine fibroblast cell lines.

The short stature in Turner syndrome occurs because only one copy of a homeobox gene (SHOX) is present. This is a gene on the pseudoautosomal region of both the X and Y chromosome so the gene is not inactivated and two copies are required for normal stature [23]. If no copies are present, the severe short stature syndrome of dyschondrosteosis or Leri–Weill syndrome emerges and there is marked mesomelic short stature and severe forearm abnormalities (Madelung deformity), with high arched palate and sometimes scoliosis. The short metacarpal and abnormal radio-ulnar angle at the wrist are milder abnormalities found in Turner syndrome. There may also be a high arched palate. The importance of the SHOX abnormality is that approximately 2.5% of children with idiopathic short stature have some features of SHOX insufficiency, including short forearms, a wide carrying angle, a muscular build and abnormalities of the gene which may be confirmed on genetic testing.

Short stature is almost invariable in Turner syndrome and tends to progress so that approximately 50% of girls are outside the normal range at 5 years of age, 75% at 9 years but almost all by the time puberty should have started. There is a 20-cm height deficit from that expected from the genetic potential so that, if both parents are tall, the girl's height may fall well into the normal centile range, especially in early childhood but will be outside her predicted genetic height. A disease-specific growth chart is available and should be used to monitor growth once the diagnosis is established [24,25].

A list of the physical characteristics is given in Table 6.5(a) with the risks they pose in early and later life. Table 6.5(b) gives a suggested surveillance program for the adult woman [26,27].

In the neonate, a baby born with lymphedema of the back of the feet, hands and the neck should be suspected as having Turner syndrome. Likewise any female baby with coarctation has Turner

Table 6.5 (a) Phenotypic features and risks of Turner syndrome in the adult and child.

System	In child	In adult	Other
Short (90%+)	GH treatment	Unknown long-term risks	Deficit 20 cm compared to MPH – if very tall parents then in normal range
Weight		Tend to put on easily	Type 2 diabetes General health risks
Type 1 diabetes	Rare	Increased risk	35% overall type 1 and 2 lifelong risk
Thyroid	±20% hypo	±40% hypo	Pick up early TSH and antithyroid antibodies
Eyesight	Eyes – (myopia)	Myopia, macular degeneration	
Hearing	Glue ear (60%+)	Nerve problems in older (50%)	Audiology
Blood pressure	Common	Common Stroke (Lipids + BP + CVS abnormalities)	Treat early Worse if weight problem
Kidney problems (30%)	USS (horseshoe)	Fairly common	May relate to BP
Osteoporosis		Delayed puberty, inadequate oestrogens	Diet adequate in calcium
Fertility, ovarian dysgenesis 90%	USS ovaries	Egg donation (?oocytes in future)	
Periods	USS uterus	Dysfunctional uterine bleeding	Patch or "pill"
Heart (±30%)	ECG, echo at diagnosis (? Coarctation; aortic stenosis)	Dilated aorta (total 5–10% – dissects 60%) MRI aorta 5 yearly	Other "silent" problems Lipids Bicuspid valves
Back	Scoliosis (15%)		
Feet	Hypoplastic nails (60%) –shoe fitting	Chiropody	75% have foot problems
Skin	Naevi (60%+)	Melanoma risk	Keloid risk increased
Lymphedema	Feet (40%), back, neck	Feet	Shoe fitting difficult
Orthodontic	High palate (50%) and orthodontic	Orthodontic	
Liver	Abnormal tests	Tests abnormal	Significance unknown
Psychology	"Different," Fertility Height Cosmetic Visuospatial problems	"Different," Fertility Height Cosmetic Visuospatial problems	Support groups Leg lengthening Plastic surgery
Education	Visuospatial problems Handwriting	May need more time at exams	Rarely major deficit
Rarities	Gonadoblastoma related to Y chromosome	Cancers and ulcers? IBD	? Slight increase colon cancer Possibly risk

BP, blood pressure; CVS, cardiovascular system; ECG, electrocardiogram; GH, growth hormone; IBD, irritable bowel disorder/disease; MPH, midparental height; MRI, magnetic resonance imaging; TSH, thyroid stimulating hormone; USS, ultrasound.

Table 6.5 (b) Surveillance of Turner syndrome required in adult woman.

	Frequency
Weight	Yearly
Blood pressure	Yearly
Glucose	Yearly
TSH	Yearly
U&E, creatinine	Yearly
DEXA	At transfer +5 yearly
Heart USS (MRI)	At transfer +5 yearly
Eye test	Regular optician review
Audiology	5 yearly
Fertility	As needed
Psychology – peer support	As needed but ask each visit

DEXA, bone densitometry; TSH, thyroid stimulating hormone; MRI, magnetic resonance imaging; U&E, urea and electrolytes.

syndrome until proved otherwise because about 30% of Turner girls are affected. Some girls with the condition have a broad chest, abnormal carrying angle, low set hairline and ptosis from birth and may be diagnosed with these features. The ears are often rather low set and malformed but usually not as markedly as in Noonan syndrome.

Glue ear is extremely common and short girls with the condition attending ENT clinics should be screened for Turner syndrome. Eighth nerve hearing loss may also be present, especially in later life. Myopia may be severe and produce a squint. However, in approximately 40% of girls, the physical features are insufficient to make an early diagnosis and they present only with short stature. Thus, Turner syndrome should be suspected in all short girls.

Stature will be on a centile lower than the height predicted from the parents. The girls are usually proportionate, although the upper limbs may be slightly short if span is measured. Relatively invariable mild features are multiple pigmented naevi and hypoplastic nails, especially on the foot, ptosis, a low posterior hairline and high arched palate. It is particularly important to identify the presence of mild coarctation of the aorta by assessment of the cardiovascular system, measuring blood pressure and palpating the peripheral pulses. Mild lymphedema may still persist into later life, particularly between the shoulder blades and on the back of the feet.

The other cardinal feature of Turner syndrome is pubertal failure secondary to ovarian failure. The "rule of diminishing 10s" says that about 10% of Turner syndrome girls develop spontaneous puberty (most commonly the mosaic forms); of these 10% will finish puberty and menstruate and 10% of those will ovulate and be able to conceive, although successful full-term pregnancy is uncommon. Girls with no signs of breast development after the age of 12 should have their gonadotropins measured and chromosomes checked if the follicle stimulating hormone (FSH) is raised. Pelvic ultrasound will show a small uterus and absent or streak ovaries with few or no follicular development.

Hypothyroidism occurs in 40% of Turner girls due to autoimmune thyroiditis, becoming more common with age, so the neck should be examined for a goiter and thyroid stimulating hormone (TSH) measured annually. Celiac disease and diabetes (types 1 and 2) also are more common than in normal girls but rarely present symptomatically at diagnosis.

Abnormalities of the renal tract should be assessed by ultrasound at diagnosis and 5-yearly thereafter. Most common are an asymptomatic horseshoe kidney or a duplex system but urinary infections may lead to scarring and hypertension, although renal artery stenosis also contributes. In older Turner girls, hypertension is common and there may be progressive dilatation of the aortic root. All girls with Turner syndrome should have an annual assessment of blood pressure and a 5-yearly magnetic resonance imaging (MRI) of the heart and aorta.

Most girls with the condition function well in normal schools, although there are commonly subtle abnormalities of visuospatial coordination, slow handwriting and sometimes isolated learning difficulties in mathematics.

Multiple gonadal dysgenesis 45X/46XY or 45X/47XYY produces highly variable genital abnormalities (including normality) but failure of pubertal growth occurs in those individuals not diagnosed because of a disorder of sexual development.

Down syndrome and other numerical chromosomal abnormalities

These conditions present antenatally or in the immediate neonatal period. Down syndrome (trisomy 21) is the most common chromosomal abnormality, although increasingly picked up on antenatal screening. Like Turner syndrome it produces a height deficit of approximately 20 cm but there is no relation to parental size. The pubertal growth spurt is blunted. Ten to 20% of cases have biochemical evidence of mild growth hormone insufficiency probably caused by hypothalamic dysregulation and/or obesity. Coexistent thyroid disease and celiac disease make the height deficit more marked and are common enough for routine screening. Individuals are typically more heavy than short in comparison to the normal centile range and syndrome-specific growth charts should be used to monitor growth after diagnosis [27]. Almost all individuals with Down syndrome present because of their dysmorphic features and learning difficulties in early life.

Edward syndrome (trisomy 18) and Patau syndrome (trisomy 13), both related to increasing maternal age, also result in extreme short stature in the relatively few individuals who survive the neonatal period. Survival beyond the neonatal period reflects tissue mosaicism.

Other mosaic trisomies are well described and these individuals are usually diagnosed because of their severe physical malformations or learning disability long before they present at a growth clinic. Triploidy (66 XXY or XYY) may occasionally be compatible with survival in chimeric/mosaic individuals in whom bulbous nose and wide simian creases on the feet are usually associated with short stature.

Clinically defined syndromes with no known chromosomal abnormality

Noonan syndrome

Noonan syndrome may present antenatally with its marked nuchal edema, in the neonatal period with a heart abnormality or with pronounced physical features but often presents later in childhood or puberty. This syndrome is slightly more common than Turner syndrome and can occur in both sexes. It has some superficial similarities to Turner syndrome but no major structural abnormality of the chromosomes. The most common physical features are seen in the head and neck, with a short neck, webbing, wide spaced eyes, ptosis, abnormal ears and occasional deafness. In boys there may be cryptorchidism and testicular abnormalities. Impaired fertility is a feature in both sexes.

Short stature is almost invariable and disease-specific charts are available once the diagnosis has been established [28]. The height deficit is approximately 15 cm with a delay in pubertal growth which can be more severe in boys with hypogonadism. Because one parent may be affected, it is important to examine the parents before concluding from the mid-parental height that the child has constitutional short stature.

Pectus carinatum may be present. The heart defect, if present, is more commonly on the right side of the heart, in contrast to Turner syndrome. Hypertropic cardiomyopathy may occur. Before any surgery, clotting factors should be measured because about 40% of patients have a bleeding diathesis. The low set abnormal ears are more marked than in Turner syndrome, as is the ptosis. School difficulties are also more common than in Turner syndrome.

Noonan syndrome is caused by a mutation in several genes on different chromosomes and at least five subtypes are described, including NS2, an autosomal recessive form; NS3 with a mutation in *KRAS* gene; NS4 with a mutation on chromosome 2 of *SOS1* gene (and more frequent heart abnormalities) and NFNS with neurofibromatosis-like features. The most commone abnormality, inherited in an autosomal dominant fashion, which occurs in about 50% cases, is in the *PTPN11* gene on the long arm of chromosome 12, which codes for tyrosine phosphatase, a non-receptor protein [29].

Imprinting disorders

Imprinting is an inactivation of some of the normal maternal or paternal gene copies (about 80 in the human) by methylation during the formation of gametes. Because of duplication of one parental chromosome (parental isodisomy) or duplication of the gene or structural damage to the other copy, only copies of the same parental gene may be expressed, resulting in abnormalities [30].

Russell–Silver syndrome

Russell–Silver syndrome presents antenatally with poor fetal growth or in the neonatal period, when feeding difficulties are a prominent (some would say obligatory) feature. Diagnosis is often delayed until the failure of catch-up growth is noticed. The syndrome includes facial abnormalities with a large forehead and a small triangular lower face. There is hemihypertrophy and a bending of the fifth finger (clinodactyly). The short stature persists after the first 2 years of life and the bone age is delayed. Final height prognosis is poor (−3 to −4 SD) because these individuals experience adrenarche and puberty at an age- but not height-appropriate time, resulting in a worse final height than would otherwise be anticipated. Several genetic abnormalities have been described, on different chromosomes but two copies of the maternal chromosome 7 have been described in approximately 10% of cases, implicating imprinting as one mechanism [31,32].

Prader–Willi syndrome

Prader–Willi syndrome (PWS) may present in the neonatal period because of the extreme hypotonia and feeding difficulties sometimes requiring nasogastric tube or gastrostomy feeding. Milder cases can present later in childhood or occasionally with failure of puberty.

PWS affects approximately 1 in 15 000 live births. Short stature is almost invariable (adult height 147 cm female; 155 cm male) but most children are diagnosed in the neonatal period because of extreme floppiness. Hypogonadism may also be a presenting feature in the neonatal period with a small penis and small or impalpable testes. Infertility is almost invariable in females (Prader, personal communication).

Milder cases can present with short stature in mid-childhood and there may be a history of poor feeding and hypotonia in the neonatal period to be gathered in retrospect. The children are short, have small hands and feet and almond-shaped eyes with myopia or esotropia. Increasingly obsessive behavior regarding feeding develops with age and the typical older child with PWS is short with severe and progressive obesity and pubertal delay. Behavioral problems include skin self-mutilation. Scoliosis is common in late childhood or in puberty. Adult females have oligomenorrhea and males usually need testosterone supplementation. Type 2 diabetes and cardiovascular disease occur early secondary to obesity. The mean developmental quotient (DQ) is 65 but developmental delay is very variable. Syndrome-specific growth charts are available [33].

The most common abnormality resulting in PWS is an imprinting of several genes on the long arm of chromosome 15. Loss of the paternal copy or duplication of the maternal copy results in the syndrome: the opposite imprinting of the same gene with duplication of the paternal copy causes the Angelman syndrome. Individuals with this disorder have abnormalities in the secretion of ghrelin from the stomach which usually precedes ingestion of food. This peptide usually releases GH in a delayed manner and stimulates appetite in the short term. In PWS the high basal concentrations are associated with increased appetite but low/low-normal GH concentrations [34].

Other syndromes

There are almost 2000 other syndromes associated with short stature. Some of the more common conditions presenting to a growth clinic are listed in Table 6.6 along with their major features and genetic abnormality when known. A computerized search engine such as the London Dysmorphology Database [35] can be used to narrow down possible diagnoses. The key to accurate syndrome diagnosis of often exceptionally rare disorders lies in a structured approach to assessment.

Every time an abnormality is found, it should be noted and quantified if possible using data from Hall *et al.* [36]. At the end of the examination, the features can be arranged with the most abnormal "handles" first and which of them are "mandatory" in the search can be listed. A list of possible diagnoses can then be obtained from the search engine and refined by eliminating some disorders (e.g. a diagnosis of Seckel syndrome is not tenable if microcephaly is *not* present) and looking at the supplied photographs and references. The Online Mendelian Inheritance in Man

website (OMIM) [37] can be used to retrieve full up-to-date information.

Intrauterine growth retardation and small for gestational age

Made in relation to appropriate standards for gestational age, IUGR should be a prenatal diagnosis and small for gestational age (SGA) a postnatal one. Apart from SGA secondary to the Russell–Silver syndrome, other syndromes with well-defined physical abnormalities also produce marked IUGR with later sometimes extreme short stature, including Seckel syndrome, microcephalic osteodysplastic primordial dwarfism types 1–3 (MOPD), neonatal progeria and other conditions which may be lumped together under the headings "primordial short stature" (Table 6.7).

Table 6.6 Some important syndromes associated with short stature.

Syndrome	Features	Genes
CHARGE	An association of iris coloboma, heart defects, choanal atresia, retarded growth and development, genital and ear abnormalities GHD not uncommon finding along with hypogonadotropic hypogonadism	Chromodomain helicase DNA-binding protein-7 (*CHD7*) 8q12.1 also by mutation in the semaphorin-3E gene 7q21.1
SHORT	Short stature, hyperextensibility and hernia, ocular depression, Rieger anomaly and teething delay	Isolated Rieger syndrome can be caused by mutation in the *PITX2* gene chromosome 4q25
Fanconi	Proximal tubular defect producing failure to thrive, polydipsia and polyuria. Renal loss of electrolytes produces symptomatic acidosis, paralysis, fractures, etc. There is a high (50%) incidence of growth hormone and thyroid abnormalities (35%) on testing	Mutation of one of several Fanconi "complementation" genes at 16q24.3
Bartter & Gitelman	Renal tubular abnormalities with electrolyte loss producing short stature – more marked in Bartter syndrome – and hypokalemic alkalosis	Bartter several subtypes, the most common type 3 caused by mutation in the kidney chloride channel B gene, 1p36 Gitelman, thiazide sensitive Na-Cl co-transporter on 16q13
Bloom	Autosomal recessive with a predisposition to easy DNA damage from sunlight producing skin lesions, internal malignancy and chromosomal breakage	Mutations in the gene encoding DNA helicase RecQ protein-like-3 15q26.1
Aarskog (Aarskog–Scott)	Shawl scrotum, cryptorchidism (variable) prominent finger pads and joints, wide spaced eyes	Some X-linked with mutation of *FDG1* but likely heterogeneous
Kabuki make-up	Developmental delay, long eyes with everted lateral one-third of lower lids, broad nose, large earlobes. Spinal, hip and hand abnormalities	Sporadic. Exact gene abnormality currently not known
3M syndrome	Autosomal recessive, hatchet-shaped face from side, prominent heels and relatively preserved head circumference. The bones are slender and the vertebrae relatively tall	Mutation of *CUL7* on chromosome 6p21.1 that controls ubiquitination a process of protein modification and degradation
Mulibrey nanism	Muscle liver brain and eye; large head with triangular face reminiscent of Russell–Silver syndrome. Liver enlarged due to constrictive pericarditis	Also probably due to a disorder of ubiquitination, a mutation of the *TRIM37* gene, which encodes a peroxisomal protein. 17q22-23
Cornelia de Lange syndrome (Brachmann–de Lange)	Low hairline with fused eyebrows (synophrys) downturned mouth and anteverted nostrils. Developmental delay	Several forms with a similar phenotype but different genes on several chromosomes have been implicated. 50% due to mutation of 5p13.1 encoding a component of the cohesin complex

Table 6.7 Primordial short-stature syndromes.

Seckel syndrome	Average birth weight 1.5 kg and eventual height −7 SD, average head circumference −8 SD forehead and chin slope backwards leaving mid-face prominent with protruding eyes and nose. Developmental delay
Microcephalic osteodysplastic primordial dwarfism (Majewski syndrome) has three subtypes, MOPD 1–3	All resemble Seckel syndrome but with different skeletal and dental abnormalities. Type 2 individuals have generally normal developmental progress. The head circumference becomes more abnormal with age. With time they develop truncal obesity and insulin resistance. They produce the most severe short stature described in humans with a height SDS of −10 SD and a final height of around 100 cm
Neonatal progeria	Recognizable at birth with small size, aged appearance, lipoatrophy, pseudohydrocephalus and developmental delay
Other	Small numbers of cases of primordial dwarfing syndromes have been described in individuals or isolated kindreds. Some of these affected individuals die in the neonatal period, some are associated with immunodeficiency and some with major skeletal abnormalities (such that they more correctly represent unknown forms of skeletal dysplasia)

Table 6.8 Investigation of disproportionate short stature.

Limited skeletal survey
(Lateral skull, chest, AP and lateral spine; pelvis and hips, one long bone, bone age)
Full blood count (for vacuolated white cells – non-specific finding in some storage disorders)
Urine and white cell enzyme concentrations for mucopolysaccharidosis/mucolipidosis
Calcium, phosphate and alkaline phosphatase
PTH

PTH, parathyroid hormone.

SGA affects 2.5% of all births and can be subdivided into those babies who are short and thin, those who are merely underweight and those who are short but of normal weight. When taken as a whole, approximately 80% of children catch up during the first 2 years of life and attain a height in their predicted genetic range but 15–20% of children remain small as adults [13]. Prenatal infection or exposure to alcohol, drugs of abuse and heavy smoking may sometimes be likely culprits but no cause is found in most cases. Attempts to force-feed such infants to promote catch-up should be resisted because of the latter effects of rapid weight gain on cardiovascular risk factors.

SGA individuals are often thin and there is increasing evidence that there may be related metabolic consequences of being born small both with and without catch-up growth [38].

Children born prematurely are often short in the first 5 years of life, with more extreme shortness being produced by more extreme prematurity. These children also show late adverse metabolic consequences (hyperlipidemia, hypertension, insulin resistance) of catch-up growth if it occurs, and some children with the most extreme prematurity are short as adults.

Skeletal dysplasias

Skeletal dysplasias can present at any age and the diagnostic assessment of these depends partly on the age of onset. There are approximately 120 different skeletal dysplasias. Each is rare and any dysmorphology search would include the skeletal radiographs needed for a diagnosis. The "International nosology and classification of constitutional disorders of bone" ([39] and online) defines 33 groups of dysplasia, based increasingly on genetic understanding of the basic defects. Few present to an endocrine clinic and there are increasing numbers of specialist bone dysplasia clinics held jointly between physicians, geneticists and surgeons.

The approach to skeletal dysplasias is determined first by the age of presentation: neonatal, childhood or later. Accurate measurement of head circumference, length and limb length is needed with, if possible, measurement of the individual segments of the limbs using an anthropometer or tape measure. This allows the determination of the segment of the limb most affected by the dysplasia, the upper section of the limbs (rhizomelia), the middle (mesomelia) or the lower part (acromelia). Whether the skull and/or spine are involved is relevant because the modeling of the membranous bones of the skull and the ossification of spinal growth centers are under separate genetic control. Skeletal radiographs allow full determination of the involvement of the epiphyses, metaphyses or shaft of the bones. In some skeletal dysplasias, there are additional specific abnormalities of the pelvis or of bone morphology for instance. The basic radiographs required for a limited skeletal survey are given in Table 6.8. What matters is not who takes the films but who reads them and few radiologists have the necessary expertise.

In this manner, dysplasias may be classified as of neonatal, childhood or late onset. Acromelic, mesomelic or rhizomelic can be used in conjunction with "cranio" if there is involvement of the head and "spondylo" for spinal involvement. A compound description such as "neonatal rhizomelic cranio metaphyseal dysplasia" might be obtained and the diagnosis confirmed using a textbook or a dysmorphology database.

Hypochondroplasia

The most common skeletal dysplasia presenting primarily to a growth clinic is hypochondroplasia. In mild cases without a recognized family history, it often presents at or near puberty because the absence of a pubertal growth spurt is characteristic. Hypochondroplasia results in short stature of variable severity with a mean final height in the range 145–165 cm for males and 130–150 cm for females. Disease-specific growth charts are available [40]. The condition is often dominantly inherited and is one of the situations where the genetic potential must be interpreted with care. If a parent is affected, the mean parental height will appear to be low and one may therefore erroneously assume that the child has constitutional short stature, particularly if the child presents early and disproportion is not clinically so evident. One should always measure the parents to establish whether one of them has short legs. It is often easier to establish a diagnosis in a parent with more mature bones on X-ray if there is doubt about the diagnosis.

Hypochondroplasia is caused by a mutation in the FGF3 gene similar to achondroplasia but of the intracellular tyrosine kinase domain rather than the trans-membrane receptor.

Achondroplasia

Achondroplasia results in much more severe short stature and patients rarely present primarily to the growth clinic. Affected individuals have macrocephaly and rhizomelia. Specific growth charts are published for head circumference, height and limb length in this disorder [41]. The mean final height is between 100 and 140 cm.

Achondroplasia is caused by mutation in the trans-membrane portion of the same FGF3 receptor affected in hypochondroplasia. In most cases, it is the father's allele that carries a mutation related to age. As in hypochondroplasia, the condition is inherited in an autosomal dominant manner but new mutations are the most common cause.

In both hypochondroplasia and achondroplasia there is a lack of widening of the lumbo-sacral spine and a relatively longer fibula than tibia, which may be used in the milder cases of hypochondroplasia to help establish the diagnosis if genetic testing is not available.

Some other skeletal dysplasias can produce extremely severe short stature, especially those with spinal as well as limb involvement. In the spondylo-epiphyseal dysplasias, for instance, the spine is severely shortened and often has a scoliosis that further diminishes height.

Disorders of calcium and phosphate, metabolic disorders and primary disorders of bone (see Chapter 20)
Hypophosphatemic rickets

Hypophosphatemic rickets is usually carried on the X chromosome and the disease is thus more severe in boys. Presentation is with early-onset vitamin D unresponsive rickets, short stature and marked bowing of the legs that reduces stature further. Mutations in the gene for a fibroblast growth factor (FGF-23) leads to autosomal dominant hypophosphatemic rickets by causing relative overexpression of this phosphaturic compound. FGF-23 is itself metabolized by an endopeptidase and PHEX mutations (which code for this protein) cause the classic X-linked form.

Pseudohypoparathyroidism

Pseudohypoparathyroidism presents at any age through childhood to adult life, depending on the severity of the features. Type 1a pseudohypoparathyroidism (Albright hereditary osteodystro-

Table 6.9 Osteogenesis imperfecta subtypes.

Type I	Dominantly inherited	Blue sclerae	COL1A1 or 1A2 17q21-22
Type II	Perinatal lethal form	Type a	COL1A1 or 1A2 17q21-22
		Type b	CRTAP, 3p22
Type III	Progressively deforming form with normal sclerae		COL1A1 or 1A2 17q21-22
Type IV	Dominantly inherited	Normal sclerae	COL1A1 or 1A2 17q21-22
Types V & VI –		Described in small numbers of kindreds	
Types VII & VIII		Autosomal recessive	

phy) produces short stature and usually obesity. The fourth (and sometime third and fifth) metacarpal is usually short and there may be subcutaneous calcification. Hypocalcemia with raised PTH concentrations implies a resistance at the serpentine guanine nucleotide binding protein alpha subunit (GNAS) linked receptor but this is variable even within families, possibly due to imprinting effects. Pseudopseudohypoparathyroidism is a description of the abnormal phenotype with normal calcium concentrations (see Chapter 20).

Conditions with a relatively short back
Osteogenesis imperfecta

Osteogenesis imperfecta has many subtypes (Table 6.9). The severe forms present as neonatal death and severe recurrent fractures but milder forms may occasionally present to a growth clinic with short stature.

Metabolic conditions

Metabolic conditions affecting growth are all rare and most present because of their major skeletal abnormalities or developmental delay. They include mucopolysaccharidoses (MPS), mucolipidoses and osteogenesis imperfecta. Some of the milder mucopolysaccharidoses (e.g. juvenile Hunter syndrome – type 2 MPS) can present primarily with short stature in the growth clinic. These individuals have a limitation of movement of the fingers producing a claw-like hand deformity and they may have mild clouding of the cornea. Heart abnormalities develop in young adult life.

Morquio syndrome (type 4 MPS) and mucolipidosis type 3 may also present first to the growth clinic with features similar to juvenile Hunter syndrome.

Disorders in specific systems

The secretion of growth hormone can be modified by input from higher centers. Its peripheral action can be decreased by inflammatory cytokines. Poor nutrition will also result in high concentrations of insulin-like growth factor binding proteins, in an evolutionarily adaptive manner that further inhibits growth. The good growth response to treatment with anti-TNF antibodies (e.g. etanercept) in some children with juvenile rheumatoid arthritis implies that high concentrations of inflammatory cytokines are directly involved in the poor growth seen in these disorders [42]. For this reason, systemic illness in any system is a potent cause of growth suppression.

Children with major symptomatic disease will be under the care of other clinics before they will be referred to a growth clinic but it is important to rule out the possibility of undiagnosed systemic disease in any child presenting with short stature. The "silent" causes of short stature include renal disease and late-onset celiac disease. Gluten enteropathy in susceptible populations may present very late in childhood, although it is more usual to present in infancy with anemia and failure to thrive, and have poor growth as its only feature. There may be abdominal distension and wasting of the buttocks and hypocalcemia may be present but a high index of suspicion is required for the diagnosis. Chronic anemia, chronic infections (HIV and TB in particular) and chronic inflammatory bowel disease all have a major effect on growth. Inflammatory bowel disease produces a particular delay or failure of the pubertal growth spurt and the inflammation seen in this group of disorders and in juvenile rheumatoid arthritis (JRA) can be especially pronounced. For this reason joint management with a systems specialist and an endocrinologist is recommended.

Chronic asthma produces short stature and delayed puberty, usually with later catch-up but the treatment of asthma with inhaled steroids can produce growth suppression in some individuals.

All of the above will tend to produce thinness which may be even more pronounced than the short stature or poor growth rate. If there is no direct clue as to the diagnosis, screening investigations in this group of children are given in Table 6.10.

Endocrine disorders causing short stature
Growth hormone deficiency

GHD can present in the neonatal period as one element of panhypopituitarism but the average age of diagnosis and treatment is 6–8 years (Tables 6.11 and 6.12) [43]. GHD may be complete, for instance after surgical removal of the pituitary gland (e.g. with a craniopharyngioma) or with deletion of the GH gene, but is more often a relative lack that may be defined in terms of response to provocation tests. Tests may give different results when repeated or analyzed in different laboratories. The more minor degrees of deficiency merge with the lower end of the normal range and idiopathic short stature; in other words, GHD is rarely an absolute diagnosis but part of a spectrum defined arbitrarily.

Growth hormone secretion from the pituitary gland is controlled by the interactions of its releasing hormones, GHRH and ghrelin and its inhibitor SS. These are under the control of higher CNS centers. Hypothalamic damage or dysfunction may result in a lack of pulsatile growth hormone secretion, particularly noticeable on overnight sampling. This, tertiary, GHD may be caused by genetic disorders of the GHRH gene and its receptor or secondary to other hypothalamic abnormalities including tumors.

Table 6.10 Investigation of the short, thin child.

Full blood count	Anemia in inflammatory bowel disease, celiac disease and renal failure, severe prolonged illness
ESR or other inflammatory marker	Inflammatory bowel disease, juvenile rheumatoid
MCV	Microcytosis is an indication of nutritional deficiency or blood loss and macrocytosis may indicate malabsorption
Acid–base status, urea and electrolytes, creatinine	Occult renal failure and Bartter syndrome (hypochloremic alkalosis)
Liver function, calcium, phosphate and alkaline phosphatase	Metabolic bone disease, hypocalcemia in celiac disease
Urine analysis, (simple biochemistry and microscopy)	Diabetes; renal "leak"; Occult urinary infection
Stool analysis	Giardiasis (can produce growth retardation and may only be picked up if the stool is inspected microscopically for cysts). Fat globules in malabsorption Reducing substances present in lactose (and rarely other sugar) intolerance Red blood cells may indicate cow's milk protein intolerance or celiac disease and thus the need for a jejunal biopsy
Antigliadin/endomysial antibody screen or tissue transglutaminase	Celiac disease
Chromosome analysis	Unexpected ring chromosomes occasionally associated with failure to thrive; Turner syndrome
Early morning testosterone (or inhibin B)	Serves as a marker of impending puberty in the male with probable delay

ESR, erythrocyte sedimentation rate; MCV, mean cell volume.

Table 6.11 Endocrine disorders causing short stature.

Growth hormone deficiency and resistance
Hypothyroidism
Hypogonadism with delayed puberty
Cushing syndrome

Primary GHD is caused by defective GH secretion from the pituitary gland. Idiopathic GHD is still the most common diagnosis but, with increasingly good scans, tests and genetic analysis, this group is shrinking.

The pituitary may not have formed normally in embryogenesis. It is dependent upon a sequence of genetic events (Table 6.13).

Table 6.12 Suggested screening investigations in the short child with relative overweight.

Wrist for bone age (short metacarpals in PHP and Turner syndrome)
U&E, osmolarity (plasma and urine)
TSH and FT4 with antithyroid antibodies
IGF-1 and IGFBP3
Chromosome analysis

If short and IGF-1 and IGFBP3 not in normal range then:
GH stimulation test (see protocol below)
+TRH/LHRH test (as part of stimulation test)
+Synacthen test (or as part of ITT)
Prolactin
ACTH at start of test

If Cushing syndrome is suspected then three sequential 24-h urinary free cortisol measurements and/or an overnight dexamethasone suppression test.
ACTH, adenocorticotropic hormone; FT4, free thyroxine; GH, growth hormone; ITT, insulin tolerance test; LHRH, Luteinizing hormone releasing hormone; PHP, pseudohypoparathyroidism; TRH, thyroid releasing hormone; TSH, thyroid stimulating hormone; U&E, urea and electrolytes.

Table 6.13 Genetic disorders affecting pituitary formation.

PAX 6	Aniridia; Peters anomaly (defect of anterior chamber of the eye); anophthalmia
HESX-1	Familial septo-optic dysplasia, rare AR, variable hypopituitarism
PIT-1/POU1F1	AR and AD forms. Combined GH, TSH and prolactin deficiencies. Posterior pituitary normal
PROP-1	AR, variable congenital hypopituitarism (with possible late ACTH deficiency), posterior pituitary normal. Gland may become hyperplastic
LHX-3 & 4	AR, variable anterior hypopituitarism plus head and neck abnormalities
SOX3	GH deficiency, central brain abnormalities, developmental delay
SHH	Homeobox gene abnormality causing some cases of holoprosencephaly/single central incisor
PITX2	Rieger abnormality (hypodontia, peg-like teeth, small mid-face with short philtrum, prognathism. Iris hypoplasia. Occasional abdominal abnormalities)

ACTH, adenocorticotropic hormone; AD, autosomal dominant; AR, autosomal recessive; GH, growth hormone; TSH, thyroid stimulating hormone.

The GH gene may be abnormal and GHD may be inherited in several distinct genetic ways (Table 6.14). In all cases where the pituitary gland is abnormal, there may be lack of other pituitary hormones resulting in partial or complete panhypopituitarism. The pituitary may be damaged by infection (e.g. meningitis or congenital rubella), tumor or vascular abnormalities, trauma and anoxia (e.g. following breech delivery).

Ectopic posterior pituitary bright spot (Fig. 6.4) is a common finding on MRI. Most cases are idiopathic but it may be seen in conjunction with a hypoplastic pituitary or following trauma or infection.

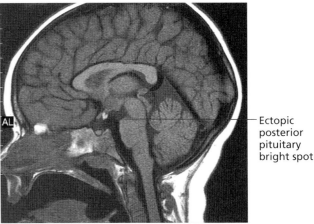

Ectopic posterior pituitary bright spot

Figure 6.4 Ectopic posterior pituitary and absent pituitary stalk. Patient with hypopituitarism but normal posterior pituitary function.

Table 6.14 Genetic defects of growth hormone (GH) formation.

GHD1a	AR	Deletion, no GH. Antibodies form against GH on treatment
GHD1b	AR	Partial GHD
GHD2	AD	Partial GHD
GHD3	X-linked	Partial GHD

AD, autosomal dominant; AR, autosomal recessive; GHD, growth hormone deficiency.

Table 6.15 Clinical features of growth hormone deficiency.

Short stature for parents
Low height velocity
Normal body proportions
Larger head than height centile
Small mid-face
High voice
Dimpled, excess truncal fat
Thin, dry skin wrinkles with age
Neonatal hypoglycemia and prolonged jaundice (especially in the hypopituitary patient)
Delayed dentition and bone age
Delayed puberty

Craniopharyngioma is a tumor formed by cystic accumulation of gelatinous fluid within remnants of Rathke's pouch. There is peripheral calcification of the tumor. The tumors are usually intrasellar but expand superiorly and may occasionally be entirely hypothalamic. The majority present with symptoms related to tumor expansion and compression of the optic chiasm (bilateral homonymous hemianopia) and aqueduct (hydrocephalus with raised intracranial pressure). Almost always there are retrospective signs and symptoms of pituitary dysfunction (anterior or posterior) but occasionally small tumors may present with isolated growth failure. After surgical or radiotherapy, pituitary failure is usual.

Increasing numbers of survivors of childhood malignancy who have received cranial irradiation subsequently develop GHD and evolving hypopituitarism.

Clinical features

GHD from an early age produces severe short stature (adult height 130–140 cm) and occurs in around 1 in 4000 to 1 in 20 000 of the population depending on the definition of severity. Idiopathic forms may present late with marked short stature but more commonly present with relatively mild short stature and a slow rate of growth (Table 6.15).

The biochemical diagnosis is made by assessing response of GH to various provokers of secretion, such as insulin, clonidine or glucagon. Measurement of spontaneous overnight secretion is used in some centers to assess hypothalamic neurosecretion. Neurosecretory dysfunction is a situation with normal provoked release of GH but inadequate spontaneous release. It may be seen after cranial irradiation but some apparently normal children with normal growth rates can also have periods of poor spontaneous overnight secretion. The existence of the phenomenon as a diagnosis is increasingly doubted [44]. Some of these children have demonstrable defects in the promoter region of the GH gene resulting in decreased expression of GH [45].

Bio-inactive GH (Kowarski syndrome 17q22-24) is a rare situation that presents with clinical features of GHD but normal GH concentrations and low IGF-1/IGFBP3 concentrations that respond to exogenous GH [46,47].

An abnormally low response of GH to provocation is defined as a peak of <20 mIU/L or approximately <7 μg/L. In idiopathic GHD, it is good practice to repeat the test before starting treatment to try to reduce errors of diagnosis because of laboratory assay problems or lack of sex-hormone priming.

The GH axis should be tested if height is <−2.5 SD below the mean, <−1.5 SD below target height centile, if height is <−2 SD below the mean and height velocity over 1 year is <1 SD below the mean for 2 years (or less than 2 SD over 1 year) or if there are signs of other pituitary hormone deficiency or intracranial pathology. Normal concentrations of IGF-1 or IGFBP3 largely exclude GH deficiency, although normal concentrations of IGFBP3 in particular may be seen in post-irradiation GHD [48], whereas low concentrations may be a result of inflammation or poor nutrition and do not prove GH deficiency. Thus, one or two GH provocation tests should be performed in children with low IGF-1 and IGFBP3 concentrations or after treatment for malignancy.

MRI of the pituitary should be performed for all cases where GHD (±other pituitary hormones) is confirmed. Structural abnormalities of the midline and optic nerves (Fig. 6.5), reduced anterior pituitary height, an attenuated or interrupted pituitary stalk and/or an ectopically positioned posterior pituitary are all associated with pituitary dysfunction. Craniopharyngiomas may be small and intrasellar, although the majority present with CNS effects secondary to secondary nerve compression or obstructive hydrocephalus. Germinomas may occur in the hypothalamic

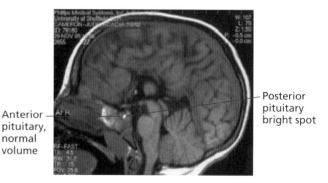

Figure 6.5 Absent corpus callosum, anatomically normal anterior and posterior pituitary [patient with growth hormone deficiency (GHD), hypothalamic hypothyroidism].

region and tumor marker concentrations (α-fetoprotein and β-hCG) are helpful in the diagnosis of these tumors. Cysts of Rathke's cleft can occasionally expand and produce hypopituitarism.

Most children with congenital GHD have normal birthweight but some of them have mild growth restriction and grow poorly from birth, even in the infantile "GH-independent" phase of growth [7].

Testing for growth hormone deficiency

Because normal GH secretion is pulsatile, with four to six pulses per 24 h, random single GH estimations are rarely helpful in diagnosing or excluding GHD. Hence, a variety of provocation tests have been used. It can be argued that pharmacological testing is non-physiological and may bear no resemblance to endogenous secretion and that provocative tests are reliable only in patients in whom the clinical signs and symptoms are clear and hence that they should be abandoned. Indeed, in countries where idiopathic short stature is a licensed indication for treatment, testing for GH secretion is obsolete. All GH provocation tests have limitations [49] and there is no "gold standard" test against which alternative protocols can be evaluated.

GH concentrations are highly assay dependent. The number of GH variants, isoforms and molecular states in human plasma is considerable. Ability to quantify each of these variants depends on assay design, antibody specificity and the composition of the standard used [50]. Competitive immunoassays employing polyclonal antibodies are better at averaging or integrating the multiple epitopes involved but the precision of such assays is poor and their sensitivity inadequate. They have now been largely superseded by non-competitive two-site assays employing monoclonal antibodies specific for 22 kDa GH. Continued use of pituitary GH standard (80/505), a heterogeneous material, rather than recombinant GH standard (88/624), inhibits progress towards agreement between laboratories. Immunoassays show poor comparability, with up to threefold differences and poor correlation, despite improvement in technology [51].

All provocation tests have poor specificity (50–80%) with a high incidence of false positives. In an attempt to overcome this problem, it has been common practice to carry out two tests separately or sequentially but the outcome of this is merely to compound the errors. Alternative approaches to assessing GH secretion have proved either too demanding (e.g. 12- or 24-h GH profiles) or to offer no advantage in terms of predictive value (e.g. urinary GH). However, guidelines on the use of human GH in children with growth failure recommend the performance of provocation tests to support the clinical diagnosis of GH deficiency [52].

Sex steroid priming

In pre- and peripubertal children who have a subnormal response to provocative testing, sex steroid priming may increase the response to that seen in late puberty and should be considered. The rationale for this is the estrogen-induced rise in GH during puberty. There is no consensus on the appropriate age for priming but it should be considered in patients with a bone age greater than 10 years and possibly younger in obese children. Oral ethinylestradiol should be given (20 μg in the evening) to girls and boys less than 11 years, daily for 3 days and the test carried out on day 4. Be aware that ethinylestradiol will almost certainly cause nausea. In boys older than 11 years, Sustanon (100 mg intramuscularly) is given as a single injection 5–7 days before the test.

GH provocation tests (Table 6.16 [53])
Insulin tolerance test
Background

Insulin-induced hypoglycemia suppresses the somatostatin tone and stimulates the α-adrenergic receptors. It induces not only GH but also ACTH release and a rise in serum cortisol concentra-

Table 6.16 Other growth hormone (GH) provocation tests.

Glucagon stimulation test
The test is particularly useful for the assessment of GH and cortisol reserve in children <2 years and others in whom the insulin tolerance test is contraindicated

Arginine stimulation test
Arginine stimulates GH secretion by reducing somatostatin tone and possibly by stimulation of α-adrenergic receptors with GHRH release

Clonidine stimulation test
Clonidine is a selective α-receptor agonist, causes GH release via GHRH secretion [15]

Levodopa stimulation test
Levodopa increases GH secretion through dopaminergic and α-adrenergic pathways

Growth hormone-releasing hormone (GHRH) stimulation test
GHRH can be used to distinguish hypothalamic from pituitary causes of GH deficiency in patients who have previously demonstrated a subnormal response to the standard provocation tests

tions. The advantage of the insulin tolerance test (ITT) is that, in addition to stimulating GH secretion, it also tests the integrity of the entire HPA axis. This test has been associated with morbidity and mortality, mainly because of the use of inappropriate amounts of hyperosmolar fluid to correct hypoglycemia. The decision to undertake an ITT should be considered carefully and carried out only in a specialized pediatric endocrine investigation unit.

Precautions

1 The test is contraindicated in children with diagnosed epilepsy or a history of unexplained blackouts and in children <2 years of age, for whom a glucagon provocation test may be more appropriate.

2 Hypothyroidism impairs the GH and cortisol response. Patients with adrenal and thyroid insufficiency should have corticosteroid replacement commenced before thyroxine, as thyroxine may precipitate an adrenal crisis. The insulin provocation test may need to be repeated after 3 months of thyroxine therapy in patients with confirmed thyroid or dual insufficiency.

3 Special precautions are required in children suspected of having panhypopituitarism.

4 Intravenous 10% dextrose (never 50%) must be immediately available.

5 A glucose meter with acceptable performance in the hypoglycemic range must be available, and staff performing the test must be certified competent to use it.

Preparation

1 Check that thyroid function tests are normal.

2 Prime with sex steroids if indicated.

3 The child should be fasted for 8 h before the test, only water is allowed.

4 The child should be weighed prior to the test, in order to calculate accurately the dose of insulin to be administered.

5 Insert IV cannula (see section on blood collection) and maintain patent with heparinized normal saline. The stress of cannulation can cause an increase in GH, making interpretation of the test difficult. After cannulation, wait for 30–60 min before commencing the test and take a blood sample at −30 min to aid interpretation if the basal sample is found to be elevated.

Protocol

1 $t = -30$ min; take blood (plain tube) for GH and cortisol estimation.

2 $t = 0$ min; give soluble insulin 0.10–0.15 U/kg IV, using the lower dose if there is a strong suspicion of panhypopituitarism or if the child has had previous cranial surgery or radiotherapy. The dose may need to be increased in patients with diabetes mellitus, insulin resistance or obesity.

3 Take samples as shown in Table 6.17. Measure glucose concentrations on the glucose meter but also send a sample to the laboratory for urgent analysis.

Table 6.17 Sampling for insulin tolerance test.

Time (min)	Meter glucose	Lab glucose (fluoride oxalate tube)	GH (plain tube)	Cortisol (plain tube)
−30 (before insulin)	+	+	+	+
0 (before insulin)	+	+	+	+
30	+	+	+	+
45	+	+	+	+
60	+	+	+	+
90	+	+	+	+
120	+	+	+	+

4 Observe child closely for clinical signs and symptoms of hypoglycemia (e.g. sweating and drowsiness).

5 The results can be interpreted only if adequate hypoglycemia has been achieved. This is defined as a laboratory glucose half the fasting value or <2.2 mmol/L. If there have been no clinical signs of hypoglycemia by 45 min, the dose of insulin should be repeated and the test continued with blood samples timed again from 0 min.

6 Once hypoglycemia has occurred, the child should be given glucose drinks. If the child remains persistently hypoglycemic or loses consciousness or fits, he/she should be treated with an IV bolus of 200 mg/kg glucose (2 mL/kg 10% dextrose) over 3 min followed by an IV infusion using 10% dextrose at 2.4–4.8 mL/kg/h (4–8 mg/kg/min glucose). Check glucose concentrations on the glucose meter after 4–5 min and adjust dextrose infusion to maintain blood glucose at 5–8 mmol/L. If there is no improvement in conscious concentration after normal glucose concentration is restored, an alternative explanation should be sought. Do not stop sampling.

7 If panhypopituitarism is suspected, give 100 mg hydrocortisone IV at the end of the test or earlier if recovery from hypoglycemia is slow.

8 The child must not be sent home until an adequate high-carbohydrate meal has been eaten without vomiting and the blood glucose has been maintained at 4 mmol/L for a minimum of 2 h.

9 This test may be conducted as part of a combined ITT/thyrotrophin-releasing hormone (TRH)/gonadotropin-releasing hormone (GnRH) pituitary function test, in which case the sampling protocol is shown in Table 6.18.

Interpretation

Interpretation is not possible unless adequate hypoglycemia (glucose <2.2 mmol/L) has been achieved.

A GH concentration of >20 mU/L (7 μg/L) excludes GH deficiency. However, the precise cutoff applied varies between centers and is dependent on the bias of the assay used by the local laboratory. Biochemical data must be interpreted in conjunction with clinical and auxological data in order to make decisions about GH treatment in an individual patient. Combining the test with mea-

Table 6.18 Sampling for combined insulin tolerance/ thyrotropin releasing hormone/gonadotropin releasing hormone (ITT/TRH/GnRH) test.

	Glucose	Cortisol	GH	LH	FSH	TSH
−30	+	+	+			
0	+	+	+	+	+	+
Give soluble insulin 0.10–0.35 U/kg, GnRH 2.5 μg/kg, TRH 5 μg/kg IV						
30	+	+	+	+	+	+
45	+	+	+			
60	+	+	+	+	+	+
90	+	+	+			
120	+	+	+			

Additional samples at 0 min: prolactin, free thyroxine, testosterone or estradiol. FSH, follicle stimulating hormone; GH, growth hormone; GnRH, gonadotropin releasing hormone; LH, luteinizing hormone; TRH, thyrotropin releasing hormone; TSH, thyroid stimulating hormone.

surement of IGF-1 and its binding proteins is one approach that has been recommended to aid the decision in patients with peak GH concentrations in the partially deficient range (>7.5 but <15 mU/L, >2.5 but <5 μg/L) [5]. GH concentrations are increasingly being expressed in ng/mL or mg/L, and mass units may replace the current international unit.

Interpretation of the cortisol response is possible only if hypothyroidism has been excluded. An adequate cortisol response is defined as a peak concentration of >550 nmol/L. Patients with peak concentrations <550 but >400 nmol/L may only need steroid cover for major illnesses and stresses.

Glucagon stimulation test

Background

Glucagon stimulates the release of GH and ACTH by a hypothalamic mechanism and therefore indirectly stimulates cortisol secretion [12]. The precise mechanism of the stimulation is unclear, particularly in cases where rebound hypoglycemia does not occur [13]. The test is particularly useful for the assessment of GH and cortisol reserve in children <2 years and others in whom the ITT is contraindicated. The timing of the peak GH response depends on whether the glucagon is injected intravenously or intramuscularly. Glucagon has also been administered subcutaneously, but this is not recommended as absorption is unreliable [2].

Precautions

1 The test is contraindicated in patients suspected of having pheochromocytoma or hyperinsulinism and is unreliable in patients with diabetes mellitus.

2 As for the ITT, hypothyroidism impairs the GH and cortisol response.

3 Glucagon may cause nausea, vomiting and abdominal pain.

Preparation

As for the ITT.

Protocol

1 $t = -30$ min; take blood (plain tube) for GH and cortisol estimation.

2 $t = 0$ min; give 20 mg/kg glucagon IV or IM up to a maximum of 1 mg.

3 Take samples as shown in Table 6.19.

4 In children with suspected hypopituitarism, prolonged fasting may induce hypoglycemia. Blood glucose should be checked using a glucose meter in these patients whenever a sample is taken for GH/cortisol. If the patient shows signs or symptoms of hypoglycemia, send an urgent sample to the laboratory for glucose analysis.

5 If hypoglycemia is confirmed, treatment should be instigated as described for the ITT.

6 This test may be performed as a combined glucagon/TRH/GnRH pituitary function test. The sampling protocol is shown in Table 6.20

Interpretation

For interpretation of GH and cortisol concentrations, see ITT. There are conflicting reports in the literature [12,14,15] regarding the sensitivity of this test relative to the ITT.

Table 6.19 Sampling for glucagon stimulation test.

Time (min)	Meter glucose	GH (plain tube)	Cortisol (plain tube)
−30 (before glucagon)	+	+	+
0 (before glucagon)	+	+	+
60	+	+	+
90	+	+	+
120	+	+	+
150	+	+	+
180	+	+	+

Table 6.20 Sampling for combined glucagon/TRH/GnRH test.

Time (min)	Meter glucose	Cortisol	GH	LH	FSH	TSH
−30	+	+	+			
0	+	+	+	+	+	+
Give glucagon 20 µg/kg, GnRH 2.5 µg/kg, TRH 5 µg/kg IV						
20				+	+	+
60	+	+	+	+	+	+
90	+	+	+			
120	+	+	+			
150	+	+	+			
180	+	+	+			

Additional samples at 0 min: as for combined ITT/TRH/GnRH test.

Arginine stimulation test

Background

The injection of various amino acids (e.g. ornithine, arginine) is followed by an increase in GH concentrations in blood. Arginine stimulates GH secretion by reducing somatostatin tone and possibly by stimulation of α-adrenergic receptors with GHRH release.

Precautions

Hypothyroidism impairs the GH response. Arginine may cause nausea and some irritation at the infusion site. Vomiting has been described in a few patients.

Preparation

As for the ITT.

Protocol

1 $t = -30$ min: take blood (plain tube) for GH estimation.

2 $t = 0$ min; give 0.5 g/kg arginine up to a maximum of 30 g. This is given by infusion IV of a 10% solution of arginine monochloride in 0.9% NaCl at a constant rate over 30 min.

3 Take samples as shown in Table 6.21

4 In children with suspected hypopituitarism, blood glucose should be checked as described in the glucagon stimulation test protocol.

5 This test may be performed as a combined arginine/TRH/GnRH/synacthen dynamic function test. The sampling protocol is shown in Table 6.22

Interpretation

For interpretation of peak GH concentrations, see ITT. Usually, the peak GH concentration is reached about 60 min after staring the arginine infusion.

Clonidine test

Background

Clonidine, a selective α-receptor agonist, causes GH release via GHRH secretion [15].

Table 6.21 Sampling for arginine, clonidine and levodopa stimulation tests.

Time (min)	Arginine	Clonidine	Levodopa
−30	+ (Before infusion)		
0	+ (At end of infusion)	+ (Before clonidine)	+ (Before levodopa)
15	+		
30	+	+	+
45	+		
60	+	+	+
90	+	+	+
120	+	+	+
150	+		

Table 6.22 Sampling for combined arginine/TRH/GnRH/synacthen test.

Time (min)	Meter glucose	Cortisol	GH	LH	FSH	TSH
−30	+		+			
Give arginine 0.5 g/kg by IV infusion over 30 min						
0	+	+	+	+	+	+
Give GnRH 2.5 μg/kg, TRH 5 μg/kg IV, synacthen 36 μg/kg IV						
30	+	+	+	+	+	+
45	+		+			
60	+	+	+	+	+	+
90	+		+			
120	+		+			

Additional samples at 0 min: as for combined ITT/TRH/GnRH test.

Precautions

Clonidine causes hypotension and drowsiness, although the former is rarely severe enough to require treatment.

Preparation

1 Check thyroid function tests.
2 Prime with sex steroids if indicated.
3 Fast child for 8 h prior to the test (only water is allowed).
4 Measure height and weight of child and calculate surface area (see patient preparation section).

Protocol

1 Give 0.15 mg/m² clonidine, orally.
2 Take samples as shown in Table 6.21.
3 Measure blood pressure every 30 min until 1 h after the test.
4 In children with suspected hypopituitarism, blood glucose should be checked as described in the glucagon stimulation test protocol.
5 Child may be safely discharged 1 h after the test if fully awake.

Interpretation

For interpretation of peak GH concentrations, see ITT. Studies in normal children [16] have indicated a higher GH response to clonidine compared with other provocative agents.

Levodopa stimulation test
Background

Levodopa increases GH secretion through dopaminergic and α-adrenergic pathways.

Precautions

Levodopa may cause nausea and occasionally vomiting, vertigo, fatigue and headache.

Preparation

1 Check thyroid function tests.
2 Prime with sex steroids if indicated.

3 Fast child for 8 h prior to the test (only water is allowed).
4 Weigh child and select appropriate dose of levodopa.

Protocol

1 Give levodopa orally: <15 kg body weight, 125 mg; <35 kg body weight, 250 mg; >35 kg body weight, 500 mg.
2 Take samples as shown in Table 6.21.
3 In children with suspected hypopituitarism, blood glucose should be checked as described in the glucagon stimulation test protocol.

Interpretation

For interpretation of peak GH concentrations, see ITT. The timing of peak response to levodopa varies widely.

Growth hormone-releasing hormone stimulation test
Indications

The GHRH stimulation test is not a front-line diagnostic test. It can be used to distinguish hypothalamic from pituitary causes of GH deficiency in patients who have previously demonstrated a subnormal response to the standard provocation tests. Hypothalamic dysfunction is a common occurrence in isolated GH deficiency.

In adults, GHRH (1 mg/kg IV) has been used in combination with somatostatin antagonists arginine (0.5 g/kg IV) or hexarelin (0.25 mg/kg). Such combinations provide a potent and reproducible test of pituitary GH secretion without side effects, which may eventually replace traditional provocative agents. It has been suggested that these combination tests directly explore the pituitary GH-releasable pool, while testing with GHRH alone explores more the integrity of hypothalamic mechanisms involved in the control of somatotroph function [17]. However, the use of these tests has not been studied extensively in children.

Precautions

GHRH commonly causes facial flushing, but there are no other side effects.

Patient preparation

1 Check thyroid function tests.
2 Prime with sex steroids if indicated.
3 Fast child for 8 h prior to the test (only water is allowed).
4 Weigh child and select appropriate dose of GHRH.
5 Insert IV cannula (see section on blood collection) and maintain patent with heparinized normal saline. After cannulation, wait for 30 min before commencing the test and take a blood sample at −15 min to aid interpretation if the basal sample is found to be elevated.

Protocol

1 $t = -15$ min: take blood (plain tube) for GH estimation.
2 $t = 0$ min; give IV bolus of GHRH (1 mg/kg diluted in 10 mL normal saline).
3 Take further samples at 0 (before GHRH), 5, 15, 30, 60, 90, 120 min.

4 In children with suspected hypopituitarism, blood glucose should be checked as described in the glucagon stimulation test protocol.

Interpretation

A good response to GHRH (but not to ITT or glucagon) suggests a hypothalamic cause of GHD. Failure to respond suggests an abnormality in the pituitary gland or in the GHRH receptor. However, because GHRH is required for both the synthesis and the release of GH, a single bolus of GHRH may also fail to elicit a response in hypothalamic disease. The pituitary somatotroph cells may be sensitized by priming the pituitary gland with daily GHRH injections over several days, after which time the GHRH test should be repeated.

Growth hormone insensitivity

GH insensitivity usually presents after birth with failure of the childhood component of growth. If there is an abnormality of IGF formation or action, there will be SGA, although an exact diagnosis is likely to take some time outside of kindreds with a known genetic defect.

The growth-promoting actions of GH are mediated by the generation of IGF-1 at the epiphyseal level. GH acts on its receptor to allow generation of IGF-1 that then promotes growth. This sequence of events from GH generation to receptor action then IGF-1 action is complex (Fig. 6.6). Defects at almost all these steps have now been described and are listed in the legend.

Severe GH insensitivity produces a height deficit of <−2.5 SD. The question of whether more minor disorders of insensitivity secondary to milder mutations and polymorphisms can produce some cases of idiopathic short stature remains to be determined.

Secondary GH insensitivity may be seen in severe nutritional restriction, liver disease, chronic illness (Crohn disease, cystic fibrosis, rheumatoid). In secondary deficiency, the IGFBP3 concentration is usually normal. Secondary insensitivity may rarely be secondary to antibodies against GH, formed after treatment of total GH gene deletion with recombinant GH.

Point mutations and occasionally deletions of the gene coding the extracellular portion of the GH receptor result in Laron syndrome. The extracellular portion of the GH receptor is identical with circulating GH binding protein, so deletion will result in low concentrations of GHBP and high concentrations of GH with low IGF-1 and IGFBP3 [54].

Laron syndrome is commonly found within consanguineous kindreds. Affected individuals have a birth size in the normal range but show progressive growth failure. They are extremely short (usually >−3 SD), usually proportionate (although some populations have minor disproportion) with normal head circumference, prominent forehead and a small mid-face. There is often gross motor delay secondary to poor muscle bulk in infancy. Body fat is increased and dimpled on the abdomen. Hypoglycemia and hypercholesterolemia are common because there is no direct action of GH to promote lipolysis.

A similar phenotype is seen with abnormalities of the transmembrane and intracellular signaling pathway from the GH receptor. Here the GHBP concentrations will be normal or high. Some individuals with STAT5b (Fig. 6.6) abnormalities and IκB and abnormalities of GH signal transduction also have immunodeficiency because they are implicated in cytokine responsiveness. This manifests with interstitial pneumonia and severe chickenpox. STAT5b mutations are associated with hyperprolactinemia [55,56].

In almost all cases of IGF-1 deficiency or insensitivity there is SGA and a reduced head circumference because GH independent IGF-1 action is required for growth *in utero* although insulin and IGF-2 are the main prenatal growth factors [57].

IGF-1 deficiency is extremely rare [58]. Because of the importance of IGF-1 for organ growth as well as statural growth, it results in IUGR, severe short stature with microcephaly, deafness, abnormal facies (micrognathia, deep eyes) and delayed development. Heterozygous family members are shorter than unaffected siblings.

IGFBP3 production depends on intact GH signaling. It binds with IGF-1 and an ALS to deliver IGF-1 to the tissues and promote growth. Individuals with ALS deficiency have IUGR, are moderately short (−2 SD), proportionate and have delayed puberty. They have low IGF-1 and IGFBP3 concentrations and do not show a good response to GH treatment [59].

IGF-1 acts on a receptor and some rare individuals with IGF-1R mutations are described with IUGR and short stature – here GH, IGF-1 and IGFBP3 concentrations may be normal or high in the presence of normal nutrition [60].

Iatrogenic short stature

Glucocorticoids (GC) are used extensively in many diseases, including autoimmune and inflammatory conditions and it is estimated that 10% of children may require some form of GC treatment during childhood. Improved survival from a number of chronic and life-threatening illnesses has been bought at the expense of adverse growth and skeletal development. In pharmacological doses, GCs affect most systems within the body that summate to cause detrimental effects on bone health. These effects include obesity, myopathy, hypogonadism, increased urinary calcium loss from the kidneys, impaired vitamin D metabolism from the gut, thus leading to a reduced bone quality and increased incidence of fractures (e.g. osteopenia and osteoporosis). Steroids have also been shown to affect most cell types within the skeleton including osteoblasts, osteoclasts, osteocytes and chondrocytes. Children are prone to all the systemic effects of steroids but additionally also show a reduction in growth rate attributed to the direct effect of steroids on the chondrocytes within the growth plate. Dexamethasone is more potent than prednisolone at suppressing short-term growth and bone turnover. Replacement doses of hydrocortisone in adrenal insufficiency rarely produce adverse effects but some children seem very prone to the growth suppressive effects of steroids and can show poor growth in response to quite small doses of inhaled or topical

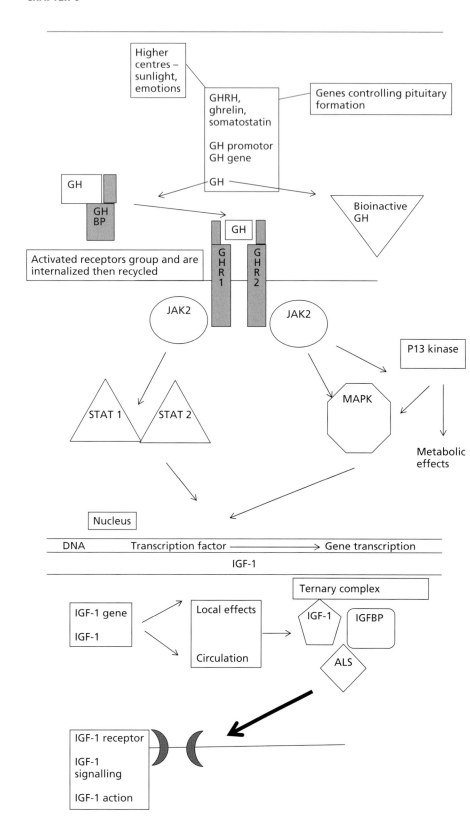

Figure 6.6 Cascade of growth promotion and described abnormalities. Growth hormone (GH) is secreted from a normal pituitary at peaks of GHRH and ghrelin secretion and troughs of somatostatin. GH circulates bound to the extracellular part of the GH receptor. GH binds 2 receptor elements (GHR 1 & 2). The dimerized receptors aggregate and are internalized. This leads to the association of JAK2, a receptor associated tyrosine kinase to the activated receptors. JAK2 in turn activates transcription factors on DNA either through the MAPK (directly or indirectly) or STAT pathways.

IGF-1 production results in local and circulating IGF-1 in association with IGF binding proteins and acid labile subunit that delivers IGF-1 to its receptor with subsequent signalling and IGF-1 induced genetic transcription. Abnormalities of this complex process resulting in short stature have been described at all levels. IGF binding is increased in inflammatory states and poor nutrition resulting in less IGF-1 available for growth.

steroids. Detrimental effects on local action of GH and IGF-1 are also effected by a number of different mechanisms including alterations in the activity of the GH binding protein, downregulation of GH receptor expression and a reduction in local IGF-1 production and activity [61].

Growth rate is improved on alternate day steroid regimens. Bone age is usually delayed and growth potential may be preserved unless there has been such severe steroid-induced osteoporosis that spinal collapse occurs or the high dose is maintained through puberty.

Methylphenidate and related amphetamine-like compounds used to treat attention deficit disorder interfere with growth and appetite in some children if used long-term: children attending these behavior clinics should have regular measurements of height and weight.

Cancer treatment with chemo- or radiotherapy, including spinal irradiation and total body irradiation pre-bone-marrow transplant, causes epiphyseal damage which is made worse by chronic inflammation, graft versus host disease, poor nutrition and precocious puberty.

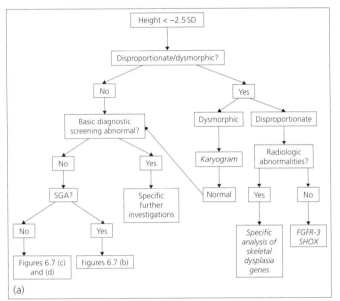

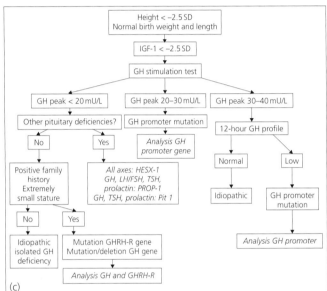

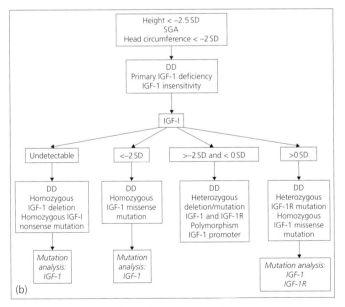

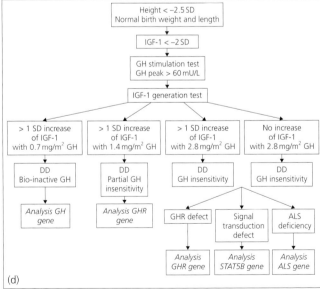

Figure 6.7 (a) Flow chart for the diagnostic approach of a child with short stature (−2.5 SD). (b) Flow chart for the evaluation of a child with proportionate short stature, born small for gestational age (SGA) and a head circumference <−2 SD. (c) Flow chart for the evaluation of a child with proportionate short stature, normal birth weight and length, low IGF-1 levels (<−2 SD) and a GH peak in a stimulation test <40 mU/L. (d) Flow chart for the analysis of a child with proportionate short stature, normal birth weight and length, low IGF-1 levels (<−2 SD) and a GH peak in a stimulation test >60 mU/L.

Psychosocial short stature

Deprivation and unhappiness can produce growth failure at any age. Anorexia and bulimia often induce marked delay of puberty and menstruation. Short stature with complete but reversible GHD can occur secondary to psychosocial deprivation. Although there is usually relative thinness this is not always the case because comfort eating may occur and there can be considerable diagnostic confusion between deprivation dwarfism and GHD. A rapid catch-up growth and a change of behavior is seen on a change of caregiver or hospitalization. There is commonly a preservation of more infantile body proportions than may be expected from the age of the child [62].

Constitutional short stature

In the context of a familial pattern of short stature there may be little concern for many years and these children often present in later childhood when their sporting and career aspirations or bullying provokes a referral. Sometimes parental anxiety is produced by their own negative experiences and then help will be sought at an earlier age. In delayed puberty, abnormalities and polymorphisms are described in a number of genes that control normal gonadotropin secretion.

Stature may be short in comparison to the centile range but normal compared to the parent's centile range. If the child is young, it is difficult to be sure whether there will be added delay of puberty. Clues would be a positive family history (usually of the same-sex parent) and relatively mild disproportion with longer leg than sitting height centiles, a situation seen several years before secondary sexual characteristic appear. There is often deceleration of height velocity in the late prepubertal years but the history, auxology and a skeletal age may give reassurance. If in doubt it is wise to exclude other causes of poor growth.

Non-familial short stature with and without pubertal delay or idiopathic short stature is a descriptive term after other causes of short stature have been excluded. Many cases are in retrospect children with a delayed tempo of growth who may again have a strong family history (usually of the same-sex parent) and relative mild disproportion with longer leg than sitting height centiles and a delayed bone age. Non-paternity should also be considered. Some of these individuals will eventually prove to have a SHOX abnormality, mild GH insensitivity, heterozygote expression of a GH signaling abnormality or a polymorphism of the GH promoter.

Summary

A scheme for diagnosing severe short stature is shown in Fig. 6.7, which is adapted from Walenkamp 2007 [63].

Tall stature

Tall stature may be classified as [1]:

(a) *Primary tall stature*
Sex chromosome abnormalities
Dysmorphic syndromes due to metabolic or connective tissue abnormality
Other dysmorphic syndromes (babies and children)
Dysmorphic syndromes with symmetrical overgrowth
Dysmorphic syndromes with partial or asymmetrical overgrowth.
(b) *Secondary causes of large size*
Growth hormone excess
Hyperinsulinism
Isolated ACTH insensitivity
Thyrotoxicosis
Precocious puberty
Other endocrine abnormalities.
(c) *Constitutional tall stature*
Familial tall stature
Non-familial tall stature with or without advance in growth and adolescence.

As well as the diagnostic classification used above, there is a useful clinical approach to tall stature based on the presence or absence of disproportion and the time of onset of the tall stature (Fig. 6.8).

Primary tall stature
Sex chromosome abnormalities

Sex chromosome abnormalities usually present late with behavioral and/or schooling difficulties or pubertal failure. An increasing number are picked up on coincidental amniocentesis. Klinefelter (XXY, XXYY, XXXY and mosaic forms) and the XYY syndromes usually produce disproportionate tall stature with intellectual or behavioral abnormalities. The legs are relatively long compared to the back, especially with late diagnosis or after failure of puberty. Three copies (or more) of the SHOX gene probably increase the height of these individuals [64].

In birth karyotype surveys these conditions occur more than twice as frequently as the Turner syndrome, 1 in 500 to 1 in 1000 male births, but many individuals are not diagnosed until adult life, if ever.

The testes are small and firm at all ages with hypergonadotropic hypogonadism sometimes. Gynecomastia may be seen from late childhood to the early teens. There is an increased risk of type 1 diabetes mellitus and hypothyroidism and many men have central obesity with metabolic markers of increased adverse cardiovascular risk.

Homocystinuria is associated with disproportionate tall stature but usually presents because of marked learning difficulties, ectopia lentis (downward dislocation) and severe myopia with later thromboembolic and cardiovascular problems.

Dysmorphic syndromes

The diagnosis of *Marfan syndrome* can be made at birth when there is a family history but, because tall individuals tend to assort non-randomly, the diagnosis can be delayed if the tall stature is attributed to constitutional familial tall stature. Many children present only when an undiagnosed parent has a sudden cardiac event.

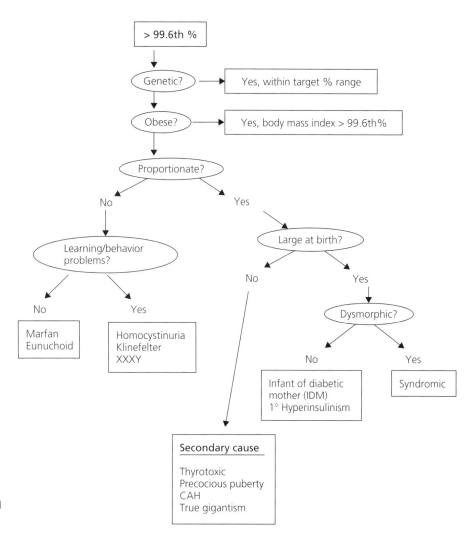

Figure 6.8 Clinical algorithm for assessment of tall stature.

Table 6.23 Marfan syndrome diagnostic criteria. If there is no family history there should be *at least two major* (underlined) features *in two systems* with involvement in one other system. If the family history is positive (± proven abnormality of the fibrillin gene) then one major feature plus involvement in one other system allows the diagnosis.

Skeleton	<u>Long span</u> (span >5 cm more than Ht). <u>Long legs</u> compared to the back, <u>arachnodactyly</u>, <u>joint laxity</u>, <u>scoliosis</u> and chest deformities (<u>pectus excavatum or carinatum</u>). High arched palate. <u>Flat feet</u>
Eyes	Myopia, upward <u>dislocation or poor fixation of the lens</u>, flat cornea and hypoplastic iris
CVS	Mitral and aortic valve incompetence, peripheral pulmonary stenosis, <u>aortic dilatation</u> and <u>dissection</u>
Chest	Spontaneous pneumothorax
Skin	Herniae, striae
MRI spine	Lumbosacral dural ectasia

CVS, cardiovascular system; MRI, magnetic resonance imaging.

Marfan syndrome is a dominantly inherited disorder characterized by disproportionate tall stature. There are many 'marfanoid' children with some of the features of the condition (and presumably more mild mutations) but, because of the important genetic and cardiac implications, it should be diagnosed only if the criteria given in Table 6.23 are met [65]. Syndrome-specific height centiles are available [66]. In Marfan syndrome there is usually a mutation of one of the copies of the fibrillin gene *FBN1* on chromosome 17q.

Beals contractual arachnodactyly is a rarer dominantly inherited disorder of another copy of a fibrillin gene on chromosome 15q and has some similarities with the Marfan syndrome. There are contractures at the knees, elbows and hands and micrognathia. The ears may be "crumpled" and there may be kyphoscoliosis.

Dysmorphic syndromes with symmetrical overgrowth

Most of these syndromes are associated with developmental delay and present in the neonatal period because of the dysmorphic features or when the delay is noted. The important causes are Sotos, Weaver, Marshall–Smith, Beckwith–Wiedemann syndrome and Simpson–Golabi–Behmel syndromes.

In Sotos syndrome, also called cerebral gigantism, early rapid growth with a tall forehead, large head circumference, a high arched palate and large chin is seen. The finger nails are concave at the base. Individuals are taller as children than adults because the bone age is usually in advance of chronological age and mean adult heights are 173 cm female, 184 cm male. There may be developmental delay of variable severity.

Marshall–Smith syndrome is the association of tall stature and thinness with developmental delay secondary to CNS malformation, blue sclerae and a small jaw. There is a tendency to respiratory infections. The bone age is very advanced with abnormal phalanges.

Weaver syndrome consists of tall stature, hypertonia, developmental delay, claw hands with unusual nails, and odd face. There is an advanced bone age with less radiographic abnormalities in the hand than Marshall–Smith syndrome although the maturation of the carpal bones is in advance of the small bones of the hand.

Beckwith–Wiedemann syndrome includes macrosomia (often more marked on one side of the body), with other dysmorphic features and hypoglycemia. The pancreas is hyperplastic and the liver and kidneys may be enlarged. There may be associated intellectual deficit as a result of the hypoglycemia. There is evidence of relative overexpression of the *in utero* growth factor IGF-2 because of a maternal imprinting defect possibly dually expressed with a paternal growth-suppressing H19 gene. There is a tendency to Wilms tumour as a result of this genetic imbalance.

Simpson–Golabi–Behmel syndrome (or "bulldog" syndrome) has overlapping features with Beckwith–Wiedemann syndrome but presents with a characteristic large mouth and tongue and is due to a deleting mutation of glypican 3, a membrane bound proteoglycan that usually sequesters IGF-2 to make it unavailable to its receptor.

The main distinguishing features of dysmorphic syndromes with partial or asymmetrical overgrowth are given in Table 6.24.

Secondary causes of large size
Early causes
Intrauterine hyperinsulinemia due to primary inherited disorders of pancreatic beta cell function or secondary to maternal diabetes causes early macrosomia, because insulin is a potent fetal growth factor. Persistent hyperinsulinemic hypoglycemia of infancy (PHHI; previously called pancreatic endocrine dysregulation syndrome or nesidioblastosis) may be secondary to somatic or germline mutations in the insulin-regulating potassium ATP channel of the beta cell on 11p. The germline mutations result in diffuse hyperinsulinism, whereas the somatic mutations may produce localized disease. Hyperinsulinism can also be secondary to mutations in the glucokinase, glutamate dehydrogenase and short chain 3-hydroxyacyl CoA dehydrogenase genes [67]. Once the abnormal insulin-secreting environment is removed after birth there is "catch-down" growth to normal genetic centiles by 2 years of age.

Table 6.24 Dysmorphic syndromes with partial or asymmetrical overgrowth.

Klippel–Trenaunay–Weber	Tissue overgrowth due to a somatic mutation in association with cutaneous vascular naevi
Proteus	Caused by a somatic mutation or chimeric tissue abnormality resulting in progressive overgrowth, lipomas and deformity in a typical "streak" pattern
Bannayan–Riley–Ruvacalba	Prenatal overgrowth, developmental delay, macrocephaly and developmental delay. Multiple mesodermal angiolipomas and macules on the penis. Caused by mutation in PTEN gene
Elejalde	Polydactyly, craniosynostosis organomegaly and renal dysplasia
Nevo	Kyphosis, abnormal hands and feet, hypotonia – related to Ehlers–Danlos syndrome kyphoscoliosis subtype may be associated with overgrowth
Beckwith–Wiedemann	The overgrowth in this syndrome may sometimes be asymmetrical producing hemihypertrophy

Table 6.25 Features of McCune–Albright syndrome.

"Coast of Maine" irregular café-au-lait patches
Polyostotic fibrous dysplasia of bone
Gonadotropin independent sexual precocity (autonomous ovarian cysts, testicular activation, isolated macro-orchidism)
Thyrotoxicosis
Parathyroid adenomas
Cushing (adrenal or pituitary disease)
GH adenomas
Prolactinomas
Pulmonary stenosis
Hepatitis
Activating post-somatic mutation of Gsα-subunit of the G-protein linked receptor

Late causes
Pituitary gigantism caused by a GH-producing adenoma in the pituitary or even less commonly GHRH excess from hypothalamic tumors is extremely rare. Forty percent of sporadic somatotrophinomas are caused by acquired activating mutations in the Gsα subunit of the transmembrane receptor. Pituitary hyperplasia with excess GH secretion may be seen as part of the McCune–Albright syndrome (Table 6.25).

Carney complex is a rare disorder [myxomas, spotty skin pigmentation (lentigenes), endocrine and non-endocrine tumors] in which somatotroph cell hyperplasia and GH excess may also be found. Although the most common pituitary tumors in multiple endocrine neoplasia type 1 are prolactinomas, GH secreting adenomas may also occur. Familial acromegaly and familial isolated pituitary adenomas are rare conditions of GH excess due to dominantly inherited mutations in aryl hydrocarbon interacting protein.

In all these conditions, proportionate, worsening tall stature with a rapid height velocity occurs but bone age is usually not markedly advanced, except in McCune–Albright syndrome with coexistent sexual precocity. All children with height velocity >97th centile over 1 year or >75th centile over 2 years require investigation. GH excess causes prominent soft tissues, prognathism and signs and symptoms resulting from optic chiasm compression caused by the pituitary tumor. There may be increased sweating and a yellowish discoloration of the palms. In the absence of treatment, adult heights up to 247 cm in the female and 274 cm in the male may be found because the tumor causes variable hypogonadotropic hypogonadism and thereby a lack of epiphyseal fusion. Acromegaly in the adult is the same disease after the fusion of the epiphyses but a number of patients with a late childhood onset share features of both conditions and 10% of acromegalics are tall. Concentrations of GH, IGF-1 and IGFBP3 are high and the GH does not suppress in response to a glucose load. An MRI of the brain may show an obvious adenoma.

Obesity and other causes of hyperinsulinism

Excess calorie intake is available for growth and may produce hyperinsulinism and relatively tall stature (at upper end of predicted target range). There is early puberty secondary to overproduction of leptin, a satiety hormone produced from white fat that has a key role in the initiation and maintenance of normal puberty. Striae and a high cheek color may mimic mild Cushing syndrome but with contrasting rapid growth compared to the universal growth failure of steroid excess. Insulin acting at the IGF-1 receptor in the skin produces acanthosis nigricans.

Mutations of the insulin receptor produce extreme primary hyperinsulinism with insulin resistance. This can cross-react at the IGF-1 receptor producing tall stature. In the HAIR-AN syndrome of type A or type B insulin resistance the facial features are described as "acromegaloid". The other features are hirsutism, acrochordons (skin-tags), insulin resistance and acanthosis nigricans [68].

Isolated ACTH insensitivity

Outside of known affected families, these individuals present in mid to late childhood.

Autosomal recessive familial glucocorticoid resistance results from mutations of the ACTH receptor (MC2-R). Patients present with Addison disease (hyperpigmentation, weakness and collapse), an increased height and head circumference (with frontal bossing) for the parental size and hypertelorism with epicanthic folds.

Other endocrine abnormalities

Thyrotoxicosis if relatively mild, and thus recognized and treated late, produces an acceleration of growth rate and relative tall stature in mid-childhood. The bone age is markedly advanced so the post-treatment height is only modestly elevated.

Early or precocious puberty causes an early onset of the pubertal phase of growth. The height velocity accelerates but skeletal maturation advances rapidly and there is early epiphyseal fusion. The child is therefore tall for his/her age initially but may end up as a short adult.

Multiple endocrine adenomatosis or neoplasia (MEA or MEN) type 2b is a familial condition where the occurrence of medullary carcinoma of the thyroid and pheochromocytoma is associated with mild tall stature and a marfanoid habitus along with neuromas of the mucous membranes, bowel and conjunctiva.

Hypogonadism for any cause or Kallmann syndrome (hypogonadotropic hypogonadism and anosmia) results in a modestly increased adult height secondary to late closure of the epiphyses and a prolonged childhood phase of growth of long bones. Absence of the sex hormone mediated growth of the spine produces disproportion in a similar fashion to that seen in delayed puberty.

Aromatase deficiency resulting from mutation of the CYP19 gene prevents the conversion of testosterone to estrogen in the male and hence there is no stimulus for epiphyseal fusion. These rare males continue growing into adulthood and have osteoporosis and infertility in association with massively raised FSH concentrations. Estrogen receptor mutations produced a similar pattern of continuing adult growth (204 cm) in a single case report [69,70].

Administration of anabolic steroids to enhance athletic performance is widespread in some societies. This may produce rapid growth in height and muscle bulk at the same time as hirsutism in females and testicular atrophy in males.

Constitutional tall stature

In the context of a tall family, there is often little concern about tall stature, which is often seen as socially advantageous. This may sometimes result in the delay of diagnosis of Marfan syndrome in particular (see above). Sometimes one parent, often the mother, has had adverse experiences related to her own size and may seek early assessment of their (usually female) child.

Familial tall stature results in tall stature during the childhood phase of growth and an increased final height within the range defined by parental size. The rate of growth varies around the 75th height velocity centile. Bone age approximates to chronological age and there is a normal age of onset of puberty. The legs are often relatively long in comparison to sitting height.

Investigations of tall stature

A bone age determination allows estimation of predicted height and may also reveal dysmorphic bones. Arachnodactyly may be measured by estimation of the metacarpal index (the average length to width ratios of the metacarpal bones) although this rarely adds anything to clinical examination. In Marfan syndrome the metacarpal index exceeds a value of >8.5.

In the presence of genital abnormalities, behavioral or learning difficulties a karyotype should be performed. Uniparental isodisomy of 11p may help confirm Beckwith–Wiedemann syndrome.

Pelvic and abdominal ultrasound examination for ovary and uterine size and estradiol (E2), luteinizing hormone (LH), FSH allow further delineation of physiological maturity and remaining growth potential. In boys testicular damage will produce menopausal FSH concentrations (e.g. Klinefelter syndrome). In both sexes, hypothalamic or pituitary hypogonadism will produce low LH and FSH concentrations that will also be suppressed by peripheral testosterone production or anabolic steroid administration. Familial glucocorticoid resistance will produce an elevated 0900 h ACTH concentration with a low cortisol concentration. TSH will be suppressed with a raised T3 and T4 in thyrotoxicosis.

If there is any possibility of MEN2b, either because of a positive family history or the presence of mucosal neuromas in a child with a marfanoid habitus, it is essential to measure calcitonin concentration and to confirm the diagnosis by analysis of the ret-proto-oncogene.

If pituitary gigantism is a possibility, an elevated IGF-1 concentration may be a useful screening test followed by a GH suppression test and pituitary imaging.

Glucose suppression test (GTT) for growth hormone

Precautions
1 Test is unnecessary in diabetic patients who demonstrate a suppressed GH in the presence of hyperglycemias.
2 Patients may feel nauseous.

Preparation
The diet for the 3 days preceding the test should contain adequate carbohydrate (approximately 60% of calories).

The patient should be fasted overnight for 10–14 h (plain water allowed) and should rest throughout the test.

Prepare the glucose load 1.75 g/kg anhydrous glucose (maximum 75 g) or 1.92 g/kg glucose monohydrate (maximum 82.5 g) dissolved in 100–200 mL water. It is not recommended to use Lucozade® or other sweetened fluids as the formulations may vary.

Insert IV cannula (see section on blood collection) and maintain patent with heparinized normal saline.

Protocol
1 0 min: take blood samples for GH (plain tube) and glucose (fluoride oxalate tube) estimation.
2 The child should drink the glucose load within 5 min.
3 Take further samples for GH and glucose at 30, 60, 90 and 120 min.

Interpretation
GH suppresses to <2 mIU/L (0.7 µg/L) in normal individuals. Failure to suppress and sometimes a paradoxical rise in GH concentrations is characteristic of GH hypersecretion.

References

1 Wit JM, Ranke MB, Kelnar CJH. ESPE classification of paediatric endocrine diagnoses. *Horm Res* 2007; **68** (Suppl 2): 1–120.

2 Karlberg J, Engstrom I, Karlberg P, Fryer JG. Analysis of linear growth using a mathematical model. I. From birth to three years. *Acta Paediatr Scand* 1987; **76**: 478–488.

3 Karlberg J, Fryer JG, Engstrom I, Karlberg P. Analysis of linear growth using a mathematical model. II. From 3 to 21 years of age. *Acta Paediatr Scand Suppl* 1987; **337**: 12–29.

4 Tanner JM. *Fetus into Man: Physical Growth from Conception to Maturity*, 2nd edn. Cambridge, MA: Harvard University Press, 1978.

5 Forbes K, Westwood M. The IGF axis and placental function: a mini review. *Horm Res* 2008; **69**: 129–137.

6 Cutfield WS, Hofman PL, Vickers M, Breier B, Blum WF, Robinson EM. IGFs and binding proteins in short children with intrauterine growth retardation. *J Clin Endocrinol Metab* 2002; **87**: 235–239.

7 Wit JM, van Unen H. Growth of infants with neonatal growth hormone deficiency. *Arch Dis Child* 1992; **67**: 920–924.

8 Strobl JS, Thomas MJ. Human growth hormone. *Pharmacol Rev* 1994; **46**: 1–34.

9 Lazarczyk MA, Lazarczyk M, Grzela T. Ghrelin: a recently discovered gut-brain peptide (review). *Int J Mol Med* 2003; **12**: 279–287.

10 Waters MJ, Hoang HN, Fairlie DP, Pelekanos RA, Brown RJ. New insights into growth hormone action. *J Mol Endocrinol* 2006; **36**: 1–7.

11 Hwa V, Oh Y, Rosenfeld RG. The insulin-like growth factor-binding protein (IGFBP) superfamily. *Endocr Rev* 1999; **20**: 761–787.

12 Breunlin DC, Desai VJ, Stone ME, Swilley JA. Failure-to-thrive with no organic etiology: a critical review of the literature. *Int J Eat Disord* 2006; **2**: 25–49.

13 Karlberg J, Albertsson-Wikland K. Growth in full-term small-for-gestational age infants: from birth to final height. *Pediatr Res* 1995; **38**: 733–739.

14 Hauspie RC, Vercauteren M, Susanne C. Secular changes in growth and maturation: an update. *Acta Paediatr* 1997; **423** (Suppl): 20–27.

15 Wales JK. Practical auxology and skeletal maturation. In: Kelnar CJH, Savage MO, Saegner P, Cowell CT, eds. *Growth Disorders*, 2nd edn. London: Edward Arnold, 2007.

16 Freeman JV, Cole TJ, Chinn S, Jones PR, White EM, Preece MA. Cross-sectional stature and weight reference curves for the UK, 1990. *Arch Dis Child* 1995; **73**: 17–24.

17 Wales JKH. A brief history of the study of human growth dynamics. *Ann Hum Biol* 1998; **25**: 175–184.

18 Lindsay R, Feldkamp M, Harris D, Robertson J, Rallison M. Utah Growth Study: growth standards and the prevalence of growth hormone deficiency. *J Pediatr* 1994; **125**: 29–35.

19 Voss LD, Mulligan J, Betts PR, Wilkin TJ. Poor growth in school entrants as an index of organic disease. *Br Med J* 1992; **305**: 1400–1402.

20 Ullrich O. Uber typische Kombinationsbilder multipler Abartung. *Z Kinderheilkd* 1930; **49**: 271–276.

21 Turner H. A syndrome of infantilism, congenital webbed neck and cubitus valgus. *Endocrinology* 1938; **23**: 566–574.

22 Chu CE. A clinical and molecular study of Turner's syndrome. MD thesis, University of Sheffield, 1994.

23 Ross JL, Scott C Jr, Marttila P, Kowal K, Nass A, Papenhausen P, *et al.* Phenotypes associated with SHOX deficiency. *J Clin Endocrinol Metab* 2001; **86**: 5674–5680.

24 Lyon A, Preece M, Grant D. Growth curves for girls with Turner syndrome. *Arch Dis Child* 1985; **60**: 932–935.

25 Ranke M, Stubbe P, Majewski F, *et al.* Spontaneous growth in Turner's syndrome. *Acta Paediatr Scand* 1988; **343** (Suppl): 22–30.

26 Saenger P, Albertsson-Wikland K, Conway G, *et al.* Recommendations for the diagnosis and management of Turner syndrome. *J Clin Endocrinol Metab* 2001; **86**: 3061–3069.

27 Styles M, Cole T, Dennis J, *et al.* New cross-sectional stature, weight and head circumference references for Down's syndrome in the UK and Republic of Ireland. *Arch Dis Child* 2002; **87**: 104–108.

28 Ranke M, Heidemann P, Knupfer C. Noonan syndrome: growth and clinical manifestations in 144 cases. *Eur J Pediatr* 1988; **148**: 220–227.

29 Tartaglia M, Martinelli S, Stella L, Bocchinfuso G, Flex E, Cordeddu V, *et al.* Diversity and functional consequences of germline and somatic PTPN11 mutations in human disease. *Am J Hum Genet* 2006; **78**: 279–290.

30 Butler M. Imprinting disorders: non-Mendelian mechanisms affecting growth. *J Pediatr Endocrinol Metab* 2002; **15** (Suppl 5): 1279–1288.

31 Preece M. The genetics of the Silver–Russell syndrome. *Rev Endocr Metab Disord* 2002; **3**: 369–379.

32 Wollmann H, Kirchner T, Enders H, *et al.* Growth and symptoms in Silver–Russell syndrome: review on the basis of 386 patients. *Eur J Pediatr* 1995; **154**: 958–968.

33 Butler M, Brunschwig A, Miller LK, *et al.* Standards for selected anthropometric measurements in Prader–Willi syndrome. *Paediatrics* 1991; **88**: 853–860.

34 Cummings DE, Karine Clement K, Purnell JQ, Vaisse C, Foster KE, Frayo RS, *et al.* Elevated plasma ghrelin concentrations in Prader–Willi syndrome. *Nat Med* 2002; **8**: 643–644.

35 Winter RM, Baraitser M. *The Winter–Baraitser Dysmorphology Database*. London Medical Databases Ltd, 38 Chalcot Crescent, London, NW1 8YD, UK: 2008.

36 Hall JG, Froster-Iskenius UG, Allanson JE. *Handbook of Normal Physical Measurements*, 1st edn. Oxford: Oxford University Press, 1990.

37 http://www.ncbi.nlm.nih.gov/sites/entrez?db=omim

38 Ibáñez L, DiMartino-Nardi J, Neus Potau N, Saenger P. Premature adrenarche: normal variant or forerunner of adult disease? *Endocr Rev* 2000; **21**: 671–696.

39 Superti-Furga A, Unger S and the Nosology Group of the International Skeletal Dysplasia Society. Nosology and Classification of Genetic Skeletal Disorders: 2006 Revision. *Am J Med Genet* 2007 (Part A) **143A**: 1–18 & http://www.csmc.edu/pdf/International NosologyandCla.pdf.

40 Appan S, Laurent S, Chapman M, Hindmarsh PC, Brook CG. Growth and growth hormone therapy in hypochondroplasia. *Acta Paediatr Scand* 1990; **79**: 796–803.

41 Horton W, Rotter J, Rimoin D, *et al.* Standard growth curves for achondroplasia. *J Pediatr* 1978; **93**: 435–438.

42 Tynjälä P, Lahdenne P, Vähäsalo P, Hannu Kautiainen H, Honkanen V. Impact of anti-TNF therapy on growth in severe juvenile idiopathic arthritis. *Ann Rheum Dis* 2006; **65**: 1044–1049.

43 Ranke M, Reiter EO, Price DA. Idiopathic growth hormone deficiencey in KIGS: selected aspects. In: Ranke M, Price DA, Reiter EO, eds. *Growth Hormone Therapy in Pediatrics: 20 Years of KIGS*. Basel: Karger, 2007: 116–135.

44 Darzy KH. Pezzoli SS. Thorner MO, Shalet SM. Cranial irradiation and growth hormone neurosecretory dysfunction: a critical appraisal. *J Clin Endocrinol Metab* 2007; **92**: 1666–1672.

45 Horan M, Millar DS, Hedderich J, Lewis G, Newsway V, Mo N, *et al.* Human growth hormone 1 (GH1) gene expression: complex haplotype-dependent influence of polymorphic variation in the proximal promoter and locus control region. *Hum Mutat* 2003; **21**: 408–423.

46 Takahashi Y, Kaji H, Okimura Y, Goji K, Abe H, Chihara K. Brief report: short stature caused by a mutant growth hormone. *N Engl J Med* 1996; **334**: 432–436.

47 Kowarski AA, Schneider JJ, Ben-Galim E, Weldon VV, Daughaday WH. Growth failure with normal serum RIA-GH and low somatomedin activity: somatomedin restoration and growth acceleration after exogenous GH. *J Clin Endocrinol* 1978; **47**: 461–464.

48 Tillmann V, Shalet SM, Price DA, Wales JKH, Pennels L, Soden J, *et al.* Serum insulin-like growth factor-1, IGF binding protein-3 and IGFBP-3 protease activity after cranial irradiation. *Horm Res* 1998; **50**: 71–77.

49 Butler J. Role of biochemical tests in assessing the need for growth hormone therapy in children with short stature: Royal College of Pathologists' Clinical Audit Project. *Ann Clin Biochem* 2001; **38**: 1–2.

50 Bristow AF. International standards for growth hormone. *Horm Res* 1999; **51** (Suppl 1): 7–12.

51 Seth J, Ellis A, Al-Sadie R. Serum growth hormone measurements in clinical practice: an audit of performance from the UK National External Quality Assessment Scheme. *Horm Res* 1999; **51** (Suppl 1): 13–19.

52 National Institute for Clinical Excellence. Guidance on the use of human growth hormone (somatotropin) in children with growth failure. *Technology Appraisal Guidance* 2002: 42.

53 Ranke M. *Diagnostics of Endocrine Function in Children and Adolescents*, 3rd edn. Basel: Karger, 2003.

54 Godowski PJ, Leung DW, Meacham LR, Galgani JP, Hellmiss R, Keret R, *et al.* Characterization of the human growth hormone receptor gene and demonstration of a partial gene deletion in two patients with Laron-type dwarfism. *Proc Natl Acad Sci U S A* 1989; **86**: 8083–8087.

55 Kofoed EM, Hwa V, Little B, Woods KA, Buckway CK, Tsubaki J, *et al.* Growth hormone insensitivity associated with a STAT5b mutation. *N Engl J Med* 2003; **349**: 1139–1147.

56 Walenkamp MJE, Lankester A, Oostdijk W, Wit JM. Partial growth hormone insensitivity and immunodeficiency caused by a disturbance in the NF-B signaling pathway. *Horm Res* 2004; **62** (Suppl 2):103.

57 Netchine I, Azzi S, Houang M, Seurin D, Daubas C, Ricort J, *et al.* Partial IGF-1 deficiency demonstrates the critical role of IGF-I in growth and brain development. *Horm Res* 2006; **65** (Suppl 4): 29.

58 Woods KA, Camacho-Hubner C, Savage MO, Clark AJ. Intrauterine growth retardation and postnatal growth failure associated with deletion of the insulin-like growth factor 1 gene. *N Engl J Med* 1996; **335**: 1363–1367.

59 Hwa V, Haeusler G, Pratt KL, Little BM, Frisch H, Koller D, *et al.* Total absence of functional acid labile subunit, resulting in severe insulin-like growth factor deficiency and moderate growth failure. *J Clin Endocrinol Metab* 2006; **91**: 1826–1831.

60 Abuzzahab MJ, Schneider A, Goddard A, Grigorescu F, Lautier C, Keller E, *et al*. IGF-1 receptor mutations resulting in intrauterine and postnatal growth retardation. *N Engl J Med* 2003; **349**: 2211–2222.

61 Mushtaq T, Ahmed SF. The impact of corticosteroids on growth and bone health. *Arch Dis Child* 2002; **87**: 93–96.

62 Wales JKH, Herber SM, Taitz LS. Height and body proportions in child abuse. *Arch Dis Child* 1992; **67**: 632–635.

63 Walenkamp M-J. Genetic disorders in the growth hormone – 1GF1 axis. Doctoral thesis, University of Leiden, 2007. Pasmans offset-drukerij BV, Der Haag, Netherlands.

64 Ogata T, Matsuo N, Nishimura G. SHOX haploinsufficiency and overdosage impact of gonadal function status. *J Med Genet* 2001; **38**: 1–6.

65 Beighton P, de Paepe A, Danks D, *et al*. International nosology of heritable disorders of connective tissue. *Am J Med Genet* 1988; **29**: 581–594.

66 Pyeritz RE. Growth and anthropometrics in the Marfan syndrome. In: Papadatos CJ, Bartsocas CS, eds. *Endocrine Genetics and Genetics of Growth*. New York: Liss, 1985.

67 Glaser B, Thornton P, Otonkoski Tunien C. Genetics of neonatal hyperinsulinism. *Arch Dis Child Fetal Neonatal Ed* 2000; **82**: 79–86.

68 Krentz AJ. Insulin resistance. *Br Med J* 1996; **313**: 1385–1389.

69 Bulun SE. Aromatase deficiency in women and men: would you have predicted the phenotypes? *J Clin Endocrinol Metab* 1996; **81**: 867–871.

70 Smith EP, Boyd J, Frank GR, Takahashi H, Cohen RM, Specker B, *et al*. Estrogen resistance caused by a mutation in the estrogen-receptor gene in a man. *N Engl J Med* 1994; **331**: 1056–1061.

7 Management of Disordered Growth

Steven D. Chernausek

Department of Pediatrics, University of Oklahoma Health Sciences Center, Oklahoma City, OK, USA

Disordered growth, which reflects an aberration in genes, hormones, nutrients and environment at any point during the first two decades of human life, is the most common problem in pediatric endocrinology. The number of diagnoses is vast and management options are varied because of the wide variety of body systems that regulate growth. Short stature and/or growth failure is more common than overgrowth and has the greater number of diagnostic possibilities.

The management of children with disorders of growth involves more than making a diagnosis and administering a drug. They always entrain psychosocial issues, the impact on school performance and behavior before and during therapy should not be underestimated. Apart from encouragement and guidance from the treating physician, serious distress and/or psychopathology require referral to mental health professionals.

Short stature

Why treat?
Treatment of short stature has gained wide acceptance among Western societies. The use of human growth hormone (hGH) has spread from hormone replacement of growth hormone deficiency (GHD) to pharmacological treatment of Turner syndrome, short children born small for gestational age (SGA) and idiopathic short stature. Regulatory approvals have been based on efficacy (an increased growth rate with or without evidence of an increase in adult stature) and relative safety in the short term. Worldwide sales of hGH approximate US$ 2 billion.

Individuals with GHD require replacement treatment for stature but also for beneficial effects on metabolic status, bone mineral content and body composition. There are other conditions where growth is so severely reduced that the ability to

function is impaired and physical appearance so abnormal that there is little disagreement that treatment should be offered but the benefits of increasing height in less severe conditions are largely presumed and treatment of such children is controversial.

There is a belief that individuals with short stature suffer bias and discrimination in society and that they may be unable to perform as well or achieve a status equivalent to that of their normal-sized peers. There is a suspicion that they are unhappy and have diminished self-esteem, issues that may provoke the initial referral to the clinic. It is hoped that treatment with hGH will ameliorate these problems. In reality, most of the data show that individuals with heights that borderline on normal have measurable but modest differences in social standing, educational achievement, income, etc. but also that they are just as happy as their peers [1,2].

The hard questions are:
- How short is too short?
- What will be the outcome if a short child is left untreated?
- How much height will be gained if a specific treatment is employed?
- Who should make the decision regarding this expensive and potentially hazardous therapy?

How to treat
Growth hormone
hGH is the most abundant hormone produced by the pituitary, comprising up to 25% of the dry weight of the gland. The secretory rate of growth hormone in the prepubertal period approximates $0.6 \, \mu g/m^2/day$, increasing twofold during puberty [3]. hGH has been used to treat GHD for 50 years. Because only hGH is effective in humans (in contrast to insulin, where porcine and bovine forms are bioactive), initial preparations were derived from human pituitary glands obtained postmortem. Because of the recognition of iatrogenic Creutzfeldt–Jakob disease, production changed to biosynthetic methods in 1985, which led to an unlimited supply and the opportunity to consider treatment of a wider range of conditions.

Brook's Clinical Pediatric Endocrinology, 6th edition. Edited by C. Brook, P. Clayton, R. Brown. © 2009 Blackwell Publishing, ISBN: 978-1-4051-8080-1.

Clinical use

hGH produces few adverse effects in children over the short or intermediate term [4,5]. The therapeutic window is wide, allowing a substantial range of doses to be given safely. When supplies of hGH were limited, many individuals with GHD were given incomplete replacement. Greater abundance of hGH for treatment now allows optimization of dosage for the condition being treated, the age of the child and the desired response.

Growth hormone use can be categorized as replacement (for GHD) or pharmacologic (for most other conditions) therapy. In the latter situation, hGH is used to stimulate growth-promoting pathways that are dampened by disease or underperforming because of normal variation. hGH is used in such cases to overcome relative GH or insulin-like growth factor (IGF) insensitivity. Only a few studies have systematically evaluated a variety of doses and recommended dosage usually reflects the dosage used during licensing trials for the condition in question rather than the optimal regimen (Table 7.1). An individual with neonatally diagnosed or recently acquired GHD should be started on a dosage that approximates daily production. A child with a non-GHD condition will need a higher dosage but in both situations there should be modifications based on desired and expected response, age, degree of short stature and anticipated duration of therapy. For example, a short child born SGA who is diagnosed late and far behind in terms of height may be served better by a relatively high hGH dosage.

The response to treatment is dictated by the sensitivity of the disease in question to hGH, the dosage and the age of the patient. The growth response is usually best in the first year of therapy and usually declines slightly thereafter but most patients increase growth velocity by at least 2 cm/year (usually more) over their baseline growth velocity. This should be evident during the first 6 months of therapy. When this does not occur or the growth velocity wanes more than expected later in the course of therapy, an explanation must be sought. Things to consider are:
• Is the diagnosis correct?
• Is the dosage appropriate for the diagnosis?
• Is all the hGH be given as prescribed?
• Has another condition, such as inadequate nutrition, hypothyroidism or an excessive dosage of glucocorticoid, developed that impedes response?

If no explanation is forthcoming, a trial at a higher hGH dosage with monitoring of circulating IGF-1 is reasonable.

Safety

hGH is well-tolerated in children and complications rarely arise. Adverse events are listed in Table 7.2. Allergy is very uncommon. Some patients develop antibodies to hGH but these rarely affect response. The exception is the patient who is homozygous for a GH gene deletion who develops high titers that neutralize exogenous hGH. The development or worsening of scoliosis has been reported in association with hGH treatment, as has slipped capital femoral epiphysis. Intracranial hypertension, a rare complication, typically responds to brief withdrawal from hGH treatment with resumption at a lower dosage.

The possible role hGH treatment might have in *de novo* neoplasm formation or in the growth of existing tumors has been of concern [6] because of data that show GH and IGF-1 promote tumor growth. Epidemiological studies that indicate higher than average circulating levels of IGF-1 are associated with an increased incidence of some common adult tumors, such as carcinoma of the colon. Also many children develop GHD because of a tumor or its treatment.

Pre-existing malignancies should be inactive and treatment complete before instituting hGH. Treating patients with craniopharyngioma and other CNS tumors with hGH does not appear to influence recurrence [7]. Administering hGH to patients treated for one tumor may modestly increase the risk of a second primary, frequently a meningioma [8]. Because the data suggest that the increased risk conferred by adding hGH is low, most children with GHD and adequately treated stable neoplasms should be offered treatment. The risk of tumor formation in normal, short or GHD children given hGH is extremely low.

Table 7.1 Suggested dosing of human growth hormone (hGH) for treatment of short stature of various etiologies.

Diagnosis	Approximate dose (µg/kg/day)	Comments
Growth hormone deficiency: childhood	25–50; 100 during puberty	Secretory rate is approx 20 µg/kg/day
Growth hormone deficiency: adulthood	6–12	Based on studies of middle-aged adults
Prader–Willi syndrome	25–50	Consider dosing by m² or ideal body weight in obese patients
Turner syndrome	50–60	Some studies use higher doses or combined with oxandrolone
Short stature with small for gestational age	35–70	Response can vary significantly among patients
Noonan syndrome	Up to 66	*PTNP11* status may influence response
SHOX gene abnormality	50	Not all patient have typical Leri–Weill features
Idiopathic short stature	50	

Table 7.2 Adverse events associated with human growth hormone (hGH) therapy. Data from Blethen *et al.* [4] and Clayton and Cowell [5].

Event	Frequency	Management	Comments
Peripheral edema		None or short course diuretic	Resolves with time
Insulin resistance/hyperglycemia	1 : 1000	None to blood glucose lowering drugs	Increased insulin : glucose common, overt DM rare
Slipped capital femoral epiphysis	1–5 : 1000	Orthopedic fixation	Due to underlying condition?
Scoliosis	1–10%	Bracing/surgery	Due to underlying condition?
Benign intracranial hypertension	1–2 : 1000	Suspend hGH, reintroduce at lower dose when resolved	More common in patients with predisposing CNS anomalies

DM, diabetes mellitus.

Monitoring

Periodic assessment of safety and efficacy are predominantly based on review of history and physical findings. A reasonable approach is to examine patients every 3–6 months, depending on the phase of treatment, to measure IGF-1 once or twice annually and to measure skeletal age radiographically every 1–3 years. The principal measure of efficacy is growth velocity, which must be interpreted in light of the patient's diagnosis, pubertal status, bone age and degree of growth retardation. Even though hGH administration always reduces insulin sensitivity, routine measures of carbohydrate status are not indicated, unless there are significant risk factors for diabetes in the patient.

The Growth Hormone Research/IGF Society recommends that circulating IGF-1 be monitored as part of ongoing surveillance and adjustments made to avoid IGF-1 concentrations above normal because of the association of these with cancers in adulthood [9]. It makes sense in GHD to use all parameters (growth rate, skeletal maturation and IGF-1 concentration) to assess the adequacy of GH replacement. Monitoring IGF-1 is helpful for detecting non-compliance. When both the growth velocity and circulating IGF-1 are lower than expected, non-compliance is almost always the problem. The use of IGF-1 to avoid hazard in non-GHD conditions remains to be determined. Resistance to IGF may underlie some conditions. If so, avoiding higher IGF-1 concentrations could be counterproductive.

Recombinant human insulin-like growth factor 1

Insulin-like growth factor 1 (IGF-1) induces growth by promoting cell division, inhibiting apoptosis and stimulating protein synthesis. It was originally recognized as "sulfation factor," the putative mediator of GH's growth-promoting actions in cartilage but it was quickly recognized that its growth regulatory role involves most organs and tissues. IGF-1 is structurally homologous with insulin and possesses both insulin-like and growth-promoting properties. Both features have been exploited therapeutically (clinical trials show improved glycemic control in diabetes mellitus) but only the treatment of short stature has obtained regulatory approval.

In the circulation IGF-1 is complexed with IGF binding protein 3 (IGFBP3) and the acid labile subunit (ALS), which are also produced by the liver in response to GH. The roles of IGFBP3 and ALS are to stabilize IGF-1, protect it from degradation and prolong its circulation. The three components form a ternary complex, which serves as a reservoir of IGF-1 within the bloodstream. In addition to this endocrine role, IGF-1 is also synthesized by multiple organs and stimulates growth within tissues of origin in a paracrine/autocrine manner.

Clinical use

Recombinant human IGF-1 (rhIGF-1) was developed as a therapeutic agent in the early 1990s. Initial trials tested the response in children with growth hormone insensitivity syndrome (GHIS, Laron syndrome), a condition with severe short stature most commonly caused by defects in the GH receptor gene [10–12] and unresponsive to GH. Clinical trials conducted in a few subjects demonstrated reasonable safety and efficacy, which led to licensing of rhIGF for a condition termed "severe primary IGF deficiency" [13].

Most individuals with GHIS lack not only IGF-1 but other components of the ternary complex as well. This results in a more rapid clearance of the hormone so twice daily dosing just before a meal in order to avoid hypoglycemia is recommended for most patients with primary IGF deficiency/GHIS. A starting dose is 40–60 µg/kg, with increases up to 120 µg/kg as tolerated. When administered thus, there is a trebling of the baseline growth velocity on average and sustained growth for several years in patients with GHIS (Fig. 7.1) but the response is not as robust as is typically observed in GH deficient individuals treated with hGH. The reasons for this have not been established but may reflect inadequate dosing, the lack of IGFBP3 and ALS or the inability of subcutaneous injections to restore the IGF-1 content of peripheral tissues.

Safety

Experience with rhIGF-1 as a therapeutic agent is limited compared to that with hGH. Although patients have been treated successfully for more than 10 years now, the total number of patients treated is few and low frequency adverse events may come to light only with more exposure (Table 7.3). Hypoglycemia in conjunction with rhIGF-1 therapy is the most common

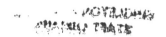

adverse event. Many GHIS patients have spontaneous hypoglycemia because of their underlying condition (GHIS) and rhIGF-1 might, in theory, exacerbate this but, as it turns out, symptomatic hypoglycemia resulting from rhIGF-1 is largely avoided when adequate calories are consumed in conjunction with the injection. Nonetheless, episodes of severe hypoglycemia can occur, especially in patients who do not consume sufficient carbohydrate before an injection.

Other adverse effects of IGF-1 are those attributable to lymphoid tissue overgrowth. Tonsillectomy and/or adenoidectomy along with tympanostomy tube placement were very common in initial trials. The extent to which this reflects lymphoid tissue growth versus the relatively small mid-face structure in GHIS patients is not clear. Intracranial hypertension may occur during either hGH or rhIGF therapy. Although too few patients have been treated to judge accurately the incidence of intracranial

hypertension during rhIGF-1 therapy, the preliminary indication suggests it may be more common than with hGH. As with hGH, it should respond to transient withdrawal of the rhIGF-1 and reintroduction at a lower dosage. Concerns about the role of IGF-1 in malignancy probably are just as applicable with rhIGF-1 as with hGH [14].

Monitoring

There must be periodic assessment of safety and efficacy by interim history and physical findings, i.e. growth response. There is no demonstrated utility of measurement of circulating IGF-1 during treatment. Home blood glucose monitoring is not formally recommended but can be helpful in some situations. The signs and symptoms of tonsillar or adenoidal hypertrophy should be sought and if present evaluated by audiometry and other measures. Symptoms of headache, nausea, changes in visual status and/or irritability should prompt an evaluation for intracranial hypertension.

Sex steroids

Androgens were the first growth-promoting hormones used clinically. They act by stimulating bone growth directly and by enhancing pituitary GH secretion. Their use is limited to older patients because of the effects on secondary sex characteristics and the propensity to accelerate skeletal maturation. This is especially true for estrogens. Androgens are used mostly to treat constitutional delay of growth and adolescence (CGDA) or as an adjunct to hGH. The available forms include testosterone, modified androgens such as oxandrolone and estrogenic compounds. Testosterone preparations are used only in males and estrogens in females. Oxandrolone has been used in both.

Clinical use

Testosterone is usually administered intramuscularly in a long-acting form (testosterone enanthate or cypionate) at monthly intervals. A typical starting dosage is 50 mg/month, with increases every 3–6 months depending on the clinical situation. Transcutaneous preparations are available but are more expensive and

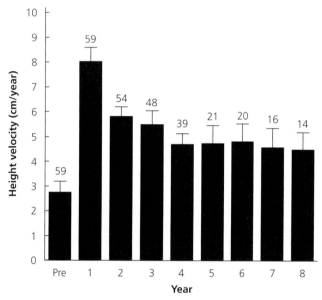

Figure 7.1 Linear growth in response to rhIGF-1 treatment in GH insensitivity. (From Chernausek *et al.* [13] with permission.)

Table 7.3 Adverse events associated with rhIGF-1 therapy in growth hormone insensitivity syndrome (GHIS). (After Chernausek *et al.* [13].)

Event	Frequency	Management	Comments
Hypoglycemia	50%	Give rhIGF-1 with meal, avoid prolonged fast	Most hypoglycemic episodes due to GHIS, not medication administration
Hypoglycemic seizure	5%	Give rhIGF-1 with meal, avoid prolonged fast	Younger patients possibly more at risk
Tonsillar/adenoidal hypertrophy	22%	Removal if obstructive symptoms	Snoring may be first sign
Hypoacusis	22%	Tympanostomy tube placement	Usually conductive
Injection site lipodystrophy	32%	Rotate sites	
Benign intracranial hypertension	4%	Suspend rhIGF-1, reintroduce at lower dose when resolved	Seen with hGH also, ? more common with rhIGF-1

SINGLETON
STAFF LIBRARY Management of Disordered Growth

the regimen for pubertal initiation or growth promotion is not established. The dose of oxandrolone, a non-aromatizable androgen administered orally, is typically in the range 0.05–0.1 mg/kg/day. Because it is not metabolized to estrogen, it may produce less bone age advancement. Some studies suggest that administering estrogens at very low (sub-feminizing) dosage may promote growth without untoward skeletal maturation but the data are limited [15]. At the present time it is hard to recommend any estrogen regimen as yielding a significant net gain in height.

Safety

Intramuscular testosterone given to males in the adolescent age range at recommended dosage is very safe. Large doses of androgens are not given orally because of adverse hepatic effects. Oxandrolone at recommended dosage is generally safe for both boys and girls. It reduces insulin sensitivity and therefore could theoretically cause carbohydrate intolerance in susceptible individuals [16]. Estrogens may produce hyperlipidemia and rarely induce thrombotic adverse events but this is very uncommon in pediatric practice.

Monitoring

No special testing is indicated other than periodic radiographs for skeletal age. Blood pressure should be measured before and after staring estrogen, and lipid profiles obtained in those with risk factors beginning estrogen therapy.

GnRH agonists and aromatase inhibitors

Adult height may be increased by extending the time for growth, which means influencing puberty to attenuate skeletal maturation. This can be achieved by delaying puberty with a gonadotropin releasing hormone (GnRH) agonist or by reducing estrogen, the main hormone driving skeletal maturation, with an aromatase inhibitor. Neither treatment is approved by regulatory agencies for height augmentation but there are several reports of clinical trials and probably limited use in clinical practice.

The effect of GnRH agonists appears modest because, when puberty is blocked completely, the growth rate slows because of the lack of sex steroid exposure. In one randomized trial of GnRH agonist in short but otherwise normal children, there was about a 5-cm gain in final height when puberty was delayed by 3 years [17].

Aromatase inhibition would theoretically allow the beneficial growth effects of androgens while negating the growth plate maturation resulting from estrogens but data on aromatase inhibition are limited. Studies do show that skeletal maturation is slowed by the treatment with growth continuing, implying that final height will be increased [18], but the actual effect on final height remains to be determined.

Clinical use

When puberty is far advanced, no medical therapy improves height outcome. GnRH agonists can be given as daily injections, intranasally or in a depot form, which lasts 1–12 months, by injection or implantation. They are effective at suppressing pituitary gonadotropin secretion but treatment dosage or frequency may need to be individualized.

Trials of aromatase inhibitors enrolled only boys because the therapy may induce ovarian cysts in girls. Although the results are encouraging, using aromatase inhibitors for improving height should be considered experimental at this time because of the small number of subjects treated and the scant data on final height.

Safety

There has been concern that delaying puberty or lowering estrogen exposure might lead to decreased bone mineral accretion but there is no evidence that this would be clinically significant. Most adverse events associated with GnRH agonists are injection site reactions and local abscess formation, which are uncommon. The drug is otherwise well-tolerated and puberty appears to be re-established normally following withdrawal. Aromatase inhibitors also appear well-tolerated but experience is much more limited. Testosterone concentrations increase substantially because of the reflex increase in gonadotropin secretion. The impact of this is unknown.

Monitoring

It is important that pituitary suppression be verified at the initiation of treatment and periodically thereafter when using GnRH agonists. Skeletal maturation should be assessed once or twice a year. It is premature to discuss monitoring for aromatase inhibition given the experimental nature of its use.

Cost effectiveness of growth-promoting therapies

With the possible exception of depot testosterone, most growth-promoting therapies are expensive and debates as to cost–benefit ratios are inevitable. At present, only effectiveness, i.e. growth response, can be assessed because the true benefit of additional height has not been measured.

Take, for example, "pubertal dosing" of hGH for GHD. A controlled trial showed that a dose twice that of the standard resulted in greater final height [19] but the cost would approximate $100 000 for each extra inch in stature. A therapeutic maneuver combining GnRH agonist therapy (e.g. leuprolide) with hGH when the onset of puberty threatens to curtail the "window of opportunity" for intervention could easily exceed $50 000 per year but its effectiveness is questionable.

A recent assessment of the cost-effectiveness of treating children with idiopathic short stature (ISS) estimated that each inch gained cost approximately $50 000 [20]. Because the number of patients with ISS is vast, the potential for a significant burden on health care systems with indiscriminant use of hGH is obvious. Solving the problem involves getting better at determining who will benefit most from treatment by identifying the patients and conditions that will yield the best growth response when treated and determining who needs the intervention to improve their well-being in the long run.

Management of specific conditions

Growth hormone deficiency

The diagnosis of GHD in children is clinical, based on the combination of medical history, auxology and laboratory testing. Reliance solely on the results of stimulation testing will misclassify many patients with short stature, especially if those with peak values <10 ng/mL are considered GH deficient. When growth is impaired because of moderate to severe GHD, the response to hGH is predictably robust with dosage in the lower ranges. When this does not occur one must assess compliance, seek other conditions that might explain a poor response (e.g. concurrent central hypothyroidism, excessive glucocorticoid replacement) and reconsider the diagnosis of true GHD.

Infancy and childhood

Most patients diagnosed as infants or young children have congenital GHD, frequently associated with other pituitary tropic hormone deficiencies. Treatment is justified as soon as the diagnosis is made in order to prevent hypoglycemia and to normalize growth. Weight-based regimens may undertreat some infants so surface area-based regimens may be preferable. Suggested dosage is 25–50 µg/kg/day or 0.7–1.4 mg/M^2/day. Monitoring growth response and documenting the prevention of hypoglycemia are important.

Adolescence

Growth hormone secretion naturally increases during puberty in boys and girls so it seems logical to increase GH dosage, at least in GHD, to mimic the natural processes. In the USA, a higher dosage (100 µg/kg/day) is approved for children during puberty. Administration of the "pubertal dose" does result in an increase in final height in individuals but at considerable expense [19]. Because this dosage exceeds the GH secretory rate of most individuals and results in a supra-normal circulating concentration of IGF in many, it is the author's practice to increase the dosage at puberty only for those patients on relatively low dosage at pubertal onset and/or who are showing a less than desirable growth response.

Adulthood

Maintaining GH dosage in pediatric ranges may help the young adult or adolescent patient to achieve normal peak bone mass. For older adults with severe GHD, hGH is indicated in order to avoid the complications of adult GHD which include decreased bone mineral and lean body mass along with increased fat mass and an unfavorable lipid profile [21]. Adults appear much more sensitive to hGH and develop arthralgias and other symptoms when given dosage easily tolerated in the pediatric population. Most of the initial studies of adults were conducted in middle-aged individuals: GH secretion normally declines gradually with age, which perhaps explains the increased sensitivity. The hGH dosage required to reverse the phenotype of adult GHD and to restore circulating concentrations of IGF-1, is much lower than that proposed for children and adolescents.

In managing patients at or near the end of the growing period, the persistence of GHD should be verified because up to 40% of patients with isolated childhood-onset GHD will retest normally as young adults. Typically, GH stimulation testing with insulin-induced hypoglycemia or arginine and growth hormone-releasing hormone (GHRH) is employed [22]. This might be bypassed for patients with organic hypothalamic-pituitary disease, multiple pituitary tropic hormone deficiencies or very low serum IGF-1 concentrations after hGH is withdrawn. Treatment at dosage approximating the pediatric range during the transitional period makes sense, with a reduction in dosage into the adult range thereafter, dictated largely by circulating IGF-1 concentrations.

Special considerations

Some patients with congenital disease limited to a subset of pituitary hormones develop additional deficiencies over time, such as those with *PROP1* mutations, in whom central adrenal insufficiency can manifest late [23]. Such patients need periodic reassessment of their pituitary function.

Prader–Willi syndrome

Prader–Willi syndrome (PWS), caused by deletions or imprinting abnormalities within regions of several genes located in the long arm of chromosome 15, is characterized by intellectual deficit, hypotonia and poor feeding that leads to failure to thrive during infancy. This is followed by an insatiable appetite and the development of morbid obesity. Many features are caused by a generalized hypothalamic defect that includes GHD and hypogonadotropic hypogonadism. Replacement of these deficits has been shown to improve the patients' condition and hGH is approved for use in children with growth failure resulting from PWS [24,25].

Whether all PWS patients should undergo GH stimulation testing is debatable. Those with the expected genetic defect and a moderate to severe abnormality of growth almost all have GHD, especially if the IGF-1 concentration is in the lower range. PWS patients in whom the growth failure is less obvious would perhaps benefit from documentation of GHD to help determine whether the treatment is indicated. As with most syndromes, there are variable expressions of the phenotype.

Infancy and childhood

During infancy, growth may be limited in PWS because of insufficient caloric intake. Once this is addressed, the GH secretory status of the individual can be evaluated. Growth hormone therapy can be initiated using the same guidelines as for typical GHD. For the markedly obese, dosing on a surface area basis to avoid overdosing is preferred. Any PWS patient with symptoms of disordered sleep breathing or sleep apnea should have full evaluation and institution of any required treatment before giving hGH. Patients with PWS are predisposed to diabetes mellitus

(DM). Because GH reduces insulin sensitivity, there has been concern that hGH therapy might induce carbohydrate intolerance or make existing DM worse. Conversely, hGH increases lean body mass and decreases fat mass, which should ameliorate abnormalities of carbohydrate homeostasis. Thus far it appears that hGH therapy does not have adverse metabolic consequences for patients with PWS. Given the predisposition for DM, periodic measures of glucose should be performed whether or not individuals are receiving hGH.

Adolescence

Treatment with hGH should continue, with adjustments based on growth rate and IGF-1 concentration, etc. For patients with hypogonadotropic hypogonadism, sex steroid therapy may be indicated. Continued assessment of glycemic status is particularly important during this time.

Adulthood

Although hGH was originally intended to treat the short stature associated with PWS, the persistence of GHD and aberrant body composition abnormalities has led to consideration of its use in adults. A recent study evaluated the effect of hGH in adults with PWS and documented GHD who were on average 30 years of age [26]. Lean body mass increased and fat mass decreased in response to a typical adult dosage of 1 mg/day. There were no additional abnormalities of carbohydrate status that resulted from the hGH and no worsening of glycemic control in patients with concomitant DM. These data suggest that the benefits of GH replacement in other adults with GHD may also be found in adults with PWS and that the improvement in body composition and other metabolic parameters outweigh the change in insulin sensitivity induced by hGH.

Special considerations

After approval of hGH for PWS, there were isolated cases of sudden death occurring in PWS patients receiving hGH [27]. This led the US FDA to state that hGH was contraindicated for "patients with Prader–Willi syndrome who are severely obese or who have respiratory impairment." Although it is not clear whether hGH treatment was a factor in these deaths, there are plausible mechanisms that could be invoked. Stimulation of tonsillar or adenoidal growth could have led to upper airway compromise in an already morbidly obese PWS patient. In addition, a recent study reported that 60% of patients with PWS may have central adrenal insufficiency [28]. Because hGH treatment increases the risk of adrenal crisis in patients with undiagnosed adrenal insufficiency, this too is a potential explanation. Careful consideration of the PWS patient's respiratory and adrenal status should take place before commencing hGH.

Turner syndrome

Turner syndrome was the first non-GHD condition for which hGH was demonstrated to be safe and effective at treating the short stature. Several published trials indicate that hGH treatment increases final height by 8–10 cm depending on dosage and age at initiation of treatment [29]. Early studies tested hGH alone and in combination with low dose oxandrolone: the combination yielded greater height gain in a shorter time period without virilization [30] but combination therapy does not appear to be in common practice.

Infancy and childhood

The first studies enrolled children as young as 4 years of age but a recent multicenter trial reports favorable results in girls with Turner syndrome treated as young as 9 months [31]. Based on this it is reasonable to initiate hGH therapy once postnatal growth failure is evident.

Adolescence

The most common question is the timing and form of estrogen introduction. When estrogen is given at feminizing doses, there is a period of growth acceleration but skeletal maturation accelerates with subsequent growth attenuation. A trial that tested the effect of age at estrogen introduction showed that girls in whom estrogen was delayed from 12 to 15 years were 4.5 cm taller on average and that the most important predictor of height gain was the number of years of hGH before estrogen introduction [32]. Therefore, the goal is to use growth-promoting therapy effectively to bring the patient into the normal height range by the normal age of puberty so that puberty can be induced concurrently with her peers.

Estrogen can be given orally, by injection or transdermally. Recommended starting dosage is 0.25 mg/day micronized ethinyl estradiol by mouth or 0.2–0.4 mg/month ethinyl estradiol by depot [33]. There are suggestions that lower dosage of estrogen might improve outcome but the data are preliminary. hGH is continued until near epiphyseal closure or the height reached is satisfactory. There is no indication for hGH treatment following this.

Special considerations

Patients with Turner syndrome have associated conditions that must be periodically assessed, as delineated in recently published guidelines (Table 7.4) [33]. Scoliosis is common and should be monitored by physical examination, radiographs and orthopedic consultation as necessary. It is not generally a contraindication to hGH treatment but may need attention. Autoimmune thyroiditis is more common and periodic screening with thyroid stimulating hormone (TSH) is required. Aortic root dilatation and fatal rupture are rare but blood pressure must be monitored and hypertension treated. Periodic imaging of the aorta is recommended. Growth hormone increases cardiac output but the potential relationship between hGH treatment and aortic root abnormalities is unclear.

The short child born small for gestational age

Ten to 30% of those born SGA show little catch-up growth as infants and remain short for the rest of their lives. Studies examining

Table 7.4 Monitoring for complications of Turner syndrome. (After Bondy [33].)

System	Concern	Monitoring
Cardiovascular	Congenital heart defects, aortic root dilatation	MRI, echocardiography at diagnosis and every 5–10 years. Blood pressure annually
Thyroid	Autoimmune thyroiditis	T4, TSH annually beginning age 4 years
Gastrointestinal	Autoimmune hepatitis, celiac disease	Liver function testing annually and celiac screen every 2–5 years starting age 4 years
Metabolic	Diabetes mellitus, hyperlipidemia	Fasting lipid panel and plasma glucose in postpubertal girls and women annually

the potential use of hGH enrolled individuals who had short stature associated with being born SGA demonstrated that hGH results in sustained improvement in growth rate, albeit at relatively high doses [34]. Based on this, hGH was licensed for treatment of short children with birth weights <−2 SD and no catch-up growth. Recommendations for treatment by regulatory agencies differ slightly, with higher recommended dosage (70 µg/kg/day) and younger allowable age (2 years) in the USA than Europe. Higher dosage does lead to increased growth and may be necessary to overcome GH or IGF-1 resistance associated with SGA.

Infancy and childhood
Most patients born SGA show catch-up growth within the first 6 months of life. By age 2, any catch-up growth that is going to occur will have occurred so monitoring is usually indicated only during the first 2 years. Thereafter, treatment may be considered in those remaining small and showing no catch-up. Most studies show that the younger patients respond better, so instituting treatment early is better, once the growth pattern is established. Regimens of 35–70 µg/kg/day are acceptable: although most studies show benefit with the higher doses, one study showed little difference in height gained whether 33 or 66 µg/kg/day were given [35]. The growth response should be monitored and adjustments in dosage made accordingly: some short SGA patients require relatively high dosage of hGH to reach acceptable final heights.

Adolescence
There are no special considerations during adolescence. Most SGA patients reach puberty at the expected age. If hGH treatment is delayed until puberty, height gain will be modest. There is no evidence to support the continuation of hGH beyond epiphyseal closure.

Special considerations
The causes of fetal growth retardation are varied and so are the responses to hGH treatment. Most clinical trials excluded individuals with syndromic features and response to treatment may be more difficult to predict in those individuals.

Bloom and Fanconi syndromes are disorders with a predisposition for malignancy that occasionally present with SGA birth and short stature. Treatment with hGH at high dosage is probably contraindicated. Although there is evidence that some short children born SGA have concomitant GHD, GH stimulation testing does not predict the response to treatment and is not recommended unless there are additional features of GHD, e.g. low circulating IGF-1 concentrations.

Idiopathic short stature and SHOX deficiency
ISS, defined as height <−2 SD without evident cause after adequate diagnostic evaluation, represents 60–80% of the population of short children seen by pediatric endocrinologists. It is a mixture of various conditions including familial short stature. Although SHOX deficiency is rare (<5% of short children), it is discussed here because hGH is approved for both conditions with similar treatment approaches. Not all patients with *SHOX* gene anomalies display the Leri–Weill phenotype (mesomelic dwarfism with Madelung deformity) [36] and a small fraction of the ISS population probably has undocumented *SHOX* gene abnormalities. SHOX deficiency is thought partly to explain the short stature of Turner syndrome and has recently been approved for hGH treatment [37].

Management is controversial: studies have shown that 4–7 years of hGH will increase heights 3.5–7.5 cm, with variable responses among patients. Those with better outcomes are treated younger, have taller parents and have the better first year growth response to hGH. Opinions differ as to value of the therapy and the severity of short stature needed to justify treatment. A recent consensus conference addressed these questions and provides some guidance [38].

Infancy and childhood
hGH is approved for treatment of ISS in the USA and other countries for children who stand below −2.25 SD (1.2 percentile) and for SHOX deficiency with short stature. Treatment could begin as young as age 5 years in ISS according to the consensus group. Patients should be seen at 3–6 month intervals for assessment of efficacy and adverse events. Periodic measurement of circulating IGF-1 is recommend for assessment of compliance, efficacy and safety. No other laboratory surveillance is routinely indicated.

Adolescence
There are no special considerations during adolescence. Treatment should be stopped near adult height (growth rate <2 cm/year and skeletal age ≥14 for girls, ≥16 for boys) or when a height in the normal range for adults has been reached.

Noonan syndrome

Noonan syndrome is characterized by short stature, right-sided cardiac anomalies, web-neck and a typical facial appearance. Although reminiscent of Turner syndrome in certain aspects of the phenotype, it is caused by a different set of genetic abnormalities and probably has a different mechanism underlying the growth problem. Median height is around −2 SD for adults and children [39,40]. Pubertal delay may extend the growing period, allowing catch-up for some patients. Although short stature is common, around 30% of adults have a height within the normal range. Mutations in *PTPN 11*, which encodes a tyrosine phosphatase, are found in about 50% of patients.

Several trials of hGH show stimulation of growth in the short term and an apparent net gain with chronic therapy of 1.3–1.7 SD [41,42]. In the USA, hGH therapy is approved for short stature associated with Noonan syndrome at a dosage of up to 66 μg/kg/day.

Infancy and childhood

Once growth failure has become evident with no obvious cause other than Noonan syndrome, there is little chance that the growth pattern will change in the near future so it is reasonable to consider intervention in the very short patient showing no improvement in growth. No special studies are required before initiation of therapy.

Adolescence

hGH is continued with the monitoring typical for any child receiving the treatment. A delay in puberty may assist in achieving a satisfactory height. Adding testosterone for males could be beneficial if pubertal delay is significant.

Special considerations

There is evidence that patients with mutations in *PTPN 11* are shorter and less responsive to GH than the other Noonan syndrome patients [41] but there appears no reason to exclude such patients from treatment or alter the initial dosage. Hypertrophic cardiomyopathy is found in 10–20% of patients with Noonan syndrome [39]. Although hGH does not appear to have an adverse effect on this, the myocardium is a target of GH and IGF-1. Monitoring and input from a cardiologist is advised for any patient with significant cardiac disease receiving hGH.

Constitutional delay of growth and adolescence

CDGA is a common clinical diagnosis typically made in a male with moderate short stature, delay in bone age and pubertal signs and a family history of pubertal delay. Height at time of presentation is usually below the 3rd centile but most end up with adult stature in the low-normal range. There is undoubtedly overlap with idiopathic and familial short stature, hypogonadotropic hypogonadism and partial GHD. Most patients with this condition need only observation and reassurance or a short course of sex steroids at pubertal age to stimulate growth and to induce puberty.

Infancy and childhood

During childhood it is impossible to distinguish ISS from CDGA and a recent consensus statement includes children with CDGA within the larger population of ISS [38]. After the exclusion of other potential causes of short stature, the modestly short child with a normal steady growth rate and suggestive family history can be observed.

Adolescence

Boys with CDGA distressed by their size or lack of pubertal development may benefit from a short course of androgens. Testosterone enanthate or cypionate, 50–75 mg/month IM for 4–6 months, works well. There is no untoward advancement of bone age nor evidence of final height compromise with such a regimen given to boys 14 years and older. Growth stimulation and the appearance of sexual hair, comedone formation and body odor should be evident following the third injection. Following a single course there is usually evidence for spontaneous puberty with testicular enlargement. If not, or if testosterone blood levels remain prepubertal, a second course may be beneficial. Oxandrolone has also been used successfully in the management of CDGA. Transdermal androgen preparations represent a theoretic option but appropriate dose schedules have not been developed and depot testosterone is cheap, simple, safe and effective [43].

CDGA appears less common is girls and there is no equivalent therapy to that used for boys. Possible virilization precludes androgen use and the greater skeletal advancement associated with estrogen therapy is probably to be counterproductive. Observation and reassurance are required [44].

Special considerations

The proof of the diagnosis of CDGA is made when the patient eventually reaches full sexual maturity. Patients should be followed until this is evident clinically or until puberty is progressing at a near normal rate. Some cases of hypogonadotropic hypogonadism, complete or partial, masquerade as CDGA. This should be suspected in cases that require more than a single course of testosterone or when testicular growth falters.

Miscellaneous conditions: skeletal dysplasias, chondrodystrophies

These comprise a heterogeneous group of conditions that affect bone growth and/or formation. Originally thought to be generally resistant to growth stimulants, studies have shown that some patients with specific diagnoses respond to hGH. Most studies have been of limited scope but provide general information about response and safety. Patients with achondroplasia and hypochondroplasia grow significantly faster when given hGH, which is well-tolerated and induces an improvement in height SD score over several years of treatment [45–47] but hGH may accentuate the disproportion of patients by causing a greater increase in the spine growth and the ultimate effect of treatment on final height is not clear. Individuals with pseudoachondroplasia and spondyloepiphyseal dysplasia respond poorly [48]. Based on these data, treatment of individuals with these conditions is not recommended.

GH insensitivity syndrome/primary IGF-1 deficiency

GHIS caused by major defects in the GH receptor is rare and usually easily diagnosed. The patients have the phenotype of severe GHD and very low serum concentrations of IGF-1 but show elevated GH secretion. Other forms of GHIS include post GH receptor defects (e.g. STAT5b deficiency), hypomorphic GH receptor anomalies and other genetic conditions such as Alagille syndrome (syndromic cholestasis). These patients and others have been categorized as having "primary IGF-1 deficiency" based on centrality of IGF-1 in growth control and the parallel with other pituitary-glandular axes.

This new terminology has generated controversy because specific diagnoses that have distinct phenotypes are lumped together (e.g. GH receptor deficiency with lesions of the *IGF-1* gene) and there has been concern that the somewhat vague definition might lead to indiscriminant use of rhIGF-1 treatment. The approved indication for rhIGF-1 treatment is short stature caused by severe primary IGF-1 deficiency, defined as height and IGF-1 serum concentrations both <−3 SD for age and sex in the face of normal GH secretion and normal nutrition [49]. More complex tests of GH response or the demonstration of diagnostic genetic abnormalities are not necessarily required, although they may be helpful in selecting patients for therapy. In cases of severe GHIS or null lesions of the *IGF-1* gene, only rhIGF-1 will stimulate growth. Some forms of partial GH resistance might respond to hGH. Whether rhIGF-1 or hGH is the better therapy in this situation is not known.

Infancy

Patients with GH receptor deficiency are near normal size at birth but growth failure manifests immediately and affected children are already short by 1 year of age. Clinical trials have not included children less than 1 year old. The frequency of hypoglycemia, which is increased with rhIGF-1, is of serious concern.

Childhood

Early childhood is perhaps the best age to initiate treatment with rhIGF-1. In clear-cut cases, beginning treatment at 60–80 µg/kg/dose and advancing to 120 µg/kg/dose as tolerated is recommended. Children should be seen at 3–4 month intervals at the onset for review of regimen and to be certain no untoward effects (e.g. hypoglycemia) are occurring. Spontaneous hypoglycemia is common because of the defect in GH action. Regular meals and snacks can help and giving the rhIGF-1 only before a meal with adequate carbohydrate content is necessary to avoid provoking a severe hypoglycemic episode. Growth rates in the 8–10 cm/year range would be considered a good response for the first 1–2 years. Thereafter 5–6 cm/year is typical [12,13,50].

Adolescent and young adult

Treatment is continued in the same dosing range as for the younger child and maintained through puberty. There are few data on final height of individuals treated with rhIGF-1. Many have not reached heights within the normal range. This will probably improve with better regimens and younger institution of treatment but the ultimate effect on final height for these patients as a group is not known.

Special considerations

Experience with rhIGF-1 is limited and there must be careful monitoring of treated patients. Subtle symptoms and signs of hypoglycemia and of intracranial hypertension should be sought at each visit. Periodic evaluation of hearing and examination for tonsillar or adenoidal hypertrophy is also recommended. Some patients gradually develop a coarsening of facial features over time as a result of soft tissue changes. These resolve, at least partially, following withdrawal of treatment. In addition, there are metabolic abnormalities that are part of GHIS which include carbohydrate intolerance and hyperlipidemia. Patients should be screened for these, particularly during adolescence and in obese subjects.

Another question is how to approach patients with several features of GHIS, who, for one reason or another, do not fit the classic picture. These might be patients with low IGF-1 levels who responded poorly to hGH administration or patients with surprisingly robust GH stimulation tests and no other pituitary abnormality. When hGH treatment fails, patients should be examined carefully for compliance and concomitant conditions that might limit growth (e.g. hypothyroidism). One must be certain that nutrition is adequate because malnutrition results in GH resistance.

Tall stature and overgrowth

Patients with disorders leading to overgrowth and tall stature (excluding those brought about by obesity) are not frequent. The majority comprise familial or constitutional tall stature, GH excess or an overgrowth syndrome (e.g. Sotos and Weaver syndromes). There is no treatment for the syndromic patients.

GH excess and pituitary gigantism

GH secreting adenomas may arise *de novo* or be part of a genetic syndrome (e.g. McCune–Albright, multiple endocrine neoplasia 1, Carney complex). The data describing diagnosis and treatment response are derived from adult practice, because the conditions are rare in childhood. The goal is to reduce or remove the tumor mass and achieve a biochemical cure defined as a circulating IGF-1 concentration in the normal range for age and sex and a GH level of <1 ng/mL 2 h after oral glucose load. Initial treatment is almost always by trans-sphenoidal surgery [51]. The incidence of postoperative hypopituitarism is low in the hands of an experienced neurosurgeon but the cure rate is approximately 90% in patients with microadenomas and 50% in those with macroadenomas so a significant proportion need additional surgery, radiation or medication.

Radiation is only partially effective and may take 5–10 years to reduce GH secretion to normal. The somatostatin analogs octreotide or lanreotide are usually tried first in patients not cured by surgery. Octreotide is available in a short-acting form given every 8 h or in long-acting forms, some of which may be administered monthly. When used as primary therapy, approximately half of patients have normalization of circulating IGF-1 concentrations and shrinkage of the tumor. Somatostatin analogs are fairly well-tolerated, the most common side effects being gastrointestinal with bloating, nausea and fat malabsorption. Asymptomatic gallstones or bile abnormality occurs in 25% of cases.

Pegvisomant, a GH receptor antagonist, is the most effective medical therapy, more than 90% of patients achieving normalization of plasma IGF-1 concentrations. Because pegvisomant blocks GH action not secretion, GH concentrations cannot be used to assess response to therapy and tumor shrinkage does not occur. GH concentrations may increase with tumor size and the tumor should be monitored annually by magnetic resonance imaging (MRI). Abnormal liver function tests have been observed in 2–10% of patients. Pegvisomant is contraindicated in patients with active liver disease. Liver function tests should be monitored monthly during the first 6 months of treatment and somewhat less frequently thereafter. Dopamine agonists (bromocriptine, carbergoline) are less effective. They may be used as adjunctive therapy in patients receiving somatostatin analogs who do not achieve treatment goals [52].

Constitutional tall stature

Very tall stature may be as distressing to some children as short stature is to others but it is usually tall parents who are concerned to prevent excessively tall stature in their children who bring the condition to attention. The use of sex steroids to stimulate bone maturation and cause earlier epiphyseal fusion has been a popular treatment for these individuals [53] if the height prediction is >180 cm for girls and >200 cm for boys. The demand for such intervention appears to have declined, perhaps because tall stature is more accepted and sometimes reaps rewards in athletic endeavors.

The accuracy of adult height prediction when treatment is contemplated is obviously important. Methods for height prediction, such as the Bayley–Pinneau tables that accompany the Greulich and Pyle atlas and the Tanner and Whitehouse (TW) prediction equations applicable to a TW bone age rating, are inaccurate when applied to individuals at the extremes of stature. For example, height prediction for tall males is overestimated by Bayley–Pinneau but seems accurate for tall girls. De Waal et al. [54] have developed more precise equations that may be useful in predicting height in these children:

$$\text{Boys final height} = 213.66 + 0.62 \times H + 0.25 \times TH - 10.49 \times CA - 12.98 \times BA_{GP} + 0.72 \times (CA \times BA_{GP})$$

$$\text{Girls final height} = 129.42 = 0.74 \times H + 0.17 \times TH - 7.70 \times BA_{GP} - 5.90 \times CA + 041(CA \times BA_{GP})$$

where H is height, TH target height, CA chronological age and BA bone age using Greulich and Pyle.

In the past, high doses of testosterone in boys and estrogen in girls have been used and, although these treatments have been well-tolerated by most, one reports suggests that fertility may be reduced in girls given high-dose estrogen to reduce adult stature [55]. Treatment is more effective when given before the onset of puberty and is related to bone age at start of therapy. One study found that girls with a bone age of 10 years had a reduction in final height of 6 cm, whereas in those with a bone age of 13 years the reduction was about 2 cm [56].

There also remain questions as to the effectiveness of treatment as previously practised and true benefit, i.e. making life better. No large randomized controlled trials are available but cohorts of Australian girls treated in the past have been compared with untreated tall girls and reveal the following. Height reduction in 279 girls given estrogen was 2.5 cm compared to controls [57]. There was no difference in psychological outcomes in between groups; both groups showed increased prevalence of depression [58] and 42% of those treated were unhappy about the decision to be treated, whereas 99% of untreated girls were glad that they had not received therapy [59].

Because the puberty growth spurt adds 25–30 cm to the height attained at the start of puberty, a more logical approach is to decide on an acceptable final height for an individual and their family and work backwards because intervention after the onset of puberty has such a small effect. For example, taking 180 cm as an appropriate final height for a girl means that she needs to be in Tanner breast stage 2 when she reaches 150 cm. If she were not and puberty were induced at this height, using physiological dosage of estrogen, the end point will be achieved without using heroic doses of sex steroids. The same principle can be applied equally effectively to boys and to patients with Marfan syndrome, for example.

Future directions in the management of disordered growth

Individualization of treatment based on genetic and other parameters that determine hormone sensitivity can be expected. The growth response to hGH has been mathematically modeled in several conditions [60] and such data can be used to identify whether an individual is meeting growth expectation and to select better treatment regimens. Response to hGH may relate to whether or not the individual expresses a common GH receptor variant [61]. Studies comparing the selection of hGH regimen based on circulating IGF-1 concentrations during treatment (a measure of GH sensitivity) to standard therapy showed that the amount of hGH required to achieve circulating IGF-1 target concentrations varied widely among subject, suggesting substantial variation in GH sensitivity [62]. Patients in future may be able to have more scientifically based, safer and effective therapies, be they hGH, rhIGF-1 or a combination. At the same time, the pool of patients with "idiopathic short stature" will dwindle because of novel molecular diagnostics that will identify the abnormalities restricting growth. New knowledge of the basis of growth disorders should lead to better understanding of them and of their outcomes leading to selection of improved therapies which can be directed to those who most need treatment.

References

1 Sandberg DE, Colsman M. Growth hormone treatment of short stature: status of the quality of life rationale. *Horm Res* 2005; **63**: 275–283.

2 Visser-van Balen H, Geenen R, Kamp GA, Huisman J, Wit JM, Sinnema G. Long-term psychosocial consequences of hormone treatment for short stature. *Acta Paediatr* 2007; **96**: 715–719.

3 Martha PM Jr, Gorman KM, Blizzard RM, Rogol AD, Veldhuis JD. Endogenous growth hormone secretion and clearance rates in normal boys, as determined by deconvolution analysis: relationship to age, pubertal status and body mass. *J Clin Endocrinol Metab* 1992; **74**: 336–344.

4 Blethen SL, Allen DB, Graves D, August G, Moshang T, Rosenfeld R. Safety of recombinant deoxyribonucleic acid-derived growth hormone: The National Cooperative Growth Study experience. *J Clin Endocrinol Metab* 1996; **81**: 1704–1710.

5 Clayton PE, Cowell CT. Safety issues in children and adolescents during growth hormone therapy: a review. *Growth Horm IGF Res* 2000; **10**: 306–317.

6 Cohen P, Clemmons DR, Rosenfeld RG. Does the GH-IGF axis play a role in cancer pathogenesis? *Growth Horm IGF Res* 2000; **10**: 297–305.

7 Swerdlow AJ, Reddingius RE, Higgins CD, Spoudeas HA, Phipps K, Qiao Z, et al. Growth hormone treatment of children with brain tumors and risk of tumor recurrence. *J Clin Endocrinol Metab* 2000; **85**: 4444–4449.

8 Ergun-Longmire B, Mertens AC, Mitby P, Qin J, Heller G, Shi W, et al. Growth hormone treatment and risk of second neoplasms in the childhood cancer survivor. *J Clin Endocrinol Metab* 2006; **91**: 3494–3498.

9 Ho KK, 2007 GH Deficiency Concensus Workshop Participants. Consensus guidelines for the diagnosis and treatment of adults with GH deficiency II: a statement of the GH Research Society in association with the European Society for Pediatric Endocrinology, Lawson Wilkins Society, European Society of Endocrinology, Japan Endocrine Society and Endocrine Society of Australia. *Eur J Endocrinol* 2007; **157**: 695–700.

10 Guevara-Aguirre J, Vasconez O, Martinez V, Martinez AL, Rosenbloom AL, Diamond FB Jr, et al. A randomized, double blind, placebo-controlled trial on safety and efficacy of recombinant human insulin-like growth factor-I in children with growth hormone receptor deficiency. *J Clin Endocrinol Metab* 1995; **80**: 1393–1398.

11 Klinger B, Laron Z. Three year IGF-I treatment of children with Laron syndrome. *J Pediatr Endocrinol Metab* 1995; **8**: 149–158.

12 Ranke MB, Savage MO, Chatelain PG, Preece MA, Rosenfeld RG, Wilton P. Long-term treatment of growth hormone insensitivity syndrome with IGF-I. Results of the European Multicentre Study. The Working Group on Growth Hormone Insensitivity Syndromes. *Horm Res* 1999; **51**: 128–134.

13 Chernausek SD, Backeljauw PF, Frane J, Kuntze J, Underwood LE. Long-term treatment with recombinant insulin-like growth factor (IGF)-I in children with severe IGF-I deficiency due to growth hormone insensitivity. *J Clin Endocrinol Metab* 2007; **92**: 902–910.

14 Furstenberger G, Senn HJ. Insulin-like growth factors and cancer. *Lancet Oncol* 2002; **3**: 298–302.

15 Ross JL, Long LM, Skerda M, Cassorla F, Kurtz D, Loriaux DL, et al. Effect of low doses of estradiol on 6-month growth rates and predicted height in patients with Turner syndrome. *J Pediatr* 1986; **109**: 950–953.

16 Wilson DM, Frane JW, Sherman B, Johanson AJ, Hintz RL, Rosenfeld RG. Carbohydrate and lipid metabolism in Turner syndrome: effect of therapy with growth hormone, oxandrolone and a combination of both. *J Pediatr* 1988; **112**: 210–217.

17 Yanovski JA, Rose SR, Municchi G, Pescovitz OH, Hill SC, Cassorla FG, et al. Treatment with a luteinizing hormone-releasing hormone agonist in adolescents with short stature. *N Engl J Med* 2003; **348**: 908–917.

18 Shulman DI, Francis GL, Palmert MR, Eugster EA. Use of aromatase inhibitors in children and adolescents with disorders of growth and adolescent development. *Pediatrics* 2008; **121**: e975–983.

19 Mauras N, Attie KM, Reiter EO, Saenger P, Baptista J. High dose recombinant human growth hormone (GH) treatment of GH-deficient patients in puberty increases near-final height: a randomized, multicenter trial. Genentech Inc, Cooperative Study Group. *J Clin Endocrinol Metab* 2000; **85**: 3653–3660.

20 Bryant J, Cave C, Mihaylova B, Chase D, McIntyre L, Gerard K, et al. Clinical effectiveness and cost-effectiveness of growth hormone in children: a systematic review and economic evaluation. *Health Technol Assess* 2002; **6**: 1–168.

21 Molitch ME, Clemmons DR, Malozowski S, Merriam GR, Shalet SM, Vance ML, et al. Evaluation and treatment of adult growth hormone deficiency: an Endocrine Society Clinical Practice Guideline. *J Clin Endocrinol Metab* 2006; **91**: 1621–1634.

22 Ghigo E, Aimaretti G, Corneli G. Diagnosis of adult GH deficiency. *Growth Horm IGF Res* 2008; **18**: 1–16.

23 Bottner A, Keller E, Kratzsch J, Stobbe H, Weigel JF, Keller A, et al. PROP1 mutations cause progressive deterioration of anterior pituitary function including adrenal insufficiency: a longitudinal analysis. *J Clin Endocrinol Metab* 2004; **89**: 5256–5265.

24 Burman P, Ritzen EM, Lindgren AC. Endocrine dysfunction in Prader–Willi syndrome: a review with special reference to GH. *Endocr Rev* 2001; **22**: 787–799.

25 Myers SE, Whitman BY, Carrel AL, Moerchen V, Bekx MT, Allen DB. Two years of growth hormone therapy in young children with Prader–Willi syndrome: physical and neurodevelopmental benefits. *Am J Med Genet A* 2007; **143**: 443–448.

26 Mogul HR, Lee PD, Whitman BY, Zipf WB, Frey M, Myers S, et al. Growth hormone treatment of adults with Prader–Willi syndrome and growth hormone deficiency improves lean body mass, fractional body fat and serum triiodothyronine without glucose impairment: results from the United States multicenter trial. *J Clin Endocrinol Metab* 2008; **93**: 1238–1245.

27 Stevenson DA, Anaya TM, Clayton-Smith J, Hall BD, Van Allen MI, Zori RT, et al. Unexpected death and critical illness in Prader–Willi syndrome: report of ten individuals. *Am J Med Genet A* 2004; **124A**: 158–164.

28 de Lind van Wijngaarden RF, Otten BJ, Festen DA, Joosten KF, de Jong FH, Sweep FC, et al. High prevalence of central adrenal insuffi-

ciency in patients with Prader–Willi syndrome. *J Clin Endocrinol Metab* 2008; **93**: 1649–1654.

29 Sas TC, Muinck Keizer-Schrama SM, Stijnen T, Jansen M, Otten BJ, Hoorweg-Nijman JJ, *et al.* Normalization of height in girls with Turner syndrome after long-term growth hormone treatment: results of a randomized dose–response trial. *J Clin Endocrinol Metab* 1999; **84**: 4607–4612.

30 Rosenfeld RG, Frane J, Attie KM, Brasel JA, Burstein S, Cara JF, *et al.* Six-year results of a randomized, prospective trial of human growth hormone and oxandrolone in Turner syndrome. *J Pediatr* 1992; **121**: 49–55.

31 Davenport ML, Crowe BJ, Travers SH, Rubin K, Ross JL, Fechner PY, *et al.* Growth hormone treatment of early growth failure in toddlers with Turner syndrome: a randomized, controlled, multicenter trial. *J Clin Endocrinol Metab* 2007; **92**: 3406–3416.

32 Chernausek SD, Attie KM, Cara JF, Rosenfeld RG, Frane J. Growth hormone therapy of Turner syndrome: the impact of age of estrogen replacement on final height. Genentech Inc, Collaborative Study Group. *J Clin Endocrinol Metab* 2000; **85**: 2439–2445.

33 Bondy CA. Care of girls and women with Turner syndrome: a guideline of the Turner Syndrome Study Group. *J Clin Endocrinol Metab* 2007; **92**: 10–25.

34 Clayton PE, Cianfarani S, Czernichow P, Johannsson G, Rapaport R, Rogol A. Management of the child born small for gestational age through to adulthood: a consensus statement of the International Societies of Pediatric Endocrinology and the Growth Hormone Research Society. *J Clin Endocrinol Metab* 2007; **92**: 804–810.

35 Van Pareren Y, Mulder P, Houdijk M, Jansen M, Reeser M, Hokken-Koelega A. Adult height after long-term, continuous growth hormone (GH) treatment in short children born small for gestational age: results of a randomized, double-blind, dose–response GH trial. *J Clin Endocrinol Metab* 2003; **88**: 3584–3590.

36 Rappold G, Blum WF, Shavrikova EP, Crowe BJ, Roeth R, Quigley CA, *et al.* Genotypes and phenotypes in children with short stature: clinical indicators of SHOX haploinsufficiency. *J Med Genet* 2007; **44**: 306–313.

37 Blum WF, Crowe BJ, Quigley CA, Jung H, Cao D, Ross JL, *et al.* Growth hormone is effective in treatment of short stature associated with short stature homeobox-containing gene deficiency: two-year results of a randomized, controlled, multicenter trial. *J Clin Endocrinol Metab* 2007; **92**: 219–228.

38 Cohen P, Rogol AD, Deal CL, Saenger P, Reiter EO, Ross JL, *et al.* Consensus statement on the diagnosis and treatment of children with idiopathic short stature: a summary of the Growth Hormone Research Society, the Lawson Wilkins Pediatric Endocrine Society and the European Society for Paediatric Endocrinology Workshop. *J Clin Endocrinol Metab* 2008; **93**: 4210–4217.

39 Shaw AC, Kalidas K, Crosby AH, Jeffery S, Patton MA. The natural history of Noonan syndrome: a long-term follow-up study. *Arch Dis Child* 2007; **92**: 128–132.

40 Noonan JA, Raaijmakers R, Hall BD. Adult height in Noonan syndrome. *Am J Med Genet A* 2003; **123A**: 68–71.

41 Limal JM, Parfait B, Cabrol S, Bonnet D, Leheup B, Lyonnet S, *et al.* Noonan syndrome: relationships between genotype, growth and growth factors. *J Clin Endocrinol Metab* 2006; **91**: 300–306.

42 Noordam K, Peer N, Francois I, De Schepper J, Burgt I, Otten B. Long-term growth hormone treatment improves adult height in children with Noonan syndrome with and without mutations in PTPN11. *Eur J Endocrinol* 2008; **159**: 203.

43 Richmond EJ, Rogol AD. Male pubertal development and the role of androgen therapy. *Nat Clin Pract* 2007; **3**: 338–344.

44 Brook CG. Treatment of late puberty. *Horm Res* 1999; **51** (Suppl 3): 101–103.

45 Ramaswami U, Rumsby G, Spoudeas HA, Hindmarsh PC, Brook CG. Treatment of achondroplasia with growth hormone: six years of experience. *Pediatr Res* 1999; **46**: 435–439.

46 Mullis PE, Patel MS, Brickell PM, Hindmarsh PC, Brook CG. Growth characteristics and response to growth hormone therapy in patients with hypochondroplasia: genetic linkage of the insulin-like growth factor I gene at chromosome 12q23 to the disease in a subgroup of these patients. *Clin Endocrinol (Oxf)* 1991; **34**: 265–274.

47 Hertel NT, Eklof O, Ivarsson S, Aronson S, Westphal O, Sipila I, *et al.* Growth hormone treatment in 35 prepubertal children with achondroplasia: a 5-year dose–response trial. *Acta Paediatr* 2005; **94**: 1402–1410.

48 Kanazawa H, Tanaka H, Inoue M, Yamanaka Y, Namba N, Seino Y. Efficacy of growth hormone therapy for patients with skeletal dysplasia. *J Bone Min Metab* 2003; **21**: 307–310.

49 Collett-Solberg PF, Misra M. The role of recombinant human insulin-like growth factor-I in treating children with short stature. *J Clin Endocrinol Metab* 2008; **93**: 10–18.

50 Laron Z. The essential role of IGF-1: lessons from the long-term study and treatment of children and adults with Laron syndrome. *J Clin Endocrinol Metab* 1999; **84**: 4397–43404.

51 Abe T, Tara LA, Ludecke DK. Growth hormone-secreting pituitary adenomas in childhood and adolescence: features and results of transnasal surgery. *Neurosurgery* 1999; **45**: 1–10.

52 Melmed S. Medical progress: acromegaly. *N Engl J Med* 2006; **355**: 2558–2573.

53 Drop SL, De Waal WJ, De Muinck Keizer-Schrama SM. Sex steroid treatment of constitutionally tall stature. *Endocr Rev* 1998; **19**: 540–558.

54 de Waal WJ, Stijnen T, Lucas IS, van Gurp E, de Muinck Keizer-Schrama S, Drop SL. A new model to predict final height in constitutionally tall children. *Acta Paediatr* 1996; **85**: 889–893.

55 Venn A, Bruinsma F, Werther G, Pyett P, Baird D, Jones P, *et al.* Oestrogen treatment to reduce the adult height of tall girls: long-term effects on fertility. *Lancet* 2004; **364**: 1513–1518.

56 de Waal WJ, Greyn-Fokker MH, Stijnen T, van Gurp EA, Toolens AM, de Munick Keizer-Schrama SM, *et al.* Accuracy of final height prediction and effect of growth-reductive therapy in 362 constitutionally tall children. *J Clin Endocrinol Metab* 1996; **81**: 1206–1216.

57 Venn A, Hosmer T, Hosmer D, Bruinsma F, Jones P, Lumley J, *et al.* Oestrogen treatment for tall stature in girls: estimating the effect on height and the error in height prediction. *Clin Endocrinol (Oxf)* 2008; **68**: 926–929.

58 Bruinsma FJ, Venn AJ, Patton GC, Rayner JA, Pyett P, Werther G, *et al.* Concern about tall stature during adolescence and depression in later life. *J Affect Disord* 2006; **91**: 145–152.

59 Pyett P, Rayner J, Venn A, Bruinsma F, Werther G, Lumley J. Using hormone treatment to reduce the adult height of tall girls: are women satisfied with the decision in later years? *Soc Sci Med* 2005; **61**: 1629–1639.

60 Vosahlo J, Zidek T, Lebl J, Riedl S, Frisch H. Validation of a mathematical model predicting the response to growth hormone treatment in prepubertal children with idiopathic growth hormone deficiency. *Horm Res* 2004; **61**: 143–147.

61 van der Klaauw AA, van der Straaten T, Baak-Pablo R, Biermasz NR, Guchelaar HJ, Pereira AM, *et al.* Influence of the d3-growth hormone (GH) receptor isoform on short-term and long-term treatment response to GH replacement in GH-deficient adults. *J Clin Endocrinol Metab* 2008; **93**: 2828–2834.

62 Cohen P, Rogol AD, Howard CP, Bright GM, Kappelgaard AM, Rosenfeld RG. Insulin growth factor-based dosing of growth hormone therapy in children: a randomized, controlled study. *J Clin Endocrinol Metab* 2007; **92**: 2480–2486.

8 Evaluation and Management of Late Effects of Cancer Treatment

Helena K. Gleeson[1] & Stephen M. Shalet[2]

[1] Department of Paediatric Endocrinology, Royal Manchester Children's Hospital, Manchester, UK
[2] Department of Endocrinology, Christie Hospital NHS Trust, Manchester, UK

Survival rates for childhood cancer have increased from 25% for those patients diagnosed in the 1960s to 75% today (Fig. 8.1). This has resulted in a growing cohort of survivors, estimated at 1 in 715 of the current young adult population in the UK [1]. Leukemia and brain tumors represent 50% of childhood cancers.

The improvement in survival is a therapeutic achievement but it is not without cost. The majority of children who survive childhood cancer will experience a late effect of treatment. This is defined as a late-occurring or chronic outcome, either physical or psychological, that persists or develops beyond 5 years from diagnosis.

Two large cohort studies, one of 10 397 survivors in the USA [Childhood Cancer Survival Study (CCSS)] [2] and the other of 1362 from a single center in the Netherlands [3], identified a similar prevalence of morbidity in this population. Three of four childhood cancer survivors experienced one or more late effect and in 40% this was severe, disabling or life-threatening. Eighty percent of brain tumor survivors had a significant medical condition compared to 50% of leukemia survivors [3]. An additional survey by the CCSS revealed that 43% of brain tumor survivors had an endocrine late effect and 18% had symptomatic cardiovascular disease [4].

The evaluation and management of endocrine late effects of childhood cancer therapy reaches beyond the specialty of pediatric endocrinology but pediatric endocrinologists must be aware of the ongoing impact of late effects into adulthood so that appropriate long-term follow-up is arranged and, when possible, preventative measures are introduced in childhood.

Endocrine late effects of cancer therapy are diverse. Evolving growth hormone deficiency (GHD) can occur after cranial irradiation (CI) through damage to the hypothalamic-pituitary (HP) axis which has implications in childhood for growth, adolescence

for achieving peak bone mass and adulthood for quality of life (Table 8.1). Radiation is the predominant cause of damage to the thyroid gland resulting in abnormal thyroid function and the development of thyroid nodules and malignancy. Gonadal damage occurs after chemotherapy, particularly alkylating agents and irradiation, especially total body irradiation (TBI), affecting sex steroid production and future fertility. Finally, as a consequence of cancer therapy itself, endocrine abnormalities, genetic predisposition or lifestyle, cancer survivors are at increased risk of cardiovascular disease and osteoporosis and fractures in adult life.

There are few longitudinal prospective studies, with published work being mostly retrospective and cross-sectional. Many study groups comprise heterogeneous subsets of patients who have received a range of treatment modalities, making it difficult to determine the etiology of damage observed. The continually changing nature of therapy and the evolutionary nature of endocrine damage mean that evaluation of a treatment regimen is not possible until sufficient children are several years (or more for evaluation of effects in adulthood) from the end of therapy. By this time, treatment for the same condition may well have been modified. Despite these problems, a considerable body of evidence is available to inform prognostic discussion with parents and children, screening for endocrinopathy and therapeutic intervention.

Principles of treatment for childhood cancer

Treatments for childhood cancer include surgery, radiotherapy and chemotherapy. Increasing intensity of treatment has contributed to improved survival rates but is likely to result in increased incidence and severity of both early and late effects. Increased recognition of sequelae of cancer therapy has led to treatment modifications aimed at reducing late effects.

For example, whereas all children previously received prophylactic CI (18–24 Gy) as central nervous system (CNS) prophylaxis in leukemia, this is now reserved for those with CNS disease and

Brook's Clinical Pediatric Endocrinology, 6th edition. Edited by C. Brook, P. Clayton, R. Brown. © 2009 Blackwell Publishing, ISBN: 978-1-4051-8080-1.

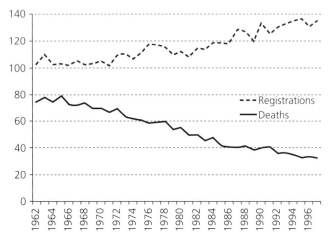

Figure 8.1 Cumulative trends in age standardized (uniform population) cancer registration and death rates, children 0–14 years, UK, 1962–1998/2001, demonstrating decreasing death rates and increasing registration. (From UK Childhood Cancer Research Group. National Registry of Childhood Tumours with permission.)

Table 8.1 Likely endocrine deficit according to cranial irradiation (CI) dose (brain tumors distant from the pituitary).

Dose (Gy)	Endocrinopathy
55–70	Hypopituitarsim, hyperprolactinemia, adult GHD
30–55	GHD, evolving endocrinopathy, early puberty, adult GHD
18–24	GHD, early puberty (girls); adult GHD
10–15	GH neurosecretory disturbance, adult GHD (uncommon)

GHD, growth hormone deficiency.

has not been routine therapy since 1990 in the UK and earlier in other parts of the world.

The burden of a chronic medical condition is highest in those who had received radiation (55%) compared with chemotherapy (15%) [3]. Children treated with surgery alone are least likely to experience long-term side effects, apart from those directly attributable to surgery. Both radiotherapy and chemotherapy have the potential to cause late endocrine problems.

Radiobiology

The radiosensitivity of a tissue is directly proportional to its mitotic activity and inversely proportional to its differentiation: poorly differentiated, rapidly dividing tumors are more likely to be radiosensitive than slowly growing, well-differentiated ones. In terms of normal tissue, this means that rapidly dividing, highly active tissues, such as skin and bone marrow, are radiosensitive, whereas more specialized, mature, quiescent cells, such as brain or bone, are relatively radioresistant.

In spite of relative radioresistance by more mature cell types, all cells are damaged by radiotherapy and, once a quiescent cell is stimulated to divide, the radiation dose required to cause chro-

mosomal damage, mitotic delay and inhibition of DNA synthesis is similar in all cells. This means that all organ systems will be damaged by radiation but explains why effects on slowly or non-proliferating cell populations may only become obvious over time.

For any given tissue, the shape of the radiation dose–effect curve for a given effect that most accurately fits *in vitro*, *in vivo* and clinical data can be described by the linear quadratic model [5]. According to this model, the effect of radiation on a given tissue is determined by the number of fractions (n), the dose of each fraction (d) and specific characteristics of the tissue in question (a/b). The a exponent refers to a "single-hit" (linear) component; the b exponent refers to the "multihit" (quadratic) component. This consists of the cumulative effect of sublethal injuries and/or the progressive destruction of the cell's ability to repair itself resulting in cell depletion. Early-reacting tissues, such as bone marrow, mucosa and most tumors, are susceptible to single-hit injury and have a high a:b ratio (typically a/b = 10). In contrast, late-reacting tissue, such as neural tissue, is particularly susceptible to multihit injury and has a low a:b ratio (2 assumed for CNS). The biological effective dose (BED) for each tissue can be calculated by the following equation (n, number of fractions; d, fraction size) and allows quantification of the different radiation schedules on the development of late effects:

$$BED = nd(1 + d/(a/b))$$

In the context of radiation-induced neurotoxicity, fraction size is important. By reducing the fraction size (d) the BED is decreased on late-reacting (neural) tissue by a greater magnitude than on early-responding (tumor) tissue for the same total dose of radiation (nd). Tissue repair also depends on the time allowed between fractions.

Hyperfractionation of the dose (dividing the total dose into smaller fractions) over the same time may reduce late effects without compromising tumor control. Hyperfractionation has the potential preferentially to increase the antitumor effect without an equivalent increase in CNS late effects. A randomized trial of treatment for medulloblastoma in Europe (PNET4) comparing standard fractionation with hyperfractionation has been instituted.

Newer radiation techniques, particularly stereotactic radiosurgery, may also have potential for disease control with less toxicity because of the highly focused nature of the irradiation but experience in children is limited to date.

Chemotherapy

A number of mechanisms have been proposed for the pathogenesis of chemotherapy-induced endocrine damage [6]. Cytotoxic drugs can induce cell death or injury (including endocrine cell death/injury) through effects on DNA replication, protein synthesis, transcription or microtubule function. They can disturb the synthesis or processing of a hormone at the transcriptional, translational or post-translational levels. Chemotherapy can enhance or inhibit the secretion of hormones through effects on receptors or messengers. Effects on signal transduction pathways are a further mechanism by which chemotherapy can affect hormone action.

Radiotherapy and chemotherapy combined

Cumulative damage from treatment with both chemotherapy and radiotherapy can occur because of additive effects, with insufficient time for regeneration between treatments. When adjuvant chemotherapy containing gonadotoxic agents is combined with radiotherapy, for instance, gonadal damage is more likely.

Treatment of common childhood cancers

Brain tumors

Brain tumors are the second most common childhood cancer. CNS tumors are diverse, representing many histological types and arising in a variety of anatomical sites. The overall 5-year survival rate for all pediatric CNS tumors is 67% but varies widely depending on histological type. Therapy depends on a range of factors, including histological type, position of the tumor and age of the child. CI (30–50 Gy) is widely used for the treatment of malignant brain tumors, increasingly in combination with adjuvant chemotherapy. In young children, in whom toxicity of radiotherapy is greatest, chemotherapy is increasingly used to delay or, if possible, avoid radiation.

Medulloblastoma is the most common malignant tumor, accounting for 15–20% of all childhood primary malignant CNS tumors. Standard therapy consists of surgery, craniospinal irradiation (CSI) and adjuvant chemotherapy. These combined modalities achieve an average survival rate of 70%. Significant long-term morbidity is almost universal, with endocrine and neurocognitive consequences being particularly common (Table 8.2).

Leukemia

Acute lymphoblastic lymphoma (ALL) is the most common childhood malignancy with a high cure rate. Treatment consists of combination chemotherapy and cranial prophylaxis to prevent CNS recurrence of leukemia. Before 1990, this prophylaxis was given as low-dose CI (18–24 Gy). Because of increasing concern about neuropsychological and, to a lesser extent, endocrine late effects, CI was discontinued and CNS prophylaxis is provided by intrathecal therapy, radiotherapy being reserved for children with proven CNS disease. Chemotherapy alone has important late effects, including obesity, increased cardiovascular risk and changes in bone mineral density (BMD). Standard treatment for ALL does not contain significant dosage of gonadotoxic chemotherapy.

Lymphoma

The incidence of Hodgkin lymphoma increases in adolescence. The original treatment regimens employed either radiation or alkylating agent based chemotherapy regimens [e.g. mustine, vincristine, procarbazine, prednisolone (MOPP)], which were associated with significant long-term morbidity, including infertility and secondary malignancies. Consequently, treatment has altered to reduce radiation fields and to introduce alternative chemotherapy regimens containing fewer alkylating agents.

In early stage disease, combined modality treatment with short duration chemotherapy such as ABVD (doxorubicin, bleomycin, vinblastine, dacarbazine) followed by involved field radiotherapy has produced good survival rates of 70–90% with less potential for long-term toxicity than with the previous approach of extended field radiotherapy alone. In advanced stage disease, combination chemotherapy is the primary modality. The ABVD regimen is now recognized as the standard. High dose chemotherapy and autologous bone marrow transplant are now widely used in patients with relapsed or refractory disease.

Bone marrow transplant

Bone marrow transplant (BMT) may be undertaken for resistant, high-risk or relapsed leukemia or lymphoma. Conditioning for BMT is undertaken with either TBI plus chemotherapy (usually including cyclophosphamide) or chemotherapy alone [most commonly busulfan and cyclophosphamide (Bu/Cy)]. Fractionation of TBI is used in an attempt to reduce late sequelae. Conditioning for BMT formerly employed 10 Gy in a single fraction. Current practice is to give 14 Gy as eight fractions over 3 days. Reduced intensity conditioning is used where possible, which may have less long-term morbidity. BMT, particularly where TBI is used as part of the conditioning regimen, is associated with significant endocrine morbidity (Table 8.3).

Patients with leukemia having BMT will usually have been pretreated with a number of chemotherapeutic agents, and those treated in the 1970s and 1980s will have received prior CI with the associated endocrine late effects.

Following BMT, immunosuppression is required as prophylaxis against chronic graft versus host disease (cGvHD), usually for about 6 months. cGvHD and its treatment with immunosuppression, which usually includes corticosteroids, results in problems associated with growth and bone mineral deficits.

Acute effects of therapy

In addition to the well-described late endocrine effects of radiation and chemotherapy, a number of chemotherapeutic agents cause acute endocrine disturbance.

Disorders of fluid balance

The syndrome of inappropriate antidiuretic hormone (SIADH) is well described in association with the vinca alkaloid chemotherapy agents, vincristine (VCR) and vinblastine [6]. During maintenance therapy for ALL, VCR is given 4-weekly. The occurrence of SIADH is idiosyncratic rather than dose related. Paired urine and plasma electrolytes and osmolalities confirm the diag-

Table 8.2 Endocrinopathy after treatment for childhood brain tumor.

Endocrinopathy	Risk factors	Assessment
Short stature	CI – increasing dose CSI Adjuvant chemotherapy Younger age at treatment GHD Early puberty	Regular 3–6 monthly assessments Height including sitting height, weight, BMI Pubertal staging
GHD	CI – increasing dose – nearly universal with doses >30 Gy Increasing time from treatment	Evaluate GH status 2 years from primary treatment Hypothalamically mediated test of GH status preferable If normal, retest at 2-yearly intervals or earlier if concern re growth Consider trial of GH therapy if poor growth without confirmed GHD if at high risk of GHD GH therapy – monitor IGF-1
Panhypopituitarism	CI >50–70 Gy Hypothalamic/pituitary tumors Increasing time from treatment	Assessment of ACTH status usually undertaken at same time as GH status Baseline TSH, fT4 and prolactin annually Evaluate gonadotropins if pubertal delay or arrest with baseline gonadotropins and sex steroid concentrations and GnRH test
Early puberty	CI Female gender Younger age at treatment	Evaluate if signs of early puberty with baseline gonadotropins and sex steroid concentrations and GnRH test In GHD combine GnRH analog with GH therapy
Thyroid dysfunction	CSI/CI Younger age at treatment Female gender Increasing time from treatment	Annual assessment Baseline TSH and fT4 Palpation of thyroid Thyroxine replacement if TSH persistently elevated after excluding ACTH deficiency
Gonadal dysfunction	CSI (girls) Gonadotoxic chemotherapy especially alkylating agents Increasing time from treatment	Evaluate if: pubertal delay or arrest or concern re gonadal failure with baseline gonadotropins and sex steroid concentrations
Reduced BMD	GHD or hypogonadism	Evaluate 2 years from primary treatment DXA scanning with assessment of volumetric BMD Repeat if abnormal or ongoing GHD or hypogonadism
Overweight/obesity	Hypothalamic damage; tumor, surgery, radiation >50 Gy Physical inactivity Endocrinopathy	Lifestyle advice

ACTH, adenocorticotropic hormone; BMD, bone mineral density; BMI, body mass index; CI, cranial irradiation; CSI, craniospinal irradiation; DXA, dual energy X-ray absorptiometry; GHD, growth hormone deficiency; GnRH, gonadotropin releasing hormone; TSH, thyroid stimulating hormone.

nosis and should be measured in any child who has received VCR and is hyponatremic. Management consists of fluid restriction until the SIADH resolves. Other chemotherapy agents that have been associated with SIADH include the alkylating agents, chlorambucil, cyclophosphamide and platinum compounds, cisplatin and carboplatin.

Nephrogenic diabetes insipidus (DI) may occur as a result of tubular toxicity, particularly from the alkylating agent ifosfamide. Proximal renal tubular defects are much more common than distal, and nephrogenic DI is rare. Hypomagnesemia, which may be severe, is common in association with ifosfamide tubulopathy.

Disorders of glucose metabolism

L-Asparaginase, a drug used in the treatment of leukemia, may cause hyperglycemia and glycosuria without ketonuria. Frequency is estimated at 1–14%. Insulin may be required during treatment with asparaginase but the hyperglycemia is reversible once treatment with asparaginase is discontinued. Asparaginase may also cause pancreatitis, and diabetes, transient or permanent, may be associated with this.

Treatment for ALL and some lymphomas includes 4-weekly pulses of corticosteroids. Historically, prednisolone was given, but there is a survival advantage in using dexamethasone, so standard therapy for ALL now includes dexamethasone as the

Table 8.3 Endocrinopathy after bone marrow transplant (BMT).

Endocrinopathy	Risk factors	Assessment
Short stature	TBI Previous CI Younger age at treatment GHD	Regular 3–6 monthly assessments Height including sitting height, weight, BMI Pubertal staging Testicular volume not a useful indicator of pubertal progression
GHD	TBI Previous CI Increasing time from treatment	Evaluate if previous CI or persistent poor growth Hypothalamically mediated test of GH status preferable If normal, repeat if concern re growth and consider retesting at 2-yearly intervals GH therapy – monitor IGF-1
Thyroid dysfunction	*Hypothyroidism* TBI Bu/Cy conditioning (lower risk than TBI) *Thyroid nodules/cancer* Female gender Younger age at treatment Increasing time from treatment	Annual assessment Baseline TSH and fT4 Palpation of thyroid Thyroxine replacement if TSH persistently elevated
Gonadal dysfunction	*Female* (infertility and sex steroid deficiency) Older age at treatment TBI Busulfan *Male* (infertility but clinical sex steroid deficiency infrequent) Effect of age unclear Radiation ≥4 Gy – azoospermia very likely Radiation ≥20 Gy-Leydig cell failure likely (testicular boost for testicular relapse is 24 Gy) Busulfan	Baseline LH, FSH, estradiol/testosterone annually Consider pelvic USS in females; uterine size, endometrial thickness, Doppler studies Semen studies in males as requested by patient Ovarian function may recover – trial off estrogen for 6–8 weeks every 2 years recommended
Reduced BMD	Hypogonadism CGvHD/steroids Inactivity Poor nutrition	Evaluate 2 years from primary treatment DXA scanning with assessment of volumetric BMD Repeat if abnormal or ongoing cGvHD/steroids or hypogonadism
Metabolic syndrome	Risk factors unknown TBI probably important GHD	Fasting glucose and lipid profile annually

BMD, bone mineral density; BMI, body mass index; CGvHD, chronic graft versus host disease; CI, cranial irradiation; DXA, dual energy X-ray absorptiometry; FSH, follicle stimulating hormone; GH, growth hormone; GHD, growth hormone deficiency; LH, luteinizing hormone; TBI, total body irradiation; TSH, thyroid stimulating hormone.

corticosteroid. Five-day courses of 6 mg/m²/day are given 4-weekly during the maintenance phase of therapy (with VCR on day 1 of the 5-day course). In a small number of susceptible children, this produces glucose intolerance and insulin therapy may be required.

Recombinant interferon has also been associated with hyperglycemia in non-diabetic patients and worsening of existing diabetes.

Adrenal suppression following corticosteroids

Although adrenal insufficiency is rare after treatment for childhood leukemia, a small number of children treated for ALL show persistent suppression of endogenous adrenal function as a consequence of corticosteroid therapy. While this usually recovers over time, it has been suggested that it may rarely be permanent.

There was initial concern that adrenal function would be adversely affected after TBI and BMT but this has not been observed in the majority of studies. The adrenal gland is relatively radioresistant. Patients who require prolonged corticosteroid therapy for cGvHD are at risk of adrenal suppression and although recovery is usual, it is not universal.

Evaluation of the adrenal axis should be undertaken after discontinuation of corticosteroids and replacement therapy administered if necessary.

Late effects of cancer therapy

Cranial irradiation and hypothalamo-pituitary damage

Children treated with CI that includes the HP axis within the radiation field are at risk of developing neuroendocrine abnormalities that evolve with time.

Growth hormone deficiency

GHD is the most frequent and often only neuroendocrine abnormality to occur following CI. The speed of onset and the degree of severity of GHD is dependent on the dose of irradiation. For example, 100% of children who receive greater than 30 Gy of CI, as in the treatment of brain tumors, develop moderate GHD (peak GH <7 μg/L) to the insulin tolerance test (ITT), while 35% of those who receive less than 30 Gy will still show a normal peak GH response to the ITT 2–5 years after radiotherapy [7]. Children who have received a radiation dose of >20 Gy are more likely to develop severe GHD (peak GH <3 μg/L) in adulthood than after lower doses of CI [8].

The threshold radiation dose at which damage occurs is not known. There is some evidence to suggest that the threshold dose for TBI causing moderate GHD (peak GH <7 μg/L) is 8–10 Gy, while doses of 10–12 Gy clearly induce moderate GHD. It is possible that 7–8 Gy may induce moderate GHD but not until many years after therapy. Doses of radiation used in TBI are unlikely to cause severe GHD (peak GH <3 μg/L) unless the patient has received prior CI [8–10]. Severe GHD is more frequent after higher doses of CI as previously used in ALL for CNS prophylaxis (24 Gy) [11,12] and currently used in brain tumors (30–50 Gy) [13,14].

Prospective studies suggest that impaired GH responses to provocative testing can occur as early as 3 months and certainly within the first 12 months following CI for brain tumors.

There is some evidence to suggest that the HP axis in children may be more sensitive because GH concentrations were lower in children after TBI (10–14 Gy) than in adults [15].

Growth hormone neurosecretory profile and dysfunction

Spontaneous GH secretion in patients who are GHD following CI has rarely been studied. However, recently Darzy *et al.* [16] examined GH profiles in GHD adult survivors of childhood cancer following CI using a sensitive chemiluminescent GH assay. GH profile was affected quantitatively but not qualitatively – only amplitude and not pulse frequency was affected. In addition, a clear augmentation of GH secretion in GHD patients in response to fasting similar to that in normal subjects was observed, emphasizing that GH neuroregulation is preserved [17].

GH neurosecretory dysfunction (GHNSD) has been described after radiation and is characterized biochemically by reduced physiological GH secretion with preserved responses to pharmacological stimuli [9]. The few longitudinal studies of GH secretion in children treated with radiotherapy, whether TBI (10 Gy), CI for leukemia or brain tumors distant from the HP axis, all suggest an evolving neurosecretory disturbance. The majority of studies were performed during puberty [18]. A study to investigate whether the phenomenon persisted into adulthood found no evidence of radiation-induced GHNSD [18].

Other pituitary hormones

At higher doses of radiation (>50 Gy), multiple pituitary hormone deficits can occur. In a study of 31 adult patients following irradiation for nasopharyngeal tumors followed over 5 years with estimated doses to the hypothalamus and pituitary of 40–62 Gy, 63.5% were found to be GHD and 30.7%, 26.7% and 14.9% of the patients were deficient in gonadotropins, adenocorticotropic hormone (ACTH) and thyroid stimulating hormone (TSH), respectively [19]. Children treated for head and neck rhabdomyosarcomas also have a high incidence of endocrinopathy [20]. The presence of tumor affecting the HP axis increases the likelihood of evolving multiple pituitary hormone deficiencies even after a lower dose of radiation (Fig. 8.2a) [21].

There appears to be a hierarchical loss of pituitary hormones after GH is affected; gonadotropins and ACTH are the next most sensitive to radiation, followed by TSH. The radiosensitivity of GH in comparison to other pituitary hormones has been confirmed by *in vivo* and *in vitro* animal work [22,23].

Although other pituitary hormone deficits are infrequent at the lower doses of CI (30–50 Gy) used to treat children with brain tumors, a small percentage of children will be affected. For instance, a study of 16 survivors of posterior fossa tumors treated with CI found that all but two demonstrated adequate cortisol responses to ITT 10 years after completion of therapy (Fig. 8.2b) [24]. In contrast, a study of 73 children treated with radiotherapy and chemotherapy demonstrated a suboptimal cortisol response to ITT or standard dose ACTH test in 14 (19%) of the patients using the same criteria (peak above 500 nmol/L, 18 μg/dL) [25]. A peak cortisol of 500 nmol/L or more was reached in the rest of the cohort but they still had significantly lower peak cortisol concentrations than control subjects. Median follow-up in the latter study was longer (15 years) than in the former (11 years), suggesting the possibility of evolving defects over time in line with other abnormalities of the HP axis. Dose of radiation and time from treatment were identified as risk factors for ACTH deficiency, with no evidence of an additive effect of adjuvant chemotherapy. Reassuringly a recent study examining physiological cortisol profiles and 24-h cortisol production rates in adult cancer survivors following CI for brain tumors found no evidence of discordancy with provocative tests [26]. On the contrary, cortisol concentrations were significantly higher than controls suggesting activation of the HP adrenal axis. The explanation for this finding remains speculative.

Central hypothyroidism is much less common than primary hypothyroidism after treatment for brain tumors. Estimates of the frequency of HP thyroid dysfunction range 4–6% (Fig. 8.2b) [24,27,28]. This may well increase over time and is likely to be an underestimate in the very long-term survivors in the adult population treated many years earlier for a childhood brain tumor.

Figure 8.2 (a) 10-year life table analysis in 37 adults with intrasellar or anatomically adjacent tumors and normal postoperative hypothalamo-pituitary (HP) function, indicating the likelihood of an evolving endocrinopathy after 37.5–42.4 Gy pituitary irradiation. (From Littley *et al.* [21]). (b) 10-year probability of an evolving endocrinopathy occurring after a median estimated HP irradiation dose (DXR) of 40 Gy in 16 survivors of resected posterior fossa tumors, tested twice (at the onset of growth failure and at completion of growth) [24]. ACTH, adenocorticotropic hormone; DXR, ; FSH, follicle stimulating hormone; GH, growth hormone; LH, luteinizing hormone; TSH, thyroid stimulating hormone.

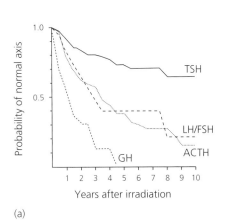

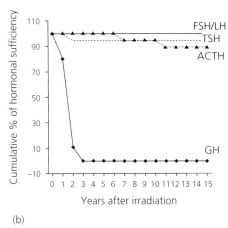

(a) (b)

Because thyroid function is commonly evaluated using basal TSH and free T4 concentrations, subtle deficits of HP thyroid axis function may be missed. One investigator has advocated the assessment of nocturnal TSH surge and/or thyrotropin releasing hormone (TRH) test in cancer survivors to ensure that cases of central hypothyroidism are not overlooked by relying on baseline thyroid function tests [29]. However, a study by Darzy *et al.* [30] in 37 euthyroid survivors including 24-h TSH profiles and TRH tests found no evidence of missed central hypothyroidism.

Gonadotropin deficiency occurs infrequently (Fig. 8.2b) [24]. Elevated concentrations of prolactin, particularly in females, can occur because of reduced dopamine release but this is rarely of clinical significance.

Early or precocious puberty

CI is associated with early puberty which is more likely the younger the age at treatment. Girls are more susceptible than boys at lower doses of radiation (18–24 Gy). At higher doses of radiation (30–50 Gy), both boys and girls are affected [31–34]. In a study of 46 children previously irradiated for brain tumors, all of whom had GHD, onset of puberty occurred at 8.51 years in girls and 9.21 years in boys (Fig. 8.3) [35]. The likely mechanism for early puberty is disinhibition of cortical influences on the hypothalamus, resulting in increased amplitude and frequency of gonadotropin releasing hormone (GnRH) pulsatile secretion. After higher doses of irradiation early puberty may be followed several years later by gonadotropin deficiency.

Site of radiation damage

Radiation-induced damage is believed to be neuronal rather than vascular, with the hypothalamus as the primary site of radiation damage, particularly with radiation doses of less than 50 Gy.

This hypothesis is supported by the presence of other abnormalities consistent with hypothalamic dysfunction. These include the presence of typically hypothalamic (delayed peak or delayed decline of peak) gonadotropin and/or TSH responses to GnRH or TRH stimulation and elevated prolactin concentrations.

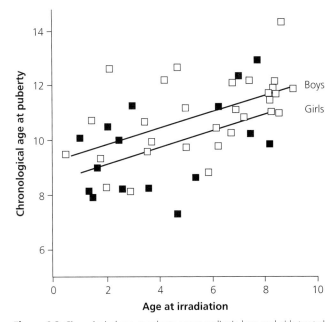

Figure 8.3 Chronological age at puberty occurs earlier in boys and girls treated at a younger age with cranial irradiation (CI; 25–47.5 Gy) as demonstrated by this study in 46 brain tumor survivors. (From Ogilvy-Stuart *et al.* [35].)

From a diagnostic perspective, the site of damage may influence the GH response to stimuli used for provocative GH testing which work through either hypothalamic or pituitary pathways, depending on the test.

A study performed in adult survivors of cancer demonstrated a discordancy between the GHRH + arginine stimulation test (a provocative test which partially involves stimulating the pituitary directly) and the ITT (a provocative test stimulating hypothalamic pathways) within 5 years of radiation with the ITT inducing significantly lower concentrations of GH. It was not until 10 years after radiation that the two tests demonstrated similar GH results [36].

From a therapeutic perspective, the administration of hypothalamic releasing factors has been shown to restore pituitary hormone secretion. Intermittent pulsatile subcutaneous GnRH therapy can successfully induce puberty in both sexes, with resultant ovulatory cycles in girls and fertility in hypogonadotropic females. Continuous subcutaneous GHRH therapy promotes growth in children with GH deficiency of presumed hypothalamic origin after irradiation for periods up to 1 year [37]. The response depends on the integrity of somatostatin secretion and is generally less than that seen with GH alone.

The change in response over time to provocative tests with hypothalamic releasing factors and the progressive nature of hormonal deficits following radiation damage have been attributed to secondary pituitary atrophy as a consequence of lack of hypothalamic releasing/tropic factors or delayed direct effects of radiotherapy on the pituitary. At higher doses of CI (>50 Gy) there may be a direct effect of irradiation on the pituitary gland [19].

A recent study in adult cancer survivors has challenged the hypothesis of pure hypothalamic damage at lower doses of radiation because normal physiological GH secretion was observed in the setting of reduced somatotroph reserve in response to two provocative tests, suggesting compensatory overdrive by the hypothalamus [18], at least in a subset of irradiated patients.

Growth and growth promoting therapies

Poor growth may be a feature at presentation or it may occur either directly due to the effects of cancer therapy or indirectly secondarily to GHD following CI. Studies to final height (FH) are essential to clarify the effect of cancer therapy on growth and growth promoting therapies.

Chemotherapy alone

Studies examining the effect of chemotherapy alone in patients treated for ALL have reported reduced growth velocity during cancer therapy followed by catch-up growth [38–43]. However, catch-up growth has not been consistently observed [44,45]. A recent report from the CCSS found that, in a cohort of survivors of ALL, the observed risk of significant short stature in adulthood (<−2.5 SD) was >3 in those that had received chemotherapy alone compared with sibling controls [46]. Although the mean FH of the chemotherapy-alone group was significantly lower than sibling controls, the actual difference was only around 0.2 SD [46].

The cause of short stature in the chemotherapy group remains a subject of debate [41,44,45,47]. It is likely that corticosteroids and methotrexate play a part, because both affect growth and influence physiological bone turnover, especially osteoclast activity.

The effect of chemotherapy-only conditioning for BMT on growth is less clear. Studies have demonstrated no disruption in growth with cyclophosphamide alone [48] or cyclophosphamide in combination with busulfan [49,50], but one study demonstrated a reduction in growth in patients receiving Bu/Cy, attributed to a large number of patients receiving prior CI with cGvHD [48]. Studies to FH are lacking. Other factors contributing to

poor growth in BMT patients include cGvHD which may cause malabsorption and necessitates treatment with corticosteroids.

Radiotherapy

Patients who have received CI for brain tumors, lymphoma or leukemia [38–42,44,45,47,51–58] or as part of TBI in preparation for BMT, particularly if they have received CI previously, are more likely to be short in adult life than those who received chemotherapy alone. The cause of short stature is multifactorial but includes the development of GHD, particularly after higher doses of CI, spinal irradiation and the onset of early puberty. Patients treated at a younger age are more likely to have a greater height deficit [32,59–62], particularly if they have received spinal irradiation, and this probably reflects a more prolonged period of disordered growth than age-specific vulnerability.

Spinal radiation is an essential component of treatment of brain tumors with a propensity to metastasize to the spine, such as medulloblastoma and ependymoma, and also as part of radiation to the CNS in the treatment of leukemia or lymphoma. The impact of this on growth is considerable in terms of both FH and disproportion, particularly after higher doses as used in the treatment of brain tumors. The greatest reduction in FH and more marked disproportion is observed in children treated at a younger age. A study of the effects of spinal irradiation on FH in 79 brain tumor patients (not treated with GH) estimated the radiation-related spinal height loss to be at least 9 cm versus 7 cm versus 5.5 cm when irradiation was given at the age of 1 year versus 5 years versus 10 years [63]. This is thought to be secondary to direct inhibition of vertebral growth [47].

Another factor, often encountered in ALL and brain tumor survivors treated with CI, is early puberty. In contrast to idiopathic early pubertal onset, when duration of puberty is often prolonged, early puberty in this population is usually of normal duration. This results in reduced potential for spinal growth and limits the time available for growth promotion. FH studies in survivors of ALL frequently demonstrate that females are at increased risk of short stature, often attributed to early puberty, which occurs only in girls after lower doses of CI [46].

Adjuvant chemotherapy has also been reported to be associated with an increased risk of short stature [64–66].

Growth promoting therapies

The first study of the effects of GH therapy in GHD childhood cancer survivors was reported in 1981. Six children who had survived a brain tumor demonstrated improved growth rates of 6.0–10.1 cm during the first year of GH therapy. Analysis of auxological data of the last 25 years of GH therapy (1975–2000) in brain tumor survivors in the same single center revealed a gradual improvement in FH outcome for both CI and CSI patients (r = 0.5, P = 0.03 and r = 0.6; P < 0.001) (Fig. 8.4) [66].

The main factors contributing to that success were the improved and higher GH regimens, the earlier introduction of GH therapy after completion of radiotherapy and the additional use of GnRH analog therapy for early puberty in selected patients.

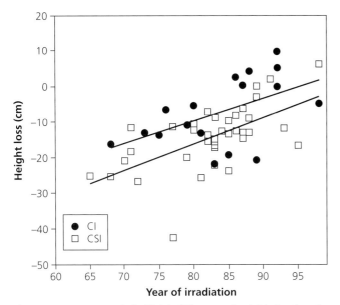

Figure 8.4 Improvements in final height (FH) measured as height loss (actual height – target height) with growth hormone (GH) therapy in 58 growth hormone deficient (GHD) brain tumor survivors treated with cranial irradiation (CI) or craniospinal irradiation (CSI) between 1965 and 2000. (From Gleeson *et al.* [66] with permission.)

To manage the detrimental effects of early puberty on growth, few studies have explored the use of GnRH analog therapy in childhood cancer survivors [66,67]. GnRH analog therapy conferred additional height benefits in selected patients, particularly those who had received CI alone without spinal irradiation, although FH gains were often achieved at the expense of increased segmental disproportion between sitting height and leg length.

Younger children with GHD following TBI treated with GH therapy have an improved FH outcome (+0.86 SD) compared with younger children with GHD not treated with GH therapy [62].

Growth hormone, relapse/recurrence and secondary malignant neoplasms

In vitro studies demonstrate that IGF-1 can act as both a mitogen and an anti-apoptotic agent in a variety of cancers so there is concern that GH therapy may increase the risk of relapse or secondary malignant neoplasms (SMNs) in patients previously treated for cancer. These include the association between acromegaly and risk of colon cancer and the positive correlation between the exact placing of the IGF-1 level within the normal range and an increased risk of common cancers of adulthood, such as breast, prostate, colon and lung.

Evidence to date is reassuring, although there are a number of methodological concerns in relation to the data: all the studies are retrospective; most are small; many focus only on subjects previously treated for intracranial tumors.

The largest UK study comparing recurrence rate in 180 GH-treated and 891 GH-naive survivors of childhood brain tumors did not demonstrate any difference in recurrence rates between the two groups [68]. The CCSS, which is a survey-based follow-up of 14 000 pediatric cancer survivors, reported its findings in relation to GH therapy and SMNs [69]. The study group included 361 children treated with GH. GH therapy did not appear to increase the risk of disease recurrence or death in survivors. However, there did appear to be a small excess of SMNs (relative risk 3.21) in GH-treated survivors, mainly because of an increased risk of SMNs in survivors of acute leukemia. A subsequent follow-up analysis 32 months after the first demonstrated that the increased risk reduced with time [70].

These data should be interpreted with caution because the number of events (15 SMNs) was small and the confidence limits wide. In addition, the study is retrospective and methodologically less than ideal. Even if the results were correct, the absolute number of excess tumors that would occur as a result of GH therapy is only three or four per 1000 person-years at 15 years from diagnosis. This small risk needs to be balanced against potential benefits of GH therapy, which may be considerable. It also needs to be taken into consideration that GH doses in the USA are generally higher than those used in Europe [71].

Evaluation

Auxology and pubertal staging should be assessed every 3–6 months from the time of diagnosis until the completion of growth and puberty in all patients. In a patient who has had spinal irradiation, leg length growth is a better indicator of height velocity than spinal growth because of the direct effect of radiation on spinal epiphyses. Be aware in a male patient previously treated with gonadotoxic therapy that testicular enlargement may not be a reliable indicator of the onset or normal progression of puberty.

Diagnosing growth hormone deficiency

In patients treated with CI, pituitary testing should be performed routinely 2 years after the completion of therapy and repeated 1–2 years thereafter to monitor for evolving GHD, even if growth is unaffected. The rationale for testing before a decline in growth velocity is the evidence that the early introduction of GH therapy results in better outcomes [66]. It is also possible that the onset of early puberty or obesity may promote growth and mask evolving GHD. Testing before 2 years after the completion of therapy should be considered if there are concerns about growth or ACTH deficiency, for instance, following higher doses of radiation for head and neck cancers or radiation for a brain tumor affecting the HP axis.

Although IGF-1 should be measured, there are concerns that it may discriminate poorly in radiation-induced GHD. Normal IGF-1 and IGFBP3 concentrations have been documented in GHD survivors, thus limiting their usefulness in this setting but IGF-1 concentrations <−2 SD in 95% of GHD cancer survivors have also been reported [14].

Choice of GH test is often decided locally. In our practice the arginine stimulation test is used and also the ITT in those without a history of seizures; otherwise this is substituted by a glucagon stimulation test. The ITT and glucagon stimulation test have the advantage of also assessing ACTH secretion. The GHRH + arginine stimulation test is also being used more frequently in the pediatric and adolescent population but this test may have limitations soon after CI [36,72]. Appropriate priming with sex steroids should be considered in prepubertal patients with a bone age in excess of 10 years.

As there is uncertainty about which test is most appropriate to diagnose radiation-induced GHD, with the high possibility of false-negative tests, one commonly used approach is that if two provocative tests produce discordant results in a child who is growing poorly with a high presumptive likelihood of GHD, a trial of GH therapy is justified. In nearly all centers 24-h GH profiling is a research tool and not part of routine investigation.

Retesting growth hormone status at final height

The severity of GHD required for consideration of GH replacement is more strict in adolescence (peak GH <5 μg/L) and adulthood (peak GH <3 μg/L) than childhood (peak GH <7–10 μg/L). Retesting of GH status in those treated with GH during childhood is therefore essential at FH, utilizing the current consensus guidelines to identify which patients will be eligible for ongoing GH therapy [73]. One study has shown that only 70% of patients previously treated for GHD secondary to CI would be eligible for GH in adolescence (peak GH <5 μg/L) and 50% in adulthood [8]. The majority of these patients were brain tumor survivors [8].

Assessing other pituitary hormones

Although ACTH deficiency is rare following CI, it is potentially life-threatening. Provocative testing of the HP-adrenal axis should be performed in children treated with doses of CI >30 Gy. There is ongoing debate as to which test is the most appropriate because of concerns that patients may have an adequate response to a standard ACTH test but suboptimal response to ITT. When ACTH deficiency has been demonstrated, hydrocortisone replacement should be instituted. It may also be necessary to provide cover just for illness and surgery in patients with subtle disturbance of the HP-adrenal axis.

Assessment of TSH deficiency relies on baseline thyroid function tests but it is important that both TSH and free thyroxine are checked. If reducing concentrations of free thyroxine are observed longitudinally in the setting of a low-normal, normal or even mildly raised TSH, the diagnosis of central hypothyroidism should be considered, particularly if the patient has multiple pituitary hormone deficits. If a diagnosis of central hypothyroidism is made, ensure ACTH status is determined because hydrocortisone should be introduced before thyroxine replacement. Thyroxine replacement should aim to achieve free thyroxine concentrations in the high-normal range. There is no role for the TRH test or assessment of the TSH nocturnal surge in the diagnosis of central hypothyroidism.

Baseline prolactin concentrations should also be checked.

Early or delayed puberty

In children presenting with early puberty (girls before the age of 9 and boys before the age of 10) in the setting of GHD, a baseline estradiol or testosterone and a GnRH test should be performed for biochemical confirmation. If additional information is required a pelvic ultrasound in girls may also be useful.

In children with delayed puberty (girls no breast development by the age of 12 and boys no testicular enlargement by the age of 13, unless previous BMT when testicular enlargement may not occur despite otherwise normal progression through puberty) with normal or low concentrations of gonadotropins, a baseline estradiol or testosterone and a GnRH test would help to diagnose gonadotropin deficiency. Puberty should be induced with sex steroids in conventional fashion.

Management
In childhood: growth hormone therapy and GnRH analogs

In children diagnosed with GHD, GH therapy should be considered. Despite the absence of evidence to support an increase in recurrence as a result of GH therapy, the risk of relapse is greatest within the first 2 years from primary treatment and it is common to delay initiation of GH therapy until 2 years after treatment.

Biochemical monitoring using IGF-1 concentrations compared to normative age-matched data is recommended. This allows optimization of GH dose if growth is poor and may provide information about the patient's adherence to GH therapy.

Children receiving GH therapy should be monitored for side effects, particularly scoliosis and glucose intolerance. Neuroimaging for brain tumor survivors or patients at risk of meningiomas following CI is not necessary routinely while on GH therapy but should be performed if clinically indicated.

Early puberty is common after CI. The combination of early puberty and GHD carries a particularly poor height prognosis. There is an argument for combining treatment with a GnRH analog and GH to maximize growth potential and some evidence to suggest that this is beneficial [66,67]. The height benefits are greater in those treated with CI alone compared with CSI [66]. Decision to start GnRH analogs in combination with GH therapy is a clinical one based on the patient's current height potential and tempo of puberty.

Reduction in BMD is a recognized side effect of treatment with GnRH analog and, in a population who are already known to be at risk of reduced BMD, this is clearly a concern. Published studies examining impact on BMD are few but do not suggest a sustained deleterious effect following combination therapy with GnRH analog and GH therapy [74].

In adolescence: growth hormone therapy

Young adults with childhood onset GHD have lower BMD and lean body mass (LBM) than young adults with adult onset GHD [75]. This led to the hypothesis that the discontinuation of GH therapy at the end of linear growth did not allow the completion of somatic growth and, in particular, the achievement of peak bone mass which occurs in early to mid-twenties. This prompted studies examining the impact of GH therapy in the so-called "transition period" from late adolescence into young adulthood. The majority of studies demonstrated that the reintroduction of GH therapy soon after completion of linear growth resulted in an improvement in BMD and LBM [75]. Although similar studies have not been exclusively performed in GHD cancer survivors, the recommendation would be that GH therapy should either be continued or restarted as recommended by the consensus statement in those fulfilling the criteria for GHD in adolescence [73].

In adulthood : growth hormone therapy

Many survivors of childhood brain tumors and ALL who received CI (>20 Gy) will have severe GHD in adult life. GH therapy has the potential to improve quality of life, reduce cardiovascular risk and normalize bone mass. Studies to date in childhood cancer survivors have demonstrated improvements in quality of life with GH therapy [76] and also improvements in cardiac systolic function and reduction in prevalence of metabolic syndrome [77].

Cancer therapy and thyroid damage

The thyroid gland is radiosensitive and radiation fields that either include or result in scatter to the neck can cause thyroid dysfunction, nodules and cancer. Patients receiving TBI conditioning for BMT, CSI/CI for brain tumors or neck irradiation as part of mediastinal irradiation for Hodgkin lymphoma or irradiation for head and neck tumors are at risk of thyroid damage [78–88]. Age at irradiation is a clear factor in the development of thyroid dysfunction, thyroid nodules or cancer regardless of primary cancer diagnosis or dose of radiation, with more thyroid abnormalities detected in children <10 years than >10 years of age at treatment [89–93]. Thyroid abnormalities are more frequently seen in females than males [80,85,91].

Thyroid dysfunction

Thyroid dysfunction is common after BMT with both chemotherapy alone (Bu/Cy) [89,94–96] and TBI conditioning [15,97–99]. Following TBI, a lower incidence of thyroid dysfunction has been reported after hyperfractionation (14.7% [89] compared with 30% after standard fractionation [100]). In the latter study, 147 patients were prospectively followed for a median of 11 years and a minimum of 5 years. A total of 3.4% developed overt thyroid dysfunction (four had primary hypothyroidism, one had hyperthyroidism), which developed between 1 and 5 years; 26.5% had subclinical compensated hypothyroidism which developed between 1 and 10 years following BMT [100]. The same group also identified a high prevalence of sick euthyroid syndrome at 3 months following BMT [101] which has also been described after chemotherapy conditioning and was associated with a poorer outcome [95].

Frequency of primary hypothyroidism following CSI for the treatment of brain tumors varies from 24% to 68% [28,102]; an increased incidence after CI is less well substantiated but has been reported. In 73% of patients primary hypothyroidism is subclinical compensated hypothyroidism (elevated TSH with normal T4 and T3); overt hypothyroidism occurs in 27% [28].

The frequency of hypothyroidism after mediastinal radiation for Hodgkin lymphoma was 25% for all patients but 50% after 20 years of follow-up for those receiving 45 Gy, demonstrating a clear increased likelihood of thyroid dysfunction at higher radiation doses (Fig. 8.5) [80]. Five percent of patients also developed hyperthyroidism [80].

Two studies suggested that patients receiving chemotherapy with radiotherapy in the treatment of brain tumors were more likely to develop thyroid dysfunction [27,103], but more recent studies in brain tumor and Hodgkin lymphoma survivors have failed to confirm this [28,80,104].

There is a debate as to the clinical significance of subclinical hypothyroidism [99]. The claim that normalizing TSH diminishes the incidence of thyroid nodules is unproven [78,105,106]. Following TBI for BMT, one study observed that subclinical compensated hypothyroidism resolved spontaneously [100], and similar recovery has been observed in other studies [107,108].

Thyroid nodules and cancer

Thyroid nodules occur frequently after neck irradiation for childhood cancer [80,92,109,110]. The reported risk of developing

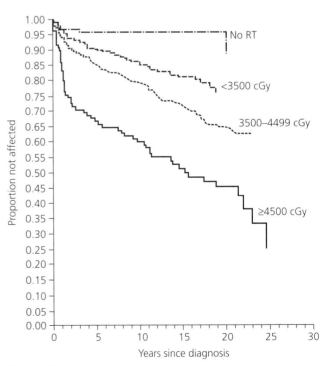

Figure 8.5 Probability of developing an underactive thyroid after diagnosis of Hodgkin lymphoma. Patients are grouped according to dose of thyroid irradiation. RT, radiation therapy. (From Sklar *et al.* [80] with permission.)

thyroid nodules varies widely because of differences in the study population (age, gender, radiation dose and length of follow-up) and factors that impact on the rate of detection (e.g. palpation versus ultrasound). In a study from a single center that used palpation as the method of detection, 39% of thyroid nodules were malignant [85] which is in agreement with other smaller series (10–33%) [109,111–115]. In contrast, only 5% of thyroid nodules among adults in the general population are likely to be malignant. Thyroid nodules may not become evident for decades after radiation therapy, with 5 years being the minimum latency period [80,92,109,110].

Once a thyroid nodule has been detected, fine needle aspiration biopsy (FNAB) is the diagnostic procedure of choice but the accuracy of FNAB in a previously irradiated population is unclear [116,117]. In one study [85] the sensitivity and specificity was similar to that described in the general population, with 19% of FNAB yielding inadequate samples. However, false-negative rates have been reported as either higher in the irradiated population at 33% [85] or similar [116,117] compared with 1–11% in the general population.

Although low doses of radiation cause thyroid nodules and cancer [118], it was previously believed that higher doses of radiation increased the risk only of developing hypothyroidism [119]. The CCSS recently explored the dose–response by performing a nested case–control study of 69 pathologically confirmed cases of thyroid cancer and 265 matched controls [91]. The risk of thyroid cancer increased with radiation doses up to 20–29 Gy but reduced thereafter, consistent with a cell killing effect (Fig. 8.6).

The majority of thyroid cancers were diagnosed 10–19 years after the first diagnosis of cancer [85,86,91,92,120]. After low dose radiation, the increased incidence of thyroid cancer continued for at least 40 years after thyroid irradiation [121]. There was no increased risk with chemotherapy alone or in combination with irradiation [91].

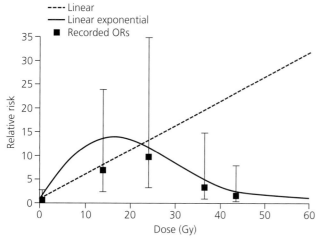

Figure 8.6 Thyroid-cancer risk by radiation dose in cases and controls after adjustment for first cancer, data from the Childhood Cancer Survival Study (CCSS). (From Sigurdson *et al.* [91] with permission.)

Most of these thyroid cancers do not behave in an aggressive fashion after a median follow-up of 6.5 years [85]. Two large case–control studies comparing thyroid cancer in patients who did and did not receive irradiation in childhood concluded that the risks of recurrence and death were similar [122,123], but others have cited evidence of more aggressive behavior [124,125].

The pathogenesis of thyroid cancer following radiotherapy is not well understood, although recent molecular genetic studies have yielded some interesting findings. Rearrangements of the RET proto-oncogene (RET/PTC) appear with greater frequency in thyroid cancer developing after ionizing radiation and after both low and high dose external radiotherapy compared with *de novo* thyroid cancer [126–128]; these may be responsible for the development of radiation induced papillary carcinoma [129] but no correlation with clinical characteristics or behavior has been made [126–128,130].

These data highlight the importance of yearly examination of the neck and thyroid gland in all survivors given radiation to the mediastinum or head and neck [80,131]. However, there is controversy surrounding the most appropriate modality for thyroid cancer screening [85,132]. The argument against the routine use of ultrasound is that the increased identification of small thyroid nodules causes an unnecessary number of surgical procedures with the associated patient anxiety and that the impalpable nodules containing malignant cells are clinically insignificant. In addition, there is no evidence that the outcome in terms of survival is worse if thyroid palpation is used as the method of screening.

Evaluation and management

All patients who have received either a BMT or irradiation near or including the thyroid require annual thyroid screening throughout life.

Annual thyroid function tests are essential and if overt primary hypothyroidism occurs, thyroxine should be started. If a patient has subclinical compensated hypothyroidism, TSH should be rechecked on two occasions; if it remains even only mildly elevated, thyroxine should be started.

The recommendation in the UK is that thyroid cancer screening should be performed by annual thyroid palpation to detect thyroid nodules. On palpation of a thyroid nodule, FNAB should be performed. If the histology is inconclusive, there should be a low threshold for proceeding to surgery. The treatment of thyroid cancer in cancer survivors is identical to that if it had occurred *de novo*.

Cancer therapy and gonadal damage

Gonadal function may be directly affected as a consequence of radiation or gonadotoxic chemotherapy. Patients who have received TBI or chemotherapy conditioning for BMT, localized pelvic or testicular radiotherapy or treatment with alkylating agents for Hodgkin lymphoma are at high risk (>80%) of gonadal damage. Patients treated for brain tumors with CSI are at medium risk compared to patients with brain tumors treated with CI alone or acute lymphoblastic leukemia who are at low risk of gonadal damage [133].

The extent of damage by radiotherapy depends on gender, field of treatment, total dose and fractionation [134–136]. In contrast to the HP axis, the same dose fractionated is more damaging for spermatogenesis than when delivered as a single dose; the reverse is true for ovarian damage.

The impact of combination cytotoxic chemotherapy on gonadal function is dependent on gender and age of child and the nature and dose of drugs received. Drugs known to cause gonadal damage include alkylating agents (cyclophosphamide, ifosfamide, chlormethine, busulfan, mephalan, chlorambucil), procarbazine, cisplatin, carboplatin and doxorubicin [137–146].

Gonadal damage in males

In males, doses as low as 0.1–1.2 Gy can damage dividing spermatogonia and disrupt cell morphology resulting in oligospermia [134,135]. Permanent azoospermia has been reported following single fraction radiation with 4 or 1.2 Gy fractionated [134,135].

Leydig cells are more resistant to radiation damage. Testicular irradiation at doses greater than 20 Gy is associated with Leydig cell dysfunction in prepubertal boys, while Leydig cell function is usually preserved up to 30 Gy in adults [136]. Biochemical compensation occurs with normal testosterone concentrations associated with elevated luteinizing hormone (LH) concentrations and there is often normal progression through puberty despite severe impairment of spermatogenesis.

Treatment for Hodgkin lymphoma in the UK with "ChlVPP" (chlorambucil, vinblastine, procarbazine, prednisolone) is known to cause gonadal damage particularly in the male. In a recent long-term study, 89% of males treated before puberty had evidence of severe damage to the germinal epithelium and recovery of spermatogenesis would be unlikely [140]. The use of ABVD is significantly less gonadotoxic [139]. However, this regimen carries the potential of cardiotoxicity from the use of anthracyclines. Current treatment in the UK involves alternate courses of ChlVPP and ABVD. This regimen is likely to result in less gonadotoxicity [147].

Testosterone replacement in male survivors with compensated primary hypogonadism is a subject under study [148]. A recent cross-sectional analysis of young adult male cancer survivors who had received gonadotoxic therapy found that 14% had a testosterone level of <10 nmol/L (below the lower limit of normal range) [149]. Cancer survivors had higher body fat and insulin concentrations than controls and a lower quality of life [149]. An earlier study also found a trend towards lower BMD in those cancer survivors who had an elevated LH compared with a LH level within the normal range [148]. It remains to be determined whether these patients would benefit from testosterone replacement.

Gonadal damage in females

Total body, abdominal or pelvic irradiation may cause ovarian and uterine damage [137,150–152]. The human oocyte is sensitive to irradiation with an estimated median lethal dose (LD50) of 2 Gy [150]. The younger the child at the time of radiotherapy the larger the number of primordial follicles present; hence, for a given radiation exposure, the longer the window of fertility before premature menopause ensues. The effective sterilizing dose of radiation (fractionated) at which premature ovarian failure occurs immediately is 20.3 Gy at birth, 18.4 Gy at 10 years, 16.5 Gy at 20 years and 14.3 Gy at 30 years [153].

It is possible that even in the setting of preserved ovarian function, radiation damage to the uterus may have occurred. Uterine irradiation in childhood increases the incidence of nulliparity, spontaneous miscarriage and intrauterine growth retardation [137,152]. The mechanism underlying uterine damage is not understood.

Ovarian dysfunction following chemotherapy resulting in premature ovarian failure is well described [154]. Following ChlVPP treatment for Hodgkin lymphoma, 50% of girls treated prepubertally had raised gonadotropin concentrations but longer follow-up would be needed to determine whether these women have recovery of function or go on to develop premature menopause [140]. Current treatment in the UK involves alternate courses of ChlVPP and ABVD. This regimen is likely to result in less ovarian damage [147].

There appears to be no lasting effect of multiagent chemotherapy regimens on uterine function. Successful pregnancies with no increased risk of miscarriage and healthy offspring have been reported.

Preservation of fertility

Preservation of fertility must be considered in all patients at high risk of infertility. The challenges differ depending on whether patients are sexually mature at the time of diagnosis. There are also ethical and legal issues to be considered [133].

Practical measures exist to shield the gonads from unnecessary radiation in males and females. In females laparoscopic removal of the ovary from the radiation field, oophoropexy, is a possibility [155] but uterine damage may still be present.

In sexually mature males, cryopreservation of spermatozoa is the only established option. This may be achieved by the production of a semen sample or, if spermatogenesis is established, sperm can be retrieved after testicular or epididymal aspiration. For patients who have not yet started puberty, the options for fertility are experimental. One area of current research is the harvesting of testicular cells for orthotopicic transplantation after the completion of cancer therapy or *in vitro* maturation [156,157]. Proof of principle exists for the mouse model [156] but whether this success can be achieved in primates is unclear [157].

In young sexually mature females with partners, the collection of mature oocytes for fertilization and subsequent embryo cryopreservation is an established option. Cryopreservation of oocytes, usually 5–10 oocytes per patient, is an alternative for females without a partner but is less successful, with fewer than one baby born per 100 oocytes. In addition, the time needed for ovarian stimulation may be unacceptable for many patients awaiting the initiation of cancer therapy [133]. The options for preserving fertility in prepubertal females remain experimental. The removal of ovarian tissue consisting of germ cells is a potential future option with the possibility of transplantation or *in vitro* maturation.

The feasibility of autologous transplantation has been demonstrated in animals [158]. Reports of successful autologous transplantation have been reported in humans. After orthotopic transplantation of ovarian tissue, spontaneous ovulation in a woman has occurred [159] and also a reported live birth [160]; in addition, human embryonic development has been reported after heterotopic transplantation [161]. The removal and storage of ovarian tissue is a promising option for prepubertal girls and young women.

One approach that has been explored clinically is the use of GnRH analogs based on the hypothesis that prepubertal gonads were quiescent and therefore likely to be less vulnerable to the cytotoxic effects of chemotherapy and radiotherapy which destroy rapidly dividing cells. Despite positive results in rodents, clinical studies in humans have been poorly designed or inadequately powered to produce conclusive results [133].

Research is ongoing into ways of inhibiting the apoptotic pathway that results in oocyte loss with positive results in mice for the use of sphingosine-1-phosphate (S1P) [162].

Predicting fertility

Predicting future fertility in patients who have undergone gonadotoxic therapy is challenging, particularly as patients who have undergone sterilizing cancer therapy can show recovery of spermatogenesis or ovulatory cycles [163,164].

In postpubertal males, semen analysis provides an assessment of spermatogenesis. As modern techniques for assisted conception using intracytoplasmic sperm injection (ICSI) have improved, even men with relatively poor semen quality can be helped to achieve parenthood [165]. In patients reluctant to provide a semen sample, reduced fertility may be predicted by elevated concentrations of follicle stimulating hormone (FSH) and the presence of reduced testicular volumes [166].

In postpubertal females, amenorrhea secondary to premature ovarian failure is strongly suggestive of significant depletion of ovarian follicles, although intermittent ovulation and the risk or chance of conception remain a possibility in a minority of such patients [164]. In females with a menstrual cycle, assessment of fertility potential is more complicated. Ovarian volumes have been reported as being reduced in size in menstruating women previously treated with cancer therapy [167]. The assessment of ovarian volume may allow the prediction of ovarian reserve in menstruating females in the future [168]. Impaired fertility is associated with elevated concentrations of FSH in the early follicular phase despite regular ovulatory cycles.

Inhibin B could be a potential marker of gonadotoxicity. This glycoprotein is secreted from Sertoli cells in males and developing antral follicles in females. It is important in adult spermatogenesis and folliculogenesis and in the regulatory feedback of FSH secretion from the pituitary. Low inhibin B concentrations have been observed in adult males after gonadotoxic chemotherapy [169] and more closely reflect sperm concentration than FSH in males following treatment for childhood Hodgkin lymphoma [170]. Its usefulness in the assessment of children and adolescence is less clear [171].

In females, anti-Mullerian hormone (AMH) concentrations correlate with age and ovarian follicular reserve [172]. AMH concentrations are lower in female survivors of cancer [167] and could potentially have a role in fertility prediction in the future.

Children of cancer survivors

Concerns have been raised that the offspring of childhood cancer survivors may be more at risk of congenital abnormalities or cancer itself [133]. In a large epidemiological study of children resulting from natural conception these fears were unfounded, except in those with familial malignant diseases [173]. Ongoing surveillance is required, particularly for children born as a result of assisted conception.

Evaluation and management

Pubertal staging should be undertaken at 3–6 month intervals until completion of growth and puberty. Testes may be inappropriately small for the stage of pubertal development therefore testicular enlargement cannot be used to monitor pubertal progression in this population. FSH, LH and estradiol/testosterone should be monitored annually in both males and females at risk of gonadal damage. Pelvic ultrasound to monitor uterine size may also provide useful information in females who have received pelvic irradiation.

Testosterone deficiency rarely occurs but patients showing evidence of testicular damage and difficulties progressing through puberty and/or symptoms of testosterone deficiency may need testosterone replacement to complete pubertal maturation.

Ovarian failure requires estrogen replacement in doses appropriate for pubertal stage. As recovery of ovarian function is well documented, estrogen replacement should be discontinued for 6–8 weeks every 2 years to determine whether ovarian recovery has occurred.

In addition, even in patients who have received significant doses of gonadotoxic therapy, recovery of spermatogenesis and ovarian function has been reported [163,164] so it remains important to discuss contraception with patients whose fertility status is uncertain. Close links with fertility services are important both at the time of cancer diagnosis and when the patient reaches sexual maturity and is considering fertility.

Cancer therapy and bone health

Altered bone metabolism during treatment may interfere with attainment of peak bone mass, potentially predisposing to an increased fracture risk. Bone mineral deficits have been reported after treatment of childhood cancers and represent a late effect that is possibly modifiable by attention to lifestyle changes and by optimization of hormone replacement for hypogonadism and GHD [174–178].

The causes of bone loss, diminished bone growth and decreased mineral accrual are secondary to direct and indirect effects of cancer therapy. Direct effects include malignant infiltration, irradiation and certain chemotherapy agents, such as prednisolone and methotrexate [175,179–182]. In addition, suboptimal nutrition and decreased physical activity may also be a factor. Indirect effects include GHD and hypogonadism.

Decreased BMD and reduced markers of bone formation have been demonstrated at diagnosis of ALL [179,183]. Leukemic infiltration is hypothesized to have a direct effect on vitamin D metabolism [179,182]. The treatment of leukemia includes high cumulative doses of corticosteroids, methotrexate and the potential use of CI or BMT and testicular radiation [176,177,181]. High doses of corticosteroids are likely to induce a reduction in BMD which may not recover fully after treatment [176,177,181]. It is possible that the use of dexamethasone has a more deleterious effect than prednisolone on BMD and fracture incidence [184]. Methotrexate has a cytotoxic effect on osteoblasts resulting in reduced bone volume and formation of new bone [185]. There is a dose response, with higher doses (>40 000 mg/m^2) being associated with the highest risk of osteopenia and failure to recover BMD after completion of therapy [181,186].

BMT patients may develop bone mineral deficits secondary to medications used to maintain engraftment and treat complications of BMT, such as cGvHD, or secondary to treatment related endocrinopathies, particularly gonadal failure secondary to alkylating agents or TBI [187–191]. It is unclear if there is an effect of the BMT itself but patients undergoing a BMT are more likely to have additional risk factors such as poor nutrition, decreased physical activity and less exposure to sunshine.

Patients with brain tumors may develop GHD as a consequence of radiation, which is associated with reduced BMD [192]. The data that implicate radiation having a direct effect on the skeleton as a primary risk factor for osteopenia are conflicting. Some investigators have suggested that local radiation and TBI may directly affect BMD by damaging bone marrow stroma [193,194] but this has not been confirmed in other studies [187,189,190]. One study found that the improvement in lumbar spine BMD in response to the osteoanabolic effects of GH did not occur in patients who had received spinal irradiation [195].

Some treatment protocols have been associated with an increased fracture risk during or shortly after therapy. Strauss *et al.* [184] reported a 5-year cumulative incidence of fractures of 28% among pediatric patients with ALL (median follow-up 7.6 years since diagnosis). Halton *et al.* [179] followed 40 children with ALL and 39% developed fractures during treatment, with decreased bone mineral content predicting development of fractures. Less is known of the fracture risk in long-term survivors.

Most survivors recover bone mass with increasing time off therapy [196] but a proportion demonstrate significant bone density deficits (Z score <−2.5 SD) years after therapy [197–199].

Evaluation and management
Screening
All cancer survivors who have received methotrexate, corticosteroids or BMT or have developed an endocrinopathy associated with bone mineral deficits should undergo screening at baseline and 2 years after the completion of cancer therapy. As BMD improves in the years following the completion of cancer therapy, the baseline result will dictate whether follow-up is necessary. If the patient sustains fractures or has an ongoing risk for developing bone mineral deficits, such as corticosteroids for cGvHD or an endocrinopathy, follow-up of BMD is essential.

The International Society of Clinical Densitometry has recommended that the terms osteopenia and osteoporosis should not be used to describe low BMD in children and adolescents. The rationale for this recommendation is that the terms are defined using T scores (SD scores) which compare the patient to young adults who have already achieved peak bone mass. They are therefore appropriate for an older patient but not for children and adolescents who have yet to achieve peak bone mass. The Z score (SD score) compares the BMD of the patient with age and gender matched normal values and is a more appropriate measurement for children and adolescents.

Measuring BMD in this age group is challenging. Dual energy X-ray absorptiometry (DXA) is most frequently used but has limitations. The calculation of Z score is based on age and gender and does not take into consideration the effect of height and pubertal stage, which may not correspond with a healthy child in a cancer survivor. In addition, density is measured as mass/unit volume whereas DXA calculations are based on an area measurement (g/cm^2) and are unable to measure bone thickness to calculate a volumetric measurement (g/cm^3). Thus, for children with short stature, DXA underestimates BMD. Methods have been developed to calculate an estimated volume from DXA measurements and, as fracture risk in healthy children has been found to be associated with volumetric BMD calculated by DXA, this approach is recommended when interpreting pediatric DXA results.

An alternative is quantitative computed tomography (QCT), which provides a direct and more accurate volumetric measurement of BMD eliminating problems with interpretation in short-for-age children. This technique also assesses trabecular bone (the metabolically more active compartment) separately from cortical bone but this method is less readily available and involves increased concentrations of radiation compared to DXA, which is comparable with that of a chest radiograph. Peripheral QCT is emerging as an alternative but has yet to be validated and standardized in a pediatric population.

An awareness of the possibility of osteonecrosis in patients who have received a BMT should prompt early investigation of persistent joint pain, particularly in the hips or knees. Magnetic resonance imaging (MRI) is the investigation of choice.

Lifestyle advice

Children and adolescents should be advised to increase weight-bearing exercise as tolerated and to optimize nutritional intake of calcium and vitamin D. Advice should be given about smoking, alcohol and caffeine consumption but there is no evidence that these measures alter outcome.

Hormone replacement

In patients with endocrinopathies associated with bone mineral deficits optimization of hormone replacement is important. The dosage of sex steroid replacement should be reviewed regularly. GH therapy should be continued or reintroduced after the completion of linear growth in GHD adolescents to aid the achievement of peak bone mass.

Cancer therapy and cardiovascular risk

Cardiopulmonary disease is the third most common cause of death in childhood cancer survivors, with recurrence of primary malignancy and SMNs being the two most common causes. Although the direct cardiotoxic effects of cancer therapy, for instance, anthracycline and mediastinal irradiation, are responsible for the majority of cardiac morbidity and mortality, it is well recognized that childhood cancer survivors also have increased cardiovascular risk secondary to metabolic abnormalities which may have implications in adult life.

Following mediastinal irradiation, 10% of patients have been reported to have symptomatic coronary artery disease after a median of 9 years follow-up [200]. The risk was increased by dyslipidemia, hypertension, smoking and obesity [200,201].

Patients who have received high-dose neck irradiation for head and neck cancers are at a 10-fold increased risk of carotid artery occlusive disease and stroke [202]. In a study of long-term survivors of childhood Hodgkin disease there was a fivefold increased risk of stroke compared with sibling controls [203]. A significantly increased risk of stroke has also been reported in survivors of childhood leukemia and brain tumors, particularly in those who received >30 Gy of CI [204].

Several metabolic abnormalities have been reported in survivors of childhood cancer. In particular, survivors of ALL are at increased risk of developing metabolic syndrome. One study of adult survivors of ALL found that 30% had obesity or dyslipidemia and 20% had hypertension or insulin resistance. In another study, 16% of childhood cancer survivors, predominantly ALL, had metabolic syndrome. However, these studies reflected ALL treatment prior to 1990 when higher doses of CI were administered routinely for CNS prophylaxis and the adverse cardiovascular risk factors were more prevalent in patients with GHD following CI. Other studies have clearly linked both obesity and hypertension in this cohort with the use of CI (>20 Gy).

An examination of the effect of more contemporary regimens on 165 patients with ALL found that 17% were overweight at the completion of cancer therapy, 21.2% were obese and 15.3% had hypertension [205]. These proportions remained unchanged after 2–3 years, although no long-term follow-up data into adulthood were available. The most significant factor was higher concentrations of corticosteroid exposure with no effect of CI which in this study was at the lower dose of 18 Gy. The study confirmed that female patients and those treated at an earlier age were more at risk of elevated body mass index (BMI) and raised blood pressure. Therefore, despite reduction in the use of CI there is still an increased risk of obesity and hypertension in survivors of ALL which is predominantly related to the much higher doses of corticosteroids used in contemporary regimens, a 60–80% increase since the 1970s, and some studies have also shown that the choice of corticosteroid may also be a factor with greater weight gain during therapy with dexamethasone than prednisone. Dexamethasone is more frequently used than prednisone because of its longer duration of action and better CNS penetration.

Long-term survivors of BMT are at risk of insulin resistance, type 2 diabetes and hypertriglyceridemia [206]. Pancreatic dysfunction may occur after BMT in the setting of a normal BMI. Type 2 diabetes has also been reported following abdominal irradiation for Wilms tumors [207].

Of 148 survivors of childhood brain tumor, age at diagnosis, radiation dose to the hypothalamus (51–72 Gy) and presence of any endocrinopathy were identified as risk factors for developing obesity [208]. Additional factors when BMI was compared with the slope for the general US population included tumor location (hypothalamic, $P < 0.001$), histology (craniopharyngioma, $P < 0.009$; pilocytic astrocytoma, $P < 0.043$; medulloblastoma, $P < 0.039$) and extent of surgery (biopsy, $P < 0.03$; subtotal resection, $P < 0.018$). Hypothalamic damage from the surgery or following radiation were prime factors in the etiology of obesity. In females, the risk of obesity was associated with younger age at diagnosis (<10 years) and increased radiation dosage.

Evaluation and management
Lifestyle advice

Patient education and counseling are important. By encouraging a healthy lifestyle through diet and exercise it may be possible to modify risk factors such as obesity, dyslipidemia and hypertension. Advice about not smoking is essential.

Monitoring

Regular assessments of BMI and waist : hip ratio are recommended, as well as monitoring of blood pressure, fasting glucose and lipid profile, particularly in those who have received mediastinal irradiation.

Hormone replacement

In patients with GHD, GH therapy may aid normalization of body composition , improve lipid profile and other adverse cardiovascular risk factors.

Summary and conclusions

Late effects of cancer therapy are diverse in their effect on the endocrine system. The resultant morbidity has implications throughout life.

Clinicians should focus on growth and puberty but knowledge of the impact of CI on the HP axis and thyroid irradiation and the increased incidence of thyroid nodules and malignancy is essential. In addition, future risk to reproductive, skeletal and cardiovascular health should be reduced by early consideration of fertility options, lifestyle advice, optimization of hormone replacement and ensuring a smooth transition to an adult endocrinologist for ongoing care.

References

1 Skinner R, Wallace WH, Levitt G. Long-term follow-up of children treated for cancer: why is it necessary, by whom, where and how? *Arch Dis Child* 2007; **92**: 257–260.

2 Oeffinger KC, Mertens AC, Sklar CA, Kawashima T, Hudson MM, Meadows AT, *et al.* Chronic health conditions in adult survivors of childhood cancer. *N Engl J Med* 2006; **355**: 1572–1582.

3 Geenen MM, Cardous-Ubbink MC, Kremer LC, van den Bos C, van der Pal HJ, Heinen RC, *et al.* Medical assessment of adverse health outcomes in long-term survivors of childhood cancer. *JAMA* 2007; **297**: 2705–2715.

4 Gurney JG, Kadan-Lottick NS, Packer RJ, Neglia JP, Sklar CA, Punyko JA, *et al.* Endocrine and cardiovascular late effects among adult survivors of childhood brain tumors: Childhood Cancer Survivor Study. *Cancer* 2003; **97**: 663–673.

5 Fowler JF. The linear-quadratic formula and progress in fractionated radiotherapy. *Br J Radiol* 1989; **62**: 679–694.

6 Yeung SC, Chiu AC, Vassilopoulou-Sellin R, Gagel RF. The endocrine effects of nonhormonal antineoplastic therapy. *Endocr Rev* 1998; **19**: 144–172.

7 Clayton PE, Shalet SM. Dose dependency of time of onset of radiation-induced growth hormone deficiency. *J Pediatr* 1991; **118**: 226–228.

8 Gleeson HK, Gattamaneni HR, Smethurst L, Brennan BM, Shalet SM. Reassessment of growth hormone status is required at final height in children treated with growth hormone replacement after radiation therapy. *J Clin Endocrinol Metab* 2004; **89**: 662–666.

9 Darzy KH, Shalet SM. Radiation-induced growth hormone deficiency. *Horm Res* 2003; **59** (Suppl 1): 1–11.

10 Brennan BM, Shalet SM. Endocrine late effects after bone marrow transplant. *Br J Haematol* 2002; **118**: 58–66.

11 Dacou-Voutetakis C, Kitra V, Grafakos S, Polychronopoulou S, Drakopoulou M, Haidas S. Auxologic data and hormonal profile in long-term survivors of childhood acute lymphoid leukemia. *Am J Pediatr Hematol Oncol* 1993; **15**: 277–283.

12 Davies HA, Didcock E, Didi M, Ogilvy-Stuart A, Wales JK, Shalet SM. Growth, puberty and obesity after treatment for leukaemia. *Acta Paediatr Suppl* 1995; **411**: 45–50; discussion 51.

13 Schmiegelow M, Lassen S, Poulsen HS, Feldt-Rasmussen U, Schmiegelow K, Hertz H, *et al.* Cranial radiotherapy of childhood brain tumours: growth hormone deficiency and its relation to the biological effective dose of irradiation in a large population based study. *Clin Endocrinol (Oxf)* 2000; **53**: 191–197.

14 Adan L, Trivin C, Sainte-Rose C, Zucker JM, Hartmann O, Brauner R. GH deficiency caused by cranial irradiation during childhood: factors and markers in young adults. *J Clin Endocrinol Metab* 2001; **86**: 5245–5251.

15 Littley MD, Shalet SM, Morgenstern GR, Deakin DP. Endocrine and reproductive dysfunction following fractionated total body irradiation in adults. *Q J Med* 1991; **78**: 265–274.

16 Darzy KH, Pezzoli SS, Thorner MO, Shalet SM. The dynamics of growth hormone (GH) secretion in adult cancer survivors with severe GH deficiency acquired after brain irradiation in childhood for nonpituitary brain tumors: evidence for preserved pulsatility and diurnal variation with increased secretory disorderliness. *J Clin Endocrinol Metab* 2005; **90**: 2794–2803.

17 Darzy KH, Murray RD, Gleeson HK, Pezzoli SS, Thorner MO, Shalet SM. The impact of short-term fasting on the dynamics of 24-hour growth hormone (GH) secretion in patients with severe radiation-induced GH deficiency. *J Clin Endocrinol Metab* 2006; **91**: 987–994.

18 Darzy KH, Pezzoli SS, Thorner MO, Shalet SM. Cranial irradiation and growth hormone neurosecretory dysfunction: a critical appraisal. *J Clin Endocrinol Metab* 2007; **92**: 1666–1672.

19 Lam KS, Tse VK, Wang C, Yeung RT, Ho JH. Effects of cranial irradiation on hypothalamic-pituitary function: a 5-year longitudinal study in patients with nasopharyngeal carcinoma. *Q J Med* 1991; **78**: 165–176.

20 Paulino AC, Simon JH, Zhen W, Wen BC. Long-term effects in children treated with radiotherapy for head and neck rhabdomyosarcoma. *Int J Radiat Oncol Biol Phys* 2000; **48**: 1489–1495.

21 Littley MD, Shalet SM, Beardwell CG, Ahmed SR, Applegate G, Sutton ML. Hypopituitarism following external radiotherapy for pituitary tumours in adults. *Q J Med* 1989; **70**: 145–160.

22 Robinson IC, Fairhall KM, Hendry JH, Shalet SM. Differential radiosensitivity of hypothalamo-pituitary function in the young adult rat. *J Endocrinol* 2001; **169**: 519–526.

23 Chrousos GP, Poplack D, Brown T, O'Neill D, Schwade J, Bercu BB. Effects of cranial radiation on hypothalamic-adenohypophyseal function: abnormal growth hormone secretory dynamics. *J Clin Endocrinol Metab* 1982; **54**: 1135–1139.

24 Spoudeas HA, Charmandari E, Brook CG. Hypothalamo-pituitary-adrenal axis integrity after cranial irradiation for childhood posterior fossa tumours. *Med Pediatr Oncol* 2003; **40**: 224–229.

25 Schmiegelow M, Feldt-Rasmussen U, Rasmussen AK, Lange M, Poulsen HS, Muller J. Assessment of the hypothalamo-pituitary-adrenal axis in patients treated with radiotherapy and chemotherapy for childhood brain tumor. *J Clin Endocrinol Metab* 2003; **88**: 3149–3154.

26 Darzy KH, Shalet SM. Absence of adrenocorticotropin (ACTH) neurosecretory dysfunction but increased cortisol concentrations and production rates in ACTH-replete adult cancer survivors after cranial irradiation for nonpituitary brain tumors. *J Clin Endocrinol Metab* 2005; **90**: 5217–5225.

27 Livesey EA, Brook CG. Thyroid dysfunction after radiotherapy and chemotherapy of brain tumours. *Arch Dis Child* 1989; **64**: 593–595.

28 Schmiegelow M, Feldt-Rasmussen U, Rasmussen AK, Poulsen HS, Muller J. A population-based study of thyroid function after radiotherapy and chemotherapy for a childhood brain tumor. *J Clin Endocrinol Metab* 2003; **88**: 136–140.

29 Rose SR, Lustig RH, Pitukcheewanont P, Broome DC, Burghen GA, Li H, *et al.* Diagnosis of hidden central hypothyroidism in survivors of childhood cancer. *J Clin Endocrinol Metab* 1999; **84**: 4472–4479.

30 Darzy KH, Shalet SM. Circadian and stimulated thyrotropin secretion in cranially irradiated adult cancer survivors. *J Clin Endocrinol Metab* 2005; **90**: 6490–6497.

31 Xu W, Janss A, Moshang T. Adult height and adult sitting height in childhood medulloblastoma survivors. *J Clin Endocrinol Metab* 2003; **88**: 4677–4681.

32 Gurney JG, Ness KK, Stovall M, Wolden S, Punyko JA, Neglia JP, *et al.* Final height and body mass index among adult survivors of childhood brain cancer: Childhood Cancer Survivor Study. *J Clin Endocrinol Metab* 2003; **88**: 4731–4739.

33 Muller J. Disturbance of pubertal development after cancer treatment. *Best Pract Res Clin Endocrinol Metab* 2002; **16**: 91–103.

34 Heikens J, Michiels EM, Behrendt H, Endert E, Bakker PJ, Fliers E. Long-term neuro-endocrine sequelae after treatment for childhood medulloblastoma. *Eur J Cancer* 1998; **34**: 1592–1597.

35 Ogilvy-Stuart AL, Clayton PE, Shalet SM. Cranial irradiation and early puberty. *J Clin Endocrinol Metab* 1994; **78**: 1282–1286.

36 Darzy KH, Aimaretti G, Wieringa G, Gattamaneni HR, Ghigo E, Shalet SM. The usefulness of the combined growth hormone (GH)-releasing hormone and arginine stimulation test in the diagnosis of radiation-induced GH deficiency is dependent on the post-irradiation time interval. *J Clin Endocrinol Metab* 2003; **88**: 95–102.

37 Ogilvy-Stuart AL, Stirling HF, Kelnar CJ, Savage MO, Dunger DB, Buckler JM, *et al.* Treatment of radiation-induced growth hormone deficiency with growth hormone-releasing hormone. *Clin Endocrinol (Oxf)* 1997; **46**: 571–578.

38 Birkebaek NH, Clausen N. Height and weight pattern up to 20 years after treatment for acute lymphoblastic leukaemia. *Arch Dis Child* 1998; **79**: 161–164.

39 Bongers ME, Francken AB, Rouwe C, Kamps WA, Postma A. Reduction of adult height in childhood acute lymphoblastic leukemia survivors after prophylactic cranial irradiation. *Pediatr Blood Cancer* 2005; **45**: 139–143.

40 Hokken-Koelega AC, van Doorn JW, Hahlen K, Stijnen T, de Muinck Keizer-Schrama SM, Drop SL. Long-term effects of treatment for acute lymphoblastic leukemia with and without cranial irradiation on growth and puberty: a comparative study. *Pediatr Res* 1993; **33**: 577–582.

41 Katz JA, Pollock BH, Jacaruso D, Morad A. Final attained height in patients successfully treated for childhood acute lymphoblastic leukemia. *J Pediatr* 1993; **123**: 546–552.

42 Starceski PJ, Lee PA, Blatt J, Finegold D, Brown D. Comparable effects of 1800- and 2400-rad (18- and 24-Gy) cranial irradiation on height and weight in children treated for acute lymphocytic leukemia. *Am J Dis Child* 1987; **141**: 550–552.

43 Holm K, Nysom K, Hertz H, Muller J. Normal final height after treatment for acute lymphoblastic leukemia without irradiation. *Acta Paediatr* 1994; **83**: 1287–1290.

44 Dalton VK, Rue M, Silverman LB, Gelber RD, Asselin BL, Barr RD, *et al.* Height and weight in children treated for acute lymphoblastic leukemia: relationship to CNS treatment. *J Clin Oncol* 2003; **21**: 2953–2960.

45 Sklar C, Mertens A, Walter A, Mitchell D, Nesbit M, O'Leary M, *et al.* Final height after treatment for childhood acute lymphoblastic

leukemia: comparison of no cranial irradiation with 1800 and 2400 centigrays of cranial irradiation. *J Pediatr* 1993; **123**: 59–64.

46 Chow EJ, Friedman DL, Yasui Y, Whitton JA, Stovall M, Robison LL *et al.* Decreased adult height in survivors of childhood acute lymphoblastic leukemia: a report from the Childhood Cancer Survivor Study. *J Pediatr* 2007; **150**: 370–375.

47 Schriock EA, Schell MJ, Carter M, Hustu O, Ochs JJ. Abnormal growth patterns and adult short stature in 115 long-term survivors of childhood leukemia. *J Clin Oncol* 1991; **9**: 400–405.

48 Wingard JR, Plotnick LP, Freemer CS, Zahurak M, Piantadosi S, Miller DF, *et al.* Growth in children after bone marrow transplantation: busulfan plus cyclophosphamide versus cyclophosphamide plus total body irradiation. *Blood* 1992; **79**: 1068–1073.

49 Giorgiani G, Bozzola M, Locatelli F, Picco P, Zecca M, Cisternino M, *et al.* Role of busulfan and total body irradiation on growth of prepubertal children receiving bone marrow transplantation and results of treatment with recombinant human growth hormone. *Blood* 1995; **86**: 825–831.

50 Shankar SM, Bunin NJ, Moshang T Jr. Growth in children undergoing bone marrow transplantation after busulfan and cyclophosphamide conditioning. *J Pediatr Hematol Oncol* 1996; **18**: 362–366.

51 Cicognani A, Cacciari E, Vecchi V, Cau M, Balsamo A, Pirazzoli P, *et al.* Differential effects of 18- and 24-Gy cranial irradiation on growth rate and growth hormone release in children with prolonged survival after acute lymphocytic leukemia. *Am J Dis Child* 1988; **142**: 1199–1202.

52 Clayton PE, Shalet SM, Morris-Jones PH, Price DA. Growth in children treated for acute lymphoblastic leukaemia. *Lancet* 1988; **1**: 460–462.

53 Davies HA, Didcock E, Didi M, Ogilvy-Stuart A, Wales JK, Shalet SM. Disproportionate short stature after cranial irradiation and combination chemotherapy for leukaemia. *Arch Dis Child* 1994; **70**: 472–475.

54 Groot-Loonen JJ, van Setten P, Otten BJ, van 't Hof MA, Lippens RJ, Stoelinga GB. Shortened and diminished pubertal growth in boys and girls treated for acute lymphoblastic leukaemia. *Acta Paediatr* 1996; **85**: 1091–1095.

55 Hata M, Ogino I, Aida N, Saito K, Omura M, Kigasawa H, *et al.* Prophylactic cranial irradiation of acute lymphoblastic leukemia in childhood: outcomes of late effects on pituitary function and growth in long-term survivors. *Int J Cancer* 2001; **96** (Suppl): 117–124.

56 Robison LL, Nesbit ME Jr, Sather HN, Meadows AT, Ortega JA, Hammond GD. Height of children successfully treated for acute lymphoblastic leukemia: a report from the Late Effects Study Committee of Childrens Cancer Study Group. *Med Pediatr Oncol* 1985; **13**: 14–21.

57 Stubberfield TG, Byrne GC, Jones TW. Growth and growth hormone secretion after treatment for acute lymphoblastic leukemia in childhood. 18-Gy versus 24-Gy cranial irradiation. *J Pediatr Hematol Oncol* 1995; **17**: 167–171.

58 Uruena M, Stanhope R, Chessells JM, Leiper AD. Impaired pubertal growth in acute lymphoblastic leukaemia. *Arch Dis Child* 1991; **66**: 1403–1407.

59 Clement-De Boers A, Oostdijk W, Van Weel-Sipman MH, Van den Broeck J, Wit JM, Vossen JM. Final height and hormonal function after bone marrow transplantation in children. *J Pediatr* 1996; **129**: 544–550.

60 Cohen A, Rovelli R, Zecca S, Van-Lint MT, Parodi L, Grasso L et al. Endocrine late effects in children who underwent bone marrow transplantation: review. *Bone Marrow Transplant* 1998; **21** (Suppl 2): S64–67.

61 Nikoskelainen J, Koskela K, Katka K, Pelliniemi TT, Kulmala J, Salmi T, et al. Allogeneic bone marrow transplantation in multiple myeloma: a report of four cases. *Bone Marrow Transplant* 1988; **3**: 495–500.

62 Sanders JE, Guthrie KA, Hoffmeister PA, Woolfrey AE, Carpenter PA, Appelbaum FR. Final adult height of patients who received hematopoietic cell transplantation in childhood. *Blood* 2005; **105**: 1348–1354.

63 Shalet SM, Gibson B, Swindell R, Pearson D. Effect of spinal irradiation on growth. *Arch Dis Child* 1987; **62**: 461–464.

64 Shalet SM, Clayton PE, Price DA. Growth and pituitary function in children treated for brain tumours or acute lymphoblastic leukaemia. *Horm Res* 1988; **30**: 53–61.

65 Shalet SM, Clayton PE, Price DA. Growth impairment following treatment for childhood brain tumours. *Acta Paediatr Scand Suppl* 1988; **343**: 137–145.

66 Gleeson HK, Stoeter R, Ogilvy-Stuart AL, Gattamaneni HR, Brennan BM, Shalet SM. Improvements in final height over 25 years in growth hormone (GH)-deficient childhood survivors of brain tumors receiving GH replacement. *J Clin Endocrinol Metab* 2003; **88**: 3682–3689.

67 Adan L, Sainte-Rose C, Souberbielle JC, Zucker JM, Kalifa C, Brauner R. Adult height after growth hormone (GH) treatment for GH deficiency due to cranial irradiation. *Med Pediatr Oncol* 2000; **34**: 14–19.

68 Swerdlow AJ, Reddingius RE, Higgins CD, Spoudeas HA, Phipps K, Qiao Z, et al. Growth hormone treatment of children with brain tumors and risk of tumor recurrence. *J Clin Endocrinol Metab* 2000; **85**: 4444–4449.

69 Sklar CA, Mertens AC, Mitby P, Occhiogrosso G, Qin J, Heller G, et al. Risk of disease recurrence and second neoplasms in survivors of childhood cancer treated with growth hormone: a report from the Childhood Cancer Survivor Study. *J Clin Endocrinol Metab* 2002; **87**: 3136–3141.

70 Ergun-Longmire B, Mertens AC, Mitby P, Qin J, Heller G, Shi W, et al. Growth hormone treatment and risk of second neoplasms in the childhood cancer survivor. *J Clin Endocrinol Metab* 2006; **91**: 3494–3498.

71 Sklar C. Paying the price for cure-treating cancer survivors with growth hormone. *J Clin Endocrinol Metab* 2000; **85**: 4441–4443.

72 Ham JN, Ginsberg JP, Hendell CD, Moshang T Jr. Growth hormone releasing hormone plus arginine stimulation testing in young adults treated in childhood with cranio-spinal radiation therapy. *Clin Endocrinol (Oxf)* 2005; **62**: 628–632.

73 Clayton PE, Cuneo RC, Juul A, Monson JP, Shalet SM, Tauber M. Consensus statement on the management of the GH-treated adolescent in the transition to adult care. *Eur J Endocrinol* 2005; **152**: 165–170.

74 Mericq V, Gajardo H, Eggers M, Avila A, Cassorla F. Effects of treatment with GH alone or in combination with LHRH analog on bone mineral density in pubertal GH-deficient patients. *J Clin Endocrinol Metab* 2002; **87**: 84–89.

75 Clayton P, Gleeson H, Monson J, Popovic V, Shalet SM, Christiansen JS. Growth hormone replacement throughout life:

76 Murray RD, Darzy KH, Gleeson HK, Shalet SM. GH-deficient survivors of childhood cancer: GH replacement during adult life. *J Clin Endocrinol Metab* 2002; **87**: 129–135.

77 Follin C, Thilen U, Ahren B, Erfurth EM. Improvement in cardiac systolic function and reduced prevalence of metabolic syndrome after two years of growth hormone (GH) treatment in GH-deficient adult survivors of childhood-onset acute lymphoblastic leukemia. *J Clin Endocrinol Metab* 2006; **91**: 1872–1875.

78 Barnes ND. Effects of external irradiation on the thyroid gland in childhood. *Horm Res* 1988; **30**: 84–89.

79 Hancock SL, Cox RS, McDougall IR. Thyroid diseases after treatment of Hodgkin's disease. *N Engl J Med* 1991; **325**: 599–605.

80 Sklar C, Whitton J, Mertens A, Stovall M, Green D, Marina N, et al. Abnormalities of the thyroid in survivors of Hodgkin's disease: data from the Childhood Cancer Survivor Study. *J Clin Endocrinol Metab* 2000; **85**: 3227–3232.

81 Black P, Straaten A, Gutjahr P. Secondary thyroid carcinoma after treatment for childhood cancer. *Med Pediatr Oncol* 1998; **31**: 91–95.

82 Rubino C, Adjadj E, Guerin S, Guibout C, Shamsaldin A, Dondon MG, et al. Long-term risk of second malignant neoplasms after neuroblastoma in childhood: role of treatment. *Int J Cancer* 2003; **107**: 791–796.

83 Metayer C, Lynch CF, Clarke EA, Glimelius B, Storm H, Pukkala E, et al. Second cancers among long-term survivors of Hodgkin's disease diagnosed in childhood and adolescence. *J Clin Oncol* 2000; **18**: 2435–2443.

84 Neglia JP, Friedman DL, Yasui Y, Mertens AC, Hammond S, Stovall M, et al. Second malignant neoplasms in five-year survivors of childhood cancer: Childhood Cancer Survivor Study. *J Natl Cancer Inst* 2001; **93**: 618–629.

85 Acharya S, Sarafoglou K, LaQuaglia M, Lindsley S, Gerald W, Wollner N, et al. Thyroid neoplasms after therapeutic radiation for malignancies during childhood or adolescence. *Cancer* 2003; **97**: 2397–2403.

86 Bhatia S, Sklar C. Second cancers in survivors of childhood cancer. *Nat Rev Cancer* 2002; **2**: 124–132.

87 Moppett J, Oakhill A, Duncan AW. Second malignancies in children: the usual suspects? *Eur J Radiol* 2001; **37**: 95–108.

88 Garwicz S, Anderson H, Olsen JH, Dollner H, Hertz H, Jonmundsson G, et al. Second malignant neoplasms after cancer in childhood and adolescence: a population-based case–control study in the 5 Nordic countries. The Nordic Society for Pediatric Hematology and Oncology. The Association of the Nordic Cancer Registries. *Int J Cancer* 2000; **88**: 672–678.

89 Boulad F, Bromley M, Black P, Heller G, Sarafoglou K, Gillio A, et al. Thyroid dysfunction following bone marrow transplantation using hyperfractionated radiation. *Bone Marrow Transplant* 1995; **15**: 71–76.

90 Socie G, Curtis RE, Deeg HJ, Sobocinski KA, Filipovich AH, Travis LB, et al. New malignant diseases after allogeneic marrow transplantation for childhood acute leukemia. *J Clin Oncol* 2000; **18**: 348–357.

91 Sigurdson AJ, Ronckers CM, Mertens AC, Stovall M, Smith SA, Liu Y, et al. Primary thyroid cancer after a first tumour in childhood (the Childhood Cancer Survivor Study): a nested case–control study. *Lancet* 2005; **365**: 2014–2023.

92 Ron E, Lubin JH, Shore RE, Mabuchi K, Modan B, Pottern LM, et al. Thyroid cancer after exposure to external radiation: a pooled analysis of seven studies. *Radiat Res* 1995; **141**: 259–277.

93 Inskip PD. Thyroid cancer after radiotherapy for childhood cancer. *Med Pediatr Oncol* 2001; **36**: 568–573.

94 Michel G, Socie G, Gebhard F, Bernaudin F, Thuret I, Vannier JP, et al. Late effects of allogeneic bone marrow transplantation for children with acute myeloblastic leukemia in first complete remission: the impact of conditioning regimen without total-body irradiation. A report from the Societe Francaise de Greffe de Moelle. *J Clin Oncol* 1997; **15**: 2238–2246.

95 Toubert ME, Socie G, Gluckman E, Aractingi S, Esperou H, Devergie A, et al. Short- and long-term follow-up of thyroid dysfunction after allogeneic bone marrow transplantation without the use of preparative total body irradiation. *Br J Haematol* 1997; **98**: 453–457.

96 Al-Fiar FZ, Colwill R, Lipton JH, Fyles G, Spaner D, Messner H. Abnormal thyroid stimulating hormone (TSH) concentrations in adults following allogeneic bone marrow transplants. *Bone Marrow Transplant* 1997; **19**: 1019–1022.

97 Katsanis E, Shapiro RS, Robison LL, Haake RJ, Kim T, Pescovitz OH, et al. Thyroid dysfunction following bone marrow transplantation: long-term follow-up of 80 pediatric patients. *Bone Marrow Transplant* 1990; **5**: 335–340.

98 Ogilvy-Stuart AL, Clark DJ, Wallace WH, Gibson BE, Stevens RF, Shalet SM, et al. Endocrine deficit after fractionated total body irradiation. *Arch Dis Child* 1992; **67**: 1107–1110.

99 Borgstrom B, Bolme P. Thyroid function in children after allogeneic bone marrow transplantation. *Bone Marrow Transplant* 1994; **13**: 59–64.

100 Ishiguro H, Yasuda Y, Tomita Y, Shinagawa T, Shimizu T, Morimoto T, et al. Long-term follow-up of thyroid function in patients who received bone marrow transplantation during childhood and adolescence. *J Clin Endocrinol Metab* 2004; **89**: 5981–5986.

101 Matsumoto M, Ishiguro H, Tomita Y, Inoue H, Yasuda Y, Shimizu T, et al. Changes in thyroid function after bone marrow transplant in young patients. *Pediatr Int* 2004; **46**: 291–295.

102 Oberfield SE, Allen JC, Pollack J, New MI, Levine LS. Long-term endocrine sequelae after treatment of medulloblastoma: prospective study of growth and thyroid function. *J Pediatr* 1986; **108**: 219–223.

103 Ogilvy-Stuart AL, Shalet SM, Gattamaneni HR. Thyroid function after treatment of brain tumors in children. *J Pediatr* 1991; **119**: 733–737.

104 van Santen HM, Vulsma T, Dijkgraaf MG, Blumer RM, Heinen R, Jaspers MW, et al. No damaging effect of chemotherapy in addition to radiotherapy on the thyroid axis in young adult survivors of childhood cancer. *J Clin Endocrinol Metab* 2003; **88**: 3657–3663.

105 Field JB, Bloom G, Chou MC, Kerins ME, Larsen PR, Kotani M, et al. Effects of thyroid-stimulating hormone on human thyroid carcinoma and adjacent normal tissue. *J Clin Endocrinol Metab* 1978; **47**: 1052–1058.

106 Rivas M, Santisteban P. TSH-activated signaling pathways in thyroid tumorigenesis. *Mol Cell Endocrinol* 2003; **213**: 31–45.

107 Favre-Schmuziger G, Hofer S, Passweg J, Tichelli A, Hoffmann T, Speck B, et al. Treatment of solid tumors following allogeneic bone marrow transplantation. *Bone Marrow Transplant* 2000; **25**: 895–898.

108 Cohen A, Rovelli A, van Lint MT, Merlo F, Gaiero A, Mulas R, et al. Secondary thyroid carcinoma after allogeneic bone marrow transplantation during childhood. *Bone Marrow Transplant* 2001; **28**: 1125–1128.

109 de Vathaire F, Hardiman C, Shamsaldin A, Campbell S, Grimaud E, Hawkins M, et al. Thyroid carcinomas after irradiation for a first cancer during childhood. *Arch Intern Med* 1999; **159**: 2713–2719.

110 Tucker MA, Jones PH, Boice JD Jr, Robison LL, Stone BJ, Stovall M, et al. Therapeutic radiation at a young age is linked to secondary thyroid cancer. The Late Effects Study Group. *Cancer Res* 1991; **51**: 2885–2888.

111 Shafford EA, Kingston JE, Healy JC, Webb JA, Plowman PN, Reznek RH. Thyroid nodular disease after radiotherapy to the neck for childhood Hodgkin's disease. *Br J Cancer* 1999; **80**: 808–814.

112 Crom DB, Kaste SC, Tubergen DG, Greenwald CA, Sharp GB, Hudson MM. Ultrasonography for thyroid screening after head and neck irradiation in childhood cancer survivors. *Med Pediatr Oncol* 1997; **28**: 15–21.

113 Vane D, King DR, Boles ET Jr. Secondary thyroid neoplasms in pediatric cancer patients: increased risk with improved survival. *J Pediatr Surg* 1984; **19**: 855–860.

114 Fleming ID, Black TL, Thompson EI, Pratt C, Rao B, Hustu O. Thyroid dysfunction and neoplasia in children receiving neck irradiation for cancer. *Cancer* 1985; **55**: 1190–1194.

115 Kaplan MM, Garnick MB, Gelber R, Li FP, Cassady JR, Sallan SE, et al. Risk factors for thyroid abnormalities after neck irradiation for childhood cancer. *Am J Med* 1983; **74**: 272–280.

116 Hatipoglu BA, Gierlowski T, Shore-Freedman E, Recant W, Schneider AB. Fine-needle aspiration of thyroid nodules in radiation-exposed patients. *Thyroid* 2000; **10**: 63–69.

117 Rosen IB, Azadian A, Walfish PG, Salem S, Lansdown E, Bedard YC. Ultrasound-guided fine-needle aspiration biopsy in the management of thyroid disease. *Am J Surg* 1993; **166**: 346–349.

118 Ron E, Modan B, Preston D, Alfandary E, Stovall M, Boice JD Jr. Thyroid neoplasia following low-dose radiation in childhood. *Radiat Res* 1989; **120**: 516–531.

119 Maxon HR, Thomas SR, Saenger EL, Buncher CR, Kereiakes JG. Ionizing irradiation and the induction of clinically significant disease in the human thyroid gland. *Am J Med* 1977; **63**: 967–978.

120 Gold DG, Neglia JP, Dusenbery KE. Second neoplasms after megavoltage radiation for pediatric tumors. *Cancer* 2003; **97**: 2588–2596.

121 Schneider AB, Ron E, Lubin J, Stovall M, Gierlowski TC. Dose–response relationships for radiation-induced thyroid cancer and thyroid nodules: evidence for the prolonged effects of radiation on the thyroid. *J Clin Endocrinol Metab* 1993; **77**: 362–369.

122 Rubino C, Cailleux AF, De Vathaire F, Schlumberger M. Thyroid cancer after radiation exposure. *Eur J Cancer* 2002; **38**: 645–647.

123 Samaan NA, Schultz PN, Ordonez NG, Hickey RC, Johnston DA. A comparison of thyroid carcinoma in those who have and have not had head and neck irradiation in childhood. *J Clin Endocrinol Metab* 1987; **64**: 219–223.

124 Robinson E, Neugut AI. The clinical behavior of radiation-induced thyroid cancer in patients with prior Hodgkin's disease. *Radiother Oncol* 1990; **17**: 109–113.

125 Roudebush CP, Asteris GT, DeGroot LJ. Natural history of radiation-associated thyroid cancer. *Arch Intern Med* 1978; **138**: 1631–1634.

126 Bounacer A, Wicker R, Caillou B, Cailleux AF, Sarasin A, Schlumberger M *et al.* High prevalence of activating ret proto-oncogene rearrangements, in thyroid tumors from patients who had external radiation. *Oncogene* 1997; **15**: 1263–1273.

127 Rabes HM, Demidchik EP, Sidorow JD, Lengfelder E, Beimfohr C, Hoelzel D, *et al.* Pattern of radiation-induced RET and NTRK1 rearrangements in 191 post-chernobyl papillary thyroid carcinomas: biological, phenotypic and clinical implications. *Clin Cancer Res* 2000; **6**: 1093–1103.

128 Collins BJ, Chiappetta G, Schneider AB, Santoro M, Pentimalli F, Fogelfeld L, *et al.* RET expression in papillary thyroid cancer from patients irradiated in childhood for benign conditions. *J Clin Endocrinol Metab* 2002; **87**: 3941–3946.

129 Fagin JA. Perspective: lessons learned from molecular genetic studies of thyroid cancer – insights into pathogenesis and tumor-specific therapeutic targets. *Endocrinology* 2002; **143**: 2025–2028.

130 Elisei R, Romei C, Vorontsova T, Cosci B, Veremeychik V, Kuchinskaya E, *et al.* RET/PTC rearrangements in thyroid nodules: studies in irradiated and not irradiated, malignant and benign thyroid lesions in children and adults. *J Clin Endocrinol Metab* 2001; **86**: 3211–3216.

131 Oeffinger KC, Sklar CA, Hudson MM. Thyroid nodules and survivors of Hodgkin's disease. *Am Fam Physician* 2003; **68**: 1016, 1018–1019; discussion 1019.

132 Eden K, Mahon S, Helfand M. Screening high-risk populations for thyroid cancer. *Med Pediatr Oncol* 2001; **36**: 583–591.

133 Wallace WH, Anderson RA, Irvine DS. Fertility preservation for young patients with cancer: who is at risk and what can be offered? *Lancet Oncol* 2005; **6**: 209–218.

134 Leiper AD, Grant DB, Chessells JM. Gonadal function after testicular radiation for acute lymphoblastic leukaemia. *Arch Dis Child* 1986; **61**: 53–56.

135 Speiser B, Rubin P, Casarett G. Aspermia following lower truncal irradiation in Hodgkin's disease. *Cancer* 1973; **32**: 692–698.

136 Shalet SM, Tsatsoulis A, Whitehead E, Read G. Vulnerability of the human Leydig cell to radiation damage is dependent upon age. *J Endocrinol* 1989; **120**: 161–165.

137 Sanders JE, Hawley J, Levy W, Gooley T, Buckner CD, Deeg HJ, *et al.* Pregnancies following high-dose cyclophosphamide with or without high-dose busulfan or total-body irradiation and bone marrow transplantation. *Blood* 1996; **87**: 3045–3052.

138 Nicholson HS, Byrne J. Fertility and pregnancy after treatment for cancer during childhood or adolescence. *Cancer* 1993; **71** (Suppl): 3392–3399.

139 Viviani S, Santoro A, Ragni G, Bonfante V, Bestetti O, Bonadonna G. Gonadal toxicity after combination chemotherapy for Hodgkin's disease: comparative results of MOPP vs ABVD. *Eur J Cancer Clin Oncol* 1985; **21**: 601–605.

140 Mackie EJ, Radford M, Shalet SM. Gonadal function following chemotherapy for childhood Hodgkin's disease. *Med Pediatr Oncol* 1996; **27**: 74–78.

141 Wallace WH, Shalet SM, Lendon M, Morris-Jones PH. Male fertility in long-term survivors of childhood acute lymphoblastic leukaemia. *Int J Androl* 1991; **14**: 312–319.

142 Lendon M, Hann IM, Palmer MK, Shalet SM, Jones PH. Testicular histology after combination chemotherapy in childhood for acute lymphoblastic leukaemia. *Lancet* 1978; **2**: 439–441.

143 Wallace WH, Shalet SM, Tetlow LJ, Morris-Jones PH. Ovarian function following the treatment of childhood acute lymphoblastic leukaemia. *Med Pediatr Oncol* 1993; **21**: 333–339.

144 Sanders JE. The impact of marrow transplant preparative regimens on subsequent growth and development. The Seattle Marrow Transplant Team. *Semin Hematol* 1991; **28**: 244–249.

145 Sklar C, Boulad F, Small T, Kernan N. Endocrine complications of pediatric stem cell transplantation. *Front Biosci* 2001; **6**: G17–22.

146 Meistrich ML, Wilson G, Brown BW, da Cunha MF, Lipshultz LI. Impact of cyclophosphamide on long-term reduction in sperm count in men treated with combination chemotherapy for Ewing and soft tissue sarcomas. *Cancer* 1992; **70**: 2703–2712.

147 Anselmo AP, Cartoni C, Bellantuono P, Maurizi-Enrici R, Aboulkair N, Ermini M. Risk of infertility in patients with Hodgkin's disease treated with ABVD vs MOPP vs ABVD/MOPP. *Haematologica* 1990; **75**: 155–158.

148 Howell SJ, Radford JA, Adams JE, Shalet SM. The impact of mild Leydig cell dysfunction following cytotoxic chemotherapy on bone mineral density (BMD) and body composition. *Clin Endocrinol (Oxf)* 2000; **52**: 609–616.

149 Greenfield DM, Walters SJ, Coleman RE, Hancock BW, Eastell R, Davies HA, *et al.* Prevalence and consequences of androgen deficiency in young male cancer survivors in a controlled cross-sectional study. *J Clin Endocrinol Metab* 2007; **92**: 3476–3482.

150 Wallace WH, Thomson AB, Kelsey TW. The radiosensitivity of the human oocyte. *Hum Reprod* 2003; **18**: 117–121.

151 Wallace WH, Shalet SM, Crowne EC, Morris-Jones PH, Gattamaneni HR. Ovarian failure following abdominal irradiation in childhood: natural history and prognosis. *Clin Oncol (R Coll Radiol)* 1989; **1**: 75–79.

152 Critchley HO, Wallace WH, Shalet SM, Mamtora H, Higginson J, Anderson DC. Abdominal irradiation in childhood: the potential for pregnancy. *Br J Obstet Gynaecol* 1992; **99**: 392–394.

153 Wallace WH, Thomson AB, Saran F, Kelsey TW. Predicting age of ovarian failure after radiation to a field that includes the ovaries. *Int J Radiat Oncol Biol Phys* 2005; **62**: 738–744.

154 Chiarelli AM, Marrett LD, Darlington G. Early menopause and infertility in females after treatment for childhood cancer diagnosed in 1964–1988 in Ontario, Canada. *Am J Epidemiol* 1999; **150**: 245–254.

155 Leporrier M, von Theobald P, Roffe JL, Muller G. A new technique to protect ovarian function before pelvic irradiation: heterotopic ovarian autotransplantation. *Cancer* 1987; **60**: 2201–2204.

156 Frederickx V, Michiels A, Goossens E, De Block G, Van Steirteghem AC, Tournaye H. Recovery, survival and functional evaluation by transplantation of frozen-thawed mouse germ cells. *Hum Reprod* 2004; **19**: 948–953.

157 Schlatt S, Kim SS, Gosden R. Spermatogenesis and steroidogenesis in mouse, hamster and monkey testicular tissue after cryopreservation and heterotopic grafting to castrated hosts. *Reproduction* 2002; **124**: 339–346.

158 Baird DT, Webb R, Campbell BK, Harkness LM, Gosden RG. Long-term ovarian function in sheep after ovariectomy and transplantation of autografts stored at −196°C. *Endocrinology* 1999; **140**: 462–471.

159 Oktay K, Karlikaya G. Ovarian function after transplantation of frozen, banked autologous ovarian tissue. *N Engl J Med* 2000; **342**: 1919.

160 Donnez J, Dolmans MM, Demylle D, Jadoul P, Pirard C, Squifflet J, *et al.* Livebirth after orthotopic transplantation of cryopreserved ovarian tissue. *Lancet* 2004; **364**: 1405–1410.

161 Oktay K, Buyuk E, Veeck L, Zaninovic N, Xu K, Takeuchi T, *et al.* Embryo development after heterotopic transplantation of cryopreserved ovarian tissue. *Lancet* 2004; **363**: 837–840.

162 Morita Y, Perez GI, Paris F, Miranda SR, Ehleiter D, Haimovitz-Friedman A, *et al.* Oocyte apoptosis is suppressed by disruption of the acid sphingomyelinase gene or by sphingosine-1-phosphate therapy. *Nat Med* 2000; **6**: 1109–1114.

163 Marmor D, Duyck F. Male reproductive potential after MOPP therapy for Hodgkin's disease: a long-term survey. *Andrologia* 1995; **27**: 99–106.

164 Bath LE, Tydeman G, Critchley HO, Anderson RA, Baird DT, Wallace WH. Spontaneous conception in a young woman who had ovarian cortical tissue cryopreserved before chemotherapy and radiotherapy for a Ewing's sarcoma of the pelvis: case report. *Hum Reprod* 2004; **19**: 2569–2572.

165 Campbell AJ, Irvine DS. Male infertility and intracytoplasmic sperm injection (ICSI). *Br Med Bull* 2000; **56**: 616–629.

166 Siimes MA, Rautonen J. Small testicles with impaired production of sperm in adult male survivors of childhood malignancies. *Cancer* 1990; **65**: 1303–1306.

167 Bath LE, Wallace WH, Shaw MP, Fitzpatrick C, Anderson RA. Depletion of ovarian reserve in young women after treatment for cancer in childhood: detection by anti-Mullerian hormone, inhibin B and ovarian ultrasound. *Hum Reprod* 2003; **18**: 2368–2374.

168 Wallace WH, Kelsey TW. Ovarian reserve and reproductive age may be determined from measurement of ovarian volume by transvaginal sonography. *Hum Reprod* 2004; **19**: 1612–1617.

169 Wallace EM, Groome NP, Riley SC, Parker AC, Wu FC. Effects of chemotherapy-induced testicular damage on inhibin, gonadotropin and testosterone secretion: a prospective longitudinal study. *J Clin Endocrinol Metab* 1997; **82**: 3111–3115.

170 van Beek RD, Smit M, van den Heuvel-Eibrink MM, de Jong FH, Hakvoort-Cammel FG, van den Bos C, *et al.* Inhibin B is superior to FSH as a serum marker for spermatogenesis in men treated for Hodgkin's lymphoma with chemotherapy during childhood. *Hum Reprod* 2007; **22**: 3215–3222.

171 Crofton PM, Thomson AB, Evans AE, Groome NP, Bath LE, Kelnar CJ, *et al.* Is inhibin B a potential marker of gonadotoxicity in prepubertal children treated for cancer? *Clin Endocrinol (Oxf)* 2003; **58**: 296–301.

172 van Rooij IA, Broekmans FJ, te Velde ER, Fauser BC, Bancsi LF, de Jong FH, *et al.* Serum anti-Mullerian hormone concentrations: a novel measure of ovarian reserve. *Hum Reprod* 2002; **17**: 3065–3071.

173 Hawkins MM, Draper GJ, Smith RA. Cancer among 1,348 offspring of survivors of childhood cancer. *Int J Cancer* 1989; **43**: 975–978.

174 Vassilopoulou-Sellin R, Brosnan P, Delpassand A, Zietz H, Klein MJ, Jaffe N. Osteopenia in young adult survivors of childhood cancer. *Med Pediatr Oncol* 1999; **32**: 272–278.

175 Warner JT, Evans WD, Webb DK, Bell W, Gregory JW. Relative osteopenia after treatment for acute lymphoblastic leukemia. *Pediatr Res* 1999; **45** (Pt 1): 544–551.

176 van der Sluis IM, van den Heuvel-Eibrink MM, Hahlen K, Krenning EP, de Muinck Keizer-Schrama SM. Bone mineral density, body composition and height in long-term survivors of acute lymphoblastic leukemia in childhood. *Med Pediatr Oncol* 2000; **35**: 415–420.

177 Tillmann V, Darlington AS, Eiser C, Bishop NJ, Davies HA. Male sex and low physical activity are associated with reduced spine bone mineral density in survivors of childhood acute lymphoblastic leukemia. *J Bone Miner Res* 2002; **17**: 1073–1080.

178 Aisenberg J, Hsieh K, Kalaitzoglou G, Whittam E, Heller G, Schneider R, *et al.* Bone mineral density in young adult survivors of childhood cancer. *J Pediatr Hematol Oncol* 1998; **20**: 241–245.

179 Halton JM, Atkinson SA, Fraher L, Webber CE, Cockshott WP, Tam C, *et al.* Mineral homeostasis and bone mass at diagnosis in children with acute lymphoblastic leukemia. *J Pediatr* 1995; **126**: 557–564.

180 Pfeilschifter J, Diel IJ. Osteoporosis due to cancer treatment: pathogenesis and management. *J Clin Oncol* 2000; **18**: 1570–1593.

181 Mandel K, Atkinson S, Barr RD, Pencharz P. Skeletal morbidity in childhood acute lymphoblastic leukemia. *J Clin Oncol* 2004; **22**: 1215–1221.

182 Atkinson SA, Fraher L, Gundberg CM, Andrew M, Pai M, Barr RD. Mineral homeostasis and bone mass in children treated for acute lymphoblastic leukemia. *J Pediatr* 1989; **114**: 793–800.

183 Arikoski P, Komulainen J, Riikonen P, Voutilainen R, Knip M, Kroger H. Alterations in bone turnover and impaired development of bone mineral density in newly diagnosed children with cancer: a 1-year prospective study. *J Clin Endocrinol Metab* 1999; **84**: 3174–3181.

184 Strauss AJ, Su JT, Dalton VM, Gelber RD, Sallan SE, Silverman LB. Bony morbidity in children treated for acute lymphoblastic leukemia. *J Clin Oncol* 2001; **19**: 3066–3072.

185 Davies JH, Evans BA, Jenney ME, Gregory JW. Skeletal morbidity in childhood acute lymphoblastic leukaemia. *Clin Endocrinol (Oxf)* 2005; **63**: 1–9.

186 Holzer G, Krepler P, Koschat MA, Grampp S, Dominkus M, Kotz R. Bone mineral density in long-term survivors of highly malignant osteosarcoma. *J Bone Joint Surg Br* 2003; **85**: 231–237.

187 Baker KS, Gurney JG, Ness KK, Bhatia R, Forman SJ, Francisco L, *et al.* Late effects in survivors of chronic myeloid leukemia treated with hematopoietic cell transplantation: results from the Bone Marrow Transplant Survivor Study. *Blood* 2004; **104**: 1898–1906.

188 Bhatia S, Ramsay NK, Weisdorf D, Griffiths H, Robison LL. Bone mineral density in patients undergoing bone marrow transplantation for myeloid malignancies. *Bone Marrow Transplant* 1998; **22**: 87–90.

189 Kaste SC, Shidler TJ, Tong X, Srivastava DK, Rochester R, Hudson MM, *et al.* Bone mineral density and osteonecrosis in survivors of childhood allogeneic bone marrow transplantation. *Bone Marrow Transplant* 2004; **33**: 435–441.

190 Nysom K, Holm K, Michaelsen KF, Hertz H, Jacobsen N, Muller J, *et al.* Bone mass after allogeneic BMT for childhood leukaemia or lymphoma. *Bone Marrow Transplant* 2000; **25**: 191–196.

191 Stern JM, Chesnut CH 3rd, Bruemmer B, Sullivan KM, Lenssen PS, Aker SN, *et al.* Bone density loss during treatment of chronic GVHD. *Bone Marrow Transplant* 1996; **17**: 395–400.

192 Barr RD, Simpson T, Webber CE, Gill GJ, Hay J, Eves M, *et al.* Osteopenia in children surviving brain tumours. *Eur J Cancer* 1998; **34**: 873–877.

193 Hopewell JW. Radiation-therapy effects on bone density. *Med Pediatr Oncol* 2003; **41**: 208–211.

194 Banfi A, Bianchi G, Galotto M, Cancedda R, Quarto R. Bone marrow stromal damage after chemo/radiotherapy: occurrence, consequences and possibilities of treatment. *Leuk Lymphoma* 2001; **42**: 863–870.

195 Murray RD, Adams JE, Smethurst LE, Shalet SM. Spinal irradiation impairs the osteo-anabolic effects of low-dose GH replacement in adults with childhood-onset GH deficiency. *Clin Endocrinol (Oxf)* 2002; **56**: 169–174.

196 Brennan BM, Mughal Z, Roberts SA, Ward K, Shalet SM, Eden TO, *et al.* Bone mineral density in childhood survivors of acute lymphoblastic leukemia treated without cranial irradiation. *J Clin Endocrinol Metab* 2005; **90**: 689–694.

197 Kaste SC, Rai SN, Fleming K, McCammon EA, Tylavsky FA, Danish RK, *et al.* Changes in bone mineral density in survivors of childhood acute lymphoblastic leukemia. *Pediatr Blood Cancer* 2006; **46**: 77–87.

198 Henderson RC, Madsen CD, Davis C, Gold SH. Bone density in survivors of childhood malignancies. *J Pediatr Hematol Oncol* 1996; **18**: 367–371.

199 Hesseling PB, Hough SF, Nel ED, van Riet FA, Beneke T, Wessels G. Bone mineral density in long-term survivors of childhood cancer. *Int J Cancer Suppl* 1998; **11**: 44–47.

200 Hull MC, Morris CG, Pepine CJ, Mendenhall NP. Valvular dysfunction and carotid, subclavian and coronary artery disease in survivors of Hodgkin lymphoma treated with radiation therapy. *JAMA* 2003; **290**: 2831–2837.

201 Reinders JG, Heijmen BJ, Olofsen-van Acht MJ, van Putten WL, Levendag PC. Ischemic heart disease after mantlefield irradiation for Hodgkin's disease in long-term follow-up. *Radiother Oncol* 1999; **51**: 35–42.

202 Dorresteijn LD, Kappelle AC, Boogerd W, Klokman WJ, Balm AJ, Keus RB, *et al.* Increased risk of ischemic stroke after radiotherapy on the neck in patients younger than 60 years. *J Clin Oncol* 2002; **20**: 282–288.

203 Bowers DC, McNeil DE, Liu Y, Yasui Y, Stovall M, Gurney JG, *et al.* Stroke as a late treatment effect of Hodgkin's disease: a report from the Childhood Cancer Survivor Study. *J Clin Oncol* 2005; **23**: 6508–6515.

204 Bowers DC, Liu Y, Leisenring W, McNeil E, Stovall M, Gurney JG, *et al.* Late-occurring stroke among long-term survivors of childhood leukemia and brain tumors: a report from the Childhood Cancer Survivor Study. *J Clin Oncol* 2006; **24**: 5277–5282.

205 Chow EJ, Pihoker C, Hunt K, Wilkinson K; Friedman DL. Obesity and hypertension among children after treatment for acute lymphoblastic leukemia. *Cancer* 2007; **110**: 2313–2320.

206 Taskinen M, Saarinen-Pihkala UM, Hovi L, Lipsanen-Nyman M. Impaired glucose tolerance and dyslipidaemia as late effects after bone-marrow transplantation in childhood. *Lancet* 2000; **356**: 993–997.

207 Teinturier C, Tournade MF, Caillat-Zucman S, Boitard C, Amoura Z, Bougneres PF, *et al.* Diabetes mellitus after abdominal radiation therapy. *Lancet* 1995; **346**: 633–634.

208 Lustig RH, Post SR, Srivannaboon K, Rose SR, Danish RK, Burghen GA, *et al.* Risk factors for the development of obesity in children surviving brain tumors. *J Clin Endocrinol Metab* 2003; **88**: 611–616.

9 Evaluation and Management of Disorders of Sex Development

Ieuan A. Hughes

University of Cambridge, Addenbrooke's Hospital, Department of Paediatrics, Cambridge, UK

In discussing disorders of sexual development, there has conventionally been a focus on ambiguous genitalia, a term referring primarily to a newborn with genital anomalies rendering assignment of sex at birth problematic and synonymous with intersex. The focus on disorders of sex development reflects the fact that genital anomalies present beyond the newborn period, at pubertal and adolescent ages. The replacement of the term intersex by the more generic terminology of disorders of sex development (DSD) has resulted in a new classification of their causes.

The embryology of the reproductive system and the genetic and hormonal control of its constituent parts are described in detail in recent texts and reviews [1–3] and the clinician charged with the evaluation and management of DSD must understand reproductive tract development which underpins differential diagnosis, focused investigation and appropriate management.

Normal sex development

The constitutive sex is female: male development requires the presence of a Y chromosome, a testis and the action of its hormonal products (Fig. 9.1). The events in fetal male sex development are summarized in Figure 9.2 and the embryology of early male development is illustrated in Figure 9.3. A critical dosage threshold and timing in expression of sex-determining genes and hormones is obligatory for normal development. Many of the large group of idiopathic XY-related disorders of sex development probably result from a deficiency in this key process.

Information about the genetic control of development of the urogenital ridge and gonad determination and subsequent hormonal control of sex differentiation has been gleaned from clinicopathologic assessment of prismatic cases of DSD and rodent-based gene targeting studies (Fig. 9.4). There are addi-

tional genes relevant in rodent urogenital development for which mutations in their human homologs causing DSD have yet to be described. Common elements in the early pathway (e.g. WT1 and SF1) explain the importance of checking renal and adrenal disorders when evaluating DSD.

It is self-evident that a sex chromosome abnormality, such as XO/XY mosaicism or an XXY karyotype, may be associated with genital anomalies. For the male with a normal XY karyotype, categories of causation of DSD include defects in testis determination and androgen production or action. For the female with a normal XX karyotype, a primary defect in ovarian determination may be the cause but far more probable is masculinization by fetal adrenal androgens (e.g. congenital adrenal hyperplasia) or androgens from a maternal source (e.g. ovarian tumor).

Terminology

The complexity of evaluating DSD should not be compounded by using terms that are themselves ambiguous and confusing. Thus, the word, *intersex*, is replaced by *disorder of sex development* (DSD) [4–7] defined as a congenital condition in which development of chromosomal, gonadal or anatomic sex is atypical (Table 9.1). Early knowledge of the sex chromosomes from the ready analysis of Y and X centromeric probes by fluorescence *in situ* hybridization (FISH) techniques renders this the starting point for the evaluation of DSD. Descriptive modes, such as the masculinized female or the undermasculinized male, retain useful currency but the term *pseudohermaphroditism* is confusing and uninformative and should be consigned to history. Hermaphrodite, prefaced by the adjective *true*, defines an hermaphroditic state characterized by the presence of both ovarian and testicular tissue in the one affected individual but simpler terminology is to describe the type of DSD as ovotesticular, which can be further subtyped according to the karyotype (46XX or 46XY).

Postnatal psychosexual development and the sociocultural influences on gender have spawned their own terminology. It is important to be familiar with the following definitions when considering the evaluation and management of DSD:

Brook's Clinical Pediatric Endocrinology, 6th edition. Edited by C. Brook, P. Clayton, R. Brown. © 2009 Blackwell Publishing, ISBN: 978-1-4051-8080-1.

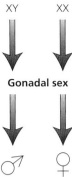

Chromosomal sex (genotype)

XY   XX

Gonadal sex

♂   ♀

Figure 9.1 Schematic of the fundamental components of sex development. **Phenotypic sex (somatotype)**

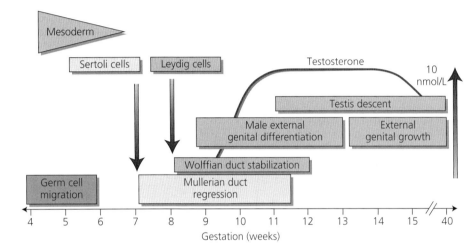

Figure 9.2 Events temporally related to sex differentiation in the male fetus. Mesoderm refers to the tissue source for Sertoli and Leydig cell formation. The continuous line depicts the rise in fetal serum testosterone, the peak concentration being around 10 nmol/L.

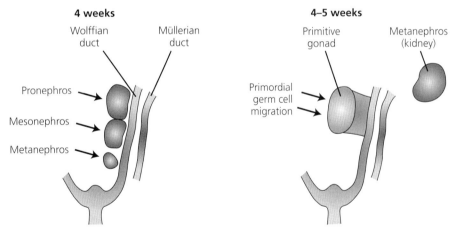

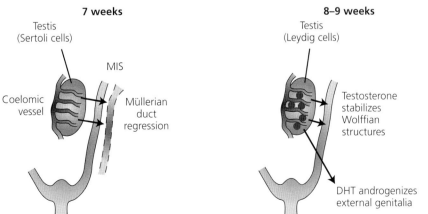

Figure 9.3 Schematic representation of the principal morphologic and functional events during early gonad/testis development in humans. DHT, dihydrotestosterone. (From Hughes & Achermann [1] with permission.)

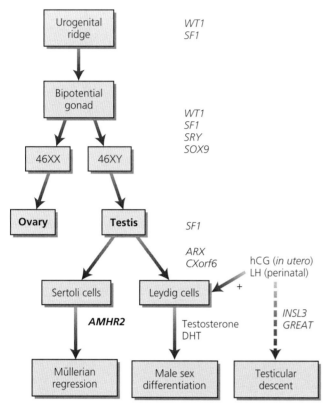

Figure 9.4 Principal genetic and hormonal factors controlling fetal sex development in humans. (Adapted from ref 1).

Table 9.1 A revised nomenclature relating to disorders of sex development (DSD).

Previous	Proposed
Intersex	*DSD*
Male pseudohermaphrodite	46XY DSD
Undervirilization of an XY male	
Undermasculinization of an XY male	
Female pseudohermaphrodite	46XX DSD
Overvirilization of an XX female	
Masculinization of an XX female	
True hermaphrodite	Ovotesticular DSD
XX male or XX sex reversal	46XX testicular DSD
XY sex reversal	46XY complete gonadal dysgenesis

• *Gender (sex) assignment:* the decisive allocation of male or female at birth, which is usually instantaneous;
• *Gender identity:* the sense of self as being male or female;
• *Gender role:* denotes aspects of behavior and preferences in which males and females differ;
• *Sexual orientation:* refers to the target of sexual arousal;
• *Gender attribution:* assigning as male or female on first encounter with a person;

• *Gender dysphoria:* a transsexual state associated with a gender identity disorder.

There is a dichotomy between the body habitus and gender identity. The process of fetal sex determination and sex differentiation appears to be normal. Transsexualism is not generally considered within the ambit of ambiguous genitalia.

In general, gender identity and gender role, together with the symbols that attribute to gender manifestations, are congruent and the subject of erotic desires is generally towards the opposite sex. It is against this background that the complex assessment of adults, who were born with ambiguous genitalia and may have been sex reassigned, must take place.

Causes of DSD

The change of nomenclature to a DSD base, subdefined according to the sex chromosomes, allows the use of three broad categories of causation (Table 9.2) covering conditions as diverse as congenital adrenal hyperplasia, androgen insensitivity, vanishing testes syndrome and cloacal extrophy but not including disorders of puberty. Whether Turner syndrome should be classified as a DSD is questionable but it merits inclusion by virtue of the sex chromosome being atypical. A functional classification of the more common causes of DSD is set out in Table 9.3.

The masculinized female: 46XX, DSD

The placenta contains an aromatase enzyme system which is generally extremely efficient in protecting a female fetus from the effects of androgens in the maternal circulation. For example, women with congenital adrenal hyperplasia (CAH) who become pregnant and have elevated testosterone concentrations throughout gestation do not have female offspring who are virilized [7], although, interestingly, there was a preponderance of male offspring in a Swedish study [8]. Androgen-secreting tumors of the adrenals and ovaries can masculinize the mother and a female fetus, presumably because the androgen substrates overwhelm the placental aromatase system.

Luteoma of pregnancy and hyperreactio luteinalis are benign tumors but produce large ovarian masses. Luteomas predominate in multiparous Afro-Caribbean women who may have a preexisting polycystic ovarian syndrome. The tumors regress postpartum but can recur in subsequent pregnancies. Other virilizing ovarian tumors include arrhenoblastoma, hilar cell tumor and Krukenberg tumor.

The use of progestational agents with some androgenic activity to prevent recurrent miscarriage is obsolete but danazol, a derivative of 17β-ethinyltestosterone, has a place in the medical treatment of endometriosis. It readily crosses the placenta and cases of masculinized female infants have been recorded [9].

Placental aromatase deficiency is a recognized cause of ambiguous genitalia in a female infant whose mother is also virilized during pregnancy [10,11]. A single *CYP19* gene is expressed through the action of tissue-specific promoters in several tissues, including the gonads, placenta and adipocytes. The aromatase

Table 9.2 Classification of disorders of sex development (DSD).

Sex chromosome DSD	46XY DSD	46,XX DSD
A: 47,XXY (Klinefelter syndrome and variants) B: 45X (Turner syndrome and variants) C: 45X/46XY (mixed gonadal dysgenesis) D: 46XX/46XY (chimerism)	A: Disorders of gonadal (testicular) development 1. Complete or partial gonadal dysgenesis (e.g. *SRY, SOX9, SF1, WT1, DHH*, etc.) 2. Ovotesticular DSD 3. Testis regression	A: Disorders of gonadal (ovary) development 1. Gonadal dysgenesis 2. Ovotesticular DSD 3. Testicular DSD (e.g. *SRY+, dup SOX9, RSPO1*)
	B: Disorders in androgen synthesis or action 1. Disorders of androgen synthesis LH receptor mutations Smith–Lemli–Opitz syndrome Steroidogenic acute regulatory protein mutations Cholesterol side chain cleavage (*CYP11A1*) 3β-hydroxysteroid dehydrogenase 2 (*HSD3B2*) 17α hydroxylase/17,20-lyase (*CYP17*) P450 oxidoreductase (*POR*) 17β-hydoxysteroid dehydrogenase (*HSD17B3*) 5α-reductase 2 (*SRD5A2*) 2. Disorders of androgen action Androgen insensitivity syndrome Drugs and environmental modulators	B: Androgen excess 1. Fetal 3β-hydroxysteroid dehydrogenase 2 (*HSD3B2*) 21-hydroxylase (*CYP21A2*) P450 oxidoreductase (*POR*) 11β-hydroxylase (*CYP11B1*) Glucocorticoid receptor mutations 2. Fetoplacental Aromatase (*CYP19*) deficiency Oxidoreductase (*POR*) deficiency 3. Maternal Maternal virilizing tumors (e.g. luteomas) Androgenic drugs
	C: Other 1. Syndromic associations of male genital development (e.g. cloacal anomalies, Robinow, Aarskog, hand-foot-genital, popliteal pterygium) 2. Persistent Müllerian duct syndrome 3. Vanishing testis syndrome 4. Isolated hypospadias (*CXorf6*) 5. Congenital hypogonadotropic hypogonadism 6. Cryptorchidism (*INSL3, GREAT*) 7. Environmental influences	C: Other 1. Syndromic associations (e.g. cloacal anomalies) 2. Müllerian agenesis/hypoplasia (e.g. MURCS) 3. Uterine abnormalities (e.g. MODY5) 4. Vaginal atresias (e.g. KcKusick–Kaufman) 5. Labial adhesions

Table 9.3 Causes of ambiguous genitalia: a functional classification.

Type/cause	Illustrative examples
Masculinized female (46XX DSD)	
Fetal androgens	CAH, placental aromatase deficiency
Maternal androgens	Ovarian and adrenal tumors
Undermasculinized male (46XY DSD)	
Abnormal testis determination	Partial (XY) and mixed (XO/XY) gonadal dysgenesis
Androgen biosynthetic defects	LH receptor inactivating mutations 17βOH-dehydrogenase deficiency 5α-reductase deficiency
Resistance to androgens	Androgen insensitivity syndrome variants
Ovotesticular DSD	
Presence of testicular and ovarian tissue	Karyotypes XX, XY, XX/XY
Syndromal	Denys–Drash, Frasier Smith–Lemli–Opitz

DSD, disorders of sex development; LH, luteinizing hormone.

enzyme is a key regulator of production of estrogens from androgens in the fetal-placental-maternal unit (Fig. 9.5).

The fetal adrenals produce large quantities of dehydroepiandrosterone sulfate (DHEAS) which is 16β-hydroxylated in both the fetal adrenal and liver. After transfer to the placenta, the sulfate moiety of 16OH-DHEAS is removed by placental sulfatase. Deficiency of this enzyme causes X-linked recessive ichthyosis and can be diagnosed by measurement of arylsulfatase C [12]. DHEA and 16OH-DHEA are converted to more potent androgens, such as androstenedione and testosterone, which are aromatized to estrone and estradiol, respectively. A large amount of estriol is also produced by aromatization of androgen substrates. Maternal urinary estriol concentrations may be low in the last trimester of a normal pregnancy as a result of either placental sulfatase or placental aromatase deficiency. Serial measurements of urinary estriol have a useful role in monitoring prenatal treatment of CAH with dexamethasone [13].

The degree of maternal and fetal masculinization can be quite profound in placental aromatase deficiency. The mother, however, may escape signs of virilization when as little as 1–2% activity of mutant enzyme is present. This illustrates the capacity of this enzyme to convert androgens to estrogens. The internal genitalia

Table 9.4 Comparative features of overlapping phenotypes in three causes of XY, disorders of sex development (DSD).

17β-hydroxysteroid dehydrogenase type 3 deficiency

Inheritance	Autosomal recessive; *HSD17B3* gene (9q22) mutations (n~20)
Genitalia	Female → ambiguous
Genital ducts	Wolffian normal; Müllerian absent
Gonads	Testes, usually undescended
Later phenotype	Virilization at puberty; gynaecomastia variable
Endocrine	↑ LH, FSH; ↑ androstenedione; ↓ testosterone: androstenedione ratio

5α-reductase type 2 deficiency

Inheritance	Autosomal recessive; *SRD5A2* gene (2p23) mutations (n~40, complete deletion in New Guinea population)
Genitalia	Usually ambiguous
Genital ducts	Wolffian normal; Müllerian absent
Gonads	Normal testes, often descended
Later phenotype	Virilization at puberty; decreased sexual hair; hypoplastic prostate
Endocrine	↑ Testosterone: DHT ratio; ↓ urinary 5α/5β C_{21} and C_{19} steroids

Partial androgen insensitivity syndrome

Inheritance	X-linked recessive; *AR* gene (Xq11.2-q12) mutations (n~280)
Genitalia	Ambiguous → isolated hypospadias → infertile male (MAIS)
Genital ducts	Wolffian often normal; Müllerian absent
Gonads	Testes, usually undescended
Later phenotype	Decreased sexual hair; gynaecomastia; rarely breast cancer
Endocrine	↑ LH, ↑ testosterone, ↑ estradiol, ↑ SHBG

DHT, dihydrotestosterone; FSH, follicle stimulating hormone; LH, luteinizing hormone; MAIS, minimal androgen insensitivity syndrome; SHBG, sex hormone-binding globulin.

of affected female infants are normal but ovarian cysts may develop in later childhood. At puberty, there is failure of breast development, onset of virilization and polycystic changes in the ovaries. A spectrum of mutations is distributed through the *CYP19* gene, including some affecting the critical heme-binding site [14]. Aromatase deficiency should be considered when CAH has been excluded in a female newborn with ambiguous genitalia.

Apparent combined deficiency of the P450 17α-hydroxylase and 21-hydroxylase enzymes can also cause mild degrees of maternal and fetal masculinization which is self-limiting after birth. Mutations are found not in the *CYP17* or *CYP21* genes but in the gene encoding for cytochrome P450 oxidoreductase [15]. This enzyme functions as an electron donor to microsomal cytochrome P450s, including the aromatase enzyme. This may partly explain the masculinization from accumulation of fetal adrenal androgens as a result of partial placental aromatase deficiency but there is also impairment of androgen biosynthesis in oxidoreductase deficiency such that affected males are undermasculinized.

The explanation for this paradox may lie with observations of steroid biosynthetic pathways in the Tammar wallaby [16], in which there is evidence that the potent androgen dihydrotestosterone (DHT) can be produced by a "backdoor" pathway involving the precursor steroid androstanediol and avoiding testosterone as an intermediary substrate. Such a pathway may exist in the human fetus only to switch to the more classic pathway of androgen biosynthesis after birth. Most patients with P450 oxidoreductase deficiency have associated skeletal malformations characteristic of the Antley–Bixler syndrome [17]. It remains to be seen whether oxidoreductase deficiency is a significant cause of non-syndromic ambiguous genitalia in newborn females and undermasculinized males of unknown diagnosis as assessed by urinary steroid analyses.

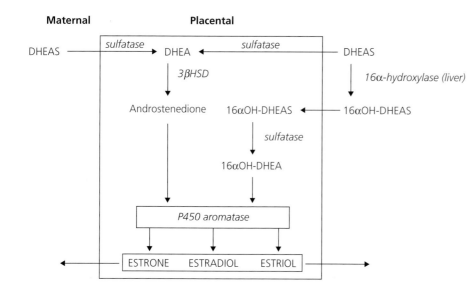

Figure 9.5 The fetal-placental-maternal steroid unit. The androgen substrate DHEAS is synthesized in both the maternal and the fetal adrenals and cleaved to DHEA by placental sulfatase. The fetal liver also hydroxylates DHEAS prior to sulfatase cleavage by the placenta. Androgen substrates are aromatized to estrogens, particularly estriol. DHEA, dehydroepiandrosterone; DHEAS, dehydroepiandrosterone sulfate; 3βHSD, 3β-hydroxysteroid dehydrogenase.

In the context of ambiguous genitalia, CAH is the most common cause and the most straightforward to diagnose. This must be undertaken promptly in view of the potential life-threatening consequences of glucocorticoid and mineralocorticoid deficiencies to the infant. Giving dexamethasone to the mother from early in pregnancy can successfully prevent masculinization of the external genitalia in an affected female infant [18,19], a unique example of preventing a major congenital malformation by prenatal medical intervention.

The under-masculinized male: 46XY, DSD

The list of causes in this category is large, not least because of inclusion of disorders such as simple hypospadias, undescended testes and isolated micropenis, which are not classic examples of ambiguous genitalia. The choice of using broad categories related to testis determination, androgen biosynthesis and androgen action stems directly from understanding the normal processes of male fetal sex development.

Defects in testis determination

Normal development and function of Sertoli cells and Leydig cells are essential for hormone-mediated sex differentiation of male internal and external genitalia. Failure of these cells to develop gives rise to a dysgenetic gonad and the clinical disorder, gonadal dysgenesis. Gonadal histology is variable and determines the sex phenotype. Thus, streak gonads are completely undifferentiated and comprised mainly of fibrous tissue with no germ cells, Sertoli cells, interstitial steroid-secreting cells, tubules or follicles. When both gonads are streaks, the phenotype is female, whatever the karyotype. Consequently, XY complete gonadal dysgenesis (Swyer syndrome) leads to complete sex reversal and no ambiguity in sex development. Some 10–15% of patients have a mutation of the *SRY* gene [20], usually in the HMG-box DNA-binding domain of the SRY protein. There are familial cases of XY complete gonadal dysgenesis in whom the genetic cause is unknown and the pattern of inheritance can be X-linked or autosomal recessive [21]. There is a high risk of gonadal tumors such as gonadoblastoma and germinoma.

Partial gonadal dysgenesis gives rise to ambiguity of the genitalia because of the preservation of some Leydig cell function. There are generally Müllerian duct remnants, reflecting inadequate Sertoli cell production of anti-Müllerian hormone (AMH). Histology shows a thin and loosely organized tunica albuginea, underdeveloped seminiferous tubules with wide intertubular spaces, abundant infantile Sertoli cells, scanty germ cells and a dense stroma containing calcified psammoma bodies [22]. These appearances are not too dissimilar from those of an early developing testis so that the dysgenetic gonads in partial gonadal dysgenesis syndromes represent a failure in gonad maturation.

Steroidogenic factor 1 (SF1) is a nuclear receptor that regulates transcription of several genes involved in both gonadal and adrenal development. The expected phenotype of XY sex reversal and adrenal failure has been observed in rare patients with inactivating SF1 mutations [23,24]. Heterozygous mutations in SF1,

often inherited from the mother in a sex-limited dominant manner, are increasingly being identified in patients with gonadal dysgenesis and normal adrenal function [25,26]. The mechanism is likely to be haploinsufficiency of SF1, the gonad being more sensitive than the developing adrenal to variations in gene–dosage effects. SF1 mutations are found in some males with bilateral anorchia or isolated micropenis [27].

A number of eponymous syndromes associated with gonadal dysgenesis should be considered in the assessment of an infant with ambiguous genitalia. Important examples are two related disorders, the Denys–Drash and Frasier syndromes [28–30], both caused by mutations in *WT1*, a gene essential for gonadogenesis and nephrogenesis. In the Denys–Drash syndrome, there are usually genital anomalies at birth in XY cases, a characteristic nephropathy caused by diffuse mesangial sclerosis and a predisposition to Wilms tumor with a median age of onset by 12 months [31]. There is a relative 'hotspot' within exon 9 of the gene where most of the heterozygous mutations occur. A *WT1* mutation can occur rarely in isolated hypospadias without evidence of a nephropathy or a Wilms tumor [32]. The rarity of this occurrence does not merit screening for *WT1* mutations in all infants with hypospadias, although there may be a case for prospective screening for nephropathy (proteinuria) and Wilms tumor (renal ultrasound) in XY infants with ambiguous genitalia.

Frasier syndrome differs with respect to a more severe gonadal dysgenesis generally resulting in XY complete sex reversal, a nephropathy characterized by focal segmental glomerulosclerosis and a predisposition to gonadoblastoma rather than Wilms tumor. Unexplained proteinuria in an adolescent girl with primary amenorrhea should prompt analysis of the *WT1* gene, particularly if the putative nephrotic syndrome is steroid-resistant [33,34]. The characteristic *WT1* abnormality in Frasier syndrome is caused by a donor splice site mutation in intron 9 which leads to an alteration in the normal ratio of WT1 protein isoforms. The WAGR syndrome (*W*ilms' tumor, *a*niridia, *g*enital anomalies, mental *r*etardation) is a contiguous gene deletion syndrome involving a chromosome 11p locus that includes the *WT1* and *PAX6* genes.

SOX9, an SRY-related protein, is a transcription factor involved in both chondrogenesis and early testis determination. Heterozygous mutations in the *SOX9* gene can cause campomelic dysplasia, a multiskeletal disorder, together with sex reversal in the majority of affected males [35]. Not all affected patients have both gonadal dysgenesis and genital anomalies which appears to be related to the function of the SOX9 protein binding to DNA either as a dimer or as a monomer [36] because dimerization is mandatory for chondrogenesis. Mutations in *SOX9* do not lead solely to genital anomalies [37] so analysis of this gene is indicated only in the investigation of XY gonadal dysgenesis associated with skeletal abnormalities.

ATRX syndrome comprises β-thalassemia, mental retardation and multiple congenital anomalies with genital anomalies caused by some form of gonadal dysgenesis [38,39]. Mutations in the *ATR-X* gene located on Xq13.3 and encoding for a protein which belongs to the SNF2 family of proteins that have chromatin remodeling activity interfere with gene expression and DNA methylation. The clinical spectrum extends to eponymous syndromes such as Juberg–Marsidi and Smith–Fineman–Myers.

The term mixed gonadal dysgenesis is used when there is associated 45XO/46XY chromosomal mosaicism. In this syndrome, gonadal morphology is typically a testis on one side and a streak gonad on the other side. The condition is not brought about by mutations in the SRY gene [40,41]. A wide spectrum of phenotypes can result from XO/XY sex chromosome mosaicism with varying degrees of sex reversal [42]. Abnormalities of the external genitalia may be in the form of a severe hypospadias with cryptorchidism but a penis of normal size. Alternatively, the degree of undermasculinization can be manifest solely as a hypertrophied clitoris. There is no correlation between the phenotype and the proportion of XO versus XY cell lines, whether this is determined in blood or fibroblasts. In later childhood, stigmata of Turner syndrome may appear.

A skewed population of XO/XY infants presents at birth with genital anomalies: >90% of fetuses with 45XO/46XY on prenatal cytogenetic studies have normal male genitalia [43,44]. There is little information about the longer term follow-up of these cases in relation to growth, puberty, fertility and risk of gonadal tumors. A set of monozygotic twins concordant for 45XO/46XY karyotype in peripheral blood but sex dimorphic for phenotype were followed to adult life [45]. The male twin had normal adult stature, genital development and Leydig cell function but was oligospermic. The female twin was short in adulthood and required pubertal induction with estrogens.

Ovotesticular DSD (true hermaphroditism) and other sex chromosome anomalies

The term ovotesticular DSD should be applied only to individuals possessing testicular and ovarian tissue that are both well differentiated; the ovaries must contain follicles and ovotestis is the most common gonad. The most frequent karyotype is 46XX followed by one-third of cases with 46XX/XY mosaicism and <10% with 46XY [46]. The prevalence of ovotesticular DSD is particularly high in black South Africans. Most patients have ambiguous genitalia with perineal hypospadias, bifid scrotum and, usually, a normal-sized phallus. The SRY gene is present in about one-third of cases with a 46XX karyotype; there is SRY mosaicism confined to the gonads in a minority of the SRY-negative cases [47]. In follow-up studies ovarian tissues remains normal while testicular tissue gradually becomes dysgenetic [48] but gonadal tumors are rare.

The XX male (1 in 20 000 male births) generally has normal differentiation of the external genitalia, although hypospadias may occur [49]. The testes are small and may be undescended; affected males are infertile; height is below average; gynecomastia is usual [50] and there is an increased risk of carcinoma of the breast. Most patients are SRY positive as a result of X–Y chromosomal interchange during paternal meiosis. SRY-negative XX males are more likely to have associated genital anomalies. The development of testes in these individuals may be the result of SRY expression confined only to the gonads or a mutation in a testis repressor gene that is autosomal or X-linked.

Coexistence of ovotesticular DSD and XX male within families and occurrence in 46XX SRY-negative monozygotic twins with genital anomalies suggests that these two conditions are varying expressions of the same underlying disorder in gonad determination [51]. The cause of XX sex reversal in SRY-negative DSD remains unknown in most cases but mutations in R-spondin1 (RSPO1) have been reported in some cases [52,53]. The R-spondin family of proteins is involved in wnt/beta-catenin signaling. It appears that RSPO1 is a specific ovarian-determining gene which results in female to male XX sex reversal, when mutated. This can be recapitulated in a Rspo1 (−/−) XX mouse model [54].

Klinefelter syndrome (47XXY) affects around 1 in 600 males and there is evidence that the birth prevalence may be increasing, based on newborn surveys, spontaneous abortions, perinatal deaths and prenatal diagnoses [55]. Genital anomalies occur in Klinefelter syndrome ranging in severity from mild anomalies such as chordee to complete sex reversal [56]. The technique of testicular sperm extraction combined with intracytoplasmic sperm injection permits some non-mosaic patients to father children [57].

Defects in androgen biosynthesis

The pathway for production of androgens by the fetal testis is shown in Figure 9.6. Fetal serum testosterone concentrations rise to the normal adult male range towards the end of the first trimester, a period when Wolffian duct stabilization occurs, followed later by growth of the external genitalia (Fig. 9.2). The timing and magnitude of the rise in androgen and AMH concentrations are critical determinants for normal male sex differentiation. Abnormalities in a number of biosynthetic steps can result in inadequate androgen production and an undermasculinized male infant. Some of these abnormalities also affect adrenal steroidogenesis.

Fetal Leydig cell androgen synthesis is initially placental human chorionic gonadotropin (hCG) dependent but is dependent on luteinizing hormone (LH) stimulation from the fetal pituitary later in pregnancy. Both ligands bind to a common LH/hCG receptor, a member of the family of G-protein-coupled receptors comprising seven transmembrane regions. Inactivating mutations in the LHR gene in XY individuals cause a wide range in severity of undermasculinization, including complete sex reversal, severe hypospadias with ambiguous genitalia, undescended testis, hypospadias or isolated micropenis [58,59].

The expected endocrine profile is low testosterone and elevated LH concentrations and no testosterone response following hCG stimulation. Testicular histology shows Sertoli cells with no Leydig cells in the interstitium. These features are difficult to confirm in the prepubertal child who may have an LHR mutation causing abnormal genital development. It is an intriguing obser-

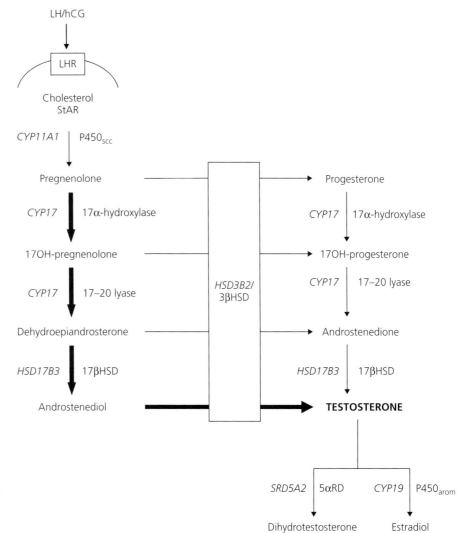

Figure 9.6 Pathways of testosterone synthesis in the human testis. The predominant pathway is indicated by the bold arrows. The enzymes encoded by their respective genes (italicized) are shown. LHR, LH receptor; P450$_{scc}$, cytochrome P450 side-chain cleavage; 17β-hydroxysteroid dehydrogenase; 3βHSD, 3β-hydroxysteroid dehydrogenase.

vation that Wolffian ducts are stabilized despite the apparent lack of normal fetal testosterone production.

The early steps of cholesterol-mediated steroidogenesis are common to both the adrenals and gonads. Thus, lipoid CAH resulting from StAR deficiency and P450 side-chain cleavage deficiency (*CYP11A1* gene mutation) in an affected male manifest as almost complete XY sex reversal. In contrast, the genitalia are either ambiguous or severely hypospadic in 3β-hydroxysteroid dehydrogenase deficiency (*HSD3B2* gene mutation) and isolated 17,20-lyase deficiency (*CYP17* gene mutation). Combined 17α-hydroxylase/17,20-lyase deficiency typically presents as a female phenotype with both XX and XY genotypes, lack of puberty, low renin hypertension and hypokalemic alkalosis. The P450 oxidoreductase deficient male may have ambiguous genitalia or isolated hypospadias.

Testis-specific defects are 17β-hydroxysteroid dehydrogenase and 5α-reductase enzyme deficiencies. A unique feature of both these enzyme defects is their presentation at birth with severe undermasculinization, often to the extent of complete sex reversal, yet a remarkable degree of virilization of the external genitalia with the onset of puberty. This phenomenon of "double sex reversal" is not fully explained, other than the suggestion that peripheral production of testosterone and DHT at puberty occurs through utilization of alternative isoenzymes of the mutant enzyme. The penultimate step in testosterone synthesis is catalyzed by the 17β-hydroxysteroid dehydrogenase type 3 enzyme using androstenedione as substrate.

A spectrum of mutations in the *HSD17B3* gene generally result in complete XY sex reversal at birth [60,61]. The disorder may be mistaken for complete androgen insensitivity syndrome. Some affected infants are more masculinized and can be raised male. Gonadectomy must be performed before puberty when sex has been assigned as female. The uterus is absent as a result of normal testicular AMH action but Wolffian ducts are stabilized, perhaps as a result of sufficient androgenic effect from locally acting high concentrations of androstenedione. Females affected with this enzyme deficiency are asymptomatic.

DHT is more potent than testosterone as an androgen because it binds more avidly to the androgen receptor. Type 2 5α-reductase enzyme is expressed in the genital anlagen so that growth of the genital tubercle and fusion of the labioscrotal folds is preferentially a DHT-dependent process. The type 2 isoenzyme in adulthood is expressed in the prostate, epididymis, seminal vesicles and liver. Type 1 isoenzyme is expressed only in skin and the liver.

Mutations in the *SRD5A2* gene have been reported worldwide, often in pockets within ethnic populations. These include the Dominican Republic, where the disorder was first characterized, New Guinea, Turkey and Egypt [62]. Affected infants are rarely completely female at birth and may be sufficiently masculinized to be sex-assigned as male. Those who are raised female but virilize profoundly at puberty often change gender [63]. Fertility can occur following artificial reproductive techniques or even spontaneously [64,65].

Defects in androgen action

Failure of development of the external genitalia in a male with a normal 46XY karyotype and testes which produce age-appropriate circulating concentrations of androgens defines a form of resistance to the action of androgens. This is the most common cause of XY DSD. Total resistance to androgens leads to complete XY sex reversal and no ambiguity of the external genitalia, the complete androgen insensitivity syndrome (CAIS), also previously known as the testicular feminization syndrome [66,67]. Some tissue response to androgens results in the partial androgen insensitivity syndrome (PAIS). The degree of response may manifest as mild clitoromegaly, true ambiguity of the genitalia, hypospadias alone or impaired fertility in an otherwise normal male [68]. The phenotypes of 17β-hydroxysteroid dehydrogenase and 5α-reductase deficiencies and PAIS can be so similar as to pose severe problems in diagnosis (Table 9.4).

Hormone concentrations in CAIS and PAIS are consistent with the definition of target resistance; typically testosterone is markedly elevated and LH concentrations are unsuppressed. Androgens are aromatized to estrogens resulting in breast development in XY males unopposed by any androgen action. Thus, the patient with CAIS has a normal female phenotype at puberty except for absent or scanty growth of pubic and axillary hair. Clinical presentation typically occurs in adolescence for assessment of primary amenorrhea but the condition may present in infancy with inguinal herniae which are found to contain testes at the time of surgical repair so it is recommended that a karyotype be performed in female infants with an inguinal hernia [69]. Another screen recommended is the measurement of vaginal length in prepubertal girls undergoing inguinal hernia repair [70]. Of premenstrual girls with inguinal hernias 1.1% have CAIS.

CAIS may present because of a mismatch between prenatal sexing and birth outcome. The patient with PAIS and a more male phenotype may develop gynecomastia at puberty and breast cancer has been reported [71]. Breast cancer does not seem to occur in CAIS, although there is one report of a juvenile fibroadenoma of the breast developing after estrogen replacement was started following gonadectomy in a young adult [72]. Breast cancer is common in women so its apparent absence in women with CAIS might indicate some protective effect associated with a mutant androgen receptor.

The pathophysiology of CAIS and PAIS is related to a defect in the intracellular action of androgens (Fig. 9.7). The androgen receptor (AR) is located in the cytoplasm of androgen target cells complexed to heat shock proteins until bound to testosterone or DHT, when the hormone-receptor complex translocates to the nucleus. Acting as a transcription factor, this complex binds as a homodimer together with co-regulator proteins to promote expression of androgen-responsive genes. It is possible to postulate a number of steps in this pathway that may result in resistance to androgens. The best characterized involves the AR itself, where mutations either affect androgen binding or disrupt interaction of the hormone receptor complex with DNA [73,74].

The AR is a member of a large family of nuclear hormone receptors that comprise four general functional domains: an N-terminal transactivation domain, a central DNA binding domain, a hinge region and a C-terminal domain to which the ligand binds (Fig. 9.8). Subdomains are involved in dimerization, nuclear localization and transcriptional regulation. The *AR* gene is located on chromosome Xq11-12. Numerous mutations have been identified throughout this 90 kb gene that cause either CAIS or PAIS. They are recorded on an international database (http://www.mcgill.ca/androgendb). More than 500 mutations are described and a selection of some of the mutations recorded on the Cambridge DSD database is shown in Figure 9.9.

Severe mutations, such as deletions and premature stop codons, predictably result in no AR function and a CAIS phenotype but most mutations are missense and located in the ligand binding domain. The same mutation may cause CAIS in one family but be manifest as PAIS in another. The factors modulating receptor activity and androgen responsiveness that result in phenotype variability are unclear but may include somatic mosaicism [75] and variation in AR trinucleotide repeat lengths [76].

A mutation is identified in the *AR* gene in about 90% of XY sex reversed females who have clinical, biochemical and histological evidence of CAIS but only 15–20% of patients with PAIS have an *AR* mutation. It is possible that resistance to androgens is not the explanation of the genital abnormality in these patients; this proportion of cases is derived following thorough evaluation and exclusion of other known causes that can cause a similar phenotype. In PAIS cases with no identifiable *AR* mutation, there is an association with low birthweight.

The ligand-activation of the AR is but one of several molecular components to androgen action. Little is known about the identity of androgen-responsive genes expressed in the developing male reproductive tract. The AR contains a polymorphic trinucleotide CAG repeat which encodes a polyglutamine tract in the

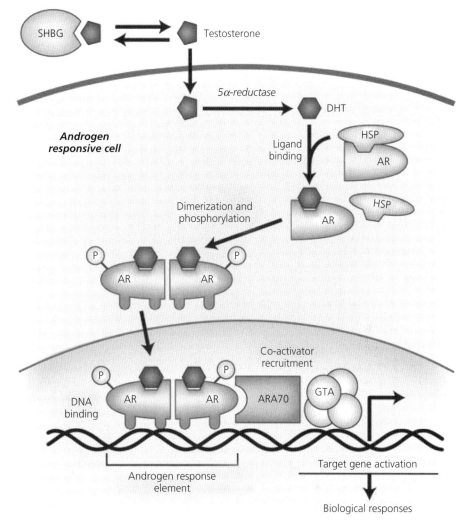

Figure 9.7 A schematic diagram of androgen action in a target cell. Circulating testosterone bound predominantly to sex hormone-binding globulin (SHBG) enters the cell in free form where it is converted to dihydrotestosterone (DHT), a more potent androgen. Both androgens bind to a single cytoplasmic androgen receptor (AR) complexed to heat-shock proteins (HSPs) and other co-chaperones such as FKBP52. Androgen binding dissociates the AR from HSPs where AR-bound androgen translocates to the nucleus, binding to DNA response elements as a homodimer. Co-activators, such as ARA70, bind to the AR complex to mediate interaction with the general transcription apparatus (GTA). This results in transcription of androgen-responsive genes and pleiotropic biologic responses; examples of such responses would include male sex differentiation, growth, muscle and bone development, spermatogenesis and prostate growth. P, phosphorylation. (From Hughes & Achermann [1] with permission.)

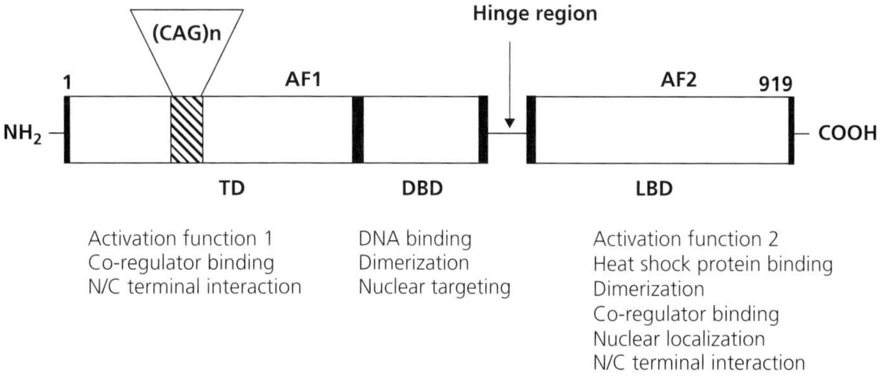

Figure 9.8 Functional domains of the androgen receptor. There are three primary domains together with the hinge region. AF1 and AF2 are subdomains and the multiple functions of the different domains are shown. (CAG)n indicates a polyglutamine tract in the N-terminal domain, which varies in length in the normal UK population within the range 11–31. Hyperexpansion of this glutamine tract causes spinobulbar muscular atrophy (Kennedy disease).

N-terminal domain. The range of repeats in the normal population is about 11–31. The tract is hyper-expanded in spinal and bulbar muscular atrophy (SBMA, Kennedy disease) [77]. Affected males display signs of mild androgen insensitivity. Transcriptional efficiency of the AR *in vitro* is inversely proportional to the number of CAG repeats. This appears to be biologically relevant as variations in the number of CAG repeats within the normal range show associations with several androgen-related disorders (Table 9.5).

Gender assignment and sex of rearing is unambiguously female in CAIS. Gender-related development in adulthood indicates that gender identity is female. There is no consensus about the timing

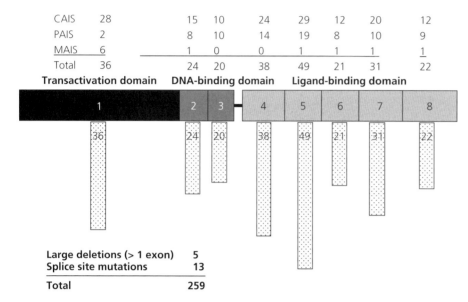

CAIS	28		15	10	24	29	12	20	12
PAIS	2		8	10	14	19	8	10	9
MAIS	6		1	0	0	1	1	1	1
Total	36		24	20	38	49	21	31	22

Transactivation domain **DNA-binding domain** **Ligand-binding domain**

Large deletions (> 1 exon)	5
Splice site mutations	13
Total	**259**

Figure 9.9 Spectrum of *AR* gene mutations identified in patients with androgen insensitivity syndrome. The frequency of mutations according to the functional domains is shown. The pattern is similar to that recorded on the international mutation database. CAIS, complete androgen insensitivity syndrome; MAIS, minimal androgen insensitivity syndrome (e.g. male factor infertility alone); PAIS, partial androgen insensitivity syndrome.

Table 9.5 Disease associations with variations in the AR glutamine repeat.

Shortened (CAG)n	Increased (CAG)n
Prostate cancer	**Above normal range**
Ovarian hyperandrogenism	SBMA (Kennedy disease)
Androgenetic alopecia	Hypospadias (one reported case)
Aspects of Klinefelter phenotype	
Response to androgen treatment	**Within normal range**
Central obesity	Male infertility
Mental retardation	Gynaecomastia
Endometrial cancer	Hypospadias
Coronary artery disease severity	Aspects of Klinefelter phenotype
	Bone density
	Breast cancer

SBMA, spinal and bulbar muscular atrophy.

of gonadectomy but it is generally delayed until young adulthood. When the gonads remain intact, puberty onset is similar to normal girls [78]. If gonadectomy is performed in infancy, low dose estrogen replacement is started at 10–11 years of age with replacement daily doses of 20 µg ethinyl estradiol reached by about 15 years of age. Delayed gonadectomy is associated with taller adult stature, the mean final height resting between the normal male and female adult heights; bone mineral density is marginally decreased in CAIS as a result of the lack of androgen effect [79,80].

Some adults with CAIS opt not to undergo gonadectomy because they consider the presence of androgens conducive to improved well-being. Even those who have had earlier gonadectomy have requested androgen replacement. The mechanism of this effect is biologically difficult to reconcile if one accepts the dogma that all androgens mediate their effect by ligand activation of a single AR ubiquitously expressed throughout the body, including the brain.

Gonadectomy is performed in CAIS because of the risk of gonadal tumor, the prevalence previously reported being as high as 25–30% in adulthood [81,82]. More recent analyses of larger series of cases indicate a prevalence of tumor development <5% for either CAIS or PAIS [83,84]. The precursor to a gonadal tumor in CAIS is the abundance of primordial germ cells in the tubules, a lesion previously labeled carcinoma *in situ* (CIS) but now referred to as intratubular germ cell neoplasia unclassified (ITGNU) by histopathologists [85]. This may subsequently result in the formation of a gonadoblastoma. The cells characteristic of the ITGNU lesion, often referred to as gonocytes, express several immunohistochemical markers which include placental-like alkaline phosphatase (PLAP), c-KIT (a receptor for stem cell factor), AP-2γ, Oct-3/4 and NANOG [86]. Stem cell factor, the ligand for c-KIT, appears to be a more specific marker that distinguishes malignant germ cells from those germ cells displaying maturational delay [87].

The initiating events that underlie the pathogenesis of testicular cancer arising from a precursor lesion such as ITGNU are unknown. A plausible hypothesis centers on testicular cancer being one component of the testicular dysgenesis syndrome which has its origin in fetal life [88], the others being cryptorchidism, hypospadias and defective spermatogenesis. The syndrome is initiated by environmental factors, such as hormone-disrupting chemicals, that act on the mother and developing fetus. The initiation of the process that results in delayed maturation of primordial germ cells and subsequent transformation to invasive malignant germ cells in adult life is against a genetic background of susceptibility. Thus, a polymorphism of the CAG repeat in the DNA polymerase gamma (POLG) gene is associated with germ cell tumors of the testis and may be a contributory factor in the pathogenesis [89].

The development of a gonadal tumor is rare before puberty in CAIS so it is reasonable to advocate later gonadectomy when the diagnosis is established in childhood. None of the aforementioned tumor markers have yet been analyzed in the circulation so, for those adults who opt not to have gonadectomy, monitoring for tumor development has to rely on ultrasound.

Management of DSD

Table 9.6 lists problems in a newborn infant that merit investigation as a possible DSD. It has been estimated that the frequency of deviation of the genital anatomy from the "ideal" male or female newborn is as high as 2% of live births [90]. The "idealized" male infant was defined as one with a penile size between 2.5 and 4.5 cm in length, normal position of the urethral meatus, testes in the scrotum and an XY karyotype. The "idealized" female infant had a clitoris ranging in size 0.2–0.85 cm, a normal female reproductive tract and an XX karyotype. Included in the "deviations" from normal were conditions such as sex chromosome aneuploidies, simple hypospadias and undescended testes.

Table 9.7 provides reference anthropometric data from the literature that provide some useful markers as to the borders of normality for undermasculinization in a male and excessive masculinization in a female [4]. There are also data available for measurements of the external genitalia in normal women, such as clitoral size, labial length and length of perineum [91]. This is important information when planning for reconstructive surgery in disorders such as CAH.

Examination

The clinical assessment of an infant born with ambiguous genitalia requires a history and physical examination. Family history and exposure to potential reproductive tract teratogens are particularly relevant. Examination of the external genitalia should record:

• *Phallus:* size and presence of chordee, is it a micropenis or clitoromegaly?
• *Site of urethral opening:* has a urine stream been observed?
• One or two external orifices on the perineum?
• *Development of labioscrotal folds:* whether there is a bifid scrotum, fused labia, rugosity and pigmentation of skin.
• Whether gonads are palpable and their position.

Table 9.6 Newborn problems that merit disorders of sex development (DSD) investigation.

Ambiguous genitalia
Apparent female genitalia with:
  Enlarged clitoris
  Posterior labial fusion
  Inguinal/labial mass
Apparent male genitalia with:
  Non-palpable testes
  Isolated perineoscrotal hypospadias
  Severe hypospadias, undescended testes, micropenis
Genital anomalies associated with syndromes
Family history of DSD, such as CAIS
Discordance between genital appearance and prenatal karyotype

CAIS, complete androgen insensitivity syndrome.

Table 9.7 Anthropometric measurements of the external genitalia.

Sex	Population	Age	Stretched penile length (PL) Mean (cm) ± SD	Penile width Mean (cm) ± SD	Mean testicular volume (cc)
M	USA	30 week GA	2.5 ± 0.4		
M	USA	Full term	3.5 ± 0.4	1.1 ± 0.1	0.52 (median)
M	Japan	Term – 14 years	2.9 ± 0.4 – 8.3 ± 0.8		
M	Australia	24–36 week GA	PL = 2.27 + (0.16 GA)		
M	Chinese	Term	3.1 ± 0.3	1.07 ± 0.09	
M	India	Term	3.6 ± 0.4	1.14 ± 0.07	
M	N America	Term	3.4 ± 0.3	1.13 ± 0.08	
M	Europe	10 years	6.4 ± 0.4		0.95–1.20
M	Europe	Adult	13.3 ± 1.6		16.5–18.2

Sex	Population	Age	Clitoral length Mean (mm) SD	Clitoral width Mean (mm) ± SD	Perineum length Mean (mm) ± SD
F	USA	Full term	4.0 ± 1.24	3.32 ± 0.78	
F	USA	Adult Nulliparous	15.4 ± 4.3		
F	USA	Adult	19.1 ± 8.7	5.5 ± 1.7	31.3 ± 8.5

GA, gestational age.

A number of grading systems have been devised to assess the degree of undermasculinization as applied to the androgen insensitivity syndrome [66] or the degree of masculinization by the Prader score as applied to female infants with CAH (Fig. 9.10a). An alternative method of assessing the degree of undermasculinization is to assign a score in relation to the presence or absence of micropenis, the position of the urethral opening (normal, glanular, penile shaft, perineal), scrotal sac fused or not and the position of the gonads (scrotal, inguinal, abdominal, absent) (Fig. 9.10b) [92].

Micropenis has been defined as a stretched penile length that is >2.5 SD below the mean for age. This equates to a lower limit of 1.9 cm for an infant up to 5 months of age [93]. A value of 2.5 cm or less for stretched penile length is often used to define micropenis, although it may be necessary to consider ethnic variations in penile size [94]. A normal range for penile length in preterm infants 24–36 weeks' gestation is available [95]. Applying some quantitative system to characterize the degree of undermasculinization in XY infants with ambiguous genitalia seems desirable, particularly if treatment with androgens is to be tried. The remainder of the assessment should include evidence of adrenal insufficiency and consideration of any congenital malformation syndromes associated with genital anomalies.

Investigation

Many schedules have been suggested for the investigation of a newborn infant with ambiguous genitalia but each unit must formulate a protocol determined by local practice and facilities [96,97]. Many centers are equipped to perform screening investigation but more detailed investigations to establish a definitive diagnosis may have to be undertaken at another center. Table 9.8 lists a range of investigations that should lead to a functional diagnosis in most newborns with ambiguous genitalia and allow early sex assignment. In reality, the leading causes are CAH, PAIS and XO/XY mixed gonadal dysgenesis. The karyotype result will be the steer to categorize the form of DSD according to the classification outlined in Table 9.2.

A provisional indication of the sex chromosomes can be obtained rapidly by FISH analysis using X chromosome centromeric probes and Y-specific SRY probe. A full karyotype is required to confirm the FISH result and a sufficient number of mitoses analyzed to exclude mosaicism. Measurement of serum 17OH-progesterone is a reliable test for CAH resulting from 21-hydroxylase deficiency. In a 46XX infant with ambiguous genitalia, elevated 17OH-progesterone (invariably >300 nmol/L) and a uterus visualized on pelvic ultrasound, the diagnosis is CAH. Ancillary biochemical tests should establish whether the infant is

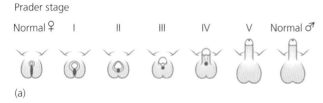

Scoring external genitalia

Prader stage

Normal ♀   I   II   III   IV   V   Normal ♂

(a)

External masculinization score

(b)

Figure 9.10 (a) Prader staging for scoring the degree of androgenization of the external genitalia in a female infant with congenital adrenal hyperplasia (CAH). (b) External masculinization score (EMS) to assess degree of underandrogenization in an individual with 46XY disorders of sex development (DSD). The score is based on the presence or absence of a micropenis and bifid scrotum, the location of the urethral meatus and the position of the testes.

Table 9.8 Investigating an infant with ambiguous genitalia.

Genetics
FISH (X centromeric and SRY probes)
Karyotype (high resolution; abundant mitoses)
Save DNA with consent

Endocrine
17OH-progesterone, 11-deoxycortisol (plus routine biochemistry; save serum) renin
ACTH, 24-h urinary steroids (also check proteinuria)
Testosterone androstenedione, DHT
LH, FSH, AMH, inhibin B
hCG stimulation test (define dose, timing)

Imaging
Pelvic, adrenal, renal US
MRI
Cystourethroscopy and sinogram

Surgical
Laparoscopy
Gonadal biopsies
Genital skin biopsy (AR studies, extract DNA and RNA)

ACTH, adenocorticotropic hormone; AMH, anti-Müllerian hormone; DHT, dihydrotestosterone; FISH, fluorescence *in situ* hybridization; FSH, follicle stimulating hormone; hCG, human chorionic gonadotropin; LH, luteinizing hormone; MRI, magnetic resonance imaging; US, ultrasound.

also a salt-loser. It may be necessary to perform an ACTH stimulation test, especially if CAH is suspected in a preterm infant or there is a possibility of one of the rarer enzyme defects. Measurement of urinary steroid metabolites by gas chromatography and mass spectrometry is the definitive test to define the type of enzyme defect [98,99]. Male infants with non-palpable testes must have a karyotype; to miss a diagnosis of CAH in a female masculinized to a Prader score V degree is unacceptable.

In the XY or XO/XY infant with ambiguous genitalia, investigations are aimed at establishing the presence and function of testicular tissue. The hCG stimulation test is pivotal in this situation, coupled with imaging and laparoscopy to identify gonad site and histological nature. There is no uniform protocol for an hCG stimulation test. One in common use is 1500 units/day IM for 3 days, with a post-hCG blood sample collected 24 h after the last injection. Occasionally, a longer test is needed using a twice-weekly injection regimen for 3 weeks. Pre- and post-hCG blood samples should be analyzed for androstenedione, testosterone and DHT. Concomitant 24-h urine collections can be performed for urinary steroid analysis but, surprisingly, this is often not reliable in the newborn for the diagnosis of disorders such as 5α-reductase deficiency and 17β-hydroxysteroid dehydrogenase deficiency. Expressing the ratio of testosterone to androstenedione following hCG stimulation is a useful screen for 17β-hydroxysteroid dehydrogenase deficiency in the differential diagnosis of XY DSD [100]. A ratio less than 0.8 is consistent with this enzyme deficiency; by contrast this is seldom the case with PAIS. Making such distinctions on biochemical criteria is an important prelude to molecular studies.

Sertoli cell function can be assessed by measurement of AMH and inhibin B. Circulating concentrations of AMH remain high until puberty when they fall in response to the effect of testosterone. AMH concentrations are elevated in DSD associated with androgen insensitivity but low in gonadal dysgenesis [101]. An undetectable value suggests anorchia, so this is a useful test in the investigation of an XY infant with ambiguous genitalia with no palpable gonads [102]. Inhibin B is also undetectable in anorchia and the concentrations correlate with the increment in testosterone following an hCG stimulation test in boys with gonadal dysgenesis and androgen insensitivity [103]. Basal measurements of AMH and inhibin B alone may be sufficient for confirming anorchia but baseline LH and FSH measurements together with a suitably performed hCG stimulation test should not be omitted from the protocol of investigations required in the XY infant with ambiguous genitalia.

Imaging with ultrasound and magnetic resonance imaging (MRI) is used to delineate the internal genital anatomy, including localizing the site and, possibly, the morphological nature of the gonads. Urogenital imaging techniques are identifying early organotypic patterns that, coupled with knowledge of genetic and hormonal pathways, can contribute to an improved understanding of phenotypic manifestations of DSD [104]. Only histology will provide precise details of the gonads and many infants with ambiguous genitalia require a laparoscopy to obtain as much detail to reach a diagnosis.

Clinical management

Ambiguous genitalia of the newborn is one of the greatest challenges a clinician has to manage. Information imparted to the parents at this early stage must be accurate, based on fact and not speculation: misinformation may be a lifelong burden for the family. Gender assignment may not be possible until a number of investigations are completed. No single professional should carry the onus of assigning gender in concert with the parents. This is a multidisciplinary team (MDT) activity which includes specialists in endocrinology, surgery, gynecology, genetics, psychology and, where appropriate, a medical ethicist, legal adviser and social worker. Each member of the team has to be competent in conveying information in a consistent manner to the parents as it becomes available.

There is consensus that all individuals with a DSD should be assigned a gender once the MDT is satisfied that sufficient information has been gleaned from an orderly set of investigations. It is not unreasonable that a short course of androgens (e.g. Sustanon 25 mg IM monthly for three injections) may be needed for an XY DSD before coming to a decision on gender assignment. Surgical procedures needed to make the genitalia concordant with gender assignment can be deferred until later, even to the extent of involving the child, if necessary, in the decision-making. There has certainly been a change in what may be regarded as the threshold for initiating clitoral reductoplasty in virilized girls with CAH. Rarely would surgery now be undertaken for less than Prader stage III clitoromegaly. This trend has been influenced by results of outcome studies in adult women with CAH showing impaired genital sensitivity and adverse effects on sexual function in those who underwent feminizing cosmetic genitoplasty [105].

Management of XY DSD is more complex and hinges on the decision reached about gender assignment. For example, an early diagnosis of 5α-reductase deficiency in a severely undermasculinized infant may guide the MDT and family towards male assignment in the knowledge that marked virilization of the external genitalia is expected at puberty. Gender role changes in those raised as female occur in about 60% of cases of 5α-reductase deficiency, raising the question that prenatal androgen exposure in this DSD is a major contributor to gender identity development [106].

Such gender role changes are not so common in 17β-hydroxysteroid dehydrogenase deficiency, an XY DSD also characterized by a predominant female phenotype at birth and profound virilization at puberty [106,107].

The infant with an XO/XY karyotype and ambiguous genitalia also poses a dilemma about gender assignment. The typical phenotype with microphallus, perineal hypospadias, unilateral descended gonad, contralateral abdominal streak gonad, the presence of a uterus and a Fallopian tube raises cogent arguments for either sex of rearing. That most XO/XY individuals are normal males may be a factor in influencing decisions towards male assignment in the minority of cases presenting with newborn ambiguous genitalia.

Transitional care

The complexity of DSD management is the result of the input of a diversity of disciplines:
• Does a single gene disorder establish a diagnosis?
• How can endocrine tests be interpreted in the newborn period?
• What options does the surgeon have for reconstructive surgery?
• What does the psychologist consider to be relevant prenatal androgen programing?
• What does the family consider to be important social and cultural issues?
• How does the MDT cope with the relative lack of outcome data, particularly in XY DSD?
Puberty and adolescence may be the time when many of these questions are resolved.

Transitional care clinics are now becoming well established in many areas of endocrinology such as pituitary disease, Turner syndrome and the multiple endocrine neoplasias. DSD, *par excellence*, is a template for such clinical care. Indeed, the professionals can be involved from the outset; the specialist gynecologist who will be caring for the adolescent girl with CAH or CAIS should be joining the pediatric urologist at the outset of any surgery for genitoplasty or gonadectomy.

Underpinning an MDT approach to the care of DSD patients from childhood to adulthood must be the registration of cases in a systematic manner which details a diagnosis, the phenotype and any identified genotype. Only then can a sufficient number of DSD cases be collated to improve diagnosis (e.g. the identification of new candidate genes in gonadal dysgenesis), the endocrine assessment of gonadal function, histological and immunohistochemical predictors of gonadal tumor risk, the optimal surgical intervention and timing and, above all, adult outcome in terms of gender identity, quality of life and reproductive potential.

A retrospective questionnaire-based study in one pediatric endocrine clinic has shown that the majority of adults with DSD seemed satisfied with their outcome in terms of gender and genital status [108]. Nevertheless, more work is needed to evaluate these parameters in larger studies conducted in several countries. To that end, a promising start has been made through the establishment of a EURO-DSD international European consortium funded through the 7th EU Framework program (http://cordis.europa.eu/fp7/home_en.html). Other resources that provided a catalyst for this international venture include the Scottish Genital Anomaly Network (http://www.sgan.nhsscotland.com), the German registry for rare diseases [109] and the Cambridge DSD Database [110]. One must also be aware that management of DSD may be influenced by criteria dictated by cultural influences in other countries. The idealized MDT and comprehensive clinical facilities may just not be available [111].

The pressing issues that need addressing in the evaluation and management of DSD include:
• An improvement in the current low success rate in establishing a diagnosis in XY DSD;
• Clearer guidelines on the weighting of the diverse factors that contribute to decision-making on gender assignment;
• How profound are the effects of prenatal androgens on gender behavior and gender identity in the DSD mosaic?
• How should the genitoplasty surgeon now function in a climate of increased frankness as to possible adverse consequences in later life of procedures undertaken in infancy?
• What is the risk of gonadal tumors where current management is tempered by a greater reluctance to perform gonadectomy? Such issues will be addressed adequately only when DSD patients are managed in MDT settings that participate in sharing knowledge at a national and international level.

Other examples of XY DSD

A number of relatively common abnormalities of male sex development come under the generic umbrella of DSD but do not present with ambiguous genitalia. These include hypospadias and cryptorchidism, the latter occasionally associated with the rare disorder, persistent Müllerian duct syndrome (PMDS).

Hypospadias

Hypospadias, incomplete fusion of the penile urethra defined by an arrest in development of the urethral spongiosum and ventral prepuce, has a birth prevalence of 3–4 per 1000 live births [112]. There is penile chordee in the more severe cases. A simple classification includes glanular, penile (mid-shaft) and perineoscrotal hypospadias (the most severe form). The etiology in most cases of isolated hypospadias is unknown.

The *CXorf6* gene located on chromosome Xq28 encodes a protein which functions as a co-activator in canonical Notch signalling [113]. Mutations of this gene have been identified in isolated hypospadias, including a series of more than 40 cases where an incidence of nearly 10% was reported [114,115].

Activating transcription factor 3 (*ATF3*), an estrogen responsive gene, is expressed in the genital tubercle and is upregulated in hypospadic genital skin [116]. Analysis of the *ATF3* gene in the foreskin of boys with hypospadias compared with controls revealed an association with a number of SNPs in intron1 and a number of nucleotide variations [117]. It is possible that *ATF3* gene variants influence the risk of hypospadias, perhaps modulated by the effects of environmental endocrine disrupters [118]. This has raised the question that hypospadias may be preventable [119]. In a genetic context, a new susceptibility locus for hypospadias on chromosome 7q32.2-q36.1 has been identified as a result of a genome-wide linkage analysis in a three-generational family with autosomal dominant inheritance of hypospadias [120]. This chromosome region contains many gene loci, some of which may be putative candidate genes for hypospadias.

Urogenital anomalies associated with apparent isolated hypospadias are sufficiently common to recommend screening of all asymptomatic hypospadias patients with urinary tract ultrasound, cystogram, urinalysis and urine culture [121]. General associations observed with hypospadias include increased maternal age, maternal vegetarian diet, maternal smoking, paternal subfertility, paternal exposure to pesticides, assisted reproductive techniques and fetal growth restriction [122].

The techniques of the surgical procedures required to relocate the urethral opening on to the glans and correct any chordee which enable satisfactory cosmetic and functional outcomes to be achieved are continuing to evolve [123]. A Pediatric Penile Perception Score has been devised based on the assessment of the meatus, glans, skin and general appearance as judged by patients, their parents and the urologist [124]. The method appears to be a reliable instrument to assess penile self-perception in children after hypospadias repair, who generally report high satisfaction with penile appearance comparable to age-matched controls. There are few outcome data on sexual function and fertility in adults who had hypospadias during childhood but a recent review provides evidence of some disturbance in psychosocial functioning during adolescence, delayed initiation of sexual activity, difficulties with ejaculation and a higher incidence of abnormal spermatogenesis [125].

Cryptorchidism

Cryptorchidism, which includes some cases of *anorchia*, is the most common congenital anomaly in boys, affecting 2–9% male live births [126]. A strong association with low birthweight, as well as associations with maternal smoking and alcohol use, gestational diabetes and possible exposure to environmental chemicals are factors to consider in etiology. A higher prevalence in hypogonadotropic hypogonadism and androgen insensitivity syndrome underwrites the role of androgens in testicular descent, particularly during the second inguinoscrotal phase. The initial transabdominal phase of testis descent is under the control of insulin-like factor 3 (INSL3) and its receptor (LGR8/GREAT), as evidenced by the effects on mouse gene knockout models [127]. By contrast, mutations in the human homologs of these two genes are found in only around 10% of boys with cryptorchidism [128].

It is apparent that an interrelationship between hormones, genes and the environment (critical fetal exposure to antiandrogenic and estrogenic compounds) underlies the multifactorial etiology of cryptorchidism [129].

Anogenital distance, a sensitive marker of androgen effect used by reproductive toxicologists in rodent experiments, is sexually dimorphic in humans; the distance is approximately twice as long in male than female infants and is inversely related to prenatal phthalate exposure [130]. Preliminary studies report a reduced anogenital distance in boys with hypospadias and cryptorchidism, perhaps suggestive of the first evidence of a direct link between environmental factors and male reproductive tract disorders [131].

Orchidopexy is generally the treatment of choice for undescended testis that is clearly distinguishable from a retractile testis. The link between testicular cancer in adulthood and previous testicular maldescent is well established and there is unequivocal evidence that performing orchidopexy before puberty significantly decreases the risk of testicular cancer [132,133]. The effect of the timing of treatment on subsequent fertility is less clear-cut but it is recommended that orchidopexy be performed before the age of 1 year in order to maximize future fertility potential [134,135].

Bilateral non-palpable testes may be the result of their maldescent and abdominal location or because they are absent (*bilateral anorchia* or the *vanishing testis syndrome*). The latter can be confirmed by a combination of endocrine tests showing elevated gonadotropins (particularly FSH), an absent testosterone response to hCG stimulation and a low or undetectable serum AMH.

The cause of this syndrome is unknown but postulated to be an intrauterine testicular torsion occurring after testis determination and the action of testosterone and AMH on internal and external genital development. Bilateral anorchia with a normal differentiated but small phallus is a recognized variant of the syndrome [136].

Surgical exploration typically shows a vas deferens disappearing into the internal inguinal ring at the end of which are nubbins of non-testicular fibrous tissue containing hemosiderin-laden macrophages and dystrophic calcification [137,138]. This has led some surgeons to consider whether laparoscopic exploration for testicular tissue is necessary if the endocrine tests are consistent with absent testes. Viable germ cell remnants and seminiferous tubules may be found occasionally [139]: because such remnants may have the potential for malignant transformation, it is generally recommended that surgical exploration be undertaken for their removal.

Persistent Müllerian duct syndrome

Maldescent of the testis in this syndrome is mechanical in nature by virtue of its attachment to a fallopian tube and uterus, retained in the male because of lack of AMH effect. This is the result of either a mutation in the *AMH* gene or the gene that encodes for the AMH type II receptor [140,141]. The range of mutations affecting these two genes is summarized in Figure 9.11. They contribute equally to cause the PMDS phenotype, a mutation being identified in more than 80% of cases. Serum AMH is low or undetectable, whereas it is in the normal range with an AMH type II receptor mutation. External male genital development is normal in this syndrome. The diagnosis may be established only at orchidopexy for an undescended testis or during an inguinal hernia repair when the sac is found to contain a uterus or fallopian tube. Sometimes the sac also contains the contralateral testis and tube. Such transverse testicular ectopia is, *de facto*, a diagnosis of PMDS.

Surgical management endeavors to resite the testis in the scrotum but there is a risk of compromising the blood supply and damaging the vas deferens. Conservative treatment may be more

AMH/MIS

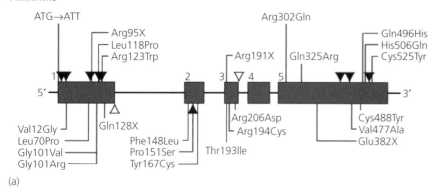

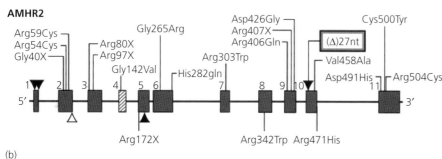

(a)

(b)

Figure 9.11 Mutations that cause persistent Müllerian duct syndrome. The numbered solid boxes depict the exons. The three-letter abbreviation for amino acids is used to indicate the position of missense mutations; X indicates a nonsense (stop) mutation; insertions and deletions resulting in frameshift and splice site mutations are shown by filled arrowheads and open arrowheads, respectively. (a) *AMH* gene mutations. (b) *AMHR2* gene mutations. D27nt (open box) is a 27-nucleotide deletion, the most common *AMHR2* mutation causing persistent Müllerian duct syndrome. (After Hughes & Achermann [1] with permission.)

appropriate in the case of transverse testicular ectopia when both testes are already sited ipsilaterally in the scrotum. There appears to be no contraindication to leaving the uterus *in situ*.

References

1 Hughes IA, Achermann JC. Disorders of sex differentiation. In: Kronenberg H, Melmed S, Polonsky K, Larsen PR, eds. *Williams' Textbook of Endocrinology*, 11th edn. Philadelphia: Saunders Elsevier, 2007: 783–748.

2 Sim H, Argentaro A, Harley VR. Boys, girls and shuttling of SRY and SOX9. *Trends Endocrinol Metab* 2008; **19**: 213–222.

3 DiNapoli L, Capel B. SRY and the standoff in sex determination. *Mol Endocrinol* 2008; **22**: 1–9.

4 Hughes IA, Houk C, Ahmed SF, Lee PA. Consensus statement on management of intersex disorders. *Arch Dis Child* 2006; **91**: 554–563.

5 Vilain E, Achermann JC, Eugster EA. We used to call them hermaphrodites. *Genet Med* 2007; **9**: 65–66.

6 Hughes IA, Nihoul-Fékété C, Thomas B, Cohen-Kettenis PT. Consequences of the ESPE/LWPES guidelines for diagnosis and treatment of disorders of sex development. *Best Pract Res Clin Endocrinol Metab* 2007; **21**: 351–365.

7 Lo JC, Schwitzgebel VM, Tyrrel JB *et al.* Normal female infants born of mothers with classic congenital adrenal hyperplasia due to 21-hydroxylase deficiency. *J Clin Endocrinol Metab* 1999; **84**: 930–936.

8 Hagenfeldt K, Janson PO, Holmdahl G, *et al.* Fertility and pregnancy outcome in women with congenital adrenal hyperplasia due to 21-hydroxylase deficiency. *Hum Reprod* 2008; **23**: 1607–1613.

9 Brunskill J. The effects of fetal exposure to Danazol. *Br J Obstet Gynecol* 1992; **99**: 212–214.

10 Conte FA, Grumbach MM, Ito Y, Fisher CR, Simpson EV. A syndrome of female pseudohermaphrodism, hypergonadotropic hypogonadism and multicystic ovaries associated with missense mutations in the gene encoding aromatase (P450arom). *J Clin Endocrinol Metab* 1994; **78**: 1287–1292.

11 Jones ME, Boon WC, McInnes K, Maffei L, Carani C, Simpson ER. Recognising rare disorders: aromatase deficiency. *Nat Clin Pract Endocrinol Metab* 2007; **3**: 414–421.

12 Oji V, Traupe H. Ichthyoses: differential diagnosis and molecular genetics. *Eur J Dermatol* 2006; **16**: 349–359.

13 Coleman MA, Honour JW. Reduced maternal dexamethasone dosage for the prenatal treatment of congenital adrenal hyperplasia. *Br J Gynaecol* 2004; **111**: 176–178.

14 Morishima A, Grumbach MM, Simpson ER, *et al.* Aromatase deficiency in male and female siblings caused by a novel mutation and the physiological role of estrogens. *J Clin Endocrinol Metab* 1995; **80**: 3689–3698.

15 Arlt W, Walker EA, Draper N, *et al.* Congenital adrenal hyperplasia caused by mutant P450 oxidoreductase and human androgen synthesis: analytical study. *Lancet* 2004; **363**: 2128–2135.

16 Auchus RJ. The backdoor pathway to dihydrotestosterone. *Trends Endocrinol Metab* 2004; **15**: 432–438.

17 Scott RR, Miller WL. Genetic and clinical features of p450 oxidoreductase deficiency. *Horm Res* 2008; **69**: 266–275.

18 Hughes IA. Prenatal treatment of congenital adrenal hyperplasia: do we have enough evidence? *Treat Endocrinol* 2006; **5**: 1–6.

19 Hirvikoski T, Nordenstrom A, Lindholm T, Lindblad F, Ritzen M, Lajic S. Long-term follow-up of prenatally treated children at risk for congenital adrenal hyperplasia: does dexamethasone cause behavioural problems? *Eur J Endocrinol* 2008; **159**: 309.

20 Harley VR, Clarkson MJ, Argentaro A. The molecular action and regulation of the testis-determining factors, SRY (sex-determining region on the Y chromosome) and SOX9 [SRY-related high-mobility group (HMG) box 9]. *Endocr Rev* 2003; **24**: 466–487.

21 Sarafoglou K, Ostrer H. Familial sex reversal: a review. *J Clin Endocrinol Metab* 2000; **85**: 483–493.

22 Chemes HE, Muzulin PM, Venara MC, *et al*. Early manifestations of testicular dysgenesis in children: pathological phenotypes, karyotype correlations and precursor stages of tumour development. *APMIS* 2003; **111**: 12–24.

23 Achermann JC, Ito M, Ito M, Hindmarsh PC, Jameson JL. A mutation in the gene encoding steroidogenic factor-1 causes XY sex reversal and adrenal failure in humans. *Nat Genet* 1999; **22**: 125–126.

24 Achermann JC, Ozisik G, Ito M, *et al*. Gonadal determination and adrenal development are regulated by the orphan nuclear receptor steroidogenic factor-1, in a dose-dependent manner. *J Clin Endocrinol Metab* 2002; **87**: 1829–1833.

25 Lin L, Philibert P, Ferraz-de-Souza B, *et al*. Heterozygous missense mutations in steroidogenic factor 1 (SF1/Ad4BP, NR5A1) are associated with 46,XY disorders of sex development with normal adrenal function. *J Clin Endocrinol Metab* 2007; **92**: 991–999.

26 Köhler B, Lin L, Ferraz-de-Souza B, *et al*. Five novel mutations in steroidogenic factor 1 (SF1, NR5A1) in 46,XY patients with severe underandrogenization but without adrenal insufficiency. *Hum Mutat* 2008; **29**: 59–64.

27 Philibert P, Zenaty D, Lin L, *et al*. Mutational analysis of steroidogenic factor 1 (NR5a1) in 24 boys with bilateral anorchia: a French collaborative study. *Hum Reprod* 2007; **22**: 3255–3261.

28 Little M, Wells C. A clinical overview of WT1 gene mutations. *Hum Mutat* 1997; **9**: 209–225.

29 Klambt B, Koziell AB, Poulat F, *et al*. Frasier syndrome is caused by defective alternative splicing leading to an altered ratio of WT1 +/− KTS splice isoforms. *Hum Mol Genet* 1998; **7**: 709–714.

30 Koziell A, Charmandari E, Hindmarsh PC, Rees L, Scambler P, Brook CGD. Frasier syndrome, part of the Denys Drash continuum or simply at WT1 gene associated disorder of intersex and nephropathy? *Clin Endocrinol* 2000; **52**: 519–524.

31 Royer-Pokara B, Beier M, Henzler M, *et al*. Twenty-four new cases of WT1 germline mutations and review of the literature: genotype/phenotype correlations for Wilms tumour development. *Am J Med Genet* 2004; **127A**: 249–257.

32 Kohler B, Schumacher V, l'Allemand D, Roger-Pokora B, Gruters A. Germline Wilms tumour suppressor gene (WT1) mutation leading to isolated genital malformation without Wilms tumour or nephropathy. *J Pediatr* 2001; **138**: 421–424.

33 Gwin K, Cajaiba MM, Caminoa-Lizarralde A, Picazo ML, Nistal M, Reyes-Múgica M. Expanding the clinical spectrum of Frasier syndrome. *J Pediatr Dev Pathol* 2008; **11**: 122–127.

34 Ismaili K, Verdure V, Vandenhoute K, Janssen F, Hall M. WT1 gene mutations in three girls with nephrotic syndrome. *Eur J Pediatr* 2008; **167**: 579–581.

35 Kwok C, Weller PA, Guioli S, *et al*. Mutations in SOX9, the gene responsible for campomelic dysplasia and autosomal sex reversal. *Am J Hum Genet* 1995; **57**: 1028–1036.

36 Bernard P, Tang P, Liu S, Dewing P, Harley VR, Vilain E. Dimerization of SOX9 is required for chondrogenesis but not for sex determination. *Hum Mol Genet* 2003; **12**: 1755–1765.

37 Kwok C, Goodfellow PN, Hawkins, JR. Evidence to exclude SOX9 as a candidate gene for XY sex reversal without skeletal malformation. *J Med Genet* 1996; **33**: 800–801.

38 Gibbons RJ, Higgs DR. Molecular-clinical spectrum of the ATR-X syndrome. *Am J Med Genet* 2000; **97**: 204–212.

39 Gibbons RJ, Wada T, Fisher CA, *et al*. Mutations in the chromatin-associated protein ATRX. *Hum Mutat* 2008; **29**: 796–802.

40 Alvarez-Nava F, Soto M, Borjas L, *et al*. Molecular analysis of SRY gene in patients with mixed gonadal dysgenesis. *Ann Genet* 2001; **44**: 155–159.

41 Canto P, Galicia N, Söderlund D, Escudero I, Méndez JP. Screening for mutations in the SRY gene in patients with mixed gonadal dysgenesis or with Turner syndrome and Y mosaicism. *Eur J Obstet Gynecol Reprod Biol* 2004; **115**: 55–58.

42 Telvi L, Lebbar A, Pino OD, Barbet JP, Chaussain JL. 45,X/46,XY mosaicism: report of 27 cases. *Pediatrics* 1999; **104**: 304–308.

43 Chang HJ, Clark RD, Bachman H. The phenotype of 45,X/46,XY mosaicism: an analysis of 92 prenatally diagnosed cases. *Am J Hum Genet* 1990; **46**: 156–167.

44 Hsu LY. Phenotype/karyotype correlations of Y chromosome aneuploidy with emphasis on structural aberrations in postnatally diagnosed cases. *Am J Med Genet* 1994; **53**: 108–140.

45 Tho SP, Jackson R, Kulharya AS, Reindollar RH, Layman LC, McDonough PG. Long-term follow-up and analysis of monozygotic twins concordant for 45,X/46,XY peripheral blood karyotype but discordant for phenotypic sex. *Am J Med Genet A* 2007; **143A**: 2616–2622.

46 Hadjiathanasiou CG, Brauner R, Lortat-Jacob S, *et al*. True hermaphroditism: genetic variants and clinical management. *J Pediatr* 1994; **125**: 738–744.

47 Queipo G, Zenteno JC, Pena R, *et al*. Molecular analysis in true hermaphroditism: demonstration of low-level hidden mosaicism for Y-derived sequences in 46,XX cases. *Hum Genet* 2002; **111**: 278–283.

48 Verkauskas G, Jaubert F, Lortat-Jacob S, Malan V, Thibaud E, Nihoul- Fékété C. The long-term follow up of 33 cases of true hermaphroditism: a 40 year experience with conservative gonadal surgery. *J Urol* 2007; **177**: 726–731.

49 Ferguson-Smith MA, Cooke A, Affara NA, *et al*. Genotype–phenotype correlations in XX males and their bearing on current theories of sex determination. *Hum Genet* 1990; **84**: 198–202.

50 Vorona E, Zitzmann M, Gromoll J, Shüring AN, Nieschlag E. Clinical, endocrinological and epigenetic features of the 46,XX male syndrome, compared with 47,XXY Klinefelter patients. *J Clin Endocrinol Metab* 2007; **92**: 3458–3465.

51 Maciel-Guerra AT, de Mello MP, Coeli FB. XX Maleness and XX true hermaphroditism in SRY-negative monozygotic twins: additional evidence for a common origin. *J Clin Endocrinol Metab* 2008; **93**: 339–343.

52 Tomaselli S, Megiorni F, De Bernardo C, *et al*. Syndromic true hermaphroditism due to an R-spondin1 (RSPO1) homozygous mutation. *Hum Mutat* 2008; **29**: 220–226.

53 Parma P, Radi O, Vidal V, *et al*. R-spondin1 is essential in sex determination, skin differentiation and malignancy. *Nat Genet* 2006; **38**: 1304–1309.

54 Tomizuka K, Horikoshi K, Kitada R. R-spondin1 plays an essential role in ovarian development through positively regulating Wnt-4 signaling. *Hum Mol Genet* 2008; **17**: 1278–1291.

55 Morris JK, Alberman E, Scott C, Jacobs P. Is the prevalence of Klinefelter syndrome increasing? *Eur J Hum Genet* 2008; **16**: 163–170.

56 Lee YS, Cheng AW, Ahmed SF, Shaw NJ, Hughes IA. Genital anomalies in Klinefelter's syndrome. *Horm Res* 2007; **68**: 150–155.

57 Wikström AM, Dunkel L. Testicular function in Klinefelter syndrome. *Horm Res* 2008; **69**: 317–326.

58 Richter-Unruh A, Martens JW, Verhoef-Post M, *et al.* Leydig cell hypoplasia: cases with new mutations, new polymorphisms and cases without mutations in the luteinising hormone receptor gene. *Clin Endocrinol* 2002; **56**: 105–112.

59 Huhtaniemi I, Alevizaki M. Gonadotrophin resistance. *Best Pract Res Clin Endocrinol Metab* 2006; **20**: 561–576.

60 Boehmer ALM, Brinkmann AO, Sandkuijl LA, *et al.* 17β-hydroxysteroid dehydrogenase-3 deficiency: diagnosis, phenotypic variability, population genetics and worldwide distribution of ancient and *de novo* mutations. *J Clin Endocrinol Metab* 1999; **84**: 4713–4721.

61 Lee YS, Kirk JM, Stanhope RG, *et al.* Phenotypic variability in 17beta-hydroxysteroid dehydrogenase-3 deficiency and diagnostic pitfalls. *Clin Endocrinol* 2007; **67**: 20–28.

62 Mazen I, Gad YZ, Hafez M, Sultan C, Lumbroso S. Molecular analysis of 5 alpha-reductase type 2 gene in eight unrelated Egyptian children with suspected 5 alpha-reductase deficiency: prevalence of the G34R mutation. *Clin Endocrinol* 2003; **58**: 627–631.

63 Cohen-Kettenis PT. Gender change in 46,XY persons with 5alpha-reductase-2 deficiency and 17beta-hydroxysteroid dehydrogenase-3 deficiency. *Arch Sex Behav* 2005; **34**: 399–410.

64 Katz MD, Kligman I, Cai LQ, *et al.* Paternity by intrauterine insemination with sperm from a man with 5alpha-reductase-2 deficiency. *N Engl J Med* 1997; **336**: 994–997.

65 Nordenskjöld A, Ivarsson SA. Molecular characterization of 5 alpha-reductase type 2 deficiency and fertility in a Swedish family. *J Clin Endocrinol Metab* 1998; **83**: 3236–3238.

66 Quigley CA, De Bellis A, Marschke KB, el-Wady MK, Wilson EM, French FS. Androgen receptor defects: historical, clinical and molecular perspectives. *Endocr Rev* 1995; **16**: 271–321.

67 Hughes IA, Deeb A. Androgen resistance. *Best Pract Res Clin Endocrinol Metab* 2006; **20**: 577–598.

68 Jääskeläinen, J, Hughes IA. Androgen insensitivity syndromes. In: Balen AH, Creighton SM, Davies MC, MacDougall J, Stanhope R, eds. *Paediatric and Adolescent Gynaecology*. Cambridge: Cambridge University Press, 2004: 253–266.

69 Deeb A, Hughes IA. Inguinal hernia in female infants: a cue to check the sex chromosomes? *BJU Int* 2005; **96**: 401–403.

70 Sarpel U, Palmer SK, Dolgin SE. The incidence of complete androgen insensitivity in girls with inguinal hernias and assessment of screening by vaginal length measurement. *J Pediatr Surg* 2005; **40**: 133–136.

71 Lobaccaro JM, Lumbroso S, Belon C, *et al.* A second instance of male breast cancer linked to a germline mutation of the androgn receptor gene. *Nat Genet* 1993; **5**: 109–110.

72 Davis SE, Wallace AM. A 19 year old with complete androgen insensitivity syndrome and juvenile fibroadenoma of the breast. *Breast J* 2001; **7**: 430–433.

73 Ahmed SF, Chang A, Dovey L, *et al.* Phenotypic features androgen receptor binding and mutational analysis in 278 clinical cases reported as androgen insensitivity syndrome. *J Clin Endocrinol Metab* 2000; **85**: 658–665.

74 Sultan C, Lumbroso S, Paris F, *et al.* Disorders of androgen action. *Semin Reprod Med* 2002; **20**: 217–228.

75 Köhler B, Lumbroso S, Leger J, *et al.* Androgen insensitivity syndrome: somatic mosaicism of the androgen receptor in seven families and consequences for sex assignment and genetic counseling. *J Clin Endocrinol Metab* 2005; **90**: 106–111.

76 Rajender S, Gupta NJ, Chakravarty B, Singh L, Thangaraj K. Androgen insensitivity syndrome: do trinucleotide repeats in androgen receptor gene have any role? *Asian J Androl* 2008; **10**: 616–624.

77 Greenland KJ, Zajac JD. Kennedy's disease: pathogenesis and clinical approaches. *Int Med J* 2004; **34**: 279–286.

78 Papadimitriou DT, Linglart A, Morel Y, Chaussain JL. Puberty in subjects with complete androgen insensitivity syndrome. *Horm Res* 2006; **65**: 126–131.

79 Danilovic DL, Correa PH, Costa EM, Melo KF, Mendonca BB, Arnhold IJ. Height and bone mineral density in androgen insensitivity syndrome with mutations in the androgen receptor gene. *Osteoporos Int* 2007; **18**: 369–374.

80 Han TS, Goswami D, Trikudanathan S, Creighton SM, Conway GS. Comparison of bone mineral density and body proportions between women with complete androgen insensitivity syndrome and women with gonadal dysgenesis. *Eur J Endocrinol* 2008; **159**: 179–185.

81 Cassio A, Cacciari E, D'Errico A, *et al.* Incidence of intratubular germ cell neoplasia in androgen insensitivity syndrome. *Acta Endocrinol (Copenh)* 1990; **123**: 416–422.

82 Rutgers JL, Scully RE. The androgen insensitivity syndrome (testicular feminization): a clinicopathologic study of 43 cases. *Int J Gynecol Pathol* 1991; **10**: 126–144.

83 Hannema SE, Scott IS, Rajpert-De Meyts E, Skakkebaek NE, Coleman N, Hughes IA. Testicular development in the complete androgen insensitivity syndrome. *J Pathol* 2006; **208**: 518–527.

84 Looijenga LH, Hersmus R, Oosterhuis JW, Cools M, Drop SL, Wolffenbuttel KP. Tumor risk in disorders of sex development (DSD). *Best Pract Res Clin Endocrinol Metab* 2007; **21**: 480–495.

85 Hannema SE and Hughes IA. Neoplasia and intersex states. In: Hay I, Wass J, eds. *Clinical Endocrine Oncology*, 2nd edn. Oxford: Blackwell Publishing, 2008: 86–96.

86 Almstrup K, Sonne SB, Hoei-Hansen CE, *et al.* From embryonic stem cells to testicular germ cell cancer: should we be concerned? *Int J Androl* 2006; **29**: 211–218.

87 Stoop H, Honecker F, van de Geijn G, *et al.* Stem cell factor as a novel diagnostic marker for early malignant germ cells. *J Pathol* 2008; **216**: 43–54.

88 Sonne SB, Kristensen DM, Novotny GW, *et al.* Testicular dysgenesis syndrome and the origin of carcinoma in situ testis. *Int J Androl* 2008; **31**: 275–287.

89 Jensen MB, Leffers H, Petersen JH, Daugaard G, Skakkebaek NE, Rajpert-De Meyts E. Association of the polymorphism of the CAG repeat in the mitochondrial DNA polymerase gamma gene (POLG) with testicular germ-cell cancer. *Ann Oncol* 2008; **19**: 1910–1914.

90 Blackless M, Charuvastra A, Derryck A, Fausto-Sterling A, Lauzanne K, Lec E. How sexually dimorphic are we? Review and synthesis. *Am J Hum Biol* 2000; **12**: 151–166.

91 Lloyd J, Crouch NS, Minto CL, Liao LM, Creighton SM. Female genital appearance: "normality" unfolds. *BJOG* 2005; **112**: 643–646.

92 Ahmed SF, Khwaja O, Hughes IA. The role of a clinical score in the assessment of ambiguous genitalia. *BJU Int* 2000; **85**: 120–124.

93 Lee PA, Mazur T, Danish R, *et al.* Micropenis. I. Criteria, etiologies and classification. *Johns Hopkins Med J* 1980; **146**: 156–163.

94 Cheng PK, Chanoine JP. Should the definition of micropenis vary according to ethnicity? *Horm Res* 2001; **55**: 278–281.

95 Tuladhar R, Davis PG, Batch J, Doyle LW. Establishment of a normal range of penile length in preterm infants. *J Paediatr Child Health* 1998; **34**: 471–473.

96 Ogilvy-Stuart AL, Brain CE. Early assessment of ambiguous genitalia. *Arch Dis Child* 2004; **89**: 401–407.

97 Peters CJ, Hindmarsh PC. Management of neonatal endocrinopathies: best practice guidelines. *Early Hum Dev* 2007; **83**: 553–561.

98 Honour JW, Brook CG. Clinical indications for the use of urinary steroid profiles in neonates and children. *Ann Clin Biochem* 1997; **34**: 45–54.

99 Wudy SA, Hartmann MF. Gas chromatography-mass spectrometry profiling of steroids in times of molecular biology. *Horm Metab Res* 2004; **36**: 415–422.

100 Ahmed SF, Iqbal A, Hughes IA. The testosterone: androstenedione ratio in male undermasculinization. *Clin Endocrinol* 2000; **53**: 697–702.

101 Rey RA, Belville C, Nihoul-Fekete C, *et al.* Evaluation of gonadal function in 107 intersex patients by means of serum antimullerian hormone measurement. *J Clin Endocrinol Metab* 1999; **84**: 627–631.

102 Lee MM, Misra M, Donahoe PK, MacLaughlin DT. MIS/AMH in the assessment of cryptorchidism and intersex conditions. *Mol Cell Endocrinol* 2003; **211**: 91–98.

103 Kubini K, Zachmann M, Albers N, *et al.* Basal inhibin B and the testosterone response to human chorionic gonadotropin correlate in prepubertal boys. *J Clin Endocrinol Metab* 2000; **85**: 134–138.

104 Wünsch L, Schober JM. Imaging and examination strategies of normal male and female sex development and anatomy. *Best Pract Res Clin Endocrinol Metab* 2007; **21**: 367–379.

105 Crouch NS, Liao LM, Woodhouse CR, Conway GS, Creighton SM. Sexual function and genital sensitivity following feminizing genitoplasty for congenital adrenal hyperplasia. *J Urol* 2008; **179**: 634–638.

106 Cohen-Kettenis PT. Gender change in 46,XY persons with 5alpha-reductase-2 deficiency and 17beta-hydroxysteroid dehydrogenase-3 deficiency. *Arch Sex Behav* 2005; **34**: 399–410.

107 Lee YS, Kirk JM, Stanhope RG, *et al.* Phenotypic variability in 17beta-hydroxysteroid dehydrogenase-3 deficiency and diagnostic pitfalls. *Clin Endocrinol (Oxf)* 2007; **67**: 20–28.

108 Meyer-Bahlburg HFL, Migeon CJ, Berkovitz GD, Gearhart JP, Dolezal C, Wisniewski AB. Attitudes of adult 46,XY intersex persons to clinical management policies. *J Urol* 2004; **171**: 1615–1619.

109 Thyen U, Lanz K, Holterhus PM, Hiort O. Epidemiology and initial management of ambiguous genitalia at birth in Germany. *Horm Res* 2006; **66**: 195–203.

110 Deeb A, Mason C, Lee YS, Hughes IA. Correlation between genotype, phenotype and sex of rearing in 111 patients with partial androgen insensitivity syndrome. *Clin Endocrinol (Oxf)* 2005; **63**: 56–62.

111 Warne GL, Raza J. Disorders of sex development (DSDs), their presentation and management in different cultures. *Rev Endocr Metab Disord* 2008; **9**: 227–236.

112 Baskin LS, Ebbers MB. Hypospadias: anatomy, etiology and technique. *J Pediatr Surg* 2006; **41**: 463–472.

113 Fukami M, Wada Y, Okada M, *et al.* Mastermind-like domain-containing 1 (MAMLD1 or CXorf6) transactivates the Hes3 promoter, augments testosterone production and contains the SF1 target sequence. *J Biol Chem* 2008; **283**: 5525–5532.

114 Fukami M, Wada Y, Miyabayashi K, *et al.* CXorf6 is a causative gene for hypospadias. *Nat Genet* 2006; **38**: 1369–1371.

115 Kalfa N, Liu B, Klein O, *et al.* Mutations of CXorf6 are associated with a range of severities of hypospadias. *Eur J Endocrinol* 2008; **159**: 453–458.

116 Liu B, Lin G, Willingham E, Ning H, Lin CS, Lue TF, Baskin LS. Estradiol upregulates activating transcription factor 3, a candidate gene in the etiology of hypospadias. *Pediatr Dev Pathol* 2007; **10**: 446–454.

117 Beleza-Meireles A, Töhönen V, Söderhäll C, *et al.* Activating transcription factor 3: a hormone responsive gene in the etiology of hypospadias. *Eur J Endocrinol* 2008; **158**: 729–739.

118 Wang MH, Baskin LS. Endocrine disruptors, genital development and hypospadias. *J Androl* 2008; **29**: 499–505.

119 Baskin LS. Can we prevent hypospadias? *Fertil Steril* 2008; **89**(2 Suppl): e39.

120 Thai HT, Söderhäll C, Lagerstedt K, *et al.* A new susceptibility locus for hypospadias on chromosome 7q32.2-q36.1. *Hum Genet* 2008; **124**: 155–160.

121 Friedman T, Shalom A, Hoshen G, Brodovsky S, Tieder M, Westreich M. Detection and incidence of anomalies associated with hypospadias. *Pediatr Nephrol* 2008; **23**: 1809–1816.

122 Brouwers MM, Feitz WF, Roelofs LA, Kiemeney LA, de Gier RP, Roeleveld N. Risk factors for hypospadias. *Eur J Pediatr* 2007; **166**: 671–678.

123 Hoag CC, Gotto GT, Morrison KB, Coleman GU, Macneily AE. Long-term functional outcome and satisfaction of patients with hypospadias repaired in childhood. *Can Urol Assoc J* 2008; **2**: 23–31.

124 Weber DM, Schönbucher VB, Landolt MA, Gobet R. The Pediatric Penile Perception Score: an instrument for patient self-assessment and surgeon evaluation after hypospadias repair. *J Urol* 2008; **180**: 1080–1084.

125 Mieusset R, Soulié M. Hypospadias: psychosocial, sexual and reproductive consequences in adult life. *J Androl* 2005; **26**: 163–168.

126 Hughes I, Acerini C. Factors controlling testis descent. *Eur J Endocrinol* 2008; **159** suppl 1: 575–582.

127 Zimmermann S, Steding G, Emmen JM, *et al.* Targeted disruption of the Insl3 gene causes bilateral cryptorchidism. *Mol Endocrinol* 1999; **13**: 681–691.

128 Ferlin A, Simonato M, Bartoloni L, *et al.* The INSL3-LGR8/GREAT ligand-receptor pair in human cryptorchidism. *J Clin Endocrinol Metab* 2003; **88**: 4273–4279.

129 Foresta C, Zuccarello D, Garolla A, Ferlin A. Role of hormones, genes and environment in human cryptorchidism. *Endocr Rev* 2008; **29**: 560–580.

130 Swan SH, Main KM, Liu F, *et al.* Decrease in anogenital distance among male infants with prenatal phthalate exposure. *Environ Health Perspect* 2005; **113**: 1056–1061.

131 Hsieh MH, Breyer BN, Eisenberg ML, Baskin LS. Associations among hypospadias, cryptorchidism, anogenital distance and endocrine disruption. *Curr Urol Rep* 2008; **9**: 137–142.

132 Pettersson A, Richiardi L, Nordenskjold A, Kaijser M, Akre O. Age at surgery for undescended testis and risk of testicular cancer. *N Eng J Med* 2007; **356**: 1835–1841.

133 Walsh TJ, Dall'Era MA, Croughan MS, Carroll PR, Turek PJ. Pre-pubertal orchiopexy for cryptorchidism may be associated with lower risk of testicular cancer. *J Urol* 2007; **178**: 1440–1446.

134 Murphy F, Paran TS, Puri P. Orchidopexy and its impact on fertility. *Pediatr Surg Int* 2007; **23**: 625–632.

135 Park KH, Lee JH, Han JJ, Lee SD, Song SY. Histological evidences suggest recommending orchiopexy within the first year of life for children with unilateral inguinal cryptorchid testis. *Int J Urol* 2007; **14**: 616–621.

136 Zenaty D, Dijoud F, Morel Y, *et al.* Bilateral anorchia in infancy: occurrence of micropenis and the effect of testosterone treatment. *J Pediatr* 2006; **149**: 687–691.

137 Law H, Mushtaq I, Wingrove K, *et al.* Histopathological features of testicular regression syndrome: relation to patient age and implications for management. *Fet Pediatr Pathol* 2006; **25**: 119–129.

138 Emir H, Ayik B, Eliçevik M, *et al.* Histological evaluation of the testicular nubbins in patients with nonpalpable testis: assessment of etiology and surgical approach. *Pediatr Surg Int* 2007; **23**: 41–44.

139 Storm D, Redden T, Aguiar M, Wilkerson M, Jordan G, Sumfest J. Histologic evaluation of the testicular remnant associated with the vanishing testes syndrome: is surgical management necessary? *Urology* 2007; **70**: 1204–1206.

140 Josso N, Belville C, de Clemente N, *et al.* AMH and AMH receptor defects in persistent müllerian duct syndrome. *Hum Reprod Update* 2005; **11**: 351–356.

141 de Clemente N, Belville C. Anti-Müllerian hormone receptor defect. *Best Pract Res Clin Endocrinol Metab* 2006; **20**: 599–610.

10 Evaluation of Disordered Puberty

Mehul T. Dattani[1], Vaitsa Tziaferi[2] & Peter C. Hindmarsh[2]

[1] Developmental Endocrinology Research Group, UCL Institute of Child Health and Great Ormond Street Hospital for Children, London, UK
[2] Developmental Endocrinology Research Group, UCL Institute of Child Health, London, UK

Puberty is a complex biological process that can be influenced by genetic, nutritional, environmental and socioeconomic factors. The physical and psychological changes occur because of orderly, sequential changes in endocrine activity. These commence towards the end of the first decade of life but it is important to realize that the axis has already been active *in utero* and during the first year of life [1]. After the first year of life, there is reduced gonadotropin secretion (restraint) until the reactivation, or rather increased amplitude, of gonadotropin pulsatility occurs at an age dictated by genetic factors determining the tempo of secondary sexual development in that individual and presumably modified by gene–environment interaction.

Normal puberty

Secular trends

The age of puberty in girls is now earlier than in past centuries, as defined by a decrease in the age of menarche in industrialized European countries and in the USA of 2–3 months per decade over the past 100–150 years [2]. This trend has generally ceased in Western Europe, at least when puberty is defined by the age of menarche. If pubertal onset is defined by the development of breast buds (breast stage 2), the secular trend is probably ongoing but because age at menarche remains constant, the duration of puberty has lengthened [3]. Unfortunately, most studies examining secular changes in puberty are susceptible to the problems inherent in the recording of the timing of puberty, not least observer variability and referral bias. As such it may be better, from an epidemiological viewpoint, to focus on menarche as the determinant because it is more robust. These observations in the Western world contrast with cultures in which the standard of living has changed little and where no trend towards earlier menarche has been documented [4], or where the standard of living has improved and events are accelerated [5].

The interaction between nutritional status and puberty is extremely important in areas of the world where food supply is limited. Chronic disease and malnutrition are common causes of delayed puberty. Strenuous physical activity in girls can also delay puberty, especially when associated with thin habitus [6]. Moderate obesity is associated with earlier menarche and advanced physical development but pathological obesity is associated with delayed menarche [7]. This may explain the current trend to earlier puberty, in that a rapid early increase in body size above that expected for parental size and secular trend does not lead to an increase in final height because of an earlier puberty.

Figure 10.1 illustrates this in Japanese children [8]. Mean length at birth has not changed in 40 years but there has been an appreciable trend of 10 mm/decade at age 2, identical to that seen in adulthood. This means that, on average, Japanese children aged 2 were 4 cm taller in 1990 than in 1950, and the same was true of young adults, in other words, the increase in height from age 2 years to adult was no different in 1950 from 1990. The secular trend occurred during the first 2 years of life and was restricted to this period.

Further support for the impact of early weight gain, either *in utero* or in early childhood influencing age at menarche or entry into puberty, comes from a series of observational studies [9–11], which imply that infant feeding practices may have an important role in determining the timing of the pubertal process and possibly impact upon size in later life [9].

The age of onset and completion of puberty in boys is less well-defined and documented than the age of menarche in girls. Overall, there has been little change with respect to the timing of onset of puberty in boys [12,13].

Genetic factors play an important part in the onset of puberty. African-American girls achieve menarche at a mean age of 12.2 years, while Caucasians do so at an average age of 12.9 years [5]. The ethnic differences in the age of secondary sexual development remain even when the effects of social or economic factors are eliminated. Further evidence for the genetic influence is

Brook's Clinical Pediatric Endocrinology, 6th edition. Edited by C. Brook, P. Clayton, R. Brown. © 2009 Blackwell Publishing,
ISBN: 978-1-4051-8080-1.

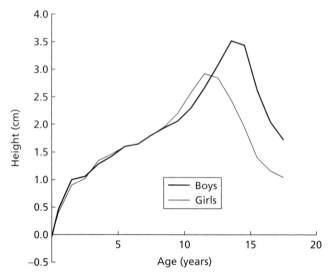

Figure 10.1 The mean secular increase in height (cm) of Japanese children by age and sex 1950–1990. (a) Lack of a trend at birth; (b) trend of 1 cm/decade at 2 and 17 years; (c) trend of 3–4 cm/decade at 12–14 years.

provided by the concordance of the age of menarche between mother–daughter pairs.

Physical changes of puberty

The physical changes of puberty in individuals are defined by the Tanner stages [14,15]. Figure 10.2 demonstrates the components and consonance of the process for girls and boys.

Breast development is controlled by ovarian estrogen secretion. It may be unilateral for several months, which may cause unfounded concern. Even though the growth of pubic and axillary hair is mainly under the influence of androgens secreted by the adrenal gland, the stage of breast development usually correlates well with the stage of pubic hair development in normal girls. However, because different endocrine organs control these two processes, the stages of each phenomenon should be classified separately. Peak height velocity is attained some 6–9 months after the appearance of breast stage 2 development.

In boys, an increase in testicular volume to 4 mL is usually the first sign and this can be easily assessed using the Prader orchidometer. Most of the increase is caused by enlargement of the Sertoli rather than the Leydig cells. In gonadotropin-independent precocious puberty (GIPP, testotoxicosis), the testes remain small in relation to the growth of the phallus and pubic hair, because the condition is caused by constitutive activation of the luteinizing hormone (LH) receptor with consequent hyperplasia of Leydig rather than Sertoli cells.

The growth of the penis and genitalia usually correlate well with pubic hair development, because both features are regulated by androgen secretion but stages of pubic hair and genital development should be determined independently because valuable clinical information can be accrued. For example, pubic hair growth without testicular enlargement suggests an adrenal rather than a gonadal source of androgens.

Peak height velocity occurs later in puberty in boys than girls, and usually coincides with a testicular volume of 10–12 mL. Voice changes in boys can be noted at 8 mL testicular volume, and become obvious by 12 mL volume.

Ovarian development in puberty

Oogonia arise from the primordial germ cells in the wall of the yolk sac near the caudal end of the embryo [16]. By the sixth month of fetal life, the cells have migrated to the genital ridge and progressed through sufficient mitoses to reach a complement of 6–7 million oogonia, which represents the maximal number of primordial follicles the individual will have throughout life. Meiosis begins but is not completed as the nucleus and chromosomes persist in prophase to mark the conversion of the oogonia to primary oocytes. Primordial follicles are composed of the primary oocyte surrounded by a single layer of spindle-shaped cells that will develop into granulosa cells and a basal lamina that will be the boundary of the theca cells later in development. As a result of apoptosis, 2–4 million primordial follicles are left at birth but only 400 000 remain at the onset of menarche [16].

At the time of the first ovulation, the first meiotic metaphase converts the primary oocyte into the secondary oocyte, which is extruded into the fallopian tubes [17]. The ovum does not form until sperm penetration, when the second polar body is eliminated. While some follicles in the fetus and child progress to the large antral stage, all developing follicles undergo atresia before puberty and few large follicles develop in the child. However, the presence of more than six follicles with a diameter of more than 4 mm indicates the presence of pulsatile gonadotropin secretion and may be seen in normal prepubertal girls, in pubertal girls before menarche and in patients recovering from anorexia nervosa. This "multicystic" appearance is considered characteristic of a phase of (mainly) nocturnal pulsatile gonadotropin secretion before positive feedback [18].

Standards for ovarian and uterine size and shape are available for normal girls and those with Turner syndrome [19–21]. The uterus lies in a craniocaudal direction in childhood without the adult flexion. The myometrium enlarges during early puberty, thereby enlarging the corpus leading to the adult corpus to cervix ratio. The cervix develops its adult shape and size just before menarche and the cervical canal enlarges.

Testicular development in puberty

The prepubertal testes consist mainly of Sertoli cells but adult testes are mostly composed of germ cells in the seminiferous tubules. The seminiferous tubules enlarge during puberty and form tight occlusive junctions leading to the development of the blood testicular junction [22]. Leydig cells are present in small numbers in prepuberty, although the interstitial tissue is mainly composed of mesenchymal tissue. At puberty, the Leydig cells become more apparent.

Spermatogenesis can be detected histologically between the ages of 11 and 15 years and sperm is found in early morning urine samples by 13.3 years of age (spermarche) [23]. Ejaculation

PUBERTAL DEVELOPMENT TIME COURSE – BOYS

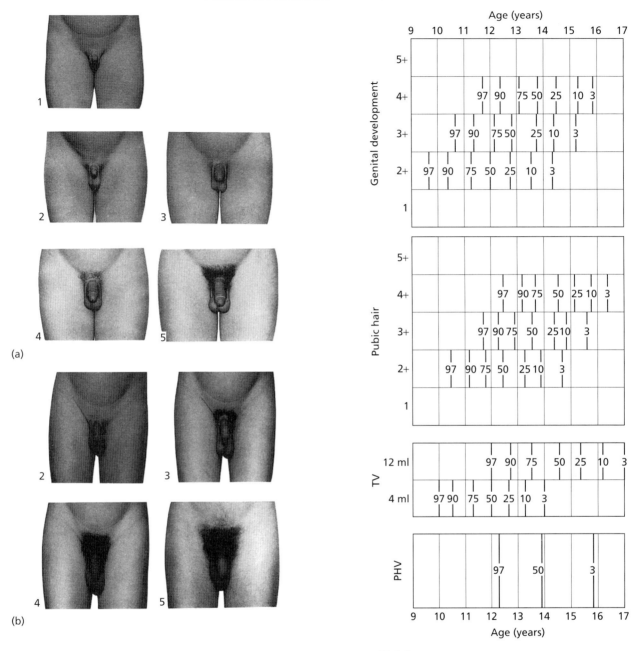

(a)

(b)

Boys: genital development

Stage 1: Preadolescent. The testes, scrotum and penis are of about the same size and proportions as in early childhood.
Stage 2: Enlargement of the scrotum and testes. The skin of the scrotum reddens and changes in texture. Little or no enlargement of the penis.
Stage 3: Lengthening of the penis. Further growth of the testes and scrotum.
Stage 4: Increase in breadth of the penis and development of the glans. The testes and scrotum are larger; the scrotum darkens.
Stage 5: Adult.

Boys: pubic hair

Stage 1: Preadolescent. No pubic hair.
Stage 2: Sparse growth of slightly pigmented downy hair chiefly at the base of the penis.
Stage 3: Hair darker, coarser and more curled, spreading sparsely over the junction of the pubes.
Stage 4: Hair adult in type, but covering a considerably smaller area than in the adult. No spread to the medial surface of the thighs.
Stage 5: Adult quantity and type with distribution of a horizontal pattern and spread to the medial surface of the thighs. Spread up linea alba occurs late, in about 80% of men, after adolescence is complete, and is rated Stage 6.

Figure 10.2 Pubertal assessment is an important component of the assessment of gondal function. Staging of each of the components is separate and should be recorded as such to allow discordance in development to be identified. The figures show the relationship in time of each of the components and each should be related to other parts of the puberty process. Note that the peak height velocity in girls takes place some 2 years before that in boys.

PUBERTAL DEVELOPMENT TIME COURSE – GIRLS

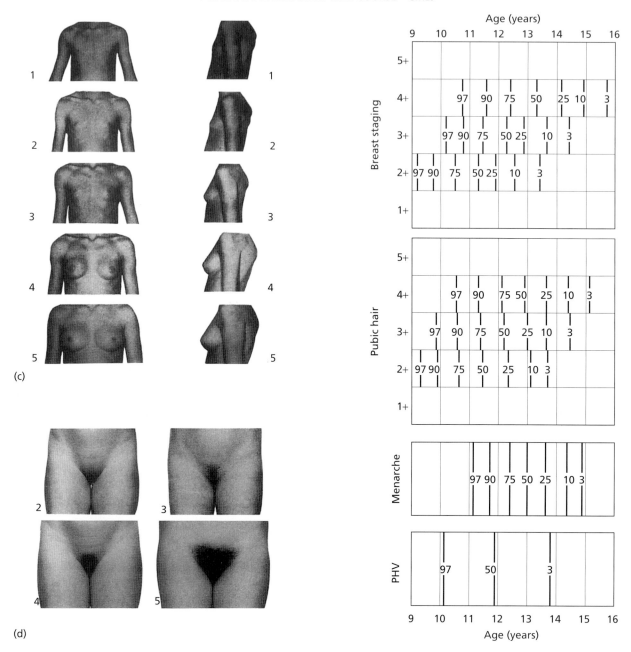

(c)

(d)

Girls: breast development

Stage 1: Preadolescent. Elevation of the papilla only.
Stage 2: Breast bud stage. Elevation of the breast and papilla as a small mound. Enlargement of the areola diameter.
Stage 3: Further enlargement and elevation of the breast and areola, with no separation of their contours.
Stage 4: Projection of the areola and papilla above the level of the breast.
Stage 5: Mature stage, projection of the papilla alone due to recession of the areola.

Girls: pubic hair

Stage 1: Preadolescent. No pubic hair.
Stage 2: Sparse growth of slightly pigmented downy hair chiefly along the labia.
Stage 3: Hair darker, coarser and more curled, spreading sparsely over the junction of the pubes.
Stage 4: Hair adult in type, but covering a considerably smaller area than in the adult. No spread to the medial surface of the thighs.
Stage 5: Adult quantity and type with distribution of a horizontal pattern and spread to the medial surface of the thighs. In about 10% of women, after adolescence is complete pubic hair spreads up the linea alba and is rated Stage 6.

Figure 10.2 *Continued*

occurs by a mean age of 13.5 years without consistent relationship to testicular volume, pubic hair development or phallic enlargement. While adult morphology, motility and concentration of sperm is not found until the bone age advances to 17 years [24], immature-appearing boys can be fertile.

Gynecomastia

Breast enlargement occurs to some degree in 39–75% of boys, usually during the first stages of puberty [25] because of an imbalance between free estrogen and free androgen actions on the breast tissue. During mid- to late puberty, more estrogen may be produced by the testes and peripheral tissues before testosterone secretion reaches adult concentrations. Other causes may include secretion of excessive estradiol from a Leydig or Sertoli cell tumor, excessive aromatization to estrogen, increased responsiveness to estrogen or the severely impaired secretion of testosterone by the testes, as in primary or secondary hypogonadism.

A number of drugs are associated with the devlopment of gynecomastia in boys, such as spironolactone and various antipsychotic agents (Table 10.1). In most cases, the tissue regresses within 2 years but occasionally in normal, often obese, boys, and frequently in pathological conditions such as Klinefelter syndrome or partial androgen insensitivity where the effective amount of bioactive testosterone is reduced, gynecomastia remains permanent. Surgery, usually through a peri-areolar incision, is the only effective mode of therapy at present, although non-aromatizable androgens or aromatase inhibitors are under study as potential treatments [25].

Table 10.1 Drugs that may cause gynecomastia.

Hormonal	Estrogens
	Aromatizable androgens
	Antiandrogens, e.g. cyproterone
Cardiac	Calcium channel blockers
	Angiotensin converting enzyme inhibitors
	Digoxin
	Amiodarone
	Spironolactone
CNS	Dopamine receptor antagonists (phenothiazines and metoclopramide)
	Tricyclic antidepressants
	Benzodiazepines
	Opiates
	Marijuana
Gastrointestinal	Omeprazole
	Cimetidine
Anti-infective	Isoniazid
	Metronidazole
	Ketoconazole
Cytotoxic	Busulfan
	Nitosureas
Alcohol	

Bone mineral density

The most important phases of bone accretion occur during infancy and puberty. Girls reach peak mineralization between 14 and 16 years of age while boys reach a peak at 17.5 years (Fig. 10.3) [26]. Both peaks are attained after peak height velocity has been achieved in either sex. Bone mineral density (BMD) is influenced not only by sex steroids but also by genetics [27], exercise [28] and GH secretion.

There is a poor correlation between calcium intake and BMD during puberty or young adulthood, suggesting that the normal age of puberty is the most significant factor in achieving peak bone mineralization [29]. It seems prudent none the less to ensure adequate calcium intake in patients with delayed or absent puberty or those treated with gonadotropin releasing hormone (GnRH) analogs to hold up puberty, until more is learned about the biology of the control of bone accretion in puberty.

Body composition

Percentages of lean body mass, skeletal mass and body fat are equal between prepubertal boys and girls but total body bone mass and fat-free mass continue to increase as boys go through puberty while only body fat and fat-free mass increase in girls [30]. The increase in lean body mass starts at 6 years in girls and 9.5 years in boys and is the earliest change in body composition in puberty [31]. At maturity, men have 1.5 times the lean body mass and almost 1.5 times the skeletal mass of women, while women have twice as much body fat as men.

Growth in puberty

The pubertal growth spurt encompasses the most rapid phase of postnatal growth after the neonatal period and follows the decreasing growth rate of the late childhood phase. It can be detected in girls before the onset of secondary sexual characteristics. In boys, the growth spurt starts on average 2 years after that in girls. Peak height velocity occurs at a mean of 13.5 years in boys and 11.5 years in girls [32], corresponding to genitalia stage 3–4 with 10–12 mL testicular volumes in boys and breast stage 2–3 in girls.

The mean difference in adult height between men and women of 12.5 cm is mainly because of the taller stature of boys at the onset of the pubertal growth spurt and also the increased height gained during the pubertal growth spurt in boys compared with girls [33]. A girl who has experienced menarche usually has no more than 2–3% of her growth remaining, because menarche closely accords to a bone age of 13 years, the only event of puberty more closely related to skeletal than chronological age. A post-menarcheal girl has 5–7.5 cm of growth remaining before adult height is reached, although the range of post-menarcheal growth extends to 11 cm.

The pubertal growth spurt is mediated by many endocrine influences. Sex steroids exert a direct effect upon the growing cartilage as well as an indirect effect mediated by increasing growth hormone (GH) secretion. Increasing sex steroid production at puberty stimulates increased amplitude (but not

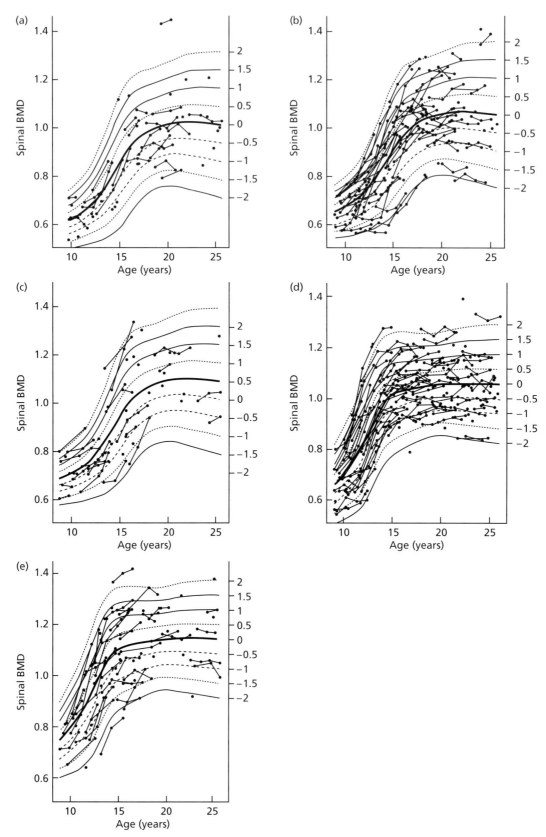

Figure 10.3 Spinal bone mineral density determined in 423 males and females showing effect of puberty in (a) Hispanic male; (b) Asian/white male: (c) black male; (d) non-black female; (e) black female.

frequency) of spontaneous GH secretion [34] as well as peak stimulated GH, and this in turn stimulates increased production of insulin-like growth factor type 1 (IGF-1).

Estrogen, either from the ovary or aromatized from testicular testosterone, is the factor that mediates the increased GH response during puberty [35]. A prepubertal child given an androgen that can be aromatized to estrogen, such as testosterone, will have augmented GH secretion whereas non-aromatizable dihydrotestosterone will not increase GH secretion. An estrogen-blocking agent such as tamoxifen will reduce GH secretion [36].

Thyroid hormone is necessary to allow the pubertal growth spurt to proceed. The rapid growth rate is accompanied by an increase in markers of bone turnover such as serum alkaline phosphatase, serum bone alkaline phosphatase, osteocalcin, Gla protein and the amino-terminal propeptide of type III procollagen; thus normal adult values of these proteins are lower than concentrations found in puberty [37].

Estrogen has a biphasic effect on growth: low concentrations stimulate growth while higher concentrations lead to cessation of growth [38]. Estrogen has a major role in the final stages of epiphyseal fusion. Patients with either estrogen receptor deficiency or aromatase deficiency have tall stature, continued growth into the third decade because of lack of fusion of the epiphyses of the long bones, increased bone turnover, reduced bone mineral density, osteoporosis and absence of a pubertal growth spurt [39]. Thus, estrogen is the main factor that fuses the epiphyses of the long bones and causes cessation of statural growth. These observations have raised the possibility of the use of aromatase inhibitors for the further management of short stature associated with a variety of conditions, with the rationale that this might allow more time for growth before epiphyseal fusion [40].

Genetic and endocrine background to the changes of puberty

Hypothalamic GnRH

The activation of pulsatile hypothalamic GnRH secretion marks the onset of puberty. Secretion arises from a network of GnRH-containing neurons which need to integrate their firing rates to generate an appropriate burst of GnRH release into the portal system [41].

Puberty arises as a result of the activation of the system after a period of quiescence from approximately 2 years of age to 8–9 years. This activation takes two forms: first, the generation of bursts of GnRH and, secondly, the orchestration of these bursts into regular events occurring on average once every 90 min. It appears that the pulse frequency changes little and that amplitude modulation of GnRH release is the predominant determinant of the activation of the pituitary-gonadal axis and progression into and through puberty. Although this is generally the situation, alterations in pulse frequency probably do take place during the menstrual cycle so that, for example, when GnRH pulse frequency is slow, follicle stimulating hormone (FSH) secretion is dominant and, as the frequency increases, LH comes to the fore. FSH concentrations are higher than LH in mid-childhood [42],

and this may reflect alterations in the frequency of neuronal firing at this stage.

The "silencing" of the GnRH pulse generator until the end of the first decade of life allows synchronization of sexual maturation with somatic growth and maturation of sexual and social behaviors in humans. Given the pivotal role that this activation has in human reproduction, single-gene mutations associated with disordered gonadotropin secretion and action are uncommon.

GnRH is a 10 amino acid peptide generated from a large 69 amino acid prohormone precursor. The gene encoding GnRH is located on chromosome 8p21-11.2 [43]. Neurons producing GnRH originate in the primitive olfactory placode early in the development of mammals and migrate to the medial basal hypothalamus [44]. The control of this migration is related to the *KAL* gene located at Xp22.3. Absence of the *KAL* gene, or rather the gene product ANOSMIN-1, causes Kallman syndrome, a decrease or lack of gonadotropin secretion with hyposmia caused by disordered development of the olfactory bulb [45].

A series of genes are also implicated in the development, migration and networking of GnRH neurons and the regulation of GnRH secretion, including *FGFR1* (fibroblast growth factor receptor 1), *GNRHR* (GnRH receptor), *GPR54* (G protein-coupled receptor 54), *LEP* (leptin) and its receptor, *SF-1* (steroidogenic factor 1), *DAX-1* (nuclear receptor subfamily 0, group B, member 1 [also known as *NR0B1*]), and *NELF* (nasal embryonic luteinizing hormone releasing hormone factor) [46–48].

The kisspeptin-GPR54 signaling complex has been proposed as a gatekeeper of pubertal activation of GnRH neurons (Fig. 10.4). The *Kiss1* gene encodes a family of peptides called kisspeptins, which bind to the G protein-coupled receptor GPR54. Kisspeptin(s) and its receptor are expressed in the forebrain and the discovery that mice and humans lacking a functional GPR54 fail to undergo puberty and exhibit hypogonadotropic

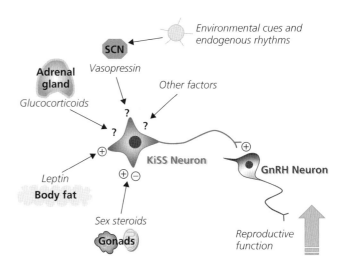

Figure 10.4 Integrative role for kisspeptin system in GnRH regulation. (From Dungan *et al. Endocrinology* 2006; **147**: 1154–1158 with kind permission of the editor.)

hypogonadism implies that kisspeptin signaling has an essential role in reproduction [49–51]. The converse, that activating mutations lead to precocious puberty, has not been as well documented [52].

Studies in several mammalian species have shown that kisspeptins stimulate the secretion of gonadotropins from the pituitary by stimulating the release of GnRH after the activation of GPR54, which is expressed by GnRH neurons [53]. Kisspeptin is expressed abundantly in the arcuate (Arc) and the anteroventral periventricular nuclei (AVPV) of the forebrain. Estradiol and testosterone both regulate the expression of the *Kiss1* gene in the Arc and AVPV but the response of the *Kiss1* gene to these steroids is exactly opposite between these two nuclei. Estradiol and testosterone downregulate *Kiss1* mRNA in the Arc and upregulate its expression in the AVPV. Thus, kisspeptin neurons in the Arc may participate in the negative feedback regulation of gonadotropin secretion, whereas kisspeptin neurons in the AVPV may contribute to generating the pre-ovulatory gonadotropin surge in the female.

GnRH is localized mainly in the hypothalamus and to a degree in the hippocampus, cingulate cortex and the olfactory bulb. There is no discrete nucleus that contains all the GnRH neurons, although the arcuate nucleus has a key role. Gonadotropins are normally released into the bloodstream in a pulsatile manner because of the pulsatile nature of GnRH secretion (Fig. 10.5). Episodic secretion appears to be an intrinsic property of the hypothalamic neurons that produce and secrete the stimulatory peptide GnRH [54]. This GnRH pulse generator, which is the basis of the CNS control of puberty and reproductive function, is also affected by biogenic amine neurotransmitters, peptidergic neuromodulators, neuroexcitatory amino acids and neural pathways; for example, epinephrine and norepinephrine increase GnRH release while dopamine, serotonin and opioids decrease GnRH release.

Testosterone and progesterone inhibit GnRH pulse frequency but the decrease in gonadotropin secretion during childhood before the onset of puberty appears to be mediated by the central nervous system (CNS). Gamma aminobutyric acid (GABA) is probably the major cause of the suppression of GnRH secretion that occurs physiologically during mid-childhood [55]. Damage to the CNS from increased intracranial pressure or tumor may release the inhibition and bring about premature pubertal development.

GnRH stimulates the production and secretion of LH and FSH from the gonadotropes by binding to a cell-surface receptor [56,57], which triggers increased intracellular calcium concentration and phosphorylation of protein kinase C in a manner similar to other peptide-receptor mechanisms. There appear to be readily releasable pools of LH which lead to a rise in serum LH within minutes after a bolus of GnRH, as well as other pools of LH which take longer to mobilize. While episodic stimulation by GnRH increases gonadotropin secretion, continuous infusion of GnRH decreases LH and FSH secretion and downregulates the pituitary receptors for GnRH. This phenomenon is utilized in the treat-

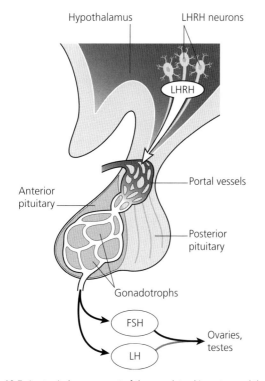
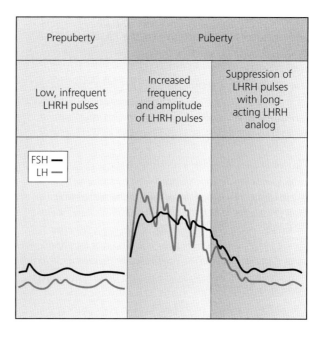

Figure 10.5 Anatomical arrangement of the gonadotrophin system and the secretory pattern of luteinizing and follicle stimulating hormone during prepuberty and puberty.

ment of central precocious puberty. Estrogens increase and androgens decrease GnRH receptors. These alterations in the GnRH receptor have an important role in regulating gonadotrope function.

Pituitary gonadotropins

FSH and LH are glycoproteins composed of two subunits, an α-subunit identical for all the pituitary glycoproteins and distinct β-subunits that confer specificity (Fig. 10.6). The β-subunits are 115 amino acids long with two carbohydrate side-chains. Human chorionic gonadotropin (hCG) produced by the placenta is almost identical in structure to LH, except for an additional 32 amino acids and additional carbohydrate groups. The LH β-subunit gene is on chromosome 19q13.32, close to the gene for β-hCG, while the FSH gene is located at 11p13.

There are rare cases of mutations in the β-subunit of gonadotropin molecules which cause pathological effects: a single case of an inactivating mutation of β LH caused absence of Leydig cells and lack of puberty, while two cases of inactivating mutations of β FSH led to lack of follicular maturation and amenorrhea and, in two males, azoospermia [58,59]. More recently, a woman with a homozygous mutation in a 5′ splice-donor site in the non-coding region of β LH displayed impaired LH secretion, normal pubertal development, secondary amenorrhea and infertility [60]. The mechanism for this is unclear. LH secretion could not be detected by two separate immunoassays suggesting that the mutant LHβ protein might be translated but unable to associate with the α-subunit, was translated but rapidly degraded or was not translated at all.

What is important from these observations is that normal pubertal maturation in women, including breast development and menarche (which indicate estrogen production sufficient for breast development and at least some tropic action on the endo-metrium), can occur in a state of LH deficiency, although normal LH secretion is obligatory for ovulation. Thus, LH is essential for the normal maturation of Leydig cells and steroidogenesis in men and its primary role in women is to induce ovulation.

The same gonadotrope cell produces both LH and FSH. The complex cascade of temporal and spatial events that lead to the formation of these cells is considered in Chapter 4. Gonadotropes are distributed throughout the anterior pituitary gland and abut upon the capillary basement membranes to allow access to the systemic circulation. Inactive gonadotrope cells that are not stimulated, e.g. because of disease affecting GnRH secretion, are small, while the gonadotrope cells of castrate individuals or those with absence of gonads such as in Turner syndrome, which are stimulated by large amounts of GnRH, are large and demonstrate prominent rough endoplasmic reticulum.

Serum gonadotropin concentrations change during pubertal development (Table 10.2). Because of the episodic nature of gonadotropin secretion, a single gonadotropin determination will be uninformative with respect to the secretory dynamics of these hormones but third-generation assays are sufficiently sensitive to indicate the onset of puberty in single basal unstimulated samples.

GnRH must stimulate gonadotropin release before other factors can affect gonadotropin secretion but, in the presence of GnRH stimulation, sex steroids and gonadal peptides can change gonadotropin secretion. Negative feedback occurs when sex steroids decrease pituitary LH and FSH secretion at the hypothalamic and pituitary levels and is exemplified in individuals with gonadal dysgenesis who have very high concentrations of LH and FSH during infancy and puberty. Inhibin, a product of both ovary and testes, and follistatin, an ovarian product, also exert direct inhibitory effects upon FSH secretion at the pituitary level. Progesterone slows LH pulse frequency.

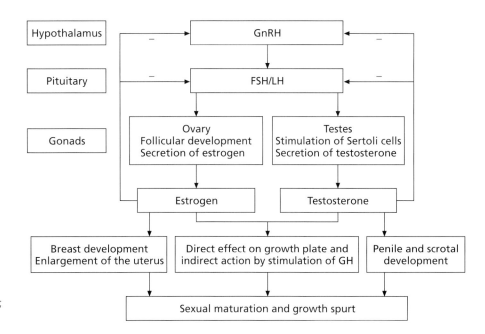

Figure 10.6 Overall feedforward and feedback loops in the hypothalamo-pituitary-gonadal axis. FSH, follicle stimulating hormone; GH, growth hormone; GnRH, gonadotropin releasing hormone; LH, luteinizing hormone.

Estradiol decreases gonadotropin secretion at low concentrations but higher values lead to positive feedback. The latter predominates in females at mid-cycle [61] when a rising concentration of estradiol greater than 200–300 pg/mL persisting for more than 48 h [62] triggers the release of a burst of LH from the pituitary gonadotropes, which stimulates ovulation about 12 h later. Several steps must prepare the hypothalamic-pituitary-gonadal axis for positive feedback, including an adequate pool of LH to release and priming of the ovary to produce adequate estrogen. Estradiol also increases pituitary gland sensitivity to GnRH which, in addition to an increase in GnRH pulse frequency, increases LH secretion. Thus, a follicle must be of adequate size to produce adequate estrogen to exert the positive feedback effect, the pituitary gland must have sufficient readily releasable LH to effect a surge of LH release and the hypothalamus must be able to secrete adequate GnRH to cause the stimulation of pituitary release. The increase in estrogen also suppresses FSH to allow luteinization of the follicle in the presence of LH.

Sex steroids

Leydig cells synthesize testosterone through a series of enzymatic conversions for which cholesterol is the precursor (Fig. 10.7). When LH binds to Leydig cell membrane receptors, the ligand–receptor complex stimulates membrane-bound adenyl cyclase to increase cyclic adenosine monophosphate (cAMP), which stimulates protein kinase, which promotes conversion of cholesterol to pregnenolone by CYP11A (side-chain cleavage enzyme). After exposure to LH, the number of receptors for LH and the post-receptor pathway decrease their responsiveness to LH for at least 24 h which explains the insensitivity to LH after daily injections of LH compared to alternate day injections. When assessing the response of testes to LH, hCG or LH must be administered at 2–3 day intervals to eliminate such downregulation.

When testosterone is secreted into the circulation, it is bound to sex hormone binding globulin and the remaining free testosterone is considered the active moiety. At the target cell, testosterone dissociates from the binding protein, diffuses into the cell and may be converted by 5α-reductase type 2 (a surface enzyme located on the genital skin and elsewhere and encoded by a gene on chromosome 2p23 [63]) to dihydrotestosterone or to estradiol by CYP19 (aromatase) [64]. Testosterone or dihydrotestosterone

binds to an androgen receptor encoded by a gene on the X chromosome (Xq11-q12) [65]. The testosterone–dihydrotestosterone receptor complex then attaches to the steroid-responsive region of genomic DNA to initiate transcription and translation.

The effects of testosterone are different from those of dihydrotestosterone because a fetus without dihydrotestosterone does not virilize fully. The androgen receptor has a greater affinity for dihydrotestosterone than for testosterone. Testosterone suppresses LH secretion, maintains Wolffian ducts and produces the male body habitus while dihydrotestosterone is mostly responsible for the virilization of the external genitalia and for much of the secondary sexual characteristics of puberty including phallic growth, prostate enlargement, androgen-induced hair loss and beard growth. Androgens exert other effects in the body: testosterone promotes muscle development, stimulates enzymatic activity in the liver and stimulates hemoglobin synthesis. Androgens must be converted to estrogen to stimulate bone maturation at the epiphyseal plate [39].

Table 10.2 Serun concentrations of luteinizing hormone (LH), follicle stimulating hormone (FSH) and the sex steroids at different pubertal stages.

Tanner stage	LH (U/L)	FSH (U/L)	Estradiol (pg/mL)
Females			
I	0.01–0.21	0.50–2.41	5–10
II	0.27–4.21	1.73–4.68	5–115
III	0.17–4.12	2.53–7.04	5–180
IV	0.72–15.01	1.26–7.37	25–345
V	0.30–29.38	1.02–9.24	25–410

Tanner stages	LH (U/L)	FSH (U/L)	Testosterone (ng/dL)
Males			
I	0.02–0.42	0.22–1.92	2–23
II	0.26–4.84	0.72–4.60	5–70
III	0.64–3.74	1.24–10.37	15–280
IV	0.55–7.15	1.70–10.35	105–545
V	1.54–7.00	1.54–7.00	265–800

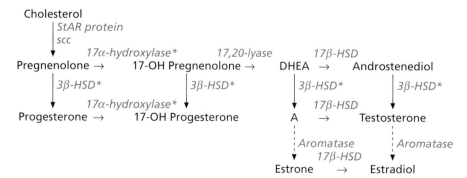

Figure 10.7 Steroid biosynthetic pathway in the gonad.

FSH binds to specific receptors on the cell surface of Sertoli cells and initiates a sequence of events that culminates in increased protein kinase in a manner similar to the stimulatory effect of LH on Leydig cells. However, FSH causes an increase in the mass of seminiferous tubules, and supports the development of sperm.

Estrogen is produced mainly by the follicle cells of the ovary using the same initial steps as testosterone production with final aromatization. LH binds to membrane receptors of ovarian cells and stimulates the activity of adenyl cyclase to produce cAMP, which stimulates the production of the low-density lipoprotein (LDL) receptor to increase binding and uptake of LDL cholesterol and the formation of cholesterol esters. LH stimulates the rate-limiting enzyme CYP11A, which converts cholesterol to pregnenolone, initiating steroidogenesis. After the onset of ovulation, LH exerts major effects upon the theca of the ovary. FSH binds to its own cell-surface receptors on the glomerulosa cells and stimulates the conversion of testosterone to estrogen.

The main active estrogen in humans is estradiol. Estrogens circulate bound to sex hormone binding globulin (SHBG) and follow the same general pattern of action at the cell level as that described for testosterone. Estradiol affects breast and uterine development, the distribution of adipose tissue and bone mineral accretion. Low concentrations of estradiol are difficult to measure in standard assays but bioassays are sensitive enough to differentiate between boys and girls in prepuberty, between prepuberty and puberty in girls and between normal girls and those with premature thelarche, who secrete only a small amount of estrogen above age-matched controls [66].

Activin and inhibin

Inhibin produced by the Sertoli cells in the male and by the ovarian granuloma cells and the placenta in the female is a heterodimeric glycoprotein member of the transforming growth factor β family [67]. Inhibin suppresses FSH secretion from the pituitary gland and provides another explanation for different serum concentrations of LH and FSH with only one hypothalamic peptide (GnRH) stimulating them. Activin, a subunit of inhibin, has the opposite effect, stimulating the secretion of FSH from the pituitary gland. Inhibin B secretion rises in early puberty in both boys and girls and reaches a steady state [68]. The infant male has concentrations of inhibin B higher than those achieved in adult males for the first 1–1.5 years after birth indicating the activity of the testes during this early period. Absence of inhibin because of gonadal failure causes a greater rise in serum FSH than LH in pubertal and adult subjects.

Anti-Müllerian hormone

Anti-Müllerian hormone (AMH) belongs to the same transforming growth factor-β family as inhibin and is produced from the Sertoli cells of the fetal testes and the granulosa cells of the fetal ovary [69]. AMH is high in the male fetus and newborn but decreases thereafter with a further drop at puberty. Patients with dysgenetic testes have decreased serum AMH while values are elevated in males with Sertoli cell tumors or females with granulosa cell tumors. AMH assays may be used to differentiate a child with congenital anorchia who has no testicular tissue from one with undescended testes who has testicular tissue that can produce AMH. Girls have low concentrations of AMH in the newborn period.

Ontogeny of endocrine pubertal development

Fetal testosterone secretion in early pregnancy is caused by placental hCG stimulation. The fetal hypothalamus contains GnRH-containing neurons by 14 weeks' gestation and the fetal pituitary gland contains LH and FSH by 20 weeks [70]. The hypothalamo-pituitary portal system develops by 20 weeks' gestation, allowing hypothalamic GnRH to reach the pituitary gonadotropes. Stimulation by GnRH causes gonadotropin secretion to rise to extremely high concentrations in mid-gestation with a decrease in responsivity thereafter. Initially unrestrained GnRH secretion by the hypothalamus comes under restraint from the CNS by mid-gestation and, probably also to some degree, from increased circulating sex steroid concentrations which exert a restraining effect upon gonadotropin secretion until after birth.

At term, gonadotropin concentrations are lower than mid-gestation but still high. Gonadotropin values rise again in an intermittent pattern after birth with episodic peaks noted up to 2–4 years after birth [71]. Estrogen and testosterone from the infantile gonads also rise episodically during this period but mean serum concentrations of gonadotropins and sex steroids during infancy remain much lower than those found in the fetus and the pubertal subject but higher than those found during mid-childhood. Because sex steroids suppress gonadotropin secretion during the first years after birth, agonadal patients, such as those with Turner syndrome, exhibit high (castrate) serum gonadotropin concentrations while maintaining the same pattern of pulsatile gonadotropin secretion as normal girls but with higher pulse amplitudes [72,73].

During the quiescent childhood phase, which reaches a nadir around 7 years of age [42], gonadotropin pulsatility and gonadal activity remain at a low level, restrained by the CNS [74]. Even in children without gonadal function, such as those with Turner syndrome, serum gonadotropin concentrations are low, demonstrating that the presence of the gonads is not necessary to suppress gonadotropin secretion during this period. Changes in gonadotropin secretion arise as a result of alterations in pulse amplitude with pulse frequency unchanged [75]. Likewise, testosterone and estrogen are measurable in the circulation using sensitive assays, demonstrating low but definite activity of the prepubertal gonads.

During the peripubertal period, before physical changes, gonadotropin secretion increases first at night (Fig. 10.5). Sequential sampling demonstrates a rise in sex steroid secretion during the late night–early morning, which follows by hours the pulses of the gonadotropins. As puberty progresses, the secretion of gonadotropins and sex steroids increases during the day until little circadian rhythm remains.

During the peripubertal period there is also a change in the response of pituitary gonadotropes to exogenous GnRH administration. The pattern of LH release increases, so that the adult pattern of response to GnRH is achieved during puberty. The release of FSH shows no such change with development, although females have more FSH release than males at all developmental stages.

Leptin, a hormone produced in the adipose cells that suppresses appetite by attaching to its receptor in the hypothalamus, has a major role in puberty in mice and rats. The leptin deficient mouse (ob/ob) will not commence puberty until leptin is replaced and leptin administration will push an immature but normal mouse through puberty. The leptin-deficient human also has pubertal delay and the introduction of leptin treatment was associated with the appearance of gonadotropin peaks [76]. These data suggest that leptin might trigger the onset of puberty but clinical studies show that leptin increases in girls during puberty in synchrony with the increase in fat mass while leptin decreases in puberty in boys with a decrease in fat mass and increase in lean mass. Leptin varies with body composition only and no sex differences are noted [77,78] and, in otherwise normal adolescents, there is no evidence that it triggers pubertal development. It appears permissive of puberty but not the cause of its onset or progression.

Adrenarche

Dehydroepiandrosterone and androstenedione, produced by the zona reticularis, increase in concentration 2 years or more before the increase in the secretion of gonadotropins and sex steroids [79]. This process (adrenarche) begins by 6–8 years of age in normal subjects, and continues until late puberty. Adrenarche occurs as a result of increased adrenal CYP17 activity [80] and causes an increase in the height velocity (the mid-childhood growth spurt), excessive secretion of apocrine sweat, the development of pubic and axillary hair and an advance in skeletal maturity.

The presence or absence of adrenarche does not influence the onset of puberty. Patients with Addison disease experience puberty at an appropriate, albeit delayed, age and children with premature adrenarche also enter gonadarche at a normal age. Thus, adrenarche is usually temporally coordinated with gonadarche during pubertal development in normal individuals but appears not to have an important role in the progression of gonadarche.

Abnormal puberty

Limits of normal pubertal development

Given the discussion on secular trends, care is needed in defining the limits of the normal timing of puberty. European data (Tables 10.3 and 10.4) suggest that precocious puberty should be considered when secondary sexual characteristics appear under 8 years of age (breast stage 2) in girls and 9 years (genitalia stage 2) in

Table 10.3 Age at stage of puberty in girls.

Stage	British girls		Swiss girls		US girls	
	Mean (years)	SD	Mean (years)	SD	Mean (years)	SD
Breast stage 2	11.50	1.10	10.9	1.2	11.2	0.7
Pubic hair stage 2	11.64	1.21	10.4	1.2	11.0	0.5
Breast stage 3	12.15	1.09	12.2	1.2	12.0	1.0
Pubic hair stage 3	12.36	1.10	12.2	1.2	11.8	1.0
Breast stage 4	13.11	1.15	13.2	0.9	12.4	0.9
Pubic hair stage 4	12.95	1.06	13.0	1.1	12.4	0.8
Menarche	13.47	1.12	13.4	1.1		
Breast stage 5	15.33	1.74	14.0	1.2		
Pubic hair stage 5	14.41	1.21	14.0	1.3	13.1	

Table 10.4 Age at stage of puberty in boys.

Stage	British boys		Swiss boys		US boys	
	Mean (years)	SD	Mean (years)	SD	Mean (years)	SD
Genitalia stage 2	11.64	1.07	11.2	1.5	11.2	0.7
Pubic hair stage 2	13.44	1.09	12.2	1.5	11.2	0.8
Genitalia stage 3	12.85	1.04	12.9	1.2	12.1	0.8
Pubic hair stage 3	13.90	1.04	13.5	1.2	12.1	1.0
Genitalia stage 4	13.77	1.02	13.8	1.1	13.5	0.7
Pubic hair stage 4	14.36	1.08	14.2	1.1	13.4	0.9
Genitalia stage 5	14.92	1.10	14.7	1.1	14.3	1.1
Pubic hair stage 5	15.18	1.07	14.9	1.0	14.3	0.8

boys [81,82]. Sexual precocity should probably more pragmatically be defined in USA by the onset of secondary sexual development before 6 years in Black girls and before 7 years in White girls. Given the fact that age at menarche remains effectively unchanged, a slightly wider definition as suggested by the US data seems reasonable but clinical evaluation outwith the European time limits probably remains the safest option [83] until sensitivity and/or specificity analysis has been undertaken using different age limits.

The definitions for pubertal delay have not changed. Boys should enter the early stages of puberty by 13.5 years (14 years is usually used for convenience) and girls by 13 years to avoid the label of delayed puberty. Puberty does not often occur spontaneously after 18 years of age. English girls complete secondary sexual development in a mean of 4.2 years (range 1.5–6 years) and boys in 3.5 years (range 2–4.5 years) [14,15].

Precocious puberty

The premature secretion of gonadal steroids in children results in the paradox of tall stature during childhood due to an accelerated rate of linear growth with eventual short stature as an adult due to early fusion of the epiphyseal growth plates. The psychological consequences of early puberty are considerable.

Etiology

The causes of early puberty can be divided into those with and without consonance of puberty (Fig. 10.8). The former include central or gonadotropin-dependent precocious puberty, in which there is premature activation of the hypothalamo-pituitary-gonadal axis, and the latter include isolated early development of breast tissue (premature thelarche/thelarche variant) or pubic/axillary hair (premature adrenarche, late-onset congenital adrenal hyperplasia, adrenal tumors). There may be activation of the ovaries or testes independently of gonadotropin secretion, so-called gonadotropin-independent precocious puberty (Table 10.5).

Precocious puberty is much more common in girls than boys [81–84] probably because activation of the hypothalamo-pituitary-gonadal axis requires a lower dose of GnRH in girls than boys [85] and suppression of sexual precocity with a GnRH analog is more difficult in girls than in boys [86].

Gonadotropin-dependent precocious puberty

In central or gonadotropin-dependent precocious puberty (GDPP), the hypothalamo-pituitary-gonadal axis is prematurely activated, the pattern of endocrine change is the same as in normal puberty and the pubertal development is consonant. Idiopathic precocious puberty accounts for the majority (>90%) of cases in girls but only 10% of cases in boys and is a diagnosis of exclusion.

Secondary GDPP is brought about by CNS lesions that can provoke premature activation of the hypothalamo-pituitary-gonadal axis, even if not in the region of the hypothalamus. These include tumors such as optic and hypothalamic

Table 10.5 Causes of premature sexual development.

I *Gonadotrophin-dependent precocious puberty*
Idiopathic central precocious puberty – most common cause in females
Secondary central precocious puberty
  congenital anomalies, e.g. septo-optic dysplasia
  brain neoplasms, e.g. optic nerve gliomas, hamartomas
  cysts
  hydrocephalus
  post-infection
  post-trauma
  post-cranial radiotherapy
  neurofibromatosis
  adoption
hCG-producing neoplasms, e.g. choriocarcinoma, hepatoblastoma, germ cell tumors of CNS or mediastinum

II *Gonadotropin-independent precocious puberty*
Ovarian cysts
Defects of LH receptor function: McCune–Albright syndrome, testotoxicosis

III *Abnormal patterns of gonadotropin secretion*
Premature thelarche (isolated breast development)
Thelarche variant and slowly progressing variants of central precocious puberty
Hypothyroidism

IV *Sexual precocity due to adrenal androgens*
Steroid secretion by the normal adrenal gland – adrenarche
Adrenal enzyme defects – congenital adrenal hyperplasia
Adrenal tumors – Cushing syndrome and virilizing tumor

V *Gonadal tumors secreting sex steroids*

VI *Exogenous sex steroids*

hCG, human chorionic gonadotropin; LH, luteinizing hormone.

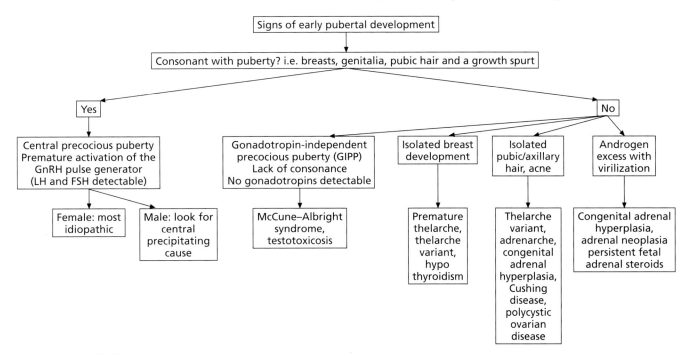

Figure 10.8 Algorithm for evaluating early puberty.

gliomas (Fig. 10.9), astrocytomas, ependymomas and pineal tumors, rare craniopharyngiomas, hydrocephalus, trauma, radiotherapy, post-CNS infection and neurofibromatosis [87]. Hamartomas of the tuber cinereum are congenital tumors composed of a heterotopic mass of GnRH neurosecretory neurones, fiber bundles and glial cells which are frequently associated with GDPP, often before 3 years of age. Gelastic epilepsy and developmental delay may be associated, and the characteristic appearance on neuroradiological imaging is that of a sessile or pedunculated mass usually attached to the posterior hypothalamus between the tuber cinereum and the mamillary bodies [88]. The tumor is thought to secrete GnRH, rather than stimulating secretion from a normal hypothalamus, and is associated with very high serum LH concentrations in response to GnRH administration.

The prevalence of GDPP is increased after cranial irradiation for local tumors or leukemia. Low dose cranial irradiation (18–24 Gy), previously employed in the CNS prophylactic treatment of acute lymphoblastic leukemia, was associated with a downward shift in the distribution of ages at pubertal onset and menarche in girls [89,90]. Moderate radiation doses (25–47.5 Gy) used for the treatment of brain tumors in children are associated with precocious puberty, with a direct relationship between ages at pubertal onset and therapy [90]. Higher doses are usually associated with gonadotropin deficiency.

Coexisting growth hormone deficiency (GHD) in those children who have received cranial radiotherapy, as well as those children with sexual precocity secondary to congenital anomalies, trauma or CNS infection, complicates the situation. Careful evaluation reveals that GH-deficient children with GDPP grow at a rate between that of children who are GH-sufficient with GDPP and that of children who have GHD without sexual precocity.

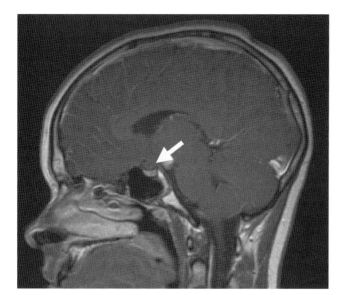

Figure 10.9 Saggital magnetic resonance image from a 8-year-old boy with clinical features of gonadotropin-dependent precocious puberty showing a hypothalamic mass with the growth characteristics of a glioma.

Because children who have received cranial irradiation are often obese, and because obesity is associated with a reduction in GH secretion, tests of GH secretion can be misleading in this group of patients and need careful interpretation.

Children adopted from developing countries and moved to a more affluent environment have an increased incidence of early and precocious puberty [3,5]. Sexual abuse has been reported as a precipitating cause of GDPP, and in these cases, the development can regress with a change in environment [91]. Sex steroid exposure has a direct maturational effect on the hypothalamus and can accelerate the onset of centrally mediated puberty (Table 10.6) [92,93].

Gonadotropin-releasing tumors (usually hCG) lead to sexual precocity. These tumors are mostly intracranial, such as pineal germ cell tumors and teratomas, or hepatoblastomas and teratomas. Tumor markers, such as α-fetoprotein and pregnancy-specific β₁-glycoprotein, are often present. Pure gonadotropin-secreting tumors of the pituitary are rare.

Gonadotropin-independent precocious puberty

In gonadotropin-independent precocious puberty (GIPP), the secretion of sex steroids is autonomous and independent of the hypothalamic GnRH pulse generator. There is loss of normal feedback regulation and sex steroid concentrations can be very high with low gonadotropin secretion. These disorders are associated with an abnormally functioning LH receptor.

The LH receptor belongs to the G-protein coupled receptor super-family characterized by the presence of seven transmembrane α-helices. The LH receptor is linked to an associated G-protein vital for signal transduction and the intracellular actions of the hormone. LH binding to its receptor activates the G-protein leading to the conversion of guanosine diphosphate (GDP) to guanosine triphosphate (GTP). An increase in intracellular cAMP follows which then sets off a chain of events culminating in the synthesis and secretion of sex steroids. Phosphorylase activity of the G-protein converts GTP to GDP which terminates the action of LH.

In boys, familial testotoxicosis or male-limited GIPP is associated with premature Leydig cell and germ cell maturation. It is inherited as an autosomal dominant condition which manifests only in males. Virilization occurs with very high concentrations of testosterone and enlargement of the testes to the early or mid-

Table 10.6 Conditions where earlier sex steroid exposure is associated with gonadotropin dependent precocious puberty.

Condition	Exposure
Congenital adrenal hyperplasia	Late diagnosis and/or poor treatment
Gonadotropin independent precocious puberty	Autonomous sex steroid secretion
Exposure to xenoestrogens	Environment
?? Premature adrenarche	Adrenal androgen secretion

pubertal range, although they seem smaller than expected in relation to the stage of penile growth. Premature Leydig and Sertoli cell maturation and spermatogenesis occur [94]. Unstimulated gonadotropin concentrations are prepubertal with a minimal prepubertal response to GnRH stimulation. There is a lack of the usual pubertal pattern of LH pulsatility. In adulthood, fertility is achieved and an adult pattern of LH secretion and response to GnRH is demonstrable.

Testotoxicosis is associated with a number of constitutively activating mutations of the LH receptor [95,96] mostly in the transmembrane domain of the receptor. Two boys have been described who have testotoxicosis with pseudohypoparathyroidism [97]. Both had a mutation in the gene encoding the Gs α-subunit of G-proteins resulting in the substitution of an alanine residue at position 366 with serine (Ala366Ser), a mutation that led to constitutive activation in the adenyl cyclase of the LH receptor. This mutation is stable at the lower temperature of the testes but degraded at 37°C, the temperature of the cAMP-dependent receptor for parathyroid hormone, which leads to parathyroid hormone resistance.

McCune–Albright syndrome (MAS) is a multisystem disorder that occurs in both boys and girls and is characterized by the classic triad of irregularly edged hyperpigmented macules or café-au-lait spots, a slowly progressive bone disorder (polyostotic fibrous dysplasia) which can involve any bone with frequent facial asymmetry and hyperostosis of the base of the skull, and, most commonly in girls, GIPP [98]. There is often a lack of consonance in pubertal development and menses may be observed with minimal breast development. Autonomous hyperfunction most commonly involves the ovary but other endocrine involvement includes thyroid (nodular hyperplasia with thyrotoxicosis), adrenal (multiple hyperplastic nodules with Cushing syndrome), pituitary (adenoma with gigantism, acromegaly or hyperprolactinemia) and parathyroid glands (adenoma or hyperplasia with hyperparathyroidism). Two of these features are required for the diagnosis. The condition is sporadic and is caused by a somatic activating missense mutation in the gene encoding the α-subunit of the G-protein (Gsα) which stimulates cAMP production (see above). The mutation results in a failure of phosphorylation of GTP to GDP and therefore constitutive activation [99]. The mutation is somatic and individuals are chimeric for the condition, hence the variability of the phenotype.

The sexual precocity in girls with MAS is caused by autonomously functioning multiple luteinized follicular cysts of the ovaries with an occasional large solitary cyst. Estrogen production is associated with a prepubertal pattern of LH secretion with an absent LH response to GnRH. GnRH-dependent puberty ensues later with ovulatory cycles. Sexual precocity is rare in boys with MAS. When it does occur, it is associated with asymmetric enlargement of the testes in addition to signs of sexual precocity. The seminiferous tubules are enlarged and exhibit spermatogenesis. Leydig cells may be hyperplastic.

Abnormal patterns of gonadotropin secretion

Premature thelarche

Premature thelarche describes the phenomenon of isolated, often fluctuating, unilateral or bilateral breast development unaccompanied by other signs of puberty. Growth velocity is normal and bone age not advanced. Premature thelarche is often present from infancy, usually occurs by the age of 2 years, and onset is rare after the age of 4. Incidence is 20 per 100 000 patient years. Sixty percent of cases occur between 6 months and 2 years of age and most regress in the period 6 months to 6 years after diagnosis. Significant nipple development is usually absent and estrogen-induced thickening and dulling of the vaginal mucosa or enlargement of the uterus on ultrasonography is uncommon. Growth in stature is normal. It is usually benign and self-limiting, although some girls progress into early or precocious puberty.

Premature thelarche is typically associated with a degree of FSH secretion and antral follicular development and ovarian function that is greater than that of prepubertal controls. Unstimulated and GnRH-stimulated plasma levels of FSH are increased, whereas those of LH are prepubertal [100].

Thelarche variant

Variations of premature thelarche occur on a spectrum towards precocious puberty. Most cases of premature thelarche present in the first 2 years of life and regress before puberty. Children who present later may demonstrate breast development that may advance with growth acceleration and skeletal maturation. The name given to this condition is thelarche variant or "a slowly progressive variant of precocious puberty in girls" [101]. The condition may be caused by a disorder of ovarian follicular maturation because mean ovarian volume exceeds the normal prepubertal size. Cyclic breast growth may be seen which does not resolve spontaneously. The condition demonstrates considerable heterogeneity in terms of gonadotropin secretion – pulsatile FSH-predominant gonadotropin secretion which is intermediate between premature thelarche and GDPP [101], LH secretory profiles more like those observed in normal puberty [102] and with a rapid but transient onset of estrogenization, suppressed responsiveness to GnRH in some girls.

Primary hypothyroidism

In primary hypothyroidism, FSH concentrations may also be increased. *In vitro* studies have demonstrated that TSH has weak agonist properties at the human FSH receptor [103]. Ovarian stimulation causes isolated breast development and testicular enlargement without other secondary sexual characteristics in boys [104]. There is no pubertal progression in the majority of cases, bone age is delayed and growth velocity poor. Nevertheless, in certain cases, normal gonadotropin-dependent puberty occurs at an inappropriately early age upon instigation of thyroxine treatment. The prognosis is excellent with reversal of puberty once treatment is commenced but final height may be affected if diagnosis is delayed or if normal puberty occurs at an early age.

Sexual precocity resulting from adrenal androgens
Adrenarche
The fetal adrenal gland secretes dehydroepiandrosterone sulfate (DHEAS) and this can manifest as pubic hair or clitoromegaly in infancy, especially in premature babies [105]. Congenital adrenal hyperplasia (CAH) and virilizing adrenal tumors need to be excluded. Adrenal androgen concentrations diminish as the fetal adrenal zone regresses and appearances return to normal.

When signs of adrenarche occur before the age of 8 years in girls and 9 years of age in boys, it is called premature adrenarche or pubarche and is more common in children from an Asian, Mediterranean or Afro-Carribean background. An association with low birthweight has been described [106]. In some populations, there appears to be an increased prevalence of minor defects of adrenal steroidogenesis in these children [107], particularly when genital enlargement is present. In spite of the increase in height velocity and advance in bone age, final height is unaffected although there may be increased prevalence of functional ovarian hyperandrogenism in the mid-teenage years [108].

Congenital adrenal hyperplasia
The classic form of CYP21 deficiency may present with salt loss and clitoromegaly in girls in the neonatal period. In boys who do not have the salt-losing form and in some very virilized girls who are not diagnosed because they are raised as boys, presentation may be with tall stature, increased height velocity, advanced bone age, clitoromegaly in girls, genital maturation in the absence of testicular enlargement in boys and the development of pubic and axillary hair in both sexes. Additionally, CYP11B1 deficiency presents similarly but also with hypertension.

The non-classic or late-onset form of CAH may present in childhood or adolescence with early pubic hair and acne or in early adulthood with menstrual irregularities, hirsutism or infertility. GDPP and the polycystic ovary syndrome are common sequelae. Final height is usually compromised. Virilization also occurs in undertreated children with CAH.

Of children with premature adrenarche, 5–10% are estimated to have late-onset CAH, although this estimate varies depending on the ethnicity of the population sampled [107]. The adrenocorticotropic hormone (ACTH) stimulation test can differentiate between children with late-onset CAH and precocious pubarche or premature adrenarche. Unstimulated and stimulated concentrations of 17α-hydroxypregnenolone (17PGN) and 17PGN:17-OHP, DHEA and androstenedione concentrations are higher in children with premature adrenarche than in control subjects or those with non-classic 21-hydroxylase deficiency.

Adrenal tumors
The characteristic picture is a short history of virilization, accelerated growth rate and advanced bone age. Cushing syndrome may be present if there is hypersecretion of cortisol. The diagnosis can be revealed by urinary steroid profile analysis. Imaging of the

adrenal glands should be performed. Treatment involves surgical resection of the tumor, with the option of adjuvant chemotherapy. The prognosis is guarded and neither operative findings nor histology help, the only factor influencing whether the lesion is likely to behave in a malignant manner or not being tumor size. Tumors less than 5 cm diameter are nearly always benign. An immediate fall in serum or urinary androgen markers of tumor secretion is encouraging and adjuvant chemotherapy or radiotherapy has not been demonstrated to improve long-term prognosis in these children. Adrenal tumors may be associated with syndromes of increased cancer risk, e.g. Li–Fraumeni syndrome.

Gonadal sex steroids
Gonadal tumors can lead to pubertal development, which is not consonant, and high sex steroid concentrations. Leydig cell tumors are associated with virilization but conversion of testosterone to estradiol leads to gynecomastia. Granulosa cell and germ cell tumors can secrete both androgens and estradiol.

Exogenous sex steroids can occasionally be the cause of sexual precocity. Hormones used in chicken rearing are occasionally implicated as a cause of "epidemics" of premature thelarche, although the relationship is unproven.

Problems associated with sexual precocity
Growth
Because puberty occurs abnormally early, the growth spurt also occurs early. GH concentrations and the increase in growth velocity are similar to those observed in normally timed puberty but, because the growth spurt has occurred abnormally early, insufficient childhood growth will have taken place so adding the fixed increment that comes with puberty (approximately 30 cm in males and 20–25 cm in females) leads to a restricted final height. Sex steroid exposure results in rapid bone age advance, in turn diminishing adult height potential.

Psychological problems
These are often the major issue for children with sexual precocity and their families because sex steroid exposure in young children results in disruptive behavior and because the child looks much older than their chronological age [109]. Most children experience problems at school, which are compounded by the difficulties that teachers and fellow pupils have in understanding them. The child and his/her family may later have problems dealing with normally timed pubertal development and are frequently apprehensive about stopping suppressive treatment. Menstruation at an early age presents practical difficulties.

Girls may be subject to sexual advances with which they are unable to deal, while boys may have erections which may be an embarrassment. Children with special educational needs as a result of a cerebral lesion or hydrocephalus are particularly vulnerable to these problems. Early maturity within the normal range correlates to some extent with an earlier onset of sexual behavior [109].

Clinical and diagnostic approach to sexual precocity

A careful history and clinical examination should be performed in the first instance, height measured and Tanner pubertal stage recorded. Bone age should be estimated. Follow-up of height velocity and pubertal progress is important for the differentiation of potentially benign, non-progressing conditions, such as premature thelarche and adrenarche, from progressive conditions, such as GDPP, GIPP, CAH and gonadal tumors. Most children presenting with sexual precocity do not require extensive investigation, although sinister underlying causes for sexual precocity such as tumors should always be considered and excluded.

Imaging

In males with GDPP, neuroradiological imaging [either computed tomography (CT) or magnetic resonance imaging (MRI)] is mandatory. In girls in the absence of neurological signs, the diagnostic return is low, with returns diminishing towards the normal timing of the onset of puberty. Interventional returns are increased in patients under 4 years of age.

At 6–8 years of age [110], intervention is not without resource implications and the closer the girl to the normal timimg of puberty the less likely is the chance of finding a lesion: under age 6, the odds of finding an abnormality are about 1 in 5 and over age 6 years 1 in 50 [111]. In the absence of data that provide robust sensitivity and specificity analysis, MRI scan should be undertaken [112–115].

All girls with early development of secondary sexual characteristics warrant transabdominal pelvic ultrasound examination. In GDPP, the ovaries are active with multiple (>6) cysts that are greater than 4 mm in diameter (Fig. 10.10a). Larger cysts are sometimes seen in premature thelarche (<3 cysts), thelarche variant (3–6 cysts) (Fig. 10.10b) and MAS (Fig. 10.10c). In prac-

tice, ovarian appearances may overlap between GDPP and premature thelarche, although children with premature adrenarche have appearances similar to controls.

The first signs of estrogenization of the uterus is a change in the shape of the uterus from a tubular structure, where the diameter of the fundus and the cervix are similar, to a pear-shaped structure, where the fundus expands so that its diameter exceeds that of the cervix. In GDPP, the changes resemble those of normal puberty, whereas in premature thelarche or thelarche variant the uterus remains prepubertal in shape. Endometrial thickening suggests that pubertal concentrations of estrogen have been attained and an endometrium around 6–8 mm implies imminent menarche.

If an adrenal tumor is suspected in patients with virilization, CT or MRI scan of the adrenal glands is indicated. Ultrasound scan of the adrenal glands is of limited use. In cases where MAS is suspected a bone scan or skeletal survey is indicated.

Biochemistry

The combination of a GnRH stimulation test and measurement of serum concentrations of sex steroids is a useful starting point. This entails the administration of a single intravenous bolus of GnRH (2.5 µg/kg to a maximum of 100 µg) with measurement of plasma LH and FSH concentrations at 0, 20 and 60 min. Normal prepubertal children have an increment of 3–4 IU/L LH and 2–3 IU/L FSH. Regardless of age, the increment is greater in puberty, although the cut-offs vary depending upon the assay. In GDPP, a pubertal LH-dominant response is observed whereas in GIPP and sexual precocity secondary to gonadal tumors or ovarian cyst formation, gonadotropin concentrations are suppressed by the autonomous sex steroid secretion. The response to GnRH in precocious adrenarche is prepubertal. In prematute

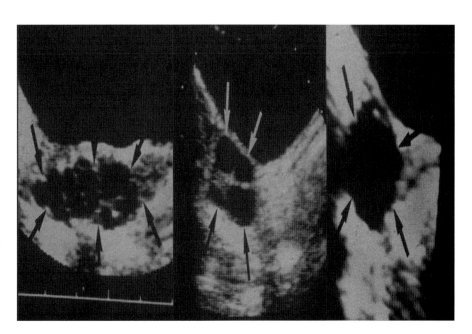

Figure 10.10 Pelvic ultrasound examinations of girls with: (a) gonadotropin-dependent precocious puberty (GDPP) showing multicystic ovary characteristic of the effects of pulstaile gonadotropin secretion; (b) the ovary in thelarche variant with several large cysts; and (c) the large single cyst present in McCune–Albright syndrome (MAS). Arrows outline ovarian structure. Marker bar depicts 1 cm intervals.

thelarche FSH tends to be dominant while in thelarche variant response is intermediate between thelarche and GDPP with FSH predominating.

In children with virilization, elevated unstimulated plasma 17OHP concentrations suggest CAH. The response to synacthen with measurement of plasma 17OHP and/or urinary steroids will confirm the diagnosis. Rapid virilization suggests the presence of an endocrine-secreting neoplasm. Testosterone, dihydrotestosterone, DHEAS and androstenedione are all elevated by adrenal virilizing tumors. Plasma cortisol may also be elevated, with a loss of the normal circadian rhythm if Cushing syndrome is a feature. There is a failure of suppression in response to dexamethasone if an adrenal tumor is present, whereas, in premature adrenarche and CAH, dexamethasone administration will lead to suppression of adrenal steroids. A urinary steroid profile is also of considerable diagnostic value if an adrenal tumor is suspected [116].

A raised serum hCG level suggests an hCG-secreting neoplasm. The response to GnRH is prepubertal. Thyroid function tests should be undertaken in a girl with premature thelarche or a boy with enlargement of the testes in the face of a lack of virilization combined with short stature, a poor growth velocity and delayed bone age to exclude primary hypothyroidism.

Delayed puberty

Assessment

A temporary delay in sexual maturation is not uncommon and resolves with time leading to normal development, optimum final height and fertility but, in patients with an underlying organic pathology, early diagnosis and treatment is essential to ensure normal pubertal progress and adequate final height. A useful algorithm is depicted in Figure 10.11.

Assessment should include a detailed history of symptoms of chronic illness, medications, symptoms suggestive of other hormone deficit or excess, previous treatment or surgery, abnormal eating patterns and a history of the family including parental heights and age at onset of puberty. Chronic illness is often associated with delayed puberty particularly asthma (and/or its treatment), eczema, cystic fibrosis and inflammatory bowel disease. The majority of those who present with delayed puberty are boys, more often because of the short stature rather than the lag in sexual development. In girls, delay is unusual and should prompt a systematic search to include eating issues and intense exercise programs.

Examination should include details of present and past heights and weights with pubertal staging. Testicular size should be measured using the Prader orchidometer. Careful documentation for body disproportion, with estimation of the upper and lower body segments, may suggest Klinefelter syndrome. Patients with Turner syndrome are short, have a low hairline, webbing of the neck, prominent ears, broad chest, renal and cardiac abnormalities with streak gonads, although presenting features in many cases may be more subtle. Presence of other dysmorphic features may reveal multisystem syndromes such as CHARGE, Prader–Willi, Bardet–Biedl or septo-optic dysplasia. Neurological examination should be performed to include visual field deficits, sense of smell and fundoscopy. Anosmia or lack of smell is suggestive of Kallmann syndrome.

Initial investigations should include a wrist radiograph to estimate skeletal age. Based on the skeletal age, it is possible to calculate a predicted adult height range and its relation to the genetic potential (mid-parental height). Further investigations and management should depend on the skeletal age, symptoms and extent of delay and stature. Laboratory measurement of serum FSH and

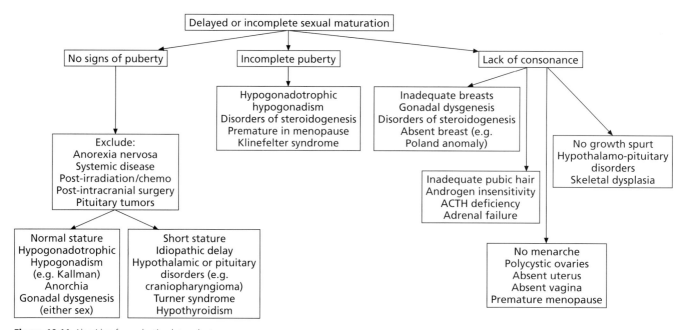

Figure 10.11 Algorithm for evaluating late puberty.

LH concentrations will help differentiate patients with hypogonadotropic and hypergonadotropic hypogonadism (Fig. 10.12). Serum gonadotropin concentrations are low in all normal children before puberty and caution must be exercised in interpretation of low serum gonadotropin concentrations, especially below a bone age of 12 years. GnRH testing has been studied extensively in pubertal delay but may not clarify whether an individual will progress in puberty or has a permanent defect [117,118]. Overnight sampling may demonstrate pulsatility but is unhelpful for prognosis. Pelvic ultrasound examination is helpful in girls, where it may reveal the multicystic pattern that is a classic feature of early puberty.

Differential diagnosis
Constitutional delay in puberty

This is the most common cause of delayed sexual maturation in males. The condition clusters in families and inheritance is complex. The presence of the condition equally in male and female relatives of subjects with the condition challenges the concept of male preponderance [119]. In addition to delayed puberty, it is characterized by short stature that is appropriate when skeletal age is taken into account. Growth velocity is normal for a prepubertal individual. As a rule, mean height velocity is 5 cm/year at 12 years of age and declines at a rate of 1 cm/year for every year thereafter that puberty is not entered. The variance on this is ±1 cm/yr. These patients demonstrate low serum gonadotropins and may occasionally be difficult to distinguish from organic gonadotropin deficiency. The rules on growth rate are important and can help prevent unnecessary investigation of the GH axis. Unless "priming" of the system is undertaken with sex steroids, low GH secretion may be documented and GH therapy instigated.

Hypogonadotropic hypogonadism

This is defined as a permanent absence of spontaneous pubertal development because of a lack of serum gonadotropin production or action, although there remains a group of individuals who appear to reverese in early adulthood (Table 10.7) [120]. The deficiency may be isolated or associated with combined pituitary hormone deficiencies, congenital or acquired [121].

Isolated gonadotropin deficiency can be idiopathic or part of X-linked Kallmann syndrome (KS) associated with anosmia [122] or in association with X-linked adrenal hypoplasia [123] or X-linked ichthyosis [124]. Additionally, gonadotropin deficiency may be associated with a number of syndromes, e.g. Bardet–Biedl and CHARGE syndrome.

Several genes have been linked to the pathogenesis of hypogonadotropic hypogonadism (HH) including *KAL1*, *FGFR1*, *GPR54*, *Kisspeptin*, *GnRHR*, *PROK2*, *PROKR2*, *NELF*, LH and FSH β-subunit genes, leptin, leptin receptor and prohormone convertase 1 (PC1), as well as a mechanism via digenic inheritance [125].

KS is characterized by HH and olfactory dysfunction ranging from hyposmia to anosmia. It is clinically and genetically heterogeneous, with an estimated prevalence in males of 1:8000 to 1:10 000 and 1:50 000 in females [45]. The olfactory dysfunction is related to olfactory bulb aplasia or hypoplasia, while the hypogonadism is caused by GnRH deficiency resulting from defective GnRH neuronal migration. Patients classically present with absent pubertal development, although it can occasionally be diagnosed in newborns on the basis of cryptorchidism, a micropenis and an absent postnatal gonadotropin and testosterone surge. Some individuals develop some spontaneous primary pubertal characteristics (testicular growth in males and a degree of breast development in females), suggesting the presence of endogenous GnRH secretion. Other variable features include high arched palate, manual synkinesia, renal aplasia/hypoplasia, sensorineural deafness, oculomotor abnormalities, dental agenesis, facial asymmetry and pes cavus.

KAL1 [126] was the first gene to be associated with KS and to date 67 mutations of *KAL1* have been described. The gene comprises 14 exons spanning approximately 210 kb on Xp22.3 and it

Figure 10.12 Conditions of pubertal delay associated with high and low gonadotropin concentrations.

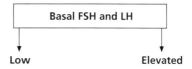

Basal FSH and LH	
Low	**Elevated**

Bone age delay
      Constitutional delay of
      growth and puberty
Investigations for reversible conditions
      Thyroid function tests
      Chronic illnesses
      Eating pattern
Evaluate sense of smell
      Kallman syndrome
LHRH test +/− HCG test (males)
MRI scan of pituitary gland
Trial of treatment
	Serum autoantibodies
	      Autoimmune disease
	Karyotype
	      Turner syndrome
	      Klinefelter syndrome
	      XY gonadal dysgenesis
	      Androgen insensitivity syndrome

Table 10.7 Causes of hypogonadotropic hypogonadism.

Developmental and genetic causes

Kallmann syndrome (HH and anosmia): X-linked (*KAL*), AD, AR
Impaired GnRH release and action (e.g. *leptin, leptin R, PC1, GnRHR*)
Multiple pituitary hormone deficiency (e.g. *HESX1, LHX3, PROP1*)
Isolated gonadotropin deficiency
Isolated LH deficiency/mutation
Congenital glycosylation disorders
Effects on multiple levels of the HPG axis (e.g. *DAX1, SF1*)
Midline defects

Chromosomal abnormalities

Deletions and rearrangements

Syndromic associations

Prader–Willi syndrome
Laurence–Moon syndrome
Gordon–Holmes spinocerebellar ataxia
CHARGE
Others

Physical causes

CNS tumors
  craniopharyngioma, germinoma, hypothalamic glioma, optic nerve glioma
  pituitary tumors
Langerhans cell histiocytosis
Post infection
Granulomatous disorders
Vascular malformations
Trauma/pituitary stalk transection
Cranial irradiation

Functional causes

Chronic renal disease
Chronic gastrointestinal disease/malnutrition
Sickle cell disease/iron overload
Chronic lung disease/cystic fibrosis/asthma
AIDS
Poorly controlled diabetes mellitus
Hypothyroidism
Cushing disease
Hyperprolactinemia
Metabolic conditions (e.g. Gaucher disease)
Anorexia nervosa
Bulimia nervosa
Psychogenic/stress
Extreme exercise
Drugs

escapes inactivation. *KAL1* encodes a protein, anosmin-1, a 100-kDa extracellular matrix N-glycosylated protein [126] consisting of 680 residues. Several components contribute to its role in axonal migration, a whey acidic protein-like (WAP) four disulfide core motif found in several protease inhibitors known to participate in axonal elongation and cell migration and large positively charged FnIII type domain essential for high-affinity

dose-dependent binding to negatively charged heparan sulfate. Heparan sulfate proteoglycan interactions have a vital role in neuronal navigation during neural development. During development, anosmin-1 confers GnRH neurons with cell-specific chemotactic responsivity as well as branch promoting and guidance functions

FGFR1 (*KAL2*) is the first gene described in association with autosomal dominant KS [127]. It is estimated that 5–10% of individuals with autosominal dominant HH have mutations in *FGFR1* [128]. The gene comprises 18 exons on chromosome 8p11.2 region and encodes the fibroblast growth factor receptor 1, a member of the FGFR family. The full length protein is a 120 kDa protein, with 822 residues. FGFR1 and anosmin-1 interact in olfactory bulb development. Sixty-four loss-of-function mutations in *FGFR1* have been described in patients with KS. There is little genotype–phenotype correlation and wide heterogeneity is found in kindreds harboring the same mutation ranging from complete absence of pubertal development to normal reproduction or even isolated anosmia [129]. This wide phenotypic variability suggests that variable degrees of endogenous GnRH release may occur. In addition, the *KAL2* phenotype frequently includes cleft lip or palate [126] and dental agenesis. Men with *KAL1* gene mutations have a more severe reproductive phenotype than those with *KAL2* gene mutations and the latter tend to have a broader spectrum of pubertal development patterns and less severe impairment of gonadotropin secretion [130].

Mutations in *Prokineticin receptor-2* (*PKOKR-2, KAL3*) and its ligand *Prokineticin-2* (*PROK-2, KAL4*) were described in patients with KS in a series of 192 patients with HH [131]. Prokineticins 1 and 2 (PROK1, PROK2) were originally described as regulators of gastrointestinal motility and genes encoding these proteins are expressed in the testes, ovaries, placenta and adrenal glands. PROK2 signaling regulates olfactory bulb morphogenesis and reproduction as shown in mice. *Pkok2*$^{-/-}$ mice have abnormal olfactory bulbs, GnRH neuron migration and hypoplasia of reproductive organs [132].

The *PROK2* gene is located on chromosome 3 (3p21.1), consists of four exons and encodes a protein of 81 amino acids in its mature form [131] sharing approximately 44% amino acid homology with PROK1. It contains two structural features: a cysteine-rich domain and a N-terminal hexapeptide sequence (AVITGA). Both PROK1 and PROK2 activate the receptors PROKR1 and PROKR2 with PROK2 showing moderately higher affinity [132]. *PROKR2* is expressed in the central nervous system while *PROKR1* is found in peripheral tissues. *PROKR2* has been mapped on chromosome 20 (20p12.3), consists of two exons and plays a role in the development of the olfactory bulb [133]. Five mutations in *PROK2* and 12 mutations in *PROKR2* have been reported.

The phenotype varies from idiopathic hypogonadotropic hypogonadism (IHH) to KS or isolated anosmia, even amongst members of same pedigree with an identical genotype. Although individuals do not manifest synkinesis, renal agenesis, cleft palate and dental agenesis are observed in patients with KS due to mutations in *KAL1* or *FGFR1*, of note is the observation that certain individuals with *PROK2* mutations are also obese.

Because by definition HH is related to gonadotropin deficiency, it would follow that the *GnRH* gene would be a suitable candidate gene for HH. To date, no human mutations have been described but 23 mutations in the gene encoding its receptor (*GnRHR*) have been reported.

The *GnRHR* gene is located on the long arm of chromosome 4 (4q21.2) and spans over 18.9 kb. The phenotype may be variable and associated with a marked delay in puberty as well as HH [49,134]. The *GnRHR* gene comprises three exons and encodes the receptor for type 1 GnRH, a 328 amino acid protein. In a cohort of 108 patients with IHH, *GnRHR* mutations were found to account for approximately 16.7% of all normosmic patients (as evaluated in a subgroup of 18 patients) and 40% of presumed autosomal recessive IHH [135]. Most of these *GnRHR* mutations are compound heterozygous changes that reduce GnRH binding and/or activation of IP3 or PLC signaling pathways [136]. There is wide phenotypic variability in *GnRHR* mutations even within the same kindred.

Kisspeptin and its receptor [GPR54 (*KISS1R*)] have been noted already to have an important role in the control of puberty [47]. GPR54 is located on chromosome 19 (19p13.3) and encodes a protein of 396 amino acids. GPR54 was previously thought to be an orphan receptor until the isolation of metastin, a 54 amino acid peptide with metastasis suppression properties. Metastin, also known as kisspeptin-54, is encoded by KISS-1 and is processed to various smaller peptides (kisspeptins 14, 13, 10) [137]. Mutations in KISS1R have been described in patients with IHH [49–51]. No human mutations in KiSS1 have yet been reported.

Nasal embryonic LHRH factor (NELF) was isolated in olfactory sensory cells and GnRH cells during embryonic development in the mouse [138]. NELF is a 530-residue protein encoded by *NELF*, located on chromosome 9 (9q34.3) and consisting of 16 exons. Five alternative splice variants have been detected; one variant (*NELF-v1*) is 93–94% similar at the amino acid level to mouse and rat and the other four are highly conserved amongst those three species. The NELF protein is a guidance molecule for the GnRH and olfactory neurons. Two mutations have been identified in patients with HH. The Y376X mutation was found in a patient heterozygous for an *FGFR1* mutation as well [125] and the other (Thr480) is highly conserved and is likely to be implicated in the pathogenesis of HH [139].

Table 10.7 depicts acquired forms of gonadotropin deficiency. Some are associated with other anterior pituitary hormone developmental abnormalities or structural problems of the brain. In addition, acquired gonadotropin deficiency may be brought about by intracranial trauma, tumors, surgery or radiotherapy. Hemochromatosis associated with transfusion can result in permanent gonadotropin deficiency [140,141].

The condition in boys is best diagnosed, or rather excluded, with a GnRH test in combination with an hCG test to stimulate the testicular release of testosterone [142]. In girls consideration needs to be given to the use of FSH to test ovarian function and

Table 10.8 Causes of hypergonadotropic hypogonadism.

Girls

Chromosomal abnormalities
Turner syndrome and variants (e.g. 45X; 46XX/45X; X chromosome abnormalities)
Mixed gonadal dysgenesis (e.g. 46XY/45X)
Deletions and rearrangements (e.g. Xq22, Xq26-28)

Abnormalities in gonadal development
Ovarian dysgenesis

Syndromic associations
Perrault, Maximilian, Quayle and Copeland, Pober, Malouf syndromes
Ataxia telangiectasia, Nijmegen, Cockayne, Rothmund–Thompson, Werner syndromes
Bletharophimosis-ptosis-epicanthus syndrome (BPES, *FOXL2*)

Disorders of steroid synthesis and action
LH resistance
FSH resistance
Pseudohypoparathyroidism 1a
SF1, StAR, CYP11a, HSD3B2, Cyp17, aromatase (CYP19) (46XX karyotype)
HSD17B2, AIS, SRD5A2 (46XY karyotype)

Other causes of primary ovarian failure
Autoimmune (e.g. AIRE)
Metabolic (e.g. galactosemia, storage disorders)
Hyperandrogenism/polycystic ovarian syndrome
Pelvic/spinal irradiation
Chemotherapy

Boys
Chromosomal causes
Klinefelter syndrome and variants (e.g. 47XXY; 46XY/47XXY)
Mixed gonadal dysgenesis (e.g. 46XY/45X)
Deletions and rearrangements

Abnormalities in gonadal development
Testicular dysgenesis (e.g. loss of functional Sry, Sox9, SF1, WT1, DMRT)

Syndromic associations
Noonan syndrome
Robinow syndrome
Others

Disorders of steroid synthesis and action
LH resistance (e.g. LHR, GNAS)
SF1, StAR, CYP11a, HSD3B2, HSD17B2, PAIS

Other causes of primary testicular (Leydig cell) failure
Anorchia
Cryptorchidism
Sertoli cell only syndrome
Testicular irradiation
Chemotherapy
Infection (e.g. mumps)

AIRE, autoimmune regulator; GNAS, guanine nucleotide protein alpha-stimulating activity polypeptide 1; LHR, luteinizing hormone receptor.

further work in this area is needed [143]. More definitive studies include the use of repeated pulses of GnRH to test more fully gonadotrope secretory potential [144]. In many cases, it is necessary also to rule out other pituitary hormone deficiencies and perform neuroimaging of the pituitary gland. In some cases the interpretation of the GnRH test is not straightforward and endocrine re-assessment may be necessary at a later time after completion of growth and puberty to ascertain the need for long-term replacement [120].

Hypergonadotropic hypogonadism

Elevated serum gonadotropin concentrations in the absence of pubertal signs at the appropriate age for puberty suggest gonadal insufficiency (Table 10.8). Radiotherapy, chemotherapy and surgery, particularly orchidopexy for very high placed testes, can all result in gonadal failure [145].

Turner syndrome (1 in 2500 live female births) should be considered in all short girls, even in the presence of pubertal signs. Patients with Turner syndrome may show markedly elevated serum gonadotropin concentrations from as early as 8–9 years of age [72,73] because of lack of negative feedback and the GnRH test is not usually needed. Pure XX and XY gonadal dysgenesis both present with delayed puberty, raised serum gonadotropins and low sex steroid concentrations. The XY gonadal dysgenesis group who are reared as females have a high risk of gonadal tumors and need early surgery for the removal of their gonads. Gonadal failure in females is also associated with autoimmune ovarian failure (which may be associated with autoimmune polyendocrinopathy syndrome) [146] and galactosemia [147].

In boys, tall stature, pubertal delay and learning difficulties are the classic features associated with Klinefelter syndrome (47XXY). Learning difficulties may be quite mild and the stature not excessive [148]. Many of the boys do enter puberty but rarely progress beyond 8 mL testicular volumes so there is a lack of consonance between the genital and pubic hair stages and small testes [149]. Other causes in boys include anorchia, torsion or infection.

References

1 Grumbach MM, Styne DM. Puberty, ontogeny, neuroendocrinology, physiology, and disorders. In: Wilson JD, Foster DW, Kronenberg MD, Larsen PR, eds. *Williams Textbook of Endocrinology*, 9th edn. Philadelphia: WB Saunders; 1998: 1509–1625.

2 Tanner JM. The trend toward earlier menarche in London, Oslo, Copenhagen, the Netherlands and Hungary. *Nature* 1973; **243**: 95.

3 Parent A-S, Teilmann G, Juul A, Skakkebaek NE, Toppari J, Bourguignon J-P. The timing of normal puberty and the age limits of sexual precocity: variations around the world, secular trends and changes after migration. *Endocrine Rev* 2003; **24**: 668–693.

4 Evelith PB. Population differences in growth: environmental and genetic factors. In: Falkner F, Tanner JM, eds. *Human Growth*. New York: Plenum Press, 1979: 373–394.

5 Proos LA, Hofvander Y, Tuvemo T. Menarcheal age and growth pattern of Indian girls adopted in Sweden. I. Menarcheal age. *Acta Paediatr Scand* 1991; **80**: 852–858.

6 Hartz AJ, Barboriak PN, Wong A. The association of obesity with infertility and related menstrual abnormalities in women. *Int J Obes* 1979; **3**: 5773.

7 Osler DC, Crawford JD. Examination of the hypothesis of a critical weight at menarche in ambulatory and bedridden mentally retarded girls. *Pediatrics* 1973; **51**: 674–679.

8 Takaishi, M. Secular changes in growth of Japanese children. *J Pediatr Endocrinol* 1994; **7**: 163–173.

9 Must A, Naumova EN, Phillips SM, Blum M, Dawson-Hughes B, Rand WM. Childhood overweight and maturational timing in the development of adult overweight and fatness: the Newton Girls Study and its follow-up. *Pediatrics* 2005; **116**: 620–627.

10 Zukauskaite S, Lasiene D, Lasas L, Urbonaite B, Hindmarsh P. Onset of breast and pubic hair development in 1231 preadolescent Lithuanian schoolgirls. *Arch Dis Child* 2005; **90**: 932–936.

11 Sloboda DM, Hart R, Doherty DA, Pennell CE, Hickey M. Age at menarche: influences of prenatal and postnatal growth. *J Clin Endocrinol Metab* 2007; **92**: 46–50.

12 Mul D, Fredriks M, van Buuren S, Oosdijk W, Verloove-Vanhorick SP, Wit JM. Pubertal development in the Netherlands 1965–1997. *Pediatric Res* 2001; **50**: 479–486.

13 de la Puente ML, Canela J, Alvarez J, Salleras L, Vicens-Calvet E. Cross-sectional growth study of the child and adolescent population of Catalonia (Spain). *Ann Hum Biol* 1997; **24**: 435–452.

14 Marshall WA, Tanner JM. Variations in pattern of pubertal changes in girls. *Arch Dis Child* 1969; **44**: 291–303.

15 Marshall WA, Tanner JM. Variations in the pattern of pubertal changes in boys. *Arch Dis Child* 1970; **45**: 13–23.

16 Baker TG. A quantitative and cytological study of germ cells in human ovaries. *Proc R Soc Lond B Biol Sci* 1999; **158**: 417–433.

17 Ross GT. Follicular development: the life cycle of the follicle and puberty. In: Grumbach MM, Sizonenko PC, Aubert MI, eds. *Control of the Onset of Puberty*. Baltimore: Williams & Wilkins, 1990: 376–386.

18 Stanhope R, Adams J, Jacobs HS, *et al.* Ovarian ultrasound assessment in normal children, idiopathic precocious puberty, and during low dose pulsatile gonadotrophin releasing hormone treatment of hypogonadotrophic hypogonadism. *Arch Dis Child* 1985; **60**: 116–119.

19 Salardi S, Orsini LF, Cacciari E, Partesotti S, Brondelli L, Cicognani A, *et al.* Pelvic ultrasonography in girls with precocious puberty, congenital adrenal hyperplasia, obesity, or hirsutism. *J Pediatr* 1988; **112**: 880–887.

20 Bridges NA, Cooke A, Healy MJ, Hindmarsh PC, Brook CG. Standards for ovarian volume in childhood and puberty. *Fertil Steril* 1993; **60**: 456–460.

21 Haber HP, Ranke MB. Pelvic ultrasonography in Turner syndrome: standards for uterine and ovarian volume. *J Ultrasound Med* 1999; **18**: 271–276.

22 Gondos B, Kogan SJ. Testicular development during puberty. In: Grumbach MM, Sizonenko PC, Aubert ML, *et al.*, eds. *Control of the Onset of Puberty*. Baltimore: Williams & Wilkins 1990: 387–402.

23 Nielsen CT, Skakkebaek NE, Richardson DW, Darling JA, Hunter WM, Jorgensen M, *et al.* Onset of the release of spermatozoa (spermarche) in boys in relation to age, testicular growth, pubic hair, and height. *J Clin Endocrinol Metab* 1986; **62**: 532–535.

24 Janczewski Z, Bablok L. Semen characteristics in pubertal boys. II. Semen quality in relation to bone age. *Arch Androl* 1985; **15**: 207–211.

25 Braunstein GD. Gynecomastia. *N Engl J Med* 2007; **357**: 1229–1237.

26 Bachrach LK, Hastie T, Wang M, *et al.* Bone mineral acquisition in healthy Asian, Hispanic, black and Caucasian youth: a longitudinal study. *J Clin Endocrinol Metab* 1999; **84**: 4702–4712.

27 Ferrari S, Rizzoli R, Slosman D, Bonjour JP. Familial resemblance for bone mineral mass is expressed before puberty. *J Clin Endocrinol Metab* 1998; **83**: 358–361.

28 Barr SI, McKay HA. Nutrition, exercise, and bone status in youth. *Int J Sport Nutr* 1998; **8**: 124–142.

29 Kardinaal AF, Ando S, Charles P, Charzewska J, Rotily M, Veaeaneanen K, *et al.* Dietary calcium and bone density in adolescent girls and young women in Europe. *J Bone Min Res* 1999; **14**: 583–592.

30 Rico H, Revilla M, Villa LF, Hernandez ER, Alvarez de Buergo M, Villa M. Body composition in children and Tanner's stages: a study with dual-energy X-ray absorptiometry. *Metabolism* 1993; **42**: 967–970.

31 Cheek DB. Body composition, hormones, nutrition and adolescent growth. In: Grumbach MM, Grave GD, Mayer FE, eds. *Control of the Onset of Puberty*. New York: John Wiley & Sons, 1974: 424–447.

32 Tanner JM, Whitehouse RH, Marubini E, Resele LF. The adolescent growth spurt of boys and girls of the Harpenden growth study. *Ann Hum Biol* 1976; **3**: 109–126.

33 Largo RH, Gasser TH, Prader A. Analysis of the adolescent growth spurt using smoothing spline functions. *Ann Hum Biol* 1978; **5**: 421–434.

34 Martha PM Jr, Rogol AD, Veldhuis JD. Alterations in the pulsatile properties of circulating growth hormone concentrations during puberty in boys. *J Clin Endocrinol Metab* 1989; **69**: 563–570.

35 Veldhuis JD, Metzger DL, Martha PMJ, Mauras N, Kerrigan JR, Keenan B, *et al.* Estrogen and testosterone, but not a nonaromatizable androgen, direct network integration of the hypothalamo-somatotrope (growth hormone)-insulin-like growth factor I axis in the human: evidence from pubertal pathophysiology and sex-steroid hormone replacement. *J Clin Endocrinol Metab* 1997; **82**: 3414–3420.

36 Metzger DL, Kerrigan JR. Estrogen receptor blockade with tamoxifen diminishes growth hormone secretion in boys: evidence for a stimulatory role of endogenous estrogens during male adolescence. *J Clin Endocrinol Metab* 1994; **79**: 513–518.

37 Calvo MS, Eyre DR, Gundberg CM. Molecular basis and clinical application of biologic markers of bone turnover. *Endocr Rev* 1996; **17**: 333–368.

38 Ross JL, Cassorla FG, Skerda MC, *et al.* A preliminary study of the effect of estrogen dose on growth in Turner's syndrome. *N Engl J Med* 1984; **309**: 1104–1106.

39 Grumbach MM, Auchus RJ. Estrogen: consequences and implication of human mutations in synthesis and action. *J Clin Endocrinol Metab* 1999; **84**: 4677–4643.

40 Cutler GB. The role of estrogen in bone growth and maturation during childhood and adolescence. *J Steroid Biochem Mol Biol* 1997; **61**: 141–144.

41 Ojeda SR, Lomniczi A, Mastronardi C, *et al.* Minireview: the neuroendocrine regulation of puberty – is the time ripe for a systems biology approach? *Endocrinology* 2006; **147**: 1166–1174.

42 Bridges NA, Matthews DR, Hindmarsh PC, Brook CGD. Changes in gonadotrophin secretion during childhood and puberty. *J Endocrinol* 1994; **141**: 169–176.

43 Adelman JP, Mason AJ, Hayflick JS, *et al.* Isolation of the gene and hypothalamic cDNA for the common precursor of gonadotropin-releasing hormone and prolactin release-inhibiting factor in human and rat. *Proc Natl Acad Sci U S A* 1986; **83**: 179–183.

44 Schwanzel-Fukada M, Jorgensen KL, Bergen HT, *et al.* Biology of normal luteinizing hormone-releasing hormone neurons during and after their migration from olfactory placode. *Endocr Rev* 1992; **13**: 623–634.

45 Seminara SB, Hayes FJ, Crowley WFJ. Gonadotropin-releasing hormone deficiency in the human (idiopathic hypogonadotropic hypogonadism and Kallmann's syndrome): pathophysiological and genetic considerations. *Endocr Rev* 1999; **19**: 521–539.

46 Seminara SB, Crowley WF Jr. The importance of genetic defects in humans in elucidating the complexities of the hypothalamic-pituitary-gonadal axis. *Endocrinology* 2001; **142**: 2173–2177.

47 Seminara SB. The first kiss: a crucial role for kisspeptin-1 and its receptor, G-protein-coupled receptor 54, in puberty and reproduction. *Natl Clin Pract Endocrinol Metab* 2006; **2**: 328–334

48 Themmen APN, Huhtaniemi IT. Mutations of gonadotropins and gonadotropin receptors: elucidating the physiology and pathophysiology of pituitary-gonadal function. *Endocr Rev* 2000; **21**: 551–583.

49 de Roux N, Genin E, Carel JC, Matsuda F, Chaussain JL, Milgrom E. Hypogonadotropic hypogonadism due to loss of function of the KiSS1-derived peptide receptor GPR54. *Proc Natl Acad Sci U S A* 2003; **100**: 10972–10976.

50 Seminara SB, Messager S, Chatzidaki EE, *et al.* The GPR54 gene as a regulator of puberty. *N Engl J Med* 2003; **349**: 1614–1627.

51 Semple RK, Achermann JC, Ellery J, *et al.* Two novel missense mutations in G protein-coupled receptor 54 in a pateint with hypogondotropic hypogonadism. *J Clin Endocrinol Metab* 2005; **90**: 1849–1855.

52 Gurgel Teles M, Bianco SDC, Nahime Brito V, *et al.* A GPR54-activating mutation in a patient with central precocious puberty. *N Engl J Med* 2008; **358**: 709–715.

53 Plant TM, Ramaswamy S, Dipietro MJ. Repetitive activation of hypothalamic G protein-coupled receptor 54 with intravenous pulses of kisspeptin in the juvenile monkey (*Macaca mulatta*) elicits a sustained train of gonadotropin-releasing hormone discharges. *Endocrinology* 2006; **147**: 1007–1013.

54 Wetsel WC, Valenca MM, Merchenthaler I, Liposits Z, Lopez FJ, Weiner RI, *et al.* Intrinsic pulsatile secretory activity of immortalized luteinizing hormone-releasing hormone-secreting neurons. *Proc Natl Acad Sci U S A* 1992; **89**: 4149–4153.

55 Mitsushima D, Hei DL, Terasawa E. Gamma-aminobutyric acid is an inhibitory neurotransmitter restricting the release of luteinizing hormone-releasing hormone before the onset of puberty. *Proc Natl Acad Sci U S A* 1994; **91**: 395–399.

56 Hazum E, Conn PM. Molecular mechanism of gonadotropin releasing hormone (GnRH) action. I. The GnRH receptor. *Endocr Rev* 1988; **9**: 379–386.

57 Huckle W, Conn PM. Molecular mechanisms of gonadotropin releasing hormone action. II. The effector system. *Endocr Rev* 1988; **9**: 387–395.

58 Huhtaniemi I, Jiang M, Nilsson C, Pettersson K. Mutations and polymorphisms in gonadotropin genes. *Mol Cell Endocrinol* 1999; **151**: 89–94.

59 Layman LC. Mutations in human gonadotropin genes and their physiologic significance in puberty and reproduction. *Fertil Steril* 1999; **71**: 201–218.

60 Lofrano-Porto A, Barcelos Barra G, Abdala Giacomini L, *et al.* Luteinising hormone beat mutation and hypogonadism in men and women. *N Engl J Med* 2007; **357**: 897–904.

61 Reiter EO, Kulin HE, Hamwood SM. The absence of positive feedback between estrogen and luteinizing hormone in sexually immature girls. *Pediatr Res* 1974; **8**: 740–745.

62 Filicori M, Butler JP, Crowley WFJ. Neuroendocrine regulation of the corpus luteum in the human. *J Clin Invest* 1999; **73**: 1638–1647.

63 Russell DW, Wilson JD. Steroid 5 a hydroxylase: two genes/two enzymes. *Annu Rev Med* 1994; **63**: 25–61.

64 Mahendroo MS, Mendelson CR, Simpson ER. Tissue specific and hormonally controlled alternative promoters regulate aromatase cyotchrome P450 gene expression in human adipose tissue. *J Biol Chem* 1993; **268**: 19463–19470.

65 Lubahn DR, Joseph DR, Sar M, *et al.* The human androgen receptor : complementary dexoribonucleic acid cloning, sequence analysis and gene expression in prostate. *Mol Endocrinol* 1988; **2**: 1265–1275.

66 Klein KO, Baron J, Colli MJ, McDonnell DP, Cutler GB. Estrogen levels in childhood determined by an ultrasensitive recombinant cell bioassay. *J Clin Invest* 1994; **94**: 2475–2480.

67 Vale W, Bilezikjian LM, Rivier C. Reproductive and other roles of inhibins and activins. In: Knobil E, Neil JD, eds. *Physiology of Reproduction*, 2nd edn. New York: Raven Press, 1994: 1861–1878.

68 Andersson AM, Toppari J, Haavisto AM, Petersen JH, Simell T, Simell O, *et al.* Longitudinal reproductive hormone profiles in infants: peak of inhibin B levels in infant boys exceeds levels in adult men. *J Clin Endocrinol Metab* 1998; **83**: 675–681.

69 Hudson PL, Dougas I, Donahoe PK, *et al.* An immunoassay to detect human mullerian inhibiting substance in males and females during normal development. *J Clin Endocrinol Metab* 1990; **70**: 16–22.

70 Gluckman PD, Grumbach MM, Kaplan SL. The neuroendocrine regulation and function of growth hormone and prolactin in the mammalian fetus. *Endocr Rev* 1981; **2**: 363–395.

71 Forest MG. Pituitary gonadotropin and sex steroid secretion during the first two years of life. In: Grumbach MM, Sizonenko PC, Aubert AU, eds. *Control of the Onset of Puberty*. Baltimore: Williams & Wilkins, 1990: 451–478.

72 Conte FA, Grumbach MM, Kaplan SL, Reiter EO. Correlation of luteinizing hormone-releasing factor-induced luteinizing hormone and follicle-stimulating hormone release from infancy to 19 years with the changing pattern of gonadotropin secretion in agonadal patients: relation to the restraint of puberty. *J Clin Endocrinol Metab* 1980; **50**: 163–168.

73 Nathwani NC, Hindmarsh PC, Massarano AA, Brook CGD. Gonadotrophin pulsatility in girls with the Turner syndrome: modulation by exogenous sex steroids. *Clin Endocrinol* 1998; **49**: 107–113.

74 Dunkel L, Alfthan H, Stenman U, *et al.* Gonadal control of pulsatile secretion of luteinizing hormone and follicle-stimulating hormone in prepubertal boys evaluated by ultrasensitive time-resolved immunofluorometric assays. *J Clin Endocrinol Metab* 1990; **70**: 107–114.

75 Mitamura R, Yano K, Suzuki N, Ito Y, Makita Y, Okuno A. Diurnal rhythms of luteinizing hormone, follicle-stimulating hormone, and testosterone secretion before the onset of male puberty. *J Clin Endocrinol Metab* 1999; **84**: 29–37.

76 Farooqi IS, Jebb SA, Langmack G, *et al.* Brief report: effects of recombinant leptin therapy in a child with congeintal leptin deficiency. *N Engl J Med* 1999; **341**: 879–884.

77 Ahmed ML, Ong KK, Morrell DJ, Cox L, Drayer N, Perry L, *et al.* Longitudinal study of leptin concentrations during puberty: sex differences and relationship to changes in body composition. *J Clin Endocrinol Metab* 1999; **84**: 899–905.

78 Arslanian S, Suprasongsin C, Kalhan SC, Drash AL, Brna R, Janosky JE. Plasma leptin in children: relationship to puberty, gender, body composition, insulin sensitivity, and energy expenditure. *Metab Clin Exp* 1998; **47**: 309–312.

79 Grumbach MM, Richards GE, Conte FA, *et al.* Clinical disorders of adrenal function and puberty: an assessment of the role of the adrenal cortex in normal and abnormal puberty in man and evidence for an ACTH-like pituitary adrenal androgen stimulating hormone. In: James VHT, Serio M, Giusti G, *et al.*, eds. *The Endocrine Function of the Human Adrenal Cortex, Serono Symposium.* New York: Academic Press, 1977: 583–612.

80 Schiebinger RJ, Albertson BD, Cassorla FG, Bowyer DW, Geelhoed GW, Cutler GB Jr, *et al.* The developmental changes in plasma adrenal androgens during infancy and adrenarche are associated with changing activities of adrenal microsomal 17-hydroxylase and 17,20-desmolase. *J Clin Invest* 1981; **67**: 1177–1182.

81 Bridges NA, Christopher JA, Hindmarsh PC, Brook CGD. Sexual precocity: sex incidence and aetiology. *Arch Dis Child* 1994; **70**: 116–118.

82 Lebrethon MC, Bourguignon JP. Management of central isosexual precocity: diagnosis, treatment and outcome. *Curr Opin Pediatr* 2000; **12**: 394–399.

83 Midyett LK, Moore WV, Jacobson JD. Are pubertal changes in girls before age 8 benign? *Pediatrics* 2003; **111**: 47–51.

84 Pescovitz OH, Comite F, Hench K, *et al.* The NIH experience with precocious puberty: diagnostic subgroups and response to short-term luteinizing hormone-releasing hormone analogue therapy. *J Pediatr* 1986; **108**: 47–54.

85 Stanhope R, Brook CGD, Pringle PJ, Adams J, Jacobs HS. Induction of puberty by pulsatile gonadotrophin-releasing hormone. *Lancet* 1987; **ii**, 552–555.

86 Donaldson MDC, Stanhope R, Lee TJ, Price DA, Brook CGD, Savage DCL Gonadotrophin responses to GnRH in precocious puberty treated with GnRH analogue. *Clin Endocrinol* 1984; **21**: 499–503.

87 Junier MP, Wolff A, Hoffman G, Ma YJ, Ojeda SR. Effect of hypothalamic lesions that induce precocious puberty on the morphological and functional maturation of the luteinizing hormone releasing hormone neuronal system. *Endocrinology* 1992; **131**: 787–798.

88 Mahachoklerwattana P, Kaplan SL, Grumbach MM The luteinizing hormone-releasing hormone-secreting hypothalamic hamartoma is a congenital malformation: natural history. *J Clin Endocrinol Metab* 1993; **77**: 118–124.

89 Quigley C, Cowell C, Jimenez M, Burger H, Kirk J, Bergin M, *et al.* Normal or early development of puberty despite gonadal damage in children treated for acute lymphoblastic leukaemia. *N Engl J Med* 1989; **321**: 143–151.

90 Ogilvy-Stuart AL, Clayton PE, Shalet SM. Cranial irradiation and early puberty. *J Clin Endocrinol Metab* 1994; **78**: 1282–1286.

91 Herman ME, Giddens AD, Sandler NE, Freidman NE. Sexual precocity in girls: an association with sexual abuse? *Am J Dis Child* 1988; **142**: 431–433.

92 Dacou-Voutetakis C, Karidis N. Congenital adrenal hyperplasia complicated by central precocious puberty: treatment with LHRH agonist analogue. *Ann N Y Acad Sci U S A* 1993; **687**: 250–254.

93 Boepple PA, Frisch LS, Wierman HE, Hoffman WH, Crowley WF. The natural history of autonomous gonadal function, adrenarche and central puberty in gonadotropin-independent precocious puberty. *J Clin Endocrinol Metab* 1992; **75**: 1550–1555.

94 Rosenthal SM, Grumbach MM, Kaplan SL. Gonadotrophin-independent familial sexual precocity with premature Leydig and germinal cell maturation (familial testotoxicosis): effects of a potent luteinizing hormone-releasing factor agonist and medroxyprogesterone acetate therapy in four cases. *J Clin Endocrinol Metab* 1983; **57**: 571–579.

95 Latronico AC, Abell AN, Arnhold IJP, Liu X, Lins TSS, Brito VN, *et al*. A unique constitutively activating mutation in third transmembrane helix of luteinizing hormone receptor causes sporadic male gonadotrophin-independent precocious puberty. *J Clin Endocrinol Metab* 1998; **83**: 2435–2440.

96 Kremer H, Martens JWM, Van Reen M, Verhoef-Post M, Wit JM, Otten BJ, *et al*. A limited repertoire of mutations of the luteinizing hormone (LH) receptor gene in familial and sporadic patients with male LH-independent precocious puberty. *J Clin Endocrinol Metab* 1999; **84**: 1136–1140.

97 Iiri T, Herzmark P, Nakamoto JM, van Dop C, Bourne HR. Rapid GDP release from Gs alpha in patients with gain and loss of endocrine function. *Nature* 1994; **371**: 164–168.

98 Lee PA, Van Dop C, Migeon CJ. McCune–Albright syndrome: long-term follow up. *JAMA* 1986; **256**: 2980–2984.

99 Weinstein LS, Shenker A, Gejman PV, Merino MJ, Freidman E, Speigel AM. Activating mutations of the stimulatory G protein in the McCune–Albright syndrome. *N Engl J Med* 1991; **325**: 1688–1695.

100 Pescovitz OH, Hench KD, Barnes KM, Loriaux DL, Cutler GB Jr. Premature thelarche and central precocious puberty: the relationship between clinical presentation and the gonadotrophin response to luteinizing hormone-releasing hormone. *J Clin Endocrinol Metab* 1988; **67**: 474–479.

101 Stanhope R, Brook CGD. Thelarche variant: a new syndrome of precocious sexual maturation? *Acta Endocrinol (Copenh)* 1990; **123**: 481–486.

102 Beck W, Stubbe P. Pulsatile secretion of luteinizing hormone and sleep-related gonadotrophin rhythms in girls with premature thelarche. *Pediatrics* 1984; **141**: 168–170.

103 Anasti JN, Flack MR, Froehlich J, Nelson LM, Nisula BC. A potential novel mechanism for precocious puberty in juvenile hypothyroidism. *J Clin Endocrinol Metab* 1995; **80**: 276–279.

104 Pringle PJ, Stanhope R, Hindmarsh PC, Brook CGD. Abnormal pubertal development in primary hypothyroidism. *Clin Endocrinol* 1988; **28**: 479–486.

105 Adams DM, Young PC, Copeland KC. Pubic hair in infancy. *Am J Dis Child* 1992; **146**: 149–151.

106 Ibanez L, Potau N, Francois I, de Zegher F. Precocious pubarche, hyperinsulinism, and ovarian hyperandrogenism in girls: relation to reduced fetal growth. *J Clin Endocrinol Metab* 1998; **83**: 3558–3562.

107 Balducci R, Boscherini B, Mangiantini A, Morellini M, Toscano V. Isolated precocious pubarche: an approach. *J Clin Endocrinol Metab* 1994; **79**: 582–589.

108 Ibanez L, Potau N, Virdis R, Zampolli M, Terzi C, Gussinye M, *et al*. Postpubertal outcome in girls diagnosed of premature pubarche during childhood: increased frequency of functional ovarian hyperandrogenism. *J Clin Endocrinol Metab* 1993; **76**: 1599–1603.

109 Ehrhardt AA, Meyer-Bahlburg HFL. Psychosocial aspects of precocious puberty. *Horm Res* 1994; **4** (Suppl 2): 30–35.

110 Grunt JA, Midyett K, Simon SD, Lowe L. When should cranial magnetic resonance imaging be used in girls with early sexual development? *J Pediatr Endocrinol Metab* 2004; **17**: 775–780.

111 Chalumeau M, Chemaitilly W, Trivin C, Adan L, Breart G, Brauner R. Central precocious puberty in girls: an evidence-based diagnosis tree to predict central nervous system abnormalities. *Pediatrics* 2002; **109**: 61–67.

112 Chemaitilly W, Trivin C, Adan L, Gall V, Sainte-Rose C, Brauner R. Central precocious puberty: clinical and laboratory features. *Clin Endocrinol* 2002; **54**: 289–294.

113 Donaldson M. Commentary. *Arch Dis Child* 2003; **88**: 417–418.

114 Ng SM, Kumar Y, Cody D, Smth C, Didi M. Cranial MRI scans are indicated in all girls with central precocious puberty. *Arch Dis Child* 2003; **88**: 414–417.

115 Brauner R. Central precocious puberty in girls: prediction of the aetiology. *J Pediatr Endocrinol Metab* 2005; **18**: 845–847.

116 Honour JW, Price DA, Taylor NF, Marsden HB, Grant DB. Steroid biochemistry of virilising adrenal tumours in childhood. *Eur J Pediatr* 1984; **142**: 165–169.

117 Lanes R, Gunczler P, Osuna JA. Effectiveness and limitations of the use of the gonadotropin-releasing hormone agonist leuprolide acetate in the diagnosis od delayed puberty in males. *Horm Res* 1997; **48**: 1–4.

118 Ghai K, Cara KF, Rosenfield RL. Gonadotropin releasing hormone agonist (nafarelin) test to differentiate gonadotropin deficiency from constitutionally delayed puberty in teen-age boys: a clinical research center study. *J Clin Endocrinol Metab* 1995; **80**: 2980–2986.

119 Wehkalampi K, Widen E, Laine T, Palotie A, Dunkel L. Patterns of inheritance of constitutional delay of growth and puberty in families of adolescent girls and boys referred to a specialist clinic. *J Clin Endocrinol Metab* 2008; **93**: 723–728.

120 Raivio T, Falardeau J, Dwyer A, *et al*. Reversal of hypogonadotropic hypogonadism. *N Engl J Med* 2007; **357**: 863–873.

121 Dattani MT, Robinson ICAF. The molecular basis for developmental disorders of the pituitary gland in man. *Clin Genet* 2000; **57**: 337–346.

122 Rugliari EI, Ballabio A. Kallman syndrome: from genetics to neurobiology. *JAMA* 1993; **270**: 2713–2716.

123 Reutens AT, Achermann JC, Ito M, Gu WX, Habiby RL, Donohoue PA, *et al*. Clinical and functional effects of mutations in the DAX-1 gene in patients with adrenal hypoplasia congenita. *J Clin Endocrinol Metab* 1999; **84**: 504–511.

124 Hernandez Martin A, Gonzalez Sarmiento R, De-Unamuno P. X-linked ichthyosis: an update. *Br J Dermatol* 1999; **141**: 617–627.

125 Pitteloud N, Quinton R, Pearce S, *et al*. Digenic mutations account for variable phenotypes in idiopathic hypogonadotropic hypogonadism. *J Clin Invest* 2007; **117**: 457–463.

126 Legouis R, Hardelin JP, Levilliers J, *et al*. The candidate gene for the X-linked Kallmann syndrome encodes a protein related to adhesion molecules. *Cell* 1991; **67**: 423–435.

127 Dodé C, Levilliers J, Dupont JM, *et al.* Loss-of-function mutations in FGFR1 cause autosomal dominant Kallmann syndrome. *Nat Genet* 2003; **33**: 463–465.

128 Albuisson J, Pêcheux C, Carel JC, *et al.* Kallmann syndrome: 14 novel mutations in KAL1 and FGFR1 (KAL2). *Hum Mutat* 2005; **25**: 98–99.

129 Trarbach EB, Silveira LG, Latronico AC. Genetic insights into human isolated gonadotropin deficiency. *Pituitary* 2007; **10**: 381–391.

130 Salenave S, Chanson P, Bry H, *et al.* Kallman's syndrome: a comparison of the reproductive phenotypes in men carrying KAL1 and FGFR1/KAL2 mutations. *J Clin Endocrinol Metab* 2008; **93**: 758–763.

131 Dodé C, Teixeira L, Levilliers J, *et al.* Kallmann syndrome: mutations in the genes encoding prokineticin-2 and prokineticin receptor-2. *PLoS Genet* 2006; **2**: e175. Epub 2.

132 Pitteloud N, Zhang C, Pignatelli D, *et al.* Loss-of-function mutation in the prokineticin 2 gene causes Kallmann syndrome and normosmic idiopathic hypogonadotropic hypogonadism. *Proc Natl Acad Sci U S A* 2007; **104**: 17447–17452.

133 Prosser HM, Bradley A, Caldwell MA. Olfactory bulb hypoplasia in Prokr2 null mice stems from defective neuronal progenitor migration and differentiation. *Eur J Neurosci* 2007; **26**: 3339–3344.

134 Lin L, Conway GS, Hill NR, Dattani MT, Hindmarsh PC, Achermann JC. A homozygous R262Q mutation in the gonadotropin-releasing hormone receptor presenting as constitutional delay of growth and puberty with subsequent borderline oligospermia. *J Clin Endocrinol Metab* 2006; **91**: 5117–5121.

135 Beranova M, Oliveira LM, Bédécarrats GY, *et al.* Prevalence, phenotypic spectrum, and modes of inheritance of gonadotropin-releasing hormone receptor mutations in idiopathic hypogonadotropic hypogonadism. *J Clin Endocrinol Metab* 2001; **86**: 1580–1588.

136 Achermann JC, Weiss J, Lee EJ, Jameson JL. Inherited disorders of the gonadotropin hormones. *Mol Cell Endocrinol* 2001; **179**: 89–96.

137 Kotani M, Detheux M, Vandenbogaerde A, *et al.* The metastasis suppressor gene KiSS-1 encodes kisspeptins, the natural ligands of the orphan G protein-coupled receptor GPR54. *J Biol Chem* 2001; **276**: 34631–34636.

138 Kramer PR, Wray S. Novel gene expressed in nasal region influences outgrowth of olfactory axons and migration of luteinizing hormone-releasing hormone (LHRH) neurons. *Genes Dev* 2000; **14**: 1824–1834.

139 Miura K, Acierno JS Jr, Seminara SB. Characterization of the human nasal embryonic LHRH factor gene, NELF, and a mutation screening among 65 patients with idiopathic hypogonadotropic hypogonadism (IHH). *J Hum Genet* 2004; **49**: 265–268.

140 Chung RT, Misdraji J, Sahani DV. Case 33-2006. A 43-year-old man with diabetes, hypogonadism, cirrhosis, arthralgias and fatigue. *N Engl J Med* 2006; **355**: 1812–1819.

141 Oerter KE, Kamp GA, Munson PJ, Nienhaus AW, Cassorla FG, Manasco PK. Multiple hormone deficiencies in children with hemochromatosis. *J Clin Endocrinol Metab* 1993; **76**: 357–361.

142 Dunkel L, Perheentupa J, Virtanen M, Maenpaa J. Gonadotropin-releasing hormone test and human chorionic gonadotropin test in the diagnosis of gonadotropin deficiency in prepubertal boys. *J Pediatr* 1985; **107**: 388–392.

143 Bouloux PM, Handelsman DJ, Jockenhovel F, Nieschlag E, Rabinovici J, Frasa WL, *et al.* First human exposure to FSH-CTP in hypogonadotrophic hypogonadal males. *Hum Reprod* 2001; **16**: 1592–1597.

144 Smals AG, Hermus AR, Boers GH, Pieters GF, Benraad TJ, Kloppenborg PW. Predictive value of luteinizing hormone releasing hormone (LHRH) bolus testing before and after 36-hour pulsatile LHRH administration in the differential diagnosis of constitutional delay of puberty and male hypogonadotropic hypogonadism. *J Clin Endocrinol Metab* 1994; **78**: 602–608.

145 Bakker B, Massa GG, Oostdijk W, Van Weel-Sipman MH, Vossen JM, Wit JM. Pubertal development and growth after total-body irradiation and bone marrow transplantation for hematological malignancies. *Eur J Pediatr* 2000; **159**: 31–37.

146 Hoek A, Schoemaker J, Drexhage HA. Premature ovarian failure and ovarian autoimmunity. *Endocr Rev* 1997; **18**: 107–134.

147 Fraser IS, Russell P, Greco S, Robertson DM. Resistant ovary syndrome and premature ovarian failure in young women with galactosaemia. *Clin Reprod Fertil* 1986; **4**: 133–138.

148 Brook CGD, Gasser T, Werder EA, Prader A, Vanderschueren-Lodewykx MA. Height correlations between parents and mature offspring in normal subjects and in subjects with Turner's and Klinefelter's and other syndromes. *Ann Hum Biol* 1977; **4**: 17–22.

149 Smyth CM, Bremner WJ. Klinefelter syndrome. *Arch Intern Med* 1998; **158**: 1309–1314.

11 Management of Disordered Puberty

Jakub Mieszczak[1], Christopher P. Houk[2] & Peter A. Lee[1,3]

[1] Indiana University School of Medicine, The Riley Hospital for Children, Indianapolis, IN, USA
[2] Medical College of Georgia, Augusta, GA, USA
[3] Penn State College of Medicine, The Milton S. Hershey Medical Center, Hershey, PA, USA

Management of disordered puberty includes any variant of normal pubertal development (Table 11.1).

Precocious puberty

Precocious puberty is categorized as **central**, which is physiologically the same as normal puberty with early activation of the hypothalamo-pituitary-gonadal (HPG) axis and **peripheral**, in which the sex steroid stimulation of development has a source other than the HPG axis.

Central precocious puberty

Precocious puberty is the onset of secondary sexual development before the normal age range [1]. The early activation of the HPG axis characteristic of central precocious puberty (CPP) results in gonadotropin-mediated gonadal activation leading to development of secondary sexual characteristics. Therapy, which involves interference with the episodic stimulation of the pituitary by gonadotropin-releasing hormone (GnRH) by continuously elevating concentrations of GnRH analog (GnRHa), should be considered after CPP has been differentiated from peripheral precocious puberty. Before deciding if treatment is warranted, distinction must be made between early progressive, non-progressive and normal puberty because the latter entities do not warrant treatment [2]. Pelvic ultrasound, including ovarian and uterine size, may be used as an aid in differentiating CPP.

General considerations of treatment

Once the most compelling clinical criterion for verifying CPP [premature breast development in girls (Fig. 11.1) and increase of testicular size in boys (Fig. 11.2)] is documented, it must be considered that not every child diagnosed requires treatment but only those with evidence of progression. GnRHa therapy should

prevent unwanted consequences of CPP, which include progression of physical changes, menstruation, the psychological impact of being physically more developed and taller than peers during childhood and diminished adult height. One factor in deciding whether or not to treat is to prevent loss of growth potential or to attempt to reclaim lost growth potential as indicated by a skeletal age which is excessive in relation to height [3]. Even though psychosexual development is generally consistent with age rather than physical maturity among children with precocious puberty, withdrawal behavior, anxiety, depression and somatic complaints may occur. Hence, therapy to preclude or ameliorate psychological problems is rarely the primary indication for therapy although enabling the child to experience pubertal changes at a similar age to peers is often a major consideration.

GnRHa therapy should therefore be considered when the natural history is leading to undesired consequences. Among families with a history of precocious puberty and normal adult height, as well as those with slowly progressive puberty, GnRHa therapy is generally not indicated.

Criteria for the diagnosis of progressive CPP and treatment include:

1 Documentation of pubertal gonadotropin secretion, either with basal concentrations above the prepubertal range using a third generation assay or a pubertal response to GnRH or GnRHa stimulation testing;
2 Documented acceleration of growth velocity;
3 An accelerating rate of skeletal age maturity or significantly advanced skeletal age;
4 Progression of early pubertal development; and
5 A need expressed by the parents or child to halt and delay further pubertal development. Parents need to comprehend what is being proposed and why and what treatment involves.

GnRHa is the only effective therapy for progressive CPP [4]. A decision not to treat may be reached if the child and parents agree that the extent of early puberty does not merit interruption. If height, growth rate and skeletal maturity all indicate that target height is likely to be realized without therapy, therapy is not

Brook's Clinical Pediatric Endocrinology, 6th edition. Edited by C. Brook, P. Clayton, R. Brown. © 2009 Blackwell Publishing, ISBN: 978-1-4051-8080-1.

Table 11.1 Forms of disordered puberty for treatment consideration.

1 Precocious and early puberty

(a) Central (GnRH-dependent) precocious puberty

    (i)   Early maturation of the HP axis, formerly called "true precocious puberty"

    (ii) Progressive precocious puberty, which may be idiopathic, the consequence of CNS abnormality, secondary to chronic exposure to sex steroids and may be reversible if increased intracranial pressure is relieved

(b) Peripheral (GnRH-independent) precocious puberty

    (i)   Resulting from hormonal stimulation from other than the HP axis, formerly called "precocious pseudopuberty"

    (ii) Numerous etiologies include genetic mutations such as LH-receptor-activating mutations, McCune–Albright syndrome and steroid producing tumors

    (iii) Partial forms are associated with primary hypothyroidism, exogenous hormones and autonomous functional ovarian cysts

(c) Partial forms of precocious puberty

    (i)   Premature thelarche – may progress to CPP

    (ii) Premature pubarche, commonly a consequence of premature adrenarche (peripubertal increased adrenal androgen secretion)

2 Delay or lack of pubertal development

(a) May occur with the potential for normal puberty

    (i)   Constitutional delay – may be treated temporarily

    (ii) Chronic systemic illness, other endocrinopathies, drug abuse, excessive energy expenditure, associated with malnutrition and psychiatric illness:
       therapy aimed at correction of underlying problem
       response to sex steroid therapy may be limited unless underlying condition under control

(b) Permanent defect with gonadal failure – hypergonadotropism

    (i)   May be associated with numerous syndromes and genetic mutations or acquired

    (ii) Sex steroid therapy to stimulate physical pubertal development:
       titered doses to mimic gradual rise with puberty to full replacement doses

    (iii) Fertility generally not possible except among those with viable germ cells that may be retrieved using assisted fertility techniques:
       Females with uterine development may carry pregnancy using donated ova. Attempts should fully consider risks, such as cardiovascular risks in Turner syndrome

(c) Hypogonadotropic hypogonadism

    (i)   Associated with hypothalamic and pituitary disorders and syndromes

    (ii) Physical puberty development can be stimulated with:
       sex steroids, gradually increasing doses to full adult replacement
       GnRH intermittent therapy or gonadotropin therapy can stimulate gonadal sex steroid response among those with adequate gonadal potential

    (iii) Fertility may be possible, such therapy limited to point of desired parenthood:
       among males with long-term gonadotropin stimulation of sperm maturation among those with adequate spermatogonia
       among females, with ovulation induction therapy

3 Inappropriate development for sex of individual

(a) Formerly called heterosexual pubertal development

(b) May occur early, at normal pubertal age, or late

(c) Among males, primary manifestation is gynecomastia

    (i)   Underlying abnormality, including hypogonadism, drugs, systemic illness, must be ruled out

    (ii) If therapy required, definitive therapy is surgical

    (iii) Pharmacologic therapy partially effective

(d) Among females, hyperandrogenism

    (i)   May manifest with acne, hirsutism, lack of menses, clitoromegaly

    (ii) Consequence of excessive ovarian or adrenal androgens

    (iii) Adrenal causes including CAH treated with glucocorticoid suppression and tumors treated with surgical resection if possible

    (iv) Ovarian hyperandrogen – PCOS treated with estrogen–progesterone suppression; rare causes: teratoma, arrhenoblastoma

CAH, congenital adrenal hyperplasia; CPP, central precocious puberty; GnRH, gonadotropin releasing hormone; HP, hypothalamic-pituitary; LH, luteinizing hormone; PCOS, polycystic ovarian syndrome.

indicated. A height prediction >155 cm in girls is evidence of a slowly progressing form of early puberty with preservation of adult height [5]. Such patients grow normally and progress slowly through puberty with early menarche.

When CPP results from a CNS abnormality that will be treated but, in most instances, the disruption of the inhibitory influences upon the hypothalamus resulting in pubertal hormone secretion is not reversible. Among those who have CPP as a consequence of successful treatment of malignancies, particularly leukemia, management involves monitoring patients for tumor recurrence, for the increased risk of developing concomitant growth hormone deficiency and subsequent gonadal failure.

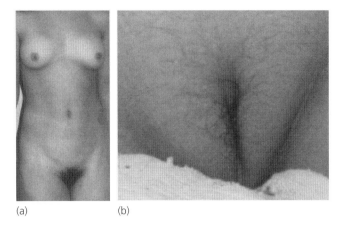

Figure 11.1 Early pubertal changes in girls: (a) 6-year-old with central precocious puberty; (b) 5-year-old female with premature pubarche.

(a)   (b)

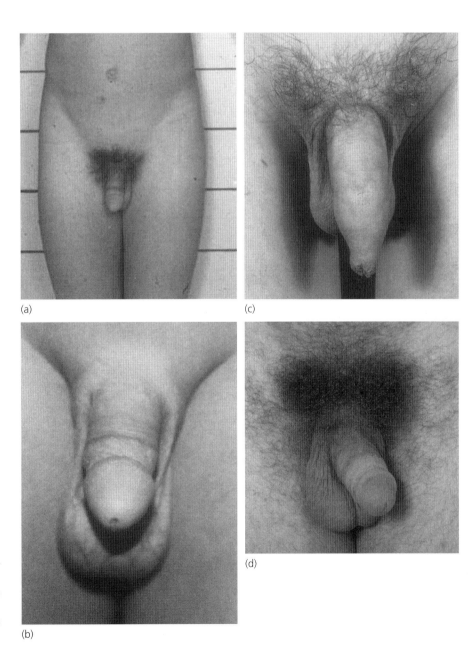

(a)   (c)

(b)   (d)

Figure 11.2 Precocious puberty in males: (a) 7-year-old with central precocious puberty; (b) 3-year-old with activating LH-receptor mutation (male-limited gonadotropin independent precocious puberty); (c) 6-year-old with 21-hydroxylase congenital adrenal hyperplasia; (d) 11-year-old with Leydig cell tumor.

GnRHa options

There are several synthetic decapeptides with amino acid substitutions of GnRH available for therapy. Different analogs have different efficacy and hence different regimens. Rapid acting formulations are listed in Table 11.2 and depots in Table 11.3. Depot formulations are generally preferred because they provide sustained suppression with decreased frequency of administration providing more assurance of compliance. Formulations used in CPP include injectable leuprolide depot and triptorelin, effective when administered subcutaneously or intramuscularly and implantable histrelin. The implant is effective for at least a year [6], while depot injections can be used at 4 or 12-week intervals.

While depot injections of leuprolide acetate are only approved for every 28 days by the Food and Drug Administration (FDA) in the USA, studies have been reported for 3-month formulations. The subcutaneous implantation of histrelin acetate may be effective for several years and a single placement will potentially be adequate for the entire therapeutic course [7]. Short-acting daily subcutaneous injections of aqueous leuprolide acetate are effective when given in adequate doses and the nasal spray is effective when applied twice daily.

Table 11.2 Rapid acting formulations of gonadotropin releasing hormone analog (GnRHa).

Administration	GnRHa	Starting dose
Subcutaneous	Leuprolide acetate	50 µg/kg/day
	Buserelin	1200–1800 µg/day
	Histrelin	8–10 µg/kg/day
	Deslorelin	4–8 µg/kg/day
	Triptorelin	20–40 µg/kg/day
Nasal spray	Nafarelin acetate	1600 µg/day
	Buserelin	20–40 µg/kg/day

Table 11.3 Depot gonadotropin releasing hormone analog (GnRHa) formulations [4,49,50].

Depot preps	Brand name	Starting dose
Goserelin	Zoladex LA	3.6 mg every months or 10.8 mg every 3 months
Buserelin	Superfact depot	6.3 mg every 2 months
Leuprolide	Enantone or Lupron-depot	3.75 mg every months or 11.25 mg every 3 months
	Prostap SR	4–8 µg/kg/day
	Lupron-depotPed	7.5 mg (0.2–0.3 mg/kg/months) or 11.25 mg every 3 months
Triptorelin	Decapeptyl, Gonapeptyl	3 or 3.75 mg every months or 11.25 every 3 months
Histrelin	Supprelin LA	50 mg implant every year

GnRHa regimen

There is no consensus concerning the degree of gonadotropin suppression for the best treatment of CPP. It can be argued that suppression of gonadotropins into the normal range of childhood rather than into the hypogonadotric range is more physiologic and beneficial. Such benefit may induce a prepubertal growth rate while not creating a hypogonadotropic status which may impact the gonad and other systems in the prepubertal child, especially growth hormone secretion, but it is very difficult to monitor therapy to attain such an endpoint.

Further, because of the stimulatory property of GnRHa, unless there is constant downregulation, inadequate doses may be accompanied by intermittent stimulation of gonadotropin release. Thus, most patients are markedly suppressed, particularly those with an implant, so they do not risk inadequate therapy. Full suppression of gonadotropin secretion is the best method of verifying that intermittent stimulation will not occur and requires less frequent monitoring. Gonadotropin secretion is then below that characteristic of prepubertal status.

As noted in Table 11.3, recommended doses for the depot form of leuprolide differ and products are packaged differently in different countries: depot Lupron is supplied for pediatric use in quantities of 7.5, 11.25 or 15 mg in the USA, 1.88 and 3.75 mg in Japan and 3.75 mg in Europe. Recommended doses in the USA are weight-based: 7.5 mg designed for those weighing <25 kg, 11.25 mg for those weighing more up to 37.5 kg and 15.0 mg being the recommended doses for those >50 kg. Rarely is there evidence of lack of suppression using the US recommended doses.

In Japan, the initial dose recommended is 30 µg/kg/4 weeks, increasing to 90 µg/kg/4 weeks to achieve suppression because many patients are not suppressed on the lowest doses. It is likely that the US doses are excessive while doses in Japan and Europe are adequate for a significant proportion of patients. While there may be racial and/or ethnic differences, it is likely that ideal doses are somewhere between these recommendations. Higher doses in the USA continue to be used partly because suppression is virtually assured and partly because much less monitoring is necessary at a time of limited medical resources. There appears to be no increased risk with excessive doses. When doses are increased, it is common to increase the frequency of administration, for example to 3 weeks rather than 4. Limited experience suggests that 3-month dosing intervals are effective.

It is possible that an initially larger dose is needed for suppression with lower doses required for maintenance. Switching patients to a 3-month formulation may be appropriate, reducing the number of injections and the intensity of medical care. Triptorelin 11.25 mg depot injection 3-monthly is adequate to suppress the pituitary-gonadal axes in most children with CPP [8] and give results comparable to monthly triptorelin depot injections [9]. Long-acting goserelin 10.8 mg depot injections at 3-month intervals showed adequate gonadotropin suppression in a majority of patients, although a subset of study patients had less inhibition before 3 months [10].

A direct comparison of three depot leuprolide doses (7.5 mg monthly, 3.75 mg monthly and 11.25 mg every 3 months) found significantly higher stimulated gonadotropin concentrations among those treated with 3.75 mg monthly or 11.25 mg every 3 months [11], while changes in gonadotropin concentrations did not correlate with those in sex steroid measurements or pubertal progression. Even though the use of every 3-month dosing of GnRHa is increasing, further dosing studies are needed.

For effective therapy, suppression of the HPG axis should occur within 2 weeks. Implantation of a 50-mg histrelin acetate implant designed to deliver 65 µg/day is followed by such suppression. Suppression was found to be greater among patients previously suppressed with depot leuprolide [6]. With this preparation, therapy involves complete suppression and using lower doses is not possible.

Monitoring GnRHa therapy

Individual monitoring of the efficacy of GnRHa is needed to ensure that goals of therapy are being met and to exclude incomplete suppression of the HPG axis, which can exacerbate CPP by intermittent stimulation of luteinizing hormone (LH) and follicle stimulating hormone (FSH) release. The initial indicator of adequacy of suppression is basal or stimulated LH concentrations, together with use of sensitive steroid assays for estradiol in girls or testosterone in boys, if available.

When suppression based on basal LH concentrations below the pubertal range using a third generation assay with defined standards occurs, GnRH or GnRHa stimulation testing is not necessary. Measurement of FSH is unnecessary because measurement of LH is more reliable. GnRH stimulation with concentrations of LH at 20 and 40 min below the pubertal response ranges is indicative of suppression. Although the peak response occurs later, subcutaneous GnRHa at a standard doses (20 µg/kg) produces a significantly lower 30-min response in the suppressed than the pubertal or non-suppressed patient. Suppression can be monitored among those receiving leuprolide acetate IM therapy by measuring LH concentration at 30–60 min after receiving their therapeutic dose [12].

Estradiol measurements in girls are generally unnecessary to verify suppression and basal concentrations are less helpful because of limits of most available assays but concentrations 24 h after GnRH or GnRHa stimulation can be used to demonstrate suppression. Basal testosterone concentrations in boys verify suppression without gonadotropin concentrations when below the usual limits of detection (<15 ng/dL). When higher concentrations are found, estimation of adrenal androgens using dehydroepiandrosterone sulfate (DHEAS) may be helpful.

Long-term suppression can be verified clinically by lack of progression or regression of physical sexual characteristics. Monitoring at 4 or 6-monthly intervals includes history of changes, including vaginal bleeding in girls and observed morning erections in boys; height, weight, growth velocity, body mass index (BMI), Tanner stages and testicular volumes, which may be static or regress, are also recorded. Sexual hair development, and hence

Tanner pubic hair staging, may advance slowly from increasing adrenal androgen secretion. This can be verified by the value or relative increase of DHEAS concentrations and the profile of androstenedione and testosterone.

Skeletal maturity is monitored after 6 months of therapy and thereafter annually. Deceleration, which may not be apparent at 6 months, should occur thereafter. Skeletal age should progress at an annual rate of 12 months per year until skeletal age associated with puberty is attained (approximately 10.5–11 years for females and 12.5 for boys). After this concentration of maturity, advancement should be very slow in the absence of sex steroids. Whenever skeletal age is checked, projected adult height can be determined to track changes with therapy. For the patient started on treatment before growth potential was lost, expected adult height should be within the target height range. For the child with loss of growth potential due to skeletal age being advanced beyond concomitant height, therapy should result in gradual increase in growth potential.

Changes in weight and body composition are not helpful in monitoring adequacy of therapy, although there is a shift in body composition toward relatively less lean body mass and more fat tissue during therapy, as is characteristic of childhood and expected as a consequence of decreasing the sex steroid concentrations. Children with precocious puberty typically have increased weight for age, related to sex steroid effects causing an increase in lean body mass. Approximately 25% of girls have increased BMI at presentation with early puberty, although the relative relationship to early puberty or the current increased incidence of childhood obesity is unclear. During and after therapy, mean BMI does not further increase and usually decreases into the normal range [13,14].

Growth rate should decelerate to an average childhood rate if bone age is prepubertal. Rate of skeletal maturity with suppression slows to that expected with removal of the sex steroid stimulus. If the skeletal age is pubertal, growth rate continues to slow to <5 cm/year. Among those with advanced skeletal age approaching epiphyseal fusion, growth rates become very slow.

Discontinuation of therapy

The decision to discontinue therapy should include consideration of chronologic age, skeletal age, height, growth rate, psychological profile and the patient's and family's desires. This decision should be individualized. Discontinuation should be discussed when the age of puberty has been reached, when data suggest that adult height will be normal or when growth rate is so slow that potential for further growth is limited. If emotional maturity or attained height is an issue, discontinuation can be earlier or later.

Long-term outcome of GnRHa therapy

Long-term experience has shown GnRHa to be effective and safe. The available data suggest that gonadal function in both sexes treated with GnRHa is not different after cessation of therapy and completion of puberty than the general population [15,16]. Suggestions of increased BMI as a consequence of GnRHa therapy have not been substantiated in a population in which obesity is prevalent [14]. Bone mineral density during GnRHa treatment may be slowed but bone mass accumulation after cessation of therapy occurs similar to peers, indicating that GnRHa therapy at this age results in no overall negative effect [17,18]. Available evidence suggests that adults who were treated with GnRHa for CPP have normal fertility [19].

Peripheral precocious puberty

Treatment of peripheral precocious puberty (PPP), the consequence of sex steroid stimulation from causes other than early activation of the HPG axis, is considerably more challenging than treatment of CPP: there is no clearly effective treatment. GnRHa are ineffective but, as a consequence of continued exposure to progression, PPP may lead to activation of the HPG axis resulting in CPP. When this occurs, GnRHa should be considered.

If PPP is a consequence of a treatable underlying defect, therapy initially involves treatment of that defect. Examples include resection of tumors, such as Leydig cell tumors of the testes, and glucocorticoid treatment of congenital adrenal hyperplasia (CAH). Androgen excess in untreated or inadequately treated classic or non-classic CAH in males and females resulting in PPP should be treated to enhance fertility, maximize growth potential and, among females, avoid secondary ovarian hyperandrogenism. Although efficacy has not been verified, growth hormone or aromatase inhibitors (AIs) are being used to stimulate linear growth. If secondary CPP has occurred, GnRHa therapy is indicated.

A variant of early puberty that can be included as a form of PPP is primary hypothyroidism associated with pubertal changes, breast development in girls and testicular enlargement in boys. Treatment with thyroxine alone is sufficient to reverse pubertal changes. The pituitary thyrotrope hyperplasia presenting with increased sellar volume will regress and requires no specific therapy.

Functional ovarian cysts may stimulate breast development and, after fluctuating concentrations, withdrawal vaginal bleeding. The cysts should be identified and followed using ultrasound. Because spontaneous regression is expected within weeks, no other therapy is indicated unless surgical intervention is needed because the cyst is so large that torsion or rupture may occur.

McCune–Albright syndrome

McCune–Albright syndrome (MAS) is a consequence of an activating mutation in exon 8 of the gene encoding $G_s\alpha$ (*GNAS*), at the codon for Arg^{201}. Constitutive ligand-free activation of affected cells in the ovary results in fluctuating autonomous estradiol secretion [20]. Endocrinopathies are just one part of the syndrome, most frequently precocious puberty, and, together with fibrous dysplasia of the bone and café-au-lait skin pigmentation, form the classic triad (Plate 11.1) [21]. Treatment involves blocking the estrogen effect to ameliorate pubertal progression and slow skeletal maturation to preserve adult stature.

Treatment in girls

Most treatments of MAS are only partially effective. Medroxyprogesterone has most frequently been used: it stopped vaginal bleeding but had no effect on skeletal maturation [22] and bone lesions. Ketoconazole, a P450 cytochrome inhibitor may decrease estrogen effect [23] but decreased cortisol production or caused hepatotoxicity [24].

AI, compounds that attach to the cytochrome P450 portion of the aromatase enzyme and prevent conversion of androgens to estrogens reducing the serum concentrations of estrogens, are being tried. A first generation AI, testolactone, trial suggested positive results [25] but a larger trial among girls did not consistently show cessation of vaginal bleeding, delay skeletal maturation or improve growth parameters [26]. A second generation AI, fadrozole, was ineffective and caused adrenal suppression [27]. A potent third generation AI, letrozole, slowed skeletal maturation but ovarian volumes increased [28]. Another third generation AI, anastrozole, failed to halt vaginal bleeding or slow skeletal maturation rates [29].

The selective estrogen receptor modulator, tamoxifen, stops pubertal progression [30] but is associated with unexplained uterine volume increase [31]. A pure estrogen receptor antagonist, fulvestrant, is currently being investigated for efficacy. Hence, there is presently no effective and safe treatment for PPP in girls with MAS.

Laparoscopic cystectomy is temporarily effective [32] but should be reserved for extreme cases of significant abdominal pain or risk of ovarian torsion. Surgical removal of the affected ovary is not a treatment option because fertility is possible and recurrence of hyperfunctioning cysts in the contralateral ovary is common [33]. As with other forms of PPP, progression to secondary CPP occurs. After this HPG activation, addition of GnRHa is beneficial [34].

Treatment in boys

MAS is less frequent in boys than in girls and tends to present at an older age, usually with enlarged testes and pubertal testosterone concentrations [35]. Current treatment options aim to slow precocious puberty and preserve adult stature and include combinations of AIs and an antiandrogen; testolactone and spironolactone effectively decreased skeletal maturation rates, thereby increasing adult height predictions [36].

Familial male-limited precocious puberty

Previously called testotoxicosis, familial male-limited precocious puberty (FMPP) results from an activating mutation of the LH receptor in males stimulating increased serum testosterone concentrations independently of gonadotropin secretion. This form of PPP may become manifest by 2 years of age (Fig. 11.2b). Therapy may impact the condition but none is completely effective. Ketoconazole, AIs such as testolactone, and spironolactone have been used together with GnRHa when secondary CPP occurs [37,38]. Ketoconazole is frequently associated with decreased testosterone, partial regression and good growth. Initial dosage is often 200 mg/day with increases to total doses up to 800 mg without morbidity. Testosterone, cortisol and liver function tests should be monitored in the morning at intervals of at least every 6 months. Treatment with the non-steroidal antiandrogen, bicalutamide, and the third generation AI, anastrozole, decreased growth velocity and skeletal maturation [39].

Treatment of gonadal tumors

Pediatric gonadal tumors are rare. Ovarian tumors include dysgerminomas secreting chorionic gonadotropin and granulosa cell and lipoid cell tumors secreting estrogens or androgens. Tumors of the adrenal cortex, either adenoma or carcinoma, cause pubertal changes in girls reflecting the magnitude and duration of androgen or estrogen secretion. Among boys, autonomous androgen secretion may result from Leydig cell tumors or androgen-secreting adrenal tumors that may be associated with glucocorticoid excess. Activating mutations of the LH receptor may cause Leydig cell tumors [40]. Rarely, tumors may secrete inappropriate sex steroids for the sex of the child, causing feminization in boys or masculinization among girls. If such tumors are untreated for long periods of time, secondary CPP may occur for which GnRHa therapy is the treatment of choice. Surgical resection of tumors is the treatment of choice.

Chorionic gonadotropin-producing tumors in males originating in the testes or liver may be associated with precocious puberty, treatment being that indicated for the tumor.

Delayed puberty

Therapy for pubertal delay may be appropriate before it can be determined whether the delay is caused by temporary or permanent lack of function of the HPG axis. When an underlying cause of the delay is identified, the cause, such as systemic illness, excessive physical activity, limitation of nutrition intake or weight loss, should be treated. If resolution occurs, puberty usually follows. Sex steroid therapy may be used if the underlying condition cannot be effectively treated or if the patient is beyond the age of normal puberty.

While assessment can identify hypergonadotropic hypogonadism, differentiating constitutional delay of puberty (Fig. 11.3a) from hypogonadotropic hypogonadism is not possible until the patient is old enough to demonstrate permanent failure to secrete gonadotropins. Constitutional delay is more frequent in males than females [41], with the majority of boys with pubertal delay having this condition.

Therapy with sex steroids should begin if there are no signs of puberty by age 14 in boys and 13 in girls in order to induce physical pubertal changes, accelerate growth and improve bone mineral density in an age and gender-appropriate fashion. Initial doses should be low to avoid unwanted side effects (e.g. unpleasant dreams and unwanted erections in boys, nausea in girls and mood changes in both) and rapid skeletal maturation, with gradual

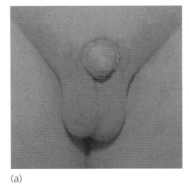 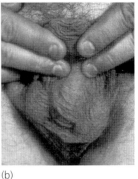

(a)   (b)

Figure 11.3 Males with delayed or incomplete pubertal development: (a) 14-year-old boy with delayed puberty; (b) 20-year-old with Klinefelter syndrome, small testes and scant pubic hair.

increases of doses as needed to stimulate pubertal maturation at a normal pace to eventual adult replacement.

Therapy should be interrupted at least twice a year to allow assessment of endogenous sex steroid and gonadotropin secretion. LH, FSH and estradiol or testosterone should be measured after exogenous hormones have been metabolized and endogenous secretion resumed, which may take 2 months off therapy, particularly if depot injections have been used. If pubertal concentrations of sex steroids and gonadotropins are found, this indicates the onset of puberty and excludes permanent hypogonadotropism. Therapy can be discontinued or, if concentrations are still low enough so that puberty does not progress (e.g. testosterone <275 ng/dL, <10 nmol/L), be continued for a further 4–6 months until another interruption. There is no evidence of detrimental effect on subsequent health or reproductive function after use of sex steroids to stimulate pubertal development.

Among patients with permanent hypogonadism, whether because of gonadotropin deficiency or gonadal failure (e.g. Klinefelter syndrome; Fig. 11.3b), it is important to use regimens adequate to maintain a eugonadal state for general and sexual health.

Males

Delay of puberty may be beneficial in a child who is neither emotionally nor socially ready for puberty or if short stature is greater than appropriate for the delay of skeletal age but, for the majority presenting with lack of development and testicular volume <4 mL by age 14, therapy is appropriate. When there are early signs of puberty indicating a high probability of constitutional delay, the patient should be given the choice of therapy or waiting for spontaneous development.

Testosterone preparations (Table 11.4) are designed to provide for adult testosterone replacement. Initial therapy to induce puberty commonly involves testosterone enanthate or cypionate 50 mg IM every 4 weeks. A dose of 25 mg may be appropriate if there is concern about lack of previous androgen exposure and 75 mg can be used if early changes are present and the patient is anxious for progression.

Table 11.4 Testosterone preparations.

Oral

Unmodified testosterone (rapidly metabolized)

17α-alkylated – hepatotoxic

Undecanoate – 17β-ester, variability in absorption, frequent dosing

Oxandrolone – non-aromatizible, too weak for replacement therapy

Transdermal

Scrotal patch – good absorption into tissue with high concentrations of 5α-reductase, daily application leads to stable concentrations of T, DHT & E_2

Skin patch – supplied in 2.5 and 5 g patches that deliver 12.2 and 24.3 mg testosterone; contains enhancers to skin passage, skin irritation for enhancer frequent

Gel packets and pumps – hydroalcoholic gel packets to deliver 25 and 50 mg from 2.5 and 5.0 g packets, each pump should deliver 12.5 mg, attains physiologic concentrations of T, DHT & E_2 into lower, middle and upper physiologic range

Injectable

Enanthate or cypionate

Indistinguishable from each other. Approximately 200–250 mg every 2 weeks leads to virtually physiologic concentrations of T with peaks slightly above the upper limit of normal and nadirs slightly below the lower limit of normal

DHT, dihydrotestosterone; E_2, estradiol; T, testosterone.

Pubertal changes with genital and sexual hair growth and an increase in linear growth rate should be monitored but because only gonadotropin, particularly FSH, stimulates testicular growth, an increase in volume is evidence of pubertal gonadotropin secretion.

If a second course of therapy is needed or when hypogonadism is permanent, the dosage can be increased by 25–50 mg at 6–12 month intervals over 2.5–4 years to the full adult replacement (equivalent of 100 mg/week). Administration at 4 or even 3 week intervals results in low circulating concentrations after 2 weeks after peak concentrations at day 3–9. Dosage can be increased by increasing the frequency of injections, rather than increasing the quantity. Intervals may be decreased to every 3 weeks and eventually to the appropriate interval for adult replacement (200 mg every 2 weeks or 100 mg/week). When adult dosage levels are reached, the preparation can be changed to the transdermal route.

Normal adult gonadotropin secretion may occur very late, even into the third decade of life. Patients diagnosed during childhood with panhypopituitarism and the rare patient with hypogonadotropic hypogonadism may acquire a eugonadal state after treatment with testosterone [42]. Such patients should be aware of the possibility of fertility. An increase in testicular volume during testosterone treatment merits a trial off therapy.

Gel and skin patches have been used to induce puberty but are not recommended because doses for induction of puberty have not been determined and preparations are designed to provide full adult replacement. Disadvantages of testosterone therapy include the need for injections which is why lower dose transdermal forms would be desirable. Side effects of excessive doses include priaprism and fluid retention manifest by weight gain and ankle swelling. The skin patch also contains absorption enhancers that may cause pruritus or erythema at the application site.

Therapy should be monitored at 4–6 month intervals. An increase in testicular volume is an indication of gonadotropin secretion. Measuring testosterone concentrations is unhelpful: adequacy of treatment can be judged only by physical examination. If the gel or patch were used, testosterone concentrations can be measured after 2–3 weeks of therapy and be used to guide dosage adjustment. Monitoring concentrations can be in morning if the gel or patch is applied at bedtime. Doses are gradually increased so that eventually adult circulating concentrations are attained.

If short stature is an issue because of diminished predicted adult height in relation to target height, aromatase inhibitors are being used concomitantly with testosterone with the goal of slowing skeletal maturation while allowing more time for linear growth [43]. Studies with measured adult heights may confirm the usefulness of AIs as adjunctive therapy [44]. Growth hormone has also been used for idiopathic short stature.

For the patient with known hypogonadotropic hypogonadism, human chorionic gonadotropin (hCG) can be used to stimulate testosterone production, thereby stimulating pubertal changes. With this therapy there is also increase in testicular volume, although there is no evidence that such therapy increases the likelihood of spermatogenesis over that attained with gonadotropin therapy later when fertility is desired. Because such therapy has to be administered at least every other day (at doses ranging 200–500 units), this modality is seldom used. It results in a disproportionate increase in estradiol production, which accelerates skeletal maturation and may cause gynecomastia.

When paternity is desired, gonadotropins can be given to stimulate spermatogenesis, beginning with hCG with later addition of human menopausal gonadotropin (hMG). Testes are more likely to function if their volume is >4 mL and in patients who do not have congenital hypogonadotropism. Because 3 months are required for maturity of sperm, many months of therapy are needed to attain a sperm density adequate for insemination. Assisted fertility can be used by taking sperm from the ejaculate; when oligospermia is present or if azoospermia persists after stimulation, germ cells can be taken from the testis without gonadotropin. Episodic delivery of GnRH stimulates pituitary gonadotropin secretion but this is time-consuming and complicated and should probably only be carried out as part of research studies.

Females

Therapy with estrogen causes development of pubertal physical characteristics and growth acceleration, all of which are monitored. In patients with Turner syndrome, height is a factor in determining the age of introduction of estrogen therapy, aiming for a balance between attaining greater height-for-age before the onset of therapy and growth stimulation that follows estrogen and growth hormone therapy. Estrogen therapy used to be delayed to improve adult height but early administration of physiologic doses of estrogen do not to have detrimental effects on adult heights in Turner girls simultaneously treated with growth hormone [45,46].

When the diagnosis of hypogonadism is known, therapy is begun between ages 10.5 and 12 years. Although constitutional delay of puberty is less common in girls, development is not considered to be delayed until 13 years of age. Therapy can be begun as soon as delay is documented. Causes of delay include chronic diseases (e.g. cystic fibrosis), anorexia nervosa and other disorders of nutrition and energy expenditure, including the adolescent triad of amenorrhea, osteoporosis and disordered eating characteristic of some girls who participate excessively in sports and fitness training. The underlying conditions must be treated, with those involving food intake and exercise expenditure requiring a multidisciplinary approach, before hormone replacement therapy is attempted. With resolution of the underlying condition, puberty may proceed spontaneously. Without amelioration of the underlying problem, therapy can be tried but there is often minimal response to treatment.

Hormone replacement therapies (Table 11.5) are designed for adults, with a lack of preparations appropriate for initiating pubertal change. Estradiol can be given orally or transdermally. Commonly available initial doses include 0.3 mg conjugated estrogens or 5 µg ethinyl estradiol orally every other day or transdermal estrogen at 12.5–25 µg/day or 25 µg twice weekly. The dosing equivalents of various estrogen preparations vary significantly: 0.1 mg transdermal 17β-estradiol equates to 2 mg oral 17β-estradiol, 20 µg oral ethinyl estradiol or 1.25 mg oral conjugated estrogen. Transdermal patches have been used overnight.

Beginning therapy with such dosage stimulates the proliferation of the endometrium. While the response varies, a progestagen should be added after a year of therapy, after substantial breast development or after breakthrough bleeding has occurred. At this point, estrogen and progesterone regimens can be given separately, adding progesterone for 10–12 days of each monthly cycle, or as combination estrogen-progesterone preparations. The latter (effectively oral contraception) should be used with forethought because of the psychological effects of giving such medication to patients who are destined to be infertile. Once withdrawal bleeding has been established, an option is to administer replacement therapy allowing withdrawal bleeding as infrequently as 3–4 times a year if the patient desires less frequent menses.

Doses are increased at 6–12 month intervals to attain full adult replacement by 3–4 years. While the dosage needed to attain and maintain adult normal bone mineral density is unknown, it would appear to be greater than that needed to maintain female sexual and physical characteristics, including appropriate withdrawal bleeding. Full replacement doses are generally considered to be 0.625 mg for conjugated estrogen and 20 µg for ethinyl

Table 11.5 Estrogen preparations.

Oral

Conjugated estrogens: supplied as 0.3, 0.45. 0.625, 0.9 or 1.25 mg tablets. 15 mg/day appears to be within range for pubertal induction, greater doses resulting in excessive skeletal age advance

Ethinyl estradiol: supplied as 10, 20 or 50 µg tablets

Estradiol tablets: supplied as 0.5, 1 or 2 mg micronized estradiol

Transdermal

Estradiol patches: supplied as 0.014, 0.025, 0.037.5, 0.050, 0.060, 0.075 or 0.100 mg/day patches

Alora®, Estraderm® & Vivelle-Dot® require 1 patch 2x per week; Climara®, Menostar® & generic require 1 patch per week

Estradiol gels

Divigel® supplied as 0.25, 0.50 or 1 g packets of 0.1% gel, 1 g of gel provides 1 mg estradiol

Estrasorb® supplied as 1.7 g packets, 3.48 g emulsion provides 0.05 mg estradiol

Oral combination therapy

Monthly preparations (monthly bleeding)

Low doses preparations can deliver as little as 0.020 mg/day estrogen with various available doses and variation of progestagens

Typical dosing preparations usually range 20–50 µg estrogen with various available doses and variations of progestagens

Ninety day preparations (infrequent bleeding)

Seasonale® & Seasonique® both deliver 0.030 mg ethinyl estradiol and 0.150 mg levonorgestrel per tablet for 84 days, followed by 7 inert tablets or 7 tablets with 0.010 mg ethinyl estradiol, respectively

Dermal combination therapy

Low dosing

Ortho Evra® delivers 0.020 mg estradiol and 0.150 mg norelgestromin per day; 1 patch per week

Typical dosing

Combipatch® delivers 0.050 mg estradiol and 0.140 or 0.250 mg norethindrone per day; 1 patch 2x week

Climara Pro® delivers 0.045 mg estradiol and 0.015 mg levonnorgestrol per day; 1 patch per week

Injectable

Estradiol

Cypionate: induction dose = 0.2 mg/month, adult dose = ~2.5 mg/month given as a monthly injection

Valerate: adult dose = 10–20 mg/month given as a monthly injection

estradiol, 5–10 mg medroxyprogesterone or 200–400 mg micronized progesterone.

While constitutional delay is more uncommon among females than males, ovulatory cycles may not become manifest until late in the teenage years. Hence, discontinuing therapy for intervals up to 4 months should be considered unless a diagnosis of hypogonadism is clear. Hormonal assessment or spontaneous menses may verify normal ovarian function.

Among patients with hyper- or hypogonadotropic hypogonadism and a developed uterus, fertility may be possible using donated ova. In those with ovarian follicles, stimulation with gonadotropins may lead to ovulation and fertility.

Treatment of other forms of disordered puberty

Girls with **premature thelarche** (Plate. 11.1b) require no interventional therapy, although the management must involve periodic assessment to assure there is not progression to CPP.

Premature pubarche resulting from premature adrenarche is usually benign unless it heralds the onset of a progressive androgen disorder, such as polycystic ovarian syndrome, CAH or an adrenal neoplasm. The screening test for adrenarche is the measurement of DHEAS to demonstrate concentrations in the early adrenarchal or early pubertal ranges. Management should involve periodic reassessment at 6-monthly intervals until it is verified that adrenal or gonadal androgen secretion is not excessive for stage of pubertal development. CAH should be excluded by measurement of 17-hydroxyprogesterone (17-OHP). To assess evidence of ovarian hyperandrogenism, LH, FSH, estradiol and testosterone can be monitored.

When **gynecomastia** is present in a pubertal male, evaluation should consider primary hypogonadism, systemic illness, recovery from malnutrition, interfering drugs and, rarely, estrogen-secreting tumors. When the gynecomastia is determined to be the variant of normal puberty but is significant in volume and has persisted without evidence of regression for more than 18 months, the definitive therapy is surgical resection using plastic surgery techniques with minimal scarring (Plate 11.2).

Pharmacologic therapy using agents that block estradiol action have been tried for pubertal gynecomastia but have not been shown to be effective [47]. A randomized double blind placebo-controlled study of 80 boys demonstrated no benefit using anastrozole, a third generation aromatase inhibitor, over placebo [48]. Future pharmacologic agents more effective at lowering estrogens in males might prove useful in treatment of gynecomastia.

Patients with Klinefelter syndrome or absent testes should be treated early with testosterone in order to prevent development or progression of gynaecomastia.

Acne may be a part of normal puberty or related to ovarian and/or adrenal androgen secretion. Most common is the development of **ovarian hyperandrogenism**, generally categorized as polycystic ovarian syndrome, which presents with hirsutism and oligomenorrhea or, less commonly, primary amenorrhea. Ovarian cysts may or may not be excessive in size and number. The relative roles of excessive LH secretion and hyperinsulinism are unclear. Treatment for ovarian hyperandrogenism usually involves suppression of the hypothalamic-pituitary-ovarian axis with combined estrogen and progesterone, sometimes, if hyperinsulinism is present, with an insulin sensitizer such as metformin.

References

1 Kaplowitz P. Pubertal development in girls: secular trends. *Curr Opin Obstet Gynecol* 2006; **18**: 487–491.

2 Palmert MR, Malin HV, Boepple PA. Unsustained or slowly progressive puberty in young girls: initial presentation and long-term follow-up of 20 untreated patients. *J Clin Endocrinol Metab* 1999; **84**: 415–423.

3 Klein KO. Precocious puberty: Who has it? Who should be treated? *J Clin Endocrinol Metab* 1999; **84**: 411–414.

4 Antoniazzi F, Zamboni G. Central precocious puberty: current treatment options. *Paediatr Drugs* 2004; **6**: 211–231.

5 Adan L, Chemaitilly W, Trivin C, Brauner R. Factors predicting adult height in girls with idiopathic central precocious puberty: implications for treatment. *Clin Endocrinol (Oxf)* 2002; **56**: 297–302.

6 Eugster EA, Clarke W, Kletter GB, Lee PA, Neely EK, Reiter EO, *et al*. Efficacy and safety of histrelin subdermal implant in children with central precocious puberty: a multicenter trial. *J Clin Endocrinol Metab* 2007; **92**: 1697–1704.

7 Hirsch HJ, Gillis D, Strich D, Chertin B, Farkas A, Lindenberg T, *et al*. The histrelin implant: a novel treatment for central precocious puberty. *Pediatrics* 2005; **116**: e798–802.

8 Carel JC, Blumberg J, Seymour C, Adamsbaum C, Lahlou N. Three-month sustained-release triptorelin (11.25 mg) in the treatment of central precocious puberty. *Eur J Endocrinol* 2006; **154**: 119–124.

9 Roger M, Chaussain JL, Berlier P, Bost M, Canlorbe P, Colle M, *et al*. Long-term treatment of male and female precocious puberty by periodic administration of a long-acting preparation of D-Trp6-luteinizing hormone-releasing hormone microcapsules. *J Clin Endocrinol Metab* 1986; **62**: 670–677.

10 Trueman JA, Tillmann V, Cusick CF, Foster P, Patel L, Hall CM, *et al*. Suppression of puberty with long-acting goserelin (Zoladex-LA): effect on gonadotrophin response to GnRH in the first treatment cycle. *Clin Endocrinol (Oxf)* 2002; **57**: 223–230.

11 Badaru A, Wilson DM, Bachrach LK, Fechner P, Gandrud LM, Durham E, *et al*. Sequential comparisons of one-month and three-month depot leuprolide regimens in central precocious puberty. *J Clin Endocrinol Metab* 2006; **91**: 1862–1867.

12 Bhatia S, Neely EK, Wilson DM. Serum luteinizing hormone rises within minutes after depot leuprolide injection: implications for monitoring therapy. *Pediatrics* 2002; **109**: E30.

13 Arrigo T, De Luca F, Antoniazzi F, Galluzzi F, Segni M, Rosano M, *et al*. Reduction of baseline body mass index under gonadotropin-suppressive therapy in girls with idiopathic precocious puberty. *Eur J Endocrinol* 2004; **150**: 533–537.

14 Palmert MR, Mansfield MJ, Crowley WF Jr, Crigler JF Jr, Crawford JD, Boepple PA. Is obesity an outcome of gonadotropin-releasing hormone agonist administration? Analysis of growth and body composition in 110 patients with central precocious puberty. *J Clin Endocrinol Metab* 1999; **84**: 4480–4488.

15 Tanaka T, Niimi H, Matsuo N, Fujieda K, Tachibana K, Ohyama K, *et al*. Results of long-term follow-up after treatment of central precocious puberty with leuprorelin acetate: evaluation of effectiveness of treatment and recovery of gonadal function. The TAP-144-SR Japanese Study Group on Central Precocious Puberty. *J Clin Endocrinol Metab* 2005; **90**: 1371–1376.

16 Antoniazzi F, Arrigo T, Cisternino M, Galluzzi F, Bertelloni S, Pasquino AM, *et al*. End results in central precocious puberty with GnRH analog treatment: the data of the Italian Study Group for Physiopathology of Puberty. *J Pediatr Endocrinol Metab* 2000; **13** (Suppl 1): 773–780.

17 Bertelloni S, Baroncelli GI, Sorrentino MC, Perri G, Saggese G. Effect of central precocious puberty and gonadotropin-releasing hormone

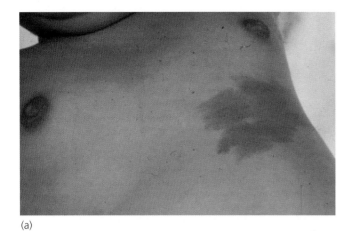

(a)

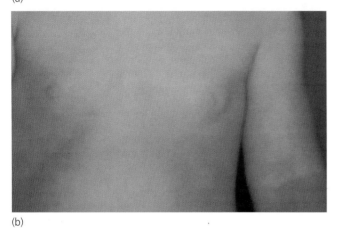

(b)

Plate 11.1 Early pubertal changes in girls: (a) 1-year-old with McCune–Albright syndrome with breast development and pigmented stimulated areolae and nipples and café-au-lait skin hyperpigmentation; (b) 1-year-old with premature thelarche.

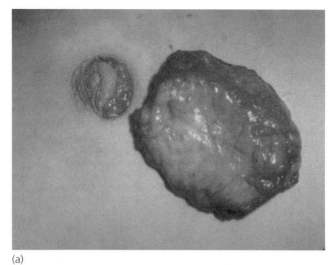

(a)

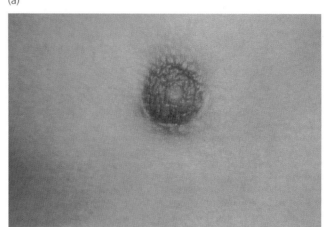

(b)

Plate 11.2 Surgical removal of gynecomastia in 15-year-old male: (a) breast tissue removed through a semicircular incision at the areolar–skin border; (b) postoperative hair-line scar barely visible.

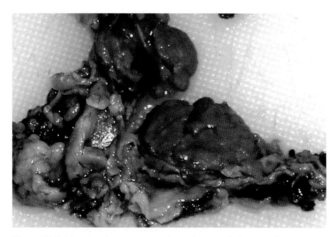

Plate 17.1 Macroscopic appearance of an adreno-cortical tumor of orange–tan color demarcated by capsule and partly replacing the adrenal gland, surrounded by mature adipose tissue. (Courtesy of Dr George Kokai.)

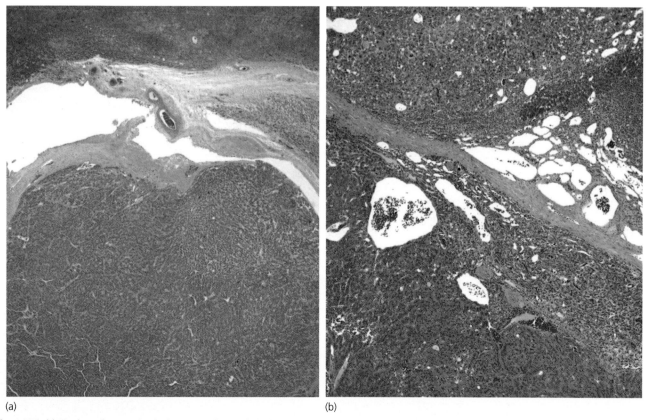

(a)

(b)

Plate 17.2 (a) Histology of encapsulated adreno-cortical tumor (below) next to normal adrenal gland (above). (b) Lobulated tumor showing variety of tumor cell population and arrangement ranging from large cells with multilobar nuclei (above) and trabecular pattern of small uniform cells (below). (Courtesy of Dr George Kokai.)

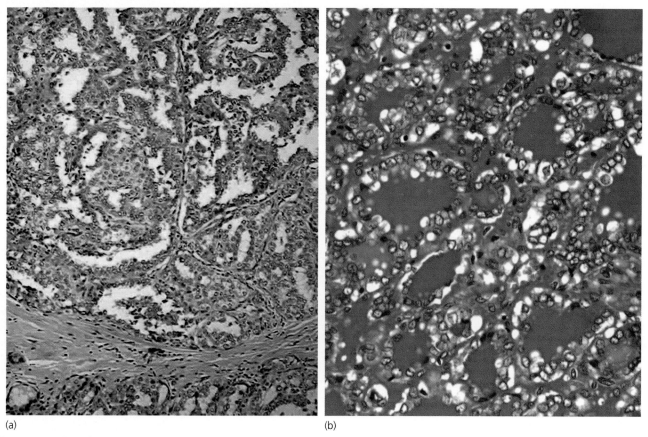

(a)

(b)

Plate 17.3 Histology of papillary carcinoma: predominantly papillary (a) and clear follicular pattern (b). Note almost entirely uniform tumour cell nuclei show characteristic "clearing" and "overlap" – regarded as diagnostic features of papillary thyroid cancer. (Courtesy of Dr George Kokai.)

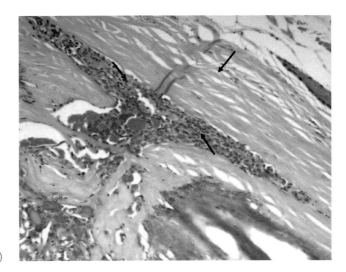

Plate 17.4 Capsular and vascular invasion in follicular carcinoma. Arrows point to the lumen of a capsular vein plugged by tumour cells. (Courtesy of Dr George Kokai.)

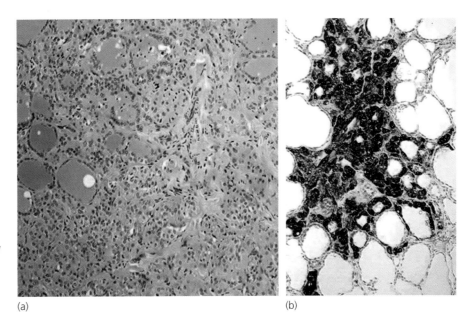

(a)

(b)

Plate 17.5 Focus of a medullary carcinoma of thyroid gland in a patient with MEN2A. (a) Ill-defined tumour nodule consisted of small elongated/spindle cells surrounded by normal-looking follicles. (b) All tumour cells are positive with immunohistochemical labeling for calcitonin (dark brown reaction). (Courtesy of Dr George Kokai.)

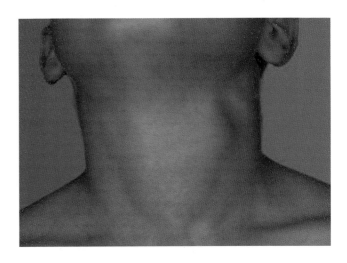

Plate 17.6 Left thyroid mass in a 12-year-old boy with papillary thyroid cancer.

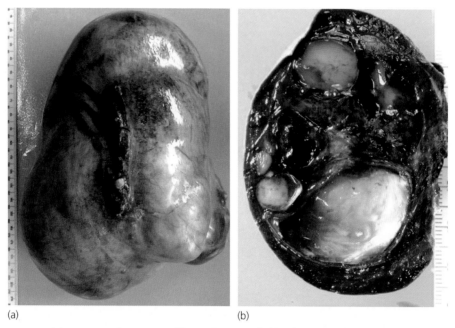

Plate 17.7 Macroscopic appearance of the mature ovarian teratoma with tense intact capsule (a) and showing different areas on cut surface reflecting wide variety of tissues present (b). (Courtesy of Dr George Kokai.)

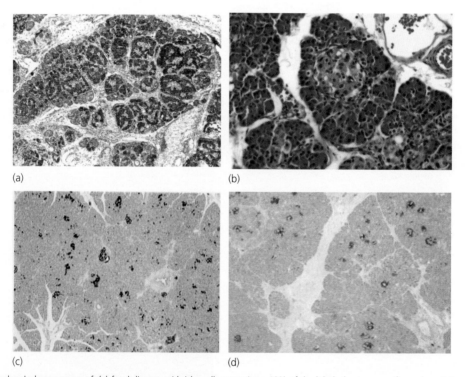

Plate 19.1 Immunohistochemical appearance of: (a) focal disease, with islet cells occupying >40% of the lobule (neuron-specific enolase stain, ×200); (b) diffuse disease, characterized by enlarged β-cell nuclei (hematoxylin and eosin stain, ×400); (c) diffuse disease at ×100. (d) Control showing, in contrast, the normal distribution of islets in the pancreatic lobules.

analogue treatment on peak bone mass and final height in females. *Eur J Pediatr* 1998; **157**: 363–367.

18 Antoniazzi F, Zamboni G, Bertoldo F, Lauriola S, Mengarda F, Pietrobelli A, *et al*. Bone mass at final height in precocious puberty after gonadotropin-releasing hormone agonist with and without calcium supplementation. *J Clin Endocrinol Metab* 2003; **88**: 1096–1101.

19 Heger S, Muller M, Ranke M, Schwarz HP, Waldhauser F, Partsch CJ, *et al*. Long-term GnRH agonist treatment for female central precocious puberty does not impair reproductive function. *Mol Cell Endocrinol* 2006; **254–255**: 217–220.

20 Weinstein LS, Shenker A, Gejman PV, Merino MJ, Friedman E, Spiegel AM. Activating mutations of the stimulatory G protein in the McCune–Albright syndrome. *N Engl J Med* 1991; **325**: 1688–1695.

21 Albright F, Butler A, Hampton A, Smith P. Syndrome characterized by osteitis fibrosa disseminate, areas of pigmentation and endocrine dysfunction, with precocious puberty in females. *N Engl J Med* 1937: **216**: 727–746.

22 Lee PA. Medroxyprogesterone therapy for sexual precocity in girls. *Am J Dis Child* 1981; **135**: 443–445.

23 Syed FA, Chalew SA. Ketoconazole treatment of gonadotropin independent precocious puberty in girls with McCune–Albright syndrome: a preliminary report. *J Pediatr Endocrinol Metab* 1999; **12**: 81–83.

24 Janssen PA, Symoens JE. Hepatic reactions during ketoconazole treatment. *Am J Med* 1983; **74**: 80–85.

25 Feuillan PP, Foster CM, Pescovitz OH, Hench KD, Shawker T, Dwyer A, *et al*. Treatment of precocious puberty in the McCune–Albright syndrome with the aromatase inhibitor testolactone. *N Engl J Med* 1986; **315**: 1115–1119.

26 Feuillan PP, Jones J, Cutler GB Jr. Long-term testolactone therapy for precocious puberty in girls with the McCune–Albright syndrome. *J Clin Endocrinol Metab* 1993; **77**: 647–651.

27 Nunez SB, Calis K, Cutler GB Jr, Jones J, Feuillan PP. Lack of efficacy of fadrozole in treating precocious puberty in girls with the McCune–Albright syndrome. *J Clin Endocrinol Metab* 2003; **88**: 5730–5733.

28 Feuillan P, Calis K, Hill S, Shawker T, Robey PG, Collins MT. Letrozole treatment of precocious puberty in girls with the McCune–Albright syndrome: a pilot study. *J Clin Endocrinol Metab* 2007; **92**: 2100–2106.

29 Mieszczak J, Lowe ES, Plourde P, Eugster EA. The aromatase inhibitor anastrozole is ineffective in the treatment of precocious puberty in girls with McCune–Albright syndrome. *J Clin Endocrinol Metab* 2008; **93**: 2751–2754.

30 Eugster EA, Shankar R, Feezle LK, Pescovitz OH. Tamoxifen treatment of progressive precocious puberty in a patient with McCune–Albright syndrome. *J Pediatr Endocrinol Metab* 1999; **12**: 681–686.

31 Eugster EA, Rubin SD, Reiter EO, Plourde P, Jou HC, Pescovitz OH. Tamoxifen treatment for precocious puberty in McCune–Albright syndrome: a multicenter trial. *J Pediatr* 2003; **143**: 60–66.

32 Gesmundo R, Guana R, Valfre L, De Sanctis L, Matarazzo P, Marzari D, *et al*. Laparoscopic management of ovarian cysts in peripheral precocious puberty of McCune–Albright syndrome. *J Pediatr Endocrinol Metab* 2006; **19** (Suppl 2): 571–575.

33 Lee PA, Van Dop C, Migeon CJ. McCune–Albright syndrome: long-term follow-up. *JAMA* 1986; **256**: 2980–2984.

34 Schmidt H, Kiess W. Secondary central precocious puberty in a girl with McCune–Albright syndrome responds to treatment with GnRH analogue. *J Pediatr Endocrinol Metab* 1998; **11**: 77–81.

35 Wasniewska M, Matarazzo P, Weber G, Russo G, Zampolli M, Salzano G, *et al*. Clinical presentation of McCune–Albright syndrome in males. *J Pediatr Endocrinol Metab* 2006; **19** (Suppl 2): 619–622.

36 Feuillan P, Merke D, Leschek EW, Cutler GB Jr. Use of aromatase inhibitors in precocious puberty. *Endocr Relat Cancer* 1999; **6**: 303–306.

37 Laue L, Kenigsberg D, Pescovitz OH, Hench KD, Barnes KM, Loriaux DL, *et al*. Treatment of familial male precocious puberty with spironolactone and testolactone. *N Engl J Med* 1989; **320**: 496–502.

38 Laue L, Jones J, Barnes KM, Cutler GB Jr. Treatment of familial male precocious puberty with spironolactone, testolactone and deslorelin. *J Clin Endocrinol Metab* 1993; **76**: 151–155.

39 Kreher NC, Pescovitz OH, Delameter P, Tiulpakov A, Hochberg Z. Treatment of familial male-limited precocious puberty with bicalutamide and anastrozole. *J Pediatr* 2006; **149**: 416–420.

40 Richter-Unruh A, Wessels HT, Menken U, Bergmann M, Schmittmann-Ohters K, Schaper J, *et al*. Male LH-independent sexual precocity in a 3.5-year-old boy caused by a somatic activating mutation of the LH receptor in a Leydig cell tumor. *J Clin Endocrinol Metab* 2002; **87**: 1052–1056.

41 Sedlmeyer IL, Palmert MR. Delayed puberty: analysis of a large case series from an academic center. *J Clin Endocrinol Metab* 2002; **87**: 1613–1620.

42 Raivio T, Falardeau J, Dwyer A, Quinton R, Hayes FJ, Hughes VA, *et al*. Reversal of idiopathic hypogonadotropic hypogonadism. *N Engl J Med* 2007; **357**: 863–873.

43 Hero M, Wickman S, Dunkel L. Treatment with the aromatase inhibitor letrozole during adolescence increases near-final height in boys with constitutional delay of puberty. *Clin Endocrinol (Oxf)* 2006; **64**: 510–513.

44 Dunkel L. Use of aromatase inhibitors to increase final height. *Mol Cell Endocrinol* 2006; **254–255**: 207–216.

45 Rosenfield RL, Devine N, Hunold JJ, Mauras N, Moshang T Jr, Root AW. Salutary effects of combining early very low-dose systemic estradiol with growth hormone therapy in girls with Turner syndrome. *J Clin Endocrinol Metab* 2005; **90**: 6424–6430.

46 Davenport ML. Evidence for early initiation of growth hormone and transdermal estradiol therapies in girls with Turner syndrome. *Growth Horm IGF Res* 2006; **16** (Suppl A): S91–97.

47 Riepe FG, Baus I, Wiest S, Krone N, Sippell WG, Partsch CJ. Treatment of pubertal gynecomastia with the specific aromatase inhibitor anastrozole. *Horm Res* 2004; **62**: 113–118.

48 Plourde PV, Reiter EO, Jou HC, Desrochers PE, Rubin SD, Bercu BB, *et al*. Safety and efficacy of anastrozole for the treatment of pubertal gynecomastia: a randomized, double-blind, placebo-controlled trial. *J Clin Endocrinol Metab* 2004; **89**: 4428–4433.

49 Lahlou N, Carel JC, Chaussain JL, Roger M. Pharmacokinetics and pharmacodynamics of GnRH agonists: clinical implications in pediatrics. *J Pediatr Endocrinol Metab* 2000; **13** (Suppl 1): 723–737.

50 Partsch CJ, Sippell WG. Treatment of central precocious puberty. *Best Pract Res Clin Endocrinol Metab* 2002; **16**: 165–189.

12 The Thyroid

Rosalind S. Brown

Endocrine Division, Childrens' Hospital Boston, Boston, MA, USA

Thyroid dysfunction in infancy and childhood results in the metabolic abnormalities found in adults but also affects growth and development. Because thyroid hormone-dependent effects on tissue maturation are developmentally regulated and organ- or tissue-specific, the clinical consequences depend on the age of the infant or child.

Untreated hypothyroidism in the fetus or newborn infant results in permanent abnormalities in intellectual and/or neurological function, reflecting the pivotal role of thyroid hormone on brain development. After the age of 3 years, when most thyroid hormone-dependent brain development is complete, hypothyroidism results in slow growth and delayed skeletal maturation but there usually is no permanent influence on cognitive or neurological development.

Thyroid hormonogenesis

The thyroid is composed of follicles that secrete thyroid hormone. They contain two types of cells that surround a central core of colloid. Thyroid hormone-secreting follicular cells, the major cellular constituent of the follicle, are interspersed with calcitonin-secreting parafollicular C cells of neurogenic origin. A basal membrane surrounds the follicle and separates it from surrounding blood and lymphatic vessels as well as nerve terminals. The major constituent of colloid is thyroglobulin (Tg), a large iodinated, dimeric glycoprotein that functions as a thyroid hormone precursor and permits storage of iodine and of iodinated tyrosyl residues covalently bound within its protein structure.

The synthesis and secretion of thyroid hormone includes a complex series of events, each proceeding simultaneously in the same cell (Fig. 12.1). Dietary iodine, I_2, is converted to iodide in the gut and concentrated 20–40 times in the thyroid by an active transport mechanism involving the Na^+/I^- symporter (NIS),

located within the basal plasma membrane. At the apical border, iodide transport into the lumen is facilitated by pendrin (PDS), an anion transporter encoded by *SLC26A4/PDS*, a gene on chromosome 7q22-31 with sequence homology to several sulfate transporters [1].

At the same time, Tg, synthesized within the follicular cell, undergoes a number of post-translational steps to attain the proper tertiary and quaternary structure. These steps include glycosylation and folding, the latter with the aid of chaperone molecules. Tg is transported by exocytosis into the follicular lumen (colloid) where, at the colloid–apical cell membrane interface, it forms the backbone for a series of reactions that result in the oxidation of I_2 to an active intermediate and the iodination of tyrosyl residues (organification) to form monoiodotyrosine (MIT) and di-iodotyrosine (DIT). Iodide oxidation and organification are both catalyzed by thyroid peroxidase (TPO), a membrane-bound glycosylated hemoprotein enzyme. TPO also catalyzes the coupling of iodotyrosines within the Tg molecule to form the thyroid hormones, triiodothyronine (T3) and tetraiodothyronine or thyroxine (T4). T3 is formed by the coupling of one DIT and one MIT molecule; the coupling of two molecules of DIT results in T4. Iodination requires hydrogen peroxide, the generation of which is regulated in part by the enzymes thyroid oxidase (DUOX1, formerly called THOX1) and DUOX2 which are inserted in the apical membrane of the thyroid follicular cell [2].

Thyroid hormones stored in the colloid are released into the circulation by a series of steps that result initially in their incorporation into the apical surface of the follicular cell by a process known as endocytosis. The ingested colloid droplets fuse with apically streaming proteolytic enzyme-containing lysosomes to form phagolysosomes, in which Tg hydrolysis occurs. Free MIT, DIT, T3 and T4 within the phagolysosomes are then released into the follicular cells. T3 and T4 released in this way diffuse from the thyroid follicular cell into the thyroid capillary blood. The released MIT and DIT are largely deiodinated by iodotyrosine deiodinase, the iodide re-entering the intracellular iodide pool to be reutilized for new hormone synthesis. Deiodination of T4 to generate T3 is a second source of T3 within the thyroid.

Brook's Clinical Pediatric Endocrinology, 6th edition. Edited by C. Brook, P. Clayton, R. Brown. © 2009 Blackwell Publishing, ISBN: 978-1-4051-8080-1.

Figure 12.1 Synthesis (left) and secretion (right) of thyroid hormones in thyroid follicular cells. These processes, which proceed simultaneously in the same cell, are drawn separately for clarity. Iodide (I⁻), amino acids (tyrosine, Tyr and others) and sugars, concentrated by follicular cells, are assembled into thyroglobulin (Tg), packaged into apical vesicles and released into the lumen. At the apical membrane, Tyr residues on the Tg backbone interact with reactive iodine (I°) species to form the iodotyrosines monoiodotyrosine (MIT) and di-iodotyrosine (DIT), a reaction catalyzed by thyroid peroxidase (TPO). MIT and DIT couple to form triiodothyronine (T3) and thyroxine (T4). These products are stored in extracellular colloid. Secretion involves invagination and formation of intracellular colloid droplets which fuse with enzyme-laden lysosomes to form phagolysosomes. Here Tg is hydrolyzed to release MIT, DIT, T3 and T4. MIT and DIT are deiodinated and the iodide reutilized; T3 and T4 are released into the circulation. Not pictured are the pendrin gene, PDS, an apical I⁻ transporter and DUOX1 and DUOX2, apical membrane-associated enzymes important in peroxidase generation. ER, endoplasmic reticulum; Go, Golgi apparatus; NIS, Na⁺/I⁻ symporter.

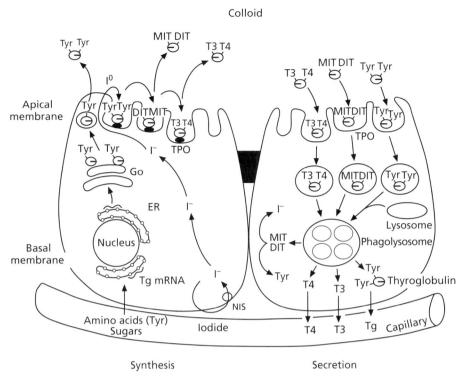

Colloid

Synthesis   Secretion

Cloning of an increasing number of genes has permitted a greater understanding of the specific events involved in thyroid hormonogenesis and of their regulation at both a molecular and cell biological level. Cloning the genes has elucidated the molecular basis for many of the inborn errors of thyroid hormonogenesis. Tg, TPO and, to a lesser extent, NIS also serve as targets of immune attack in patients with autoimmune thyroid disease. In view of the location of TPO and Tg in the interior of the cell, these proteins are unlikely to be the primary trigger of immune attack but are accessible to the immune system after the cell has been injured.

Regulation of thyroid function

Thyrotropin

Thyrotropin (TSH), a glycoprotein hormone secreted by the pituitary gland is the major regulator of thyroid function. Like other pituitary glycoprotein hormones with which TSH shares structural homology, the TSH molecule is composed of a common α subunit and a TSH-specific β subunit. TSH stimulates both thyroid gland function and growth by binding to a specific receptor located on the basal plasma membrane [3]. The TSH receptor, which is a member of the G-protein coupled receptor superfamily, is composed of a large extracellular domain, seven hydrophobic transmembrane spanning regions and a short intra-cytoplasmic tail (Fig. 12.2). The N-terminal extracellular domain appears to be sufficient for binding of hormone whereas the

cytoplasmic loops and C-terminal tail are important in signal transduction.

Through effects mediated primarily by the cyclic adenosine monophosphate (cAMP) signal-transduction pathway, TSH exhibits transcriptional control of the genes for Tg, TPO and NIS and stimulates an array of cellular events, including iodine uptake and organification, as well as thyroid hormone synthesis and secretion. TSH also stimulates follicular cell proliferation and growth. Although the effects of TSH are mediated primarily through the adenyl cyclase-protein kinase A signal transduction pathway, TSH at higher concentrations also stimulates the phosphoinositol-protein kinase-C pathway.

In view of the importance of the TSH receptor in regulating thyroid function, it is not surprising that both germline and somatic mutations can lead to abnormalities of thyroid growth and function in patients (Fig. 12.2) [4]. In addition, unlike Tg and TPO, the TSH receptor is accessible to immune attack as it is located not in the interior of the cell but at the basal plasma membrane adjacent to both the blood and lymphatic vessels. Both stimulatory and blocking TSH receptor antibodies (Abs) may occur in patients and result in stimulation and/or inhibition of TSH-induced thyroid cell growth and function.

The secretion of TSH is under positive feedback control by hypothalamic TSH releasing hormone (TRH), a small tripeptide synthesized in the hypothalamus and transported to the pituitary through the pituitary portal vascular system. TSH secretion is under negative feedback control by thyroid hormone, the latter acting both at the level of the hypothalamus and the pituitary

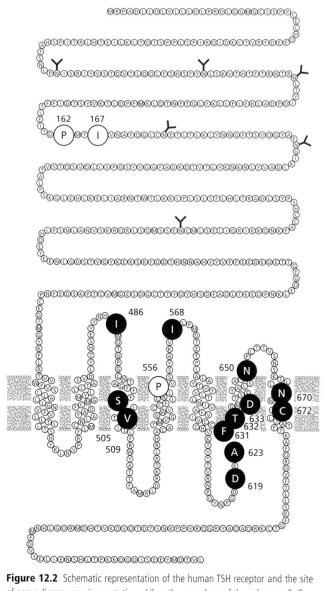

Figure 12.2 Schematic representation of the human TSH receptor and the site of some disease-causing mutations. Like other members of the subgroup 2, G-protein coupled receptor superfamily, the TSH receptor is composed of a large extracellular domain, seven hydrophobic transmembrane spanning regions and a short intracytoplasmic tail. The white symbols refer to loss-of-function mutations while the black symbols refer to gain-of-function mutations. Note the transmembrane location of the loss-of-function Pro^{556}Leu mutation in the hyt-/hyt mouse. (From Van Sande et al. [4] with permission.)

gland. Dopamine, somatostatin and high doses of corticosteroids also inhibit pituitary release of TSH. Decreasing environmental and/or body temperature increases TRH release.

Iodide

Adequacy of dietary iodine is a critical regulator of thyroid gland function through adaptive mechanisms that respond to both deficiency and excess. This is understandable because the major thyroid hormones T4 and T3 are 65% and 59% iodine by weight,

respectively. The daily iodine intake (RDA) recommended by the Food and Nutrition Board of the Institute of Medicine, USA, is 150 μg for adults, 110 μg for infants 0–6 months of age, 130 μg for infants 7–12 months of age, 220 μg for pregnant women and 290 μg for lactating women. Premature infants require 30 μg/kg/day [5].

In iodine deficiency, there is increased trapping of iodide by the thyroid gland as a result of both TSH-independent and TSH-dependent mechanisms. In addition, increased TSH secretion results in a stimulation of thyrocyte proliferation and hormonogenesis. Tg secretion is increased but, because of the reduced iodine content, there is preferential synthesis and secretion of the less iodinated compounds MIT and T3 compared with DIT and T4. Iodine deficiency also results in increased peripheral conversion of T4 to T3. The reverse is true in iodine excess.

Excess iodine inhibits a number of different steps in thyroid hormonogenesis, including organification of iodide and subsequent hormone synthesis (the Wolff–Chaikoff effect), Tg synthesis, hormone release and thyroid growth. Fortunately, under normal circumstances, the iodide-induced inhibition is transient and normal hormone synthesis resumes (adaptation to or escape from the Wolff–Chaikoff effect). The escape from the Wolff–Chaikoff effect appears to be caused, at least in part, by a decrease in NIS mRNA and protein expression, with resultant decreased iodide transport into the thyroid [6]. This adaptation lowers the intrathyroidal iodine content below a critical inhibitory threshold allowing organification of iodide to resume.

Other

Many other extracellular stimulatory signals bind to thyroid membranes and affect thyroid function and/or growth *in vitro* but their importance *in vivo* is not known. They include adrenergic agents, growth factors such as insulin-like growth factor type 1 (IGF-1) and epidermal growth factor (EGF) and purinergic agents. Thyroid cells contain thyroid hormone receptors so that thyroid hormone itself could function as a regulator of thyroid function by a short loop feedback mechanism. In addition, cytokines, produced by infiltrating lymphocytes in patients with autoimmune thyroid disease and even by the thyroid follicular cells themselves, can directly modulate both thyroid function and growth.

Thyroid hormone transport

T4 and T3 released into the circulation are transported to their target cells in non-covalent linkage with carrier proteins. These binding proteins produced in the liver include thyroxine-binding globulin (TBG), transthyretin and the secondary carrier protein, albumin. TBG, although the least abundant, is the most important carrier protein for T4. Transthyretin binds T4 but not T3 and appears to have a role in T4 transport into the brain. In the euthyroid steady state, almost all circulating thyroid hormone is bound to protein. This is especially true for T4, 99.97% of which is bound, compared to 99.7% of T3. Transport proteins function as an extrathyroidal storage pool of thyroid hormone that enables the release of free hormone on demand while at the same time protecting tissues from excessive hormone but they are not essential for normal thyroid function. Thus, the importance of thyroid hormone binding proteins clinically lies in an appreciation of how abnormalities secondary to genetic defects, drugs or illness may impact on the assessment of thyroid function.

Thyroid hormone metabolism

Thyroid hormone synthesized and secreted by the thyroid gland is activated and inactivated primarily by a series of monodeiodination steps in target tissues. Sulfation is an additional method of thyroid hormone metabolism of particular importance in the fetus. In contrast to T4, the sole source of which is the thyroid gland, only 20% of circulating T3 is derived by coupling of tyrosyl residues within the thyroid gland itself. The remainder (approximately 80%) of T3 is derived from the peripheral conversion of T4 to T3 in peripheral tissues, especially the liver, kidney, brain and pituitary gland. In certain tissues (e.g. brain), T3 is generated intracellularly from T4.

T4 and T3 are thyronine molecules, which consist of an inner (tyrosyl or α ring) and outer (phenolic or β) ring (Fig. 12.3). Monodeiodination of the outer ring of T4 results in T3 which is three or four times more metabolically active than T4 *in vivo*. Monodeiodination of the inner ring produces reverse T3 (rT3), a metabolically inactive metabolite. Nearly all rT3 is derived from peripheral conversion and only 2% from the thyroid gland. Progressive tissue monodeiodination results in a series of diiodinated, monoiodinated and non-iodinated forms of thyronine, all of which are metabolically inactive.

Three selenoprotein iodothyronine monodeiodinase enzymes have been described. Two, deiodinase (D)l and D2, are activating

enzymes because they deiodinate the outer ring; there is one inactivating deiodinase, D3, which deiodinates the inner ring (Fig. 12.3) [7]. Dl is also capable of inner-ring monodeiodination, particularly of sulfated iodothyronines.

The deiodinases are developmentally regulated and differ in both their tissue distribution and properties. In the cerebral cortex, for example, >50% of the intracellular T3 is derived from the intracellular conversion of T4 to T3. In contrast, in liver, only 25% of the intracellular T3 is generated from T4, the remainder being derived from plasma. As a consequence of these variations in deiodinase activity, the relative amounts of T4 and T3 in the serum do not necessarily correspond to their intracellular proportions.

D1, responsible for much of the circulating T3, is expressed predominantly in liver and kidney. The highest concentration of D2 is in brain, pituitary, placenta and brown adipose tissue. D3 is present predominantly in fetal tissues and the utero-placental unit, emphasizing the importance of protecting the fetus from the effects of thyroid hormone excess. Adaptive mechanisms in the activity of the deiodinases at a cellular level is an important pre-receptor level of control that results in the preferential shunting of thyroid hormone to areas of need. For example, increased conversion of T4 to T3 by the fetal brain in the presence of hypothyroidism is a protective mechanism that accounts, in part, for the normal or near-normal cognitive outcome of babies with congenital hypothyroidism as long as postnatal therapy is early and adequate.

Thyroid hormone action

Thyroid hormone has multiple effects in cells, including stimulation of thermogenesis, water and ion transport and acceleration of substrate turnover and amino acid and lipid metabolism. Thyroid hormone also potentiates the action of catecholamines,

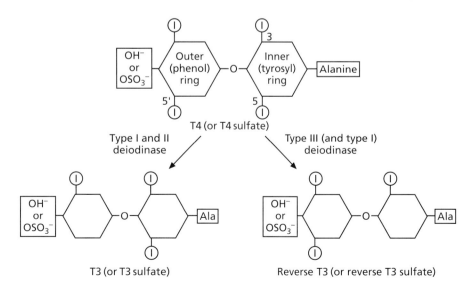

Figure 12.3 Structure of the major thyroid hormones and the action of the monoiodothyronine deiodinase enzymes. The type I and II deiodinases deiodinate the outer (phenol) ring, while the type III (and type I) deiodinases deiodinate the inner (tyrosyl) ring.

an effect responsible for many of the clinical manifestations seen in patients with hyperthyroidism. Unique to infants and children is the stimulation of growth and development of various tissues, including the brain and skeleton.

Thyroid hormone is actively transported into the cell with a number of families of solute carriers, including organic anion transporting polypeptides, amino acid transporters and monocarboxylate transporters (MCTs) [8]. Within the cell, thyroid hormone initiates its action by binding to specific receptors located in the cell nucleus. The binding of T3 to the thyroid hormone receptor (TR) is 10 times higher than T4 [9]. In addition to the four classic TRs, α1, α2, β1 and β2, multiple transcripts that encode protein products have been identified [10]. The gene encoding the TR α-subtype is located on chromosome 17 while the gene encoding the TR β-subtype is on chromosome 3; the respective isoforms (1 and 2) result from alternative splicing of the initial mRNA transcripts.

The TRs are composed of a carboxy-terminal portion important for ligand binding and interactions between receptors, a DNA binding domain with two loop structures known as "zinc fingers" and an amino-terminal domain with no known function (Fig. 12.4). TRα2 and other splice variants, such as TRvα2 and TRvα3, do not bind T3 and may inhibit the binding of the other TRs to DNA (dominant negative inhibition). The TRα gene produces an orphan receptor, Rev-erbAα that has a role in cerebellar development [11].

TRs exist as monomers, homodimers or heterodimers with other nuclear proteins such as the retinoid X-receptors. The heterodimeric structure is the active form of the receptor. TRα1, TRβ1 and TRβ2 stimulate or suppress responsive genes. This requires the interaction of numerous co-activators and co-repressors. In the unliganded state, TRs repress gene function.

Tissue specificity of thyroid hormone action derives from multiple factors, including the predominant TR isoform expressed, the cofactor(s) involved and the type of receptor with which the TR partners. As a result, different genes are stimulated or inhibited in different tissues.

Like the iodothyronine deiodinases, the various TRs are expressed differentially in tissues and are developmentally regulated. TRα1 and TRα2 are widely distributed: the highest concentration of TRβ1 mRNA is found in brain, developing ear, liver, kidney and heart, whereas TRβ2 mRNA expression is restricted to pituitary and brain tissues.

Ontogenesis and regulation of thyroid function

The ontogeny of thyroid function involves hypothalamo-pituitary and thyroid gland organogenesis and maturation, as well as the development of each of the component systems required for mature activity, thyroid hormone transport, metabolism and action. In addition, the placenta plays a part not only by regulating the transport of essential factors and hormones, particularly T4 and iodide, but by synthesizing and metabolizing hormones.

Hypothalamo-pituitary development
Hypothalamic development involves a cascade of transcription factors, including sonic hedgehog (SHH) and ZIC-2 (a homolog of the *Drosophila* odd-paired gene). SF-1 and the LIM class homeodomain factors LHX-3 and LHX-4 also have a role. Transcription factors involved in pituitary development include the pituitary homeobox gene (PTX-1), TITF1/NKX2-1 (formerly called thyroid transcription factor, TTF-1, also called T/EBP) and the LIM class homeodomain transcription factors LHX-3 and LHX-4. NKX2-1 is also involved in thyroid gland and lung development. The terminal factors in the cascade are PROP1 and POU1F1 (formerly called PIT-1). POU1F1 is essential for the differentiation of thyrotrophs, lactotrophs and somatotrophs; PROP1, a homeodomain protein expressed briefly in the embryonic pituitary, is necessary for POU1F1 expression.

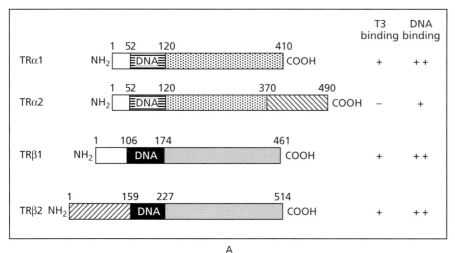

Figure 12.4 The deduced amino acid structure and functional domains of the known thyroid hormone receptor (TR) subtypes (α and β) and isoforms (1 and 2). Note that unlike the other TRs, TRα2 does not bind thyroid hormone. (From Brent [9] with permission.)

Thyroid gland development

The thyroid gland is derived from the fusion of a medial outpouching from the floor of the primitive pharynx, the precursor of the T4-producing follicular cells and bilateral evaginations of the fourth pharyngeal pouch, which give rise to the parafollicular calcitonin (C) secreting cells. Commitment towards a thyroid-specific phenotype, as well as the growth and descent of the thyroid anlage into the neck, results from the coordinate action of transcription factors which include TITF1/NKX2-1, FOXE1 (formerly called TTF-2, also called FKHL15) and PAX 8 [12]. TITF1/NKX2-1 and PAX8 also have a role in the survival of thyroid cell precursors and regulate thyroid-specific gene expression. FOXE1 is important in cellular migration. Because these transcription factors are also expressed in a limited number of other cell types, it appears to be the specific combination of transcription factors and possibly non-DNA binding cofactors acting coordinately that determine the phenotype of a cell.

Other transcription factors and growth factors that have a role in early thyroid gland organogenesis include HHEX1, HOXA3 and members of the fibroblast growth factor family, e.g. FGF10 acting through its receptor, but the initial inductive signal is unknown. A role of the neighbouring heart primordium in the specification of the thyroid anlage has been postulated. Studies of cadherin expression suggest that the caudal translocation of the thyroid anlage may also arise indirectly as a result of the growth and expansion of adjacent tissues, including the major blood vessels [13]. In addition, mice deficient in the T box transcription factor (Tbx1), the gene implicated in cardiac outflow tract abnormalities observed in patients with the 22q11 deletion syndrome, have a severely hypoplastic thyroid gland [14]. In late organogenesis, the *SHH* gene appears to have an important role in the symmetric bilobation of the thyroid; SHH also suppresses the ectopic expression of thyroid follicular cells [15].

During caudal migration, the pharyngeal region of the thyroid anlage contracts to form a narrow stalk known as the thyroglossal duct, which subsequently atrophies so that no lumen is left. An ectopic thyroid and persistent thyroglossal duct or cyst may occur as a consequence of abnormalities of thyroid descent.

In the rat, at fetal day 15, despite early evidence of Tg, TPO and TSH receptor gene expression, the thyroid gland is difficult to distinguish from the surrounding structures and iodine organification, thyroid hormonogenesis and evidence of a follicular structure are absent. This suggests that TITF1/NKX2-1 and PAX8 are necessary but not sufficient for the expression of the fully differentiated thyroid phenotype. On fetal day 17, TSH receptor gene expression is significantly upregulated and this is accompanied by significant growth and by rapid development in both structural and functional characteristics [16].

Expression of Tg and TPO mRNA is increased at this time, thyroid follicles first appear on morphological examination, TPO function can be demonstrated and there is evidence of thyroid hormonogenesis. These findings suggest that the TSH receptor has an important role only at this later stage of development but not earlier in gestation. In support of this interpretation, hyt/hyt

mice, which have a loss-of-function (Pro556-Leu) mutation in the transmembrane domain of the TSH receptor, have severe hypothyroidism and hypoplastic but normally located thyroid glands with a poorly developed follicular structure [17]. Similar findings are detected in babies born to mothers with potent TSH receptor-blocking Abs as well as in babies with severe loss-of-function mutations of the TSH receptor. The genes for factors regulating iodide metabolism (e.g., NIS and TPO) are the ones primarily regulated by TSH; regulation of Tg is more complex.

Developmental events in humans parallel those in rodent species but the timing of maturation differs (Fig. 12.5). Embryogenesis is largely complete by 10–12 weeks' gestation, equivalent to fetal day 15–17 in the rat. At this stage, tiny follicle precursors are first seen, Tg can be detected in follicular spaces and evidence of iodine uptake and organification is first obtained. Low concen-

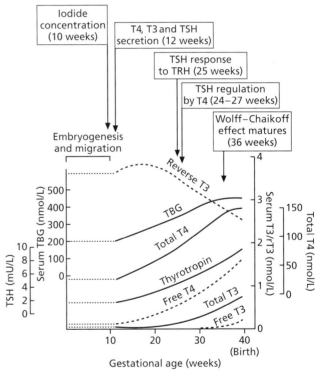

Figure 12.5 Maturation of thyroid gland development and function during gestation. Note that embryogenesis and migration of the thyroid anlage are complete by the end of the first trimester of pregnancy. Serum levels of T4, free T4 and TSH remain low until mid-gestation, however, when the hypothalamic-pituitary axis starts to mature and the pituitary does not begin to respond to stimulatory or inhibitory signals until the end of the second trimester. For this reason, during the first half of pregnancy the fetus is dependent on maternal T4. Throughout gestation, the serum level of T3 remains low and the concentration of reverse T3 is high, a consequence of low D1 activity. In the fetus, like in the older child, high iodine exposure results in inhibition of thyroid hormone synthesis (Wolff–Chaikoff effect) but the ability to escape from this inhibition does not mature until late in gestation. For this reason, the premature infant is unusually susceptible to iodine overload. (From Brown & Larson [99] with permission.)

trations of T4 and T3 are detectable in fetal serum at 10–12 weeks, although it is likely that a fraction of the thyroid hormone measurable at this early stage of the development is maternal in origin.

Tg, first identified in the follicular spaces by 10–11 weeks, can be identified in the human fetal circulation at gestational age 27–28 weeks but when Tg can first be detected in serum is not known. The secretion of a poorly iodinated thyroid hormone precursor and impaired clearance of this glycoprotein from the circulation by the immature liver results in a higher serum concentration of Tg in the premature fetus than at term.

Despite the fact that iodide uptake by the thyroid can be demonstrated at 10–11 weeks' gestation, the capacity of the fetal thyroid to reduce iodide trapping in response to excess iodide (escape from the Wolff–Chaikoff effect) does not appear until 36–40 weeks' gestation (Fig. 12.5). Thus, premature infants are much more likely to develop hypothyroidism when exposed to excess iodine than full-term babies.

Maturation of the hypothalamo-pituitary-thyroid axis

TSH is detectable in fetal serum at levels of 3–4 mIU/L at 12 weeks' gestation and increases from 18 weeks to levels of 10 mU/L at term. This is accompanied by a parallel increase in fetal thyroid radioiodine uptake and by a progressive increase in the serum concentrations of both total T4 and free T4. The serum concentration of TBG also increases during gestation as a consequence of placental estrogen effects on the fetal liver. There is a progressive increase in the ratio of free T4:TSH concentration during the second half of gestation, suggesting changes in both the sensitivity of the pituitary thyrotroph to the negative feedback effect of thyroid hormones and the thyroid follicular cell sensitivity to TSH.

Maturation of hypothalamo-pituitary-thyroid feedback control is first observed early in the third trimester, as indicated by an elevated fetal serum TSH in response to hypothyroxinemia and a suppressed TSH in fetuses with hyperthyroidism brought about by maternal Graves disease. Similarly, a fetal TSH response to exogenously administered TRH has been demonstrated as early as 25 weeks' gestation.

Serum levels of TRH are higher in the fetal circulation than in maternal blood, the result both of extra-hypothalamic TRH production (placenta and pancreas) and the decreased TRH degrading activity in fetal serum. The physiological significance of these increased levels of TRH in the fetal circulation is not known.

Maturation of thyroid hormone metabolism

Activity of D1, an important activating deiodinase in the adult, is low throughout gestation. In contrast, D3, the major inactivating deiodinase, is highly expressed in fetal tissues and in the placenta. As a result, circulating T3 concentrations in the fetus are quite low, approximately 50–60 ng/dL (approximately 1 nmol/L) at birth. In addition, the concentrations of the specific substrates metabolized by D1, rT3 and the sulfate conjugates of T4 are markedly elevated in the fetal circulation as well as in amniotic

fluid. The physiological rationale for the maintenance of reduced circulating T3 concentrations throughout fetal life is still unknown but it has been suggested that its function may be to avoid tissue thermogenesis and premature tissue maturation while at the same time potentiating the anabolic state of the rapidly growing fetus. Despite the low circulating T3 levels, precise temporal and spatial maturation of thyroid hormone metabolism occurs at the local level. This, coupled with receptor activation, permits the coordination of the complex gene networks required for orderly development of thyroid hormone-responsive tissues and organ systems.

For example, in contrast to D1, D2, highly expressed in brain and pituitary, is detectable by mid-gestation. As a consequence, fetal brain T3 levels are 60–80% those of the adult by fetal age 20–26 weeks, despite the low levels of circulating T3. In the presence of fetal hypothyroidism, D2 increases while D3 decreases. These coordinate adjustments are of critical importance and preserve near-normal brain T3 levels providing that maternal T4 levels are maintained at normal concentrations.

The ontogeny of thyroid hormone metabolism is closely associated with maturation of thyroid hormone action both temporally and spatially. This is best illustrated with the example of the cochlea where D2 activity in the mouse rises dramatically to reach a peak level at postnatal day 6, a few days before the onset of hearing [18]. D2 expression is localized to connective tissue immediately adjacent to the sensory epithelium and spiral ganglion where thyroid hormone receptors (TRs) are found. This suggests that D2 containing cells in the connective tissue take up T4 from the circulation, convert T4 to T3 and then release T3 to the adjacent responsive cells. A similar paracrine relationship is found in the cerebral cortex where D2 is expressed predominantly in glial cells whereas TRs are found in the adjacent neurons and oligodendrocytes [19]. In other areas of the brain, such as the pituitary gland, hippocampus and caudate nucleus, D2 and TRs are coexpressed. Unlike D2, D3 is coexpressed with TRs in neurons, perhaps underlying the importance of protecting affected tissues from the effects of excess thyroid hormone.

Maturation of thyroid hormone action

Like thyroid hormone metabolism, the ontogenesis of thyroid hormone-mediated responsiveness is tissue specific and developmentally regulated. Whereas thyroid hormone-mediated effects in the pituitary, brain and bone can be detected prenatally, thyroid hormone-dependent action in brown adipose tissue, liver, heart, skin and carcass are apparent only postnatally. Three examples illustrate the complexity and specificity of thyroid hormone action in different target organs or tissues.

Thyroid hormone and brain development

In the brain, the action of thyroid hormone and its developmental regulation are complex and only beginning to be understood [19,20]. At a functional level, thyroid hormone provides the induction signal for the differentiation and maturation of a diverse array of processes that lead to the establishment of neural circuits during a critical window of brain development. These processes include neurogenesis and neural cell migration (occurring predominantly between 5 and 24 weeks), neuronal differentiation, dendritic and axonal growth, synaptogenesis, gliogenesis (late fetal to 6 months postpartum), myelination (second trimester to 24 months postpartum) and neurotransmitter enzyme synthesis. The absence of thyroid hormone appears to delay rather than eliminate the timing of critical morphological events or gene products, resulting in a disorganization of intercellular communication.

TRs are found in highest concentration in developing neurons and in multiple areas of the fetal brain, including the cerebrum, cerebellum, auditory and visual cortex. Consistent with a nuclear receptor-mediated mode of action, thyroid hormone stimulates numerous developmentally regulated genes, including genes for myelin, neurotropins and their receptors, cytoskeletal components, transcription factors, extracellular matrix proteins and adhesion molecules, intracellular signaling molecules, as well as mitochondrial and cerebellar genes. In some cases these genes appear to be direct targets of thyroid hormone action as thyroid hormone response elements can be detected in the DNA regulatory region and/or the genes are stimulated in cell culture. In other cases, thyroid hormone control may occur secondarily as a consequence of effects on terminal differentiation. In addition, thyroid hormones regulate some genes at the level of mRNA stability or mRNA splicing.

For some time, the surprising lack of developmental abnormalities seen in mutant mice lacking TRβ1, TRα or both, in contrast to the severe abnormalities observed in hypothyroid animals, was unexplained. It is now apparent that the reason for the abnormal brain development observed after thyroid hormone deficiency but not TR deficiency is transcriptional repression by the unliganded TR. This was demonstrated by experiments in which mutant mice lacking the TRα1 receptor were made hypothyroid: no effects on cerebellar development were seen, contrary to findings in wild-type animals [19]. It is relevant that deafness, found in the TRβ1 knockout mouse, is also a frequent finding in patients with severe endemic cretinism and in some patients with thyroid hormone resistance brought about by a deletion in the TRβ1 gene.

It is likely that the complexity of maturational control of thyroid hormone action involves developmental regulation of a myriad of factors that affect TR activity. These factors include co-repressors and co-activators as well as transcription factors that compete with TRs for thyroid hormone response elements (TREs) on target genes, providing further levels of modulation [19].

It is also possible that the action of T4 on the developing CNS may involve, in part, a non-nuclear mechanism. T4-regulated actin polymerization has been shown to have an integral role in the regulation of deiodinase activity and it has been proposed that the action of T4 on the actin cytoskeleton might be important in cellular migration, neurite outgrowth and dendritic spine formation [21].

Thyroid hormone and bone

A second important thyroid hormone target in the perinatal period is bone, as evidenced by the striking growth retardation, decreased growth velocity and delayed ossification of the epiphyseal growth plate characteristic of long-standing untreated hypothyroidism in infancy and childhood. Thyroid hormone-mediated bone maturation involves both direct and indirect actions, the latter mediated by regulation of growth hormone gene expression and the IGF system [22,23]. At a direct level, T3 regulates endochondral ossification and controls chondrocyte differentiation in the growth plate both *in vitro* and *in vivo* [22,24]. Osteoblasts and growth plate chondrocytes both express TRs and several T3-specific target genes have been identified in bone [25]. T3 also stimulates closure of the skull sutures *in vivo*, the basis for the enlarged anterior and posterior fontanelle characteristic of infants with congenital hypothyroidism [26]. Analogous to findings in the brain, the growth retardation observed in hypothyroid mice is more severe than that seen in TR $\alpha^{0/0}\beta^{-/-}$ double knockout mice. This is consistent with the effect of the unliganded aporeceptor in mediating the deleterious effects of thyroid hormone deficiency.

Thyroid hormone and brown adipose tissue

During the perinatal period, brown adipose tissue is essential for non-shivering thermogenesis. In this tissue, thyroid hormone stimulates transcription of thermogenin [also called uncoupling protein (UCP-1)], a unique protein that uncouples nucleotide phosphorylation and the storage of energy as ATP. As the child matures, shivering thermogenesis assumes greater importance and brown adipose tissue disappears.

Role of the placenta

The placenta has an important role in fetal thyroid development and function by regulating the passage of certain maternal hormones, substrates and drugs and by serving as an important site of thyroid hormone metabolism. Although the placenta also synthesizes hormones that can affect the fetal thyroid (e.g. human chorionic gonadotropin, TRH), these appear to have little influence on the fetus.

Thyroid hormone

Under normal circumstances, the placenta has only limited permeability to thyroid hormone and the fetal hypothalamo-pituitary-thyroid system develops relatively independently of maternal influence [27]. This relative barrier to thyroid hormone transport is primarily because of the high placental content of D3, which inactivates most of the thyroid hormone presented from the maternal circulation. The iodide released in this way can then be used for fetal thyroid hormone synthesis.

When a significant T4 gradient between the maternal and fetal compartment exists, however, there is an increased net flux of maternal thyroid hormone to the fetus. Such a situation occurs when the fetus is hypothyroid, as illustrated by infants with the complete inability to synthesize T4 because of an inherited absence of the TPO enzyme. These infants have cord T4 concentrations between 25 and 50% of normal. Similar results are obtained in retrospective studies of cord serum in infants with sporadic congenital athyreosis.

There is also accumulating evidence that maternal–fetal T4 transfer occurs in the first half of pregnancy, when fetal thyroid hormone levels are low [28]. Low concentrations of T4, presumably of maternal origin, have been detected in human embryonic coelomic fluid as early as 6 weeks' gestation and in fetal brain as early as 10 weeks' gestation before the onset of fetal thyroid function. Furthermore, both D2 and D3 activity as well as TR isoforms are present in human fetal brain from the mid first trimester, indicating that the machinery to convert T4 to T3 and to respond to T3 are present.

The transplacental passage of maternal T4 (coupled with the coordinate adjustments in brain deiodinase activity) has a critical role in minimizing the adverse effects of fetal hypothyroidism. Not only may it help to explain the normal or near-normal cognitive outcome of hypothyroid fetuses as long as postnatal treatment is early and adequate, it also may provide a partial explanation for the relatively normal clinical appearance at birth of over 90% of infants with congenital hypothyroidism. By contrast, when both maternal and fetal hypothyroidism occurs, whether this is caused by severe iodine deficiency, potent TSH receptor blocking Abs or maternal–fetal POU1F1 deficiency, there is a significant impairment in neurointellectual development despite the initiation of early and adequate postnatal thyroid replacement [29–31]. Even maternal hypothyroidism and hypothyroxinemia alone have been reported to cause significant cognitive and/or motor delay in the offspring, although the magnitude

of the deficit is not as great as when both fetal and maternal hypothyroidism are present [32,33]. Unlike fetal hypothyroidism, the effects of maternal hypothyroidism are not reversible by early postnatal therapy.

Other hormones and factors

In contrast to thyroid hormone, the placenta is freely permeable to TRH and iodide, the latter being essential for fetal thyroid hormone synthesis. The placenta also is permeable to certain drugs and to immunoglobulins of the immunoglobulin g (IgG) class. Thus, the administration to the mother of excess iodide, drugs (especially propylthiouracil or methimazole) or the transplacental passage of TSH receptor Abs from mothers with severe Graves disease or primary myxedema may have significant effects on fetal and neonatal thyroid function.

Maternal TSH does not cross the placenta. Similarly, Tg is undetectable in the serum of athyreotic infants, indicating the absence of any transplacental passage of this large protein.

Thyroid function in the full-term and premature neonate, the infant and during childhood

The neonate

Marked changes occur in thyroid physiology at the time of birth in the full-term newborn (Fig. 12.6). One of the most dramatic is an abrupt rise in serum TSH that occurs within 30 min of delivery, reaching concentrations of 60–70 mU/L. This causes a marked stimulation of the thyroid, resulting in an approximate

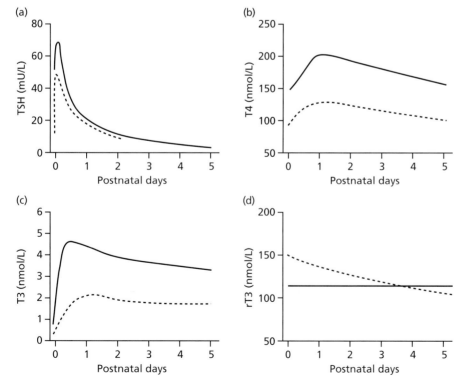

Figure 12.6 Postnatal changes in the serum concentration of TSH, T4, T3 and rT3 in term babies, (continuous line) as compared with premature infants (discontinuous line) in the first week of life. Note that the postnatal surge in TSH is followed by a transient increase in the T4 and T3 concentration in the first few days of life. Changes in premature infants are similar to those seen in term babies but are much less marked. (From Fisher & Klein [98] as modified by Brown & Larson [99] with permission.)

50% increase in the serum T4 and an increase of three- to four-fold in the concentration of serum T3 within 24 h. Studies in experimental animals suggest that the increase in TSH is a consequence of the relative hypothermia of the ambient extrauterine environment. The marked increase in T3 is due not only to the increase in TSH but also to maturation of D1 activity and the loss of placental D3 at the time of delivery. The elevated concentrations of the other substrates of D1, rT3 and T3 sulfate, decrease relatively rapidly during the newborn period. Increased activity of D2 in brown adipose tissue at birth leads to an increase in T3, which is required for optimal uncoupling protein synthesis and thermogenesis.

The premature infant

Thyroid function in the premature infant reflects the relative immaturity of the hypothalamo-pituitary-thyroid axis found in comparable gestational age infants *in utero*. In cord blood samples obtained by umbilical cord sampling (cordocentesis), there is a progressive increase in the TSH, TBG, T4 and T3 concentrations in fetuses with increasing degrees of maturity [34]. Following delivery, there is a surge of TSH and T4 as observed in term infants but the magnitude of the increase is less in premature neonates and there is a more dramatic fall in the T4 concentration over the subsequent 1–2 weeks (Fig. 12.7) [35,36].

The decrease in the T4 concentration is particularly significant in very low birthweight infants (<1.5 kg, approximately equivalent to <30 weeks' gestation) in whom the serum T4 may occa-

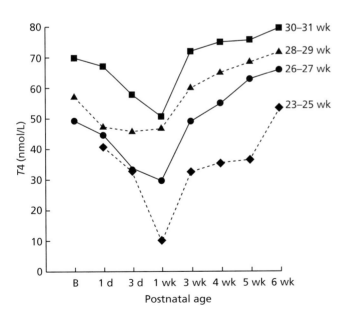

Figure 12.7 Postnatal changes in the serum T4, concentration in premature babies in the first 6 weeks of life. Note that in very premature infants, no postnatal increase in the T4, concentration in the first few days of life is observed. Instead, the T4, concentration decreases with a nadir at 1 week of life. Often the free T4 is not as affected as the total T4 (not pictured). Values subsequently normalize by 3–6 weeks. (From Mercado *et al.* [35] with permission.)

sionally be undetectable. In most cases, the total T4 is more affected than the free T4, a consequence of abnormal protein binding and/or the decreased TBG in these babies with immature liver function [36,37]. In addition to these changes in TSH and T4 concentrations, the serum rT3 tends to stay higher and serum T3 reduced for a longer period, reflecting the greater immaturity of the type 1 deiodinase system.

The causes of the decrease in T4 observed postnatally in premature infants are complex. In addition to clearance of maternal T4 from the neonatal circulation, preterm babies have decreased thyroidal iodide stores and are less able to regulate iodide balance [38], particularly in borderline iodine-deficient areas of the world. Preterm infants are frequently sicker than their more mature counterparts and may be treated by drugs that affect neonatal thyroid function (e.g. dopamine and steroids). In addition, because the capacity of the immature thyroid to adapt to exogenous iodide is reduced, there is an increased sensitivity to the thyroid-suppressive effects of excess iodide found in certain skin antiseptics and drugs to which these babies are frequently exposed.

Despite the reduced total T4 observed in some preterm babies, the TSH concentration is not significantly elevated in most of them. Transient elevations in TSH are seen in some, the finding of a TSH concentration >40 mU/L being more frequent the greater the degree of prematurity. In one study the prevalence of a TSH concentration >40 mU/L in very low birthweight (<1.5 kg) premature infants was eightfold higher and in low birthweight (1.5–2.5 kg) neonates twofold higher than in term babies [39].

Although an elevated TSH concentration may reflect true primary hypothyroidism, the increase in TSH seen in preterm infants at several weeks of age may also reflect the elevated TSH observed in adults who are recovering from severe illness. Such individuals may develop transient TSH elevations, which are associated with still reduced serum T4 and T3 concentrations. These have been interpreted as reflecting a "reawakening" of the illness-induced suppression of the hypothalamo-pituitary axis. As the infant recovers from prematurity associated illnesses such as respiratory distress syndrome (RDS), a recovery of the illness-induced suppression of the hypothalamo-pituitary-thyroid axis would also occur.

Infants and children

After the neonatal period there is a slow and progressive decrease in the concentrations of T4, free T4, T3 and TSH during infancy and childhood. Age and gender-specific normative values in a large population of children have been published [40]. The higher concentrations of TSH and of T3 in children than in adults are particularly noteworthy. Adult normative data are frequently provided clinically and apparent abnormalities in these values are not infrequent reasons for referral to a pediatric endocrinologist.

The serum concentration of rT3 remains unchanged or increases slightly. Radioactive iodine uptake is higher, particularly in the newborn period, and there is a markedly higher T4 turnover in this age group relative to that in the adult. In early infancy, T4 production rates are estimated to be of the order of 7–9 μg/kg/day, decreasing slowly over the first few years of life to about 3–5 μg/kg/day at 1–3 years and 2–3 μg/kg/day at ages 3–9 years. This is to be contrasted with the production rate of T4 in the adult, which is about 1–1.5 μg/kg/day. Serum Tg levels also fall over the first year of life, reaching concentrations typical of adults by about 6 months of age.

The size of the thyroid gland increases slowly by about 1 g/year from approximately 1 g in the newborn to about 15–20 g at age 15 when it has achieved its adult size. The thyroid lobe is comparable to the terminal phalanx of the infant or child's thumb.

Thyroid disease in infancy

Congenital hypothyroidism

Congenital hypothyroidism (CH) is the most common treatable cause of mental retardation. Worldwide, the most common cause of CH is iodine deficiency, a problem that continues to affect almost 1 billion people despite international efforts aimed at its eradication. In areas where iodine deficiency is severe, CH is endemic (endemic cretinism) and characterized by mental retardation, short stature, deaf mutism and specific neurological abnormalities. Endemic cretinism and iodine deficiency have been the subject of several excellent reviews [41,42]. Babies with CH have an increased incidence of cardiac anomalies, particular atrial and ventricular septal defects.

Screening for congenital hypothyroidism

In iodine-sufficient areas and in areas of borderline iodine deficiency, CH is usually sporadic and occurs in 1 in 2500–4000 infants. In order to achieve optimal neurologic outcome, treatment must be initiated soon after birth before affected infants are recognizable clinically. Neonatal screening programs have therefore been introduced in most industrialized areas of the world. Elsewhere, such as Eastern Europe, South America, Asia, Oceania and Africa, neonatal screening programs are under development.

By 1992, some 50 million infants worldwide had been screened for CH with 6000 cases detected annually. There continues to be disagreement whether minor neuro-intellectual sequelae remain in the most severely affected infants and what constitutes the best treatment strategy, but accumulating evidence suggests that a normal outcome is possible, even in the latter group of babies as long as treatment is started sufficiently early and is adequate. Certainly, the main objective of screening, the eradication of mental retardation due to CH, has been achieved and it has been estimated that the financial benefit–cost ratio of a neonatal screening program is approximately 10 : 1, a ratio that does not include the loss of tax income that would result from impaired intellectual capacity in the untreated but non-institutionalized person. Newborn screening has also permitted elucidation of the prevalence of the various causes of CH, including a series of transient disorders found predominantly in premature infants. CH has been found to be 4–5 times more common than phenylketonuria for which screening programs were developed first.

Screening strategies for congenital hypothyroidism

Measurement of T4 and/or TSH is performed on an eluate of dried whole blood collected on filter paper by skin puncture on day 1–4 of life. Two principal strategies for the detection of CH have evolved. A two-tiered approach is used in both. In much of North America, primary screening is of T4, with TSH reserved for specimens T4 in (usually) the lowest 10–20th centiles. In most of Europe and in Japan, a primary TSH approach is employed. With the development of more sensitive, non-radioisotopic TSH assays, Canada and some states in the USA have switched to a primary TSH program. A few programs measure both T4 and TSH.

Whatever method is used, babies whose initial TSH is >50 mU/L are most likely to have permanent CH while a TSH of 20–49 mU/L may be a false-positive or represent transient hypothyroidism. Transient CH is particularly common in premature infants in borderline iodine-deficient areas.

Each screening strategy has advantages and disadvantages but primary T4/backup TSH and primary TSH approaches appear to be equal in the detection of babies with permanent primary CH. The T4/backup TSH program detects primary, secondary or tertiary hypothyroidism, babies with a low initial T4 but delayed rise in the TSH, TBG deficiency and hyperthyroxinemia but may miss compensated hypothyroidism. The primary TSH strategy detects overt and compensated hypothyroidism but misses secondary or tertiary hypothyroidism, a delayed TSH rise, TBG deficiency and hyperthyroxinemia. There are fewer false-positives with a primary TSH strategy.

Since 1995 the Netherlands has employed a novel multistep screening strategy that includes, in addition to primary T4/backup TSH, the measurement of thyroxine binding globulin (TBG) in the filter paper specimens with the lowest 5% of T4 values [43]. The T4 : TBG ratio is used as an indirect reflection of the free T4, which cannot be measured directly in dried blood spots. For a relatively small incremental cost, this approach has resulted in increased sensitivity and specificity in the detection of milder cases of primary congenital hypothyroidism that might otherwise be missed. It has identified >90% of infants with central hypothyroidism, compared with 22% with primary T4 screening and none with a primary TSH approach.

The incidence of central hypothyroidism detected on screening was 1 in 16 000–21 000, much higher than a recent estimate of 1 in 95 933 obtained in the USA [44]. More than 80% of these babies had multiple pituitary hormone deficiencies [45]. Given the high morbidity and mortality of congenital hypopituitarism, the availability of effective therapy and an apparent frequency similar to that of phenylketonuria (1 in 18 000), the disorder for which neonatal screening began, the goals of newborn thyroid screening could be extended to include the detection of babies with central hypothyroidism.

In New York State and to a lesser extent the USA in general, an increased frequency of CH (1 in 2500 versus the original estimate of 1 in 3000–4000) has been noted in recent years, a trend that is not adequately explained by changes in the screening strategy or other likely contributing factors, such as differences in gestational age, ethnicity, multiple births or maternal age [46]. A similar prevalence has been reported in the Netherlands [47]. It is possible that some of these cases represent infants with transient CH that have been misclassified as permanent.

All screening strategies miss the rare infant whose T4 and TSH levels on initial screening are normal but who later develops low T4 and elevated TSH concentrations (<0.5% of infants). This pattern has been termed "atypical"' CH or "delayed TSH rise" and is observed most commonly in premature babies with transient hypothyroidism or in infants with less severe forms of permanent disease.

Some programs have responded by performing a second screen on all infants at the time of their return visit to their pediatrician at 2–6 weeks of age. In addition, some of these programs request follow-up serum on any baby with a very low T4 value (<3rd percentile) on two occasions or a very low filter paper T4 below a critical value (<3 µg/dL, 40 nmol/L) on one occasion. Some programs that perform a second screen report the detection of an additional 10% of CH cases but this practice greatly increases the cost of screening [48].

Other programs routinely perform a second screen only on patients at high risk of delayed TSH elevation, such as very low birthweight infants and babies in the neonatal intensive care unit. These programs report a 14-fold increased incidence of this problem in very low birthweight infants [49]. As noted previously, it may not be certain in some of these cases whether the elevated TSH level is pathological or represents an appropriate compensatory response following hypothyroxinemia secondary to sick euthyroid syndrome. Other groups at high risk of delayed TSH rise are babies with cardiovascular anomalies, patients with Down syndrome and monozygotic twins [50]. In the last group of infants, fetal cord mixing may occur and initially mask the presence of CH.

In all strategies there is the very real possibility for human error failing to identify an affected infant because of poor communication, lack of receipt of requested specimens or the failure to test an infant who is transferred between hospitals during the neonatal period.

Newborn screening was performed initially at 3–4 days of life and the normal values that were derived reflected this postnatal age. The practice of early discharge of otherwise healthy full-term infants from the hospital has resulted in a greater proportion of babies being tested before this time. It has been estimated that 25% or more of newborns in North America are discharged within 24 h of delivery and 40% in the second 24 h of life. Because of the neonatal TSH surge and the dynamic changes in T4 and T3 concentrations that occur within the first few days of life, early discharge increases the number of false-positive results. In California, the ratio of false-positive to confirmed CH has doubled from 2.5:1 to approximately 5:1. Some programs have responded by increasing the threshold value for TSH within the first day of life but this increases the possibility of missing infants with a slowly rising TSH.

Another complicating factor is the dramatically increased survival of very premature infants. They greatly increase the cost of screening programs because blood T4 concentrations are lower and the incidence of transient hypothyroidism is much higher than in full-term babies. It has been estimated that very low birthweight infants constitute 0.8% of the population but increase the number of T4 assays in a primary TSH program by 9%. Very low birthweight infants account for 8% of all TSH assays performed in a primary T4 program.

In the last decade, normal values have been published according to gestational age (and/or birthweight) for cord blood [34,36], filter paper at the time of screening [39] and serum in the first 6 weeks of life [36,51], the latter using newer more sensitive assay techniques.

Thyroid dysgenesis

The most common cause of non-endemic CH, accounting for 85–90% of cases, is thyroid dysgenesis, almost always a sporadic disease. Thyroid dysgenesis may result in the complete absence of thyroid tissue (agenesis) or it may be partial (hypoplasia); the latter is often accompanied by a failure to descend into the neck (ectopy). Unilateral agenesis or hypoplasia may also occur but this does not usually affect thyroid function in the newborn period. Females are affected more often than males. Thyroid dysgenesis, is less frequent among African-Americans and more common among Asians and Hispanics in the USA.

Genetic and environmental factors have been implicated in the etiology of thyroid dysgenesis but the cause is unknown in most patients. The 2% familial occurrence, the reported gender and ethnic differences, as well as the increased incidence in babies with Down syndrome, all suggest that genetic factors might have a role in some cases. The transcription factors TITF1/NKX2-1, FOXE1 and PAX8 appear to be obvious candidate genes in view of their important role in thyroid organogenesis and thyroid-specific gene expression but, to date, abnormalities have been found in only a small proportion of patients with isolated thyroid dysgenesis [52]. A heterozygous loss-of-function mutation of the *PAX8* gene has been identified and affected patients have had thyroid hypoplasia with or without ectopy. It is possible that thyroid dysgenesis is a polygenic disease with variable penetrance, depending on the genetic background. Alternately, epigenetic modifications, early somatic mutations or stochastic developmental events may have a role. Table 12.1 summarizes known molecular defects in transcription factors and other causes of CH.

In contrast to the rarity of germline mutations of *TITF1/NKX2-1, FOXE1* and *PAX8* in patients with isolated thyroid dysgenesis, heterozygous germline mutations in these genes may be a more common cause of abnormal thyroid gland development when thyroid dysgenesis or abnormal thyroid function is associated

Table 12.1 Genetic disorders of thyroid gland development, hormonogenesis and action.

Abnormality	Gene	Gene locus	Characteristic picture	Inheritance
Transcription factor			**Thyroid usually dysgenetic**	
	TITF1/NKX2-1	14q13	Choreoathetosis, respiratory problems, thyroid hypoplasia/agenesis	AD
	FOXE1	9q22	Thyroid agenesis, cleft palate, spiky hair, choanal atresia, bifid epiglottis	AR
	PAX8	2q12-q14	Thyroid hypoplasia	AD
	Tbx1	22q11.2	Thyroid hemiagenesis, DiGeorge syndrome	AD
	SHH	7q11	Thyroid hemiagenesis, William syndrome	AD
↓ TSH synthesis			**Thyroid gland eutopic, not enlarged**	
Combined pituitary deficiencies	PROP1	5q	Anterior pituitary hormone deficiencies (GH, PRL, TSH, LH/FSH, evolving ACTH)	AR
	POU1F1	3p11	Anterior pituitary hormone deficiencies (GH, PRL, TSH)	AR, AD
	LHX3	9q34.3	Anterior pituitary hormone deficiencies (GH, PRL, TSH, LH/FSH), limited neck rotation	AR
	LHX4	1q25	Anterior pituitary hormone deficiencies (GH, TSH, ACTH), cerebellar abnormalities	AR, AD
	HESX1	3p21.2-p21.1	Anterior and posterior pituitary hormone deficiencies (GH, TSH, LH/FSH, ACTH, ADH, septo-optic hypoplasia	AR, AD
Isolated ↓ TSH	TRH	3p	↓ TSH	AR
	TRH receptor	14q31	↓ TSH, (↓ PRL)	AR
	TSH β-subunit	1p13	↓ TSH	AR
↓ TSH response			**Thyroid gland eutopic ± hypoplastic**	
	TSH receptor	14q31	Thyroid hypoplasia/apparent aplasia	AR
	Gsα	20q13.2	Thyroid hypoplasia, pseudohypoparathyroidism 1a (Albright hereditary osteodystrophy)	AD
↓ T4 synthesis			**Thyroid gland eutopic, ± goiter**	
	NIS	19p12–13.2	↓I_2 uptake	AR
	TPO	2p25	Abnormal I_2 organification	AR
	DUOX2	15q15.3	Abnormal I_2 organification 2° to ↓ H_2O_2 generation; heterozygotes may have transient CH	AR
	Thyroglobulin	8q24		AR,AD
	Dehalogenase	6q24–25	Abnormal Tg synthesis, abnormal plasma/urinary iodoprotein	AR
	SLC26A4/PDS	7q31	Defective iodine recycling, ↑ MIT and DIT in plasma/urine Congenital deafness, partial organification defect	AR
↓ T4 action			**Inappropriately ↑ TSH**	
Thyroid hormone resistance	TRβ	3p24.3	↑ T4, ↑ T3, inappropriately ↑ TSH; tachycardia, ADH, failure to thrive, small goiter	AD
↓ T4 transport	MCT8	Xq13.2	Slightly ↓ T4, ↑ T3, inappropriately ↑ TSH) severe mental retardation, deafness	X-linked
↓ Deiodinase 2 activity	SECISBP2	9q22.2	Slightly ↑ T4, ↓T3, ↑ rT3 inappropriately ↑ TSH	AR

ACTH, adrenocorticotropic hormone; AD, autosomal dominant; ADH, antidiuretic hormone; AR, autosomal recessive; DIT, di-iodotyrosine;
FSH, follicle stimulating hormone; GH, growth hormone; LH, luteinizing hormone; MIT, monoiodotyrosine; PRL, prolactin; TSH, thyroid stimulating hormone.
Note that considerable phenotypic variability may be found and abnormal function often develops over time.

with other dysmorphic findings. This is consistent with the important role of these transcription factors in non-thyroid tissues during embryonic development. Heterozygous deletions of *TITF1/NKX2-1* have been reported in a number of patients with CH, neurological manifestations (particularly choreoathetosis) and unexplained neonatal respiratory distress. Abnormal thyroid, lung, pituitary and forebrain development is found in mice with a targeted disruption of this gene. The thyroid phenotype in these patients has varied from compensated hypothyroidism with a eutopic thyroid gland on scintiscan to overt hypothyroidism associated with thyroid gland hypoplasia or aplasia (Table 12.1) [12].

Homozygous missense mutations in the *FOXE1* gene have been associated with the syndrome of thyroid agenesis, bifid epiglottis, cleft palate, kinky hair and choanal atresia.

It has been suggested that the thyroid hemiagenesis sometimes observed in patients with 22q11.2 deletion (DiGeorge/velocardiofacial syndrome) might be related to defects in the genes for

SHH (or sonic hedgehog signaling) [15]. Mice with a targeted disruption in both the *Shh* and *Tbx1* genes, an important downstream target of sonic hedgehog, also have thyroid hemiagenesis [15].

Inborn errors of thyroid hormonogenesis

Decreased T4 synthesis due to an inborn error is responsible for most of the remaining cases (10–15%) of CH. Defects include failure to concentrate iodide, defective organification of iodide due to an abnormality in the TPO enzyme or in the H_2O_2 generating system, defective Tg synthesis or transport and abnormal iodotyrosine deiodinase activity.

The association of a partial organification defect with sensorineural deafness is known as Pendred syndrome. Affected patients have a goiter and characteristic enlargement of the vestibular aqueduct on magnetic resonance imaging (MRI) but the phenotype is variable. Thyroid function is characteristically normal in the newborn period and, in some patients, a hearing defect is the only finding [53].

All inborn errors of thyroid hormonogenesis are associated with a normally placed (eutopic) thyroid gland of normal or increased size which distinguishes them clinically from thyroid dysgenesis. Inborn errors tend to have an autosomal recessive form of inheritance consistent with a single gene mutation and a molecular basis for many of them has been identified (Table 12.1) [54], including mutations in the genes for NIS, TPO and Tg, respectively. Pendred syndrome has been shown to be caused by a defect in the pendrin (*SLC26A4/PDS*) gene [1] and mutations in *DUOX2*, important in hydrogen peroxide generation, have been shown to underly many cases of apparent organification defect [2]. Missense mutations and deletions in *DEHAL1*, the gene encoding iodotyrosine deiodinase, underly the hypothyroidism in patients with clinical evidence of this abnormality [55]. Considerable phenotypic variability has been observed.

TSH resistance

Decreased T4 synthesis due to resistance to TSH is a less common cause of CH. Babies have a normal or hypoplastic gland and, in rare cases, no thyroid gland at all is discernible on thyroid imaging, a picture indistinguishable from thyroid agenesis. Because the TSH receptor gene is expressed only after the thyroid gland has migrated to the neck, loss-of-function mutations could explain the finding of hypoplasia or apparent aplasia but not ectopy. Clinical findings in TSH resistance vary from compensated to overt hypothyroidism, depending on the severity of the defect. Some patients have a loss-of-function mutation of the TSH receptor, usually involving the extracellular domain [4]. Rarely, a loss-of-function mutation involves the transmembrane domain, analogous to the hyt/hyt mouse (Fig. 12.2). In a few infants, a discrepancy between presumed "athyreosis" on thyroid scintigraphy and the detection of either a "normal" serum Tg concentration or glandular tissue on ultrasound examination has been noted but this has not been consistent.

The relative frequency of TSH receptor gene mutations as a cause of TSH resistance is not known. In one study, inactivating mutations of the TSH receptor gene were found in 1 of 100 patients with CH associated with thyroid hypoplasia or aplasia. TSH receptor gene mutations may be more common in certain ethnic groups, e.g. in Wales [56]. Most familial cases of TSH resistance due to a loss-of-function mutation of the TSH receptor have an autosomal recessive form of inheritance. Some of the remaining patients with TSH resistance are likely to have a post-receptor defect, possibly involving a signal transduction pathway.

TSH resistance may rarely be brought about by an inactivating mutation of the stimulatory guanine nucleotide-binding protein (Gs_{α}-gene). This syndrome, pseudohypoparathyroidism type Ia or Albright hereditary osteodystrophy, is characterized by variable resistance to G-protein coupled receptors, most commonly the parathyroid hormone receptor. Unlike loss-of-function mutations of the TSH receptor, Albright hereditary osteodystrophy has an autosomal dominant inheritance with variable expression. The hypothyroidism at birth is usually mild.

Decreased TSH synthesis or secretion

CH due to TSH deficiency is detected only by newborn screening programs that utilize a primary T4 strategy. The most recent data in USA indicate a prevalence of 1 in 95 933, <5% of all cases of CH [44]; in the Netherlands, where a T4 : TBG ratio is added to the screening strategy, the reported prevalence is five- to sixfold higher (1 in 16 400–21 000) [43,45].

TSH deficiency may be isolated or associated with other pituitary hormone deficiencies. Causes of isolated TSH deficiency include mutations in the genes for TSHβ and TRH, both of which may be familial. TRH resistance due to a mutation in the TRH receptor gene has been described in a child in whom secondary hypothyroidism was missed on newborn screening. In this patient, the diagnosis was suspected because of an absent TSH and prolactin response to TRH despite a normal pituitary gland on imaging [57].

TSH deficiency in association with other pituitary hormone deficiencies may be associated with abnormal midline facial and brain structures (particularly cleft lip and palate with absent septum pellucidum and/or corpus callosum) and should be suspected in any male infant with microphallus and hypoglycemia. A mutation in the *HESX-1* homeobox gene has been demonstrated in some patients with septo-optic dysplasia. Non-dysmorphic causes of CH include pituitary hypoplasia, often associated with an ectopic posterior pituitary gland and molecular defects in the genes for the transcription factors LHX, POU1F1 or PROP1.

Decreased thyroid hormone action

Although the classic cause of thyroid hormone resistance is a loss-of-function mutation of the thyroid hormone receptor (TR), in recent years two additional causes of decreased thyroid hormone action have been identified. These include defective cellular T4 transport and abnormal conversion of T4 to T3.

Thyroid hormone resistance

Resistance to the action of thyroid hormone, although usually diagnosed later in life, may be identified by neonatal screening programs that determine primarily TSH. Affected babies are not usually symptomatic. Most cases result from a mutation in the TRβ gene and follow an autosomal dominant pattern of inheritance. The incidence has been estimated to be 1 in 50 000.

Decreased T4 cellular transport

Decreased T4 transport into target cells is another congenital abnormality of thyroid hormone action [58] and mutations in the monocarboxylate transporter 8 (*MCT8*) gene, located on the X chromosome, have been associated with male-limited hypothyroidism and severe neurological abnormalities, including global developmental delay, dystonia, central hypotonia, spastic quadriplegia, rotary nystagmus and impaired gaze and hearing. Heterozygous females had a milder thyroid phenotype and no neurological defects.

Abnormal thyroid hormone metabolism

Decreased T4 action has been described in patients with a homozygous missense mutation in *SECISBP2*, a gene required for the incorporation of selenocysteine into D2, a selenoprotein [59]. Affected patients have abnormal thyroid function but are otherwise normal.

Transient congenital hypothyroidism

Estimates of the frequency of transient CH vary greatly depending on how this condition is defined, whether transient hypothyroidism is to be considered in all infants with a single elevated blood TSH concentration or only babies in whom a low T4 and elevated TSH are found in both the screening and confirmatory serum samples, associated with disappearance of the condition within a few weeks with or without replacement therapy (Table 12.2). In North America, the original incidence was 1 in 40 000 neonates but the condition appears now to be threefold more common (1 in 11 000–12 000) [44,47], probably caused, at least partly, by the survival of increasingly premature infants.

Iodine deficiency, iodine excess and drugs are common causes of transient hypothyroidism in premature babies but often the cause is unknown. Transient TSH elevation may represent a compensatory response in infants recovering from sick euthyroid syndrome.

Iodine deficiency and iodine excess

Transient hypothyroidism resulting from iodine deficiency or excess is more common in iodine-deficient areas of Europe than in North America, an iodine-sufficient region. In Belgium, for example, transient hypothyroidism used to be eightfold higher than in North America but administration of potassium iodide was successful in significantly reducing the incidence. Because newborn infants are so susceptible to the adverse effects of iodine deficiency, serum TSH on newborn screening has been shown to reflect the prevalence of iodine deficiency in a population. Pre-

Table 12.2 Differential diagnosis of transient congenital hypothyroidism.

Primary hypothyroidism
Prenatal or postnatal iodine deficiency or excess
Maternal antithyroid medication
Maternal TSH receptor blocking antibodies

Secondary or tertiary hypothyroidism
Prenatal exposure to maternal hyperthyroidism
Prematurity (particulary <27 weeks' gestation)
Drugs:
  steroids
  dopamine

Miscellaneous
Isolated TSH elevation
Low T4 with normal TSH:
  prematurity
  illness
  undernutrition

TSH, thyroid stimulating hormone.

mature infants are particularly at risk, not only because of decreased thyroidal iodine stores accumulated *in utero* but also because of immaturity of the capacity for thyroid hormonogenesis, the hypothalamo-pituitary-thyroid axis and the ability to convert T4 to T3. Furthermore, premature infants are in negative iodine balance for the first 1–2 weeks of postnatal life.

In addition to iodine deficiency, the fetus and infant are sensitive to thyroid-suppressive effects of iodine administered to the mother during pregnancy or lactation or directly to the baby. This occurs because the fetus is unable to decrease thyroidal iodine uptake in response to an iodine load before 36 weeks' gestation but increased skin absorption and decreased renal clearance of iodine are likely to play a part. Sources of iodine include drugs (e.g. potassium iodide or amiodarone), radiocontrast agents (e.g. iopanoic acid or sodium ipodate) and antiseptic solutions (e.g. povidone-iodine) used for skin cleansing or vaginal douches. Iodine-induced transient hypothyroidism is much less common in North America than in Europe [60].

Maternal antithyroid medication

Transient neonatal hypothyroidism may develop in babies whose mothers are treated with propylthiouracil (PTU), methimazole (MMI) or carbimazole for Graves disease. The fetus appears to be particularly sensitive to antithyroid drugs, even when the doses used in the mother are within recommended guidelines. Babies with antithyroid drug-induced hypothyroidism develop an enlarged thyroid gland which may be large enough to cause respiratory embarassment, especially with higher doses. Both the hypothyroidism and goiter resolve with clearance of the drug from the baby's circulation and replacement therapy is rarely required.

Maternal thyrotropin receptor antibodies

TSH receptor blocking Abs, a population of Abs closely related to the TSH receptor stimulating Abs in Graves disease, may be transmitted to the fetus in sufficient titer to cause transient CH. The incidence of this disorder has been estimated to be 1 in 180 000 in North America, equivalent to 20% of transient cases [61]. TSH receptor blocking Abs are found most often in mothers who have been treated previously for Graves disease or who have the non-goitrous form of chronic lymphocytic thyroiditis (primary myxedema). Occasionally, mothers are unaware that they are hypothyroid and the diagnosis is made in them only after CH has been recognized in their infant. Unlike TSH receptor stimulating Abs that mimic the action of TSH, TSH receptor blocking Abs inhibit both binding and action of TSH. Because TSH-induced growth is inhibited, babies do not have a goiter; if the blocking Ab activity is sufficiently potent, no thyroid tissue may be identified. More often, babies are misdiagnosed with thyroid agenesis because TSH-stimulated radioactive iodine uptake is inhibited. In contrast to findings on scintiscan, a normally placed thyroid gland can usually be visualized on ultrasound. The hypothyroidism generally resolves in 3–4 months when Abs are cleared from the neonatal circulation.

Babies with TSH receptor blocking-Ab-induced hypothyroidism are difficult to distinguish from thyroid dysgenesis but differ in a number of ways (Table 12.3). They do not require lifelong therapy but there is a high recurrence rate in subsequent offspring because of the tendency of these maternal Abs to persist for many years. Unlike babies with thyroid dysgenesis, in whom cognitive outcome is normal if postnatal therapy is early and adequate, babies with maternal blocking-Ab-induced hypothyroidism may have permanent intellectual deficit if feto-maternal hypothyroidism was present *in utero* [31].

Transient secondary and/or tertiary hypothyroidism

Babies born to mothers who were hyperthyroid during pregnancy may develop transient hypothalamo-pituitary suppression. This is usually self-limited but may last for years and require replacement therapy. In general, the titer of TSH receptor stimulating Abs in this population of infants is lower than in those who develop transient neonatal hyperthyroidism.

Other causes of transient secondary and tertiary hypothyroidism include prematurity (<27 weeks' gestation) and drugs used in the neonatal intensive care unit (e.g. steroids, dopamine).

Other abnormalities of thyroid function discovered on newborn screening

Isolated hyperthyrotropinemia

Persistent mild hyperthyrotropinemia has been detected primarily by screening programs that utilize a primary TSH method but also in some infants in whom mild hypothyroidism (e.g. T4 <10th percentile, TSH <40 μU/mL on screening) is first detected in the newborn period. The condition is most common in premature infants and has many potential causes. Babies diagnosed with hyperthyrotropinemia in infancy have a slightly higher serum TSH compared to control children when re-examined in early childhood, suggesting a mild permanent abnormality of thyroid function or a higher setpoint [62]. These infants have a higher prevalence of thyroid morphological abnormalities, antithyroid antibodies and mutations in thyroperoxidase and TSH receptor genes than do controls [63]. In babies whose blood specimen is obtained within the first day or two of life because of early discharge, isolated hyperthyrotropinemia may be due to the cold-induced TSH surge observed postnatally. Maternal heterophile Abs that cross-react in the TSH radioimmunoassay have been implicated in some cases. Isolated hyperthyrotropinemia of unknown etiology has been reported in Japan. Because some affected babies had a normal TSH and T3 response to TRH and the TSH normalized without treatment, the hyperthyrotropinemia was thought to have represented immaturity of the hypothalamo-pituitary-thyroid axis.

Hypothyroxinemia

Hypothyroxinemia with a "normal" TSH is found in 50% of babies with <30 weeks' gestation. Free T4 is often less affected than the total T4. In addition to hypothalamo-pituitary immaturity, premature infants frequently have TBG deficiency due to both immature liver function and undernutrition and may have "sick euthyroid syndrome".

Abnormalities in thyroid binding proteins, particularly TBG, may cause hypothyroxinemia with hyperthyrotropinemia. The incidence of TBG deficiency is 1 in 5000–12 000.

Clinical manifestations

Clinical evidence of hypothyroidism is usually difficult to appreciate in the newborn period. Many of the classic features (large tongue, hoarse cry, facial puffiness, umbilical hernia, hypotonia, mottling, cold hands and feet and lethargy) develop only with the passage of time. Figure 12.8 shows a baby with untreated CH diagnosed clinically compared with an infant in whom the diagnosis was made at 3 weeks of age in the early days of newborn screening. Non-specific signs that suggest the diagnosis of CH include prolonged unconjugated hyperbilirubinemia, gestation

Table 12.3 Comparison of clinical features of thyroid dysgenesis and TSH receptor blocking Ab-induced congenital hypothyroidism (CH).

Clinical feature	Thyroid dysgenesis	Blocking Ab-induced CH
Severity of CH	+ to ++++	+ to ++++
Palpable thyroid	No	No
Ultrasound	No/ectopic thyroid	Eutopic thyroid
123I uptake	None to low	None to normal
Clinical course	Permanent	Transient
Familial risk	No	Yes
TPO Abs	Variable	Variable
TSH receptor Abs	Absent	Potent
Prognosis	Normal	May be delayed

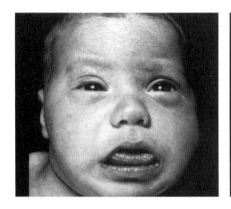 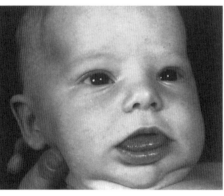

Figure 12.8 Infant with severe untreated congenital hypothyroidism diagnosed clinically before the advent of newborn screening (left), compared with an infant with congenital hypothyroidism identified through newborn screening (right). Note the striking difference in the severity of the clinical features.

>42 weeks, feeding difficulties, delayed passage of stools, hypothermia or respiratory distress in an infant weighing >2.5 kg. A large anterior fontanelle and/or a posterior fontanelle >0.5 cm is frequently present in affected infants.

The extent of clinical findings depends on the cause, severity and duration of the hypothyroidism. Babies in whom severe feto-maternal hypothyroidism was present *in utero* tend to be the most symptomatic at birth. Babies with athyreosis or a complete block in thyroid hormonogenesis tend to have more signs and symptoms than infants with an ectopic thyroid, the most common cause of CH.

Babies with CH are of normal size at birth but subsequent linear growth is impaired if the diagnosis is delayed. Palpable thyroid tissue suggests that the hypothyroidism is caused by an abnormality in thyroid hormonogenesis or thyroid hormone action or that it will be transient.

Laboratory evaluation

Infants detected by newborn screening should be evaluated without delay, preferably within 24 h. The diagnosis is confirmed by the demonstration of a decreased concentration of free T4 and an elevated TSH concentration. Most infants with permanent abnormalities have serum TSH concentration >50 mU/L but infants with less severe CH at birth have a higher incidence of permanent thyroid abnormalities than do babies whose thyroid function is initially normal. Serum T4 concentration is much higher in full-term infants in the first 2 months of life (6.5–16.3 μg/dL; 84–210 nmol/L) than in adults for whom reference values are given by many laboratories; TSH values depend on gestational age and day of life. Measurement of T3 is of little value in the diagnosis of CH.

A bone age X-ray is often performed as a reflection of the duration and severity of the hypothyroidism *in utero*. Thyroid imaging provides information about the location and size of the thyroid gland and is helpful in genetic counseling. A normally placed thyroid gland is likely to represent either transient CH or a defect in thyroid hormonogenesis, almost always an autosomal recessive condition. However, thyroid dysgenesis is usually sporadic, so subsequent offspring have no increased risk as compared with the general population. A radionuclide scan (^{123}I or [99m]pertechnetate)

reflects metabolic activity and is more sensitive than ultrasound in detecting ectopic thyroid tissue, the most common cause of permanent CH, although color Doppler ultrasonography may be better than grayscale [64].

Ectopic thyroid glands may be located anywhere along the pathway of thyroid descent from the foramen caecum to the anterior mediastinum. If scintigraphy is performed, ^{123}I is the preferred isotope because of the greater sensitivity and because ^{123}I, unlike technetium, is organified. Imaging with this isotope allows quantitative uptake measurements and tests for both iodine transport defects and abnormalities in thyroid oxidation. The lowest possible dose of [123]I (usually 25 μCi) should be used. If an organification defect is suspected, a perchlorate discharge test can be performed, sodium perchlorate 10 mg/kg being administered intravenously 2 h after ^{123}I; radioactive iodine uptake is measured before and 1 h later. A normal result is the release of <10% of the radioactive iodine uptake; 10–20% is borderline, >20% is abnormal.

Pertechnetate is cheaper and more widely available than [123]I. There has been is disagreement as to whether thyroid imaging by scintiscan should be performed in all babies because of the unknown risk of radiation exposure, particularly in centers where ^{131}I is used in large doses. For optimal resolution, scintiscan should be performed when the TSH is elevated (>30 μU/mL) but therapy should never be postponed for this procedure. In most babies with classic CH this is not a problem as the TSH remains elevated for at least a week but definitive diagnosis can be postponed until after 3 years of age when most thyroid hormone-dependent brain development is complete. The usual approach is temporarily to discontinue therapy but recombinant hTSH is a promising alternative [65].

Unlike scintiscan, ultrasound does not involve irradiation and can be performed irrespective of thyroid function. Ultrasound will reveal the presence of a eutopic thyroid gland in patients misdiagnosed with agenesis on scintiscan because of decreased RAI uptake, e.g. resulting from iodine excess, TSH potent receptor blocking Abs, a loss-of-function mutation in the TSH receptor or an iodine trapping defect. Ultrasound may also reveal the presence of other structural abnormalities, e.g. hemiagenesis or cysts, but care should be taken not to mistake the ultimobranchial bodies for thyroid tissue.

Autoimmune thyroid disease in the mother or a history of a previously affected sibling should alert the physician to the possibility of TSH receptor-blocking Ab-induced CH but such information is not always reliable. A binding assay is appropriate for screening; bioassay can be performed later to demonstrate the biological action of the Abs. In cases of TSH receptor Ab-induced CH, the blocking activity is extremely potent, half-maximal TSH binding-inhibition being reported with as little as a 1:20 to 1:50 dilution of serum; a weak or borderline result should cause reconsideration of this diagnosis. TPO Abs, although frequently detectable in babies with blocking Ab-induced CH, are neither sensitive nor specific in predicting the presence of transient CH.

Potential clues to the diagnosis of a loss-of-function mutation of the TSH receptor include a normal or decreased serum Tg concentration and/or evidence of a thyroid gland on ultrasound examination despite the failure to visualize thyroid tissue on imaging studies. Verification of the diagnosis requires the demonstration of a genetic abnormality in the TSH receptor gene.

Measurement of urinary iodine is helpful if a diagnosis of iodine-induced hypothyroidism is suspected. An iodide-concentrating defect should be suspected in patients with a family history of CH, particularly if an enlarged thyroid gland is present. The diagnosis is confirmed by the demonstration of a decreased ^{123}I uptake on scan and by a salivary:blood ^{123}I ratio approaching unity. The detailed evaluation of infants suspected of having this and other abnormalities in thyroid hormonogenesis has been described elsewhere [66].

Measurement of Tg is most helpful in distinguishing a defect in Tg synthesis or secretion from other causes of thyroid dyshormonogenesis (iodide trapping defect organification defect). In the former, the serum Tg concentration is low or undetectable despite the presence of an enlarged eutopic thyroid gland but it is high in the latter. Serum Tg concentration reflects the amount of thyroid tissue present and the degree of stimulation and is helpful, in association with ultrasound or scintiscan, to distinguish patients with thyroid agenesis from dysgenesis. Tg is undetectable in most patients with thyroid agenesis and intermediate in babies with an ectopic thyroid gland.

In babies in whom hypothyroxinemia unaccompanied by TSH elevation is found, free T4 should be measured, preferably by a direct dialysis method and the TBG concentration should also be evaluated. A low free T4 in the presence of a normal TBG may suggest secondary or tertiary hypothyroidism, particularly if the patient has microphallus or a midline facial abnormality. In these cases, TRH testing has been recommended to distinguish between pituitary and hypothalamic defects but the utility of this test has been questioned [67]; TRH is not available in the USA. Pituitary function testing and brain imaging should also be performed in these infants.

In premature, low birthweight or sick babies in whom a low T4 and "normal" TSH are found, the free T4 when measured by a direct dialysis method frequently is not as low as the total T4. In these infants, T4 (and/or free T4) and TSH should be repeated every 1–2 weeks until the T4 normalizes because of the rare occurrence of delayed TSH rise. Thyroid function should also be monitored in other infants at risk for delayed TSH rise, such as severely ill babies in an intensive care setting and monozygotic twins in whom fetal blood mixing may initially mask the presence of CH in one of them. Even though many such babies have transient hypothyroidism, treatment should be considered if values do not normalize within 1–2 weeks because a prolonged period of neonatal hypothyroidism, even if transient, could have adverse effects on cognitive development. In any infant, if signs or symptoms suggestive of hypothyroidism are present, thyroid function testing should be repeated because of the possibility of delayed onset of hypothyroidism and because of rare errors in the screening program.

An approach to the investigation of infants with abnormal results on newborn thyroid screening is shown in Fig. 12.9.

Treatment

Replacement therapy with L-T4 should begin as soon as the diagnosis of CH is confirmed. Parents should be counseled regarding the causes of CH, the importance of compliance and the excellent prognosis in most babies if therapy is initiated early. Educational materials should be provided. Treatment need not be delayed in anticipation of performing a thyroid scan as long as the latter is performed within 5–7 days of initiating treatment before suppression of the serum TSH.

An initial dose of 10–15 μg/kg is currently recommended but 50 μg, equivalent to 12–17 μg/kg/day, will result in more rapid normalization of serum T4 and TSH concentrations [68]. Babies with compensated hypothyroidism may be started on the lower dose, while those with severe CH [e.g. T4 < 5 μg/dL (64 nmol/L)], such as those with thyroid agenesis, should be started on the higher dose. Thyroid hormone may be crushed and administered with water, juice or breast milk but care should be taken that all the medicine has been swallowed. Thyroid hormone should not be given with substances that interfere with its absorption, such as iron (including iron-supplemented formula), soy or fiber. Many babies will swallow the pills whole or chew the tablets with their gums before they have teeth. Liquid preparations are unstable and not available commercially in the USA, although they are available elsewhere, e.g. Germany. They should be used only if prepared by a reputable pharmacy.

The aims of therapy are to normalize serum T4 concentration in 3 days and TSH in 2 weeks, to avoid hyperthyroidism and to promote normal growth and development. Adjustments in the dosage are made according to the results of thyroid function tests and the clinical picture. Some infants develop supraphysiologic serum T4 values but the serum T3 concentration usually remains normal; most affected infants are not symptomatic and these short-term T4 elevations are not associated with adverse effects.

Normalization of TSH may be delayed because of relative pituitary resistance but this appears to be less common now than in the past. In such cases, characterized by a normal or increased serum T4 and an inappropriately high TSH, the T4 value is used

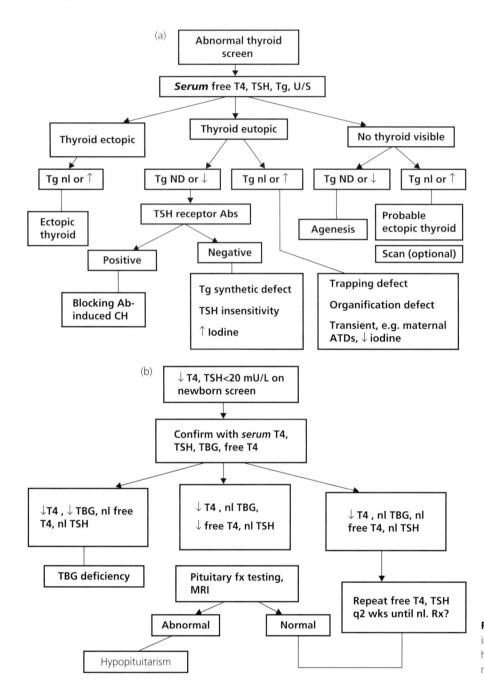

Figure 12.9 Suggested initial approach to the investigation of an infant with congenital hypothyroidism: (a) if TSH is elevated; (b) if TSH is normal. See text for details.

to titrate the dose of medication but non-compliance is the most common cause and should be excluded.

Measurement of T4 and TSH should be repeated every 1–2 weeks until thyroid function tests are normalized, every 1–2 months during the first year of life, every 2–3 months between 1 and 3 years of age and every 3–12 months until growth is complete. In hypothyroid babies in whom an organic basis was not established at birth and in whom transient disease is suspected, a trial off replacement therapy can be initiated after the age of 3 years when most thyroid hormone-dependent brain maturation has occurred. Recombinant hTSH may prove useful in the future, without the need to withdraw T4.

Whether premature infants with hypothyroxinemia should be treated remains controversial [5]. Early retrospective investigations failed to document a difference in cognitive outcome in premature infants with hypothyroxinemia compared with controls but numbers were small. Later a relationship was shown between severe hypothyroxinemia and both developmental delay and disabling cerebral palsy in preterm infants <32 weeks' gestation. Whether the poorer prognosis in these infants was causal or coincidental could not be determined but the serum T4 in premature infants, like in adults, has been shown to reflect the severity of illness and risk of death. There are conflicting results on the effect of therapeutic intervention with T4 or T3 on neurocognitive outcome, mortality rate and respiratory function.

In a placebo-controlled double-blind trial of T4 treatment, 8 µg /kg/day for 6 weeks carried out in 200 infants less than 30 weeks' gestation, no difference in cognitive outcome was found overall but there was an 18-point increase in the Bayley Mental Development Index score in the subgroup of T4-treated infants <27 weeks' gestation when first studied at 2 years of age [69]. Of some concern was the additional finding that treatment with T4 was associated with a 10-point decrease in mental score ($P = 0.03$) in infants >27 weeks' gestation. When these children were restudied at 10 years of age, the mental gap had disappeared but there remained a small insignificant difference in the need for special education and in motor impairment [70]. There remains insufficient evidence to treat premature infants whose serum TSH concentration is normal. In premature babies whose TSH is persistently elevated, 8 µg/kg/day has been recommended.

Prognosis

In early reports, the intellectual quotient (IQ) of affected infants was 6–19 points lower than control babies despite the eradication of severe mental retardation. Although this IQ deficit was small, it was significant as judged by a fourfold increase in the need for special education in affected children. In addition, sensorineural hearing loss, sustained attention problems and various neuropsychological variables were noted, although the frequency and severity of these abnormalities were less than in the prescreening era. Babies most likely to have permanent intellectual sequelae were infants with the most severe *in utero* hypothyroidism as determined by initial T4 level (<5 µg/dL (64 nmol/L) and skeletal maturation at birth. These findings led to the widely held conclusion that some cognitive deficits in most severely affected babies might not be reversible by postnatal therapy.

In the initial programs, a thyroxine dose of 5–8 µg/kg was used and treatment was not initiated until 4–5 weeks of age. Accumulating data from a number of different studies have demonstrated that when a higher initial treatment dose is used (10–15 µg/kg) and treatment is initiated earlier (before 2 weeks), the "developmental gap" can be closed, irrespective of the severity of the CH at birth. An even higher starting dose of 50 µg daily for a full-term infant (corresponding to 12–17 µg/kg) may be even better [71]; dose and timing of onset of therapy are independent variables [72]. Whether or not the higher starting dose is associated with increased behavioral difficulties and attention problems, particularly in less severely affected infants, remains controversial [73]. Therapy with T4 and T3 offers no advantage to T4 alone [74].

Neonatal hyperthyroidism

Transient neonatal hyperthyroidism (neonatal Graves disease)

Unlike CH, which is usually permanent, neonatal hyperthyroidism is almost always transient. It results from the transplacental passage of maternal TSH receptor-stimulating Abs. Hyperthyroidism develops in babies born to mothers with the most potent stimulatory activity in serum, corresponding to 2–3% of mothers with Graves disease or 1 in 50 000 newborns. The incidence is four times higher than that for transient neonatal hypothyroidism caused by maternal TSH receptor-blocking Abs. TSH receptor Ab potency, severity and duration of *in utero* hyperthyroidism and maternal antithyroid medication are all important determinants of neonatal thyroid status (Table 12.4). Most babies born to mothers with Graves disease have normal thyroid function (Table 12.5 [75]).

Some mothers have stimulating and blocking Abs in their circulation, the proportions of which may change. Not surprisingly, the clinical picture in the fetus and neonate of these mothers is complex and depends not only on the relative proportion of each activity in the maternal circulation at any one time but also on the rate of their clearance from the neonatal circulation. Thus, one affected mother gave birth in turn to a normal infant, a baby with transient hyperthyroidism and one with transient hypothyroidism.

In another neonate, the onset of hyperthyroidism did not become apparent until 1–2 months postpartum when the higher affinity blocking Abs had been cleared from the neonatal circulation. In the last case, multiple monoclonal TSH receptor stimulating and blocking Abs were cloned from peripheral lymphocytes in the mother's blood. Each monoclonal Ab recognized different antigenic determinants (epitopes) on the receptor and had different functional properties.

Table 12.4 Situations that should prompt consideration of fetal or neonatal hyperthyroidism.

Fetus or neonatae has unexplained tachycardia
Mother has persistently high TRAb* titer
Mother requires persistently high dose of antithyroid medication
Mother has undergone thyroid ablation
Previous sibling was affected

*TRAb, TSH receptor Ab.

Table 12.5 Thyroid function of neonates born to mothers with Graves disease ($n = 230$). (After Mitsuda *et al.* [75].)

	n	%
Thyrotoxicosis		
Clinical (↑ T4, ↓ TSH)	6	2.6
Chemical (nl T4, ↓ TSH)	7	3.0
Hypothyroidism		
Overt (↓ T4, ↑ TSH)	5	2.2
Subclinical (nl T4, ↑ TSH)	18	7.8
Central hypothyroidism	2	0.9
Euthyroid	192	83.5

Neonatal hyperthyroidism may occur in infants born to hypothyroid mothers, the maternal thyroid having been destroyed by radioablation, surgery or autoimmune processes so that potent thyroid-stimulating Abs present in the maternal circulation are silent in contrast to the neonate whose thyroid gland is normal.

Clinical manifestations

Although maternal TSH receptor Ab-mediated hyperthyroidism may present *in utero*, its onset is usually towards the end of the first week of life both because of the clearance of maternally administered antithyroid drugs from the infant's circulation and the increased conversion of T4 to T3 after birth. The onset of neonatal hyperthyroidism may be delayed if higher-affinity blocking Abs are also present.

Fetal hyperthyroidism is suspected in the presence of fetal tachycardia (pulse >160/min), especially if there is evidence of failure to thrive. Fetal hyperthyroidism does not usually occur before the third trimester when the fetal TSH receptor is upregulated and the concentration of maternal IgG in the fetal circulation increases. The diagnosis is more often appreciated only towards the end of the first week of postnatal life when maternal antithyroid drug is cleared from the baby's circulation. Characteristic signs and symptoms include tachycardia, irritability, poor weight gain and prominent eyes. Goiter may be related to maternal antithyroid drug treatment as well as to the neonatal Graves disease. Infants with neonatal Graves disease may present with thrombocytopenia, hepatosplenomegaly, jaundice and hypoprothrombinemia, a picture that may be confused with congenital infections. Dysrhythmias and cardiac failure may develop and cause death if treatment is delayed or inadequate. In addition to a significant mortality rate that approximates 20% in some older series, untreated fetal and neonatal hyperthyroidism is associated with deleterious long-term consequences, including premature closure of the cranial sutures (cranial synostosis), failure to thrive and developmental delay.

The half-life of TSH receptor Abs is 1–2 weeks. The duration of neonatal hyperthyroidism, a function of Ab potency and metabolic clearance rate, is usually 2–3 months but may be longer.

Laboratory evaluation

Because of the importance of early diagnosis and treatment, fetuses and infants at risk for neonatal hyperthyroidism should undergo clinical and biochemical assessment. A high index of suspicion is necessary in babies of women who have had thyroid ablation because a high titer of TSH receptor Abs would not be evident clinically. Similarly, women with persistently elevated TSH receptor Abs and a high requirement for antithyroid medication during pregnancy are at increased risk of having an affected child.

The diagnosis is confirmed by an increased concentration of T4, free T4, T3 and free T3 accompanied by a suppressed TSH. Fetal ultrasonography may help detect a goiter and monitors fetal growth. Blood can be obtained by cordocentesis and results compared with normal values during gestation. A high titer of TSH receptor Abs in the baby or mother will confirm the etiology of the hyperthyroidism and, in babies whose thyroid function tests are initially normal, indicate the degree to which the baby is at risk. Babies likely to become hyperthyroid have the highest TSH receptor Ab titer, whereas the baby is most unlikely to become hyperthyroid if TSH receptor Abs are not detectable. In this case, it can be anticipated that the baby will be euthyroid, have transient hypothalamo-pituitary suppression or have a transiently elevated TSH, depending on the relative contribution of maternal hyperthyroidism versus the effects of maternal antithyroid medication. Antithyroid drug therapy is rarely necessary. If TSH receptor Ab potency is intermediate, it is likely that the baby will be euthyroid, have a transiently elevated T4 or have transient hypothalamo-pituitary suppression.

The sensitivity of different TSH receptor Ab assays varies, so specific values that are recommended in the literature should be interpreted with caution. In the author's experience, bioassays performed in clinical laboratories are less sensitive than those reported in the literature. Close follow-up of all babies with abnormal thyroid function tests or detectable TSH receptor Abs is mandatory.

Therapy

Treatment of the fetus is accomplished by administration of antithyroid medication to the mother using the minimal dose of PTU or MMI necessary to normalize the fetal heart rate and render the mother euthyroid or slightly hyperthyroid. Treatment is expectant in the neonate. PTU (5–10 mg/kg/day) or MMI (0.5–1.0 mg/kg/day) can be used initially in three divided doses. If the hyperthyroidism is severe, a strong iodine solution (Lugol solution or SSKI, 1 drop every 8 h) is added immediately to block the release of thyroid hormone because the effect of PTU and MMI may be delayed for several days. Therapy with PTU and iodine is adjusted depending on the response. Propranolol (2 mg/kg/day in two or three divided doses) is added if sympathetic overstimulation is severe, particularly in the presence of pronounced tachycardia. If cardiac failure develops, treatment with digoxin should be initiated and propranolol be discontinued.

Prednisone (2 mg/kg/day) may be added for immediate inhibition of thyroid hormone secretion and decreased generation of T3 from T4 in peripheral tissues. Sodium ipodate (0.5 g every 3 days), an iodine-containing radiocontrast material that inhibits thyroid hormone secretion and the conversion of T4 to T3, has been used successfully as the sole treatment. Measurement of TSH receptor Abs in treated babies may be helpful in predicting when antithyroid medication can safely be discontinued. Lactating mothers on antithyroid medication can continue nursing as long as the dose of PTU or MMI does not exceed 400 or 40 mg, respectively. As the milk:serum ratio of PTU is one-tenth that of MMI, a consequence of pH differences and increased protein binding, PTU is preferable to MMI, although relatively low doses of MMI can be given to nursing mothers with no adverse effects on the baby. Higher doses of antithyroid medication require close supervision of the infant.

Permanent neonatal hyperthyroidism

Neonatal hyperthyroidism can be permanent due to a germline mutation in the TSH receptor resulting in its constitutive activation. A gain-of-function mutation of the TSH receptor should be suspected if persistent neonatal hyperthyroidism occurs in the absence of detectable TSH receptor Abs in the maternal circulation. Most cases result from a mutation in exon 10 which encodes the transmembrane domain and intracytoplasmic tail (Fig. 12.2) [4]. Less frequently, a mutation encoding the extracellular domain has been described. Autosomal dominant inheritance has been noted in many of these infants but other cases have been sporadic, arising from a *de novo* mutation. Early recognition is important because the thyroid function of affected infants is frequently difficult to manage medically. When diagnosis and therapy are delayed, irreversible sequelae, such as cranial synostosis and developmental delay, may result. For this reason, early aggressive therapy with thyroidectomy or radioablation has been recommended.

Thyroid disease in childhood and adolescence

Hypothyroidism

Chronic lymphocytic thyroiditis

The causes of hypothyroidism after the neonatal period are listed in Table 12.6. The most frequent cause is chronic lymphocytic thyroiditis (CLT), an autoimmune disease closely related to Graves disease. In both CLT and Graves disease a background inherited predisposition to autoimmunity and additional environmental and hormonal factors that trigger and modulate the disease process appear to be involved [76]. In CLT, lymphocyte and cytokine-mediated thyroid apoptosis predominates, whereas Ab-mediated thyroid stimulation occurs in Graves disease but overlap may occur. Goitrous (Hashimoto thyroiditis) and non-goitrous (primary myxedema; Fig. 12.10) variants of thyroiditis have been distinguished. The disease has a striking predilection for females, and a family history of autoimmune thyroid disease (both CLT and Graves disease) is found in 30–40% of patients. The most common age at presentation is adolescence but the disease may occur at any age, even infancy.

Patients with insulin-dependent diabetes mellitus, 20% of whom have positive thyroid Abs and 5% of whom have an elevated serum TSH level, have an increased prevalence of CLT, which may also occur as part of an autoimmune polyglandular syndrome (APS). In APS 1, also called APECED (autoimmune polyendocrinopathy, candidiasis, ectodermal dystrophy) syndrome, CLT is found in 10% of patients. APS 1 is associated with defective cell-mediated immunity and presents in childhood. It results from a mutation in the AIRE (autoimmune regulator) gene. CLT and diabetes mellitus with or without adrenal insufficiency (APS 2, also referred to as Schmidt syndrome) tends to occur later in childhood or in adults. In addition to the polyglandular syndromes, there is an increased incidence of CLT in patients with Down, Turner, Klinefelter and Noonan syndromes.

Table 12.6 Differential diagnosis of juvenile hypothyroidism.

Primary hypothyroidism

Chronic lymphocytic thyroiditis
Goitrous (Hashimoto)
Atrophic (primary myxedema)

Congenital abnormality
Thyroid dysgenesis
Inborn error of thyroid hormonogenesis

Iodine deficiency (endemic goiter)

Drugs or goitrogens
Antithyroid drugs (PTU, MMI, carbimazole)
Anticonvulsants
Other (lithium, thionamides, aminosalicylic acid, amiodarone, aminoglutethimide)
Goitrogens (cassava, water pollutants, cabbage, sweet potatoes, cauliflower, broccoli, soya beans)

Miscellaneous
Cystinosis
Histiocytosis X
Iatrogenic:
  radioactive iodine
  external irradiation of non-thyroid tumors
  surgery
Mitochondrial disease
Infantile hemangioma

Secondary or tertiary hypothyroidism

Congenital abnormality
Acquired:
  hypothalamic or pituitary tumor (especially craniopharyngioma)
  infiltrative or infectious disease
  trauma
Iatrogenic:
  surgery
  radiation

MMI, methimazole; PTU, propylthiouracil.

CLT may be associated with chronic uriticaria and with immune-complex glomerulonephritis.

Antibodies to Tg and TPO (microsomal), the thyroid Abs measured in routine clinical practice, are detectable in over 95% of patients with CLT. They are useful markers of underlying autoimmune thyroid damage, TPO Abs being more sensitive and specific. TSH receptor Abs are found in a small proportion of patients. When stimulatory TSH receptor Abs are present, they may give rise to a clinical picture of hyperthyroidism, the coexistence of CLT and Graves disease being known as hashitoxicosis. Blocking Abs, however, have been postulated to underlie both the hypothyroidism and the absence of goiter in some patients with primary myxedema but are detectable in only a minority of children. The disappearance of blocking Abs has sometimes been associated with a normalization of thyroid function in previously hypothyroid patients.

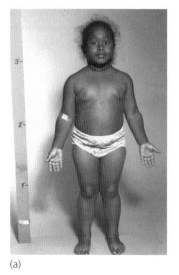
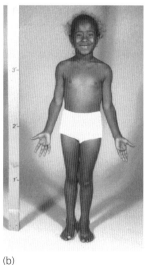

(a)   (b)

Figure 12.10 Ten-year-old female with severe primary hypothyroidism caused by primary myxedema before (a) and after (b) treatment. Presenting complaint was poor growth. Note the dull facies, relative obesity and immature body proportions before treatment. At age 10 years she had not lost a deciduous tooth. After treatment was initiated she lost six teeth in 10 months and had striking catch-up growth. Bone age was 5 years at a chronologic age of 10 years. TSH receptor blocking antibodies were negative.

Goiter, present in approximately two-thirds of children with CLT, results primarily from lymphocytic infiltration and, in some patients, from a compensatory increase in TSH. The role of Abs in goitrogenesis is controversial. Contrary to previous belief, evidence now suggests that primary myxedema arises as a result of independent immune mechanisms and does not represent the "burned out" phase of CLT.

Children with CLT may be euthyroid or may have compensated or overt hypothyroidism. Rarely, they may experience an initial thyrotoxic phase because of the discharge of preformed T4 and T3 from the damaged gland. Alternatively, as indicated above, thyrotoxicosis may be caused by concomitant thyroid stimulation by TSH receptor stimulatory Abs (hashitoxicosis).

Long-term follow-up has suggested that, while most children who are hypothyroid initially remain hypothyroid, spontaneous recovery of thyroid function may occur, particularly in those with initial compensated hypothyroidism. However, some initially euthyroid patients become hypothyroid with observation. Therefore, whether or not treatment is initiated, follow-up is necessary.

Other causes of acquired hypothyroidism
Thyroid dysgenesis and inborn errors of thyroid hormonogenesis
Some patients with thyroid dysgenesis escape detection by newborn screening and present later in childhood with non-goitrous hypothyroidism or with an enlarging mass at the base of the tongue or along the course of the thyroglossal duct. Children with inborn errors of thyroid hormonogenesis may be recognized later in childhood because of the detection of a goiter.

Iodine and other micronutrient deficiency; natural goitrogens
Iodine deficiency is a major public health problem. Endemic cretinism, the most serious consequence, occurs only in areas where the problem is most severe. Hypothyroidism in older infants, children and adults is seen in regions of moderate iodine deficiency. It develops when adaptive mechanisms fail and may be exacerbated by the coincident ingestion of goitrogen-containing foods, such as cassava, soya beans, broccoli, cabbage, sweet potatoes and cauliflower or by water pollutants. Iodine deficiency can be caused by dietary restriction (for multiple food allergies), vegan diet or the result of a fad. Thiocyanate-containing foods (broccoli, sweet potatoes and cauliflower) block trapping and subsequent organification of iodine. Iodine deficiency may be exacerbated by lack of selenium, a component of the selenocysteine thyroid hormone deiodinases.

Drugs
Drugs used in childhood that may affect thyroid function include antithyroid medication, some anticonvulsants, lithium, amiodarone, aminosalicylic acid and aminoglutethimide.

Secondary or tertiary hypothyroidism
Secondary or tertiary hypothyroidism may be recognized later in childhood as a result of damage to the pituitary or hypothalamus by tumours (particularly craniopharyngioma), granulomatous disease, head irradiation, infection (meningitis), surgery or trauma. Other pituitary hormones are often affected, particularly growth hormone and gonadotropins.

Thyroid hormone resistance
Children with thyroid hormone resistance usually come to attention when thyroid function tests are performed because of poor growth, hyperactivity, a learning disability or other non-specific signs or symptoms. A small goiter may be present. The presentation is variable with symptoms of thyroid hormone deficiency or excess but it may be asymptomatic.

In the past, some individuals have been classified as having selective pituitary resistance as distinct from generalized resistance to thyroid hormone because they appeared to have evidence of peripheral hypermetabolism in response to the elevated thyroid hormone levels. Variable levels of expression of the mutant allele have not been demonstrated, so it has been suggested that the variable clinical manifestations of the syndrome are a result of the genetic heterogeneity of the many cofactors that modulate TR expression.

Thyroid hormone resistance is caused most frequently by a point mutation in the hinge region or ligand binding domain of the TRβ gene (Fig. 12.4). As a consequence, there is a dramatic reduction in T3 binding. Less frequently, it results from impaired interaction with one of the cofactors involved in the mediation of thyroid hormone action. Because these mutant TRs interfere with the function of the normal TRs, a dominant pattern of inheritance is seen. In contrast, in the single family with a deletion of all coding sequences of the TRβ gene, only homozygotes manifested resistance.

Rarely, thyroid hormone resistance may be found in patients with cystinosis.

Miscellaneous causes of acquired hypothyroidism

The thyroid gland may be involved in generalized infiltrative (cystinosis), granulomatous (histiocytosis X) or infectious disease processes of sufficient severity to disturb thyroid function. Hypothyroidism may also occur in patients with mitochondrial disease [77]. In infancy, a large hemangioma with high D3 activity can be associated with rapid inactivation of T4 and severe hypothyroidism [78]. Extremely high replacement doses of T4 may be required.

Mantle irradiation for Hodgkin disease or lymphoma and craniospinal irradiation in the treatment of brain tumors may result in hypothyroidism. In the former, primary hypothyroidism develops; in the latter, primary and secondary hypothyroidism may occur.

Clinical manifestations

The onset of hypothyroidism in childhood is insidious. Affected children are usually recognized because of the detection of a goiter or because of poor growth, sometimes for several years before diagnosis. Because height is affected more than weight, affected children are relatively overweight for height, although they rarely are significantly obese. If the hypothyroidism is severe and long-standing, immature facies with an underdeveloped nasal bridge and immature body proportions (increased upper : lower body ratio) may be noted. Dental and skeletal maturation are delayed, the latter often >3 years. Patients with secondary or tertiary hypothyroidism tend to be less symptomatic than those with primary hypothyroidism.

Classic clinical manifestations can be elicited but they are often not the presenting complaints. These include lethargy, cold intolerance, constipation, dry skin or hair texture and periorbital edema. School performance is not usually affected, in contrast to the severe irreversible neuro-intellectual sequelae that occur in inadequately treated babies with CH.

Causes of hypothyroidism associated with a goiter (CLT, inborn errors of thyroid hormonogenesis) should be distinguished from non-goitrous causes (primary myxedema, thyroid dysgenesis, secondary or tertiary hypothyroidism). The typical thyroid gland in CLT is diffusely enlarged and rubbery. Although the surface is classically described as "pebbly" or bosselated, asymmetric enlargement can occur and must be distinguished from thyroid neoplasia. An enlarged pyramidal lobe or Delphian lymph node superior to the isthmus can be found and may be confused with a thyroid nodule. A delayed relaxation time of the deep tendon reflexes may be appreciated in more severe cases.

In patients with severe hypothyroidism of long-standing duration, the sella turcica may be enlarged due to thyrotrope hyperplasia. There is an increased incidence of slipped femoral capital epiphyses. The combination of severe hypothyroidism and muscular hypertrophy, which gives the child a "Herculean" appearance, is known as the Kocher–Debré–Sémélaigne syndrome.

Puberty tends to be delayed in hypothyroid children, although sexual precocity has been described in long-standing severe hypothyroidism. Females may menstruate but commonly have breast development with little sexual hair. Ovarian cysts may be demonstrated on ultrasonography due to follicle-stimulating hormone (FSH) secretion. Galactorrhea due to hyperprolactinemia may occasionally occur. In boys, testicular enlargement may be inappropriate for the stage of puberty.

Laboratory evaluation

Measurement of TSH is the best screening test for primary hypothyroidism. If TSH is elevated, measurement of free T4 will distinguish subclinical (normal free T4) from overt (low free T4) hypothyroidism.

Measurement of TSH is not helpful in secondary or tertiary hypothyroidism, which is demonstrated by a low free T4 with a low TSH. A hypothalamic versus pituitary origin of the hypothyroidism can sometimes be distinguished by TRH testing but the value of this procedure has been questioned. In hypopituitarism, there is little or no TSH response to TRH. TRH is no longer available in the USA. Mild TSH elevation can be seen in individuals with hypothalamic hypothyroidism, a consequence of the secretion of a TSH molecule with impaired bioactivity but normal immunoreactivity.

Thyroid hormone resistance is characterized by elevated levels of free T4 and T3 with an inappropriately normal or elevated TSH concentration. In obese children, a slightly elevated serum T3 concentration that is clinically insignificant may be noted, the consequence of increased T4 to T3 conversion.

CLT is diagnosed by elevated titers of Tg and/or TPO Abs. Ancillary investigations (thyroid ultrasonography and/or thyroid scintigraphy) may be performed if thyroid Ab tests are negative or if a nodule is palpable but are rarely necessary. The typical picture of spotty uptake of radioactive iodine that is seen in adults is rare in children. If thyroid Ab tests are negative and no goiter is present, thyroid ultrasonography and/or scan identify the presence and location of thyroid tissue and thereby distinguish primary myxedema from thyroid dysgenesis. Inborn errors of thyroid hormonogenesis beyond a trapping defect are usually suspected by an increased radioiodine uptake and a large gland on scan.

Therapy

In contrast to CH, rapid replacement is not essential in the older child. This is particularly true in children with long-standing severe thyroid underactivity in whom rapid normalization may result in unwanted side effects (deterioration in school performance, short attention span, hyperactivity, insomnia and behavior difficulties). Replacement doses should be increased slowly over several weeks to months. Severely hypothyroid children should be observed for complaints of headache when therapy is initiated because of the rare development of pseudotumor cerebri.

Full replacement can be initiated at once without much risk in children with mild hypothyroidism. Treatment does not reduce the body mass index (BMI) in most children, except in those with severe hypothyroidism.

Treatment of children with subclinical hypothyroidism (normal T4, elevated TSH) is controversial. Some physicians treat all such patients while others reassess thyroid function in 3–6 months before initiating therapy because of the possibility that the thyroid abnormality will be transient.

Compensated hypothyroidism in adults has been associated with a variety of systemic hypothyroid or neuropsychiatric complaints and with mild lipid abnormalities [79]. Treatment has been advocated for symptom relief and because of the risk of progression to overt hypothyroidism, a risk particularly in older individuals with a positive titre of anti-TPO Abs [80]. An expert US panel recently recommended observation without treatment of adult patients whose TSH level was <10 mU/L regardless of Ab titer [81]. When signs or symptoms suggestive of hypothyroidism are present, L-T4 therapy can be tried.

The typical replacement dose of L-T4 in childhood is $100\ \mu g/M^2$ or 4–6 $\mu g/kg$ for children 1–5 years of age, 3–4 $\mu g/kg$ for those ages 6–10 years and 2–3 $\mu g/kg$ for those 11 years of age and older. In patients with a goiter, a somewhat higher dose to keep the TSH in the low-normal range (0.3–1.0 mU/L in an ultrasensitive assay) is used to minimize its goitrogenic effect. Whether and how patients with thyroid hormone resistance should be treated is controversial [82].

After the child has received the recommended dose for at least 6–8 weeks, T4 and TSH should be measured. Once a euthyroid state has been achieved, patients should be monitored every 6–12 months. Close attention is paid to interval growth and bone age as well as to the maintenance of a euthyroid state. Some children with severe long-standing hypothyroidism at diagnosis may not achieve their adult height potential even with optimal therapy, emphasizing the importance of early diagnosis and treatment. Therapy is usually lifelong.

Asymptomatic goiter

Goiter occurs in 4–6% of schoolchildren in iodine-sufficient areas and is more common (>10%) in areas of iodine deficiency. Like thyroid disease in general, there is a female preponderance of 2–3:1. Patients with goiter are usually euthyroid but may be hypothyroid or hyperthyroid. The most frequent cause of asymptomatic goiter in iodine sufficient areas is CLT.

Non-toxic (simple or colloid) goiter

Non-toxic (colloid) goiter is another cause of euthyroid thyroid enlargement in childhood. There is often a family history of goiter, CLT or Graves disease, leading to the suggestion that non-toxic goiter might also be an autoimmune disease. Thyroid growth immunoglobulins have been identified in some patients with simple goiter but their etiological role is controversial. The cause of non-toxic goiter is unknown but may represent unrecognized borderline iodine deficiency or CLT. Whereas many colloid goiters regress spontaneously, others undergo periods of growth and regression, resulting, ultimately, in the large nodular thyroid glands observed later in life.

Clinical manifestations and laboratory investigation
Clinical examination reveals a diffusely enlarged thyroid gland. Measurement of the serum TSH concentration is the initial approach to diagnosis. In euthyroid patients, TPO and Tg Abs should be measured to exclude CLT; ultrasound examination or thyroid scintiscan can be performed to look for evidence of lymphocytic infiltration in Ab-negative patients but this is rarely indicated. All patients with initially negative thyroid Abs should have repeat examinations because some children with CLT develop positive titers.

Therapy
Thyroid suppression of a euthyroid goiter in children is controversial. A small reduction in the size of the gland [83] in pediatric patients with CLT can be detectable on ultrasonography but is not appreciable clinically [84]. Whether this small effect is sufficient to warrant lifetime therapy is not clear. There is no evidence that treatment affects the underlying thyroiditis and no long-term studies are available in children with colloid goiter. A therapeutic trial may be tried when the goiter is large. In some cases, surgery may be required for cosmesis.

Painful thyroid

Painful thyroid enlargement is rare and suggests either acute (suppurative) or subacute thyroiditis. Occasionally, CLT may be associated with intermittent pain and be confused with the latter disorder. In acute thyroiditis, progression to abscess formation may occur rapidly so prompt recognition and antibiotic therapy is essential. Recurrent attacks and involvement of the left lobe suggest a pyriform sinus fistula between the oropharynx and the thyroid as the route of infection. A pyriform sinus can usually be demonstrated by barium swallow; surgical extirpation will frequently prevent further attacks.

Subacute thyroiditis is characterized by fever, malaise, thyroid enlargement and tenderness. Serum thyroxine may be normal or elevated, the result of the release of preformed T4 and T3 into the circulation. Unlike Graves disease, radioactive iodine uptake is low or absent. A low titer of TPO and Tg Abs may be found and the sedimentation rate is elevated. The thyrotoxic phase generally lasts 1–4 weeks followed by transient hypothyroidism as the thyroid gland recovers. Treatment is supportive and includes large doses of acetylsalicylic acid or other anti-inflammatory drugs. Corticosteroid medication may be helpful in severe cases. Antithyroid medication is not indicated.

Hyperthyroidism

Graves disease

The causes of hyperthyroidism in childhood and adolescence are indicated in Table 12.7. Ninety-five percent are caused by Graves disease, an autoimmune disorder that, like CLT, occurs in a genetically predisposed population. There is a strong female predisposition (6–8:1) and a higher concordance of disease in monozygotic as compared with dizygotic twins. Graves disease is much less common in children than adults, although it can occur at any age, especially in adolescence. Prepubertal children, especially <4 years of age, tend to have more severe disease, require longer medical therapy and achieve a lower rate of remission as compared with pubertal children.

Susceptibility genes and environmental triggers (e.g. viruses, stress, iodine) appear to interact to initiate the characteristic immunologic response. Genetic factors, estimated to account for 70% of the risk for Graves disease, consist of a series of interacting susceptibility alleles of genes important in antigen recognition and/or immune modulation which include HLA-DR3, cytotoxic T lymphocyte-associated factor 4 (CTLA-4), protein tyrosine phosphatase 22 (PTPN22) and CD40. The genes located on the major histocompatibility complex (MHC) influence the presentation of the immunogenic peptide to T cells [76], while CTLA-4 and PTPN22 are inhibitors of T-lymphocyte activation. CD40, a member of the TNF-R receptor family, has an important role in B-cell activation [85].

Polymorphisms of putative antigens, e.g. the TSH receptor and Tg, have also been demonstrated. A specific HLA polymorphism (DRb1-Arg 74) has been demonstrated in the peptide binding pocket of HLA and a potential role in affecting its affinity to putative thyroidal antigens, such as Tg has been hypothesized [86]. Some polymorphisms, e.g. HLA-DR3, CD40 and the TSH receptor, are specific for Graves disease, while others, e.g. CTLA-4, PTPN22 and Tg, are found in patients with Graves disease and CLT.

Graves disease has been described in children with other endocrine and non-endocrine autoimmune diseases which include diabetes mellitus, Addison disease, vitiligo, systemic lupus erythematosus, rheumatoid arthritis, myasthenia gravis, periodic paralysis, idiopathic thrombocytopenia purpura and pernicious anemia. There is an increased risk of Graves disease in children with Down syndrome (trisomy 21) and, perhaps, DiGeorge syndrome (22q11 deletion).

Unlike CLT in which thyrocyte apoptosis is predominant, the major clinical manifestations of Graves disease are hyperthyroidism and goiter. Graves disease is caused by TSH receptor Abs that mimic the action of TSH. Binding of ligand results in stimulation of adenyl cyclase with subsequent thyroid hormonogenesis and growth. TSH receptor-blocking Abs inhibit TSH-induced stimulation of adenyl cyclase. Both stimulatory and blocking TSH receptor Abs bind to the extracellular domain of the receptor and recognize apparently discrete linear epitopes antigen in

the context of a three-dimensional structure but the specific epitope(s) with which they interact continues to be controversial. In some studies, stimulatory Abs bind to the amino-terminal portion of the extracellular domain, while blocking Abs bind to a more carboxy-terminal domain but there is considerable overlap.

The generation of human monoclonal TSH receptor stimulating and blocking Abs and crystyllographic studies of their interaction with the TSH receptor at a molecular level should enhance understanding of binding domains important in TSH action [87]. Studies using monoclonal TSH receptor Abs cloned from patients' peripheral lymphocytes and recombinant mutant TSH receptor have demonstrated that multiple TSH receptor Abs exist each with different specificities and functional activities. In general, blocking Abs are more potent inhibitors of TSH binding than stimulatory ones.

The clinical assessment of TSH receptor Abs (TRAbs) takes advantage of their ability to inhibit the binding of TSH to its receptor [binding assay, e.g. radioreceptor assay, coated tube chemiluminescent assay or enzyme-linked immunosorbent assay (ELISA)] or to stimulate (or inhibit) TSH-induced stimulation of adenyl cyclase (bioassay). TSH receptor Abs measured by binding assay are generally referred to as TRAbs or TSH binding inhibitory immunoglobulins (TBII), whereas those that are measured by bioassay are called thyroid-stimulating Abs (TSAbs) or thyroid stimulating immunoglobulins (TSI). Porcine thyroid membranes or human TSH receptor that has been transfected on Chinese hamster ovary (CHO cells) are used as the source of receptor for binding assays. "Second generation" assays utilize receptors in solid phase ELISA and are more sensitive than the first generation assays in which solubilized porcine membranes were used. Labeled monoclonal TSH receptor Ab has been been substituted for TSH in a "third generation" assay.

Commercial TRAb assays are extremely sensitive and specific, being positive in up to 99% of pediatric patients with Graves disease, but they provide no information about biologic activity, i.e. whether the Abs are stimulators or blockers. Bioassays, although theoretically preferable, are more expensive and more technically demanding. Technical improvements have included the use of CHO cells transfected with hTSH receptor in place of the immortalized rat thyroid FRTL-5 cell line and the development of luminescent bioassays in which a cAMP response element is transfected upstream of a luciferase reporter. Despite these improvements, bioassays that are available clinically tend to be less sensitive than either binding assays or results obtained in research laboratories. In particular, results of assays that utilize the rat FRTL-5 cell line, commonly used in the past, should be interpreted with caution as these cells lose sensitivity with repeated passage.

Seventy percent of children with Graves disease also have TPO and/or Tg Abs in their sera but measurement of these Abs is much less sensitive and specific for the diagnosis of Graves' disease than measurement of TSH receptor Abs [88].

Rarer causes of hyperthyroidism

Hyperthyroidism may be caused by a functioning thyroid adenoma, by constitutive activation of the TSH receptor or be part of the McCune–Albright syndrome. Other rare causes are listed in Table 12.7.

Hyperthyroidism may be caused by inappropriately elevated TSH secretion, the result of a TSH-secreting pituitary adenoma or pituitary resistance to thyroid hormone.

Miscellaneous causes of thyrotoxicosis without hyperthyroidism include the toxic phase of CLT, subacute thyroiditis and thyroid hormone ingestion (thyrotoxicosis factitia). Thyroxine may be abused by adolescents trying to lose weight or be inadvertently eaten by toddlers. When the resultant thyrotoxicosis is severe, treatment with iopanoic acid may be effective [89].

Clinical manifestations

All but a few children with Graves disease present with some degree of thyroid enlargement and most have symptoms and signs of excessive thyroid activity, such as headache, tremor, inability to fall asleep (and fatigue as a result), weight loss despite an increased appetite, proximal muscle weakness, heat intolerance and tachycardia. Often the onset is insidious. Shortened attention span and emotional lability may lead to behavioral and school difficulties. Some patients complain of polyuria and nocturia, the result of an increased glomerular filtration rate. Acceleration in linear growth may occur, often accompanied by advancement in skeletal maturation but adult height is not affected. In the adolescent child, puberty may be delayed. If menarche has occurred, secondary amenorrhea is common.

Physical examination reveals a diffusely enlarged, soft or "fleshy" thyroid gland, smooth skin and fine hair texture, excessive activity and a fine tremor of the tongue and fingers. A thyroid bruit may be audible. A thyroid nodule suggests the possibility of a toxic adenoma. The hands are often warm and moist. Tachy-

Table 12.7 Causes of thyrotoxicosis in childhood.

Hyperthyroidism
Diffuse toxic goiter (Graves disease)
Functioning thyroid adenoma
Toxic multinodular goiter
Gain of function mutation of TSH receptor
McCune–Albright disease
Hydatidiform mole

TSH-induced hyperthyroidism
TSH producing pituitary tumour
"Selective pituitary resistance" to thyroid hormone

Thyrotoxicosis without hyperthyroidism
Chronic lymphocytic thyroiditis
Subacute thyroiditis
Thyroid hormone ingestion

cardia, a wide pulse pressure and a hyperactive precordium are common. Café-au-lait spots, particularly in association with precocious puberty, suggests McCune–Albright syndrome, but if a goiter is absent thyrotoxicosis factitia should be considered. Severe ophthalmopathy is considerably less common in children than in adults, although a stare and mild proptosis are frequent.

Laboratory evaluation

The clinical diagnosis is confirmed by increased concentrations of circulating thyroid hormones. A suppressed TSH excludes TSH-induced hyperthyroidism and pituitary resistance to thyroid hormone in which the TSH is inappropriately "normal" or slightly elevated. If these diseases are suspected, the free α-subunit, which is elevated in patients with a pituitary TSH secreting tumor, should be measured. Elevated levels of T4 in association with inappropriately "normal" levels of TSH may be due to an excess of TBG (either familial or acquired) or to increased T4 binding by a mutant albumin (familial dysalbuminemic hyperthyroxinemia). In the latter cases, free T4, total and free T3 and serum TBG concentration will be normal. An important acquired cause of TBG excess is estrogen excess, e.g. secondary to oral contraceptive use or pregnancy.

If the diagnosis of Graves disease is unclear, TSH receptor Abs should be measured. A binding assay utilizing one of the second or third generation assays is appropriate for initial screening because they are sensitive and technically simple, rapid and reproducible. Bioassay may occasionally be useful in the Graves disease patient who is negative in the binding assay or in treated patients whose clinical picture is discordant with results in the binding assay. Some individuals, initially negative in the binding assay, become positive several weeks later. It has been hypothesized that TSH receptor Ab synthesis in these patients is restricted at first to lymphocytes residing within the thyroid gland itself or, alternately, that TSH receptor Abs escape detection because of binding by soluble TSH receptor circulating in serum. Negative results may also have been due to relative assay insensitivity.

Measurement of TSH receptor Abs may be particularly useful in distinguishing the toxic phase of CLT and subacute thyroiditis (TSH receptor Ab negative) from patients with CLT and Graves disease (hashitoxicosis, TSH receptor antibody positive). As noted above, Tg and/or TPO Abs are often present but are less sensitive and specific than TSH receptor Abs in the diagnosis of Graves disease in childhood. Radioactive iodine uptake and scan are necessary to confirm the diagnosis of Graves disease only in atypical cases (e.g. if measurement of TSH receptor Abs is negative or if the thyrotoxic phase of either CLT or subacute thyroiditis or a functioning thyroid nodule were suspected).

Therapy

The choice of medical therapy, radioactive iodine or surgery should be individualized. Each approach has advantages and disadvantages.

Medical therapy

Thiouracil derivatives (PTU or MMI) are the initial choice of most pediatricians, although radioiodine is gaining increasing acceptance, particularly in non-compliant adolescents, in children who are mentally retarded and in those about to leave home (e.g. to go to college).

PTU, MMI and carbimazole (converted to MMI) exert their antithyroid effect by inhibiting the organification of iodine and the coupling of iodotyrosine residues on the Tg molecule to generate T3 and T4. MMI may be preferred because an equivalent dose requires fewer tablets and has a longer half-life, an advantage in non-compliant adolescents. MMI is associated with a more rapid resolution of hyperthyroidism and the rate of minor side effects appears to be dose-related; severe side effects are seen almost exclusively in patients taking PTU [90]. However, PTU but not MMI inhibits the conversion of T4 to T3, an advantage if the thyrotoxicosis is severe.

The usual initial dose of MMI is 0.5 mg/kg/day given once or twice daily and that of PTU is 5 mg/kg/day given thrice daily. Carbimazole is best given in a dose of 10–20 mg twice or thrice daily, depending on the concentration of the free T4. A European multicentre trial has demonstrated that a low initial MMI dose (10 mg/day) in adults is almost as effective as a high dose (40 mg/day) in normalizing thyroid function tests within 3–6 weeks but whether or not a similar approach would be effective in children who tend to have more severe persistent disease has not been evaluated. In view of the apparent relationship between dose of MMI and side effects, the smallest effective dose necessary to control the hyperthyroidism should be used. In severe cases, a beta-adrenergic blocker (propranolol 0.5–2.0 mg/kg/day given every 8 h) can be added to control cardiovascular hyperactivity.

Concentrations of T4 and T3 normalize in 3–6 weeks but TSH may not return to normal for several months. Measurement of TSH is useful as a guide to therapy only after it has normalized. Once T4 and T3 have fallen by >50% and/or normalized, the dose of thioamide drug can be reduced by 30–50% or a supplementary dose of L-thyroxine be added in a block-replacement regimen when the TSH begins to rise. Advocates of the block-replacement regimen cite fewer hospital visits but a larger MMI dose is required, perhaps resulting in a higher incidence of side effects. Studies suggesting that combined therapy might be associated with an improved rate of remission have not been confirmed. Maintenance doses of PTU have to be given twice daily and of MMI once daily.

As long as patients are compliant, hyperthyroidism is readily controlled with drugs in 90% of individuals. The major difficulty relates to the persistence of the disease in pediatric patients as compared with their adult counterparts. Unlike most adults, in whom TSH receptor Abs disappear from the circulation within 6 months of initiating treatment, TSH receptor Abs remain elevated in >80% of children and adolescents with Graves disease even after 1–2 years of treatment (Fig. 12.11) [91]. The median time to remission is 3–4 years and in one study only 25% of pediatric patients remitted after 2 years, with an additional 25% remitting every 2 years for up to 6 years of ATD therapy [92]. Prepubertal children, especially those <4 years of age, have particularly severe and persistent disease [93]. Thus, treatment for a fixed duration of time, e.g. 1–2 years, as recommended in adults, is likely to result in relapse in many children. In patients who are compliant and in whom the hyperthyroidism can be controlled readily and tapered to a relatively small dose of medication, medical therapy is reasonable and is well tolerated. Lack of eye signs, small goiter and a small drug requirement suggest that drug therapy can be tapered and withdrawn.

Persistence of TSH receptor Abs predicts a high likelihood of relapse. It is not possible to predict at diagnosis which patient is likely to undergo a sustained remission. Lower initial hyperthyroxinemia [T4 <20 μg/dL (257.4 nmol/L); T3 : T4 ratio <20], body mass index, older age (pubertal versus prepubertal age) and lower TRAbs have been associated with an increased likelihood

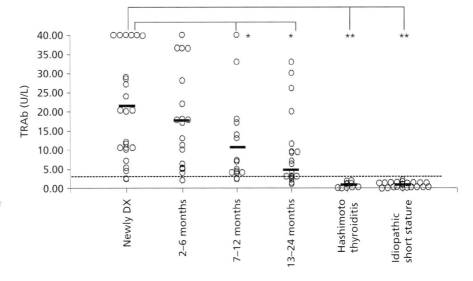

Figure 12.11 Persistence of TSH receptor Abs (TRAbs) in pediatric patients with Graves disease treated with antithyroid medication (cross-sectional analysis). Dashed line (------) indicates upper limit of normal. *$P < 0.05$; **$P < 0.001$. Note that even after 13–24 months, TRAbs had only normalized in <20% of patients. (From Smith & Brown [91] with permission.)

of permanent remission in most studies. Drug withdrawal is usually carried out during school vacation so as to minimize potential interference with school performance. After cessation of ATD therapy, relapses usually occur within 6 months.

Toxic drug reactions (erythematous rashes, urticaria, arthralgias, transient granulocytopenia – <1500 granulocytes/mm³) appear more commonly in children than in adults but the incidence varies depending on the series. These minor side effects, considered to be allergic reactions, are more common in the first few months of therapy and, in patients treated with MMI, appear to be dose-related. Usually they subside spontaneously or with substitution of an alternative thionamide drug; they can be treated with antihistamine therapy so do not warrant discontinuation of the drug. A 20–30% incidence of transient abnormalities in liver enzymes and of mild leukopenia was quoted in one review [94] but, in a review of 651 children from 10 centers treated with antithyroid drugs, the incidence of granulocytopenia was 5.0% and of abnormal liver function 1.9% [95]. The higher estimate probably reflects the use of PTU and/or the underlying Graves disease itself. Transient elevations of SGOT/SGPT (1.1–6 times the upper range of normal) occur frequently in untreated patients and in those treated with PTU; they resolve spontaneously and are not predictive of liver damage [90].

Major side effects [agranulocytosis (<500 granulocytes/mm³), hepatitis, a lupus-like syndrome and thrombocytopenia] are rare. The most serious complication is agranulocytosis, occurring in 0.1–0.5% of cases. Agranulocytosis should be distinguished from the mild granulocytopenia (absolute granulocyte count <1500/mm³) that occurs in patients with Graves disease and resolves spontaneously. This life-threatening complication is more common in the first 3 months of therapy and close monitoring of the white blood cell count during this initial time period was shown to be useful in identifying agranulocytosis before the development of a fever and infection in one study. However, agranulocytosis can occur a year or more after therapy is initiated, even after a prior uneventful course. It occurs more often in adults over the age of 40 years and in patients given larger doses of MMI (>40 mg/day). Because the onset is often abrupt and unpredictable, routine monitoring of the white blood cell count is not usually recommended.

Patients should stop their medication immediately and consult their physician should they develop unexplained fever, sore throat or gingival sores. Medication should also be discontinued if the granulocyte count is <1000/mm³; if the granulocyte count is 1–5000 the patient should be monitored but medication need not be discontinued. Patients who develop agranulocytosis should be hospitalized immediately and ATDs discontinued. Treatment with broad-spectrum antibiotics that include coverage for *Pseudomonas* should be administered intravenously. Granulocyte colony-stimulating factor (G-CSF) is usually recommended, although its benefit is controversial. Because cross-reactivity between MMI and PTU for agranulocytosis is well documented, further treatment with ATDs is contraindicated and affected patients should be treated with radioactive iodine or surgery.

Hepatitis, the second major, potentially fatal, complication of ATD therapy, is more commonly observed with PTU, whereas cholestatic hepatitis typically occurs with MMI [90]. Signs and symptoms include nausea, vomiting, anorexia, malaise and jaundice. Routine liver function tests are not helpful in predicting the development of hepatitis and are not recommended. The risk of hepatitis, like agranulocytosis, appears to be greater within the first 3 months of therapy. Treatment includes discontinuation of ATDs and, frequently, glucocorticoids; rarely liver transplantation has been required.

Systemic vasculitis, the third and rarest side effect of ATD therapy, is also more common with PTU and appears to occur more frequently in Asians. Clinical features include fever, arthritis, hematuria, proteinuria, acute renal failure, vasculitic rash, skin ulcerations and hemorrhage. Antineutrophil cytoplasmic antibody (ANCA) and serologic evidence consistent with systemic lupus erythematosus may be demonstrated. Treatment consists of discontinuation of ATDs. Glucocorticoids, cyclophosphamide and hemodialysis have been required in more severe cases.

Ten percent of children treated medically develop hypothyroidism later in life, a consequence of coincident cell and cytokine-mediated destruction and/or the development of TSH receptor blocking Abs.

Radioactive iodine

Radioactive iodine (RAI; or surgical thyroid ablation) is usually reserved for patients who have failed drug therapy, developed a toxic drug reaction or are non-compliant. RAI is favored increasingly in some centers as the initial approach to therapy [94] because of the ease of administration, the reduced need for follow-up and the lack of adverse effects. However, because the goal of therapy is thyroid ablation, daily medication with thyroxine is being substituted for MMI and continued follow-up is necessary.

RAI should be used with caution in children <10 years of age and particularly in those <5 years of age because of the increased susceptibility of the thyroid gland to the proliferative effects of ionizing radiation. Almost all patients who developed papillary thyroid cancer after the Chernobyl disaster were children <10 years at the time of the accident. The risk of benign thyroid nodules following RAI therapy for Graves disease is also greatest in the first decade of life.

A dose of 50–250 µCi of ^{131}I/estimated gram of thyroid tissue has been used but the higher dose is recommended, particularly in younger children, to ablate the thyroid and thereby reduce the risk of future neoplasia. The size of the thyroid gland is estimated, based on the assumption that the normal gland is 0.5–1.0 g/year of age, maximum 15–20 g. The formula used is:

$$\frac{\text{Estimated thyroid weight in grams} \times 50\text{–}200 \times \mu\text{Ci }^{131}\text{I}}{\text{fractional }^{131}\text{I 24-h uptake}}$$

Some centers administer a fixed dose to all children. Pretreatment with antithyroid drugs before RAI therapy is not necessary unless the hyperthyroidism is very severe.

Thyroid hormone concentrations may rise transiently 4–10 days after RAI administration owing to the release of preformed hormone from the damaged gland. Beta-blockers may be useful. Analgesics may be necessary for the discomfort of radiation thyroiditis. Other acute complications of RAI therapy (nausea, significant neck swelling) are rare. A therapeutic effect within 6 weeks to 3 months is seen.

Worsening of ophthalmopathy described in adults after RAI does not appear to be common in childhood but RAI therapy should be used with caution and treatment with corticosteroids for 6–8 weeks after RAI administration may be wise if significant ophthalmopathy is present; alternatively surgery should be considered.

In 1200 children with Graves disease treated with RAI and followed for 5 to >20 years, there does not appear to be an increased rate of leukemia, thyroid cancer or congenital anomalies in offspring [94] but only a few children were ≤11 years and even fewer were <5 years of age, the population of patients who are most at risk [96]. Given the rarity of thyroid cancer in children (1 in a million) and adults (1 in 100 000), as well as the long latency period, small increases would not be detectable in such a small series.

Surgery

The major advantage of surgery is immediate resolution of hyperthyroidism. Because the goal is to prevent future relapses and because complications of partial and near-total thyroidectomy are similar, near-total thyroidectomy is generally preferred. Surgery is appropriate for patients who have failed medical management, have a markedly enlarged thyroid (>60–80 g), refuse RAI or have significant eye disease.

Pretreatment with antithyroid medication for 4–6 weeks until the hyperthyroidism is controlled followed by iodide (Lugol solution, 5–10 drops daily) for 1–2 weeks to decrease the vascularity of the gland is usually recommended, although successful surgery has been reported after pretreatment with β-adrenergic antagonist drug alone or in combination with iodide for only 10–14 days. Surgery has been associated with a higher morbidity rate than medical therapy or RAI, greatly limiting its popularity.

When the results of six separate studies involving more than 2000 children treated with surgery were pooled, the most common complication (aside from temporary pain and discomfort, present in all patients) was transient hypocalcemia (10%). Keloid formation occurred in 2.8% of patients. Less common side effects were recurrent laryngeal nerve paralysis (2%), permanent hypoparathyroidism (2%) and death (0.08%) [94]. However, in a recent review of 82 children and adolescents from one institution, no instances of either recurrent laryngeal paralysis or permanent hypoparathyroidism were recorded and no patients died [97]. Thus, when an experienced thyroid surgeon is available and modern methods of anesthesia and pain control are used, this therapeutic option is safe and effective. Unfortunately, with the increased use of RAI, there has been a reduction in the number of experienced surgeons.

After RAI or surgical ablation, most patients become hypothyroid and require lifelong thyroid replacement. Inadequate therapy may result in recurrence of hyperthyroidism.

Thyroid storm

This rare, potentially life-threatening manifestation of thyrotoxicosis is characterized by fever (usually >38.5 °F), tachycardia out of proportion to the fever, vomiting, diarrhea and confusion. Untreated patients can develop high output heart failure, coma and die. A number of precipitating factors have been implicated, including infection, stress (e.g. trauma, surgery), non-compliance with ATDs and RAI therapy.

Initial treatment consists of supportive measures to treat infection, rapid reduction of serum and tissue concentrations of thyroid hormones and interference with the peripheral action of thyroid hormones. PTU is preferred to MMI because of its ability in high doses to block the conversion of T4 to T3. PTU 100–200 mg every 4–6 h can be administered orally, rectally or by nasogastric tube. Iodides (e.g. SSKI, five to six drops every 8 h) are recommended to inhibit the release of preformed hormone from the gland but should be given at least 1 h after PTU. Propranolol (2 mg/kg/day orally) will block the adrenergic effects of thyroid hormone while glucocorticoids (e.g. hydrocortisone, 2 mg/kg given as an IV bolus, followed by 36–45 mg/m²/day given in divided doses every 6 h) block the release of thyroid hormone from the thyroid gland; propranolol and glucocorticoids also inhibit T4 to T3 conversion.

Thyrotoxic periodic paralysis

Thyrotoxic periodic paralysis (TPP) is characterized by sudden weakness, hypokalemia and hyperthyroidism. It affects proximal limb muscles ranging from mild weakness to total paralysis. TPP is most common in males of Asian descent. Characteristic electrocardiographic (ECG) findings have been described. TPP is more common in the early morning and can be precipitated by exercise, high carbohydrate intake, alcohol ingestion and stress. The disorder is thought to be related to abnormal plasma membrane permeability to sodium and potassium, a function linked to Na^+-K^+ ATPase activity. Affected patients should be hospitalized for cardiac monitoring, treatment of hypokalemia (maximum 10 mmol/h potassium IV) and initiation of antithyroid medication. Once the patient is stable, thyroid ablation should be performed. In the interim, precipitating factors should be avoided.

References

1 Everett LA, Glaser B, Beck JC, Idol JR, Buchs A, Heyman M, et al. Pendred syndrome is caused by mutations in a putative sulphate transporter gene (PDS). *Nat Genet* 1997; **17**: 411–422.

2 Moreno JC, Bikker H, Kempers MJ, van Trotsenburg AS, Baas F, de Vijlder JJ, et al. Inactivating mutations in the gene for thyroid oxidase 2 (THOX2) and congenital hypothyroidism. *N Engl J Med* 2002; **347**: 95–102.

3 Vassart G, Dumont JE. The thyrotropin receptor and the regulation of thyrocyte function and growth. *Endocr Rev* 1992; **13**: 596–611.

4 Van Sande J, Parma J, Tonacchera M, Swillens S, Dumont J, Vassart G. Somatic and germline mutations of the TSH receptor gene in thyroid diseases. *J Clin Endocrinol Metab* 1995; **80**: 2577–2785.

5 Williams FL, Visser TJ, Hume R. Transient hypothyroxinaemia in preterm infants. *Early Hum Dev* 2006; **82**: 797–802.

6 Eng PH, Cardona GR, Fang SL, Previti M, Alex S, Carrasco N, *et al.* Escape from the acute Wolff–Chaikoff effect is associated with a decrease in thyroid sodium/iodide symporter messenger ribonucleic acid and protein. *Endocrinology* 1999; **140**: 3404–3410.

7 Bianco AC, Salvatore D, Gereben B, Berry MJ, Larsen PR. Biochemistry, cellular and molecular biology and physiological roles of the iodothyronine selenodeiodinases. *Endocr Rev* 2002; **23**: 38–89.

8 Hennemann G, Docter R, Friesema EC, de Jong M, Krenning EP, Visser TJ. Plasma membrane transport of thyroid hormones and its role in thyroid hormone metabolism and bioavailability. *Endocr Rev* 2001; **22**: 451–476.

9 Brent GA. The molecular basis of thyroid hormone action. *N Engl J Med* 1994; **331**: 847–853.

10 O'Shea PJ, Williams GR. Insight into the physiological actions of thyroid hormone receptors from genetically modified mice. *J Endocrinol* 2002; **175**: 553–570.

11 Bernal J. Action of thyroid hormone in brain. *J Endocrinol Invest* 2002; **25**: 268–288.

12 De Felice M, Di Lauro R. Thyroid development and its disorders: genetics and molecular mechanisms. *Endocr Rev* 2004; **25**: 722–746.

13 Fagman H, Grande M, Edsbagge J, Semb H, Nilsson M. Expression of classical cadherins in thyroid development: maintenance of an epithelial phenotype throughout organogenesis. *Endocrinology* 2003; **144**: 3618–3624.

14 Fagman H, Liao J, Westerlund J, Andersson L, Morrow BE, Nilsson M. The 22q11 deletion syndrome candidate gene Tbx1 determines thyroid size and positioning. *Hum Mol Genet* 2007; **16**: 276–285.

15 Fagman H, Grande M, Gritli-Linde A, Nilsson M. Genetic deletion of sonic hedgehog causes hemiagenesis and ectopic development of the thyroid in mouse. *Am J Pathol* 2004; **164**: 1865–1872.

16 Brown RS, Shalhoub V, Coulter S, Alex S, Joris I, De Vito W, *et al.* Developmental regulation of thyrotropin receptor gene expression in the fetal and neonatal rat thyroid: relation to thyroid morphology and to thyroid-specific gene expression. *Endocrinology* 2000; **141**: 340–5.

17 Stein SA, Shanklin DR, Krulich L, Roth MG, Chubb CM, Adams PM. Evaluation and characterization of the hyt/hyt hypothyroid mouse. II. Abnormalities of TSH and the thyroid gland. *Neuroendocrinology* 1989; **49**: 509–519.

18 Campos-Barros A, Amma LL, Faris JS, Shailam R, Kelley MW, Forrest D. Type 2 iodothyronine deiodinase expression in the cochlea before the onset of hearing. *Proc Natl Acad Sci U S A* 2000; **97**: 1287–1292.

19 Bernal J, Guadano-Ferraz A, Morte B. Perspectives in the study of thyroid hormone action on brain development and function. *Thyroid* 2003; **13**: 1005–1012.

20 Anderson GW, Schoonover CM, Jones SA. Control of thyroid hormone action in the developing rat brain. *Thyroid* 2003; **13**: 1039–1056.

21 Farwell AP, Dubord-Tomasetti SA. Thyroid hormone regulates the expression of laminin in the developing rat cerebellum. *Endocrinology* 1999; **140**: 4221–4227.

22 Robson H, Siebler T, Stevens DA, Shalet SM, Williams GR. Thyroid hormone acts directly on growth plate chondrocytes to promote hypertrophic differentiation and inhibit clonal expansion and cell proliferation. *Endocrinology* 2000; **141**: 3887–3897.

23 Robson H, Siebler T, Shalet SM, Williams GR. Interactions between GH, IGF-I, glucocorticoids and thyroid hormones during skeletal growth. *Pediatr Res* 2002; **52**: 137–147.

24 Ball SG, Ikeda M, Chin WW. Deletion of the thyroid hormone beta1 receptor increases basal and triiodothyronine-induced growth hormone messenger ribonucleic acid in GH3 cells. *Endocrinology* 1997; **138**: 3125–3132.

25 O'Shea PJ, Harvey CB, Suzuki H, Kaneshige M, Kaneshige K, Cheng SY, *et al.* A thyrotoxic skeletal phenotype of advanced bone formation in mice with resistance to thyroid hormone. *Mol Endocrinol* 2003; **17**: 1410–1424.

26 Akita S, Nakamura T, Hirano A, Fujii T, Yamashita S. Thyroid hormone action on rat calvarial sutures. *Thyroid* 1994; **4**: 99–106.

27 Roti E, Gnudi A, Braverman LE. The placental transport, synthesis and metabolism of hormones and drugs which affect thyroid function. *Endocr Rev* 1983; **4**: 131–149.

28 Morreale de Escobar G, Obregon MJ, Escobar del Rey F. Is neuropsychological development related to maternal hypothyroidism or to maternal hypothyroxinemia? *J Clin Endocrinol Metab* 2000; **85**: 3975–3987.

29 Cao XY, Jiang XM, Dou ZH, Rakeman MA, Zhang ML, O'Donnell K, *et al.* Timing of vulnerability of the brain to iodine deficiency in endemic cretinism. *N Engl J Med* 1994; **331**: 1739–1744.

30 de Zegher F, Pernasetti F, Vanhole C, Devlieger H, Van den Berghe G, Martial JA. The prenatal role of thyroid hormone evidenced by fetomaternal Pit-1 deficiency. *J Clin Endocrinol Metab* 1995; **80**: 3127–3130.

31 Matsuura N, Konishi J. Transient hypothyroidism in infants born to mothers with chronic thyroiditis: a nationwide study of twenty-three cases. The Transient Hypothyroidism Study Group. *Endocrinol Jpn* 1990; **37**: 369–379.

32 Haddow JE, Palomaki GE, Allan WC, Williams JR, Knight GJ, Gagnon J, *et al.* Maternal thyroid deficiency during pregnancy and subsequent neuropsychological development of the child. *N Engl J Med* 1999; **341**: 549–555.

33 Pop VJ, Kuijpens JL, van Baar AL, Verkerk G, van Son MM, de Vijlder JJ, *et al.* Low maternal free thyroxine concentrations during early pregnancy are associated with impaired psychomotor development in infancy. *Clin Endocrinol (Oxf)* 1999; **50**: 149–155.

34 Thorpe-Beeston JG, Nicolaides KH, McGregor AM. Fetal thyroid function. *Thyroid* 1992; **2**: 207–217.

35 Mercado M, Yu VY, Francis I, Szymonowicz W, Gold H. Thyroid function in very preterm infants. *Early Hum Dev* 1988; **16**: 131–141.

36 Williams FL, Simpson J, Delahunty C, Ogston SA, Bongers-Schokking JJ, Murphy N, *et al.* Developmental trends in cord and postpartum serum thyroid hormones in preterm infants. *J Clin Endocrinol Metab* 2004; **89**: 5314–5320.

37 Deming DD, Rabin CW, Hopper AO, Peverini RL, Vyhmeister NR, Nelson JC. Direct equilibrium dialysis compared with two non-dialysis free T4 methods in premature infants. *J Pediatr* 2007; **151**: 404–408.

38 Ares S, Escobar-Morreale HF, Quero J, Duran S, Presas MJ, Herruzo R, *et al.* Neonatal hypothyroxinemia: effects of iodine intake and premature birth. *J Clin Endocrinol Metab* 1997; **82**: 1704–1712.

39 Frank JE, Faix JE, Hermos RJ, Mullaney DM, Rojan DA, Mitchell ML, *et al.* Thyroid function in very low birth weight infants: effects on neonatal hypothyroidism screening. *J Pediatr* 1996; **128**: 548–554.

40 Zurakowski D, Di Canzio J, Majzoub JA. Pediatric reference intervals for serum thyroxine, triiodothyronine, thyrotropin and free thyroxine. *Clin Chem* 1999; **45**: 1087–1091.

41 Delange FM. Iodine Deficiency. In: Braverman LE, Utiger RD, eds. *Werner & Ingbar's The Thyroid*, 8th edn. Philadelphia: Lippincott Williams & Wilkins; 2000.

42 Boyages SC. Clinical review 49: iodine deficiency disorders. *J Clin Endocrinol Metab* 1993; **77**: 587–591.

43 Lanting CI, van Tijn DA, Loeber JG, Vulsma T, de Vijlder JJ, Verkerk PH. Clinical effectiveness and cost-effectiveness of the use of the thyroxine/thyroxine-binding globulin ratio to detect congenital hypothyroidism of thyroidal and central origin in a neonatal screening program. *Pediatrics* 2005; **116**: 168–173.

44 Fisher D. Next generation newborn screening for congenital hypothyroidism? *J Clin Endocrinol Metab* 2005; **90**: 3797–3799.

45 van Tijn DA, de Vijlder JJ, Verbeeten B Jr, Verkerk PH, Vulsma T. Neonatal detection of congenital hypothyroidism of central origin. *J Clin Endocrinol Metab* 2005; **90**: 3350–3359.

46 Harris KB, Pass KA. Increase in congenital hypothyroidism in New York State and in the United States. *Mol Genet Metab* 2007; **91**: 268–277.

47 Kempers MJ, Lanting CI, van Heijst AF, van Trotsenburg AS, Wiedijk BM, de Vijlder JJ, *et al.* Neonatal screening for congenital hypothyroidism based on thyroxine, thyrotropin and thyroxine-binding globulin measurement: potentials and pitfalls. *J Clin Endocrinol Metab* 2006; **91**: 3370–3376.

48 Hunter MK, Mandel SH, Sesser DE, Miyabira RS, Rien L, Skeels MR, *et al.* Follow-up of newborns with low thyroxine and non-elevated thyroid-stimulating hormone-screening concentrations: results of the 20-year experience in the Northwest Regional Newborn Screening Program. *J Pediatr* 1998; **132**: 70–74.

49 Larson C, Hermos R, Delaney A, Daley D, Mitchell M. Risk factors associated with delayed thyrotropin elevations in congenital hypothyroidism. *J Pediatr* 2003; **143**: 587–591.

50 Perry R, Heinrichs C, Bourdoux P, Khoury K, Szots F, Dussault JH, *et al.* Discordance of monozygotic twins for thyroid dysgenesis: implications for screening and for molecular pathophysiology. *J Clin Endocrinol Metab* 2002; **87**: 4072–4077.

51 Adams LM, Emery JR, Clark SJ, Carlton EI, Nelson JC. Reference ranges for newer thyroid function tests in premature infants. *J Pediatr* 1995; **126**: 122–127.

52 Brown RS, Demmer LA. The etiology of thyroid dysgenesis: still an enigma after all these years. *J Clin Endocrinol Metab* 2002; **87**: 4069–4071.

53 Kopp P. Pendred's syndrome: identification of the genetic defect a century after its recognition. *Thyroid* 1999; **9**: 65–69.

54 Gillam MP, Kopp P. Genetic defects in thyroid hormone synthesis. *Curr Opin Pediatr* 2001; **13**: 364–372.

55 Moreno JC, Klootwijk W, van Toor H, Pinto G, D'Alessandro M, Leger A, *et al.* Mutations in the iodotyrosine deiodinase gene and hypothyroidism. *N Engl J Med* 2008; **358**: 1811–1818.

56 Jordan N, Williams N, Gregory JW, Evans C, Owen M, Ludgate M. The W546X mutation of the thyrotropin receptor gene: potential major contributor to thyroid dysfunction in a Caucasian population. *J Clin Endocrinol Metab* 2003; **88**: 1002–1005.

57 Djemli A, Van Vliet G, Delvin EE. Congenital hypothyroidism: from paracelsus to molecular diagnosis. *Clin Biochem* 2006; **39**: 511–518.

58 Dumitrescu AM, Liao XH, Best TB, Brockmann K, Refetoff S. A novel syndrome combining thyroid and neurological abnormalities is associated with mutations in a monocarboxylate transporter gene. *Am J Hum Genet* 2004; **74**: 168–175.

59 Dumitrescu AM, Liao XH, Abdullah MS, Lado-Abeal J, Majed FA, Moeller LC, *et al.* Mutations in SECISBP2 result in abnormal thyroid hormone metabolism. *Nat Genet* 2005; **37**: 1247–1252.

60 Brown RS, Bloomfield S, Bednarek FJ, Mitchell ML, Braverman LE. Routine skin cleansing with povidone-iodine is not a common cause of transient neonatal hypothyroidism in North America: a prospective controlled study. *Thyroid* 1997; **7**: 395–400.

61 Brown RS, Bellisario RL, Botero D, Fournier L, Abrams CA, Cowger ML, *et al.* Incidence of transient congenital hypothyroidism due to maternal thyrotropin receptor-blocking antibodies in over one million babies. *J Clin Endocrinol Metab* 1996; **81**: 1147–1151.

62 Daliva AL, Linder B, DiMartino-Nardi J, Saenger P. Three-year follow-up of borderline congenital hypothyroidism. *J Pediatr* 2000; **136**: 53–56.

63 Calaciura F, Motta RM, Miscio G, Fichera G, Leonardi D, Carta A, *et al.* Subclinical hypothyroidism in early childhood: a frequent outcome of transient neonatal hyperthyrotropinemia. *J Clin Endocrinol Metab* 2002; **87**: 3209–3214.

64 Ohnishi H, Sato H, Noda H, Inomata H, Sasaki N. Color Doppler ultrasonography: diagnosis of ectopic thyroid gland in patients with congenital hypothyroidism caused by thyroid dysgenesis. *J Clin Endocrinol Metab* 2003; **88**: 5145–5149.

65 Tiosano D, Even L, Shen Orr Z, Hochberg Z. Recombinant thyrotropin in the diagnosis of congenital hypothyroidism. *J Clin Endocrinol Metab* 2007; **92**: 1434–1437.

66 Gruters A, Finke R, Krude H, Meinhold H. Etiological grouping of permanent congenital hypothyroidism with a thyroid gland *in situ*. *Horm Res* 1994; **41**: 3–9.

67 Mehta A, Hindmarsh PC, Stanhope RG, Brain CE, Preece MA, Dattani MT. Is the thyrotropin-releasing hormone test necessary in the diagnosis of central hypothyroidism in children. *J Clin Endocrinol Metab* 2003; **88**: 5696–5703.

68 Selva KA, Mandel SH, Rien L, Sesser D, Miyahira R, Skeels M, *et al.* Initial treatment dose of L-thyroxine in congenital hypothyroidism. *J Pediatr* 2002; **141**: 786–792.

69 van Wassenaer AG, Kok JH, de Vijlder JJ, Briet JM, Smit BJ, Tamminga P, *et al.* Effects of thyroxine supplementation on neurologic development in infants born at less than 30 weeks' gestation. *N Engl J Med* 1997; **336**: 21–26.

70 van Wassenaer AG, Westera J, Houtzager BA, Kok JH. Ten-year follow-up of children born at <30 weeks' gestational age supplemented with thyroxine in the neonatal period in a randomized, controlled trial. *Pediatrics* 2005; **116**: e613–618.

71 Selva KA, Harper A, Downs A, Blasco PA, Lafranchi SH. Neurodevelopmental outcomes in congenital hypothyroidism: comparison of initial T4 dose and time to reach target T4 and TSH. *J Pediatr* 2005; **147**: 775–780.

72 Bongers-Schokking JJ, Koot HM, Wiersma D, Verkerk PH, de Muinck Keizer-Schrama SM. Influence of timing and dose of thyroid hormone replacement on development in infants with congenital hypothyroidism. *J Pediatr* 2000; **136**: 292–297.

73 Rovet JF. In search of the optimal therapy for congenital hypothyroidism. *J Pediatr* 2004; **144**: 698–700.

74 Cassio A, Cacciari E, Cicognani A, Damiani G, Missiroli G, Corbelli E, *et al.* Treatment for congenital hypothyroidism: thyroxine alone or thyroxine plus triiodothyronine? *Pediatrics* 2003; **111** (5 Pt 1): 1055–1060.

75 Mitsuda N, Tamaki H, Amino N, Hosono T, Miyai K, Tanizawa O. Risk factors for developmental disorders in infants born to women with Graves disease. *Obstet Gynecol* 1992; **80** (3 Pt 1): 359–364.

76 Vaidya B, Kendall-Taylor P, Pearce SH. The genetics of autoimmune thyroid disease. *J Clin Endocrinol Metab* 2002; **87**: 5385–5397.

77 Chinnery PF, Turnbull DM. Mitochondrial medicine. *Q J Med* 1997; **90**: 657–667.

78 Huang SA, Tu HM, Harney JW, Venihaki M butte AJ, Kozakewich HP, *et al.* Severe hypothyroidism caused by type 3 iodothyronine deiodinase in infantile hemangiomas. *N Engl J Med* 2000; **343**: 185–189.

79 Danese D, Sciacchitano S, Farsetti A andreoli M, Pontecorvi A. Diagnostic accuracy of conventional versus sonography-guided fine-needle aspiration biopsy of thyroid nodules. *Thyroid* 1998; **8**: 15–21.

80 Cooper DS. Antithyroid drugs in the management of patients with Graves' disease: an evidence-based approach to therapeutic controversies. *J Clin Endocrinol Metab* 2003; **88**: 3474–3481.

81 Surks MI ortiz E, Daniels GH, Sawin CT, Col NF, Cobin RH, *et al.* Subclinical thyroid disease: scientific review and guidelines for diagnosis and management. *JAMA* 2004; **291**: 228–238.

82 Weiss RE, Refetoff S. Treatment of resistance to thyroid hormone: primum non nocere. *J Clin Endocrinol Metab* 1999; **84**: 401–404.

83 Svensson J, Ericsson UB, Nilsson P, Olsson C, Jonsson B, Lindberg B, *et al.* Levothyroxine treatment reduces thyroid size in children and adolescents with chronic autoimmune thyroiditis. *J Clin Endocrinol Metab* 2006; **91**: 1729–1734.

84 Rother KI, Zimmerman D, Schwenk WF. Effect of thyroid hormone treatment on thyromegaly in children and adolescents with Hashimoto disease. *J Pediatr* 1994; **124**: 599–601.

85 Jacobson EM, Tomer Y. The genetic basis of thyroid autoimmunity. *Thyroid* 2007; **17**: 949–961.

86 Jacobson EM, Huber A, Tomer Y. The HLA gene complex in thyroid autoimmunity: from epidemiology to etiology. *J Autoimmun* 2008; **30**: 58–62.

87 Smith BR, Sanders J, Furmaniak J. TSH receptor antibodies. *Thyroid* 2007; **17**: 923–938.

88 Botero D, Brown RS. Bioassay of thyrotropin receptor antibodies with Chinese hamster ovary cells transfected with recombinant human thyrotropin receptor: clinical utility in children and adolescents with Graves disease. *J Pediatr* 1998; **132**: 612–618.

89 Brown RS, Cohen JH 3rd, Braverman LE. Successful treatment of massive acute thyroid hormone poisoning with iopanoic acid. *J Pediatr* 1998; **132**: 903–905.

90 Cooper DS. Antithyroid drugs. *N Engl J Med* 2005; **352**: 905–917.

91 Smith J, Brown RS. Persistence of thyrotropin (TSH) receptor antibodies in children and adolescents with Graves' disease treated using antithyroid medication. *Thyroid* 2007; **17**: 1103–1107.

92 Lippe BM, Landaw EM, Kaplan SA. Hyperthyroidism in children treated with long term medical therapy: twenty-five percent remission every two years. *J Clin Endocrinol Metab* 1987; **64**: 1241–1245.

93 Segni M, Leonardi E, Mazzoncini B, Pucarelli I, Pasquino AM. Special features of Graves' disease in early childhood. *Thyroid* 1999; **9**: 871–877.

94 Rivkees SA, Sklar C, Freemark M. Clinical review 99: The management of Graves' disease in children, with special emphasis on radioiodine treatment. *J Clin Endocrinol Metab* 1998; **83**: 3767–3776.

95 Zimmerman D, Lteif AN. Thyrotoxicosis in children. *Endocrinol Metab Clin North Am* 1998; **27**: 109–126.

96 Read CH, Jr., Tansey MJ, Menda Y. A 36-year retrospective analysis of the efficacy and safety of radioactive iodine in treating young Graves' patients. *J Clin Endocrinol Metab* 2004; **89**: 4229–4233.

97 Sherman J, Thompson GB, Lteif A, Schwenk WF 2nd, van Heerden J, Farley DR, *et al.* Surgical management of Graves disease in childhood and adolescence: an institutional experience. *Surgery* 2006; **140**: 1056–1061; discussion 61–62.

98 Fisher DA, Klein AH. Thyroid development and disorders of thyroid function in the newborn. *N Engl J Med* 1981; **304**: 702–712.

99 Brown RS, Larson, PR. Thyroid gland development and disease in infancy and childhood. In: *Thyroid Disease Manager*, 1999: http://thyroidmanager.org

13 The Adrenal Cortex and its Disorders

Walter L. Miller

Department of Pediatrics, University of California, San Francisco, CA, USA

Embryology, anatomy and history

The adrenal cortex produces three categories of steroid hormones. *Mineralocorticoids*, principally aldosterone, regulate renal retention of sodium, which influences electrolyte balance, intravascular volume and blood pressure. *Glucocorticoids*, principally cortisol, are named for their carbohydrate-mobilizing activity but influence a wide variety of bodily functions. *Adrenal androgens* modulate the mid-childhood growth spurt and regulate some secondary sexual characteristics in women; their overproduction may result in virilism.

Embryology

The cells of the adrenal cortex are mesodermal, in contrast to the ectodermal adrenal medulla. Between 5 and 6 weeks post-conception, the "gonadal ridge" develops near the rostral end of the mesonephros. These cells give rise to the steroidogenic cells of the gonads and the adrenal cortex. The adrenal and gonadal cells separate, with the adrenal cells migrating retroperitoneally and the gonadal cells migrating caudally. Between the seventh and eighth weeks, the adrenal cells are invaded by sympathetic neural cells that give rise to the adrenal medulla. By the end of the eighth week, the adrenal has become encapsulated and is clearly associated with the upper pole of the kidney, which is much smaller than the adrenal.

The fetal adrenal cortex consists of an outer "definitive" zone, the principal site of glucocorticoid and mineralocorticoid synthesis and a much larger "fetal" zone that makes androgenic precursors for the placental synthesis of estriol. The fetal adrenal gland is huge in proportion to other structures. At birth, the adrenals weigh 8–9 g, roughly the size of adult adrenals and represent 0.5% of total body weight, compared with 0.0175% in the adult.

Brook's Clinical Pediatric Endocrinology, 6th edition. Edited by C. Brook, P. Clayton, R. Brown. © 2009 Blackwell Publishing, ISBN: 978-1-4051-8080-1.

Anatomy

The adrenals derive their name from their anatomical location, located on top of the upper pole of each kidney. Unlike most other organs, the arteries and veins serving the adrenal do not run in parallel. Arterial blood is provided by several small arteries arising from the renal and phrenic arteries, the aorta and, sometimes, the ovarian and left spermatic arteries. The veins are more conventional, with the left adrenal vein draining into the left renal vein and the right adrenal vein draining directly into the vena cava. Arterial blood enters the sinusoidal circulation of the cortex and drains toward the medulla, so that medullary chromaffin cells are bathed in high concentrations of steroid hormones. High concentrations of cortisol are needed for expression of phenylethanolamine-N-methyltransferase, which converts norepinephrine to epinephrine, linking the steroidal and catecholamine responses to stress.

The adrenal cortex consists of three histologically recognizable zones: the *glomerulosa* is immediately below the capsule, the *fasciculata* is in the middle and the *reticularis* lies next to the medulla, constituting 15%, 75% and 10%, respectively, of the adrenal cortex in the older child and adult. The zones appear to be distinct functionally as well as histologically but considerable overlap exists, and immunocytochemical data show that the zones physically interdigitate. After birth, the large fetal zone begins to involute and disappears by 1 year of age. The definitive zone enlarges simultaneously but two of the adult zones, the glomerulosa and the fasciculata, are not fully differentiated until about 3 years of age and the reticularis may not be fully differentiated until about 15 years of age.

History

The adrenal glands were first described in 1563 by the Italian anatomist Bartolomeo Eustaccio, better known for the eustachian tube of the ear. Medical interest in them as something other than an anatomical curiosity began in the mid-19th century with Addison's classic description of adrenal insufficiency and Brown-Séquard's experimental creation of similar disorders in animals subjected to adrenalectomy. The signs and symptoms of glucocorticoid excess due to adrenal tumors were well known by 1932, when Cushing described the pituitary tumors that cause what is now known as Cushing syndrome. Effects of adrenalectomy on salt and water metabolism were reported in 1927 and, by the late 1930s, Selye had proposed the terms "glucocorticoid" and "mineralocorticoid" to distinguish the two broad categories of actions of adrenal extracts.

Numerous adrenal steroids were painstakingly isolated and their structures determined during the 1930s in the laboratories of Reichstein and Kendall, leading to their sharing the 1950 Nobel Prize for Medicine. Many of these steroids were synthesized chemically, providing pure material for experimental purposes. The observation in 1949 that glucocorticoids ameliorated the symptoms of rheumatoid arthritis greatly stimulated interest in synthesizing new pharmacologically active analogs of naturally occurring steroids. The structures of the various adrenal steroids suggested precursor–product relationships, leading in 1950 to the first treatment of congenital adrenal hyperplasia (CAH) with cortisone. This opened a vigorous era of clinical investigation of the pathways of steroidogenesis in a variety of inherited adrenal and gonadal disorders. The association of cytochrome P450 with 21-hydroxylation was made in 1965 and some of the steroidogenic enzymes were then isolated in the 1970s. It was not until the genes for most of these enzymes were cloned in the 1980s that it became clear which proteins participated in which steroidal transformations. The identification of these genes (Table 13.1) then led to an understanding of the genetic lesions causing heritable disorders of steroidogenesis. At the same time, studies of steroid hormone action led to the discovery of steroid hormone receptors in the 1960s but it was not until they were cloned that their biology was understood.

Steroid hormone synthesis

Early steps: cholesterol uptake, storage and transport

The adrenal gland can synthesize cholesterol *de novo* from acetate but most of its cholesterol comes from plasma low-density lipoproteins (LDL) derived from dietary cholesterol. Adequate concentrations of LDL will suppress 3-hydroxy3-methylglutaryl coenzyme A (HMGCoA) reductase, the rate-limiting enzyme in cholesterol synthesis. Adrenocorticotropic hormone (ACTH), which stimulates adrenal steroidogenesis, also stimulates the activity of HMGCoA reductase, LDL receptors and uptake of LDL-cholesterol. LDL-cholesterol esters are taken up by receptor-mediated endocytosis and are then stored directly or converted to free cholesterol and used for steroid hormone synthesis. Storage of cholesterol esters in lipid droplets is controlled by the action of two opposing enzymes: cholesterol esterase (cholesterol ester hydrolase) and cholesterol ester synthetase. ACTH stimulates the esterase and inhibits the synthetase, thus increasing the availability of free cholesterol for steroid hormone synthesis.

Steroidogenic enzymes
Cytochrome P450

Most steroidogenic enzymes are members of the cytochrome P450 group of oxidases [1]. Cytochrome P450 is a generic term for a large number of oxidative enzymes, all of which have about 500 amino acids and contain a single heme group. They are termed P450 (pigment 450) because all absorb light at 450 nm in their reduced states. It is sometimes stated that certain steroidogenic enzymes are P450-dependent enzymes. This is a misnomer, because it implies a generic P450 cofactor to a substrate-specific

Table 13.1 Physical characteristics of human genes encoding steroidogenic enzymes.

Enzyme	Number of genes	Gene size (kb)	Chromosomal location	Exons (n)	mRNA size (kb)
P450scc	1	>20	15q23–q24	9	2.0
P450c11	2	9.5	8q21–22	9	4.2
P450c17	1	6.6	10q24.3	8	1.9
P450c21	2	3.4	6p21.1	10	2.0
P450aro	1	>52	15q21.2	10	3.5, 2.9
3β-HSD-I and -II	2	8	1p13	4	1.7
11β-HSD-I	1	7	1	6	1.6
11β-HSD-II	1	6.2	16p22	5	1.6
17β-HSD-I	2	3.3	17q21	6	1.4, 2.4
17β-HSD-II	1	>40	16q24	5	1.5
17β-HSD-III	1	>60	9q22	11	1.4
Adrenodoxin	1	>30	11q22	5	1.0, 1.4, 1.7
Adrenodoxin reductase	1	11	17q24–q25	12	2.0
P450 oxidoreductase	1	69	7q11.2	16	2.5
5α-Reductase – type 1	1	>35	5p15	5	2.4
5α-Reductase – type 2	1	>35	2p23	5	2.4

enzyme; the P450 *is* the enzyme binding the steroidal substrate and catalyzing the steroidal conversion on an active site associated with the heme group. Most cytochrome P450 enzymes are found in the endoplasmic reticulum of the liver, where they metabolize countless endogenous and exogenous toxins, drugs, xenobiotics and environmental pollutants. Despite this huge variety of substrates, the Human Genome Project has shown that humans have only 57 distinct P450 genes. The overwhelming majority of drugs that undergo hepatic degradation are metabolized by only eight P450 enzymes. Thus, P450 enzymes can metabolize multiple substrates, catalyzing a broad array of oxidations. This theme recurs with each adrenal P450 enzyme.

Five distinct P450 enzymes are involved in adrenal steroidogenesis (Fig. 13.1). P450scc, found in adrenal mitochondria, is the cholesterol side-chain cleavage enzyme catalyzing the series of reactions formerly termed 20,22-desmolase. Two distinct isozymes of P450c11, P450c11β and P450c11AS, also found in mitochondria, catalyze 11β-hydroxylase, 18-hydroxylase and 18-methyl oxidase activities. P450c17, found in the endoplasmic reticulum, catalyzes both 17α-hydroxylase and 17,20-lyase activities and P450c21 catalyzes the 21-hydroxylation of both glucocorticoids and mineralocorticoids. In the gonads (and elsewhere), P450aro in the endoplasmic reticulum catalyzes aromatization of androgens to estrogens and four other P450 enzymes, P450c1α, P450c24, P450c27 and P4502R1, are responsible for the activation and degradation of vitamin D [2].

Hydroxysteroid dehydrogenases

In addition to the cytochrome P450 enzymes, a second class of enzymes termed hydroxysteroid dehydrogenases (HSDs) is also

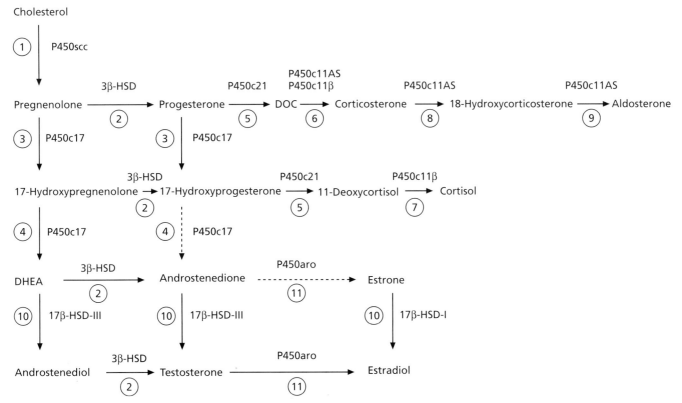

Figure 13.1 Principal pathways of human adrenal steroid hormone synthesis. Other quantitatively and physiologically minor steroids are also produced. The names of the enzymes are shown by each reaction and the traditional names of the enzymatic activities correspond to the circled numbers. Reaction 1, mitochondrial cytochrome P450scc mediates 20α-hydroxylation, 22-hydroxylation and cleavage of the C20–22 carbon bond. Reaction 2, 3β-HSD mediates 3β-hydroxysteroid dehydrogenase and isomerase activities, converting Δ⁵ steroids to Δ⁴ steroids. Reaction 3, P450c17 catalyzes the 17α-hydroxylation of pregnenolone to 17-OH pregnenolone and of progesterone to 17-OH progesterone. Reaction 4, the 17,20-lyase activity of P450c17 converts 17-OH pregnenolone to dehydroepiandrosterone (DHEA); only insignificant amounts of 17-OH progesterone are converted to Δ⁴ androstenedione by human P450c17, although this reaction occurs in other species. Reaction 5, P450c21 catalyzes the 21-hydroxylation of progesterone to deoxycorticosterone (DOC) and of 17-OH progesterone to 11-deoxycortisol. Reaction 6, DOC is converted to corticosterone by the 11-hydroxylase activity of P450c11AS in the zona glomerulosa and by P450c11β in the zona fasciculata. Reaction 7, 11-deoxycortisol undergoes 11β-hydroxylation by P450c11β to produce cortisol in the zona fasciculata. Reactions 8 and 9, the 18-hydroxylase and 18-oxidase activities of P450c11AS convert corticosterone to 18-OH corticosterone and aldosterone, respectively, in the zona glomerulosa. Reactions 10 and 11 are found principally in the testes and ovaries. Reaction 10, 17β-HSD-III converts DHEA to androstenediol and androstenedione to testosterone, while 17β-HSD-I converts estrone to estradiol. Reaction 11, testosterone may be converted to estradiol and androstenedione may be converted to estrone by P450aro.

involved in steroidogenesis [3]. These enzymes have molecular masses of about 35–45 kDa, do not have heme groups and require NAD^+ or $NADP^+$ as cofactors. Whereas most steroidogenic reactions catalyzed by P450 enzymes result from the action of a single form of P450, each of the reactions catalyzed by HSDs can be catalyzed by at least two, often very different, isozymes. Members of this family include the 3α- and 3β-hydroxysteroid dehydrogenases, the two 11β-hydroxysteroid dehydrogenases and a series of 17β-hydroxy-steroid dehydrogenases; the 5α-reductases are unrelated to this family.

P450scc

Conversion of cholesterol to pregnenolone in mitochondria is the first, rate-limiting and hormonally regulated step in the synthesis of all steroid hormones. This involves three distinct chemical reactions: 20α-hydroxylation, 22-hydroxylation and cleavage of the cholesterol side-chain to yield pregnenolone and isocaproic acid. Early studies showed that 20-hydroxycholesterol, 22-hydroxycholesterol and 20,22-hydroxycholesterol could all be isolated from adrenals in significant quantities, suggesting that three separate and distinct enzymes were involved. However, protein purification studies and *in vitro* reconstitution of enzymatic activity show that a single protein, termed P450scc (where scc refers to the *side-chain cleavage* of cholesterol), encoded by a single gene on chromosome 15, catalyzes all the steps between cholesterol and pregnenolone [1]. These three reactions occur on a single active site that is in contact with the hydrophobic bilayer membrane. Deletion of the gene for P450scc in animals eliminates all steroidogenesis, indicating that all steroidogenesis is initiated by this one enzyme.

Transport of electrons to P450scc: adrenodoxin reductase and adrenodoxin

P450scc functions as the terminal oxidase in a mitochondrial electron transport system [4]. Electrons from NADPH (reduced form of nicotinamide adenine dinucleotide phosphate) are accepted by a flavoprotein, termed adrenodoxin reductase, that is loosely associated with the inner mitochondrial membrane. Adrenodoxin reductase transfers the electrons to an iron–sulfur protein termed adrenodoxin, which is found in the mitochondrial matrix or loosely adherent to the inner mitochondrial membrane. Adrenodoxin then transfers the electrons to P450scc (Fig. 13.2). Adrenodoxin reductase and adrenodoxin serve as generic electron transport proteins for all mitochondrial P450s and not just for those involved in steroidogenesis; hence, these proteins are also termed ferredoxin oxidoreductase and ferredoxin. Adrenodoxin forms a 1:1 complex with adrenodoxin reductase, then dissociates and subsequently reforms an analogous 1:1 complex with P450scc or P450c11, thus functioning as an indiscriminate electron shuttle mechanism. Adrenodoxin reductase is a membrane-bound mitochondrial flavoprotein that receives electrons from NADPH. The human adrenodoxin reductase gene and the functional adrenodoxin gene are expressed in all human tissues.

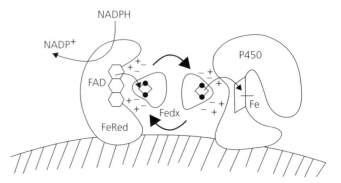

Figure 13.2 Electron transfer to mitochondrial P450 enzymes. A pair of electrons from nicotinamide adenine dinucleotide phosphate (NADPH) is taken up by adrenodoxin reductase on the inner mitochondrial membrane (FeRed), which then passes them to adrenodoxin (Fedx); these two proteins interact by electrostatic charge. Adrenodoxin then dissociates from adrenodoxin reductase, diffuses through the mitochrondrial matrix and docks with the redox-partner binding-site of the P450; electrostatic interactions again coordinate the protein–protein interaction. The electrons from the adrenodoxin then travel through the P450 protein to reach the heme ring; the heme iron then mediates catalysis with substrate bound in the P450. © WL Miller.

Cholesterol transport into mitochondria

The chronic regulation of steroidogenesis by ACTH is at the level of gene transcription but the acute regulation, in which cortisol is released within minutes of a stimulus, is at the level of cholesterol access to P450scc. When either steroidogenic cells or intact rats are treated with inhibitors of protein synthesis, such as cycloheximide, the acute steroidogenic response is eliminated, suggesting that a short-lived cycloheximide-sensitive protein acts at the level of the mitochondrion as the specific trigger to the acute steroidogenic response. This "acute trigger" of steroidogenesis is the steroidogenic acute regulatory protein (StAR) [5].

StAR was first identified as short-lived 30- and 37-kDa phosphoproteins that were rapidly synthesized when steroidogenic cells were stimulated with trophic hormones. Mouse StAR was then cloned from MA-10 Leydig cells. The central role of StAR was definitively proven by showing that it promoted steroidogenesis in non-steroidogenic COS-1 cells co-transfected with StAR and the cholesterol side-chain cleavage enzyme system and by finding that mutations of StAR caused the most severe disorder of human steroidogenesis, congenital lipoid adrenal hyperplasia [6]. Thus, StAR is the acute trigger that is required for the rapid flux of cholesterol from the outer to the inner mitochondrial membrane, which is needed for the acute response of aldosterone to angiotensin II, of cortisol to ACTH and of sex steroids to a luteinizing hormone (LH) pulse.

Some steroidogenesis is independent of StAR; when non-steroidogenic cells are transfected with the P450scc system, they convert cholesterol to pregnenolone at about 14% of the StAR-induced rate. Furthermore, some steroidogenic tissues, including the placenta, utilize mitochondrial P450scc to initiate steroidogenesis but do not express StAR. The mechanism of StAR-independent steroidogenesis is unknown. It is possible that it occurs spontaneously, without any triggering protein or that some other protein may exert StAR-like activity to promote cholesterol flux without StAR's rapid kinetics. The mechanism of StAR's action is unclear but StAR acts exclusively on the outer mitochondrial membrane where it undergoes structural changes while interacting with the outer mitochondrial membrane [7]. Substantial data indicate that the action of StAR requires its interaction with the peripheral benzodiazepine receptor on the outer mitochondrial membrane [8].

3β-Hydroxysteroid dehydrogenase/$\Delta^5 \rightarrow \Delta^4$ isomerase

Once pregnenolone is produced from cholesterol, it may undergo 17α-hydroxylation by P450c17 to yield 17-hydroxy-pregnenolone or it may be converted to progesterone, the first biologically important steroid in the pathway. A single 42-kDa microsomal enzyme, 3β-hydroxysteroid dehydrogenase (3β-HSD), catalyzes both the conversion of the hydroxyl group to a keto group on carbon 3 and the isomerization of the double bond from the B ring (Δ^5 steroids) to the A ring (Δ^4 steroids). Thus, a single enzyme converts pregnenolone to progesterone, 17α-hydroxypregnenolone to 17α-hydroxyprogesterone, dehydroepiandrosterone (DHEA) to androstenedione and androstenediol to testosterone. As is typical of hydroxysteroid dehydrogenases, there are two isozymes of 3β-HSD, encoded by separate genes. The enzyme catalyzing 3β-HSD activity in the adrenals and gonads is the type II enzyme; the type I enzyme, encoded by a closely linked gene with identical intron/exon organization, catalyzes 3β-HSD activity in placenta, breast and "extraglandular" tissue.

P450c17

Both pregnenolone and progesterone may undergo 17α-hydroxylation to 17α-hydroxypregnenolone and 17α-hydroxyprogesterone (17-OHP) respectively. 17α-Hydroxyprogesterone may also undergo cleavage of the C17,20 carbon bond to yield DHEA; however, very little 17-OHP is converted to androstenedione because the human P450c17 enzyme catalyzes this reaction at only 3% of the rate for conversion of 17α-hydroxypregnenolone to DHEA. These reactions are all mediated by P450c17. This P450 is bound to smooth endoplasmic reticulum, where it accepts electrons from P450 oxidoreductase. As P450c17 has both 17α-hydroxylase activity and C-17,20-lyase activity, it is the key branch point in steroid hormone synthesis. If neither activity of P450c17 is present, as in the zona glomerulosa, pregnenolone is converted to mineralocorticoids; if 17α-hydroxylase activity is present but 17,20-lyase activity is not, as in the zona fasciculata, pregnenolone is converted to cortisol; if both activities are present, as in the zona reticularis, pregnenolone is converted to precursors of sex steroids (Fig. 13.1).

17α-Hydroxylase and 17,20-lyase were once thought to be separate enzymes. The adrenals of prepubertal children synthesize ample cortisol but virtually no sex steroids (i.e. they have 17α-hydroxylase activity but not 17,20-lyase activity) until adrenarche initiates the production of adrenal androgens (i.e. turns on 17,20-lyase activity). Furthermore, patients have been described lacking 17,20-lyase activity but retaining normal 17α-hydroxylase activity. However, purification of P450c17 to homogeneity and *in vitro* reconstitution of enzymatic activity show that both 17α-hydroxylase and 17,20-lyase activities reside in a single protein and cells transformed with a vector expressing P450c17 cDNA acquire both 17α-hydroxylase and 17,20-lyase activities. P450c17 is encoded by a single gene on chromosome 10q24.3 that is structurally related to the genes for P450c21 (21-hydroxylase).

Thus, the distinction between 17α-hydroxylase and 17,20-lyase is functional and not genetic or structural. The factors involved in determining whether a steroid molecule will remain on the single active site of P450c17 and undergo 17,20 bond cleavage after 17α-hydroxylation remain unknown. P450c17 prefers Δ^5 substrates, especially for 17,20 bond cleavage, consistent with the large amounts of DHEA secreted by both fetal and adult adrenal. Furthermore, the 17α-hydroxylase reaction occurs more readily than the 17,20-lyase reaction. An additional important factor is the abundance of electron donors for P450c17.

Electron transport to P450c17: P450 oxidoreductase and cytochrome b_5

All microsomal forms of cytochrome P450, including P450c17 and P450c21, receive electrons from a membrane-bound flavoprotein, termed P450 oxidoreductase, which is a different protein from the mitochondrial flavoprotein, adrenodoxin reductase. P450 oxidoreductase receives two electrons from NADPH and transfers them one at a time to the P450 [4]. Electron transfer for the lyase reaction is promoted by the action of cytochrome b_5 as an allosteric factor rather than as an alternative electron donor. 17,20-Lyase activity also requires the phosphorylation of serine residues on P450c17 by a cyclic adenosine monophosphate (cAMP)-dependent protein kinase (Fig. 13.3). Because the adrenal

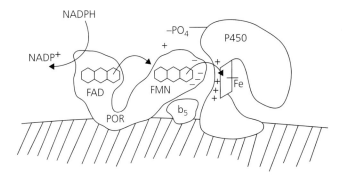

Figure 13.3 Electron transfer to microsomal P450 enzymes. A pair of electrons from NADPH is taken up by P450 oxidoreductase (POR), which is bound to the endoplasmic reticulum. The electrons are received by the FAD moiety and passed to the FMN moiety of POR. The FMN domain of POR then interacts with the redox-partner binding site of the P450 and electrons reach the heme iron as described in Fig. 13.2. The interaction of POR and the P450 is coordinated by electrostatic interactions. In the case of human P450c17, this interaction is facilitated by the allosteric action of cytochrome b_5 and by the serine phosphorylation of P450c17. © WL Miller.

endoplasmic reticulum contains many more molecules of P450c17 and of P450c21 than of P450 oxidoreductase, the P450s compete with one another for the reducing equivalents provided by the reductase.

The availability of electrons determines whether P450c17 performs only 17α-hydroxylation or also performs 17,20 bond cleavage. Thus, the regulation of 17,20-lyase activity and consequently of DHEA production, depends on factors that facilitate the flow of electrons to P450c17. These are high concentrations of P450 oxidoreductase, the presence of cytochrome b_5 and serine phosphorylation of P450c17 [4]. The essential role of P450 oxidoreductase in mammalian biology is underscored by the demonstration that mice lacking a functional gene for P450 oxidoreductase are malformed and die *in utero*. Nevertheless, mutations in human P450 oxidoreductase can cause a picture of combined 17α-hydroxylase and 21-hydroxylase deficiencies, often in combination with the Antley–Bixler skeletal malformation syndrome [9].

P450c21

After the synthesis of progesterone and 17-hydroxyprogesterone, these steroids are hydroxylated at the 21 position to yield deoxycorticosterone (DOC) and 11-deoxycortisol, respectively (Fig. 13.1). The nature of the 21-hydroxylating step has been of great clinical interest because disordered 21-hydroxylation causes more than 90% of all cases of CAH. The clinical symptoms associated with this common genetic disease are complex and devastating. Decreased cortisol and aldosterone synthesis often leads to sodium loss, potassium retention and hypotension, which may lead to cardiovascular collapse and death within the month after birth if not treated appropriately. Decreased synthesis of cortisol *in utero* leads to overproduction of ACTH and consequent overstimulation of adrenal steroid synthesis; as the 21-hydroxylase step is impaired, 17-OHP accumulates because P450c17 converts only miniscule amounts of 17-OHP to androstenedione. However, 17-hydroxypregnenolone also accumulates and is converted to DHEA and subsequently to androstenedione and testosterone, resulting in severe prenatal virilization of female fetuses.

CAH has been studied extensively [10]. Characterization of the P450c21 protein and gene cloning show that there is only one 21-hydroxylase encoded by a single functional gene on chromosome 6p21. As this gene lies in the middle of the major histocompatibility locus, disorders of adrenal 21-hydroxylation are closely linked to specific human leukocyte antigen (HLA) types.

Adrenal 21-hydroxylation is mediated by P450c21 found in smooth endoplasmic reticulum. P450c21 uses the same P450 oxidoreductase used by P450c17 to transport electrons from NADPH. 21-Hydroxylase activity has also been described in a broad range of adult and fetal extra-adrenal tissues. However, extra-adrenal 21-hydroxylation is not mediated by the P450c21 enzyme found in the adrenal. Several hepatic P450 enzymes are responsible for extra-adrenal 21-hydroxylation. As a result, patients with absent adrenal 21-hydroxylase activity may still have appreciable concentrations of 21-hydroxylated steroids in their plasma.

P450c11β and P450c11AS

Two closely related enzymes, P450c11β and P450c11AS, catalyze the final steps in the synthesis of both glucocorticoids and mineralocorticoids [11]. These two isozymes have 93% amino acid sequence identity and are encoded by tandemly duplicated genes on chromosome 8q21–22. Like P450scc, the two forms of P450c11 are found on the inner mitochondrial membrane and use adrenodoxin and adrenodoxin reductase to receive electrons from NADPH. By far the more abundant of the two isozymes is P450c11β, which is the classic 11β-hydroxylase that converts 11-deoxycortisol to cortisol and 11-deoxycorticosterone to corticosterone. The less abundant isozyme, P450c11AS, is found only in the zona glomerulosa, where it has 11β-hydroxylase, 18-hydroxylase and 18-methyl oxidase (aldosterone synthase) activities; thus, P450c11AS is able to catalyze all the reactions needed to convert DOC to aldosterone.

P450c11β, which is principally involved in the synthesis of cortisol, is encoded by a gene (*CYP11B1*) primarily induced by ACTH via cAMP and suppressed by glucocorticoids such as dexamethasone. The existence of two distinct functional genes is confirmed by the identification of mutations in each that cause distinct genetic disorders of steroidogenesis. Thus, patients with disorders in P450c11β have classic 11β-hydroxylase deficiency but can still produce aldosterone, whereas patients with disorders in P450c11AS have rare forms of aldosterone deficiency (so-called corticosterone methyl oxidase deficiency) while retaining the ability to produce cortisol.

17β-Hydroxysteroid dehydrogenase

Androstenedione is converted to testosterone, DHEA to androstenediol and estrone to estradiol by a series of short-chain dehydrogenases called 17β-hydroxysteroid dehydrogenases (17β-HSDs), sometimes also termed 17oxidoreductase or 17-ketosteroid reductase [1,3]. The terminology for these enzymes varies, depending on the direction of the reaction being considered, which is regulated by cofactor availability. There are several different 17β-HSD enzymes encoded by distinct genes: some are preferential oxidases, whereas others are preferential reductases; they differ in their substrate preference and sites of expression; and some proteins termed 17β-HSD actually have very little 17β-HSD activity and are principally involved in other reactions.

Type I 17β-HSD (17β-HSD-I), also known as estrogenic 17β-HSD, is a cytosolic protein first isolated and cloned from the placenta, where it produces estriol and is expressed in ovarian granulosa cells, where it produces estradiol. 17β-HSD-I is not reversible and does not participate in androgen metabolism. 17β-HSD-I uses NADPH as its cofactor to catalyze its reductase activity. The three-dimensional structure of human 17β-HSD-I has been determined by X-ray crystallography. No genetic deficiency syndrome for 17β-HSD-I has been described.

17β-HSD-II is a microsomal oxidase that uses NAD$^+$ to inactivate (oxidize) estradiol to estrone and testosterone to Δ^4 androstenedione. 17β-HSD-II is found in the placenta, liver, small intestine, prostate, secretory endometrium and ovary. In contrast to 17β-HSD-I, which is found in placental syncytiotrophoblast cells, 17β-HSD-II is expressed in endothelial cells of placental intravillous vessels, consistent with its apparent role in defending the fetal circulation from transplacental passage of maternal estradiol or testosterone. No deficiency state for 17β-HSD-II has been reported.

17β-HSD-III, the androgenic form of 17β-HSD, is a microsomal enzyme that is apparently expressed only in the testis where it converts androstenedione to testosterone. This is the enzyme that is disordered in the classic syndrome of male pseudohermaphroditism, which is often termed 17-ketosteroid reductase deficiency.

An enzyme termed 17β-HSD-IV was initially identified as an NAD$^+$-dependent oxidase with activities similar to 17β-HSD-II but this peroxisomal protein is primarily an enoyl-CoA hydratase and 3-hydroxyacyl-CoA dehydrogenase.

17β-HSD-V originally cloned as a 3α-hydroxysteroid dehydrogenase, catalyzes the reduction of Δ^4 androstenedione to testosterone but its precise role is unclear and no deficiency state has been described. It is widely expressed in peripheral tissues and is probably the enzyme responsible for "peripheral conversion" of androstenedione to testosterone and of DHEA to androstenediol, accounting for the efficacy of those steroids as anabolic agents.

Steroid sulfotransferase and sulfatase

Steroid sulfates may be synthesized directly from cholesterol sulfate or may be formed by sulfation of steroids by cytosolic sulfotransferases [12]. The principal sulfotransferase of the adrenal, termed SULT2A1, sulfates the 3β-hydroxyl group of pregnenolone, 17OH-pregnenolone, DHEA and androsterone but not cholesterol. Mutations of human sulfotransferase enzymes have not been described but African-Americans have a high rate of polymorphism in SULT2A1, apparently influencing plasma ratios of DHEA to DHEAS. Steroid sulfates may also be hydrolyzed to the native steroid by steroid sulfatase. Deletions in the steroid sulfatase gene on chromosome Xp22.3 cause X-linked ichthyosis. In the fetal adrenal and placenta, diminished or absent sulfatase deficiency reduces the pool of free DHEA available for placental conversion to estrogen, resulting in low concentrations of estriol in the maternal blood and urine. The accumulation of steroid sulfates in the stratum corneum of the skin causes the ichthyosis. Steroid sulfatase is also expressed in the fetal rodent brain, possibly converting peripheral DHEA sulfate (DHEAS) to active DHEA.

Aromatase: P450aro

Estrogens are produced by the aromatization of androgens, including adrenal androgens, by a complex series of reactions catalyzed by a single microsomal aromatase, P450aro [13]. This typical cytochrome P450 is encoded by a single, large gene on chromosome 15q21.1. This gene uses several different promoter sequences, transcriptional start sites and alternatively chosen first exons to encode aromatase mRNA in different tissues under different hormonal regulation. Aromatase expression in the extraglandular tissues, especially adipose tissue, can covert adrenal androgens to estrogens. Aromatase in the epiphyses of growing bone can convert testosterone to estradiol, accelerating epiphyseal maturation and terminating growth. Although it has traditionally been thought that aromatase activity is needed for embryonic and fetal development, infants and adults with genetic disorders in this enzyme have been described, showing that fetoplacental estrogen is not needed for normal fetal development.

5α-Reductase

Testosterone is converted to dihydrotestosterone by 5α-reductase in testosterone's target tissues. There are two distinct forms of 5α-reductase. The type I enzyme, found in the scalp and other peripheral tissues, is encoded by a gene on chromosome 5; the type II enzyme, the predominant form found in male reproductive tissues, is encoded by a gene on chromosome 2p23. The syndrome of 5α-reductase deficiency, a disorder of male sexual differentiation, results from a wide variety of mutations in the gene encoding the type II enzyme [14]. The type 1 and 2 genes show an unusual pattern of developmental regulation of expression. The type 1 gene is not expressed in the fetus; it is expressed briefly in the skin of the newborn and then remains unexpressed until its activity and protein are again found after puberty. This probably explains the lack of peripheral virilization of male fetuses despite the presence of testosterone concentrations equivalent to adult male levels. The type 2 gene is expressed in fetal genital skin, in the normal prostate and in prostatic hyperplasia and adenocarcinoma. Thus, the type I enzyme may be responsible for the pubertal virilization seen in patients with classic 5α-reductase deficiency and the type II enzyme may be involved in male pattern baldness.

11β-Hydroxysteroid dehydrogenase

Although certain steroids are categorized as glucocorticoids or mineralocorticoids, the "mineralocorticoid" (glucocorticoid type II) receptor has equal affinity for both aldosterone and cortisol. However, cortisol does not act as a mineralocorticoid *in vivo*, even though cortisol concentrations can exceed aldosterone concentrations by 100- to 1000-fold. In kidney and other mineralocorticoid-responsive tissues, cortisol is converted to cortisone, a metabolically inactive steroid. The interconversion of cortisol and cortisone is mediated by two isozymes of 11β-hydroxysteroid dehydrogenase (11β-HSD), each of which has both oxidase and reductase activity [15].

The type I enzyme (11β-HSD-I) is expressed mainly in glucocorticoid-responsive tissues, such as the liver, testis, lung and proximal convoluted tubule. 11β-HSD-I can catalyze the oxidation of cortisol to cortisone using NADP$^+$ as its cofactor (K_m 1.6 μmol/L) or the reduction of cortisone to cortisol using NADPH as its cofactor (K_m 0.14 μmol/L); the reaction catalyzed depends on which cofactor is available but the enzyme can only function with high (micromolar) concentrations of steroid. 11β-HSD-II catalyzes only the oxidation of cortisol to cortisone using NADH and can function with low (nanomolar) concentrations of steroid (K_m 10–100 nmol/L). 11β-HSD-II is expressed in mineralocorticoid-responsive tissues and thus serves to "defend" the mineralocorticoid receptor by inactivating cortisol to cortisone, so that only "true" mineralocorticoids, such as aldosterone or deoxycorticosterone, which are not substrates for 11β-HSD-II, can exert a mineralocorticoid effect. Thus, 11β-HSD-II prevents cortisol from overwhelming renal mineralocorticoid receptors. In the placenta and other fetal tissues, 11β-HSD-II also inactivates cortisol. The placenta also has abundant $NADP^+$, favoring the oxidative action of 11β-HSD-I, so that, in the placenta, both enzymes protect the fetus from high maternal concentrations of cortisol, thus ensuring that the fetus develops in an environment with very little glucocorticoid. 11β-HSD-I is not in contact with the cytoplasm but lies inside the endoplasmic reticulum, where it receives NADPH provided by the action of hexose-6-phosphate dehydrogenase. This links 11β-HSD-I to the pentose monophosphate shunt, linking glucocorticoid production and energy storage as fat.

Fetal adrenal steroidogenesis

Adrenocortical steroidogenesis begins early in embryonic life, probably around 6 weeks' gestation (8 weeks after the mother's last menstrual period). Fetuses affected with genetic lesions in adrenal steroidogenesis can produce adrenal androgen sufficient to virilize a female fetus to a nearly male appearance and this masculinization of the genitalia is complete by 12 weeks' gestation. The definitive zone of the fetal adrenal produces steroid hormones according to the pathways in Figure 13.1. In contrast, the large fetal zone of the adrenal is relatively deficient in 3β-HSD-II activity because it contains very little mRNA for this enzyme [16]. The fetal adrenal has relatively abundant 17,20-lyase activity of P450c17; low 3β-HSD and high 17,20-lyase activity account for the huge amount of DHEA and DHEAS produced by the fetal adrenal for conversion to estrogens by the placenta.

The fetal adrenal has considerable sulfotransferase activity but little steroid sulfatase activity, which favors conversion of DHEA to DHEAS. The resulting DHEAS cannot be a substrate for adrenal 3β-HSD-II; instead, it is secreted, 16α-hydroxylated in the fetal liver and then acted on by placental 3β-HSD-I, 17β-HSD-I and P450aro to produce estriol; the substrates can also bypass the liver to yield estrone and estradiol. Placental estrogens inhibit adrenal 3β-HSD activity, providing a feedback system to promote the production of DHEAS. Fetal adrenal steroids account for 50% of the estrone and estradiol and 90% of the estriol in the maternal circulation.

Although the fetoplacental unit produces huge amounts of DHEA, DHEAS and estriol, as well as other steroids, they do not appear to serve an essential role. Successful pregnancy is dependent on placental synthesis of progesterone, which suppresses uterine contractility and prevents spontaneous abortion, but fetuses with genetic disorders of adrenal and gonadal steroido-genesis develop normally, reach term gestation and undergo normal delivery.

Mineralocorticoid production is required postnatally, estrogens are not required and androgens are needed only for male sexual differentiation. It is not clear whether human fetal development requires glucocorticoids but, if so, the small amount of maternal cortisol that escapes placental inactivation suffices.

The regulation of steroidogenesis and growth of the fetal adrenal are not fully understood but both are related to ACTH. ACTH stimulates steroidogenesis by fetal adrenal cells *in vitro* and excess ACTH is clearly involved in the adrenal growth and overproduction of androgens in fetuses affected with CAH. Prenatal treatment of such fetuses by administering dexamethasone orally to the mother at 6–10 weeks' gestation can significantly reduce fetal adrenal androgen production and thus reduce the virilization of female fetuses.

The hypothalamo-pituitary-adrenal axis functions very early in fetal life but anencephalic fetuses, which lack pituitary ACTH, have adrenals that contain a fairly normal complement of steroidogenic enzymes and retain their capacity for steroidogenesis. Thus, it appears that fetal adrenal steroidogenesis is regulated by both ACTH-dependent and ACTH-independent mechanisms.

Regulation of steroidogenesis

The hypothalamic-pituitary-adrenal axis

The principal steroidal product of the human adrenal is cortisol, which is mainly secreted in response to ACTH (corticotropin) produced in the pituitary; secretion of ACTH is stimulated mainly by corticotropin-releasing factor (CRH) from the hypothalamus. Hypothalamic CRH is a 41-amino-acid peptide synthesized mainly by neurons in the paraventricular nucleus. These same hypothalamic neurons also produce arginine vasopressin (AVP, also known as antidiuretic hormone or ADH). CRH and AVP travel through axons to the median eminence, which releases them into the pituitary portal circulation, although most AVP axons terminate in the posterior pituitary. Both CRH and AVP stimulate the synthesis and release of ACTH but they appear to do so by different mechanisms. CRH functions principally by receptors linked to the protein kinase A pathway, stimulating production of intracellular cAMP, whereas AVP appears to function via protein kinase C and intracellular Ca^{2+}. CRH is the more important physiological stimulator of ACTH release, although maximal doses of AVP can elicit a maximal ACTH response. When given together, CRH and AVP act synergistically, as would be expected from their independent mechanisms of action.

ACTH and pro-opiomelanocortin

Pituitary ACTH is a 39 amino acid peptide derived from pro-opiomelanocortin (POMC), a 241 amino acid protein. POMC undergoes a series of proteolytic cleavages, yielding several biologically active peptides (Fig. 13.4). The N-terminal glycopeptide (POMC 1–75) can stimulate steroidogenesis and may function as

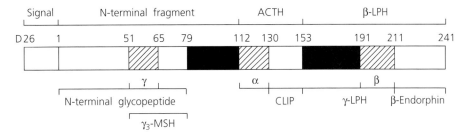

Figure 13.4 Structure of human prepro-opiomelanocortin. The numbers refer to amino acid positions, with no. 1 assigned to the first amino acid of POMC after the 26 amino acid signal peptide. The α-, β- and γ-MSH regions, which characterize the three "constant" regions, are indicated by diagonal lines; the "variable" regions are solid. The amino acid numbers shown refer to the N-terminal amino acid of each cleavage site; because these amino acids are removed, the numbers do not correspond exactly to the amino acid numbers of the peptides as used in the text. CLIP, corticotrophin-like intermediate lobe peptide.

an adrenal mitogen. POMC 112–150 is ACTH 1–39; POMC 112–126 and POMC 191–207 constitute α- and β-MSH (melanocyte stimulating hormone), respectively. POMC 210–241 is β-endorphin. POMC is produced in small amounts by the brain, testis and placenta but this extrapituitary POMC does not contribute significantly to circulating ACTH. Malignant tumors will commonly produce "ectopic ACTH" in adults and rarely in children; this ACTH derives from ectopic biosynthesis of the same POMC precursor. Only the first 20–24 amino acids of ACTH are needed for its full biological activity and synthetic ACTH 1–24 is widely used in diagnostic tests of adrenal function. The shorter forms of ACTH have a shorter half-life than native ACTH 1–39. POMC gene transcription is stimulated by CRH and is inhibited by glucocorticoids.

Actions of ACTH

ACTH stimulates steroidogenesis by interacting with the melanocortin-2 receptor (MC2R) that stimulates the production of cAMP, which elicits acute and long-term effects. ACTH, acting via cAMP, stimulates the biosynthesis of LDL receptors and the uptake of LDL, which provides most of the cholesterol used for steroidogenesis. ACTH via cAMP also stimulates transcription of the gene for HMGCoA reductase, the rate-limiting step in cholesterol biosynthesis but adrenal biosynthesis of cholesterol is quantitatively much less important than the uptake of LDL-cholesterol.

Cholesterol is stored in steroidogenic tissues as cholesterol esters in lipid droplets. ACTH stimulates the activity of cholesterol esterase while inhibiting cholesterol ester synthetase, thus increasing the intracellular pool of free cholesterol, the substrate for P450scc. The esterase is similar to gastric and lingual lipases. Finally, ACTH facilitates transport of cholesterol into mitochondria by stimulating the synthesis and phosphorylation of StAR, thus increasing the flow of free cholesterol into the mitochondria. All these actions occur within minutes and constitute the acute effect of ACTH on steroidogenesis. The adrenal contains relatively modest amounts of steroid hormones; thus, release of preformed cortisol does not contribute significantly to the acute response to ACTH, which occurs by the rapid provision of large supplies of cholesterol to mitochondrial P450scc.

Long-term chronic effects of ACTH are mediated directly at the level of the steroidogenic enzymes. ACTH via cAMP stimulates the accumulation of the steroidogenic enzymes and their mRNAs by stimulating the transcription of their genes. Thus, ACTH increases both the uptake of the cholesterol substrate and its conversion to steroidal products. The stimulation of this steroidogenesis occurs at each step in the pathway, not only at the rate-limiting step, P450scc.

The role of ACTH and other peptides derived from POMC in stimulating growth of the adult adrenal remains uncertain. However, in the fetal adrenal, ACTH stimulates the local production of insulin-like growth factor (IGF) II, basic fibroblast growth factor and epidermal growth factor. These, and possibly other factors, work together to mediate ACTH-induced growth of the fetal adrenal [16].

Diurnal rhythms of ACTH and cortisol

Plasma concentrations of ACTH and cortisol are high in the morning and low in the evening. Peak ACTH levels are usually seen at 04.00–06.00 h and peak cortisol levels follow at about 08.00 hours. Both ACTH and cortisol are released episodically in pulses every 30–120 min throughout the day but the frequency and amplitude are greater in the morning. The basis of this diurnal rhythm is complex and incompletely understood. The hypothalamic content of CRH itself shows a diurnal rhythm, with peak content at about 04.00 h. At least four factors appear to have a role in the rhythm of ACTH and cortisol. These interdependent factors include intrinsic rhythmicity of synthesis and secretion of CRH by the hypothalamus, light–dark cycles, feeding and inherent rhythmicity in the adrenal, possibly mediated by adrenal innervation.

Dietary rhythms may have as large a role as light–dark cycles, as animal experiments show that altering the time of feeding can overcome the ACTH/cortisol periodicity established by a light–dark cycle. In normal human subjects, cortisol is released before lunch and supper but not at these times in persons eating continuously during the day. Thus, glucocorticoids, which increase blood glucose, appear to be released at times of fasting and are inhibited by feeding.

As all parents know, infants do not have a diurnal rhythm of sleep or feeding. They acquire such behavioral rhythms in response to the environment long before they acquire a rhythm of ACTH and cortisol. The diurnal rhythms begin to be established at 6–12 months but are often not well established until after 3 years of age. Once the rhythm is well established in the older child or adult, it is changed only with difficulty. When people move time zones, ACTH/cortisol rhythms may take 15–20 days to adjust.

Physical stress (major surgery, severe trauma, blood loss, high fever or serious illness) increases the secretion of both ACTH and cortisol but minor surgery and minor illnesses (upper respiratory infections) have little effect. Infection, fever and pyrogens can stimulate the release of interleukin 1 (IL-1) and IL-6, which stimulate secretion of CRH and also IL-2 and tumor necrosis factor (TNF), which stimulate release of ACTH, providing further stimulus to cortisol secretion during inflammation [17]. Most psychoactive drugs, such as anticonvulsants, neurotransmitters and antidepressants, do not affect the diurnal rhythm of ACTH and cortisol, although cyproheptidine (a serotonin antagonist) suppresses ACTH release.

Adrenal–glucocorticoid feedback

The hypothalamo-pituitary-adrenal axis is a classic example of an endocrine feedback system. ACTH increases the production of cortisol and cortisol decreases the production of CRH and ACTH. Like the acute and chronic phases of the action of ACTH on the adrenal, there are acute and chronic phases of the feedback inhibition of ACTH. The acute phase, which occurs within minutes, inhibits release of ACTH (and CRH) from secretory granules. With prolonged exposure, glucocorticoids inhibit ACTH synthesis by directly inhibiting the transcription of the gene for POMC. Some evidence also suggests that glucocorticoids can inhibit steroidogenesis at the level of the adrenal fasciculata cell itself but this appears to be a physiologically minor component of the regulation of cortisol secretion.

Mineralocorticoid secretion: the renin-angiotensin system

Renin is a serine protease enzyme synthesized primarily by the juxtaglomerular cells of the kidney. It is also produced in a variety of other tissues, including the glomerulosa cells of the adrenal cortex. Adrenally produced renin appears to maintain basal levels of P450c11AS but it is not known whether angiotensin II is involved in this action. Renin is synthesized as a precursor (406 amino acids) that is cleaved to pro-renin (386 amino acids) and, finally, to the 340 amino acid protein found in plasma. Decreased blood pressure, upright posture, sodium depletion, vasodilatory drugs, kallikrein, opiates and β-adrenergic stimulation all promote the release of renin. Renin enzymatically attacks angiotensinogen, the renin substrate, in the circulation.

Angiotensinogen is a highly glycosylated protein and therefore has a highly variable molecular weight, from 50 000 to 100 000 Da. Renin proteolytically releases the aminoterminal 10 amino acids

of angiotensinogen, referred to as angiotensin I. This decapeptide is biologically inactive until converting enzyme, an enzyme found primarily in the lungs and blood vessels, cleaves off its two carboxy-terminal amino acids to produce an octapeptide termed angiotensin II. Converting enzyme can be inhibited by captopril and related agents useful in the diagnosis and treatment of hyper-reninemic hypertension.

Angiotensin II has two principal actions, both of which increase blood pressure. It directly stimulates arteriolar vasoconstriction within a few seconds and it stimulates the synthesis and secretion of aldosterone within minutes. Increased plasma potassium is a powerful and direct stimulator of aldosterone synthesis and release.

Aldosterone, secreted by the adrenal glomerulosa cells, has the greatest mineralocorticoid activity of all naturally occurring steroids. It causes renal sodium retention and potassium loss, with a consequent increase in intravascular volume and blood pressure. Angiotensin II functions through receptors that stimulate the production of phosphatidylinositol, mobilize intracellular and extracellular Ca^{2+} and activate protein kinase C. These intracellular second messengers then stimulate transcription of the P450scc gene by means independent of those used by ACTH and cAMP. Potassium ions increase uptake of Ca^{2+}, with consequent hydrolysis of phosphoinositides to increase phosphatidylinositol. Thus, angiotensin II and potassium work at different levels of the same intracellular second messenger pathway but these differ fundamentally from the action of ACTH.

Although the renin-angiotensin system is clearly the major regulator of mineralocorticoid secretion, ACTH and possibly other POMC-derived peptides such as γ_3-MSH, can also promote secretion of aldosterone when used in high concentrations in animal systems. The relevance of physiological concentrations in human beings has not been established. Ammonium ions, hyponatremia, dopamine antagonists and some other agents can also stimulate secretion of aldosterone; atrial natriuretic factor is a potent physiological inhibitor of aldosterone secretion.

Adrenal androgen secretion and the regulation of adrenarche

DHEA, DHEAS and androstenedione, which are almost exclusively secreted by the adrenal zona reticularis, are generally referred to as adrenal androgens because they can be converted peripherally to testosterone. These steroids have little if any capacity to bind to and activate androgen receptors and are hence only androgen precursors, not true androgens. The fetal adrenal secretes large amounts of DHEA and DHEAS and these steroids are abundant in the newborn; their concentrations fall rapidly as the fetal zone of the adrenal involutes after birth.

After the first year of life, the adrenals of young children secrete small amounts of DHEA, DHEAS and androstenedione until the onset of adrenarche, usually around age 7–8 years, preceding the onset of puberty by about 2 years. Adrenarche is independent of puberty, the gonads or gonadotropins and the mechanism by which its onset is triggered remains unknown. The secretion of

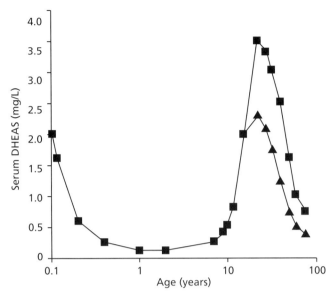

Figure 13.5 Concentrations of dehydroepiandrosterone sulfate (DHEAS) as a function of age. Note that the x-axis is on a log scale. Squares, males; triangles, females.

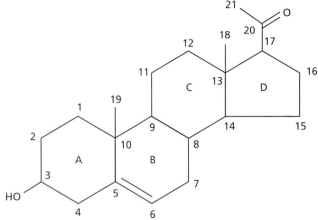

Figure 13.6 Structure of pregnenolone. The carbon atoms are indicated by numbers and the rings are designated by letters according to standard convention. Pregnenolone is derived from cholesterol, which has a six-carbon side-chain attached to carbon 21. Pregnenolone is a "Δ^5 compound," having a double bond between carbons 5 and 6; the action of 3β-hydroxysteroid dehydrogenase/isomerase moves this double bond from the B ring to carbon numbers 4 and 5 in the A ring, forming Δ^4 compounds. All the major biologically active steroid hormones are Δ^4 compounds.

DHEA and DHEAS continues to increase during and after puberty and reaches maximal values in young adulthood, after which there is a slow gradual decrease in the secretion of these steroids in elderly people ("adrenopause") (Fig. 13.5). Despite the increases in the adrenal secretion of DHEA and DHEAS during adrenarche, circulating concentrations of ACTH and cortisol do not change with age. Thus, ACTH has a permissive role in adrenarche but does not trigger it. Searches for hypothetical polypeptide hormones that might specifically stimulate the zona reticularis have been unsuccessful.

Recent studies of adrenarche have focused on the roles of 3β-HSD and P450c17. The abundance of 3β-HSD protein in the zona reticularis appears to decrease with the onset of adrenarche and the adrenal expression of cytochrome b_5, which fosters the 17,20-lyase activity of P450c17, is confined almost exclusively to the zona reticularis [16]. Both these factors would strongly favor the production of DHEA. Exaggerated adrenarche has been found in association with insulin resistance and girls with this condition appear to be at a much higher risk of developing the polycystic ovarian syndrome as adults. Recent evidence suggests that infants born small for gestational age may be at increased risk of this syndrome. Evidence is accumulating to suggest that replacement of DHEA after adrenopause may improve memory and a sense of well-being in elderly people [18].

Plasma steroids and their disposal

Structure and nomenclature

All steroid hormones are derivatives of pregnenolone (Fig. 13.6). Pregnenolone and its derivatives that contain 21 carbon atoms are often termed C_{21} steroids. Each carbon atom is numbered,

indicating the location at which the various steroidogenic reactions occur (e.g. 21-hydroxylation, 11-hydroxylation). The 17,20-lyase activity of P450c17 cleaves the bond between carbon atoms 17 and 20, yielding C_{19} steroids, which include all the androgens. P450aro converts C_{19} androgens to C_{18} estrogens. With the exception of estrogens, all steroid hormones have a single unsaturated carbon–carbon double bond. Steroids having this double bond between carbon atoms 4 and 5, including all the principal biologically active steroids, are termed Δ^4 steroids; their precursors, having a double bond between carbon atoms 5 and 6, are termed Δ^5 steroids. The two isozymes of 3β-HSD convert Δ^5 to Δ^4 steroids.

A rigorous, logically systematic and unambiguous chemical terminology accurately describes the structure of all the steroid hormones and their derivatives. However, this terminology is cumbersome (e.g. cortisol is 11β,17α,21-trihydroxy-pregn4-ene-3,20-dione and dexamethasone is 9α-fluoro-11β,17α, 21-trihydroxyprena-1,4-diene-3,20-dione). Therefore, we use only the standard trivial names.

Before the structures of the steroid hormones were determined in the 1930s, Reichstein, Kendall and others identified them as spots on paper chromatograms and designated them A, B, C, etc. Unfortunately, some persist in using this outmoded terminology more than 70 years later, so that corticosterone is sometimes termed "compound B," cortisol "compound F" and 11-deoxycortisol "compound S." This archaic terminology obfuscates the precursor–product relationships of the steroids and should not be used.

Circulating steroids

Although over 50 different steroids have been isolated from adrenocortical tissue, the main pathways of adrenal steroidogenesis include only a dozen or so steroids, of which only a few are secreted in sizable quantities. The adult secretion of DHEA and cortisol is each about 20 mg/24 h and the secretion of corticosterone, a weak glucocorticoid, is about 2 mg/24 h. Although glucocorticoids, such as cortisol and mineralocorticoids, such as aldosterone, are both needed for life and hence are of "equivalent" physiological importance, diagrams such as Fig. 13.1 fail to indicate that these steroids are not secreted in molar equivalents. The adult secretion rate of aldosterone is only about 0.1 mg/24 h. This 100- to 1000-fold molar difference in the secretory rates of cortisol and aldosterone must be borne in mind when considering the effects of steroid-binding proteins in plasma and when conceptualizing the physiological manifestations of incomplete defects in steroidogenesis due to single amino acid changes causing the partial loss of activity of a steroidogenic enzyme.

Most circulating steroids are bound to plasma proteins, including corticosteroid-binding globulin (CBG, also termed transcortin), albumin and α_1-acid glycoprotein. CBG has a very high affinity for cortisol but a relatively low binding capacity; albumin has a low affinity and high capacity; α_1-acid glycoprotein is intermediate for both variables. The result is that about 90% of circulating cortisol is bound to CBG and a little more is bound to other proteins. These steroid-binding proteins are not transport proteins, as the biologically important steroids are water soluble in physiologically effective concentrations and absence of CBG does not cause a detectable physiological disorder. However, these plasma proteins do act as a reservoir for steroids. This insures that all peripheral tissues will be bathed in approximately equal concentrations of cortisol, which greatly diminishes the physiological effect of the great diurnal variation in cortisol secretion.

Synthetic glucocorticoids do not bind significantly to CBG and bind poorly to albumin, partially accounting for their increased potencies, which are also associated with increased receptor-binding affinities. Aldosterone is not bound well by any plasma protein; hence, changes in plasma protein concentration do not affect plasma aldosterone concentrations but greatly influence plasma cortisol concentrations. Estradiol and testosterone bind strongly to a different plasma protein termed sex steroid-binding globulin and also bind weakly to albumin.

Because steroids are hormones, it is often thought that the concentration of "free" (i.e. unbound) circulating steroids determines biological activity. However, the target tissues for many steroid hormones contain enzymes that modify those steroids. Thus, many actions of testosterone are actually due to dihydrotestosterone produced by local 5α-reductase; cortisol will have differential actions on various tissues as a result of the presence or absence of 11β-HSD, which inactivates cortisol to cortisone. Similar peripheral metabolism occurs via "extraglandular" 21-hydroxylase, P450aro, 3β-HSD and 17β-HSD. Thus, circulating steroids are both classic hormones and precursors to locally acting autocrine or paracrine factors.

Steroid catabolism

Only about 1% of circulating plasma cortisol and aldosterone is excreted unchanged in the urine; the remainder is metabolized by the liver. A large number of hepatic metabolites of each steroid is produced, most containing additional hydroxyl groups and linked to a sulfate or glucuronide moiety, rendering them more soluble and readily excretable by the kidney. A great deal is known about the various urinary metabolites of the circulating steroids because their measurement in pooled 24-h urine samples has been an important means of studying adrenal steroids. Although the measurement of urinary steroid metabolites by modern mass spectrometric techniques remains an important research tool, the development of separation techniques and of specific and highly sensitive radioimmunoassays for each of the steroids in plasma has greatly reduced the need to measure their excreted metabolites in clinical practice.

Clinical and laboratory evaluation of adrenal function

Clinical evaluation

Primary adrenal deficiency or hypersecretion is generally evident before performing laboratory tests. Patients with chronic adrenal insufficiency have weakness, fatigue, anorexia, weight loss, hypotension and hyperpigmentation. Patients with acute adrenal insufficiency have hypotension, shock, weakness, apathy, confusion, anorexia, nausea, vomiting, dehydration, abdominal or flank pain, hyperthermia and hypoglycemia.

Early signs of glucocorticoid excess include increased appetite, weight gain and growth arrest without a concomitant delay in bone age. Chronic glucocorticoid excess in children results in typical cushingoid facies but the buffalo hump and centripetal distribution of body fat characteristic of Cushing disease in adults are seen only in long-standing undiagnosed disease.

Mineralocorticoid excess is characterized by hypertension but patients receiving very low sodium diets (e.g. the newborn) are not hypertensive, as mineralocorticoids increase blood pressure primarily by retaining sodium and thus increasing intravascular volume.

Deficient adrenal androgen secretion will compromise the acquisition of virilizing secondary sexual characteristics (pubic and axillary hair, comedones, axillary odor) in female adolescents. Moderate hypersecretion of adrenal androgens is characterized by mild signs of virilization, whereas substantial hypersecretion of adrenal androgens is characterized by accelerated growth with a disproportionate increase in bone age, increased muscle mass, acne, hirsutism, deepening of the voice and more profound degrees of virilism. A key feature of any physical examination of a virilized male is careful examination and measurement of the testes. Bilaterally enlarged testes suggest true (central) precocious puberty; unilateral testicular enlargement suggests testicular tumor; prepubertal testes in a virilized male indicate an extratesticular source of androgen, such as the adrenal.

Imaging studies are of limited use in adrenocortical disease. Computed tomography (CT) rarely detects pituitary tumors secreting ACTH, although recent advances in magnetic resonance imaging (MRI) may detect many of these with gadolinium enhancement. The small size, odd shape and location near other structures compromise the use of imaging techniques for the adrenals. Patients with Cushing disease or CAH have modestly enlarged adrenals but these are often not detectable by imaging with any useful degree of certainty. The gross enlargement of the adrenals in congenital lipoid adrenal hyperplasia, their hypoplasia in adrenal hypoplasia congenita or in the hereditary ACTH unresponsiveness syndrome can be imaged, as can many malignant tumors but most adrenal adenomas are too small to be detected. Thus, imaging studies may establish the presence of pituitary or adrenal tumors but never exclude them.

Laboratory evaluation

Steroid measurements

Plasma cortisol is measured by a variety of techniques including radioimmunoassay, immunoradiometric assay and high-performance liquid chromatography (HPLC). Other procedures, such as fluorimetric assays and competitive protein-binding assays, are useful research tools but are not in general clinical use. It is of considerable importance to know what procedure one's laboratory is using and precisely what it is measuring, because laboratories may have different normal values and most central hospital and commercial laboratories are designed primarily to serve adult, rather than pediatric, patients. Tables 13.2 and 13.3 summarize the normal plasma concentrations for a variety of steroids.

All immunoassays have some degree of cross-reactivity with other steroids and most cortisol immunoassays detect cortisol and cortisone, which are readily distinguished by HPLC. As the newborn's plasma contains mainly cortisone rather than cortisol during the first few days of life, comparison of newborn data obtained by HPLC with published standards obtained by immunoassays may incorrectly suggest adrenal insufficiency.

With the notable exception of DHEAS, most adrenal steroids exhibit a diurnal variation based on the diurnal rhythm of ACTH. Because the stress of illness or hospitalization can increase adrenal steroid secretion and because diurnal rhythms may not be well established in children <3 years of age, it is best to obtain two or more samples for the measurement of any steroid.

Table 13.2 Mean sex steroid concentration in infants and children. Data adapted from Endocrine Sciences, Tarzana, CA, USA.

	PROG	17-OHP	DHEA	DHEAS	Δ4 A	E1	E2	T		DHT	
								M	F	M	F
Cord blood	1100	62	21	6400	3.0	52	30	1.0	0.9	0.2	0.2
Premature babies	11	8.1	28	11000	7.0			4.2	0.4	1.0	0.1
Term newborns		1.1	20	4400	5.2			6.9	1.4	0.9	0.3
Infants	1.0	1.0	3.8	820	0.7	<0.1	<0.1	6.6	<0.4	1.4	<0.1
Children											
1–6 years			1.0	270	0.9	<0.1	<0.1	0.2	0.1		
6–8 years			3.1	540	0.9	<0.1	<0.1	0.2	0.1		
8–10 years			5.6	1400	0.9	<0.1	<0.1	0.2	0.1		
Males											
Pubertal stage I	0.6	1.3	5.6	950	0.9	0.0	0.0	0.2		<0.1	
Pubertal stage II	0.6	1.6	10	2600	1.6	0.1	0.0	1.4		0.3	
Pubertal stage III	0.8	2.0	14	3300	2.4	0.1	0.1	6.6		0.7	
Pubertal stage IV	1.1	2.6	14	5400	2.8	0.1	0.1	13		1.2	
Pubertal stage V	1.3	3.3	17	6300	3.5	0.1	0.1	19		1.6	
Adult	1.1	3.3	16	7300	4.0	0.1	0.1	22		1.7	
Females											
Pubertal stage I	0.6	1.0	5.6	1100	0.9	0.1	0.0		0.2		0.1
Pubertal stage II	1.0	1.6	11	1900	2.3	0.1	0.1		0.7		0.3
Pubertal stage III	1.3	2.3	14	2500	4.2	0.1	0.1		0.9		0.3
Pubertal stage IV	9.2	2.9	15	3300	4.5	0.1	0.2		0.9		0.3
Pubertal stage V	5.1	3.6	19	4100	6.0	0.2	0.4		1.0		0.3
Adult											
Follicular	1.0	1.5	16	4100	5.8	0.2	0.2		1.0		0.3
Luteal	24	5.4	16	4100	5.8	0.4	0.5		1.0		0.3

Δ4 A androstenedione; DHEA, dehydroepiandrosterone; DHEAS, DHEA sulfate; DHT, dihydrotestosterone; E1, estrone; E2, estradiol; F, female; M, male; PROG, progesterone; 17-OHP, 17-hydroxyprogesterone; T, testosterone.
All values are in nmol/L.

Table 13.3 Mean glucocorticoid and mineralocorticoid concentrations.

	Cortisol	DOC	Corticosterone	18-OH corticosterone	Aldosterone	Plasma renin activity
Cord blood	360	5.5	19		2.4	50
Premature babies	180			5.5	2.8	222
Newborns	140		6.6	9.7	2.6	58
Infants	250	0.6	16	2.2	0.8	33
Children (08.00 h)						
1–2 years	110–550			1.8	0.8	15
2–10 years	As adults	0.3		1.2	0.3→0.8*	8.3
10–15 years	As adults			0.7	0.1→0.6*	3.3
Adults (08.00 h)	280–550	0.2	12	0.6	0.2→0.4*	2.8→4.0*
Adults (16.00 h)	140–280		3.8			

DOC, deoxycorticosterone.

All values in nmol/L except plasma renin activity (µg/L/s).

*Two values separated by an arrow indicate those in supine and upright posture.

Plasma renin

Renin is not generally measured directly but is assayed by its enzymatic activity. Plasma renin activity (PRA) is simply an immunoassay of the amount of angiotensin I generated per milliliter of serum per hour at 37 °C. In normal serum, the concentration of both renin and angiotensinogen (the renin substrate) is limiting. Therefore, another test, plasma renin content (PRC), measures the amount of angiotensin I generated in 1 h at 37 °C in the presence of excess concentrations of angiotensinogen. Immunoassays for renin itself are beginning to enter clinical practice.

PRA is sensitive to dietary sodium intake, posture, diuretic therapy, activity and sex steroids. Because PRA values can vary widely, it is best to measure renin twice, once in the morning after overnight supine posture and then again after maintenance of upright posture for 4 h. A simultaneous 24-h urine for total sodium excretion is generally needed to interpret PRA results. Decreased dietary and urinary sodium, decreased intravascular volume, diuretics and estrogens will increase PRA. Sodium loading, hyperaldosteronemia and increased intravascular volume decrease PRA.

Renin measurements are commonly used in the evaluation of hypertension and in the management of CAH. However, several additional situations require assessment of the renin-angiotensin system. Children with simple virilizing adrenal hyperplasia who do not have clinical evidence of urinary salt wasting (hyponatremia, hyperkalemia, acidosis, hypotension, shock) may nevertheless have increased PRA, especially when dietary sodium is restricted. This was an early clinical sign that this form of 21-hydroxylase deficiency (21-OHD) was simply a milder form of the more common, severe, salt-wasting form. Treatment of simple virilizing 21-OHD with mineralocorticoid sufficient to suppress PRA into the normal range will reduce the child's requirement for glucocorticoids, thus maximizing final adult height. Children with CAH need to have their mineralocorticoid

replacement therapy monitored routinely by measuring PRA. Measurement of angiotensin II is also possible in some research laboratories but most antibodies to angiotensin II cross-react strongly with angiotensin I. Thus, PRA remains the most useful way of evaluating the renin-angiotensin-aldosterone system.

Urinary steroid excretion

The measurement of 24-h urinary excretion of steroid metabolites is one of the oldest procedures for assessing adrenal function and is still useful. Examination of the total 24-h excretion of steroids eliminates the fluctuations seen in serum samples as a function of time of day, episodic bursts of ACTH and steroid secretion and transient stress (such as a visit to the clinic or difficult venepuncture). Collection of a complete 24-h urinary sample can be difficult in the infant or small child. Two consecutive 24-h collections should be obtained. Because of the diurnal and episodic nature of steroid secretion, one should never obtain 8- or 12-h collections and attempt to infer the 24-h excretory rate from such partial collections.

Urinary 17-hydroxycorticosteroids, assayed by the colorimetric Porter–Silber reaction, measures 17,21-dihydroxy-20-ketosteroids by the generation of a colored compound after treatment with phenylhydrazine. The reaction is highly specific for the major urinary metabolites of cortisol and cortisone. It will also measure metabolites of 11-deoxycortisol.

Measurement of 17-hydroxycorticosteroids is being replaced by measurement of urinary free cortisol, thus avoiding the nonspecificity and drug interference problems inherent in 17-hydroxycorticosteroids. In adults, the test is highly reliable in the diagnosis of Cushing syndrome. Free cortisol is extracted from the urine and measured by immunoassay or HPLC, providing the advantage of specificity; furthermore, unlike 17-hydroxycorticosteroids, urinary free cortisol is not increased in exogenous obesity. The upper limit of normal for urinary free cortisol excretion for children is 80 µg/m²/day and that for 17-hydroxycorticosteroids is 5 mg/m²/day. Some clinical experience indicates that urinary 17-hydroxycorticosteroids may be more reliable for the diagnosis of Cushing disease in children, possibly because of greater experience with 17-hydroxycorticosteroids.

Urinary 17-ketosteroids, assayed by the Zimmerman reaction, measure 17-ketosteroids by the generation of a colored compound after treatment with *meta*-dinitrobenzine and acid. The reaction principally measures metabolites of DHEA and DHEAS and thus correlates with adrenal androgen production. Androstenedione will contribute significant 17-ketosteroids and, if an alkali extraction is not used, estrone will also contribute. The principal androgens, testosterone and dihydrotestosterone, have hydroxyl rather than keto groups on carbon 17; hence, their metabolic products are not measured as 17-ketosteroids. A wide variety of drugs, including penicillin, nalidixic acid, spironolactone and phenothiazines, as well as non-specific urinary chromogens can spuriously increase values of 17-ketosteroids. Measurement of urinary 17-ketosteroids remains a useful inexpensive screening test and some clinicians prefer to follow 17-ketosteroids to monitor therapy of CAH but measurements of plasma steroids have now replaced the use of urinary 17-ketosteroids in most centers.

Urinary 17-ketogenic steroids are occasionally confused with urinary 17-ketosteroids because of the similarity of the names; however, 17-ketogenic steroids are used to measure urinary metabolites of glucocorticoids, not sex steroids. Although some laboratories continue to perform measurements of 17-ketogenic steroids, this obsolete assay no longer has a place in modern pediatric practice.

Plasma ACTH and other POMC peptides

Accurate immunoassay of plasma ACTH is available in most centers but its measurement remains more difficult and variable than the assays for most other pituitary hormones. Samples must be drawn into a plastic syringe containing heparin or ethylenediamine tetraacetic acid (EDTA) and transported quickly in plastic tubes on ice, as ACTH adheres to glass and is quickly inactivated. Elevated plasma ACTH concentrations can be informative but most assays cannot detect low or low-normal values and such values can be spurious if the samples are handled badly. In adults and older children with well-established diurnal rhythms of ACTH, normal 08.00 h values rarely exceed 50 pg/mL, whereas 20.00 h values are usually undetectable. Patients with Cushing disease often have normal morning values but consistently elevated afternoon and evening ones can suggest the diagnosis. Patients with the ectopic ACTH syndrome have values from 100 to 1000 pg/mL.

Secretory rates

The secretory rates of cortisol and aldosterone (or other steroids) can be measured by administering a small dose of tritiated cortisol or aldosterone and measuring the specific activity of one or more known metabolites in a 24-h urine collection. This procedure permitted the measurement of certain steroids, such as aldo-

sterone, before specific immunoassays became available. The procedures have provided much information about the normal rate of production of various steroids. On the basis of this procedure, most authorities previously concluded that children and adults secrete about 12 mg cortisol per square meter of body surface area per day. More recent studies indicate a rate of 6–9 mg/m² in children and adults. Such differences are of considerable importance in estimating physiological replacement doses of glucocorticoids.

Dexamethasone suppression test

Administration of small doses of dexamethasone, a potent synthetic glucocorticoid, will suppress secretion of pituitary ACTH and of adrenal cortisol. Originally described by Liddle in 1960, the dexamethasone suppression test remains the most useful procedure for distinguishing whether glucocorticoid excess is caused primarily by pituitary or adrenal disease. As dexamethasone also suppresses adrenal androgen secretion, this test is useful for distinguishing between adrenal and gonadal sources of sex steroids. A dexamethasone suppression test requires the measurement of basal values and those obtained in response to both low- and high-dose dexamethasone. Variations of the test are common, notably the single 1.0-mg dose in adults or 0.3 mg/m² in children. This is a useful outpatient screening procedure for distinguishing Cushing syndrome from exogenous obesity. It can be useful for the same purpose in adolescents and older children but is otherwise of limited utility in pediatrics. An overnight high-dose dexamethasone suppression test is probably more reliable than the standard 2-day high-dose test in differentiating adults with Cushing disease from those with the ectopic ACTH syndrome. The usefulness of this test in pediatric patients has not been established.

Stimulation tests

Direct stimulation of the adrenal with ACTH is a rapid, safe and easy way to evaluate adrenocortical function. The original ACTH test consisted of a 4- to 6-h infusion of 0.5 units/kg of ACTH (1–39) to stimulate adrenal cortisol secretion maximally. It diagnoses primary adrenal insufficiency (Addison disease). In secondary adrenal insufficiency, some steroidogenic capacity is present and some cortisol is produced in response to the ACTH.

This ACTH test has been replaced in clinical practice by the 60-min test, in which a single bolus of ACTH (1–24) is administered intravenously and cortisol values are measured at 0 and 60 min. Normal responses are shown in Table 13.4 [19]. Synthetic ACTH (1–24) (cosyntropin) is preferred as it has a more rapid action and shorter half-life than ACTH (1–39). The usual dose is 0.1 mg in newborns, 0.15 mg in children up to 2 years of age and 0.25 mg for children over the age of 2 years and adults. All these doses are pharmacological.

A very low-dose (1 µg) test may be useful in assessing adrenal recovery from glucocorticoid suppression. Newer data show that maximal steroidal responses can be achieved after only 30 min but the best available standards are for a 60-min test.

	Infants		Prepubertal		Pubertal	
	Basal	Stimulated	Basal	Stimulated	Basal	Stimulated
17-OH-pregnenolone	6.8		1.7	9.6	3.6	24
17-OHP	0.8	5.8	1.5	5.8	1.8	4.8
DHEA	1.4		2.4	4.3	9.0	19
11-Deoxycortisol	2.3		1.8	5.8	1.7	4.9
Cortisol	280	830	360	830	280	690
DOC	0.6	2.4	0.2	1.7	0.2	1.7
Progesterone	1.1	3.2	1.1	4.0	1.9	4.8

Table 13.4 Responses of adrenal steroids to a 60-min ACTH test. Data adapted from Endocrine Sciences, Tarzana, CA, USA.

All values are mean values in nmol/L.

One of the widest uses of intravenous ACTH tests in pediatrics is in diagnosing CAH. Stimulating the adrenal with ACTH increases steroidogenesis, resulting in the accumulation of steroids proximal to the disordered enzyme. For example, inspection of Fig. 13.1 shows that impaired activity of P450c21 (21-hydroxylase) should lead to the accumulation of progesterone and 17-hydroxyprogesterone (17-OHP). However, progesterone does not accumulate in appreciable quantities, because it, too, is converted to 17-OHP. Measuring the response of 17-OHP to a 60-min or 6-h challenge with ACTH is the single most powerful and reliable means of diagnosing 21-OHD. Comparing the patient's basal and ACTH-stimulated values of 17-OHP against those from large numbers of well-studied patients usually permits the discrimination of normal persons, heterozygotes, patients with non-classic CAH and patients with classic CAH, although there is inevitably some overlap between groups (Fig. 13.7). Measurement of testosterone or Δ^4 androstenedione in response to ACTH can distinguish normal persons from patients with classic CAH but heterozygotes and patients with cryptic CAH have values overlapping both normal and classic CAH.

Longer ACTH tests of up to 3 days have also been used to evaluate adrenal function but it is important to remember that ACTH has both acute and chronic effects. Thus, short tests measure only the acute effects of ACTH, the maximal stimulation of pre-existing steroidogenic machinery. A 3-day test will examine the more chronic effects of ACTH to stimulate increased capacity for steroidogenesis by increasing the synthesis of steroidogenic machinery. Few situations exist in which a 3-day intramuscular ACTH test is indicated, although it is useful in diagnosing the rare syndrome of hereditary unresponsiveness to ACTH [20].

Insulin-induced hypoglycemia is another commonly used test. The hypoglycemia stimulates the release of counter-regulatory hormones (ACTH and cortisol, growth hormone, epinephrine and glucagon) that have actions to increase plasma glucose concentrations. Most patients experience hunger, irritability, diaphoresis and tachycardia; when these are followed by drowsiness or sleep, blood sugar levels are probably below acceptable limits. If this occurs, a blood sample should be obtained and 2 mL/kg 25% glucose given intravenously to a maximum of 100 mL.

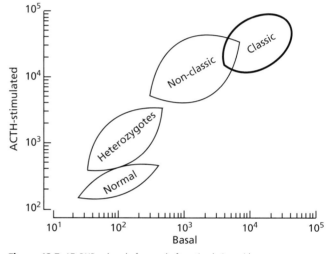

Figure 13.7 17-OHP values before and after stimulation with adrenocorticotropic hormone (ACTH) in normal subjects, patients with congenital adrenal hyperplasia (CAH) and heterozygotes.

Metyrapone test

Metyrapone blocks the action of P450c11β and, to a much lesser extent, P450scc. It is thus a chemical means of inducing a transient deficiency of 11-hydroxylase activity, which results in decreased cortisol secretion and subsequent increase in ACTH secretion. Metyrapone testing is carried out to assess the capacity of the pituitary to produce ACTH in response to a physiological stimulus. This test is useful in evaluating the hypothalamo-pituitary axis in the presence of central nervous system lesions after neurosurgery or long-term suppression by glucocorticoid therapy. Patients with a previous history of hypothalamic, pituitary or adrenal disease or those who have been withdrawn from glucocorticoid therapy should be re-evaluated with a metyrapone test or with an insulin tolerance test. A normal response indicates recovery of the hypothalamo-pituitary-adrenal axis and predicts that the patient will respond normally to the stress of surgery.

Metyrapone is generally given orally as 300 mg/m² every 4 h for a total of six doses (24 h). Unlike many other drugs, it is appropriate to continue to increase the dose in older or overweight patients but the total dose should not exceed 3.0 g. Blood should be obtained for cortisol, 11-deoxycortisol and ACTH before and after the test and a 24-h urine collection should be obtained before and during the test for 17-hydroxycorticosteroids. In a normal response to metyrapone, cortisol decreases, ACTH increases and 11-deoxycortisol (the substrate for P450c11β) increases greatly to about 5 μg/dL. Metabolites of 11-deoxycortisol result in a doubling in urinary 17-hydroxycorticosteroid excretion. Adults and older children can be tested with the administration of a single oral dose of 30 mg/kg at midnight, given with food to reduce the gastrointestinal irritation. Blood samples are drawn at 08.00 h on the mornings before and after administering the drug.

CRH testing

CRH is now generally available as a test of pituitary ACTH reserve. It remains experimental in adults and little experience has been gained from children. Early data suggest that it may be useful for distinguishing hypothalamic from pituitary causes of ACTH deficiency and may also be a useful adjunct in establishing the diagnosis of Cushing disease.

Genetic lesions in steroidogenesis

Autosomal recessive disorders disrupt each of the steps in the pathway shown in Fig. 13.1. Most cause diminished cortisol synthesis. In response to adrenal insufficiency, the pituitary synthesizes increased amounts of POMC and ACTH, which promotes increased steroidogenesis; ACTH and possibly other peptides derived from the amino-terminal end of POMC also stimulate adrenal hypertrophy and hyperplasia. Thus, the term congenital adrenal hyperplasia (CAH) refers to a group of diseases traditionally grouped together on the basis of the most prominent finding at autopsy.

In theory, CAH is easy to understand. A genetic lesion in one of the steroidogenic enzymes interferes with normal steroidogenesis. The signs and symptoms of the disease derive from deficiency of the steroidal end product and the effects of accumulated steroidal precursors proximal to the blocked step. Thus, reference to the pathways in Fig. 13.1 and a knowledge of the biological effects of each steroid should permit one to deduce the manifestations of the disease.

In practice, CAH can be confusing, both clinically and scientifically. The key clinical, laboratory and therapeutic features of each form are summarized in Table 13.5. Because each steroidogenic enzyme has multiple activities and many extra-adrenal tissues contain enzymes that have similar activities, the complete elimination of a specific adrenal enzyme may not result in the complete elimination of its steroidal products from the circulation. In the past, disorders of steroidogenic enzymes had to be studied by examining their steroid metabolites in serum and urine, an indirect approach that led to numerous misconceptions about the steroidogenic processes. The cloning of the genes for the steroidogenic enzymes has now permitted the direct study of these diseases, altering traditional views substantially.

Congenital lipoid adrenal hyperplasia – defects in StAR

Lipoid CAH, the most severe genetic disorder of steroid hormone synthesis, is characterized by the absence of significant concentrations of all steroids, high basal ACTH and plasma renin activity. Steroid responses to long-term treatment with high doses of ACTH or human chorionic gonadotropin (hCG) are absent. The adrenals are usually grossly enlarged with cholesterol and cholesterol esters, although some cases have normal-sized adrenals. These findings indicate a lesion in the first step in steroidogenesis, the conversion of cholesterol to pregnenolone. However, the P450scc gene is normal in these patients. The normal P450scc system plus the accumulation of cholesterol esters in the affected adrenal suggested that the lesion lay in a factor involved in cholesterol transport to the mitochondria. The steroidogenic regulatory protein (StAR) was cloned in 1994 and was quickly identified as the disordered step in lipoid CAH [6]. Thus, lipoid CAH was the first disorder in steroid hormone biosynthesis identified that is not caused by a disrupted steroidogenic enzyme.

Lipoid CAH provided a gene knockout of nature, elucidating the complex physiology of the StAR protein. StAR promotes steroidogenesis by increasing the movement of cholesterol into mitochondria; in the absence of StAR, steroidogenesis proceeds at about 14% of the StAR-induced level. This observation led to the two-hit model of lipoid CAH [21]. The first hit is the loss of StAR itself, leading to a loss of most but not all steroidogenesis, with a compensatory rise in ACTH and LH. These hormones increase cellular cAMP, which increases biosynthesis of LDL receptors, their uptake of LDL-cholesterol and *de novo* synthesis of cholesterol. In the absence of StAR, this increased intracellular cholesterol accumulates as in a storage disease causing the second hit, which is the mitochondrial and cellular damage caused by the accumulated cholesterol, cholesterol esters and their auto-oxidation products.

The two-hit model explains the unusual clinical findings in lipoid CAH. In the fetal testis, which is steroidogenically very active under the trophic stimulation of hCG, the Leydig cells are destroyed early in fetal life, eliminating testosterone biosynthesis. An affected 46XY fetus does not undergo normal virilization and is born with female external genitalia and a blind vaginal pouch. The Sertoli cells remain undamaged and continue to produce Müllerian inhibitory hormone, so that the phenotypically female 46XY fetus has no cervix, uterus or fallopian tubes. The steroidogenically active fetal zone of the adrenal is similarly affected, eliminating most fetal adrenal DHEA biosynthesis and the feto-placental production of estriol; mid-gestation maternal and fetal estriol levels are thus very low.

The definitive zone of the fetal adrenal, which differentiates into the zonae glomerulosa and fasciculata, normally produces very little aldosterone and, as fetal salt and water metabolism are maintained by the placenta, stimulation of the glomerulosa by angiotensin II generally does not begin until birth. Consistent

Table 13.5 Clinical and laboratory findings in the congenital adrenal hyperplasias.

Enzyme	Presentation	Laboratory findings	Therapeutic measures
Lipoid CAH (StAR, P450scc)	Salt-wasting crisis Male pseudohermaphroditism	Low/absent levels of all steroid hormones Decreased/absent response to ACTH Decreased/absent response to hCG in male pseudohermaphroditism ↑ACTH and PRA	Glucocorticoid and mineralocorticoid replacement and salt supplementation Estrogen replacement at age 12 years Gonadectomy of male pseudohermaphrodite
3β-HSD	Salt-wasting crisis ↑Δ⁵/Δ⁴ serum steroids Male and female pseudohermaphroditism	↑Δ⁵ steroids before and after ACTH Suppression of elevated adrenal steroids after glucocorticoid administration ↑ACTH and PRA	Glucocorticoid and mineralocorticoid replacement Salt supplementation Surgical correction of genitalia Sex hormone replacement as necessary
P450c21	*Classic form:* Salt-wasting crisis Female pseudohermaphroditism Pre- and postnatal virilization *Non-classic form:* Premature adrenarche, menstrual irregularity, hirsutism, acne, infertility	↑17-OHP before and after ACTH ↑Serum androgens and urine 17-ketosteroids Suppression of elevated adrenal steroids after glucocorticoid treatment ↑ACTH and PRA	Glucocorticoid and mineralocorticoid replacement Salt supplementation Surgical repair of female pseudohermaphroditism
P450c11β	Female pseudohermaphroditism Postnatal virilization in males and females	↑11-deoxycortisol and DOC before and after ACTH ↑Serum androgens and urine 17-ketosteroids Suppression of elevated steroids after glucocorticoid administration ↑ACTH and ↓PRA Hypokalemia	Glucocorticoid administration Surgical repair of female pseudohermaphroditism
P450c11AS	Failure to thrive Weakness Salt loss	Hyponatremia, hyperkalemia ↑Corticosterone ↓Aldosterone and ↑PRA	Mineralocorticoid replacement Salt supplementation
P450c17	Male pseudohermaphroditism Sexual infantilism Hypertension	↑DOC, 18-OH-DOC, corticosterone, 18-hydroxycorticosterone Low 17α-hydroxylated steroids and poor response to ACTH Poor response to hCG in male pseudohermaphroditism Suppression of elevated adrenal steroids after glucocorticoid administration ↑ACTH and ↓PRA Hypokalemia	Glucocorticoid administration Surgical correction of genitalia and sex steroid replacement in male pseudohermaphroditism consonant with sex of rearing Estrogen replacement in female at 12 years Testosterone replacement if reared as male (rare)
POR	Infants with Antley–Bixler syndrome plus genital anomaly and adrenal insufficiency; maternal aromatase deficiency. Adults with infertility.	↑Prog, 17-OHP, ACTH ↓DHEA androstenedione testosterone, estradiol Poor cortisol response to ACTH Normal mineralocorticoids	Glucocorticoid, mineralocorticoid and sex steroid replacement.

ACTH, adrenocorticotropic hormone; CAH, congenital adrenal hyperplasia; DHEA, dehydroepiandrosterone; DOC, deoxycorticosterone; hCG, human chorionic gonadotropin; PRA, plasma renin activity.

with this, many newborns with lipoid CAH do not have a salt-wasting crisis until after several weeks of life, because StAR-independent aldosterone synthesis initially suffices but chronic stimulation by angiotensin II eventually leads to cellular damage [21].

The two-hit model also explains the spontaneous feminization of affected 46XX females who are treated in infancy and reach adolescence. The fetal ovary makes no steroids and contains no steroidogenic enzymes; consequently, the ovary remains undamaged until it is first stimulated by gonadotropins at the time of puberty, when it produces some estrogen by StAR-independent steroidogenesis. Continued stimulation results in cholesterol accumulation and cellular damage, so that biosynthesis of progesterone in the latter part of the cycle is impaired. Because gonadotropin stimulation recruits individual follicles and does not promote steroidogenesis in the whole ovary, most follicles remain undamaged and available for future cycles. Cyclicity is determined by the hypothalamo-pituitary axis and remains normal. With each new cycle, a new follicle is recruited and more estradiol is produced by StAR-independent steroidogenesis. Although net ovarian steroidogenesis is impaired, enough estrogen is produced (especially in the absence of androgens) to induce breast development, general feminization, monthly estrogen withdrawal and cyclic vaginal bleeding. However, progesterone synthesis in the latter half of the cycle is disturbed by the accumulating cholesterol esters so that the cycles are anovulatory. Measurements of estradiol, progesterone and gonadotropins throughout the cycle in affected adult females with lipoid CAH confirm this model. Similarly, examination of StAR knockout mice confirms the two-hit model. Thus, examination of patients with lipoid CAH has elucidated the physiology of the StAR protein in each steroidogenic tissue.

Genetic analysis of patients with lipoid CAH has revealed numerous mutations in the StAR gene. These data reveal several genetic clusters. Lipoid CAH is common in Japan; about 65–70% of affected Japanese alleles and virtually all affected Korean alleles carry the mutation Q258X. The carrier frequency for this mutation appears to be about 1 in 300, so that 1 in every 250 000–300 000 newborns in these countries is affected, giving a total of about 500 patients in Japan and Korea. Other genetic clusters are found among Palestinian Arabs, most of whom carry the mutation R182L, Saudis, who carry R182H and Swiss, who carry L260P.

Many other mutations have been found throughout the gene but all amino acid replacement (missense) mutations are found in the carboxy-terminal 40% of the protein, which is the biologically important domain. Deletion of only 10 carboxy-terminal residues reduces StAR activity by half and deletion of 28 carboxy-terminal residues by the common Q258X mutation eliminates all activity. In contrast, deletion of the first 62 amino-terminal residues has no effect on StAR activity, even though this deletes the entire mitochondrial leader sequence and forces StAR to remain in the cytoplasmic compartment. Studies of StAR's mitochondrial import show that StAR acts exclusively on the outer mitochondrial membrane and that its level of activity is proportional to the length of time it resides there [22]. Although lipid CAH typically presents in early infancy, some patients with wholly inactivating mutations have survived without therapy for a year and patients with mutations retaining partial activity may present at age 2–4 years with normal male genitalia, a disorder termed "non-classical lipoid CAH" [23]. Treatment of lipoid CAH is straightforward if the diagnosis is made. Physiological replacement with glucocorticoids, mineralocorticoids and salt permit survival to adulthood. The differential diagnosis includes P450scc deficiency, 3β-HSD deficiency and adrenal hypoplasia congenita (AHC). The glucocorticoid requirement is less than in the virilizing adrenal hyperplasias because it is not necessary to suppress excess adrenal androgen production. Growth in these patients should be normal. Genetic males with female external genitalia should undergo orchidectomy and be raised as females.

P450scc and SF1 deficiencies

Fetoplacental P450scc is needed for placental synthesis of progesterone, which is required to suppress uterine contractility and maintain pregnancy in the first trimester. This observation led to the presumption that human P450scc deficiency is incompatible with term gestation. However, a few reports have now described patients with mutations in P450scc. Like patients with lipoid CAH, P450scc-deficient patients have a severe deficiency in the production of all steroid hormones but their adrenals are not enlarged [24]. Affected infants have either had some residual P450scc activity permitting survival to term or have been born prematurely, apparently when the maternal corpus luteum of pregnancy is no longer able to make sufficient progesterone to suppress uterine contractility. A similar clinical presentation has been described in three patients with mutations in steroidogenic factor 1 (SF1), a transcription factor required for the adrenal and gonadal (but not for placental) expression of all steroidogenic enzymes. Thus, the hormonal findings of lipoid CAH may be caused by mutations in factors other than StAR.

3β-Hydroxysteroid dehydrogenase deficiency

3β-HSD deficiency is a rare cause of glucocorticoid and mineralocorticoid deficiency that is fatal if not diagnosed early. Genetic females may have mild cliteromegaly and virilization because the fetal adrenal overproduces large amounts of DHEA, a small portion of which is converted to testosterone by extra-adrenal 3β-HSD type I and 17β-HSD-V. Genetic males also synthesize some androgens by peripheral conversion of adrenal and testicular DHEA but the concentrations are insufficient for complete male genital development so that these males have a small phallus and severe hypospadias. Thus, 3β–HSD deficiency can lead to genital ambiguity in both sexes.

There are two functional human genes for 3β-HSD: the type I gene is expressed in the placenta and peripheral tissues and the type II gene in the adrenals and gonads. Genetic and endocrine studies of 3β-HSD deficiency show that both the gonads and the adrenals are affected as a result of a single mutated 3β-HSD-II gene that is expressed in both tissues. However, considerable hepatic 3β-HSD activity persists in the face of complete absence of adrenal and gonadal activity as a result of the enzyme encoded by the 3β-HSD-I gene, thus complicating the diagnosis of 3β-HSD deficiency. Numerous mutations causing 3β-HSD deficiency have been identified, all in the type II gene [25]. Mutations have never been found in 3β-HSD-I, presumably because this would prevent placental biosynthesis of progesterone, resulting in a spontaneous first-trimester abortion.

The presence of peripheral 3β-HSD activity complicates the diagnosis of this disease. Affected infants should have low concentrations of 17-OHP but some newborns with 3β-HSD deficiency have high concentrations of serum 17-OHP, approaching those seen in patients with classic 21-OHD. These are due to extra-adrenal 3β-HSD-I. The adrenal of a patient with 3β-HSD-II deficiency will secrete very large amounts of the principal Δ^5 compounds, pregnenolone, 17-hydroxypregnenolone and DHEA.

Some of the secreted 17-hydroxypregnenolone is converted to 17-OHP by 3β-HSD-I. This 17-OHP is not effectively picked up by the adrenal for subsequent conversion to cortisol because the circulating concentrations are below the K_m of P450c21. The ratio of the Δ^5 to the Δ^4 compounds remains high, consistent with the adrenal and gonadal deficiency of 3β-HSD. Thus, the principal diagnostic test in 3β-HSD deficiency is intravenous administration of ACTH with measurement of the three Δ^5 compounds and their corresponding Δ^4 compounds.

Mild or "partial" defects of adrenal 3β-HSD activity have been reported on the basis of ratios of Δ^5 steroids to Δ^4 steroids after an ACTH test that exceed 2 or 3 standard deviations (SD) above the mean. The patients are typically young girls with premature adrenarche or young women with a history of premature adrenarche and complaints of hirsutism, virilism and oligomenorrhea. The 3β-HSD-II genes are normal in these patients and even patients with mild 3β-HSD-II mutations have ratios of Δ^5 to Δ^4 steroids that exceed 8 SD above the mean [26]. The basis of the mildly elevated ratios of Δ^5 to Δ^4 steroids in these hirsute individuals with normal 3β-HSD genes is unknown. These patients prove that hormonal studies alone may be insufficient to make a diagnosis of a specific form of CAH. In adult women, the hirsutism can be ameliorated and regular menses restored by suppressing ACTH with 0.25 mg/day dexamethasone given orally but such treatment is contraindicated in girls who have not yet reached final height.

17α-Hydroxylase/17,20-lyase deficiency

P450c17 is a single enzyme that has both 17α-hydroxylase and 17,20-lyase activities. Deficient 17α-hydroxylase activity and deficient 17,20-lyase activity have been described as separate genetic diseases but it is now clear that they represent different clinical manifestations of different lesions in the same gene. P450c17 deficiency is fairly rare, although this disorder is common in Brazil, due to genetic founder effects, with the mutation R362C predominating among individuals of Portuguese ancestry and W406R predominating among those of Spanish descent. Deficient 17α-hydroxylase activity results in decreased cortisol synthesis, overproduction of ACTH and stimulation of the steps proximal to P450c17. The patients may have mild symptoms of glucocorticoid deficiency but this is not life-threatening as the lack of P450c17 results in the overproduction of corticosterone, which also has glucocorticoid activity. This is similar to the situation in rodents, the adrenals of which lack P450c17 and consequently produce corticosterone as their glucocorticoid. Affected patients overproduce DOC in the zona fasciculata, which causes sodium retention, hypertension and hypokalemia and also suppresses plasma renin activity and aldosterone secretion from the zona glomerulosa. When P450c17 deficiency is treated with glucocorticoids, DOC secretion is suppressed and plasma renin activity and aldosterone concentrations rise to normal [27].

The absence of 17α-hydroxylase and 17,20-lyase activities in complete P450c17 deficiency prevents the synthesis of adrenal and gonadal sex steroids. As a result, affected females are phenotypically normal but fail to undergo adrenarche and puberty; genetic males have absent or incomplete development of the external genitalia. The classic presentation is a teenage female with sexual infantilism and hypertension. The diagnosis is made by finding low or absent 17-hydroxylated C_{21} and C_{19} plasma steroids and low urinary 17-hydroxycorticosteroids and 17-KS, which respond poorly to stimulation with ACTH. Serum levels of DOC, corticosterone and 18-hydroxy-corticosterone are elevated, show hyper-responsiveness to ACTH and are suppressible with glucocorticoids.

The single gene for P450c17 is located on chromosome 10q24.3. The molecular basis of 17α-hydroxylase deficiency has been determined in many patients by cloning and sequencing of the mutated gene, identifying nearly 40 distinct mutations.

Selective deficiency of the 17,20-lyase activity P450c17 has been reported in about a dozen cases, which initially led to the incorrect conclusion that 17α-hydroxylase and 17,20-lyase are separate enzymes. One of the original patients had two wholly inactivating mutations, which led to a corrected diagnosis of the patient as having complete 17α-hydroxylase deficiency. Thus, because both 17α-hydroxylase and 17,20-lyase activities of P450c17 are catalyzed by the same active site, it was not clear that a syndrome of isolated 17,20-lyase deficiency could exist until two patients with genital ambiguity, normal excretion of 17-hydroxycorticosteroids and markedly reduced production of C_{19} steroids were studied [28]. One was homozygous for the P450c17 mutation R347H and the other homozygous for R358Q. Both mutations changed the distribution of surface charges in the redox partner binding site of P450c17. When expressed in transfected cells, both mutants retained nearly normal 17α-hydroxylase activity but had no detectable 17,20-lyase activity. Enzymatic competition experiments proved that the mutations did not affect the substrate binding site. When an excess of both P450 oxidoreductase and cytochrome b_5 was provided, some 17,20-lyase activity was restored, demonstrating that the loss of lyase activity was caused by impaired electron transfer. The diagnosis of isolated 17,20 lyase deficiency is difficult, requiring accurate hormonal assays and sophisticated cell biology approaches. Three additional well-characterized patients have been reported carrying mutations in R347 or R358 and one family has been described carrying E305G.

Computational modeling of P450c17 accurately predicts the effects of all known mutations, including those with partial retention of both activities and those causing selective 17,20-lyase deficiency. The model identifies both Arg-347 and Arg-358 and several other arginine and lysine residues in the redox partner binding site; mutations of these residues all cause varying degrees of selective loss of 17,20-lyase activity. Another example of the critical nature of redox partner interactions comes from the sole reported case of cytochrome b_5 deficiency; this patient was a male pseudohermaphrodite but was not evaluated hormonally. The central role of electron transfer in 17,20-lyase activity is now well established.

21-Hydroxylase deficiency

21-OHD results from mutations in the gene encoding adrenal P450c21. It is one of the most common inborn errors of metabolism and accounts for about 95% of CAH cases. Because of success in diagnosis and treatment in infancy, many patients with severe forms of 21-OHD have reached adulthood, so management issues in CAH concern physicians dealing with all age groups. Detailed reviews of the complex physiology and molecular genetics of this disorder have appeared [29] and a consensus statement on its management has been endorsed by the world's leading pediatric endocrine societies [30].

Pathophysiology

For patients with a complete absence of P450c21, the clinical manifestations can be deduced from Fig. 13.1. Inability to convert progesterone to DOC results in aldosterone deficiency causing severe hyponatremia (Na^+ often below 110 mmol/L), hyperkalemia (K^+ often above 10 mmol/L) and acidosis (pH often below 7.1) with concomitant hypotension, shock, cardiovascular collapse and death. As the control of fluids and electrolytes in the fetus can be maintained by the placenta and the mother's kidneys, the salt-losing crisis develops only after birth, usually during the second week of life.

The inability to convert 17-OHP to 11-deoxycortisol results in cortisol deficiency, which impairs postnatal carbohydrate metabolism and exacerbates cardiovascular collapse because a permissive action of cortisol is required for full pressor action of catecholamines. Although a role for cortisol in fetal physiology is not established, cortisol deficiency is also manifested prenatally. Low fetal cortisol stimulates ACTH secretion, which stimulates adrenal hyperplasia and transcription of the genes for all the steroidogenic enzymes, especially for P450scc, the rate-limiting enzyme in steroidogenesis. This increased transcription increases enzyme production and activity, with consequent accumulation of non-21-hydroxylated steroids, especially 17-OHP. As the pathways in Fig. 13.1 indicate, these steroids are converted to testosterone.

In the male fetus, the testes produce large amounts of mRNA for the steroidogenic enzymes and concentrations of testosterone are high in early to mid-gestation. This testosterone differentiates external male genitalia from the pluripotential embryonic precursor structures. In the male fetus with 21-OHD, the additional testosterone produced in the adrenals has little if any phenotypic effect. In a female fetus, the ovaries lack steroidogenic enzyme mRNAs and are hormonally quiescent; no sex steroids or other factors are needed for differentiation of the female external genitalia. The testosterone inappropriately produced by the adrenals of the affected female fetus causes varying degrees of virilization of the external genitalia. This can range from mild cliteromegaly, with or without posterior fusion of the labioscrotal folds, to complete labioscrotal fusion that includes a urethra traversing the enlarged clitoris (Fig. 13.8). These infants have normal ovaries, fallopian tubes and a uterus but have ambiguous external genitalia or may be sufficiently virilized that they appear to be male, resulting in errors of sex assignment at birth.

The diagnosis of 21-OHD is suggested by genital ambiguity in females, a salt-losing episode in either sex or rapid growth and virilization in males. Plasma 17-OHP is markedly elevated and hyper-responsive to stimulation with ACTH (Fig. 13.7). Measurement of 11-deoxycortisol, 17-OHP, DHEA and androstenedione is important to distinguish it from other forms of CAH and because adrenal or testicular tumors can also produce 17-OHP. High newborn 17-OHP values that rise further after ACTH can also be seen in 3β-HSD and P450c11 deficiencies. 17-OHP is

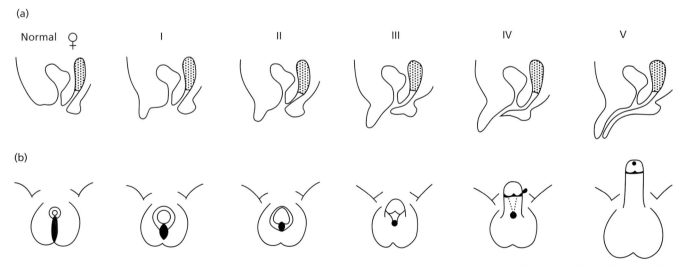

Figure 13.8 Virilization of the external genitalia. A continuous spectrum is shown from normal female to normal male in both sagittal section (a) and perineal views (b), using the staging system of Prader. Disorders of external genitalia can occur either by the virilization of a normal female, as in congenital adrenal hyperplasia or because of an error in testosterone synthesis in the male. In females with congenital adrenal hyperplasia due to 21-OHD, the degree of virilization correlates poorly with the presence or absence of clinical signs of salt loss.

normally high in cord blood but falls to normal newborn levels after 12–24 h (Fig. 13.9) so that assessment of 17-OHP should not be made in the first 24 h of life. Premature infants and term infants under severe stress (e.g. with cardiac or pulmonary disease) may have persistently elevated 17-OHP concentrations with normal 21-hydroxylase. Newborn screening programs measuring 17-OHP have improved the ascertainment of newborns with CAH. The technologies and age-adjusted normal values vary substantially in different health care systems, thus each endocrinologist must become familiar with the local assays and the values found in premature infants, which may otherwise be suspected of having CAH.

Clinical forms of 21-OHD

The broad spectrum of clinical manifestations of 21-OHD depends on the mutations of the P450c21 alleles. The different forms are not different diseases but a spectrum of manifestations, ranging from severe salt wasting to clinically unapparent forms that may be normal variants. Thus, the disease forms described are mainly for clinical convenience.

Salt-wasting 21-OHD

Salt wasting is caused by a complete deficiency of P450c21 activity, effectively eliminating both glucocorticoid and mineralocorticoid synthesis. Females are frequently diagnosed at birth because of masculinization of the external genitalia. After appropriate resuscitation of the cardiovascular collapse, acidosis and electro-

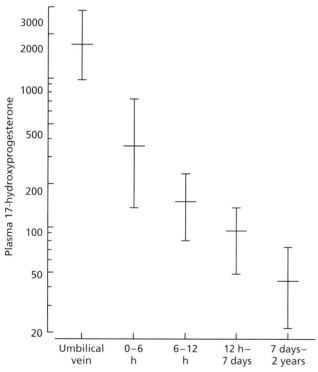

Figure 13.9 Means and ranges of 17-OHP in normal newborns (ng/100 mL). Note that values can be very high and quite variable for the first 24 h of life.

lyte disorders, the mineralocorticoids and glucocorticoids can be replaced orally and the ambiguous genitalia can be corrected with plastic surgical procedures. The management of steroid replacement is difficult because of the rapidly changing needs of a growing infant or child. Drug doses must be adjusted frequently and there is considerable individual variability in what constitutes physiological replacement. As underdosage of glucocorticoids can be life-threatening, especially during illness, most pediatricians have tended to err on the safe side, so children have received inappropriately large doses. It is not possible to compensate for growth lost during the first 2 years of life, when it is fastest, so these children almost always end up short. Female survivors may have sexual dysfunction, marry with a low frequency and have decreased fertility. Males are not generally diagnosed at birth and they come to medical attention either during the salt-losing crisis that follows 5–15 days later or they die, invariably having been diagnosed incorrectly.

Simple virilizing 21-OHD

Virilized females with elevated concentrations of 17-OHP but who do not suffer a salt-losing crisis have long been recognized as having the simple virilizing form of CAH. The existence of this clinical variant first led to the incorrect belief that there were distinct 21-hydroxylases in the zona glomerulosa and in the zona fasciculata. Males often escape diagnosis until age 3–7 years, when they develop pubic, axillary and facial hair and phallic growth. The testes remain of prepubertal size in CAH, whereas gonadotropic stimulation in true precocious puberty results in pubertal-sized testes. The children grow rapidly and are tall for age when diagnosed but their bone age advances at a disproportionately rapid rate so that adult height is compromised.

Untreated or poorly treated children may fail to undergo normal puberty and boys may have small testes and azoospermia because of the feedback effects of the adrenally produced testosterone. When treatment is begun at several years of age, suppression of adrenal testosterone secretion may remove tonic inhibition of the hypothalamus, occasionally resulting in true central precocious puberty requiring treatment with a gonadotropin-releasing hormone (GnRH) agonist. High concentrations of ACTH in some poorly treated boys may stimulate enlargement of adrenal rests in the testes. These enlarged testes are usually nodular, unlike the homogeneously enlarged testes in central precocious puberty. Because the adrenal normally produces 100–1000 times as much cortisol as aldosterone, mild defects (amino acid replacement mutations) in P450c21 are less likely to affect mineralocorticoid than cortisol secretion. Thus, patients with simple virilizing CAH simply have a less severe disorder of P450c21. This is reflected by increased plasma renin activity seen after moderate salt restriction.

Non-classic 21-OHD

Many people have very mild forms of 21-OHD. These may be evidenced by mild to moderate hirsutism, virilism, menstrual irregularities and decreased fertility in adult women (so-called late-onset CAH) but there may be no phenotypic manifestations at all, other than an increased response of plasma 17-OHP to an intravenous ACTH test (so-called cryptic CAH). Despite the minimal manifestations of this disorder, these individuals have hormonal evidence of a mild impairment in mineralocorticoid secretion, as predicted from the existence of a single adrenal 21-hydroxylase.

There has been considerable debate about how to classify patients, principally because each diagnostic category represents a picture in a spectrum of disease resulting from a spectrum of lesions in the P450c21 gene. Furthermore, because many different mutant P450c21 alleles are common in the general population, most patients are compound heterozygotes, carrying a different mutation in the alleles inherited from each parent. Finally, many factors other than the specific mutations found in P450c21 influence the clinical phenotype, including the presence of extra-adrenal 21-hydroxylases (other than P450c21), undiagnosed P450c21 promoter mutations and variations in androgen sensitivity. Discordances between genotype and phenotype are to be expected.

Incidence of 21-OHD

Perinatal screening for elevated concentrations of serum 17-OHP in several countries yields an incidence of 1 in 14 000 for salt-wasting and simple virilizing CAH and 1 in 60 for heterozygous carriers. This calculation has been confirmed through the screening of 1.9 million newborns in Texas [31]. The overall incidence was 1 in 16 000 and, because of the large numbers involved, an ethnic breakdown was possible showing an incidence of 1 in 15 600 Caucasians, 1 in 14 500 Hispanics (primarily Mexican Americans of indigenous American ancestry) and 1 in 42 300 African-Americans. Because about 20% of the African-American gene pool is of European descent, the calculated incidence in individuals of wholly African ancestry is about 1 in 250 000.

Non-classic 21-OHD is much more common but the data vary from 1 in 27 for Ashkenazi Jews, 1 in 53 for Hispanics, 1 in 63 for Yugoslavs, 1 in 333 for Italians to 1 in 1000 for other Whites. This indicates that one-third of Ashkenazi Jews, one-quarter of Hispanics, one-fifth of Yugoslavs, one-ninth of Italians and one-fourteenth of other Caucasians are heterozygous carriers. However, carrier rates of 1.2–6% for Caucasian populations that were not subdivided further have been recorded. These differences reflect the small populations examined, the restricted and geographic localities involved and the errors that arise when hormonal data are used to distinguish individuals with non-classic CAH from heterozygous carriers of classic CAH. This error can be ameliorated by careful measurement of 17-OHP before and after stimulation with ACTH (Fig. 13.7).

In homozygotes for both classic and non-classic CAH, serum concentrations of 21-deoxycortisol rise in response to ACTH but ACTH-induced 21-deoxycortisol remains normal in heterozygotes for both classic and non-classic CAH. However, these studies have classified individuals by hormonal phenotype without examining the P450c21 genes directly to establish these incidences. Therefore, the diagnosis of non-classic CAH requires family studies, as the hormonal data (17-OHP responses to ACTH) in these individuals may be indistinguishable from those for unaffected heterozygous carriers of the more severe forms. The high incidence, lack of mortality and lack of decreased fertility in most individuals with non-classic CAH indicate that this is probably a variant of normal and not a disease in the classic sense. Nevertheless, patients may seek help for virilism and menstrual disorders.

Genetics of the 21-hydroxylase locus
21-Hydroxylase genes

There are two 21-hydroxylase loci, containing a functional gene (formally termed *CYP21A2*) and a non-functional pseudogene (formally termed *CYP21A1P*). These genes, P450c21B (functional gene) and P450c21A (pseudogene), are duplicated in tandem with the *C4A* and *C4B* genes encoding the fourth component of serum complement (Fig. 13.10). Although the P450c21A locus is transcribed, the resulting RNA does not encode a protein; only the P450c21B gene encodes adrenal 21-hydroxylase. The P450c21 genes consist of 10 exons, are about 3.4 kb long and differ in only 87 or 88 of these bases. This high degree of sequence similarity indicates that the two genes are evolving in tandem through intergenic exchange of DNA. The P450c21 genes of mice and cattle are also duplicated and linked to leukocyte antigen loci but only P450c21B functions in humans, only P450c21A functions in mice but both function in cattle. Sequencing of the gene duplication boundaries shows that the human locus, duplicated after mammalian speciation, is consistent with data indicating that other mammals have single P450c21 gene copies.

HLA linkage

The 21-hydroxylase genes lie within the class III region of the human major histocompatibility complex (MHC) (Fig. 13.10). The P450c21 locus lies about 600 kb from HLA-B and about 400 kb from HLA-DR. HLA typing has been used for prenatal diagnosis and to identify heterozygous family members. Statistical associations (linkage disequilibrium) are well established between CAH and certain specific HLA types. Salt-losing CAH is associated with HLA-B60 and HLA-40 in some populations and the rare HLA type Bw47 is very strongly associated with salt-losing CAH. HLA-Bw51 is often associated with simple virilizing CAH in some populations and 30–50% of haplotypes for non-classic CAH carry HLA-B14. HLA-B14 is often associated with a duplication of the *C4B* gene. In contrast, all HLA-B alleles can be found linked to CAH. HLA-identical individuals in a single family may have different clinical features of 21-OHD despite HLA identity, possibly representing extra-adrenal 21-hydroxylation, *de novo* mutations or multiple genetic crossover events.

C4 genes

The tandemly duplicated *C4A* and *C4B* loci produce proteins that can be distinguished functionally and immunologically; the C4B protein has substantially more hemolytic activity, despite greater

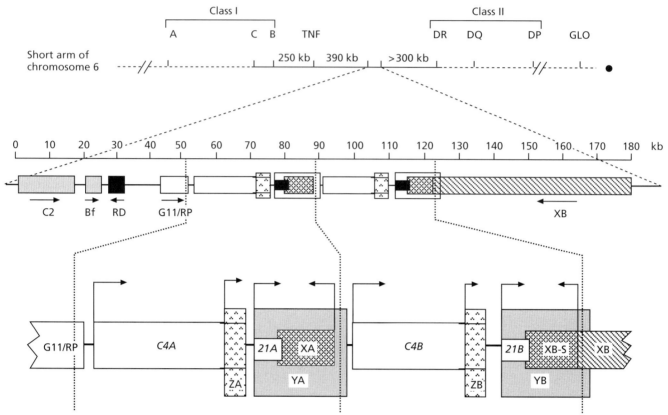

Figure 13.10 Genetic map of the human leukocyte antigen (HLA) locus containing the genes for P450c21. The top line shows the p21.1 region of chromosome 6, with the telomere to the left and the centromere to the right. Most HLA genes are found in the class I and II regions; the class III region containing the P450c21 genes lies between these two. The second line shows the scale (in kilobases) for the diagram immediately below, showing (from left to right) the genes for complement factor C2, properedin factor Bf, the RD gene of unknown function and the G11/RP gene encoding a nuclear serine/threonine kinase; arrows indicate transcriptional orientation. The bottom line shows the 21-hydroxylase locus on an expanded scale, including the C4A and C4B genes for the fourth component of complement, the inactive *CYP21A* gene (21A) and

the active *CYP21B* gene (21B) that encodes P450c21. XA, YA and YB are adrenal-specific transcripts that lack open reading frames. The *XB* gene encodes the extracellular matrix protein tenascin-X; *XB-S* encodes a truncated adrenal-specific form of the tenascin-X protein whose function is unknown. ZA and ZB are adrenal-specific transcripts that arise within the *C4* genes and have open reading frames but it is not known whether they are translated into protein; however, the promoter elements of these transcripts are essential components of the CYP21A and CYP21B promoters. The arrows indicate transcriptional orientation. The vertical dotted lines designate the boundaries of the genetic duplication event that led to the presence of A and B regions.

than 99% sequence identity with C4A. The *C4A* gene is always 22 kb long but there are long (22 kb) and short (16 kb) forms of *C4B* because of a variation in one intron. The 3′ ends of the *C4* genes are only 2466 bp upstream from the transcriptional start sites of the P450c21 genes. Promoter sequences needed for the transcription of the human P450c21B gene lie within intron 35 of the *C4B* gene.

Other genes in the 21-hydroxylase locus

In addition to the P450c21 and C4 genes, there are numerous other genes within 100 kb of the P450c21 gene (Fig. 13.10). XA and XB genes are duplicated with the C4 and P450c21 genes. These lie on the strand of DNA opposite the C4 and P450c21 genes and overlap the 3′ end of P450c21. The last exon of XA and XB lies within the 3′ untranslated region of exon 10 in P450c21A and P450c21B, respectively. Although the human XA locus was

truncated during the duplication of the ancestral C4–P450c21–X genetic unit, the XA gene is abundantly transcribed in the adult and fetal adrenal. In contrast, the XB gene encodes a large extracellular matrix protein (tenascin X) that is expressed in a wide variety of adult and fetal tissues, especially connective tissue [32]. The XB gene spans about 65 kb of DNA and includes 43 exons encoding a 12-kb mRNA. The XA gene also encodes a short truncated form of tenascin X with unknown function and arising from an intragenic promoter.

Identification of a patient with a "contiguous gene syndrome" comprising a deletion of both the P450c21B and XB genes demonstrated that deficiency of tenascin X results in Ehlers–Danlos syndrome (EDS). EDS from tenascin X deficiency is autosomal recessive and typically more severe than the common dominant form of EDS caused by mutations in collagen V [33]. Haploinsufficiency of tenascin X is associated with joint hypermobility.

Tenascin X is associated with and stabilizes collagen fibrils, thus explaining the related phenotype of mutations in tenascin X and collagen-associated genes. Although the various transcripts from the XA and XB genes are complementary to the mRNA for P450c21 and the other transcripts that arise from the P450c21 promoters, these RNAs do not form RNA/RNA duplexes *in vivo* and hence do not regulate P450c21.

P450c21 gene lesions causing 21-OHD

21-OHD can be caused by P450c21B gene deletions, gene conversions and apparent point mutations. Most of the point mutations in the P450c21B gene are actually small gene conversion events, so that gene conversions account for about 85% of the lesions in 21-OHD. The P450c21 genes are autosomal; hence, each person has two alleles, one contributed by each parent. Most patients with 21-OHD are compound heterozygotes, having different lesions on their two alleles. Because gene deletions and large conversions eliminate all P450c21B gene transcription, these lesions cause salt-losing 21-OHD in the homozygous state. Some microconversions, such as those creating premature translational termination, are also associated with salt-losing CAH. Milder forms (simple virilizing and non-classic 21-OHD) are associated with amino acid replacements in the P450c21 protein caused by gene microconversion events. Patients with these forms of CAH are usually compound heterozygotes bearing a severely disordered allele and a mildly disordered allele so that the clinical manifestations are based on the nature of the mildly disordered allele.

Mapping of P450c21 genes in normal subjects and in 21-OHD

Although the P450c21B and P450c21A loci differ by only 87 or 88 nucleotides, they can be distinguished by restriction endonuclease digestion and Southern blotting. Two unusual and related features of the 21-hydroxylase locus complicate its analysis. First, the gene deletions in this locus are most unusual in that they extend 30 kb from one of several points in the middle of P450c21A to the precisely homologous point in P450c21B. Thus, the 15% of alleles that carry deletions do not yield a typical Southern blotting pattern with a band that is a different size from that of the normal, unless one uses very rare cutting enzymes and analyzes the resulting large DNA fragments by pulsed-field gel electrophoresis. The second unusual feature of this locus is that gene conversions are extremely common.

Gene conversions

If a segment of gene A replaces the corresponding segment of the related gene B, the structure of recipient gene B is said to be "converted" to that of donor gene A. The hallmark of gene conversion is that the number of closely related genes remains constant but their diversity decreases. Two types of gene conversions commonly cause 21-OHD, large gene conversions that can be mistaken for gene deletions and small microconversions that resemble point mutations.

The relative frequency of large gene conversions compared with gene deletions in 21-OHD was formerly controversial, principally because initial studies used relatively small groups of patients from single locations or ethnic groups. A compilation of the world literature on the genetics of 21-OHD found that 19% of mutant alleles had gene deletions, 8% large gene conversions, 67% microconversions and 6% uncharacterized lesions (Fig. 13.11). Such statistics must be viewed with caution because there is considerable ascertainment bias in favor of the more severely affected patients and because some studies excluded mildly affected patients. Thus, the above statistics are weighted in favor of gene deletions and large conversions, which can only yield a phenotype of salt-wasting 21-OHD.

Point mutations (microconversions) causing 21-OHD

About 75% of mutated P450c21 genes appear to be structurally intact by Southern blotting and thus appear to carry point mutations. Many mutant P450c21B genes causing 21-OHD have been cloned and sequenced (Table 13.6), revealing that a relatively small number of mutations cause the condition, virtually all of which are also found in the P450c21A pseudogene. These observations indicate that most CAH alleles bearing apparent point mutations actually carry microconversions.

Effects of known point mutations on 21-hydroxylase activity

Three changes in the P450c21A pseudogene render its product non-functional. Each results in an altered reading frame and/or premature stop codon, hence eliminating all activity; all of these, the C→T transition at codon 318, the 8-bp deletion in exon 3 and the T insertion in exon 7, have been found in P450c21B alleles that cause severe salt-losing 21-OHD. Three closely clustered base changes alter the normal amino acid sequence Ile–Val–Glu–Met at codons 236–239 in exon 6 to Asn–Glu–Glu–Lys in both P450c21A and in a small number of genes causing severe

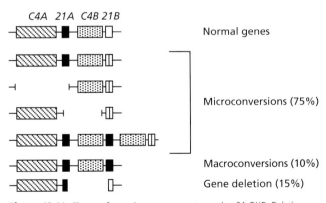

Figure 13.11 Classes of genetic rearrangements causing 21-OHD. Deletions or duplications of the *C4A* and *C4B* genes can occur with or without associated lesions in the P450c21B gene. Note that all "point mutations" in P450c21B are actually "microconversion." Many authors combine the "gene deletion" and "macroconversion" groups because these are difficult to distinguish by Southern blotting, as both result in a loss of the P450c21B gene but the genotypes are clearly distinct, as shown.

Table 13.6 Microconversions of the P450c21B gene that cause 21-hydroxylase deficiency.

Mutation	Location	Associated phenotypes	Activity
Pro-30→Leu	Exon 1	NC/SV	30–60%
A→G	Intron 2	SV/SW	Minimal
8-bp deletion	Exon 3	SW	0
Ile-172→Asn	Exon 4	SV	3–7%
Ile-236→Asp			
Val-237→Glu	Exon 6	SW	0
Met-239→Lys			
Val-281→Leu	Exon 7	NC	18 ± 9%
Gly-292→Ser	Exon 7	SW	
T insertion at 306	Exon 7	SW	0
Gly-318→Stop	Exon 8	SW	0
Arg-339→His	Exon 8	NC	20–50%
Arg-356→Trp	Exon 8	SV/SW	2%
Pro-453→Ser	Exon 10	NC	20–50%
GG→C at 484	Exon 10	SW	0

salt-losing 21-OHD. There is no assayable 21-hydroxylase activity when this sequence is expressed *in vitro*.

The most common lesion in classic 21-OHD is an A→G change in the second intron, 13 bases upstream from the normal 3′ splice acceptor site of this intron, a microconversion found in over 25% of severely affected alleles. This intronic mutation causes abnormal splicing of the mRNA precursor, destroying activity. However, a small portion of this mRNA may be spliced normally in some patients so that the phenotypic presentation is variable; most such patients are salt losers but some are not salt losing. This intron 2 microconversion is often associated with the Ser/Thr polymorphism at codon 268; this is a true polymorphism as S268T does not alter enzymatic activity. The microconversion R356W, which is found in about 10% of severely affected alleles, eliminates all detectable activity, apparently because it changes a residue in the binding site for P450 oxidoreductase. This mutation may retain slight activity and has been found in simple virilizing cases. Other, extremely rare mutations have been described in single individuals.

Missense mutations causing simple virilizing 21-OHD

The microconversion I172N is the most common cause of simple virilizing 21-OHD. Ile-172 is conserved in the other known mammalian P450c21 genes and may contribute to the hydrophobic interactions needed to maintain the correct conformation of the enzyme. When Ile-172 was changed to Asn, Leu, Gln or His and the constructed mutants were expressed in mammalian cells, the mutant constructions yielded only 3–7% of the 21-hydroxylase activity of normal P450c2. The intron 2 microconversion is occasionally seen in simple virilizing cases. The microconversion P30L is generally associated with non-classic 21-OHD but is found in some patients with the simple virilizing form.

Missense mutations causing non-classic 21-OHD

The most common mutation causing non-classic 21-OHD is V281L. This microconversion is seen in all patients with the non-classic form linked to HLA-B14 and HLA-DR1 but is also found in patients with other HLA types. This mutation does not alter the affinity of the enzyme for substrate but drastically reduces its V_{max}. The microconversion P30L is found in about 15–20% of non-classic alleles. In addition, the mutations R339H and P453S have been associated with the non-classic form. Initial surveys of the mutations in P450c21A failed to reveal these mutations, suggesting that they are bona fide point mutations rather than gene microconversions. Examination of large numbers of P450c21A pseudogenes shows that at least the P453S mutation is polymorphic in about 20% of P450c21A pseudogenes and hence also represents a microconversion event.

Structure–function inferences from P450c21 mutations

Each P450c21 missense mutation appears to occur in a functional domain of P450c21. By analogy with the computationally inferred structure of the closely related enzyme P450c17, Arg-356 may be part of the redox partner binding site, Val-281 appears to participate in coordinating the heme moiety and Cys-428 is the crucial cystine residue in the heme binding site found in all cytochrome P450 enzymes. All these mutations can arise by gene microconversions. The N-terminal region of P450c21, including Pro-30, appears to be required for membrane insertion and enzyme stability. Finding most mutations in the amino-terminal portion of P450c21 is consistent with finding most gene conversion and gene deletion events occurring in exons 1–8 of the P450c21B gene. Changes in exons 9 and 10 are very rare, possibly as a result of evolutionary pressure to retain the 3′ untranslated and 3′ flanking DNA of the P450c21B gene, as this DNA also contains the 3′ end of the XB gene.

Prenatal diagnosis of 21-OHD

The prenatal diagnosis and therapy of 21-OHD are being actively pursued but prenatal therapy remains experimental and controversial [30,34–36]. The fetal adrenal is active in steroidogenesis from early in gestation, so a diagnosis can be made by amniocentesis and measurement of amniotic fluid 17-OHP. Concentrations of Δ^4 androstenedione are also elevated in the amniotic fluid of fetuses with 21-OHD, providing a potentially useful adjunctive assay. However, amniotic fluid concentrations of 17-OHP and Δ^4 androstenedione are reliable only for identifying fetuses affected with severe salt-losing 21-OHD, because these steroids may not be elevated above the broad range of normal in the non-salt-losing or non-classic forms.

If a fetus is known to be at risk because the parents are known heterozygotes, 21-OHD can be diagnosed by HLA typing of fetal amniocytes or by analysis of fetal amniocyte DNA. However, this procedure is expensive and not wholly reliable because some HLA antigens are not expressed on fetal amniocytes, hence HLA typing is rarely used for this purpose in clinical practice.

Experimental prenatal treatment of CAH

Experimental prenatal treatment requires early and accurate prenatal diagnosis. Female fetuses affected with 21-OHD begin to become virilized at about 6–8 weeks' gestation at the same time that a normal male fetal testis produces large amounts of testosterone, causing fusion of the labioscrotal folds, enlargement of the genital tubercle into a phallus and the formation of the phallic urethra. The adrenals of affected female fetuses can produce concentrations of testosterone that may approach those in a normal male, resulting in varying degrees of masculinization of the external genitalia. If fetal adrenal steroidogenesis is suppressed in an affected fetus, the virilization can be reduced or eliminated. Several studies have reported the application of this approach by administering dexamethasone to the mother as soon as pregnancy is diagnosed. This can be done only when the parents are known to be heterozygotes by already having had an affected child. However, even in such pregnancies, only one in four fetuses will have CAH. Furthermore, as no prenatal treatment is needed for male fetuses affected with CAH, only one in eight pregnancies of heterozygous parents would harbor an affected female fetus that might potentially benefit from prenatal treatment and seven would have been treated unnecessarily.

The efficacy, safety and desirability of such prenatal treatment remain controversial [34–36]. It is not known precisely when the fetal hypothalamus begins to produce CRH, when the fetal pituitary begins to produce ACTH, whether all fetal ACTH production is regulated by CRH or whether these hormones are suppressible by dexamethasone in the early fetus. Although there is considerable evidence that pharmacological doses of glucocorticoids do not harm pregnant women, few data exist for the fetus. Pregnant women with diseases such as nephrotic syndrome and systemic lupus erythematosus are generally treated with prednisone, which does not reach the fetus because it is inactivated by placental 11β-HSD. Treatment of a fetus requires the use of fluorinated steroids that escape metabolism by these enzymes and few data are available about the long-term use of such agents throughout gestation. The available studies indicate that the response of the fetal genital anatomy to treatment is generally good if the treatment is started very early (before week 6); thereafter, the virilization is reduced but may not be eliminated, so that at least one reconstructive surgical procedure may still be needed in the infant.

Successful treatment requires dexamethasone doses of 20 μg/kg maternal body weight. For a 70-kg woman, this is 1.4 mg, which is equivalent to that in the low-dose dexamethasone suppression test. As the physiological replacement dose of dexamethasone is less than 0.2 mg/m^2 body surface area, this dose is three to six times the physiological replacement dose. The fetus normally develops in the presence of very low cortisol concentrations (less than 100 nmol/L, 3.6 μg/dL), i.e. about 10% of the corresponding maternal level. Thus, the doses used in prenatal treatment appear to achieve effective concentrations of active glucocorticoid that may be up to 60 times physiological for the fetus. Treatment of pregnant rats with 20 μg/kg dexamethasone predisposes the fetuses to hypertension in adulthood and some studies indicate that even moderately elevated concentrations of glucocorticoids can be neurotoxic. Thus, prenatal treatment of CAH remains an experimental and controversial therapy that should be performed only in research centers. Follow-up studies of very long duration are needed to evaluate its effects fully, especially on the seven fetuses treated unnecessarily.

Other non-traditional approaches to CAH have been proposed. Experimental combined treatment with an aromatase inhibitor (e.g. testolactone) and an antiandrogen (e.g. flutamide), in addition to cortisol replacement, has been reported to improve growth [37]. Inhibition of aromatase will ameliorate the rapid advancement of bone age, as it is estrogens, not androgens, that stimulate epiphyseal closure, while the antiandrogen ameliorates virilization. The advantage of this approach is that it permits the use of physiologic replacement doses of cortisol (8 mg/m^2/day) rather than the traditional supraphysiologic dose of 12–15 mg/m^2/day needed to suppress ACTH and the abnormal adrenal steroidogenesis of CAH. However, the drugs involved are expensive and not approved for this use.

Another controversial experimental approach is the performance of adrenalectomy in patients with severe salt-losing CAH. Laparascopic adrenalectomy is itself relatively low-risk. Among 18 adrenalectomized patients with CAH, five had adrenal crisis when glucocorticoid replacement therapy was insufficient and two became hypoglycemic in association with another illness [38]. It is not clear whether this represents an increased risk compared to children receiving conventional therapy without adrenalectomy.

Diagnosis

The key diagnostic maneuver in all forms of 21-OHD is the measurement of the 17-OHP response to intravenous synthetic ACTH. Individual patient responses must be compared with age- and sex-matched data from normal children (Table 13.4; Fig. 13.7). Other ancillary tests are listed in Table 13.5.

PRA and its response to salt restriction constitute an especially useful test. Most patients with simple virilizing 21-OHD have high PRA, which increases further on sodium restriction, confirming that these patients are partially mineralocorticoid deficient and can maintain a normal serum sodium only by hyperstimulation of the zona glomerulosa. Mineralocorticoid therapy in these patients returns plasma volume to normal and eliminates the hypovolemic drive to ACTH secretion. Thus, mineralocorticoid therapy often permits the use of lower doses of glucocorticoids in patients with simple virilizing CAH, optimizing growth in children and diminishing unwanted weight gain in adults.

Long-term management is difficult and requires clinical and laboratory evaluation. Growth should be measured at 3- to 4-month intervals, along with an annual assessment of bone age. Each visit should be accompanied by measurement of urinary 17-KS and serum Δ^4 androstenedione, DHEA, DHEAS and testosterone. Measurement of 3α-androstenediol glucuronide may also be useful. In general, plasma 17-OHP is a suboptimal indicator of therapeutic efficacy because of its great diurnal variation and hyperresponsiveness to stress (e.g. clinic visits).

Treatment

Although effective treatment of 21-OHD with cortisone was demonstrated in 1950, the management of this disorder remains difficult. Overtreatment with glucocorticoids causes delayed growth, even when the degree of overtreatment is insufficient to produce signs and symptoms of Cushing syndrome. Undertreatment results in continued overproduction of adrenal androgens, which hastens epiphyseal maturation and closure, again resulting in compromised growth and other manifestations of androgen excess.

Doses of glucocorticoids should be based on the expected normal cortisol secretory rate. Widely cited classic studies have reported that the secretory rate of cortisol is 12.5 ± 3 mg/m^2/day and have led most authorities to recommend doses of 10–20 mg/m^2/day hydrocortisone (cortisol). However, the cortisol secretory rate is actually substantially lower, at $6–7 \pm 2$ mg/m^2/day. Newly diagnosed patients, especially newborns, do require substantially higher initial dosages to suppress their hyperactive CRH-ACTH-adrenal axis: simple physiological replacement is usually insufficient to suppress adrenal androgens.

The glucocorticoid used is important. Most tables of glucocorticoid dose equivalences are based on their equivalence in anti-inflammatory assays. However, the growth-suppressant equivalences of various glucocorticoids do not parallel their anti-inflammatory equivalences. Thus, long-acting synthetic steroids such as dexamethasone have a disproportionately greater growth-suppressant effect and must be avoided when treating growing children and adolescents (Table 13.7). Most authorities favor the use of oral hydrocortisone or cortisone acetate in three divided daily doses in growing children. However, adults and older teen-

agers who have already fused their epiphyses may be managed very effectively with prednisone or dexamethasone.

Only one oral mineralocorticoid preparation, fludrocortisone (9α-fluorocortisol), is generally available. It must be given as crushed tablets, not as a suspension, which delivers the medication unreliably. When the oral route is not available in severely ill patients, mineralocorticoid replacement is achieved through intravenous hydrocortisone plus sodium chloride. Hydrocortisone (20 mg) has a mineralocorticoid effect of about 100 µg 9α-fluorocortisol (Table 13.7). Mineralocorticoids are unique in pharmacology in that their doses are not based on body mass or surface area. In fact, newborns are quite resistant to mineralocorticoids, as reflected by their high serum aldosterone concentrations (Fig. 13.12) and require larger doses (100–200 µg/day) than do adults. In older children, the replacement dose of 9α-fluorocortisol is 50–150 µg/day. A mineralocorticoid is useless unless adequate sodium is presented to the renal tubules. Thus, additional salt supplementation, usually 1–2 g/day NaCl in the newborn, is also needed. Patients with severe salt-losing CAH can sometimes discontinue mineralocorticoid replacement and salt supplementation as adults. They certainly need lower doses, possibly because they become more sensitive to the mineralocorticoid action of hydrocortisone via a developmental decrease in renal 11β-HSD activity, which normally inactivates cortisol to cortisone.

P450 oxidoreductase deficiency – a disorder affecting multiple P450 enzymes

P450 oxidoreductase (POR) deficiency is a newly described and surprisingly common disorder of steroidogenesis. POR is the single enzyme that donates electrons to all microsomal forms of cytochrome P450, as well as to some other enzymes. Having such a broad array of functions, it was not surprising that deletion of the P450 oxidoreductase gene in mice caused early embryonic

Table 13.7 Potency of various therapeutic steroids (set relative to the potency of cortisol).

Steroid	Anti-inflammatory glucocorticoid effect	Growth-retarding glucocorticoid effect	Salt-retaining mineralocorticoid effect	Plasma half-life (min)	Biological half-life (h)
Cortisol (hydrocortisone)	1.0	1.0	1.0	80–120	8
Cortisone acetate (oral)	0.8	0.8	0.8	80–120	8
Cortisone acetate (IM)	0.8	1.3	0.8		18
Prednisone	3.5–4	5	0.8	200	16–36
Prednisolone	4		0.8	120–300	16–36
Methyl prednisolone	5	7.5	0.5		
Betamethasone	25–30		0	130–330	
Triamcinolone	5		0		
Dexamethasone	30	80	0	150–300	36–54
9α-Fluorocortisone	15		200		
DOC acetate	0		20		
Aldosterone	0.3		200–1000		

IM, intramuscularly.

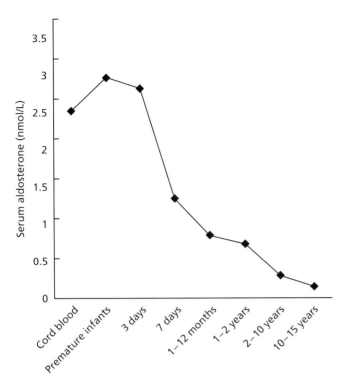

Figure 13.12 Concentrations of aldosterone as a function of age.

lethality. Thus, it was most surprising that POR deficiency was compatible with human life. The first four patients described included three infants with the Antley–Bixler skeletal malformation syndrome and one phenotypically normal adult woman with a form of polycystic ovary syndrome [9]. Antley–Bixler syndrome is characterized by craniosynostosis, radio-ulnar synostosis, bowed femora and other mild malformations. Most genetic forms of craniosynostosis are caused by autosomal dominant, gain-of-function mutations in the gene for fibroblast growth factor receptor 2 (*FGFR2*). Some patients have been described having Antley–Bixler syndrome and *FGFR2* mutations but those patients have normal steroidogenesis and normal external genitalia. By contrast, patients with severe autosomal recessive POR mutations have the Antley–Bixler phenotype plus a complex disorder of steroidogenesis characterized by partial deficiencies in the activities of P450c17, P450c21 and, in some cases, P450aro (aromatase). As a result of the disordered steroidogenesis, external genitalia in males are underdeveloped and in females are partially virilized, so that there is genital ambiguity in both genetic sexes. Other patients have milder mutations in POR, have no malformations associated with the Antley–Bixler syndrome but have reproductive disorders in both sexes. The undervirilization of severely affected male infants and the infertility in mildly affected adult males is a consequence of underproduction of testosterone associated with decreased activity of the 17,20 lyase activity of P450c17. In fact, some individuals with POR deficiency were initially thought to have 17,20 lyase deficiency.

The virilization in females is more complex and appears to involve either or both of two mechanisms. One mechanism for

the virilization of newborn females with POR deficiency is diminished activity of P450aro, which aromatizes androgens to estrogens. Patients with P450aro mutations are virilized at birth because the placental defect in P450aro results in a failure to convert androgenic precursor steroids from the fetal adrenal to estrogens, so that these fetal adrenal androgens are not inactivated and consequently partially virilize the fetus. Pregnant women carrying a fetus (and placenta) with P450aro mutations will also become virilized for the same reason: failure of placental inactivation of fetal adrenal androgens. Some but not all women who have given birth to infants with severe POR mutations have also become virilized during pregnancy, suggesting that the POR deficiency impaired the activity of the placental P45aro [9]. The other mechanism that may be involved in virilized female fetuses with POR deficiency is the diversion of accumulated 17-hydroxyprogesterone through the so-called "backdoor pathway of androgen synthesis" [39]. Current data indicate that both mechanisms are active, with their relative importance depending on the specific POR mutations involved.

Although first described in 2004 [9], about 50 patients were described by 2007, having a wide variety of disordered steroids [40]. The typical pattern includes normal basal concentrations of cortisol that respond poorly to stimulation with ACTH and increased basal and ACTH-stimulated 17-OHP; deoxycorticosterone is typically elevated while there is an irregular pattern of normal or decreased concentrations of DHEA androstenedione and testosterone. The elevated 17-OHP values may be detected on newborn screening programs but rarely reach the levels seen in 21-hydroxylase deficiency. Because there is a broad spectrum of severity among the many POR mutations to date, each patient should be evaluated with basal and ACTH-stimulated measurements of cortisol, 17-OHP and, if possible, 21-deoxycortisol. Measurements of progesterone, deoxycorticosterone, DHEA androstenedione and testosterone should be carried out in all infants. We recommend physiologic cortisol replacement therapy and the use of increased "stress doses" of glucocorticoids for surgery, major trauma or febrile illness, as with any other patient with an impaired cortisol response to ACTH.

A wide variety of mutations have been found in the gene for POR but two are especially common: A287P in patients of European ancestry and R457H in patients of Japanese ancestry. All patients described to date have had a missense mutation on at least one allele. It seems unlikely that patients will be found who are homozygous for mutations that destroy all activity, as knockout of P450 oxidoreductase in mice causes embryonic lethality. As P450 oxidoreductase is required for the activities of all hepatic drug-metabolizing P450 enzymes, it is likely that such patients will also have abnormal drug metabolism. While this issue has not yet been studied directly, reports of Antley–Bixler syndrome in some infants of mothers who ingested fluconazole (an antifungal agent that interferes with the fungal P450 catalyzing lanosterol14-demethylase activity) suggest that defective drug metabolism due to defective P450 oxidoreductase may result in abnormal metabolism of otherwise benign drugs, thus rendering them teratogenic [9,40].

Lesions in isozymes of P450c11: 11β-hydroxylase deficiency, corticosterone methyl oxidase deficiency and glucocorticoid-suppressible hypertension

There are two distinct forms of 11-hydroxylase. P450c11β mediates the 11β-hydroxylation of 11-deoxycortisol to cortisol and that of DOC to corticosterone in the zonae fasciculata and reticularis. P450c11AS, aldosterone synthase, is found only in the zona glomerulosa and mediates 11β-hydroxylation, 18-hydroxylation and 18-oxidation; thus, it is the sole enzyme required to convert DOC to aldosterone. Deficient P450c11β activity is a rare cause of CAH in persons of European ancestry but accounts for about 15% of cases in both Moslem and Jewish Middle Eastern populations. Severe deficiency of P450c11β decreases the secretion of cortisol, causing CAH and virilization of affected females. However, because one of the steroids that accumulates in P450c11β deficiency, DOC, is a mineralocorticoid, these patients can retain sodium.

Although DOC is less potent than aldosterone, it is secreted at high levels in 11β-hydroxylase deficiency, so that salt is retained and the serum sodium remains normal. Overproduction of DOC frequently leads to hypertension; as a result, 11β-hydroxylase deficiency is often termed "the hypertensive form of CAH." However, newborns often manifest mild, transient salt loss, presumably as a result of the normal newborn resistance to mineralocorticoids (Fig. 13.12); this may lead to incorrect diagnosis and treatment. Thus, there may be a poor correlation between DOC concentrations, serum potassium and blood pressure or between the degree of virilization in affected females and the electrolyte and cardiovascular manifestations. The diagnosis is established by demonstrating elevated basal concentrations of DOC and 11-deoxycortisol, which hyperrespond to ACTH; a normal or suppressed plasma renin activity is also a hallmark of this disease.

The genetic lesions causing 11β-hydroxylase deficiency are in the *CYP11B1* gene that encodes P450c11β. In a study of Sephardic Jews of Moroccan ancestry, 11 of 12 affected alleles bore the mutation R448H but at least two frameshifts, four premature stop codons and five amino acid replacement mutations have also been described in other populations [11]. A milder, non-classic form of 11β-hydroxylase deficiency, analogous to non-classic 21-OHD, has been reported in otherwise asymptomatic women with hirsutism, virilism and menstrual irregularities. However, true non-classic 11β-hydroxylase deficiency is rare; only two of five hyperandrogenemic women who had 11-deoxycortisol values more than three times higher than the 95th percentile in response to stimulation with ACTH had mutations of P450c11β, all of which retained 15–37% of normal activity. Repeated ACTH testing in two of the three women who lacked mutations showed much lower (but still elevated) 11-deoxycortisol values. Thus, just as in the case of non-classic 3β-HSD deficiency, an abnormal steroid response to ACTH is not sufficient to diagnose a genetic lesion.

P450c11AS, the isozyme of P450c11β that is 93% identical in its amino acid sequence, is expressed exclusively in the zona glomerulosa, where it catalyzes 11β-hydroxylase, 18-hydroxylase and 18-methyl oxidase activities. Both P450c11AS and P450c11β are expressed in the zona glomerulosa and both can convert DOC to corticosterone but the conversion of corticosterone to 18-hydroxycorticosterone and subsequently to aldosterone is performed exclusively by P450c11AS. Disorders of P450c11AS cause the so-called corticosterone methyl oxidase (CMO) deficiencies, in which aldosterone biosynthesis is impaired while the zonae fasciculata continues to produce corticosterone and DOC. The absence of aldosterone biosynthesis will generally result in a salt-wasting crisis in infancy, at which time the normal secretory rate of DOC is insufficient to meet the newborn's mineralocorticoid requirements (similarly to the newborn with P450c11β deficiency).

These infants typically present with hyponatremia, hyperkalemia and metabolic acidosis but the salt-wasting syndrome is typically less severe than in patients with 21-OHD or lipoid CAH because of the persistent secretion of DOC. These patients may recover spontaneously and grow to adulthood without therapy. This probably reflects the increasing sensitivity to mineralocorticoid action with advancing age in childhood, as reflected by the usual age-related decrease in serum aldosterone (Fig. 13.12). Consistent with this, plasma renin activity is markedly elevated in affected children but may be normal in affected adults.

CMO-I deficiency results from a complete loss of P450c11AS activity so that no 18-hydroxylase or 18-methyl oxidase activity persists, eliminating the biosynthesis of 18OH corticosterone and aldosterone while preserving the biosynthesis of corticosterone by P450c11β. Thus, the diagnosis for CMO-I deficiency is usually based on an increased ratio of corticosterone to 18-OH corticosterone. Only a few cases of CMO-I deficiency have been fully characterized genetically, including a frameshift mutation, a premature stop codon and the missense mutation R384P.

CMO-II deficiency results from amino acid replacement mutations in P450c11AS that selectively delete the 18-methyl oxidase activity while preserving the 18-hydroxylase activity. The diagnosis of CMO-II deficiency requires an increased 18-OH corticosterone and very low aldosterone concentration. CMO-II deficiency is common in Sephardic Jews of Iranian origin, where all affected individuals appear to be homozygous for two different mutations: R181W and V385A [11]. Family members who were homozygous for only one of these mutations were clinically unaffected; both mutations are required to cause disease. The distinction between CMO-I and CMO-II is not precise and these disorders should be regarded as different degrees of severity on a clinical spectrum, just as the various forms of 21-OHD.

Rats have four *CYP11B* genes encoding three P450c11 enzymes but there are only two *CYP11B* genes in the human genome, encoding P450c11β and P450c11AS. This genetic anatomy is reminiscent of the P450c21A and P450c21B genes. Although gene conversion can cause CMO-II deficiency, gene conversion appears to be much rarer than in the P450c21 locus. This may be due to the higher recombinational frequency in the HLA region carrying the P450c21 genes.

Although gene conversion events in the P450c11 locus are rare, an unusual gene duplication causes glucocorticoid-suppressible hyperaldosteronism [41]. This homologous recombination event creates a third P450c11 gene, which fuses the 5′ flanking DNA of the P450c11β gene on to the gene for P450c11AS. These hybrid genes produce a hybrid P450c11 that retains aldosterone synthase activity; however, as the hybrid gene has P450c11β regulatory regions, its transcription is induced by ACTH and cAMP, as is the normal P450c11β gene. Thus, these patients make P450c11AS in response to physiology that should stimulate P450c11β. The excess P450c11AS causes hyperaldosteronism and hypertension, which is then suppressible by glucocorticoid suppression of ACTH, which normally suppresses P450c11β.

It is conceivable that localized microconversions, similar to those that cause most cases of 21-OHD, could insert sequences crucial for aldosterone synthase activity into the P450c11β gene. Expression of chimeric proteins produced *in vitro* identified the residues Ser-288 and Val-320 as important for this activity. However, examination of large numbers of patients with low-renin hypertension has failed to show mutations in this gene system, other than the gene conversions that cause glucocorticoid-suppressible hypertension.

Adrenal insufficiency

Besides CAH, many other conditions cause adrenal insufficiency, including ACTH deficiency and primary adrenal disorders. Primary adrenal insufficiency is commonly termed Addison disease, a vague term that encompasses many disorders (Table 13.8). Up until World War II, most patients with "Addison

disease" had tuberculosis of the adrenal but over 80% of contemporary adult patients have autoimmune adrenalitis and the term *Addison disease* is now widely used to indicate an autoimmune or idiopathic cause.

Chronic primary adrenal insufficiency
Autoimmune adrenalitis
Autoimmune adrenalitis is most commonly seen in 25- to 45-year-old adults, about 70% of whom are women. The incidence in adults is about 1 in 25 000 [42]. The incidence in children is unknown but much less. Boys constitute about 75% of patients. Chronic adrenal insufficiency is suggested by poor weight gain or weight loss, weakness, fatigue, anorexia, hypotension, hyponatremia, hypochloremia, hyperkalemia, frequent illnesses, nausea and vague gastrointestinal complaints (Table 13.9), reflecting chronic deficiency of both glucocorticoids and mineralocorticoids. Early in the course of autoimmune adrenalitis, one may see signs of glucocorticoid deficiency (weakness, fatigue, weight loss, hypoglycemia, anorexia) without signs of mineralocorticoid deficiency [hyponatremia, hyperkalemia, acidosis, tachycardia, hypotension, low voltage on electrocardiogram (ECG), small heart on chest X-ray] or evidence of mineralocorticoid deficiency without glucocorticoid deficiency. Thus, an initial clinical presentation that spares one category of adrenal steroids does not mean it will be spared in the long run. The symptoms listed in Table 13.9 can be seen in chronic adrenal insufficiency that is either primary or secondary.

Table 13.9 Signs and symptoms of adrenal insufficiency.

Features shared by acute and chronic insufficiency
Anorexia
Apathy and confusion
Dehydration
Fatigue
Hyperkalemia
Hypoglycemia
Hyponatremia
Hypovolemia and tachycardia
Nausea and vomiting
Postural hypotension
Salt craving
Weakness

Features of acute insufficiency (adrenal crisis)
Abdominal pain
Fever

Features of chronic insufficiency (Addison disease)
Decreased pubic and axillary hair
Diarrhea
Hyperpigmentation
Low-voltage electrocardiogram
Small heart on X-ray
Weight loss

Table 13.8 Causes of adrenal insufficiency.

Primary adrenal insufficiency
Autoimmune adrenalitis
Autoimmune polyglandular syndromes (types I and II)
Tuberculosis, fungal infections
Sepsis
AIDS
Congenital adrenal hyperplasia
Adrenal hemorrhage or infarction
Congenital adrenal hypoplasia
Adrenoleukodystrophy
Primary xanthomatosis
Unresponsiveness to ACTH

Secondary adrenal insufficiency
Withdrawal from glucocorticoid therapy
Hypopituitarism
Hypothalamic tumors
Irradiation of the CNS

In primary chronic adrenal insufficiency, the low concentrations of plasma cortisol stimulate the hypersecretion of ACTH and other POMC peptides, including the various forms of MSH, which result in hyperpigmentation of the skin and mucous membranes. Such hyperpigmentation is most prominent in skin exposed to sun and in extensor surfaces such as knees, elbows and knuckles. The diagnosis is suggested by the signs and symptoms, verified by a low morning cortisol level with a high ACTH and confirmed by a minimal response of cortisol to a 60-min intravenous ACTH test. Associated findings may include the appearance of a small heart on chest X-ray, anemia, azotemia, eosinophilia, lymphocytosis and hypoglycemia. Treatment consists of physiological glucocorticoid and mineralocorticoid replacement therapy.

Autoimmune adrenalitis is associated with specific HLA haplotypes. The diagnosis of an autoimmune cause is based on finding circulating antiadrenal antibodies. In many cases, the adrenal antigens are the steroidogenic P450 enzymes, especially P450c21. It appears that the primary process is initiated by T lymphocytes and that the antibodies to steroidogenic P450 enzymes are secondary markers, analogous to the antibodies to insulin and glutamic acid decarboxylase seen in type 1 diabetes mellitus.

Type 1 autoimmune polyendocrine syndrome (APS1), also known as autoimmune polyendocrinopathy-candidiasis-ectodermal dysplasia (APECED), is characterized by chronic mucocutaneous candidiasis, autoimmune Addison disease and hypoparathyroidism. At least two of these features must be present to make the diagnosis and their age of onset can be highly variable. Chronic mucocutaneous candidiasis usually affects the mouth and nails in early childhood. Hypoparathyroidism can present with clinical hypocalcemia during mid- or late childhood, although in some cases hypocalcemia may be masked by untreated adrenal insufficiency. The adrenal insufficiency typically becomes apparent in childhood or adolescence. Other findings related to autoimmunity may also be present, including alopecia and vitiligo; gastritis, chronic diarrhea and malabsorption with or without pernicious anemia; and hypergonadotropic hypogonadism. Hepatitis, thyroiditis, interstitial nephritis, myositis, dental enamel hypoplasia and type 1 diabetes mellitus are rare. Keratoconjunctivitis may be an associated feature that requires careful monitoring and treatment to prevent blindness. Oral or esophageal squamous cell carcinoma occurs in 10% of affected adults. Although rare in most populations, APS1 is common among people of Finnish, Sardinian and Iranian Jewish ancestry. APS1 is caused by autosomal recessive mutations in a transcription factor called AIRE (for autoimmune regulator). More than 50 AIRE mutations have been described and R257X is especially common in the Finnish population. The mechanism by which these mutations result in the clinical findings of APS1 are not yet clear, although deletion of AIRE in mice results in ectopic expression of peripheral tissue antigens in thymic medullary epithelial cells, resulting in the development of an autoimmune disorder similar to APS1/APECED.

Type 2 autoimmune polyendocrine syndrome (APS2), also known as Schmidt syndrome, refers to the common association of autoimmune adrenalitis with thyroiditis and/or type 1 diabetes. APS2 is more common in females (3:1 ratio), is HLA-linked and is generally seen in young or middle-aged adults but can present at almost any age. Primary (hypergonadotropic) ovarian failure is seen in up to one-quarter of post-pubertal females with APS2 but primary testicular failure is rare. Pernicious anemia, hepatitis, vitiligo and alopecia may also be seen but the hypoparathyroidism and mucocutaneous candidiasis typical of APS1 are not seen in APS2. APS2 is associated with the same HLA markers as idiopathic autoimmune adrenalitis, which may simply be a form of APS2.

Metabolic causes

Metabolic disorders cause chronic primary adrenal insufficiency, including adrenoleukodystrophy (Schilder disease), primary xanthomatosis (Wolman disease), cholesterol ester storage disease, hereditary unresponsiveness to ACTH and adrenal hypoplasia congenita.

Adrenoleukodystrophy is caused by mutations in a gene on chromosome Xq28a termed ALDP but the mechanism by which these mutations cause the disease is unclear. ALDP encodes a peroxisomal membrane protein termed ABCD1, which belongs to the superfamily of ATP-binding cassette transporters. ALDP imports acyl CoA derivatives of very-long-chain fatty acids into peroxisomes, where they are shortened by β-oxidation, thus affected individuals and carrier females have a surplus of very-long-chain fatty acids. This X-linked disorder is seen almost exclusively in males, with an incidence of about 1 in 20 000, although a rare severe infantile autosomal recessive form also occurs. The disease is characterized by high ratios of $C_{26}:C_{22}$ very-long-chain fatty acids in plasma and tissues, permitting diagnosis of carriers and affected fetuses as well as individual patients. Symptoms commonly develop in mid-childhood but a variant of the disorder, adrenomyeloneuropathy, presents in early adulthood. Both adrenoleukodystrophy and adrenomyeloneuropathy are caused by mutations in the gene for ALDP. The same mutation causes both forms of the disease, so it is likely that other genetic loci are also involved.

Earliest findings are associated with the central nervous system leukodystrophy and include behavioral changes, poor school performance, dysarthria and poor memory, progressing to severe dementia. Symptoms of adrenal insufficiency usually appear after symptoms of white-matter disease but adrenal insufficiency may be the initial finding in up to 20% of cases. In contrast, adrenomyeloneuropathy begins with adrenal insufficiency in childhood and adolescence and signs of neurological disease follow 10–15 years later. A small number of female carriers may also develop neurologic symptoms and adrenal insufficiency with time. Measurement of C_{26} and C_{22} very-long-chain fatty acids can provide accurate early diagnosis if adrenoleukodystrophy is considered. Treatment is largely supportive. Dietary therapy with so-called Lorenzo's oil improves circulating concentrations of very-long-chain fatty acids but is ineffective in reversing established neurologic disease, although its potential role in preventing the onset of neurologic symptoms with early treatment is being evaluated [43,44].

Wolman disease (primary xanthomatosis) and cholesterol ester storage disease are two allelic variants in the secreted form of lysosomal acid lipase (cholesterol esterase) that mobilizes cholesterol esters from adrenal lipid droplets. The gene for this enzyme on chromosome 10q has been cloned and the mutations in it causing one case of Wolman disease have been identified. Because insufficient free cholesterol is available to P450scc, there is adrenal insufficiency. The disease is less severe than congenital lipoid adrenal hyperplasia with respect to steroidogenesis and patients may survive for several months after birth. However, the disease affects all cells, not just steroidogenic cells, as all cells must store and utilize cholesterol; hence, the disorder is relentless and fatal.

Vomiting, steatorrhea, failure to thrive, hepatosplenomegaly and adrenal calcification are the usual presenting findings. The diagnosis is established by bone marrow aspiration yielding foam cells containing large lysosomal vacuoles engorged with cholesterol esters and is confirmed by finding absent cholesterol esterase activity in fibroblasts, leukocytes or marrow cells. Cholesterol ester storage disease appears to be a milder defect in the same enzyme, generally presenting in childhood or adolescence among the 10 reported cases.

Hereditary unresponsiveness to ACTH (familial glucocorticoid deficiency) can present as an acute adrenal crisis precipitated by an intercurrent illness in an infant or with the signs and symptoms of chronic adrenal insufficiency in childhood [20]. Unlike patients with autoimmune adrenalitis, adrenal hypoplasia or other forms of destruction of adrenal tissue, patients with hereditary unresponsiveness to ACTH continue to produce mineralocorticoids normally because production of aldosterone by the adrenal zona glomerulosa is regulated principally by the renin-angiotensin system. Thus, the presenting picture consists of failure to thrive, lethargy, pallor, hyperpigmentation, delayed milestones and hypoglycemia (often associated with seizures) but serum electrolytes are normal and dehydration is usually seen only as part of the precipitating intercurrent illness. There are two forms of familial glucocorticoid deficiency. FGD1 is caused by mutations in the ACTH receptor (MC2R). More than 20 mutations have been found in at least 40 affected individuals [45] but these appear to account for only about 25% of all patients who appear to have familial glucocorticoid deficiency. Hypoglycemia is common and tall stature and increased head circumference may be associated findings. FGD2 is clinically indistinguishable from FGD1 but is caused by mutations in the MC2R accessory protein MRAP and accounts for about 20% of cases of ACTH resistance [20]; thus the cause of about 55% of FGD remains unknown. Both forms of FGD present with dramatically elecated concentrations of ACTH and skin hyperpigmentation. Treatment is with physiologic replacement doses of glucocorticoids; suppression of the ACTH values into the normal range requires supraphysiologic doses of glucocorticoids, which should be avoided.

Triple A (Allgrove) syndrome is a rare disorder consisting of ACTH-resistant adrenal (glucocorticoid) deficiency, achalasia of the cardia and alacrima. Each feature is seen in 80–90% of patients. The disorder is autosomal dominant and resembles ACTH resistance [20]. Many patients also have progressive neurological symptoms, including intellectual impairment, sensorineural deafness, peripheral neuropathies and autonomic dysfunction [45]. The disorder is caused by mutations in a gene called *ALADIN*, which encodes a WD-repeat protein in the nuclear pore [46]. The clinical findings in triple A syndrome may be quite variable, even within a single family. Adrenal insufficiency is rarely the presenting symptom; affected children are typically first evaluated for achalasia or failure to progress neurologically.

Adrenal hypoplasia congenita (AHC, congenital adrenal hypoplasia) generally affects males because the principal form is caused by mutations of the *DAX-1* gene on chromosome Xp21. This gene encodes a nuclear transcription factor that participates at various steps in the differentiation of adrenal and gonadal tissues, as well as in gonadotropin expression, so that successfully treated children may not enter puberty. In this disorder, the definitive zone of the fetal adrenal does not develop and the fetal zone is vacuolated and cytomegalic. Poor function of the fetal zone results in low maternal estriol concentrations during pregnancy but parturition is normal. Neonatal glucocorticoid and mineralocorticoid deficiencies manifest with a typical salt-wasting crisis and respond well to replacement therapy. Deletions of the *DAX-1* gene may also encompass adjacent genes, causing glycerol kinase deficiency, Duchenne muscular dystrophy and mental retardation [47]. Genetic 46XY males with adrenal hypoplasia have normal male external genitalia but, in 46XX females, the distinction between adrenal hypoplasia congenita and congenital lipoid adrenal hyperplasia cannot be made hormonally and requires imaging of the adrenals, which are small in adrenal hypoplasia and large in lipoid CAH. Boys with AHC respond well to glucocorticoid and mineralocorticoid replacement therapy and to testosterone replacement at the age of puberty. Female carriers of DAX1 mutations are unaffected. AHC is relatively common, having been described in over 200 families.

A rare autosomal recessive "miniature" form of AHC affects both sexes equally but the underlying defect remains unclear. A small number of patients have also been described with mutations in SF1 (steroidogenic factor 1), a transcription factor required for adrenal development, transcription of adrenal and gonadal steroidogenic enzymes and for hypothalamic induction of puberty [47].

Primary adrenal failure has also been reported in association with Smith–Lemli–Opitz syndrome, Pallister–Hall syndrome, Pena–Shoekir syndrome, Meckel syndrome, IMAGe syndrome (*i*ntrauterine growth retardation, *m*etaphyseal dysplasia, *a*drenal hypoplasia and *g*enitourinary anomalies) and mitochondrial disorders such as the Kearns–Sayre syndrome.

Other causes

Chronic adrenal insufficiency may result from causes other than these. Adrenal hypoplasia, hemorrhage and infections, all discussed below as causes of acute primary adrenal insufficiency, may spare some adrenal tissue, leaving severely compromised, rather than totally absent, adrenal function. The result, as with autoimmune adrenalitis, is a chronic disorder with insidious onset of the broad range of non-specific findings described above. Tuberculosis, fungal infections and amyloidosis may cause a similar clinical picture.

Acute primary adrenal insufficiency

Acute adrenal crisis occurs most commonly in the child with undiagnosed chronic adrenal insufficiency who is subjected to an additional stress such as major illness, trauma or surgery. The major presenting symptoms and signs include abdominal pain, fever, hypoglycemia with seizures, weakness, apathy, nausea, vomiting, anorexia, hyponatremia, hypochloremia, acidemia, hyperkalemia, hypotension, shock, cardiovascular collapse and death. Treatment consists of fluid and electrolyte resuscitation, ample doses of glucocorticoids, chronic glucocorticoid and mineralocorticoid replacement and treatment of the precipitating illness.

Massive adrenal hemorrhage with shock from blood loss can occur in large infants who have had a traumatic delivery. A flank mass is usually palpable and can be distinguished from renal vein thrombosis by microscopic rather than gross hematuria. The diagnosis is confirmed by CT or ultrasonography. Massive adrenal hemorrhage is more commonly associated with meningococcemia (Waterhouse–Friderichsen syndrome). Meningitis is often but not always present. The characteristic petechial rash of meningococcemia can progress rapidly to large ecchymoses; the blood pressure drops and respirations become labored, frequently leading rapidly to coma and death. Immediate intervention with intravenous fluids, antibiotics and glucocorticoids is not always successful. A similar adrenal crisis may also occur rarely with septicemia from *Streptococcus*, *Staphylococcus*, *Pneumococcus* or diphtheria.

Secondary adrenal insufficiency

Chronic adrenal insufficiency may result from insufficient trophic stimulation of the adrenal and tissue insensitivity to adrenal steroids. Insufficient trophic stimulation of the adrenal can be caused by idiopathic hypopituitarism, central nervous system tumors that damage the cells producing CRH and/or POMC or chronic suppression of these cells by long-term glucocorticoid therapy.

Idiopathic hypopituitarism (multiple anterior pituitary hormone deficiency) is a hypothalamic rather than a pituitary disorder. The deficient secretion of growth hormone, gonadotropins, thyroid-stimulating hormone and ACTH is caused by insufficient stimulation of the pituitary by the corresponding hypothalamic hormones. Isolated growth hormone deficiency, a common disorder and isolated ACTH deficiency, a rare disorder, are variants of this theme. In hypopituitarism from most causes, growth hormone secretion is generally lost first, followed in order by gonadotropins, thyroid-stimulating hormone (TSH) and ACTH. Combined deficiency of growth hormone and ACTH will strongly predispose the patient to hypoglycemia, as both hormones act to raise plasma glucose. Patients with ACTH deficiency, either with or without deficiency of other anterior pituitary hormones, have a relatively mild form of adrenal insufficiency. Mineralocorticoid secretion is normal, whereas cortisol secretion is reduced but not absent. However, adrenal reserve is severely compromised by the chronic understimulation of biosynthesis of the steroidogenic enzymes.

Because some cortisol synthesis continues, the diagnosis may not be apparent unless a CRH or metyrapone test of pituitary ACTH production capacity and an intravenous ACTH test of adrenal reserve are performed. This can be especially true when TSH deficiency is a component of hypopituitarism. The hypothyroidism resulting from TSH deficiency will result in slowed metabolism of the small amount of cortisol produced, which therefore protects the patient from the symptoms of adrenal insufficiency. Treatment of the hypothyroidism with thyroxine will accelerate metabolism of the small amounts of cortisol, thus unmasking adrenal insufficiency resulting from ACTH deficiency and, on occasion, precipitating an acute adrenal crisis. Careful evaluation of the pituitary-adrenal axis is required in hypopituitarism with secondary hypothyroidism. Many clinicians will choose to "cover" a patient with small doses of glucocorticoids (one-quarter to one-half of physiological replacement) during initial treatment of such secondary hypothyroidism.

Hypothalamic and pituitary tumors, such as craniopharyngioma, are associated with ACTH deficiency in about 25% of patients, perhaps more in tumors such as germinoma and astrocytoma. Adrenal insufficiency is rarely the presenting complaint but may contribute to the clinical picture. After surgery and radiotherapy, the great majority of these patients have ACTH deficiency as part of their pituitary damage and all patients should receive glucocorticoid coverage during treatment, irrespective of the status of the hypothalamo-pituitary-adrenal axis at the time the tumor is identified. Cortisol is required for the kidney to excrete free water. Treatment of secondary adrenal insufficiency in some central nervous system tumors can unmask a previously latent deficiency of antidiuretic hormone (ADH) and thus precipitate diabetes insipidus so close attention must be given to a patient's fluids and electrolytes when glucocorticoid therapy is begun.

Metabolic causes of ACTH insufficiency include disorders of the development of the hypothalamic-pituitary axis from mutations in the transcription factors HESX1, LHX4 and SOX3. HESX1 mutations are one of many causes of septo-optic dysplasia, specifically affecting optic nerve development, while LHX4 mutations are associated with cerebellar anomalies. Mutations in PROP1, a transcription factor associated with Pit1, are a frequent cause of multiple pituitary hormone deficiencies, including ACTH deficiency. Defects in POMC synthesis and processing can also cause adrenal insufficiency. Rare cases can be caused by mutations in TBX19, a transcription factor that directly regulates POMC gene transcription. Deletion or mutation of the POMC gene itself can affect multiple POMC-derived peptides, causing a distinct syndrome of red hair, pale skin, obesity and adrenal insufficiency. Defects in PC1, the prohormone convertase that cleaves POMC into its products also cause hypocortisolemia associated with obesity, malabsorptive diarrhea and hypogonadotropic hypogonadism.

Long-term glucocorticoid therapy can suppress POMC gene transcription and the synthesis and storage of ACTH. Furthermore, long-term therapy apparently decreases the synthesis and storage of CRH and diminishes the abundance of receptors for CRH in the pituitary. Therefore, recovery of the hypothalamo-pituitary axis from long-term glucocorticoid therapy entails recovery of multiple components in a sequential cascade and often requires considerable time. Patients successfully withdrawn from glucocorticoid therapy or successfully treated for Cushing disease may exhibit a fairly rapid normalization of plasma cortisol values while continuing to have diminished adrenal reserve for over 6 months.

Glucocorticoid therapy of pregnant women can suppress the fetal adrenal. Treatment of pregnant women with cortisone or prednisone will result in minimal suppression of the fetal adrenal, because placental 11β-HSD converts the biologically active form of these steroids, cortisol and prednisolone, back to their biologically inactive parent compounds. Thus, when radiolabeled cortisol or prednisolone is administered to a pregnant woman, the equilibrium concentrations in maternal plasma are 10 times higher than those in cord plasma. However, dexamethasone is a poor substrate for 11β-HSD, so that administration of low doses to a pregnant woman can affect fetal adrenal steroidogenesis.

Adrenal excess

Cushing syndrome

The term *Cushing syndrome* describes any form of glucocorticoid excess. *Cushing disease* designates hypercortisolism caused by pituitary overproduction of ACTH. The related disorder caused by ACTH of non-pituitary origin is termed the *ectopic ACTH syndrome*. Other causes of Cushing syndrome include adrenal adenoma, adrenal carcinoma and multinodular adrenal hyperplasia. All these are distinct from *iatrogenic Cushing syndrome*, which is the clinical constellation resulting from administration of supraphysiological quantities of ACTH or glucocorticoids.

Although generally described in great detail and illustrated with striking photographs in endocrine texts, Cushing disease is rare in adults but 25% of patients referred to large centers are children, so it is clear that the disorder is more common in children than generally recognized. Many patients first seen as adults actually experienced the onset of symptoms in childhood or adolescence. Harvey Cushing's original patient was a young woman of only 23 years whose history and clinical features indicated long-standing disease. In adults and children over 7 years of age,

the most common cause of Cushing syndrome is Cushing disease. Adult women have a higher incidence of Cushing disease than adult men but the sex ratio is equal in adolescence and prepubertal boys are affected more frequently than prepubertal girls. In infants and children under 7 years, adrenal tumors predominate. Among 60 infants under 1 year of age with Cushing syndrome, 48 had adrenal tumors (Table 13.10) [48].

Clinical findings

The physical features of Cushing syndrome are familiar. Central obesity, "moon facies," hirsutism and facial flushing are seen in over 80% of adults. Striae, hypertension, muscular weakness, back pain, buffalo hump fat distribution, psychological disturbances, acne and easy bruising are also very commonly described (35–80%). These are the signs of advanced Cushing disease. When annual photographs of such patients are available, it is often apparent that the features can take 5 years or longer to develop. Thus, the classic cushingoid appearance will usually not be the initial picture seen in the child with Cushing syndrome.

The earliest, most reliable indicators of hypercortisolism in children are weight gain and growth arrest (Table 13.11) [49]; any overweight child who stops growing should be evaluated for Cushing syndrome. The obesity of Cushing disease in children is initially generalized rather than centripetal and a buffalo hump is evidence of long-standing disease. Psychological disturbances, especially compulsive overachieving behavior, are seen in about 40% of children and adolescents with Cushing disease and are distinctly different from the emotional lability and depression typically seen in adults. An underappreciated aspect is the substantial degree of bone loss and undermineralization in these patients. It is likely that Cushing disease is generally regarded as a disease of young adults because the diagnosis was missed, rather than absent, during adolescence. Rarely, Cushing syndrome caused by adrenal carcinoma and the ectopic ACTH syndrome can produce a rapid fulminant course.

Cushing disease

The recent development of trans-sphenoidal surgical approaches to the pituitary has led to pituitary exploration in large numbers

Table 13.10 Etiology of Cushing syndrome in infancy. Data from Miller *et al.* [48].

	Males	Females
Adrenal tumors (*n* = 48)		
Carcinoma	5	20
Adenoma	4	16
Not defined	2	1
Ectopic ACTH syndrome	1	1
Nodular adrenal hyperplasia	1	4
Undefined adrenal hyperplasia	2	2
ACTH-producing tumor	1	0
Total	16	44

Table 13.11 Findings in 39 children with Cushing disease. Data from Devoe *et al.* [49].

Sign/symptom	Number of patients	%
Weight gain	36/39	92
Growth failure	31/37	84
Ostopenia	14/19	74
Fatigue	26/39	67
Hypertension	22/35	63
Delayed or arrested puberty	21/35	60
Plethora	18/39	46
Acne	18/39	46
Hirsutism	18/39	46
Compulsive behavior	17/39	44
Striae	14/39	36
Bruising	11/39	28
Buffalo hump	11/39	28
Headache	10/39	26
Delayed bone age	2/23	13
Nocturia	3/39	8

of patients with Cushing disease. Among adults, over 90% of such patients have identifiable pituitary microadenomas, which are generally 2–10 mm in diameter, are not encapsulated, have ill-defined boundaries and are frequently detectable with a contrast-enhanced pituitary MRI. They are often identifiable only by minor differences in their appearance and texture from surrounding tissue, so the frequency of surgical cure is correlated with the technical skill of the surgeon. Although histological techniques may not distinguish the tumor from normal tissue, molecular biological techniques confirm increased synthesis of POMC in these tissues. Among children and adolescents, about 80–85% of those with Cushing disease have surgically identifiable microadenomas. Although removal of the tumor usually appears to be curative, 20% of such "cured" patients suffer relapse and manifest Cushing disease again within about 5 years, so that the net cure rate is 65–75%. Trans-sphenoidal surgery offers the best initial approach for rapid and complete cure of most patients, thus maximizing final height, which is typically reduced by 1.5–2.0 SD by the long-term hypercortisolism. Following the removal of the excessive ACTH produced by the microadenoma, the remaining corticotropes of the pituitary respond slowly, over several months, so that postoperative patients have secondary adrenal insufficiency requiring low-dose physiologic replacement and stress coverage for up to several months.

The high cure rate of trans-sphenoidal microadenomectomy in Cushing disease indicates that the majority of patients have primary disease of the pituitary itself, rather than secondary hyperpituitarism resulting from hyperstimulation of the pituitary by CRH or other agents. In most postoperative patients, the circadian rhythms of ACTH and cortisol return to normal, ACTH and cortisol respond appropriately to hypoglycemia, cortisol is easily suppressed by low doses of dexamethasone and the other hypothalamo-pituitary systems return to normal.

Some patients with Cushing disease have no identifiable microadenoma and some "cured" patients relapse. This suggests that this smaller population of patients may have a primary hypothalamic disorder. Effective treatment of Cushing disease with cyproheptidine, a serotonin antagonist, has been reported in adults, further suggesting a hypothalamic disturbance. Thus, present clinical investigation suggests that Cushing disease is usually caused by a primary pituitary adenoma but that sometimes it is caused by hypothalamic dysfunction. Microsurgery can be curative in the former but not in the latter. Unfortunately, no diagnostic maneuver is available to distinguish the two possibilities, so trans-sphenoidal exploration remains the preferred initial therapeutic approach to the patient with Cushing disease.

Other therapeutic approaches include hypophysectomy, pituitary irradiation, cyproheptidine, adrenalectomy and drugs that inhibit adrenal function. All have significant disadvantages, especially in children. Hypophysectomy eliminates pituitary secretion of growth hormone, TSH and gonadotropins, causing growth failure, hypothyroidism, failure to progress in puberty and infertility.

Pituitary irradiation has been touted to avoid many of these problems but the deficiency of various pituitary hormones may be obscured by delayed onset and the delayed onset in elimination of the hypersecretion of ACTH will further compromise the final adult height of the child with Cushing disease. Furthermore, large doses of radiation increase the risk of cerebral arteritis, leukoencephalopathy, leukemia, glial neoplasms, bone tumors involving the skull and congenital defects in subsequent offspring.

Cyproheptidine is not useful in pediatric Cushing disease, partly because of the side effects (weight gain, irritability, hallucinations) often seen with the doses needed.

Laparascopic adrenalectomy is the preferred approach when two trans-sphenoidal procedures fail. In addition to the obvious effects of eliminating normal production of glucocorticoids and mineralocorticoids, removal of the adrenal eliminates the physiological feedback inhibition of the pituitary. In some adults, this results in the development of pituitary macroadenomas, producing very large quantities of ACTH. These can expand and impinge on the optic nerves and can produce sufficient POMC to yield enough MSH to produce profound darkening of the skin (Nelson syndrome) but this is rarely seen in children. There is little pediatric experience with ketoconazole and other drugs that inhibit steroidogenesis but these may provide a useful form of therapy for selected patients. Metyrapone is not useful for long-term therapy. *Ortho, para*-DDD (mitotane), an adrenolytic agent, may be used to effect a chemical adrenalectomy but its side effects of nausea, anorexia and vomiting are severe.

Other causes of Cushing syndrome

The ectopic ACTH syndrome is commonly seen in adults with oat cell carcinoma of the lung, carcinoid tumors, pancreatic islet cell carcinoma and thymoma. Ectopically produced POMC and ACTH are derived from the same gene that produces pituitary

POMC but it is not sensitive to glucocorticoid feedback in the malignant cells. This phenomenon permits distinction between pituitary and ectopic ACTH by suppressibility of the former by high doses of dexamethasone. Although the ectopic ACTH syndrome is rare in children, it has been described in infants younger than 1 year of age. Associated tumors have included neuroblastoma, pheochromocytoma and islet cell carcinoma of the pancreas. The ectopic ACTH syndrome is typically associated with ACTH concentrations 10–100 times higher than those seen in Cushing disease.

Adults and children with this disorder may show little or no clinical evidence of hypercortisolism, probably because of the typically rapid onset of the disease and the general catabolism associated with malignancy. Unlike patients with Cushing disease, patients frequently have hypokalemic alkalosis, presumably because the extremely high levels of ACTH stimulate the production of DOC by the adrenal fasciculata and may also stimulate the adrenal glomerulosa in the absence of hyper-reninemia.

Adrenal tumors, especially adrenal carcinomas, are the more typical cause of Cushing syndrome in infants and small children (Table 13.10). They occur with much greater frequency in girls for unknown reasons. Adrenal adenomas almost always secrete cortisol with minimal secretion of mineralocorticoids or sex steroids. In contrast, adrenal carcinomas tend to secrete both cortisol and androgens. Congenital bodily asymmetry (hemihypertrophy) may be associated with adrenal adenoma or carcinoma, with or without association with the Beckwith–Wiedemann syndrome. CT and MRI are useful in the diagnosis of adrenal tumors. The treatment is surgical, although the prognosis for adrenal carcinoma is generally poor. A few patients have done well with adjunctive therapy with *ortho, para*-DDD. The histologic distinction between carcinoma and adenoma is particularly difficult in the adrenal; size is the best guide to differentiating adenoma (<10 cm) from carcinoma.

ACTH-independent multinodular adrenal hyperplasia is a rare entity characterized by the secretion of both cortisol and adrenal androgens. It is seen in infants, children and young adults, with females affected more frequently. Familial instances have been seen and many of these have an autosomal dominant disorder (Carney complex), consisting of pigmented lentigines and blue nevi on the face, lips and conjunctivae atrial myxomas and a variety of other tumors including schwannomas and Sertoli cell tumors [50]. Carney complex, which accounts for up to 80% of patients with *bilateral* micronodular adrenal hyperplasia, is linked to two distinct genetic loci. The PRKAR1A gene on chromosome 17q22–24, which encodes regulatory subunit 1A of cyclic AMP-dependent protein kinase A (PKA), is mutated in about half of affected patients. Most other patients appear to have mutations in phosphodiesterase 11A4, identified by linkage to chromosome 2q31–2q35 [51]. Because the hypercortisolism is resistant to suppression with high doses of dexamethasone and because both glucocorticoids and sex steroids are produced, this entity was difficult to distinguish from the ectopic ACTH syndrome before plasma ACTH assays became available. Adrenalectomy is usually indicated, although some successes have been reported with subtotal resections. A form of multinodular adrenal hyperplasia is occasionally seen in the McCune–Albright syndrome, suggesting that this form of adrenal hyperfunction may be associated with a G-protein defect.

Differential diagnosis

The suspicion of Cushing syndrome in children is usually raised by weight gain, growth arrest, mood change and change in facial appearance (plethora, acne, hirsutism). The diagnosis may be subtle and difficult when it is sought early in the natural history of the disease. Absolute elevations of concentrations of plasma ACTH and cortisol are often absent. Rather than finding morning concentrations of cortisol >20 µg/dL or of ACTH >50 pg/mL, it is more typical to find mild, often equivocal elevations in the afternoon and evening values. This loss of diurnal rhythm, evidenced by continued secretion of ACTH and cortisol throughout the afternoon, evening and night-time, is usually the earliest reliable laboratory index of Cushing disease. A single plasma cortisol measurement at midnight, obtained from an indwelling venous catheter while the patient remains asleep, should be less than 2 µg/dL and is the most sensitive single test for Cushing disease. Values for ACTH and cortisol are typically extremely high in the ectopic ACTH syndrome, whereas cortisol is elevated but ACTH suppressed in adrenal tumors and in multinodular adrenal hyperplasia (Table 13.12). Inferior petrosal sinus sampling for ACTH has been widely used to distinguish pituitary Cushing disease from ectopic ACTH syndrome in adults but there are few indications for this procedure in adolescents and it is technically impractical in smaller children.

The performance of low- and high-dose dexamethasone suppression tests can be useful. Two days of baseline (control) data should be obtained. Low-dose dexamethasone (20 µg/kg/day) should be given, divided into equal doses given every 6 h for 2 days followed by high-dose dexamethasone (80 µg/kg/day) given in the same fashion. Values at 08.00 h and 20.00 h for ACTH and cortisol and 24-h urine collections for 17-OHS, 17-ketosteroids, free cortisol and creatinine (to monitor the completeness of the collection) should be obtained on each of the 6 days of the test. Because of variations due to episodic secretion of ACTH, 08.00 and 20.00 h blood values should be drawn in triplicate: on the hour and 15 and 30 min after. In patients with exogenous obesity or other non-Cushing disorders, cortisol, ACTH and urinary steroids will be suppressed readily by low-dose dexamethasone. Plasma cortisol should be less than 5 µg/100 mL, ACTH less than 20 pg/mL and 24-h urinary 17-OHS less than 1 mg/g creatinine.

Patients with adrenal adenoma, adrenal carcinoma or the ectopic ACTH syndrome have values relatively insensitive to both low- and high-dose dexamethasone, although some patients with multinodular adrenal hyperplasia may respond to high-dose suppression. Patients with Cushing disease classically respond with a suppression of ACTH, cortisol and urinary steroids during the high-dose treatment but not during the low-dose treatment.

Table 13.12 Diagnostic values in various causes of Cushing syndrome.

Test	Values	Normal	Adrenal carcinoma	Nodular adrenal	Adrenal hyperplasia adenoma	Cushing disease	Ectopic ACTH syndrome
Plasma cortisol	AM	>14	↑	↑	↑	±	↑↑
concentration	PM	<8	↑	↑	↑	↑	↑↑
Plasma ACTH	AM	<100	↓	↓	↓	↑	↑↑
concentration	PM	<50	↓	↓	↓	↑	↑↑
Low-dose dex	Cortisol	<3	No Δ	No Δ	No Δ	*	No Δ
suppression	ACTH	<30	No Δ	No Δ	No Δ	*	No Δ
	17-OHCS	<2	No Δ	No Δ	No Δ	*	No Δ
High-dose dex	Cortisol	↓↓	No Δ	No Δ	†	↓	No Δ
suppression	ACTH	↓↓	No Δ	No Δ	†	↓	No Δ
	17-OHCS	↓↓	No Δ	No Δ	†	↓	No Δ
IV ACTH test	Cortisol	>20	No Δ	±↑	±↑	↑	No Δ
Metyrapone test	Cortisol	↓	±↓	No Δ	±↓	↓	±↓
	11-Deoxycortisol	↑	±↑	No Δ	±↑	↑	±↑
	ACTH	↑	No Δ	No Δ	±↑	↑	No Δ
	17-OHCS	↑	No Δ	No Δ	±	↑	No Δ
24-h urinary excretion	17-OHCS		↑↑	↑	↑	↑	↑ (basal)
	17-Ketosteroids		↑↑	±↑	↑	↑	↑
Plasma concentration	DHEA or DHEAS		↑↑	↓	±↑	↑	↑

Dex, dexamethasone.
Cortisol concentration in mg/dL. ACTH concentration in pg/mL. 17-OHCS in mg/24 h.
*Incomplete response, i.e. ±.
†Usually no Δ.

However, some children, especially those early in the course of their illness, may exhibit partial suppression in response to low-dose dexamethasone. Thus, if the low dose exceeds 20 µg/kg/day or if the assays used are insufficiently sensitive to distinguish partial from complete suppression, false-negative tests may result. In general, the diagnosis of Cushing disease is considerably more difficult to establish in children than in adults.

Virilizing and feminizing adrenal tumors

Most virilizing adrenal tumors are carcinomas producing a mixed array of androgens and glucocorticoids. Virilizing and feminizing adrenal adenomas are rare. Virilizing tumors in boys have a presentation similar to that of simple virilizing CAH with phallic enlargement, erections, pubic and axillary hair, increased muscle mass, deepening of the voice, acne and scrotal thinning; however, testicular size will remain prepubertal. Elevated concentrations of testosterone in young boys alter behavior, with increased irritability, rambunctiousness, hyperactivity and rough play without evidence of libido. Diagnosis is based on hyperandrogenemia that is non-suppressible by glucocorticoids. The treatment is surgical; all such tumors should be handled as if they are malignant, with care exerted not to cut the capsule and seed cells onto the peritoneum. The pathological distinction between adrenal adenoma and carcinoma is difficult.

Feminizing adrenal tumors are extremely rare. P450aro, the enzyme aromatizing androgenic precursors to estrogens, is not normally found in the adrenals but is found in peripheral tissues such as fat. Expression of P450aro has been described in some feminizing adrenocortical carcinomas. Feminizing adrenal (or extra-adrenal) tumors can be distinguished from true (central) precocious puberty in girls by the absence of increased circulating concentrations of gonadotropins and by a prepubertal response of LH to an intravenous challenge of GnRH. In boys, such tumors will cause gynecomastia, which will resemble the benign gynecomastia that often accompanies puberty. However, as with virilizing adrenal tumors, testicular size and the gonadotropin response to GnRH testing will be prepubertal. The diagnosis of a feminizing tumor in a pubertal boy can be extremely difficult but is usually suggested by an arrest in pubertal progression and can be proved by the persistence of circulating plasma estrogens after the administration of testosterone.

Other disorders

Conn syndrome, characterized by hypertension, polyuria, hypokalemic alkalosis and low PRA because of an aldosterone-producing adrenal adenoma, is well described in adults but is exquisitely rare in children. The diagnostic task is to differentiate primary aldosteronism from physiological secondary hyperaldosteronism occurring in response to another physiological disturbance. Any loss of sodium, retention of potassium or decrease in blood volume will result in hyper-reninemic secondary hyperaldosteronism. Renal tubular acidosis, treatment with diuretics, salt-wasting nephritis or hypovolemia due to nephrosis, ascites or blood loss are typical settings for physiological secondary hyperaldosteronism. Primary aldosteronism is characterized by hypertension and hypokalemic alkalosis. The cause is a small adrenal adenoma, usually confined to the zona glomerulosa of one adrenal. Both adrenals need to be explored surgically because adrenal vein catheterization is not possible in children and is difficult in adults.

Familial glucocorticoid resistance is a very rare disorder caused by mutations in the glucocorticoid receptor. Decreased glucocorticoid action results in grossly increased ACTH secretion, which stimulations production of cortisol and other adrenal steroids. Thus, these patients may present with fatigue, hypertension and hypokalemic alkalosis, suggesting a mineralocorticoid excess syndrome but may also have hyperandrogenism [52]. Patients have been described who are homozygous for missense mutations or who are heterozygous for a gene deletion, so that in each case some receptor activity remains. No patients have been described with homozygous deletion of this receptor but glucocorticoid receptor-knockout mice also have disordered hepatic gluconeogenesis, absent adrenomedullary chromaffin cells and die from neonatal respiratory distress syndrome. Thus, familial glucocorticoid resistance is a syndrome of only partial resistance to the action of glucocorticoids.

Pseudohypoaldosteronism (PHA) is a rare salt-wasting disorder of infancy characterized by hyponatemia, hyperkalemia and increased plasma renin activity in the face of elevated aldosterone concentrations. The more common autosomal recessive form of PHA (pseudohypoaldosteronism type II) is caused by inactivating mutations in any of the three subunits (α, β, γ) of the amiloride-sensitive sodium channel, ENaC. This condition is often associated with lower respiratory tract disease consisting of chest congestion, cough and wheezing (but not pulmonary infections) as ENaC mutations increase the volume of pulmonary fluid. This disease persists into adulthood, requiring vigorous salt-replacement therapy throughout life. Gain-of-function mutations due to carboxy-terminal truncation of β-ENaC cause Liddle syndrome, an autosomal dominant form of salt-retaining hypertension.

Autosomal dominant type I pseudohypoaldosteronism (PHA type I) is caused by inactivating mutations in the mineralocorticoid receptor. Approximately 20 different mutations have been found in this receptor, which interfere with mineralocorticoid binding and gene transcription [53]. This disease is milder than the recessive forms of PHA caused by ENaC mutations and remits with age but requires sodium replacement therapy in infancy and childhood. Rarely, point mutations in the mineralocorticoid receptor have been found in association with an autosomal dominant form of severe hypertension, which begins in adolescence and worsens in pregnancy. In these cases, alterations in the structure of the ligand-binding domain of the mineralocorticoid receptor result in mild constitutive activation as well as permitting binding and activation of the receptor by progesterone. An acquired, transient form of PHA is often seen in infants with obstructive uropathy, especially shortly following surgical relief of the obstruction. The lesion is renal tubular so that mineralocorticoid treatment is generally ineffective; salt replacement generally suffices while the renal lesion resolves.

Glucocorticoid therapy and withdrawal

Since their introduction into clinical medicine in the early 1950s, glucocorticoids have been used to treat virtually every known disease. At present, their rational use falls into two broad categories: replacement in adrenal insufficiency and pharmacotherapeutic use. The latter category is largely related to the anti-inflammatory properties of glucocorticoids but also includes their actions to lyze leukemic leukocytes, lower plasma calcium concentrations and reduce increased intracranial pressure. Virtually all these actions are mediated through glucocorticoid receptors, which are found in most cells. Because there appears to be only one major type of glucocorticoid receptor, all glucocorticoids affect all tissues containing such receptors. Thus, with the exception of the distinction between glucocorticoids and mineralocorticoids, tissue-specific, disease-specific or response-specific analogs of naturally occurring glucocorticoids cannot be produced. The only differences among the various glucocorticoid preparations are their ratio of glucocorticoid to mineralocorticoid activity, their capacity to bind to various binding proteins, their molar potency and their biological half-life. Dexamethasone is commonly used in reducing increased intracranial pressure and brain edema. Neurosurgical experience indicates that the optimal doses are 10–100 times those that would thoroughly saturate all available receptors, suggesting that this action of dexamethasone may not be mediated through the glucocorticoid receptor.

Glucocorticoids are so termed because of their major actions to increase plasma concentrations of glucose. This occurs by their induction of the transcription of the genes encoding the enzymes of the Embden–Myerhoff glycolytic pathway and other hepatic enzymes that divert amino acids, such as alanine, to the production of glucose. Thus, the coordinated action to increase the transcription of these genes can result in increased plasma concentrations of glucose, obesity and muscle wasting. The other features of Cushing syndrome are similarly attributable to the increased transcriptional activity of specific glucocorticoid-sensitive genes.

Replacement therapy

Glucocorticoid replacement therapy is complicated by undesirable side effects with even minor degrees of overtreatment or undertreatment. Overtreatment can cause the signs and symptoms of Cushing syndrome and even minimal overtreatment can impair growth. Undertreatment will cause the signs and symptoms of adrenal insufficiency (Table 13.9) only if the extent of undertreatment (dose and duration) is considerable. However, undertreatment may impair the individual's capacity to respond to stress.

To optimize pediatric glucocorticoid replacement therapy, physicians have gauged their therapy to resemble the endogenous secretory rate of cortisol. Previous authorities recommended treatment equivalent to a secretory rate of 12.5 mg cortisol per square meter of body surface area per day, 9.5–15.5 mg/m^2/day. The time-honored value of 12.5 mg/m^2 is too high and appropriate replacement may be as low as 6 mg/m^2 in younger children and 9 mg/m^2 in older children and adolescents.

The management of the delicate balance between over- and undertreatment is confounded by considerable variation in the normal cortisol secretory rate among different children of the same size and the probability that most conventional guidelines err on the side of overtreatment. Additional factors must, however, be considered in tailoring a specific child's glucocorticoid replacement regimen.

The specific form of adrenal insufficiency influences therapy. When treating autoimmune adrenalitis or any other form of Addison disease, it is prudent to err slightly on the side of undertreatment. This will eliminate the possibility of glucocorticoid-induced iatrogenic growth retardation and permit the pituitary to continue to produce normal to slightly elevated concentrations of ACTH. This ACTH will continue to stimulate the remaining functional adrenal steroidogenic machinery and provide a convenient means of monitoring the effects of therapy. In contrast, when treating CAH, the adrenal should be suppressed more completely, as any adrenal steroidogenesis will result in the production of unwanted androgens, with their consequent virilization and rate of advancement of bony maturation that is more rapid than the rate of advancement of height.

The presence or absence of associated mineralocorticoid deficiency is important. Children with mild degrees of mineralocorticoid insufficiency, such as those with simple virilizing CAH, may continue to have mildly elevated ACTH values, suggesting insufficient glucocorticoid replacement in association with elevated PRA. In some children, the ACTH is elevated in response to chronic compromised hypovolemia, attempting to stimulate the adrenal to produce more mineralocorticoid. In these children, who do not manifest overt signs and symptoms of mineralocorticoid insufficiency, treatment with mineralocorticoid replacement may permit one to decrease the amount of glucocorticoid replacement needed to suppress plasma ACTH and urinary 17-ketosteroids. This reduction in glucocorticoid therapy reduces the likelihood that adult height will be compromised.

The specific formulation of glucocorticoid is of great importance. Potent long-acting glucocorticoids, such as dexamethasone or prednisone, are preferred in the treatment of adults but are rarely appropriate for children. Small, incremental dose changes are more easily carried out with weaker glucocorticoids. It is easy to change from 25 to 30 mg hydrocortisone but virtually impossible to change from an equivalent 0.5 to 0.6 mg dexamethasone. The efficacy of attempting to mimic the physiological diurnal variation in steroid hormone secretion remains controversial. As ACTH and cortisol concentrations are high in the morning and low in the evening, it is logically appealing to attempt to duplicate this circadian rhythm in replacement therapy but the results do not indicate clearly that better growth is achieved by giving larger doses in the morning and lower doses at night.

This probably reflects the fact that ACTH and cortisol secretion are episodic throughout the day and that this well-established circadian variation is not smooth. The pattern of high in the morning and low in the evening is only an averaged result. Furthermore, the adrenal releases cortisol episodically throughout the day in response to various physiological demands (e.g. hypoglycemia, exercise, stress); thus, under normal circumstances, the plasma concentrations are high when the clearance and disposal rates are also high. A planned program of replacement therapy cannot possibly anticipate these day-to-day variations.

Finally, dosage equivalents among various glucocorticoids can be misleading (Table 13.7) because most preparations of glucocorticoids are intended for pharmacotherapeutic use rather than replacement therapy and because the most common indication for pharmacological doses of glucocorticoids is for their anti-inflammatory properties.

All these variables explain why there is little unanimity in recommendations for designing a glucocorticoid replacement regimen. An understanding of them will permit appropriate monitoring of the patient and encourage the physician to vary the treatment according to the responses and needs of the individual child.

Commonly used glucocorticoid preparations

Numerous chemical derivatives and variants of the naturally occurring steroids are commercially available in a huge array of dosage, forms, vehicles and concentrations, all carrying confusing and uninformative brand names. Choosing the appropriate product can be simplified by considering only the most widely used steroids listed in Table 13.7. There are four relevant considerations.

First, the glucocorticoid potency of the various drugs is generally calculated and described according to the anti-inflammatory potency. The pharmaceutical industry has chosen this standard for convenience and because the majority of their sales are to physicians using pharmacological doses of these steroids to achieve anti-inflammatory effects.

Second, the growth-suppressant effect of a glucocorticoid preparation may be significantly different from its anti-inflammatory effect. This results from differences in half-life, metabolism and protein-binding and receptor affinity (potency) but it is not because of receptor specificity as all known receptor-mediated effects of glucocorticoids are mediated through a single type of receptor.

Third, the mineralocorticoid activity of various glucocorticoid preparations varies widely. Both glucocorticoid and mineralocorticoid hormones can bind to both glucocorticoid (type I) and mineralocorticoid (type II) receptors and most authorities now regard these as two different types of glucocorticoid receptors and find that there is no true specific mineralocorticoid receptor.

Mineralocorticoid activity is intimately related to the activity of 11β-HSD, which metabolizes glucocorticoids but not mineralocorticoids to a form that cannot bind the receptor. Thus, the relative mineralocorticoid potency of various steroids is determined by both their affinity for the type II receptor and their resistance to the activity of 11β-HSD. An understanding that some commonly used glucocorticoids, such as cortisol, cortisone, prednisolone and prednisone, have significant mineralocorticoid activity is especially important when large doses are used as stress doses in a patient on replacement therapy. Stress doses of the glucocorticoid preparation may provide sufficient mineralocorticoid activity to meet physiological needs, so mineralocorticoid supplementation is not needed.

Fourth, the plasma half-life and biological half-life of the various preparations may be discordant and vary widely. This is mainly related to binding to plasma proteins, hepatic metabolism and hepatic activation. For example, cortisone and prednisone are biologically inactive (and even have mild steroid antagonist actions) until they are metabolized by hepatic 11β-HSD-I to their active forms, cortisol and prednisolone. Thus, the relative glucocorticoid potency of these preparations will also be affected by hepatic function. Cortisone and prednisone are cleared more rapidly in patients receiving drugs such as phenobarbital or phenytoin, which induce hepatic enzymes and are cleared more slowly in patients with liver failure.

In addition to these chemical considerations, the route of administration is critical. Glucocorticoids are available for oral, intramuscular, intravenous, intrathecal, intra-articular, inhalant and topical use on skin, mucous membranes and conjunctivae. Each preparation is designed to deliver the maximal concentration of steroid to the desired tissue while delivering less steroid systemically. All the preparations are absorbed to varying extents, so that the widely used inhalant preparations used to treat asthma can, in sufficient doses, cause growth retardation and other signs of Cushing syndrome.

In general, and in contradistinction to many other drugs, orally administered steroids are absorbed rapidly but incompletely, whereas intramuscularly administered steroids are absorbed slowly but completely. Thus, if the secretory rate of cortisol is 8 mg/m^2 body surface area, the intramuscular or intravenous replacement dose of cortisol (hydrocortisone) would be 8 mg/m^2. However, because only about half of an oral dose is absorbed intact, the oral equivalent would be about 15 mg hydrocortisone. The efficiency of absorption of glucocorticoids can vary considerably depending on diet, gastric acidity, bowel transit time and other individual factors. Thus, the dosage equivalents listed in Table 13.7 are only general approximations. The equivalences shown are estimated biological equivalences with a broad range of variability and are not physical chemical equivalents.

ACTH can also be used for glucocorticoid therapy by its action to stimulate endogenous adrenal steroidogenesis. Although intravenous and intramuscular ACTH are useful in diagnostic tests, the use of ACTH as a therapeutic agent is no longer favored, principally because it will stimulate synthesis of mineralocorticoids and adrenal androgens as well as glucocorticoids. Furthermore, the need to administer ACTH parenterally further diminishes its usefulness.

Intramuscular ACTH (1–39) in a gel form is the treatment of choice for infantile spasms (West syndrome) and possibly also for other forms of epilepsy in infants resistant to conventional anticonvulsants. Whether this action is mediated by ACTH itself, by other peptides in the biological preparation, by ACTH-induced adrenal steroids or by ACTH-responsive synthesis of novel "neurosteroids" in the brain has not been determined. When pharmacological doses of ACTH are used therapeutically, as in infantile spasms, the patient should be given a low-sodium diet to ameliorate steroid hypertension.

Although greatly elevated concentrations of ACTH, as in the ectopic ACTH syndrome, cause pituitary suppression, treatment with daily injections of ACTH results in less hypothalamo-pituitary suppression than treatment with equivalent doses of oral glucocorticoids, presumably because the effect on the adrenal is transient. Adrenal suppression obviously does not occur in ACTH therapy. Because the effects of ACTH on adrenal steroidogenesis are highly variable, it is even more difficult to determine dosage equivalences for ACTH and oral steroid preparations than it is among the various steroids. A very rough guide from studies in adults is that 40 units of ACTH (1–39) gel is approximately equivalent to 100 mg cortisol.

Pharmacological steroid therapy

Pharmacological doses of glucocorticoids are used in an endless variety of clinical situations. The choice of glucocorticoid preparation to be used is guided by pharmacological parameters (described above and in Table 13.7) and by custom (e.g. the use of betamethasone rather than dexamethasone to induce fetal lung maturation in impending premature deliveries). There is substantial variation in the relative glucocorticoid and mineralocorticoid activities of different steroids, depending on the assay used, hence Table 13.7 is a summary from multiple studies and can only be regarded as an imprecise guide.

Pharmacological doses of glucocorticoids administered for more than 1–2 weeks will cause signs and symptoms of iatrogenic Cushing syndrome. These are similar to the glucocorticoid-induced findings in Cushing disease but may be more severe because of the high doses involved (Table 13.13). Iatrogenic Cushing syndrome is not associated with adrenal androgen effects and mineralocorticoid effects are rare.

Alternate-day therapy can decrease the toxicity of pharmacological glucocorticoid therapy, especially suppression of the hypothalamo-pituitary-adrenal axis and growth. The basic premise of alternate-day therapy is that the disease state can be suppressed with intermittent therapy, while there is significant recovery of the hypothalamo-pituitary-adrenal axis during the "off" day. Alternate-day therapy requires the use of a short-acting glucocorticoid administered once in the morning of each therapeutic day to ensure that the "off" day is truly "off." Long-acting

Table 13.13 Complications of high-dose glucocorticoid therapy.

Short-term therapy	Long-term therapy
Gastritis	Gastric ulcers
Growth arrest	Short stature
Increased appetite	Weight gain
Hypercalciuria	Osteoporosis, fractures
Glycosuria	Slipped epiphyses
Immunosuppression	Ischemic bone necrosis
Masked symptoms of infection, especially	Poor wound healing
fever and inflammation	Catabolism
Toxic psychoses	Cataracts
	Bruising (capillary fragility)
	Adrenal/pituitary suppression
	Toxic psychosis

glucocorticoids, such as dexamethasone, should not be used for alternate-day therapy; results are best with oral prednisone or methyl prednisolone.

Withdrawal of glucocorticoid therapy

Withdrawal of glucocorticoid therapy can lead to symptoms of glucocorticoid insufficiency. When glucocorticoid therapy has been used for only 1 week or 10 days, therapy can be discontinued abruptly, even if high doses have been used. Although only one or two doses of glucocorticoid are needed to suppress the hypothalamo-pituitary-adrenal axis, this axis recovers very rapidly from short-term suppression. When therapy has persisted for 2 weeks or longer, recovery of hypothalamo-pituitary-adrenal function is slower and tapered doses of glucocorticoids are indicated. Acute discontinuation of therapy in such patients will lead to symptoms of glucocorticoid insufficiency, the so-called steroid withdrawal syndrome. This symptom complex does not include salt loss, as adrenal glomerulosa function regulated principally by the renin-angiotensin system remains normal. However, blood pressure can fall abruptly, as glucocorticoids are required for the action of catecholamines in maintaining vascular tone.

The most prominent symptoms of the steroid withdrawal syndrome include malaise, anorexia, headache, lethargy, nausea and fever. In reducing pharmacological doses of glucocorticoids, it might appear logical to reduce the dosage precipitously to physiological replacement doses. This is rarely successful and occasionally disastrous. Even when given physiological replacement, patients who have been receiving pharmacological doses of glucocorticoids experience steroid withdrawal.

Although the mechanism is not known, it is most likely that long-term pharmacological glucocorticoid therapy inhibits transcription of the gene(s) for glucocorticoid receptors, thus reducing the number of receptors per cell. If this is so, physiological concentrations of glucocorticoids will elicit subphysiological cellular responses, resulting in the steroid withdrawal syndrome. Thus, it is necessary to taper gradually from the outset. The duration of glucocorticoid therapy is a critical consideration in designing a glucocorticoid withdrawal program. Therapy for a couple of months will completely suppress the hypothalamo-pituitary-adrenal axis but will not cause adrenal atrophy. Therapy of years' duration may result in almost total atrophy of the adrenal fasciculata/reticularis, which may require a withdrawal regimen that takes months.

Procedures for tapering steroids are empirical. Their success is determined by the length and mode of therapy and by individual patient responses. Patients who have been on alternate-day therapy can be withdrawn more easily than those receiving daily therapy, especially daily therapy with a long-acting glucocorticoid such as dexamethasone. In patients on long-standing therapy, a 25% reduction in the previous level of therapy is generally recommended weekly. When withdrawal is carried out with steroids other than cortisone or cortisol, measurement of morning cortisol values can be a useful adjunct. Morning cortisol values of 10 µg/dL or more indicate that the dose can be reduced safely.

Even after the successful discontinuation of therapy, the hypothalamo-pituitary-adrenal axis is not wholly normal and may be incapable of responding to severe stress for 6–12 months after successful withdrawal from long-term high-dose glucocorticoid therapy. Evaluation of the hypothalamus and pituitary by a CRH or metyrapone test and evaluation of adrenal responsiveness to pituitary stimulation with an intravenous ACTH test should be performed at the conclusion of a withdrawal program and 6 months thereafter. The results of these tests will indicate if there is a need for steroid cover in acute surgical stress or illness.

Stress doses of glucocorticoids

The cortisol secretory rate increases significantly during physiological stress such as trauma, surgery or severe illness. Patients receiving glucocorticoid replacement therapy or those recently withdrawn from pharmacological therapy need cover with stress doses. The indications for this cover and the appropriate dose are controversial and difficult to establish; most practitioners prefer to err on the safe side of steroid overdosage. This is a good tactic in the short term but can have a significant effect on growth over a period of years.

It is generally said that doses 3–10 times physiological replacement are needed for the stress of surgery. The stress accompanying a surgical procedure can vary greatly. Modern techniques of anesthesiology, better anesthetic, analgesic and muscle-relaxing drugs and increased awareness of the particular needs of children in managing intraoperative fluids and electrolytes have greatly reduced the stress of surgery. In the past, a significant portion of such stress had to do with pain and hypovolemia but these should be minimized in contemporary practice. Similarly, part of the stress of acute illness is fever and fluid loss, factors now familiar to all pediatricians. Although it remains appropriate and necessary to give about three times physiological requirements during such periods of stress, it is probably not necessary to give much higher doses. Similarly, it is not necessary to triple a child's physiological replacement regimen during simple colds, upper respiratory infection, otitis media or after immunizations.

The preparation of the hypoadrenal patient on replacement therapy for surgery is simple if planned in advance. Although stress doses of steroids can be administered intravenously by the anesthetist during surgery, this may be suboptimal. Doses administered as an intravenous bolus are short acting and may not provide cover throughout the procedure. The transition from ward to operating room to recovery room usually involves a transition among three or more teams of personnel, increasing the risk for error. Because intramuscularly administered cortisone acetate has a biological half-life of about 18 h, we recommend intramuscular administration of twice the day's physiological requirement at 18 h before surgery and again at 8 h before surgery. This provides the patient with a body reservoir of glucocorticoid throughout the surgical and immediate postoperative period. Regular therapy at two to three times physiological requirements can then be reinstituted on the day after the surgical procedure.

Mineralocorticoid replacement

Replacement therapy with mineralocorticoids is indicated in salt-losing CAH and in syndromes of adrenal insufficiency that affect the zona glomerulosa. Only one mineralocorticoid, 9α-fluorocortisol (Fluorinef), is currently available. There is no parenteral mineralocorticoid preparation, so hydrocortisone and salt must be used.

Mineralocorticoid doses used are essentially the same irrespective of the size or age of the patient. Newborns are quite insensitive to mineralocorticoids and may require larger doses than adults. The replacement dose of 9α-fluorocortisol is usually 50–100 μg/day; sodium must be available to the nephrons for mineralocorticoids to promote reabsorption of sodium.

Cortisol has significant mineralocorticoid activity and, when given in stress doses, provides adequate mineralocorticoid activity so that mineralocorticoid replacement can be interrupted. Because 9α-fluorocortisol can be administered only orally and because this may not be possible in the postoperative period, the appropriate drug for glucocorticoid replacement is cortisol or cortisone, which have mineralocorticoid activity, rather than a synthetic steroid such as prednisone or dexamethasone, which have little mineralocorticoid activity.

References

1 Auchus RJ, Miller WL. The principles, pathways and enzymes of human steroidogenesis. In: DeGroot LJ, Jameson JL, eds. *Endocrinology*. Philadelphia: WB Saunders, 2005: 2263–2285.

2 Miller WL, Portale AA. Genetics of vitamin D biosynthesis and its disorders. *Bailliere's Clin Endocrinol Metab* 2001; **15**: 95–109.

3 Penning TM. Molecular endocrinology of hydroxysteroid dehydrogenases. *Endocr Rev* 1997; **18**: 281–305.

4 Miller WL. Regulation of steroidogenesis by electron transfer. *Endocrinology* 2005; **146**: 2544–2550.

5 Stocco DM, Clark BJ. Regulation of the acute production of steroids in steroidogenic cells. *Endocr Rev* 1996; **17**: 221–244.

6 Lin D, Sugawara T, Strauss JF III, Clark BJ, Stocco DM, Saenger P, *et al.* Role of steroidogenic acute regulatory protein in adrenal and gonadal steroidogenesis. *Science* 1995; **267**: 1828–1831.

7 Miller WL. StAR search: what we know about how the steroidogenic acute regulatory protein mediates mitochondrial cholesterol import. *Mol Endocrinol* 2007; **21**: 589–601.

8 Papadopoulos V, Liu J, Culty M. Is there a mitochondrial signaling complex facilitating cholesterol import? *Mol Cell Endocrinol* 2007; **265**: 59–64.

9 Flück CE, Tajima T, Pandey AV, Arlt W, Okuhara K, Verge CF, *et al.* Mutant P450 oxidoreductase causes disordered steroidogenesis with and without Antley-Bixler syndrome. *Nat Genet* 2004; **36**: 228–230.

10 White PC, Speiser PW. Congenital adrenal hyperplasia due to 21-hydroxylase deficiency. *Endocr Rev* 2000; **21**: 245–291.

11 White PC, Curnow KM, Pascoe L. Disorders of steroid 11β-hydroxylase isozymes. *Endocr Rev* 1994; **15**: 421–438.

12 Nowell S, Falany CN. Pharmacogenetics of human cytosolic sulfotransferases. *Oncogene* 2006; **25**: 1673–1678.

13 Grumbach MM, Auchus RJ. Estrogen: consequences and implications of human mutations in synthesis and action. *J Clin Endocrinol Metab* 1999; **84**: 4677–4694.

14 Wilson JD. The role of androgens in male gender role behavior. *Endocr Rev* 1999; **20**: 726–737.

15 Draper N, Stewart PM. 11β-hydroxysteroid dehydrogenase and the pre-receptor regulation of corticosteroid hormone action. *J Endocrinol* 2005; **186**: 251–271.

16 Mesiano S, Jaffe RB. Role of growth factors in the developmental regulation of the human fetal adrenal cortex. *Steroids* 1997; **62**: 62–72.

17 Chrousos GP. The hypothalamic-pituitary-adrenal axis and immune-mediated inflammation. *N Engl J Med* 1995; **332**: 1351–1362.

18 Arlt W. Dehydroepiandrosterone replacement therapy. *Sem Reprod Med* 2004; **22**: 379–388.

19 Lashansky G, Saenger P, Fishman K, Gautier T, Mayes D, Berg G, *et al.* Normative data for adrenal steroidogenesis in a healthy pediatric population: Age and sex-related changes after ACTH stimulation. *J Clin Endocrinol Metab* 1991; **73**: 674–686.

20 Metherell LA, Chan LF, Clark AJ. The genetics of ACTH resistance syndromes. *Best Pract Res Clin Endocrinol Metab* 2006; **20**: 547–560.

21 Bose HS, Sugawara T, Strauss JF III, Miller WL. The pathophysiology and genetics of congenital lipoid adrenal hyperplasia. *N Engl J Med* 1996; **335**: 1870–1878.

22 Bose HS, Lingappa VR, Miller WL. Rapid regulation of steroidogenesis by mitochondrial protein import. *Nature* 2002; **417**: 87–91.

23 Baker BY, Lin L, Kim CJ, Raza L, Smith CP, Miller WL, *et al.* Non-classic congenital lipoid adrenal hyperplasia. A new disorder of the steroidogenic acute regulatory protein with very late presentation and normal male genitalia. *J Clin Endocrinol Metab* 2006; **91**: 4781–4785.

24 Kim CJ, Lin L, Huang N, Quigley CA, AvRuskin TW, Achermann JC, Miller WL. Severe combined adrenal and gonadal deficiency caused by novel mutations in the cholesterol side chain cleavage enzyme, P450scc. *J Clin Endocrinol Metab* 2008; **93**: 696–702.

25 Morel Y, Mébarke F, Rhéaume E, Sanchez R, Forest MG, Simard J. Structure–function relationships of 3β-hydroxysteroid dehydrogenase: Contribution made by the molecular genetics of 3β-hydroxysteroid dehydrogenase deficiency. *Steroids* 1997; **62**: 176–184.

26 Lutfallah C, Wang W, Mason JI, Chang YT, Haider A, Rich B, et al. Newly proposed hormonal criteria via genotypic proof for type II 3β-hydroxysteroid dehydrogenase deficiency. *J Clin Endocrinol Metab* 2002; **87**: 2611–2622.

27 Auchus RJ. The genetics, pathophysiology and management of human deficiencies of P450c17. *Endocrinol Metab Clin North Am* 2001; **30**: 101–119.

28 Geller DH, Auchus RJ, Mendonça BB, Miller WL. The genetic and functional basis of isolated 17,20 lyase deficiency. *Nat Genet* 1997; **17**: 201–205.

29 Merke DP, Bornstein SR. Congenital adrenal hyperplasia. *Lancet* 2005; **365**: 2125–2136.

30. Joint LWPES/ESPE CAH Working Group (Writing Committee: Clayton PE Miller WL, Oberfield SE, Ritzen EM, Sippell WG, Speiser PW). Consensus statement on 21-hydroxylase deficiency from The Lawson Wilkins Pediatric Endocrine Society and The European Society for Paediatric Endocrinology. *J Clin Endocrinol Metab* 2002; **87**: 4048–4953.

31 Therrell BL Jr, Berenbaum SA, Manter-Kapanke V, Simmank J, Korman K, Prentice L, et al. Results of screening 1.9 million Texas newborns for 21-hydroxylase-deficient congenital adrenal hyperplasia. *Pediatrics* 1998; **101**: 583–590.

32 Bristow J, Tee MK, Gitelman SE, Mellon SH, Miller WL. Tenascin-X. A novel extracellular matrix protein encoded by the human XB gene overlapping P450c21B. *J Cell Biol* 1993; **122**: 265–278.

33 Schalkwijk J, Zweers MC, Steijlen PM, Dean WB, Taylor G, van Vlijmen IM, et al. A recessive form of the Ehlers–Danlos syndrome caused by tenascin-X deficiency. *N Engl J Med* 2001; **345**: 1167–1175.

34 New MI, Carlson A, Obeid J, Marshall I, Cabrera MS, Goseco A, et al. Extensive personal experience: prenatal diagnosis for congenital adrenal hyperplasia in 532 pregnancies. *J Clin Endocrinol Metab* 2001; **86**: 5651–5657.

35 Miller WL. Dexamethasone treatment of congenital adrenal hyperplasia: an experimental therapy of unproven safety. *J Urol* 1999; **162**: 537–540.

36 Hirvikoski T, Nordenstrom A, Lindholm T, Lindblad F, Ritzén EM, Wedell A, et al. Cognitive functions in children at risk for congenital adrenal hyperplasia treated prenatally with dexamethasone. *J Clin Endocrinol Metab* 2007; **92**: 542–548.

37 Merke DP, Keil MF, Jones JV, Fields J, Hill S, Cutler GB Jr. Flutamide, testolactone and reduced hydrocortisone dose maintain normal growth velocity and bone maturation despite elevated androgen levels in children with congenital adrenal hyperplasia. *J Clin Endocrinol Metab* 2000; **85**: 1114–1120.

38 Van Wyk JJ, Ritzén EM. The role of bilateral adrenalectomy in the treatment of congenital adrenal hyperplasia. *J Clin Endocrinol Metab* 2003; **88**: 2993–2998.

39 Auchus RJ. The backdoor pathway to dihydrotestosterone. *Trends Endocrinol Metab* 2004; **15**: 432–438.

40 Scott RR, Miller WL. Genetic and clinical features of P450 oxidoreductase deficiency. *Horm Res* 2008; **69**: 266–275.

41 Dluhy RG, Lifton RP. Glucocorticoid-remediable aldosteronism. *J Clin Endocrinol Metab* 1999; **84**: 4341–4344.

42 Betterle C, Dal Pra C, Mantero F, Zanchetta R. Autoimmune adrenal insufficiency and autoimmune polyendocrine syndromes: autoantibodies, autoantigens and their applicability in diagnosis and disease prediction. *Endocr Rev* 2002; **23**: 327–364.

43 Moser HW, Raymond GV, Dubey P. Adrenoleukodystrophy: new approaches to a neurodegenerative disease. *JAMA* 2005; **294**: 3131–3134.

44 Kemp S, Wanders RJA. X-linked adrenoleukodystrophy: very long-chain fatty acid metabolism, ABC half-transporters and the complicated route to treatment. *Mol Genet Metab* 2007; **90**: 268–276.

45 Sandrini F, Farmakidis C, Kirschner LS, Wu SM, Tullio-Pelet A, Lyonnet S, et al. Spectrum of mutations of the AAAS gene in Allgrove syndrome: lack of mutations in six kindreds with isolated resistance to corticotropin. *J Clin Endocrinol Metab* 2001; **86**: 5433–5437.

46 Cronshaw JM, Matunis MJ. The nuclear pore complex protein ALADIN is mislocalized in triple A syndrome. *Proc Natl Acad Sci U S A* 2003; **100**: 5823–5827.

47 Lin L, Gu W-X, Ozisik G, To WS, Owen CJ, Jameson JL, et al. Analysis of DAX1 (*NR0B1*) and steroidogenic factor-1 (SF1/Ad4BP, *NR5A1*) in children and adults with primary adrenal failure: Ten years' experience. *J Clin Endocrinol Metab* 2006; **91**: 3048–3054.

48 Miller WL, Townsend JJ, Grumbach MM, Kaplan SL. An infant with Cushing's disease due to an adrenocorticotropin-producing pituitary adenoma. *J Clin Endocrinol Metab* 1979; **48**: 1017–1025.

49 Devoe DJ, Miller WL, Conte FA, Kaplan SL, Grumbach MM, Rosenthal SM, et al. Long-term outcome of children and adolescents following transsphenoidal surgery for Cushing disease. *J Clin Endocrinol Metab* 1997; **82**: 3196–3202.

50 Stratakis CA, Kirschner LS, Carney JA. Clinical and molecular features of the Carney complex: diagnostic criteria and recommendations for patient evaluation. *J Clin Endocrinol Metab* 2001; **86**: 4041–4046.

51 Horvath A, Boikos S, Giatzakis C, Robinson-White A, Groussin L, Griffin KJ, et al. A genome-wide scan identifies mutations in the gene encoding phosphodiesterase 11A4 (*PDE11A*) in individuals with adrenocortical hyperplasia. *Nat Genet* 2006; **38**: 794–800.

52 Charmandari E, Kino T, Chrousos GP. Familial/sporadic glucocorticoid resistance: clinical phenotype and molecular mechanisms. *Ann N Y Acad Sci* 2004; **1024**: 168–181.

53 Sartorato P, Lapeyraque AL, Armanini D, et al. Different inactivating mutations of the mineralocorticoid receptor in fourteen families affected by type I pseudohypoaldosteronism. *J Clin Endocrinol Metab* 2003; **88**: 2508–2517.

14 Polyglandular Syndromes

Catherine J. Owen[1], Tim D. Cheetham[2] & Simon H.S. Pearce[1]

[1] Institute of Human Genetics, Newcastle University, Newcastle upon Tyne, UK
[2] Department of Paediatrics, Royal Victoria Infirmary, Newcastle upon Tyne, UK

The autoimmune polyglandular endocrinopathy syndromes (APS) encompass a wide clinical spectrum of disease with monogenic and complex genetic etiologies. The first manifestation of these disorders is frequently in childhood or adolescence and their presentation is heterogeneous.

Autoimmune polyglandular syndrome type I

Definition

Autoimmune polyglandular syndrome type 1 (APS1), known as the autoimmune polyendocrinopathy–candidiasis–ectodermal dystrophy syndrome (APECED), is a rare and frequently debilitating disorder of childhood. It is inherited as an autosomal recessive condition; heterozygotes have no manifestations. The female : male ratio is close to 1. The clinical diagnosis of APS1 requires the presence of two of the three cardinal components: chronic mucocutaneous candidiasis, autoimmune hypoparathyroidism and autoimmune adrenal failure [1–6]. Only one of these manifestations is required if a sibling has the syndrome [1]. There is a spectrum of associated minor components, which include endocrine and non-endocrine manifestations.

Large cohorts of APS1 patients have been reported from several countries including Finland [2,6], Norway [5], Israel [3], Sardinia [7], northern Italy [4] and northern America [1]. Although a rare disorder in most countries (about two or three cases per million in the UK [8]), it shows a founder effect leading to a much higher prevalence in certain populations: Finns 1 in 25 000 [2], Iranian Jews 1 in 9000 [3] and Sardinians 1 in 14 500 [7]. There are also differences in the phenotype between different populations: for example, chronic mucocutaneous candidiasis and adrenal failure are among the most common manifestations in most patients of European descent but are present in only about 20% of Iranian Jews [3,6].

Brook's Clinical Pediatric Endocrinology, 6th edition. Edited by C. Brook, P. Clayton, R. Brown. © 2009 Blackwell Publishing,
ISBN: 978-1-4051-8080-1.

Clinical features and course

The first manifestation is typically mucocutaneous candidiasis, which develops in infancy or early childhood. Hypoparathyroidism characteristically develops around the age of 7 years and adrenocortical failure by the age of 13 years (Fig. 14.1) [4,8,9]. The complete evolution of the three cardinal features usually occurs in the first 20 years, with additional minor manifestations continuing to appear at least until the fifth decade [1]. Although this temporal sequence of appearance of the major manifestations is frequently observed in childhood, APS1 subjects not uncommonly present in other ways, either with one cardinal feature and several minor manifestations or with several minor manifestations and characteristic ectodermal dystrophy. This variability in the early clinical picture can make the diagnosis of APS1 challenging.

The median number of disease components is four, with up to 10 manifestations in some subjects. The cardinal triad occurs in around 60% of subjects and there may be a delay in diagnosis in the early years when rarer components may dominate the clinical picture. Patients who present initially with adrenal insufficiency rather than candidiasis tend to develop fewer components than others [2,6]. It has also been reported that the earlier the first component presents, the more likely that multiple components will develop [1,4]. Table 14.1 lists the cardinal and more common minor manifestations together with their frequency.

Cardinal manifestations
Chronic mucocutaneous candidiasis

Chronic or periodic mucocutaneous candidiasis (CMC) is commonly the first manifestation of the syndrome, occurring as early as 1 month of age but more typically in the first 2 years of life and it should alert the clinician to the possibility of APS1. It is frequently mild or intermittent and responds well to periodic systemic anticandidal treatment. In some subjects, CMC does not develop until adulthood [1,2] but it is the most frequently occurring cardinal manifestation, present in 73–100% of patients [1,2,4–6]. It is considered to be the clinical expression of dysfunctional presentation of *Candida albicans* antigens to T lympho-

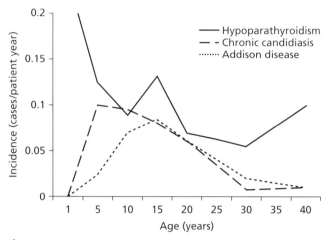

Figure 14.1 Incidence of the three most common components of APS1 according to age. (After Perheentupa [6]).

Table 14.1 Frequencies of the major and main minor components of APS1.

Disease	Frequency (%)
Main manifestations	
Chronic mucocutaneous candidiasis	72–100
Autoimmune hypoparathyroidism	76–93
Autoimmune adrenal failure	73–100
Common minor manifestations	
Autoimmune endocrinopathies	
Hypergonadotropic hypogonadism	17–69
Autoimmune thyroid disease	4–31
Type 1 diabetes mellitus	0–33
Pituitary defects	7
Gastrointestinal components	
Pernicious anemia	13–31
Malabsorption	10–22
Cholelithiasis	44
Chronic active hepatitis	5–31
Skin autoimmune diseases	
Vitiligo	8–31
Alopecia	29–40
Urticarial-like erythema with fever	15
Ectodermal dysplasia	
Nail dystrophy	10–52
Dental enamel hypoplasia	40–77
Tympanic membrane calcification	33
Other manifestations	
Keratoconjunctivitis	2–35
Hyposplenism/asplenia	15–40

Data from European and North American patients [1,2,4–6,9,12]. Iranian Jews have distinctly different frequencies from the other populations and have been excluded.

cytes. Oral candidiasis is the most common presentation but esophagitis is also found, causing substernal pain and odynophagia. Infection of the intestinal mucosa leads to abdominal discomfort and diarrhea. Candidal infection can also affect the vaginal mucosa, nails and skin.

Hypoparathyroidism

This is frequently the first endocrine feature of APS1 [1–6,10], with a peak incidence between 2 and 11 years of age. Hypoparathyroidism occurs in 75–95% [1,2,4–6,9], although there appears to be a slightly reduced penetrance and later age of onset in males [11,12]. Hypoparathyroidism may be asymptomatic but presents typically with tetany and generalized seizures. Presentation may be precipitated by factors such as fasting, low calcium or high phosphate intake. The diagnosis is confirmed by a low or undetectable plasma parathyroid hormone (PTH) concentration in the presence of hypocalcemia. Hyperphosphatemia and hypomagnesemia are common, with low urinary calcium excretion. Autopsy studies of parathyroid glands from these patients show atrophy and an infiltration of the parathyroids with mononuclear cells [10].

Adrenal failure

Autoimmune adrenal failure (Addison disease) is typically the third of the cardinal manifestations to present in APS1, with a peak incidence around 13 years [1–6,9]. In most populations of APS1 patients, it occurs less frequently than the other major components (72–100%) [1,2,4–6]. The destruction of the adrenal cortex may develop gradually and deficiencies of cortisol and aldosterone can appear in either order up to 20 years apart [6]. At autopsy, the adrenals of these patients are atrophic, with the adrenal cortex being almost completely destroyed and having an extensive inflammatory cell infiltrate. The diagnosis of adrenal insufficiency is confirmed by a normal or low cortisol concentration with increased adrenocorticotrophic hormone (ACTH) and a subnormal cortisol response to ACTH stimulation. A temporary hypermineralocorticoid-like state is seen in some patients with cortisol deficiency, paradoxically leading to hypokalemia [6,12]. Deficiency of aldosterone may be heralded by postural hypotension or salt craving and is confirmed by a raised plasma renin activity even before the development of overt electrolyte disturbance.

Minor manifestations
Autoimmune endocrinopathies
Primary hypogonadism

Primary hypogonadism is the most common minor manifestation of APS1, occurring in 17–61% of cases [1–6,9,13]. It is almost invariably accompanied by adrenal failure. About half of APS1 females with hypogonadism present with primary amenorrhea and the remainder have secondary amenorrhea. Male hypogonadism has been reported from puberty onwards [6]. One male patient has been reported with azoospermia and possible anti-sperm autoimmunity [6].

Type 1 diabetes mellitus

Type 1 diabetes mellitus is relatively infrequent in APS1 compared with other polyendocrinopathy syndromes. There is an age-related penetrance with a peak presentation towards middle age [12]. There is a wide range in the reported prevalence between different APS1 populations from 0 to 23%, depending on age of the cohort [1–6,9].

Autoimmune thyroid diseases

Destructive autoimmune thyroid diseases (Hashimoto thyroiditis or primary atrophic thyroiditis) are relatively uncommon in APS1, occurring in 4–18% of cases. The age of presentation varies from around 10 years for Hashimoto thyroiditis to 17 years for primary atrophic thyroiditis [1,2,4]. Hyperthyroidism is very rare.

Pituitary defects

Pituitary defects such as lymphocytic hypophysitis or autoimmune pituitary disease have occasionally been described (approximately 5%) and can induce single or multiple hormonal defects [9]. Cases of secondary hypogonadism [2], growth hormone deficiency [12,14] and idiopathic diabetes insipidus [4] have been reported.

Gastrointestinal components

Chronic atrophic gastritis

This affects up to one-third of patients with APS1, with a peak incidence at 10–20 years [1–6,9]. It can lead to a megaloblastic anemia due to vitamin B_{12} deficiency (pernicious anemia) or a microcytic anemia because of iron deficiency.

Malabsorption

This occurs in 10–22% of cases [1–6,9] and can be due to a variety of causes including villous atrophy, exocrine pancreatic insufficiency, intestinal infections (*Giardia lamblia* or *Candida*), defective bile acid reabsorption and intestinal lymphangiectasia [4,6,15]. Autoimmune destruction of the enterochromaffin cells of the small intestine leading to deficiency of cholecystokinin and serotonin has been implicated [16]. The malabsorption presents with periodic or chronic diarrhea, usually with steatorrhea but may be associated with constipation. It can be a characteristic feature of an early "atypical" presentation of APS1 in the first year of life, being an initial manifestation in around 10%. There is a strong association with the hypocalcemia of hypoparathyroidism, as hypocalcemia impairs the secretion of cholecystokinin leading to a failure of normal gallbladder contraction and pancreatic enzyme secretion.

Cholelithiasis

This is present in up to 40% by ultrasonography [9], is frequently asymptomatic and is thought to be secondary to disruption of the enterohepatic circulation.

Chronic active hepatitis

This develops in 5–30% of cases [1–6,9]. The clinical course varies from chronic but asymptomatic in the majority of cases to the development of cirrhosis or fulminant hepatic failure with a potentially fatal outcome [1,17]. It may present in early childhood and can be the first manifestation of APS1 but the risk of hepatitis is low after adolescence. Elevation of serum alanine aminotransferase for more than 3 months, when no other cause such as viral or drug-induced hepatitis can be found, is an indication for liver biopsy [2]. Clinicians should be particularly vigilant in the early weeks after the identification of abnormal liver function in APS1 subjects as rapid decompensation to frank liver failure may occur.

Skin autoimmune diseases

Vitiligo

Vitiligo can appear at any age but most commonly in childhood [1,9], affecting up to one-quarter of APS1 patients [1–6,9]. It is highly variable in extent and often worsens with time.

Alopecia

Alopecia affects about one-third of patients and can involve all body sites in varying degrees [1–6,9]. It can develop rapidly and at any age.

Recurrent urticaria with fever

This has been reported as an unusual manifestation in about 10% of patients during childhood. It may persist for many years and is strongly associated with uveitis. High concentrations of immunoglobulin G (IgG) and circulating immune complexes are found and skin biopsy reveals a lymphoplasmacytic vasculitis [6].

Other manifestations

Ectodermal dystrophy

This affects the nails and tooth enamel (Fig. 14.2). The pitted nails are unrelated to candidal infection and can be an important clue to the diagnosis of APS1. Dental enamel hypoplasia has been reported in 40–75% of patients [1–6,9], although deciduous teeth are never affected. Enamel hypoplasia can precede hypoparathyroidism and is unrelated to serum calcium concentrations. Even in the absence of ear infection, one-third of patients have calcified plaques on the tympanic membranes [2,6].

Keratoconjunctivitis

Incidence varies from 10% to 40% between reports [1–6,9,10]. It is the first manifestation of APS1 in some cases. The initial symptoms are intense photophobia, blepharospasm and lacrimation; permanent visual impairment and even blindness is not infrequent [6]. Some patients enter a quiescent phase around 10 years after onset.

Asplenia

Aspenia or hyposplenism has been documented by ultrasonography or suggested by hematological parameters in up to 15% of APS1 cases [6]. It may be congenital or acquired, secondary to progressive autoimmune-mediated destruction or vascular insult to the spleen. It is suspected by a typical blood smear including

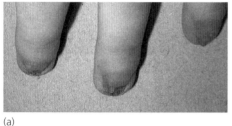 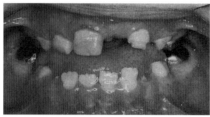

(a)   (b)

Figure 14.2 Ectodermal features of APS1 illustrating (a) nail dystrophy and (b) dental enamel hypoplasia.

Table 14.2 Rarer minor manifestations having reported association with APS1 [1–6,9].

Rare components of APS 1

Immunological	**Hematological**
Selective IgA deficiency	Pure red cell aplasia
Hypergammaglobulinemia	Autoimmune hemolytic anemia
Tuberculin anergy	
Renal	**Malignant**
Interstitial nephritis	Oral squamous cell carcinoma
Hypercalcemia-based nephrocalcinosis	Esophageal carcinoma
	Adenocarcinoma of the stomach
Neurological	**Ophthalmic**
Intracranial calcification	Iridiocyclitis
Progressive myopathy	Optic nerve atrophy
	Retinal degeneration
Connective tissue	**Other**
Sjögren syndrome	Metaphyseal dysplasia
Cutaneous vasculitis	Primary pulmonary hypertension
Scleroderma	Lymphocytic myocarditis
Rheumatoid arthritis	Bronchiolitis obliterans pneumonia
Lupus-like panniculitis	

Howell–Jolly bodies and thrombocytosis. It causes an additional secondary immunodeficiency, rendering subjects susceptible to pneumococcal sepsis.

Rarer associations

Several cases of selective IgA deficiency and hypergammaglobulinemia have been reported [15]. Many patients have tuberculin anergy but whether this indicates an abnormal susceptibility to tuberculosis is unclear. Impairment of renal function, due to interstitial nephritis or iatrogenic nephrocalcinosis, was reported in more than 5% of Finnish cases and necessitates transplantation in some cases [6]. Neoplasia, most commonly squamous carcinoma of the oral mucosa (in subjects with chronic oral *Candida* who smoke cigarettes) and adenocarcinoma of the stomach, is also seen. Other rare manifestations are listed in Table 14.2.

Sudden death

Sudden death is well recognized in established APS1 patients, their siblings and from postmortem studies of subjects in whom the diagnosis was not suspected [2,5,8]. It is presumed that these deaths result from undiagnosed adrenal failure, fulminant sepsis, hypoparathyroidism or a combination of these.

Genetics

The gene defective in APS1 was identified by positional cloning in 1997 and is located on chromosome 21q22.3. It is named the *auto*immune *re*gulator or *AIRE* gene [18,19]. *AIRE* encodes a putative nuclear protein, containing several motifs suggestive of a transcription factor, including two zinc fingers. It is expressed in a variety of tissues of the immune system but particularly in the medullary epithelial antigen-presenting cells in the thymus, where it is thought to have an important role in the central induction of self-tolerance. The molecular mechanism by which the AIRE protein induces central tolerance is still unexplained; however, it is thought to be involved in the negative selective of potentially autoreactive thymocytes by regulating expression of self-antigens in the antigen presenting cells of the thymus [5,20]. In subjects with *AIRE* mutations, autoreactive T cells escape to the periphery leading to autoimmunity in selected organs [21]. *AIRE* has also been found to be expressed in peripheral dendritic cells and so may also have an additional role in the maintenance of peripheral immune tolerance [21]. A markedly reduced number of CD4$^+$CD25$^+$ T regulatory cells have been found in the peripheral blood of APS1 subjects which could be a secondary effect of *AIRE* mutations [22].

Over 60 different disease-causing mutations have now been described in the *AIRE* gene [2,4,5,7,18,19,21,23]. These include point mutations, insertions and deletions and are spread through the whole coding region of the gene. Mutations affecting splice sites have also been reported. The most frequent *AIRE* mutations include the founder Finnish mutation in exon 6 (R257X) [18,19] and the common northern European mutation in exon 8 (964del13) [23]. This 13-bp deletion is seen frequently in Norwegian patients and in White people from the USA and UK [23], where it accounts for more than 70% of all mutant *AIRE* alleles. Many patients with this 13-bp deletion carry the same haplotype over the 21q.22 region, which is evidence for a founder effect. The common Finnish *AIRE* mutation is also fairly prevalent (5–30%) in other subjects of White European ancestry [4,5]. Additional common mutations are found in isolated populations such as a mutation in exon 3 (R139X) found in Sardinians [7] and a mutation in exon 2 (Y85C) in the Iranian Jewish population [2]. In several instances, only one mutant allele of the *AIRE* gene has been reported in typical APS1 patients, suggesting that the second mutation might be located in the regulatory regions of the gene. Most of these mutations are believed to form null alleles that lead either to the synthesis of a truncated product or to the production of a nonsense transcript with a rapidly degraded mRNA. Missense mutations in the amino terminus of the protein may inhibit function by preventing dimerization or altering the distribution of the AIRE protein [24].

It is possible that the specific manifestations that develop in a particular APS1 patient may depend on alleles at other loci such as human leukocyte antigens (*HLA*), because the same *AIRE* mutations are associated with varying phenotypes and clinical course even among affected siblings [12,25]. No consistent associations between APS1 manifestations and *HLA* alleles have been found but *HLA-A28* shows a weak association with hypoparathyroidism, keratopathy and alopecia in this disease [2] and *HLA-A3* with ovarian failure [26]. Addison disease has been associated with *HLA DRB1*03* and alopecia with *HLA DRB1*04, DQB1*0302*. Type 1 diabetes shows negative correlation with *DRB1*15, DQB1*0602* [27]. Thus, *HLA* polymorphisms may explain some of the variability in phenotype seen in APS1, although no association between HLA type and autoantibodies in APS1 patients is seen [27]. No correlation between cytotoxic T lymphocyte antigen 4 (*CTLA4*) gene polymorphisms and APS1 have been found to date [9]; however, a negative correlation has been shown between the insulin gene polymorphism and the development of type 1 diabetes in these subjects [28]. The factors determining an individual phenotype are not understood and it is likely that there are several loci involved.

Autoantibodies and pathogenesis

The pathogenesis of many of the manifestations of APS1 is unclear but autoimmunity is involved in the development of the endocrinopathies and patients have circulating autoantibodies to a variety of antigens from other affected tissues. One recently identified autoantibody is directed against interferons, in particular α-interferon (IFN-α) and IFN-ω and has almost 100% prevalence in APS1 subjects, regardless of the clinical picture or mutation type [29]. These anti-IFN autoantibodies have been found to be present at a very early stage and persist, being present after over 30 years of disease. They have not been found in any subjects with isolated AAD or APS2, so appear to be disease-specific [25,29]. This clearly provides an excellent tool to aid in the diagnosis of APS1 in the prodromal stage or in atypical cases and suggests the intriguing possibility that these autoantibodies may modulate the expression of immune responses directly.

Steroid 21-hydroxylase (P450c21) and cholesterol side-chain cleavage enzyme (P450scc) are the major adrenal autoantigens; P450scc is the major gonadal autoantigen in APS1 patients [30]. Antibodies against at least one of P450scc, steroid 17α-hydroxylase (P450c17) and P450c21 were found in 81% of APS1 patients with and in 21% of those without adrenal failure. The presence of antibodies for at least one of these three enzymes correlates significantly with gonadal failure in female but not

male patients [4,5]. This is possibly because of the blood–testis barrier protecting the Leydig cells from immunological attack. Adrenal cell autoantibodies are frequently detectable in patients with candidiasis or hypoparathyroidism without adrenal failure. These patients are almost certain to develop adrenal failure [9].

Autoantibodies to the extracellular domain of the calcium-sensing receptor have been reported in idiopathic hypoparathyroidism including up to 86% of subjects with APS1 [31,32]. This has not been replicated in several other studies [11,30], probably because of differences in assay technique and sensitivity [32,33]. In addition, antibodies against a novel parathyroid-specific antigen, NALP5, have recently been found in about half of APS1 patients with hypoparathyroidism [34]. The prognostic significance and pathophysiological role of these autoantibodies remains undetermined.

Glutamic acid decarboxylase 65 (GAD-65) autoantibodies have been found in 75% of patients with diabetes up to 8 years before the onset but these are non-specific and are also found in 40% of non-diabetic APS1 patients [35]. Antibodies against the IA-2 tyrosine phosphatase-like protein and insulin are less common in these patients compared with non-APS1-associated type 1 diabetes but have higher specificity (96–100%) [11]. Circulating antithyroid antibodies have been found to be a poor marker for predicting hypothyroidism in APS1 [4].

The main autoantigens for hepatitis in APS1 appear to be cytochrome P450 1A2 (CYP1A2), P450 2A6 (CYP2A6) and aromatic L-amino acid decarboxylase (AADC) [36]. CYP1A2 in particular appears to be a highly specific but insensitive marker for APS1 hepatitis [36]. Liver–kidney microsomal (LKM) autoantibodies have been found in 50% of APS1 patients with chronic active hepatitis and 11% of APS1 patients without increased concentrations of hepatic enzymes [36]. Other hepatic autoantigens associated with non-APS1 autoimmune hepatitis, such as smooth muscle and antinuclear antibodies, are not found [36]. Tryptophan hydroxylase autoantibodies have been found to be a sensitive predictor of autoimmune hepatitis in APS1 [30]. Although a rise in antibody titers to liver antigens may predate biochemical evidence of liver disease, raised autoantibodies are not found in all APS1 patients with autoimmune hepatitis at biopsy [17]. This, together with the broad spectrum of autoantigens found, suggests heterogeneity in pathogenesis, as well as outcome.

Antiparietal cell and intrinsic factor autoantibodies precede parietal cell atrophy. Villous atrophy is associated with endomysial and/or tissue transglutaminase (TTG) autoantibodies [4]. Gastrointestinal dysfunction has been associated with autoantibodies to tryptophan hydroxylase (48% cases), histidine decarboxylase and GAD-65 [30]. Vitiligo in APS1 is associated with the presence of complement-fixing melanocyte autoantibodies [4] and has been associated with antibodies to the transcription factors SOX9, SOX10 [37] and to AADC [30]. Antibodies to tyrosine hydroxylase are found in APS1 subjects with alopecia areata [9].

Measurement of autoantibodies may be of limited use in patients with APS1 in determining their risk of developing new components because the sensitivity of the antibody test may frequently be less than the patient's pre-existing risk of the complication. However, there are certain autoantibodies that are almost exclusive to APS1, particularly AADC, CYP1A2, tyrosine hydroxylase, tryptophan hydroxylase, IFN-α and IFN-ω. This unique spectrum of autoantibodies can thus help to differentiate APS1 and other autoimmune diseases (Table 14.3) [29,30].

Diagnosis of APS1

Perheentupa [6] found the classic criteria (two out of three cardinal manifestations) to be fulfilled by 5 years in only 22%, by 10 years in 67%, by 20 years in 89% and by 30 years in 93.5% of cases. In order to make a prompt diagnosis, all the different disease components should be considered. Suspicion should be high in patients under 30 years with mucocutaneous candidiasis, hypoparathyroidism, adrenal failure, ectodermal dystrophy, keratoconjunctivitis, prolonged diarrhea, vitiligo or non-infectious hepatitis. Such patients should be checked for other manifestations, particularly the sometimes subtle nail signs of ectodermal dystrophy oral or ophthalmic components. DNA screening for *AIRE* mutations and an autoantibody screen should be considered in subjects with an atypical presentation.

Table 14.3 The identified autoantigens in APS1 for the more common disease components.

Disease component	Autoantigens
APS1 (non-specific)	IFN-α$_2$, IFN-ω*
Major manifestations	
Addison disease	P450c21, P450scc, P450c17
Hypoparathyroidism	Calcium-sensing receptor,† NALP5*
Minor manifestations	
Gonadal failure	P450c17, P450scc
Type 1 diabetes	GAD65, insulin, 1A-2
Hashimoto thyroiditis	Thyroid peroxidase, thyroglobulin
Graves disease	TSH receptor, thyroid peroxidase
Autoimmune hepatitis	CYP1A2,* CYP2A6, AADC,* LKM
Autoimmune gastritis/pernicious anemia	H/K-ATPase of gastric parietal cells, intrinsic factor
Celiac disease	Transglutaminase, gliadin
Gastrointestinal dysfunction	TPH,* histidine decarboxylase, GAD65
Vitiligo	SOX9 and SOX10, AADC*
Alopecia	Tyrosine hydroxylase*

Those marked *are almost exclusive to APS1 and thus helpful in differentiating APS1 from other autoimmune diseases [4,5,9,11,17,29–31,34–37].
†Not unequivocally proven, detection critically dependent on assay system [32].
1A-2, tyrosine phosphatase-like protein 1A-2; AADC, aromatic L-amino acid decarboxylase; CYP1A2, cytochrome P450 1A2; CYP2A6, cytochrome P450 2A6; GAD65, glutamic acid decarboxylase 65; LKM, liver–kidney microsomal; P450c21, steroid 21-hydroxylase; P450scc, cholesterol side-chain cleaving enzyme; P450c17, steroid 17α-hydroxylase; SOX, transcription factors; TPH, tryptophan hydroxylase.

There is often no clinical value in DNA analysis in subjects with two or more cardinal features but the molecular findings in a proband will be of value in counseling and for screening siblings. All patients with established APS1 and those with one or more suspicious features need close follow-up for the development of new components. Their siblings should also be examined, as one of the cardinal manifestations or a definite ectodermal component is diagnostic.

Diagnosis is often delayed, perhaps because of the long interval between development of the first and second manifestation. Up to two-thirds of patients are not diagnosed until admission to hospital with acute adrenal insufficiency or hypocalcemic crisis and nearly half of these already have one major component of APS1 present [5]. Increased awareness of APS1 is essential to prevent fatalities. Mutational analysis has aided the early diagnosis of APS1 but it must be remembered that there are a large number of possible mutations and, in the UK, only the most common two are routinely screened. Thus, APS1 is not excluded by negative routine DNA analysis and the presence of one abnormal allele in a child with a major or minor manifestation makes the diagnosis highly likely. The use of the recently identified anti-IFN autoantibodies may well have an important role in aiding diagnosis in the future [29]. The individual disease components of APS1 should be recognized by the standard endocrine surveillance methods. The search for antibodies predicting new diseases can be an additional tool in aiding early diagnosis (Table 14.3).

Follow-up

The most important goal of this is the recognition of new disease components, which is essential as some manifestations are life-threatening. These patients should be seen three or four times a year and have rapid access to an "expert" if any new problems arise. Each visit requires a thorough history and examination, particularly for oral mucocutaneous candidiasis and signs of evolving adrenal insufficiency, such as postural change in blood pressure. Blood should be taken for basal hormone, hematological and biochemical markers and an occasional antibody screen performed (Table 14.4). This, together with a high index of clinical suspicion, allows earlier diagnosis and treatment of additional components as they develop.

The early diagnosis of Addison disease is of particular importance. Individuals at risk need an annual measurement of ACTH until adrenocortical failure develops [2]. Plasma renin activity should be measured at the same time. Adrenal failure can evolve rapidly in APS1 and annual assessment may not be sufficient to prevent acute presentations. The patient, immediate family and primary health care team must be made aware of the signs and symptoms of adrenal failure [8]. Postural blood pressure and serum electrolytes should be determined at each clinic visit, together with periodic screening for 21-hydroxylase autoantibodies.

Treatment

Treatment of the individual disorders is no different from treating patients with the isolated disorders, except that polypharmacy

Table 14.4 Investigations recommended in the routine follow-up of APS1 patients to attempt to identify early development of new complications.

Disease component	Blood screening investigation
Major manifestation	
Addison disease	U&E, ACTH, plasma renin activity, annual synacthen test
Hypoparathyroidism	Serum calcium, phosphate, and magnesium
Minor manifestation	
Hypogonadism	Gonadotropin concentrations
Type 1 diabetes	Glycosylated hemoglobin
Autoimmune thyroid disease	fT3, fT4 and TSH
Autoimmune hepatitis	Liver function tests
Atrophic gastritis/pernicious anemia	FBC*
Hyposplenism/asplenism	FBC*, blood smear†

ACTH, adenocorticotropic hormone; FBC, full blood count; TSH, thyroid stimulating hormone; U&E, urea and electrolytes.

*The presence of anemia on FBC results needs further investigation with ferritin, transferrin and serum iron concentrations if the anemia is microcytic and vitamin B$_{12}$ concentrations if macrocytic.

†A blood smear indicating hyposplenism/asplenism (Howell–Jolly bodies, anisocytes, poikilocytes, target cells and burr cells) and/or the presence of thrombocytosis needs follow-up with an abdominal ultrasound to assess spleen presence and size.

is the rule and that malabsorption may complicate therapy. The different endocrine failures are managed by conventional hormonal replacement, which may be complex when a patient has several endocrine deficiencies. Immunosuppressive treatment with glucocorticoids can also complicate matters. Professional psychological support is needed for many patients. A high rate of depression, social isolation, alcoholism and substance misuse is reported, particularly as patients reach adulthood.

Mucocutaneous candidiasis is treated with local and/or systemic antifungal drugs, dental care and oral hygiene, with expert oral surgical follow-up for refractory cases. Suppression of oral candidiasis is important because of the risk of oral carcinoma. Fluconazole or ketoconazole are indicated if topical treatments fail. Itraconazole is preferable to treat nail candidiasis but requires a course of 4–6 months [4]. These drugs can cause transient elevation of liver enzymes and occasionally hepatitis, so close monitoring is required. Ketoconazole is a global P450 cytochrome inhibitor and so can precipitate decompensation in patients with marginal adrenal reserve.

In APS1 patients with adrenal failure and/or hypoparathyroidism, serum calcium concentrations appear to be labile compared with non-APS1 hypoparathyroidism and serious hypercalcemia can occur despite previous long periods of normocalcemia. Although standard doses of calcitriol or alfacalcidol can be used initially (20–50 ng/kg/day), patients with APS1 often require much larger doses of vitamin D analogs to maintain eucalcemia (3–5 µg/day being not unusual). This is presumed to

be due to malabsorption and the intermittent nature of this can lead to marked hypercalcemia with rapid onset of renal impairment.

Our practice is to monitor serum calcium and phosphate concentrations 8-weekly with regular determinations of urinary calcium excretion. Standard treatment with vitamin D analogs often leads to hypercalciuria, so serum calcium concentrations need to be maintained at around the lower end of the normal range (2.0–2.2 mmol/L total serum calcium). The vicious cycle of hypocalcemia and malabsorption can usually be broken by an increased oral dose but parenteral therapy may be required in severe situations. Refractory cases may benefit from monthly intramuscular (IM) injections of calciferol to maintain basal concentrations, in addition to the daily use of a short-acting sterol. Hypomagnesemia may contribute to resistance and require treatment. Owing to the prevalence of nephrocalcinosis, our practice is to perform occasional (approximately 3- to 5-yearly) renal ultrasonography in subjects with hypoparathyroidism, taking the additional opportunity to assess the gallbladder and the size of the spleen. In patients with adrenal insufficiency, alteration of the cortisol dose will lead to an alteration in calcium absorption. Also of note is that unexplained hypercalcemia may be the first sign of the development of adrenal failure.

There is a lack of prospective data regarding the treatment and outcome of APS1-associated hepatitis. Autoimmune hepatitis is treated with immunosuppressive therapy, most experience being with the use of prednisolone and/or azathioprine. Liver transplantation has occasionally been reported in APS1-associated hepatitis [17]. Immunosuppressive therapy may increase the risk of *Candida*-related cancer and predispose the patient to generalized candidal infection [4]. Immunosuppressants are occasionally required for severe intestinal dysfunction with diarrhea and there can be an associated improvement in control of serum calcium concentrations. The use of prednisolone with azathioprine, methotrexate or cyclosporin A has been reported with varying symptomatic benefits [6]. Milder diarrhea has been found to respond to gut motility-reducing agents such as loperamide. Oral bile acid replacement therapy may help with fat malabsorption in patients with steatorrhea resulting from cholecystokinin deficiency [16].

Live vaccines must be avoided in view of the underlying immunodeficiency [6] but, as splenic atrophy is a common component, all APS1 patients should receive polyvalent pneumococcal vaccine with measurement of antibody response 6–8 weeks later. Nonresponders or those who are asplenic should receive prophylactic daily antibiotics [8].

Prognosis

Many patients feel chronically unwell and the physical and psychological impact of the multiple problems should not be underestimated. Despite improved survival, mortality rates are still high at 10–20% and a recent review in Finland has found the average age of death to be 34 years (range 6.8–63 years) [12]. Death is from a variety of causes including adrenal crisis, diabetic ketoacidosis, fulminant hepatic failure, oral carcinoma, septicemia, hypocalcemia, generalized candidal infection during immuno-suppressive treatment, complications of kidney failure and alco-holism [2,4,6]. Around 3% die before the diagnosis of APS1 has been made, with adrenal failure the likely cause. Depression and suicide is high among this patient group as the disease poses a great psychological burden, with the constant risk of developing life-threatening complications, disfiguring disease components and the requirement for multiple medications. Working capacity may be maintained in subjects with a limited number of mani-festations but many are significantly incapacitated [6,12].

Summary

The clinical presentation of APS1 is very variable. Diagnosis can be difficult initially when only one manifestation is present and it often takes years for others to appear. Increased awareness of the condition, combined with analysis of specific autoantibodies and mutational analysis of the *AIRE* gene, should help to diag-nose this condition earlier and prevent serious complications and fatalities.

Autoimmune polyglandular syndrome type 2 and associated disorders

Definition

APS2 is defined by the presence of primary adrenocortical insuf-ficiency with either autoimmune thyroid disease or type 1 diabe-tes in the same individual. An autoimmune origin of all the major components should be demonstrated for the correct diagnosis of APS2. The association of autoimmune Addison disease and auto-immune thyroid disease is known as Schmidt syndrome and the association of Addison disease with type 1 diabetes is also called Carpenter syndrome. Other endocrine and non-endocrine auto-immune disorders occur with increased frequency in these indi-viduals and their families [1].

APS3 is defined as the association between autoimmune thyroid disease and an additional autoimmune disease other than Addison disease [9]. Many clinical combinations can be found in APS3 and it can therefore be subdivided into 3A–D, depending on the associated conditions (Table 14.5) [9]. Some authors use the term APS4 to encompass an association of autoimmune dis-eases not falling into the categories APS1–3 [9]. Many of these patients develop more classic APS2/3 manifestations later and this classification describes an extremely heterogeneous group of patients. We feel that there is little clinical benefit in its use and that it is generally more helpful to describe the individual components.

APS2

Clinical features and course

APS2 is rare, with an estimated prevalence of 4–5 per 100 000 [38,39]. Clinical presentation can be at any age but is most fre-quently in early adulthood, with a peak onset in the fourth decade.

Table 14.5 Classification of APS3 [9].

Autoimmune thyroid disease plus	Autoimmune endocrinopathy excluding Addison disease, e.g. type 1 diabetes, POF, lymphocytic hypophysitis	3A
	Autoimmune gastrointestinal disease, e.g. pernicious anaemia, celiac disease, autoimmune hepatitis	3B
	Skin or neurological manifestations, e.g. alopecia, vitiligo, myasthenia gravis	3C
	Connective tissue disease, e.g. SLE, rheumatoid arthritis, Sjögren syndrome	3D

POF, premature ovarian failure; SLE, systemic lupus erythematosus.

It is recognized less commonly in children and adolescents. It affects both sexes, with a female : male ratio of 3 : 1 [38].

Major manifestations

By definition, Addison disease is present in 100% of APS2 cases. Autoimmune thyroid disease occurs in 70–90% and type 1 dia-betes in 20–50% [1,9,40,41]. Only about 10% have the complete triad [9,41]. Adrenal failure is the first endocrine abnormality in around 50% but several minor APS2 components are often present at the diagnosis of adrenal failure, raising the possibility of APS2. On presentation with Addison disease, type 1 diabetes already exists in around 20% and autoimmune thyroid disease in around 30% but they may present more than 20 years before the diagnosis of adrenal failure. Autoimmune thyroid disease encom-passes a variety of thyroid disorders, including Hashimoto thy-roiditis, atrophic hypothyroidism, Graves disease and postpartum thyroiditis. Hypothyroidism is more common than Graves disease but Graves disease tends to present at a younger age in the context of APS2.

Delayed diagnosis and preventable deaths still occur in patients with undiagnosed adrenal failure. Signs and symptoms are often vague and non-specific until an adrenal crisis ensues. Low morning serum cortisol concentrations and electrolyte abnor-malities (hyponatremia and hyperkalemia) represent late changes, occurring at or just before the onset of clinical adrenal insuffi-ciency. Hyperpigmentation may be observed but may be absent in fair or red-headed subjects. Adrenal insufficiency may present as hypoglycemic seizures in children.

In those who already have type 1 diabetes, deterioration of glycemic control with recurrent hypoglycemia and a decrease in total insulin requirements can be the presenting sign. The onset of autoimmune hyperthyroidism or thyroxine replacement for newly diagnosed hypothyroidism leads to enhanced cortisol clearance and can precipitate adrenal crisis in subjects with sub-clinical adrenocortical failure [42]. Clinicians should maintain a high degree of alertness for underlying adrenal failure before ini-tiating thyroid hormone replacement. Conversely, cortisol inhib-its thyrotrophin release, so thyroid stimulating hormone (TSH) concentrations are often high at the initial diagnosis of adrenal insufficiency (typically 5–10 mU/L) but return to normal after initiation of glucocorticoid replacement in the absence of coexistent thyroid disease. Adrenal insufficiency can mask the hyperglycemia of type 1 diabetes.

An increasingly recognized component of APS2 is latent autoimmune diabetes in adults (LADA). By definition, this is diabetes developing in adulthood with a delay from diagnosis in the need for insulin therapy but with the presence of diabetes-associated autoantibodies [43]. Thus, the clinician needs to remain vigilant for the development of other autoimmune conditions regardless of the age of the patient.

Minor manifestations

These are listed in Table 14.6 together with their frequency. All these associated autoimmune disorders are present at lower frequency in APS2 compared with APS1 and they are usually associated with their respective immunological markers. Primary hypogonadism is one of the most common minor manifestations in APS2/3 females, with premature ovarian failure leading to secondary amenorrhea in around 10% of women under 40 years. Testicular failure is very rare in APS2/3 [44]. Pituitary involvement is very occasionally seen in APS2/3, with lymphocytic hypophysitis leading to empty sella syndrome, panhypopituita-

Table 14.6 Minor manifestations frequently associated with APS2 [9,40,41,44].

	Frequency (%)
Minor manifestation	
Pernicious anemia	1–25
Gonadal failure:	
Females	3.5–10
Males	1–2
Vitiligo	4–12
Alopecia	2–5
Autoimmune hepatitis	4
Malabsorption (including celiac disease)	1–2
Sjögren syndrome	1
Neoplasias	3

Rarer manifestations	
Endocrine	*Neurological*
Pituitary involvement	Myositis
Hypophysitis	Myasthenia gravis
Empty sella syndrome	Neuropathy
Late-onset hypoparathyroidism	Stiff man syndrome
Gastrointestinal	*Other*
Ulcerative colitis	Sarcoidosis
Primary biliary cirrhosis	Serositis
Dermatological	Selective IgA deficiency
Granuloma annulare	Idiopathic heart block
Dermatitis herpetiformis	Idiopathic thrombocytopenia purpura
	Rheumatoid arthritis

rism or isolated failure of any of the anterior pituitary hormones [45].

In contrast to APS1, hypoparathyroidism is very rare in APS2/3. If hypocalcemia does occur in APS2, celiac disease is the most likely reason and the finding of an elevated PTH concentration in the latter will distinguish the two. Hypoparathyroidism has been described in a few adult patients with parathyroid-suppressing antibodies [31,44], often coexisting with autoimmune thyroid disease. Autoimmune hypoparathyroidism in childhood is almost pathognomic of APS1.

Incomplete APS2

Patients with autoimmune thyroid disease or type 1 diabetes and adrenal autoantibodies in the serum or patients with Addison disease and either thyroid and/or islet cell autoantibodies are sometimes classified as incomplete APS2 [9]. Self-evidently, these patients may develop APS2 in the future, particularly those with evidence of subclinical disease such as an elevated TSH or impaired glucose tolerance. Annual screening by ACTH and renin measurement, together with education about the likely presentation of adrenal failure, is recommended for such individuals. About 30% of subjects with positive adrenal antibodies progress to adrenal failure over a 6-year period [46]. Patients with either autoimmune thyroid disease or type 1 diabetes alone but who have a sibling with APS2, are also classified by some authors as having incomplete APS2, because of their possible higher risk of adrenal failure [9].

APS3

APS3 is defined as the association between autoimmune thyroid disease and autoimmune disorders other than Addison disease. Hashimoto thyroiditis is the most common form of autoimmune thyroid disease, although Graves disease and postpartum thyroiditis are also seen. Autoimmune thyroid diseases tend to increase in incidence in the teenage years, with a peak in the fourth decade for Graves disease and in the fifth and sixth decades for autoimmune hypothyroidism. Autoimmune thyroid disease is most commonly isolated and polyglandular involvement in the form of APS3 or APS2 is rare (approximately 5%). Only 1% of patients with isolated autoimmune thyroid disease have adrenal autoantibodies (with risk of APS2), whereas 3–5% have either pancreatic islet autoimmunity and/or clinical type 1 diabetes [47].

Autoimmune thyroid disease is more commonly associated with pernicious anemia, vitiligo, alopecia, myasthenia gravis and Sjögren syndrome and autoimmune thyroid disease should be sought prospectively in patients with these conditions. Around 30% of subjects with vitiligo have another autoimmune disorder, with autoimmune thyroid disease and pernicious anemia being the most common. Many patients with vitiligo are asymptomatic and other autoimmune diseases are diagnosed only by prospective screening, including evaluation of autoantibody status [44,48]. Up to 15% of patients with alopecia and nearly 30% of those with myasthenia gravis have autoimmune thyroid disease.

Genetics

APS2 is a genetically complex and multifactorial disease. It clusters in families and appears to show an autosomal dominant pattern of inheritance with incomplete penetrance in some [49]. Susceptibility is determined by multiple genetic loci that interact with environmental factors. Only two genes have shown consistent association with APS2: HLA and CTLA4. Of these, HLA appears to have the strongest gene effect [1]. Two further genes show some evidence for association in autoimmune Addison disease (ADD) and are thus likely to have a role in APS2, PTPN22 and CYP27B1.

HLA and APS2

Many of the component disorders in APS2, including autoimmune thyroid disease, type 1 diabetes, Addison disease, celiac disease, myasthenia gravis, selective IgA deficiency and dermatitis herpetiformis, are associated with the same extended HLA haplotype: HLA-A1, HLA-B8, HLA DR3, DQA1*0501, DQB1*0201 (DQ2). Thus, unsurprisingly, HLA DR3, DQB1*0201 is associated with APS2 [9,50]. Type 1 diabetes and, to a lesser extent, Addison disease also show association with HLA DR4, DQA1*0301, DQB1*0302 (DQ8) [50,51] and HLA DR5 shows association in patients with a combination of Addison disease and autoimmune hypothyroidism [9]. Some 35% of individuals with type 1 diabetes are heterozygous for the HLA DR3/DR4 combination, with about 50% of children developing type 1 diabetes under 5 years having this combination of haplotypes.

Although specific HLA haplotypes influence susceptibility to APS component disorders, others appear to be protective. The haplotype DR2 (DRB1*1501), DQA1*0102, DQB1*0602 appears to provide dominant protection against type 1 diabetes, even in the presence of insulin autoantibodies [49]. Similarly patients with P450c21 autoantibodies and DRB1* 0401 and DRB1*0402 appear to progress to adrenal failure less often [52].

CTLA4

CTLA4 encodes an important negative regulator of T-cell activation that is expressed on the surface of activated T lymphocytes. Alleles of CTLA4 have been linked primarily to autoimmune thyroid disease, both Graves disease and Hashimoto thyroiditis [53,54] but there is also a weaker effect in type 1 diabetes [51,55]. Addison disease (either isolated or as part of APS2) has been shown to be associated with CTLA4 alleles, particularly in a subgroup of patients carrying HLA DQA1*0501 [53,56,57]. Other studies have shown association with Addison disease in certain populations only [51] or failed to find association [58].

PTPN22 and CYP27B1

The PTPN22 gene encodes lymphoid tyrosine phosphatase (LYP), which has a key role in early T-cell activation. Association with a functionally significant tryptophan for arginine variant in LYP has been found in a mixed UK cohort of AAD and APS2 subjects [59] and in Norwegian subjects [60] but this was not replicated in a German AAD cohort [61]. CYP27B1, the gene encoding

vitamin D 1α-hydroxylase, is involved in immune regulation and cell proliferation. Two small studies have shown association of CYP27B1 alleles with AAD [62,63].

The association of the component disorders in APS2 is therefore, in part, related to the shared susceptibility alleles of HLA, CTLA4 and PTPN22 conferring risk to the different diseases. It is also likely that there is a complex interaction between these variants, CYP27B1 and other as yet unidentified loci and environmental factors.

Autoantibodies and pathogenesis

The pathogenesis of autoimmunity in APS2 is considered as a multifactorial or complex genetic trait, similar to that of the individual disease components. There are several hypotheses to explain why autoimmunity occurs against multiple organs in individuals with APS. It has been suggested that this may result from a shared epitope(s) between an environmental agent and a common antigen present in several endocrine tissues [64] or that the organs derived from the same germ layer expressing common germ layer-specific antigens could serve as targets for the autoimmune response in APS [65]. More likely, there is a subtle thymic defect of negative selection of autoreactive T cells, caused either by a defect in T-cell apoptosis or by a problem in presentation of self-antigens. This may be most severe for low-abundance specialist antigens, such as those needed for the biosynthesis, secretion and regulation of the various hormones. Defects in CD4$^+$CD25$^+$ regulatory T-cell suppressor function [66] and impaired caspase-3 expression by peripheral T cells [67] have also been demonstrated. Thus, loss of peripheral suppression and/or defective peripheral apoptosis could be involved in the pathogenesis of this syndrome [66,67].

At the onset of autoimmune adrenal failure, adrenal cell autoantibodies or P450c21 autoantibodies are detectable in >90% of patients [9,39]. P450c21 has been identified as the major adrenal antigen in autoimmune adrenalitis and these antibodies are present in 80–90% of patients with disease duration under 15 years, declining to 60% with disease duration over 15 years. These P450c21 autoantibodies are highly specific, being found in only 0.5% of healthy subjects and those with other autoimmune diseases. Some 40–50% of patients with such adrenal autoantibodies have abnormal ACTH stimulation tests. Thus, P450c21 autoantibodies have a high predictive value for clinical Addison disease [39]. Spontaneous disappearance of adrenal antibodies has been reported in up to 20% of cases [39] but disease is permanent in patients who have an abnormal ACTH stimulation test.

Other steroid-producing cell autoantibodies (SCA), such as P450c17 and P450scc, are present in 20–30% patients with Addison disease and are more frequent in females than males [39,68]. There is a strong association between the presence of SCA and ovarian failure in women with APS2/3 but SCA are extremely rare in women with ovarian failure with no signs of adrenal autoimmunity [39,68]. Because of the shared antigens of the steroidogenic enzymes, adrenal autoimmunity is more common (approximately 10%) in those subjects with established gonadal failure.

Autoimmune thyroid disease or type 1 diabetes is a frequent component of APS2. Thyroperoxidase (TPO) and thyroglobulin (TG) are the major thyroid antigens. In Hashimoto thyroiditis, TPO autoantibodies are found in 90–100% and TG autoantibodies in 60–70%. They are both also frequently found in Graves disease, where TSH receptor autoantibodies are found in approximately 90% of cases [44]. Many patients with thyroid autoantibodies but normal TSH progress very slowly to clinical disease [69].

Islet cell autoantibodies are found in around 80% of new-onset type 1 diabetes patients [39]. The main islet autoantigens are insulin, GAD65 and the tyrosine phosphatase-related protein IA-2. Among recently diagnosed subjects with type 1 diabetes, the prevalence of antibodies to insulin and IA-2 is dependent on age, being most frequent in children and adolescents with type 1 diabetes but less than 30% with adult onset or LADA [43]. The frequency of antibodies to GAD65 is 70–80% and is not influenced by age; this therefore gives the highest diagnostic sensitivity in LADA [43,70]. In one investigation, all APS2 patients with type 1 diabetes were positive for GAD65 antibodies but only 54% of those with antibodies had type 1 diabetes. In comparison, IA-2 antibodies are less sensitive but more specific for type 1 diabetes [39].

Gastric parietal cell autoantibodies are found in about 90% of patients with chronic autoimmune gastritis or pernicious anemia [71] and in 30% of their non-anemic first-degree relatives. The major autoantigen is gastric H/K-ATPase. Around 70% of patients with pernicious anemia are also positive for intrinsic factor autoantibodies that block the binding of vitamin B_{12} to intrinsic factor [44]. Tissue transglutaminase (TTG) is the major autoantigen in celiac disease. IgA TTG antibodies are more specific for celiac disease than IgG but both have a high diagnostic sensitivity and specificity. There is good correlation between endomysial autoantibodies and TTG antibodies [44].

Diagnosis and follow-up

Once APS2/3 is suspected, a full assessment of endocrine function is needed. The number of disorders that will develop and the age at which they will present is unpredictable, so long-term follow-up is needed. A high clinical index of suspicion needs to be maintained, particularly in those subjects who have yet to develop adrenal failure or diabetes. Presymptomatic recognition of autoimmune disease minimizes associated morbidity and mortality. There is a clear link between the presence of organ-specific autoantibodies and the progression to disease, although there is often an asymptomatic latent period of months or years. The absence of autoantibodies does not exclude the risk of a disease component.

In any patient with clinical and biochemical signs of adrenal insufficiency, determination of P450c21 autoantibodies demonstrates the autoimmune nature of the disease [44]. In those who are autoantibody "negative" on the first screen, these should be repeated and are often found to become positive within the first few months of developing adrenal failure. An etiological diagnosis should be sought in all subjects but the presence of autoimmune disorders in family members is suggestive of autoimmunity. In all patients with Addison disease, there is a need to screen for other endocrine disorders, particularly autoimmune thyroid disease and type 1 diabetes. At diagnosis, screening for TPO and GAD65 autoantibodies is worthwhile. If negative, this should be repeated occasionally, perhaps every 2–3 years. In children or adolescents with Addison disease, determination of insulin and IA-2 autoantibodies is a sensitive predictor of type 1 diabetes, particularly if both autoantibodies are present. If these β-cell autoantibodies are found, an assessment of fasting blood glucose and, in some cases, an oral glucose tolerance test are required.

The determination of thyroid function should be carried out at least annually for early recognition of thyroid disease in all subjects with type 1 diabetes and Addison disease. The determination of P450c17 and P450scc antibodies in females with Addison disease and APS2 may identify subjects at high risk from primary hypogonadism before gonadotropins become elevated. Such subjects may be suitable for cryopreservation of ovarian material.

The determination of P450c21 autoantibodies should be performed in children presenting with type 1 diabetes as positive adrenal autoantibodies are highly predictive of future adrenal insufficiency [39]. In subjects with P450c21 autoantibodies, an ACTH stimulation test, determination of electrolytes and plasma renin activity enables identification of patients with preclinical adrenal dysfunction. If normal, the ACTH stimulation test should be repeated yearly with interval determination of postural blood pressure and electrolytes. Regardless of antibody status, patients with persistent or worsening symptoms after treatment of autoimmune thyroid disease and subjects with type 1 diabetes who have brittle control or persistent lethargy or those with unexplained vague symptoms should be screened biochemically for Addison disease.

An increased frequency of IgG–TTG antibody has been found in type 1 diabetes children but the prevalence in adult Addison or type 1 diabetes patients is the same as in the healthy population. Thus, they should be included in APS2/3 screening of children but limited in adults to cases with clinical or laboratory signs of malabsorption. Positive TTG antibodies in children require follow-up with an intestinal biopsy to confirm the diagnosis of celiac disease. The predictive value of gastric parietal cell or intrinsic factor autoantibodies for autoimmune gastritis and pernicious anemia is limited by the frequent occurrence of these in healthy first-degree relatives and in the general population (approximately 5–10%). A blood count to detect macrocytosis is a more useful routine investigation, although neurological features of vitamin B_{12} deficiency can be present in the absence of anemia. Thus, vitamin B_{12} concentrations should be measured urgently if clinically suspected.

Screening for APS2-associated disorders should also be performed in women with primary or secondary amenorrhea or premature ovarian failure and young patients with vitiligo. As

APS2 shows strong familial tendencies, family members should also be checked for features of associated endocrine conditions.

Management

Hormone replacement or other therapies for the component diseases of APS2 are similar whether the disease occurs in isolation or in association with other conditions and disorders should be treated as they are diagnosed but certain combinations of diseases require specific attention. Most importantly, thyroxine therapy for hypothyroidism can precipitate a life-threatening adrenal crisis in a patient with untreated and unsuspected adrenal insufficiency [42]. Thus, to avoid adrenal crisis, clinicians should maintain a high degree of suspicion for coexisting adrenal failure in subjects who are hypothyroid. Hyperthyroidism increases cortisol clearance so, in patients with adrenal insufficiency who have unresolved hyperthyroidism, glucocorticoid replacement should be at least doubled until the patient is euthyroid. Decreasing insulin requirements or increasing occurrence of hypoglycemia in type 1 diabetes can be one of the earliest indications of adrenocortical failure. One of the most important aspects of managing these patients is to be continually alert to the possibility of the development of further endocrinopathies to insure early diagnosis and treatment.

Prognosis

Mortality in patients with primary adrenal insufficiency appears to be elevated about twofold compared to the background population [72]. Life expectancy is often reduced as a consequence of unrecognized adrenal crisis but infectious disease, cardiovascular disease and cancer also appear to be increased. Despite adequate hormonal replacement, quality of life is often impaired in these patients, with predominant complaints being unpredictable fatigue, lack of energy, depression and anxiety. It has been shown that the number of patients receiving disability pensions is two- to threefold higher than the general population in certain countries [73].

Summary

A high index of suspicion needs to be maintained whenever one organ-specific autoimmune disorder is diagnosed in order to prevent morbidity and mortality from the index disease as well as associated diseases. Further definition of susceptibility genes and autoantigens, as well as a better understanding of the pathogenesis, is required to improve the diagnosis and management of these patients.

Miscellaneous disorders with autoimmune endocrinopathies

Immune dysregulation, polyendocrinopathy and enteropathy (X-linked) syndrome

Immune dysregulation, polyendocrinopathy and enteropathy (X-linked) syndrome (IPEX) is a rare and devastating X-linked con-

dition of male infants, affecting immune regulation and resulting in multiple autoimmune disorders. The first feature is commonly intractable diarrhea and failure to thrive due to autoimmune enteropathy occurring around 3–4 months of age. Type 1 diabetes and autoimmune hypothyroidism develop in the first year of life in around 90% and 50% of males, respectively. Additional clinical features include eczema, autoimmune hemolytic anemia, autoimmune thrombocytopenia, recurrent infections, lymphadenopathy, membranous nephropathy and striking growth retardation. Other autoimmune features are less frequent [74]. Sepsis may result from a primary defect in immune regulation but is exacerbated by autoimmune neutropenia, immunosuppressive drugs, malnutrition, enteropathy and eczema.

The condition is heterogeneous in its presentation, with the occasional case not presenting until later childhood or adulthood [75]. Diabetes or eczema is a not infrequent initial presentation but any of the disease components can present first. There are no estimates of incidence but it is likely to be underdiagnosed because of the clinical variability in presentation and the presence of frequent new mutations. Intermittent eosinophilia and raised IgE concentrations are found in many patients but there is an absence of any other consistent features of immunodeficiency. The presence of autoantibodies appears to be variable. The most consistent pathological finding is total villous atrophy of the small intestine, with inflammatory cell infiltration of the lamina propria. Diagnosis relies on the clinical presentation, family history and elimination of other diagnoses with similar presentations. Genetic screening has proved useful in some cases. There is a high mortality in these infants, many succumbing to the untreatable diarrhea, malnutrition and superimposed infections by 24 months of age. Survival into adolescence is occasionally seen with the use of aggressive immunosuppression and parenteral feeding, although symptoms are rarely entirely relieved [74,76]. There are increasing reports of the use of bone marrow transplantation in these infants but experience is very limited [74].

IPEX was first reported more than 20 years ago in a large family with typical X-linked recessive inheritance [75]. IPEX appears to be mediated by an abnormality in CD4+ T-cell regulation, with evidence for increased T-cell activation and overproduction of cytokines. By recognition of a similar phenotype in a murine model, mutations in the *FOXP3* gene, located at Xp11, encoding a transcription factor belonging to the forkhead/winged-helix family, were found in IPEX boys [74]. An increasing number of mutations have been reported, mainly in the coding region of *FOXP3*, although one mutation in the regulatory region has also been found [74,76]. *FOXP3* is specifically expressed in naturally arising CD4+CD25+ regulatory T cells and appears to convert naïve T cells to this regulatory phenotype. Thus, *FOXP3* is a critical regulator of CD4+CD25+ T-cell development and function [77]. Severe autoimmunity in FOXP3 deficiency may in part therefore be caused by aggressive helper T-cells that develop from regulatory T-cell precursors that cannot mature because of a lack of FOXP3 [78]. In a few cases, no mutation has been identified. Although female carriers of *FOXP3* mutations appear to be healthy, a small number of cases of an IPEX-like syndrome have been reported recently in families with affected girls in whom no mutation was found [76]. It is likely that there may be an autosomal locus accounting for the problem in some families and mutations in the IL-2 receptor subunit CD25 have been shown to cause a similar syndrome [79]. This genetic heterogeneity may explain some of the clinical variation seen in this syndrome but, as yet, no obvious genotype–phenotype relationship has been identified and other modifying genes, such as *HLA*, as well as environmental factors may influence the outcome.

Autoimmune lymphoproliferative syndrome

Autoimmune lymphoproliferative syndrome (ALPS) was first described in 1967, although the etiology and pathogenesis of the condition were unknown [80]. Onset is usually in the first 2 years of life and the characteristic feature in all cases is massive generalized lymphadenopathy. Hepatosplenomegaly and hematological autoimmunity (hemolytic anemia and thrombocytopenia) are also frequent manifestations. Other autoimmune conditions, including thyroid autoimmunity and type 1 diabetes, have occasionally been reported as part of this syndrome [81]. Characteristically, fever, infections or immunosuppressive therapy lead to a decrease in the degree of lymphadenopathy and hepatosplenomegaly and an improvement in the autoimmune phenomena. ALPS tends to follow a chronic course, with the response to immunosuppressive drugs varying. Splenectomy is usually performed to reduce the lymphadenopathy and improve the thrombocytopenia and hemolytic anemia, although this leads to an increased risk of infections in patients who are often neutropenic. Long-term outcome is variable, although survival into adulthood has been reported, when an increase in malignancy is seen [82]. Allogenic bone marrow transplantation has been found to be a successful treatment in a few children.

Mutations of the Fas receptor or of its ligand FasL are responsible for ALPS type 1a and 1b, respectively [82]. ALPS type 2 is a clinical variant caused by mutations in the caspase-10 gene. Fas is a key receptor in the apoptotic pathway and the binding of FasL to Fas leads to apoptosis by activating a series of events involving a group of proteases called caspases. The defective apoptotic function in ALPS leads to an accumulation of lymphocytes (particularly CD3$^+$CD4$^-$CD8$^-$), including potentially autoreactive cells.

Kabuki make-up syndrome

Kabuki make-up syndrome (KMS) is a syndrome of unknown cause, although probably genetic, consisting of five characteristic manifestations:

1 Dysmorphic face with eversion of the lower lateral eyelid, arched eyebrows with sparseness of their lateral one-third, long palpebral fissures with long eyelashes, depressed nasal tip and prominent large ears (100%);
2 Unusual dermatoglyphic patterns (96%);
3 Skeletal abnormalities and hypermobile joints (88%);
4 Mild to moderate mental retardation (84%); and

5 Postnatal growth retardation with short stature (55%) [83]. Other well-recognized features include dental abnormalities, susceptibility to infections, particularly recurrent otitis media, cardiovascular anomalies, renal and urinary tract anomalies, biliary atresia, diaphragmatic hernia and anorectal anomalies. Less common associations include growth hormone deficiency, primary ovarian dysfunction, Hashimoto thyroiditis, type 1 diabetes, hypoglycaemia and vitiligo [81,83]. Other endocrine abnormalities reported in these patients include most commonly isolated premature thelarche occurring in around 25% as early as 4 months of age. True central precocious puberty is rarely seen. Elevated gonadotropin concentrations particularly follicle stimulating hormone (FSH), are found and although unknown the etiology has been postulated to be secondary to low hypothalamic sensitivity to the suppressive effects of sex hormones on gonadotropin secretion [83]. Rare endocrine findings include growth hormone deficiency, hypoglycemia, congenital hypothyroidism and type 1 diabetes [83].

It has been recognized most commonly within the Japanese population (incidence 1 in 32 000) but it is now recognized in all countries. Patients often survive with a good prognosis unless they have severe complications such as cardiovascular, hepatic or renal disease [83]. Males and females are affected equally and most cases are sporadic, although a few familial cases have been reported. KMS may be inherited as an autosomal recessive disorder. As yet, there is no evidence or clues to the underlying cause of the syndrome. The endocrinopathies should be treated along standard lines.

References

1 Neufeld M, Maclaren NK, Blizzard RM. Two types of auto-immune Addison's disease associated with different polyglandular autoimmune (PGA) syndromes. *Medicine (Baltimore)* 1981; **60**: 355–362.

2 Ahonen P, Myllärniemi S, Sipilä I, Perheentupa J. Clinical variation of autoimmune polyendocrinopathy–candidiasis–ectodermal dystrophy (APECED) in a series of 68 patients. *N Engl J Med* 1990; **322**: 1829–1836.

3 Zlotogora J, Shapiro MS. Polyglandular autoimmune syndrome type I among Iranian Jews. *J Med Genet* 1992; **29**: 824–826.

4 Betterle C, Greggio NA, Volpato M. Clinical review 93: autoimmune polyglandular syndrome type I. *J Clin Endocrinol Metab* 1998; **83**: 1049–1055.

5 Myhre AG, Halonen M, Eskelin P, *et al.* Autoimmune polyendocrine syndrome type I (APS1) in Norway. *Clin Endocrinol (Oxf)* 2001; **54**: 211–217.

6 Perheentupa J. APS-I/APECED: the clinical disease and therapy. *Endocrinol Metab Clin North Am* 2002; **31**: 295–320.

7 Rosatelli MC, Meloni A, Devoto M, *et al.* A common mutation in Sardinian autoimmune polyendocrinopathy–candidiasis–ectodermal dystrophy patients. *Hum Genet* 1998; **103**: 428–434.

8 Pearce SH, Cheetham TD. Autoimmune polyendocrinopathy syndrome type I: treat with kid gloves. *Clin Endocrinol (Oxf)* 2001; **54**: 433–435.

9 Betterle C, Dal Pra C, Mantero F, Zanchetta R. Autoimmune adrenal insufficiency and autoimmune polyendocrine syndromes: autoantibodies, autoantigens and their applicability in diagnosis and disease prediction. *Endocr Rev* 2002; **23**: 327–364.

10 Gass JD. The syndrome of keratoconjunctivitis, superficial moniliasis idiopathic hypoparathyroidism and Addison disease. *Am J Ophthalmol* 1962; **54**: 660–674.

11 Gylling M, Kääriäinen E, Väisänen R, et al. The hypoparathyroidism of autoimmune polyendocrinopathy–candidiasis–ectodermal dystrophy protective effect of male sex. *J Clin Endocrinol Metab* 2003; **88**: 4602–4608.

12 Perheentupa J. Autoimmune polyendocrinopathy-candidiasis-ectodermal dystrophy. *J Clin Endocrinol Metab* 2006; **91**: 2843–2850.

13 Sotsiou F, Bottazzo GF, Doniach D. Immunofluorescence studies on autoantibodies to steroid-producing cells and to germline cells in endocrine disease and infertility. *Clin Exp Immunol* 1980; **39**: 97–111.

14 Franzese A, Valerio G, Di Maio S, Iannucci MP, Bloise A, Tenore A. Growth hormone insufficiency in a girl with the autoimmune polyendocrinopathy–candidiasis–ectodermal dystrophy. *J Endocrinol Invest* 1999; **22**: 66–69.

15 Bereket A, Lowenheim M, Blethen SL, Kane P, Wilson TA. Intestinal lymphangiectasia in a patient with autoimmune polyglandular disease type I and steatorrhea. *J Clin Endocrinol Metab* 1995; **80**: 933–935.

16 Högenauer C, Meyer RL, Netto GJ, et al. Malabsorption due to cholecystokinin deficiency in a patient with autoimmune polyglandular syndrome type 1. *N Engl J Med* 2001; **344**: 270–274.

17 Smith D, Stringer MD, Wyatt J, et al. Orthoptic liver transplantation for acute liver failure secondary to autoimmune hepatitis in a child with autoimmune polyglandular syndrome type 1. *Pediatr Transplant* 2002; **6**: 166–170.

18 Nagamine K, Peterson P, Scott HS, et al. Positional cloning of the APECED gene. *Nat Genet* 1997; **17**: 393–398.

19 The Finnish–German APECED Consortium. An autoimmune disease, APECED, caused by mutations in a novel gene featuring two PHD-type zinc-finger domains. *Nat Genet* 1997; **17**: 399–403.

20 Liston A, Lesage S, Wilson J, Peltonen L, Goodnow CC. AIRE regulates negative selection of organ-specific T cells. *Nat Immunol* 2003; **4**: 350–354.

21 Mathis D, Benoist C. A decade of AIRE. *Nat Rev Immunol* 2007; **7**: 645–650.

22 Ryan KR, Lawson CA, Lorenzi AR, Arkwright PD, Isaacs JD, Lilic D. CD4$^+$CD25$^+$ T-regulatory cells are decreased in patients with autoimmune polyendocrinopathy candidiasis ectodermal dystrophy. *J Allergy Clin Immunol* 2005; **116**: 1158–1159.

23 Pearce SH, Cheetham T, Imrie H, et al. A common and recurrent 13-bp deletion in the autoimmune regulator gene in British kindreds with autoimmune polyendocrinopathy type I. *Am J Hum Genet* 1998; **63**: 1675–1684.

24 Pitkänen J, Doucas V, Sternsdorf T, et al. The autoimmune regulator protein has transcriptional transactivating properties and interacts with the common coactivator CREB-binding protein. *J Biol Chem* 2000; **275**: 16802–16809.

25 Wolff AS, Erichsen MM, Meager A, et al. Autoimmune polyendocrinopathy syndrome type 1 in Norway: phenotypic variation, autoantibodies and novel mutations in the autoimmune regulator gene. *J Clin Endocrinol Metab* 2007; **92**: 595–603.

26 Ahonen P, Koskimies S, Lokki ML, Tiilikainen A, Perheentupa J. The expression of autoimmune polyglandular disease type 1 appears associated with several HLA-A antigens but not with HLA-DR. *J Clin Endocrinol Metab* 1988; **66**: 1152–1157.

27 Halonen M, Eskelin P, Myhre AG, et al. AIRE mutations and human leukocyte antigen genotypes as determinants of the autoimmune polyendocrinopathy–candidiasis–ectodermal dystrophy phenotype. *J Clin Endocrinol Metab* 2002; **87**: 2568–2574.

28 Adamson KA, Cheetham TD, Kendall-Taylor P, Seckl JR, Pearce SH. The role of the *IDDM2* locus in the susceptibility of UK APS1 subjects to type 1 diabetes mellitus. *Int J Immunogenet* 2007; **34**: 17–21.

29 Meager A, Visvalingam K, Peterson P, et al. Anti-interferon autoantibodies in autoimmune polyendocrinopathy syndrome type 1. *PLoS Med* 2006; **3**: 1152–1164.

30 Söderbergh A, Myhre AG, Ekwall O, et al. Prevalence and clinical associations of ten defined autoantibodies in autoimmune polyendocrine syndrome type 1. *J Clin Endocrinol Metab* 2004; **89**: 557–562.

31 Li Y, Song Y, Rais N, et al. Autoantibodies to the extracellular domain of the calcium sensing receptor in patients with acquired hypoparathyroidism. *J Clin Invest* 1996; **97**: 910–914.

32 Gavalas NG, Kemp EH, Krohn KJ, Brown EM, Watson PF, Weetman AP. The calcium-sensing receptor is a target of autoantibodies in patients with autoimmune polyendocrine syndrome type 1. *J Clin Endocrinol Metab* 2007; **92**: 2107–2114.

33 Pearce SH, Leech NJ. Editorial: Toward precise forecasting of autoimmune endocrinopathy. *J Clin Endocrinol Metab* 2004; **89**: 544–547.

34 Alimohammadi M, Björklund P, Hallgren A, et al. Autoimmune polyendocrine syndrome type 1 and NALP5, a parathyroid autoantigen. *N Engl J Med* 2008; **358**: 1018–1028.

35 Tuomi T, Björses P, Falorini A, et al. Antibodies to glutamic acid decarboxylase and insulin-dependent diabetes in patients with autoimmune polyendocrine syndrome type I. *J Clin Endocrinol Metab* 1996; **81**: 1488–1494.

36 Obermayer-Straub P, Perheentupa J, Braun S, et al. Hepatic autoantigens in patients with autoimmune polyendocrinopathy–candidiasis–ectodermal dystrophy. *Gastroenterology* 2001; **121**: 668–677.

37 Hedstrand H, Ekwall O, Olsson MJ, et al. The transcription factors SOX9 and SOX10 are vitiligo autoantigens in autoimmune polyendocrine syndrome type 1. *J Biol Chem* 2001; **276**: 35390–35395.

38 Laureti S, Vecchi L, Santeusanio F, Falorini A. Is the prevalence of Addison disease underestimated? *J Clin Endocrinol Metab* 1999; **84**: 1762.

39 Falorni A, Laureti S, Santeusanio F. Autoantibodies in autoimmune polyendocrine syndrome type II. *Endocrinol Metab Clin North Am* 2002; **31**: 369–389.

40 Betterle C, Volpato M, Greggio AN, Presotto F. Type 2 polyglandular autoimmune disease (Schmidt's syndrome). *J Pediatr Endocrinol Metab* 1996; **9** (Suppl 1): 113–123.

41 Betterle C, Lazzarotto F, Presotto F. Autoimmune polyglandular syndrome type 2: the tip of an iceberg? *Clin Exp Immunol* 2004; **137**: 225–233.

42 Murray JS, Jayarajasingh R, Perros P. Deterioration of symptoms after start of thyroid hormone replacement. *Br Med J* 2001; **323**: 332–333.

43 Leslie RD, Williams R, Pozzilli P. Type 1 diabetes and latent autoimmune diabetes in adults: one end of the rainbow. *J Clin Endocrinol Metab* 2006; **91**: 1654–1659.

44 Schatz DA, Winter WE. Autoimmune polyglandular syndrome II: clinical syndrome and treatment. *Endocrinol Metab Clin North Am* 2002; **31**: 339–352.

45 Belvisi L, Bombelli F, Sironi L, Doldi N. Organ-specific autoimmunity in patients with premature ovarian failure. *J Endocrinol Invest* 1993; **16**: 889–892.

46 Betterle C, Volpato M, Rees Smith B, *et al.* I. Adrenal cortex and steroid 21-hydroxylase autoantibodies in adult patients with organspecific autoimmune diseases: markers of low progression to clinical Addison disease. *J Clin Endocrinol Metab* 1997; **82**: 932–938.

47 Yamaguchi Y, Chikuba N, Ueda Y, *et al.* Islet cell antibodies in patients with autoimmune thyroid disease. *Diabetes* 1991; **40**: 319–322.

48 Mandry RC ortiz LJ, Lugo-Somolinos A, Sanchez JL. Organ-specific autoantibodies in vitiligo patients and their relatives. *Int J Dermatol* 1996; **35**: 18–21.

49 Robles DT, Fain PR, Gottlieb PA, Eisenbarth GS. The genetics of autoimmune polyendocrine syndrome type II. *Endocrinol Metab Clin North Am* 2002; **31**: 353–368.

50 Huang W, Connor E, Dela Rosa T, *et al.* Although DR3-DQB1*0201 may be associated with multiple component diseases of the autoimmune polyglandular syndromes, the human leukocyte antigen DR4-DQB1*0302 haplotype is implicated only in beta-cell autoimmunity. *J Clin Endocrinol Metab* 1996; **81**: 2259–2263.

51 Vaidya B, Pearce S, Kendall-Taylor P. Recent advances in the molecular genetics of congenital and acquired primary adrenocortical failure. *Clin Endocrinol (Oxf)* 2000; **53**: 403–418.

52 Yu L, Brewer KW, Gates S, *et al.* DRB1*04 and DQ alleles: expression of 21-hydroxylase autoantibodies and risk of progression to Addison disease. *J Clin Endocrinol Metab* 1999; **84**: 328–335.

53 Donner H, Braun J, Seidl C, *et al.* Codon 17 polymorphism of the cytotoxic T lymphocyte antigen 4 gene in Hashimoto thyroiditis and Addison disease. *J Clin Endocrinol Metab* 1997; **82**: 4130–4132.

54 Yanagawa T, Hidaka Y, Guimaraes V, Soliman M, DeGroot LJ. CTLA-4 gene polymorphism associated with Graves disease in a Caucasian population. *J Clin Endocrinol Metab* 1995; **80**: 41–45.

55 Nisticò L, Buzzetti R, Pritchard LE, *et al.* The CTLA-4 gene region of chromosome 2q33 is linked to and associated with, type 1 diabetes. Belgium Diabetes Registry. *Hum Mol Genet* 1996; **5**: 1075–1080.

56 Vaidya B, Imrie H, Geatch DR, *et al.* Association analysis of the cytotoxic T lymphocyte antigen-4 (CTLA-4) and autoimmune regulator-1 (AIRE-1) genes in sporadic autoimmune Addison disease. *J Clin Endocrinol Metab* 2000; **85**: 688–691.

57 Blomhoff A, Lie BA, Myhre AG, *et al.* Polymorphisms in the cytotoxic T lymphocyte antigen-4 gene region confer susceptibility to Addison's disease. *J Clin Endocrinol Metab* 2004; **89**: 3474–3476.

58 De Nanclares GP, Martin-Pagola A, Bilbao JR, Vazquez F, Castano L. No evidence of association of *CTLA4* polymorphisms with Addison's disease. *Autoimmunity* 2004; **37**: 453–456.

59 Velaga MR, Wilson V, Jennings CE, *et al.* The codon 620 tryptophan allele of the lymphoid tyrosine phosphatase (LYP) gene is a major determinant of Graves' disease. *J Clin Endocrinol Metab* 2004; **89**: 5862–5865.

60 Skinningsrud B, Husebye ES, Gervin K, *et al.* Mutation screening of PTPN22: association of the 1858T-allele with Addison's disease. *Eur J Hum Genet* 2008; **16**: 977–982

61 Kahles H, Ramos-Lopez E, Lange B, Zwermann O, Reincke M, Badenhoop K. Sex-specific association of PTPN22 1858T with type 1 diabetes but not with Hashimoto's thyroiditis or Addison's disease in the German population. *Eur J Endocrinol* 2005; **153**: 895–899.

62 Lopez ER, Zwermann O, Segni M, *et al.* A promoter polymorphism of the CYP27B1 gene is associated with Addison's disease, Hashimoto's thyroiditis, Graves' disease and type 1 diabetes mellitus in Germans. *Eur J Endocrinol* 2004; **151**: 193–197.

63 Jennings CE, Owen CJ, Wilson V, Pearce SH. A haplotype of the CYP27B1 promoter is associated with autoimmune Addison's disease but not with Graves' disease in a UK population. *J Mol Endocrinol* 2005; **34**: 859–863.

64 Kamradt T, Mitchinson NA. Tolerance and autoimmunity. *N Engl J Med* 2001; **344**: 655–664.

65 Tadmor B, Putterman C, Naparstek Y. Embryonal germ-layer antigens: target for autoimmunity. *Lancet* 1992; **339**: 975–978.

66 Kriegel MA, Lohmann T, Gabler C, Blank N, Kalden JR, Lorenz H-M. Defective suppressor function of human CD4+CD25+ regulatory T cells in autoimmune polyglandular syndrome type II. *J Exp Med* 2004; **9**: 1285–1291.

67 Vendrame F, Segni M, Grassetti D, *et al.* Impaired caspase-3 expression by peripheral T cells in chronic autoimmune thyroiditis and in autoimmune polyendocrine syndrome-2. *J Clin Endocrinol Metab* 2006; **91**: 5064–5068.

68 Betterle C, Volpato M, Pedini B, Chen S, Rees Smith B, Furmaniak J. Adrenal-cortex autoantibodies and steroid-producing cells autoantibodies in patients with Addison disease: comparison of immunofluorescence and immunoprecipitation assays. *J Clin Endocrinol Metab* 1999; **84**: 618–622.

69 Vanderpump MP, Tunbridge WM, French JM, *et al.* The incidence of thyroid disorders in the community: a twenty-year follow-up of the Wickham Survey. *Clin Endocrinol (Oxf)* 1995; **43**: 55–68.

70 Vandewalle CL, Falorni A, Svanholm S, Lernmark A, Pipeleers DG, Gorus FK. High diagnostic sensitivity of glutamate decarboxylase autoantibodies in insulin-dependent diabetes mellitus with clinical onset between age 20 and 40 years. The Belgian Diabetes Registry. *J Clin Endocrinol Metab* 1995; **80**: 846–851.

71 Toh BH, van Driel IR, Gleeson PA. Pernicious anemia. *N Engl J Med* 1997; **337**: 1441–1448.

72 Bergthorsdottir R, Leonsson-Zachrisson M, Oden A, Johannsson G. Premature mortality in patients with Addison's disease: a population based study. *J Clin Endocrinol Metab* 2006; **91**: 4849–4853.

73 Lovas K, Husebye ES. High prevalence and increasing incidence of Addison disease in western Norway. *Clin Endocrinol (Oxf)* 2002; **56**: 787–791.

74 Wildin RS, Smyk-Pearson S, Filipovich AH. Clinical and molecular features of the immunodysregulation, polyendocrinopathy, enteropathy, X linked (IPEX) syndrome. *J Med Genet* 2002; **39**: 537–545.

75 Powell BR, Buist NR, Stenzel P. An X-linked syndrome of diarrhea, polyendocrinopathy and fatal infection in infancy. *J Pediatr* 1982; **100**: 731–737.

76 Owen CJ, Jennings CE, Imrie H, *et al.* Mutational analysis of the FOXP3 gene and evidence for genetic heterogeneity in the immunodysregulation, polyendocrinopathy, enteropathy syndrome. *J Clin Endocrinol Metab* 2003; **88**: 6034–6039.

77 Fontenot JD, Gavin MA, Rudensky AY. FOXP3 programs the development and function of CD4$^+$CD25$^+$ regulatory T cells. *Nat Immunol* 2003; **4**: 330–336.

78 Gavin MA, Torgerson TR, Houston E, *et al.* Single-cell analysis of normal and FOXP3-mutant human T cells: FOXP3 expression without regulatory T cell development. *Proc Natl Acad Sci U S A* 2006; **103**: 6659–6664.

79 Caudy AA, Reddy ST, Chatila T, Atkinson JP, Verbsky JW. CD25 deficiency causes an immune dysregulation, polyendocrinopathy, enteropathy, X-linked syndrome and defective IL-10 expression from CD4 lymphocytes. *J Allergy Clin Immunol* 2007; **119**: 482–487.

80 Canale VC, Smith CH. Chronic lymphadenopathy simulating malignant lymphoma. *J Pediatr* 1967; **70**: 891–899.

81 Dotta F, Vendrame F. Neonatal syndromes of polyendocrinopathy. *Endocrinol Metab Clin North Am* 2002; **31**: 283–293.

82 Drappa J, Vaishnaw AK, Sullivan KE, Chu J, Elkon KB. Fas gene mutations in the Canale–Smith syndrome, an inherited lymphoproliferative disorder associated with autoimmunity. *N Engl J Med* 1996; **335**: 1643–1649.

83 Adam MP, Hudgins L. Kabuki syndrome: a review. *Clin Genet* 2004; **67**: 209–219.

15 Disorders of Water Balance

David R. Repaske

Division of Endocrinology, Nationwide Children's Hospital, Ohio State University, Columbus, OH, USA

Cellular functioning depends on maintenance of extracellular tonicity within a narrow range of 275–295 mOsm/kg. Alterations in plasma tonicity affect cell shape and size and alter the concentration of both intracellular and extracellular ions and other osmolytes, which can alter action potentials, ion channel activities and other functions of the cells. Water intake and excretion varies widely in normal infants, children and adults but regulatory systems integrating thirst, vasopressin secretion and renal responses maintain tight control of osmolality under usual conditions. Serum osmolality can usually be maintained within this tight range under conditions as varied as hiking in the desert and heavy social drinking.

Two complementary systems have evolved to regulate extracellular volume and osmolality: sodium intake and excretion are the primary determinants of extracellular volume; water intake and excretion are the primary determinants of osmolality. Thirst controls water intake and arginine vasopressin (AVP) [also known as antidiuretic hormone (ADH)] secretion controls urine concentration and thereby water excretion. The renin-angiotensin-aldosterone system modulates sodium intake and excretion.

Body water and electrolytes

Throughout life, water contributes the largest mass to the human body of any of its chemical components. The relation of water to total body weight changes from birth to childhood and adulthood [1]. In term neonates and young infants, 75–80% of body weight is water, with 45–50% of body weight extracellular water and 30% of body weight intracellular water (Fig. 15.1) [2]. During the first few days of life, there is a rapid diuresis of 7% of total body water from the extracellular compartment. This trend slows but continues over the first year of life so that the adult distribution of intracellular, extracellular and total body water of 40%, 20% and 60%, respectively, is achieved during childhood.

The large and consistent contribution of water to total body weight in healthy children and adults reflects a dynamic equilibrium achieved by the balance of fluctuating water intake and excretion. Daily water intake and loss can vary 10-fold between individuals and even within a given individual due to changes in diet, environmental conditions and state of health (e.g. increased losses with febrile illness, gastroenteritis or simply living in an arid locality). Water losses occur through the respiratory tract and skin (insensible losses) and the gastrointestinal tract and urine. Urine volume depends on either the volume of free water or the amount of solute to be excreted. Excretion of free water adds to urine volume but solute excretion also requires a minimum volume of free water that depends on the degree to which the kidney can concentrate the urine.

Normal daily obligate solute excretion is approximately 500 mOsm/m²/day. To excrete this solute in urine in the middle of the concentration range (osmolality 500–600 mOsm/kg) requires approximately 900 mL/m²/day urine in adults but, in healthy infants and children, these parameters can vary over a wide range as a result of factors such as changes in the composition of infant formula, milk, juice and other dietary components introduced over the first year of life, together with improved renal concentrating capacity over the first months [3]. In the first months of life, on a relatively high solute infant formula with low urinary concentrating ability, the obligate urinary volume is much higher than in adults.

The obligatory urine volume to excrete solute of 900 mL/m²/day, combined with respiratory and skin losses of 750 mL/m²/day, gastrointestinal losses of 100 mL/m²/day and gain of total body weight due to water of oxidation generated during metabolism of energy sources of 250 mL/m²/day, yields an average net loss of approximately 1500 mL/m²/day. This is considered to be the amount of maintenance fluid to be administered to a typical adult to maintain homeostasis. Under conditions in which urine cannot be diluted or concentrated to the mid-range, this maintenance volume can lead either to overhydration or to dehydration, with resultant abnormalities in plasma osmolality.

Brook's Clinical Pediatric Endocrinology, 6th edition. Edited by C. Brook, P. Clayton, R. Brown. © 2009 Blackwell Publishing, ISBN: 978-1-4051-8080-1.

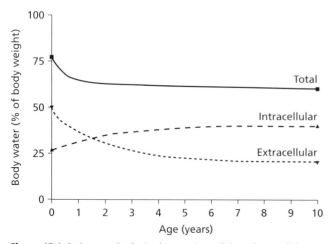

Figure 15.1 Body water distribution between intracellular and extracellular compartments as a function of body weight in infants and children. (After Friis-Hansen [1] and Fomon & Nelson [2].)

Table 15.1 Daily electrolyte requirements (additional adjustments should be made for abnormal losses).

Electrolyte	Amount
Sodium	20–50 mEq/m²/day
Potassium	20–50 mEq/m²/day
Calcium:	
Term newborns	50–75 mg/kg/day
Infants	600 mg/day
Children	800 mg/day
Adolescents	1200 mg/day

Calcium figures are for oral intake.

When considering the amounts of water needed to maintain osmotic stability, it is useful to consider daily electrolyte requirements to avoid depletion of electrolyte stores or excess solute diuresis (Table 15.1). This is particularly important when intravenous fluids are the main source of water and electrolytes. During fluid therapy of short duration (hours to a few days), sodium, potassium and associated anions are the primary electrolytes that should be administered. With intravenous fluid therapy of longer duration, additional electrolytes such as calcium, magnesium and phosphorus need to be added.

A change of osmolality in either the intracellular or the extracellular compartment at equilibrium results in a transient difference in osmolality between the compartments that is rapidly equalized. Cell membranes are impermeable to electrolytes, such as sodium and chloride, which constitute the main extracellular solutes, and potassium and phosphate, which constitute the main intracellular solutes, and they undergo active transport into and out of cells to establish their gradients. While these solutes differ in relative amounts intracellularly and extracellularly, the total solute concentration is the same at equilibrium due to the unim-

peded movement of water across most cell membranes. Thus, a change in the osmolality of one compartment results in an osmotic gradient that is removed by the rapid redistribution of water from one compartment to the other.

For example, a loss of water exceeding the loss of sodium and chloride relative to the composition of normal plasma during an episode of gastroenteritis results in a transient increase in extracellular sodium and its anions and in the osmolality of plasma and interstitial fluids. The osmotic gradient introduced between intracellular and extracellular compartments causes the net movement of water from the intracellular space to the extracellular space, evenly distributing the water loss throughout total body water and equalizing the osmotic gradient with a decrease in the osmolality of the extracellular compartment and an increase in the osmolality of the intracellular compartment. Conversely, dilution of plasma sodium and its anions by rapid administration of hypotonic fluids results in the net movement of water from the extracellular compartment to the intracellular compartment to distribute the water gain throughout total body water. Chronic, as opposed to acute, changes in cell osmolality can result in cell adaptation by reversibly increasing or decreasing intracellular, impermeable solutes. Whether these adaptive changes might have occurred has to be considered when instituting therapy designed to correct hyponatremia or hypernatremia.

Physiology of osmotic regulation

To maintain plasma osmolality in the range that allows optimal cellular function requires sensitive mechanisms for detecting deviation of osmolality from a normal set point and neural and biochemical pathways that implement a means of restoring the system to that normal set point. Osmosensors within the central nervous system modulate two effector pathways to maintain homeostasis: thirst to change water intake and posterior pituitary vasopressin secretion to alter renal water excretion.

Vasopressin and regulation of water excretion
Biochemistry

Arginine vasopressin (AVP) regulates plasma osmolality by controlling free water excretion in humans and most animals. AVP is a cyclic nonapeptide that, like its evolutionarily related counterpart oxytocin, consists of a six-member disulfide ring and a three-member tail on which the carboxy-terminal group is amidated (Fig. 15.2a). Oxytocin differs from AVP only in replacement of isoleucine for phenylalanine at position 3 and of leucine for arginine at position 8 of the molecule. These differences allow activation of receptors for either vasopressin or oxytocin and thereby separation of biological effects. While vasopressin potently activates renal V_2-type vasopressin receptors, the affinity for oxytocin is two orders of magnitude lower [4], such that it could not effectively substitute for loss of vasopressin in promoting free water reabsorption.

Vasopressin is synthesized within the cell body of neurons in the hypothalamus as a preprohormone composed of a signal peptide followed by the nonapeptide hormone, a tripeptide

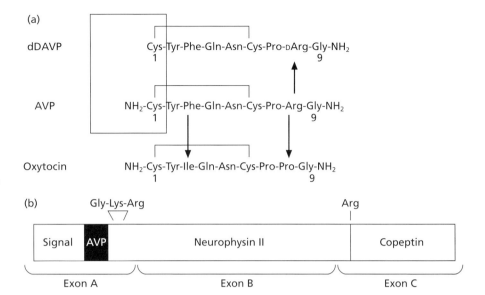

(a)

dDAVP   Cys-Tyr-Phe-Gln-Asn-Cys-Pro-DArg-Gly-NH$_2$
             1   9

AVP   NH$_2$-Cys-Tyr-Phe-Gln-Asn-Cys-Pro-Arg-Gly-NH$_2$
             1   9

Oxytocin   NH$_2$-Cys-Tyr-Ile-Gln-Asn-Cys-Pro-Pro-Gly-NH$_2$
             1   9

(b)   Gly-Lys-Arg   Arg

Signal	AVP	Neurophysin II	Copeptin

Exon A   Exon B   Exon C

Figure 15.2 Arginine vasopressin (AVP) protein and gene structure. (a) Amino acid comparison of AVP and the structurally related molecules oxytocin and dDAVP. Amino acids are numbered from the amino-terminus of each molecule and differences in amino acids between these molecules are shown by the arrows. The box indicates the deamidation of the amino-terminus in dDAVP compared with AVP. (b) Relationship of AVP to its prepro-AVP precursor. Intron–exon boundaries of the gene relative to the coding sequences are shown, as are the di- and monobasic cleavage sites essential for protein processing.

linker, a binding protein known as neurophysin II, an Arg linker and a glycosylated peptide known as copeptin (Fig. 15.2b). The vasopressin gene and oppositely oriented oxytocin gene are located adjacent to one another on chromosome 20 in humans [5,6]. The structure of the oxytocin precursor is similar to that of vasopressin, except that it lacks copeptin and encodes neurophysin I instead of neurophysin II. Despite their linkage in mammalian genomes and highest expression within the hypothalamus, the genes encoding vasopressin and oxytocin are expressed in different neurons [7].

During its synthesis, translocation of preprovasopressin into the endoplasmic reticulum is associated with cleavage of the signal peptide. The precursor molecule folds, enclosing the small vasopressin moiety into a neurophysin binding pocket, presumably to protect it from proteolysis. The neurophysin component promotes self-association during transition from the Golgi apparatus into the neurosecretory granules, initially as dimers [8].

The importance of neurophysin folding and oligomerization in the trafficking of provasopressin is highlighted by the condition of familial autosomal dominant neurohypophyseal diabetes insipidus (ADNDI), a dominantly inherited vasopressin deficiency that results from vasopressin processing abnormalities. ADNDI is most frequently brought about by mutations in neurophysin II that prevent proper targeting of the otherwise normal mature vasopressin hormone to neurosecretory granules [9]. The efficiency of neurophysin II folding, and hence vasopressin trafficking, is dependent upon pairing of its seven internal disulfides and binding of the mature hormone moiety [10]. The intermolecular interaction and oligomerization of the neurophysins is enhanced by non-covalent binding of the nonapeptide hormone region to the amino-terminal domain of the neurophysin [11].

The neurosecretory granule containing the folded vasopressin precursor travels from the cell body down the axon toward the axon terminal. During this transit, the prohormone is cleaved by endopeptidases and exopeptidases, releasing vasopressin, neuro-

physin II and copeptin. The individual cleaved prohormone components remain non-covalently bound during the transit process. The hormone is amidated at its C-terminus by a monooxygenase and lyase present as insoluble complexes with neurophysin II within granules. The vasopressin-containing granules are then stored in the nerve terminals until neuronal activation occurs causing calcium entry into the nerve terminal and subsequent exocytotic release of vasopressin bound to neurophysin II into the circulation.

Once in plasma, the vasopressin–neurophysin complex dissociates and the hormone circulates in a free form. Increases in secretion of vasopressin are coupled to increases in synthesis but this compensatory response may not always balance the increased rate of release [12]. A chronic severe stimulus, such as prolonged water deprivation or nephrogenic diabetes insipidus (NDI), may thus severely deplete posterior pituitary stores of vasopressin, as can be seen by absence of the pituitary bright spot on magnetic resonance imaging (MRI).

Detailed structure–function analyses of specific amino acids within the vasopressin and oxytocin peptides have generated new molecules that are advantageous in the management of states of vasopressin deficiency. For example, replacement of L-arginine with D-arginine at position 8 of vasopressin together with its amino-terminal deamidation resulted in a vasopressin analog with more potent and prolonged antidiuretic activity, which is now widely used clinically [desamino-D-arginine vasopressin (dDAVP), Fig. 15.2] [13].

Anatomy

Vasopressin destined for modulation of renal water handling is synthesized by neurons located in the bilateral hypothalamic supraoptic and paraventricular nuclei. The large magnocellular neurons within these nuclei send axons toward the midline at the base of the hypothalamus to terminate at various levels within the pituitary stalk or in the posterior pituitary (neurohypophysis) itself (Fig. 15.3). Vasopressin-containing neurosecretory vesicles stored in nerve terminals can be visualized as the posterior pituitary bright spot on T1-weighted MRI images. Vasopressin is released from these neurosecretory granule-rich terminals in the posterior pituitary and stalk into the systemic circulation. The superior and inferior hypophyseal arteries, distal branches of the internal carotid artery, provide the blood supply to the posterior pituitary [14]. There is a second group of smaller parvocellular neurons that also synthesize vasopressin in the paraventricular nucleus of the hypothalamus. In contrast to the magnocellular neurons, the parvocellular neurons give rise to axons that terminate at the median eminence and secrete vasopressin into the portal-hypophyseal vascular plexus to augment adrenocorticotropic hormone (ACTH) synthesis and release from anterior pituitary corticotrophs [15].

Regulation of vasopressin secretion

The release of most hormones is regulated by feedback inhibition. For instance, TSH release is limited through inhibition by the circulating level of thyroid hormone. Regulation of vasopressin secretion is not dependent on sensing circulating vasopressin levels but rather by sensing plasma osmolality. Under normal conditions, as plasma osmolality increases, more vasopressin is secreted to increase water retention and, as plasma osmolality decreases, vasopressin secretion is suppressed.

The sensing of plasma osmolality might well occur within the magnocellular neurons that produce and store vasopressin and in fact, magnocellular vasopressin-containing neurons in the supraoptic and paraventricular nuclei can depolarize and secrete vasopressin in response to a hypertonic environment. But they are not the physiologic sensors of osmolality because they are insulated from rapid changes in plasma osmolality by the blood–brain barrier. Instead, there are osmosensing neurons outside the blood–brain barrier in the organ vasculosum of the lamina terminalis and the subfornical organs [16,17] which sense and relay osmotic information both to magnocellular neurons and to the thirst center. Destruction of these centers in animal models disrupts vasopressin (and thirst) regulation of plasma osmolality.

Vasopressin is also released in response to non-osmotic stimuli. Vasopressin slows free water release from the body, so it makes physiological sense that it might be released in response to conditions where intravascular volume preservation is beneficial. Indeed, vasopressin is released in response to severe hypovolemia or hypotension and this response can override even the suppression of vasopressin release under conditions of hypo-osmolality. Vasopressin is also released in response to severe stress, nausea and some centrally acting drugs.

Osmotic regulation

In healthy individuals, the set point for initiation of vasopressin secretion occurs at a plasma osmolality of 280 mOsm/kg, although this can vary between 275 and 290 mOsm/kg based upon inter-individual genetic differences, other hormonal signals and volume status [18]. For example, during pregnancy or the luteal phase of the menstrual cycle, the osmotic threshold for vasopressin release and thirst are both decreased by 5–10 mOsm/kg (Fig. 15.4) [19]. Human chorionic gonadotropin elevation during pregnancy and alteration in luteinizing hormone (LH) secretion during the luteal phase may mediate these changes.

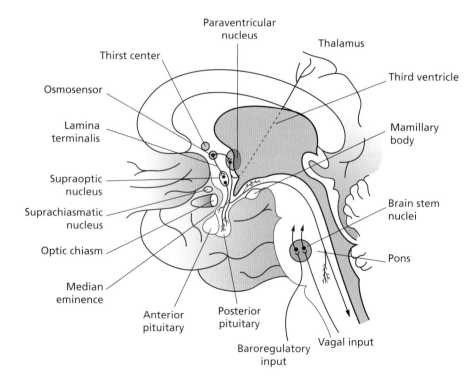

Figure 15.3 Anatomy of arginine vasopressin (AVP) producing cells in the hypothalamus and their projections to the posterior pituitary. AVP is produced by neurons in the supraoptic, paraventricular and suprachiasmatic nuclei. The magnocellular neurons located in the supraoptic and paraventricular nuclei send axonal projections to the posterior pituitary for secretion of vasopressin into the systemic circulation. (From Muglia & Majzoub [149] with permission.)

When serum osmolality falls below the osmotic threshold for vasopressin release, plasma vasopressin concentration falls below 1 pg/mL (0.92 pmol/L), the sensitivity limit of most radioimmunoassays [20,21]. This reduction signals the kidney to excrete free water and produce maximally diluted urine. The resultant loss of free water increases serum osmolality and limits further dilution of intracellular and extracellular fluids.

Once serum osmolality exceeds the threshold for vasopressin release, increasing plasma osmolality by 1% (i.e. approximately 2.8 mOsm/kg) increases plasma vasopressin by approximately

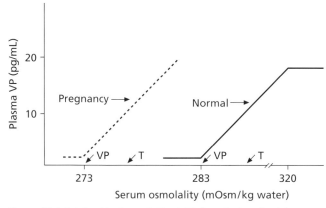

Figure 15.4 Relationship of osmotic thresholds for activation of arginine vasopressin (AVP) secretion and thirst. Note that the threshold for vasopressin release occurs at a lower osmolality than the osmolality required for the sensation of thirst. Under normal circumstances, plasma AVP increases linearly until an osmolality of approximately 320 mOsm/kg and then plateaus. In pregnancy, the set points for both vasopressin release and thirst are shifted such that induction occurs with similar sensitivity but at a lower threshold. Arrows on the x-axis indicate the threshold for AVP secretion (VP) or thirst sensation (T). (From Muglia & Majzoub [149] with permission.)

1 pg/mL (0.92 pmol/L), an amount sufficient to alter urine concentration and flow (Fig.15.5). Peak antidiuresis and production of a maximally concentrated urine occurs at a plasma vasopressin concentration of 5 pg/mL [20,21]. Osmotic stimulation linearly increases plasma vasopressin to as high as 20 pg/mL at a plasma osmolality of 320 mOsm/kg or above but this causes no further increase in urine concentration or decrease in urine volume.

Many solutes contribute to plasma osmolality but sodium and its anions constitute the majority and they modulate vasopressin release, as controlled by osmosensor neurons [22]. Increases in osmolality by sugars such as mannitol also augment vasopressin release through the osmosensors but not all solutes that contribute to plasma osmolality have the capacity to stimulate vasopressin release. Non-stimulatory solutes include glucose and urea in healthy individuals but hyperglycemia does stimulate vasopressin release in the context of insulin deficiency, which may exacerbate hyponatremia during treatment of diabetic ketoacidosis [23], although urine flow is maintained by osmotic diuresis as long as the kidneys are well-perfused. The mechanisms by which plasma solutes are differentially sensed by the osmoregulators have not yet been determined.

Non-osmotic regulation

In addition to plasma osmolality, other homeostatic and environmental factors influence vasopressin secretion. Of these, acute changes in intravascular volume and pressure are particularly important. Baroreceptors in the cardiac atria and aortic arch are activated by stretch resulting from normal blood volume and normal blood pressure, respectively, and signal to neurons within the brainstem nucleus tractus solitarius [24]. These neurons relay signals through the ventrolateral medulla to magnocellular neurons within the supraoptic and paraventricular nuclei and inhibit

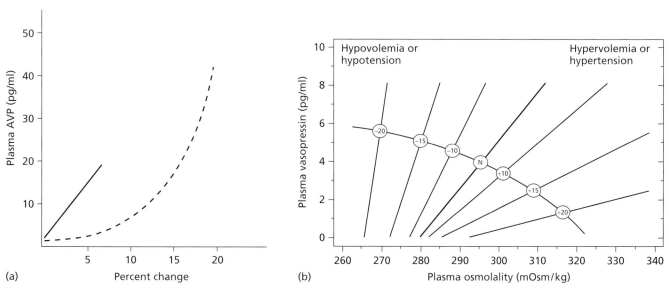

(a)   (b)

Figure 15.5 Interactions of osmolality and hemodynamic stimuli in the regulation of vasopressin secretion. (a) Plasma arginine vasopressin (AVP) concentration in relation to percentage increase in blood osmolality (solid line) or percentage decrease in blood volume (dashed line). (After Dunn *et al.* [150].) (b) Changes in hemodynamic status alter the sensitivity of AVP secretion into the plasma. Numbers in circles are % change in volume from normal. (From Robertson [151] with permission.)

vasopressin release. When blood pressure or volume decreases, inhibition of vasopressinergic neurons within the hypothalamus is diminished, resulting in augmented vasopressin release.

In contrast to the subtle changes in plasma osmolality that modulate vasopressin secretion, larger percentage decreases in intravascular volume (and even larger decreases in pressure) are needed to initiate vasopressin release. Vasopressin concentration does not increase until intravascular volume deficits exceed 8% (Fig. 15.5) [19,25]. When intravascular volume depletion exceeds this threshold, plasma vasopressin levels increase exponentially so that decreases in intravascular volume of 20–30% increase plasma vasopressin to levels far greater than those required for maximum antidiuresis and maximal levels seen with osmotic stimulation.

Osmotic and hemodynamic stimuli interact to enhance the vasopressin response generated by each independent stimulus (Fig. 15.5). For example, hypovolemia or hypotension lowers the threshold and increases the slope of the vasopressin release curve in response to osmotic signals [19]. Conversely, increased intravascular volume or hypervolemia dampens the vasopressin response to increases in plasma osmolality. This interaction suggests that the osmo- and baro-regulatory systems, although anatomically distinct, converge upon the same population of neurosecretory neurons [26].

Nausea strongly promotes vasopressin secretion [27] and resulting levels of vasopressin may exceed those associated with maximal osmotic stimulation. This is probably mediated by afferents from the area postrema of the brainstem, a key emetic center. Nicotine is also a strong stimulus for vasopressin release [28], as is 3,4-methylenedioxymethamphetamine (ecstasy) [29]. These signals probably do not directly involve osmosensors or baroreceptors, because pharmacological blockade of an emetic stimulus does not alter the vasopressin secretory response to increased plasma osmolality or hypotension.

Other non-osmotic stimuli for vasopressin release include physiological stressors, such as acute hypoglycemia, hypoxia and hypercapnia, as well as many drugs and hormones. Vasopressin secretion is inhibited by glucocorticoids. Thus, with glucocorticoid deficiency, loss of inhibition of vasopressin release may occur and contribute to hyponatremia [30,31].

Many drug effects on vasopressin secretion occur indirectly by providing hemodynamic or emetic stimuli. Psychological or physiological stress caused by pain, emotion, physical exercise or other deviations from homeostasis has long been thought to cause the release of vasopressin but this may be caused indirectly by other factors, such as the hypotension or nausea that often accompany vasovagal reactions [19].

Vasopression metabolism

Vasopressin has a half-life of 5–10 min in the circulation, being quickly degraded by vasopressinase, a cysteine aminoterminal peptidase. Because of its resistance to aminoterminal degradation, dDAVP has a much longer half-life of 8–24 h. Vasopressinase activity increases during pregnancy as it is synthesized and

secreted by the placenta [32]. Pregnant women compensate for the increased clearance of vasopressin by increasing its secretion. During pregnancy, women with subtle compensated impairment of vasopressin secretion or action [33], or those with increased concentrations of placental vasopressinase associated with liver dysfunction [34] or multiple gestations [35] may develop diabetes insipidus (DI), which resolves after delivery of the placenta [36]. This form of vasopressinase-dependent pregnancy-associated DI responds well to treatment with dDAVP but not with vasopressin.

Biological action of vasopressin

The crucial action of vasopressin in regulation of plasma osmolality or intravascular volume in cases of moderate to severe water or volume depletion is to limit the further loss of water. It does so by increasing the permeability of the distal nephron to luminal water, thereby increasing reabsorption of free water and reducing urine output. To achieve this antidiuretic effect, vasopressin acts upon receptors on the serosal surface of the distal and collecting renal tubules (Fig. 15.6). Three subtypes of vasopressin receptors have been identified, designated V_{1a}, V_{1b} (also called V_3) and V_2 [37]. Each arises from a different gene coding for a member of the seven-transmembrane G-protein coupled receptor family [38].

The V_2 receptor in the kidney accounts for the antidiuretic effects of vasopressin. The small 2-kb three exon gene (*AVPR2*)

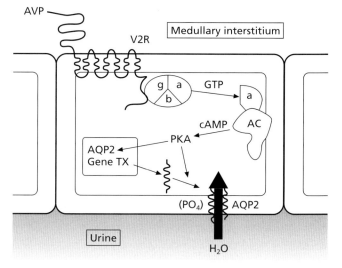

Figure 15.6 Renal actions of vasopressin. In the collecting duct epithelium, vasopressin binding to the V_2 receptor results in Gα-mediated activation of cyclic adenosine monophosphate (cAMP) production from adenylyl cyclases. The elevation in intracellular cAMP causes activation of protein kinase A (PKA), which then phosphorylates aquaporin-2 (AQP-2) at serine 256. This phosphorylation event promotes aggregation of AQP-2 homotetramers in subapical membrane vesicles and their fusion with the apical plasma membrane. The insertion of the water channels into the luminal membrane allows the flow of water from the urine within the duct lumen into the hypertonic medullary interstitium, decreasing free water clearance. (From Muglia & Majzoub [149] with permission.)

encoding the V_2 receptor maps to the distal long arm of the X chromosome (Xq28) and mutations in the gene result in X-linked NDI (Fig. 15.7a) [39]. The V_2 receptor signals by coupling to adenyl cyclase through $G_{\alpha s}$ to increase intracellular cyclic adenosine monophosphate (cAMP) concentration. In addition to the distal nephron, V_2 receptors are located in the thick ascending limb of Henle's loop and periglomerular tubules [4,41].

V_2 receptors are also found on vascular endothelial cells, where activation promotes vasodilatation [41], and on hepatocytes where activation promotes release of von Willebrand factor, factor VIIIa and tissue plasminogen activator. The prothrombotic actions of vasopressin, and specifically dDAVP, have been used to treat bleeding disorders associated with von Willebrand disease and hemophilia.

Vasopressin acting on V_{1a} receptors mediates extrarenal effects, including contraction of vascular smooth muscle, stimulation of hepatic glycogenolysis and aggregation of platelets [42]. V_{1b} (also known as V_3) receptors are primarily located on ACTH-producing corticotrophs in the anterior pituitary [43], where activation by vasopressin from parvocellular hypothalamic neurons increases ACTH release during acute and chronic stress. In addition, V_{1b} receptors in the brain may mediate behavioral actions of vasopressin [44]. In contrast to V_2, neither V_{1a} nor V_{1b} couples to $G_{\alpha s}$ to cause induction of cAMP production. Instead, both couple to phospholipase C with modulation of intracellular calcium and phosphatidylinositol signaling pathways. The substitution of the D-Arg into vasopressin makes dDAVP specific for V_2 receptors only.

In an adult, approximately 20% of the cardiac output enters the renal arteries as the renal blood flow (1.25 L/min) and 10%

of that volume becomes the renal ultrafiltrate (125 mL/min). Approximately 10% of that volume remains after passage through the proximal tubule, the loop of Henle and the distal tubule (12.5 mL/min). In the absence of vasopressin, the luminal surface of the epithelial cells that line the collecting duct (called principal cells) is largely impermeable to water and solutes. The 12.5 mL/min of dilute tubular fluid traversing from the more proximal nephron passes through the collecting duct without additional concentration and urine is maximally dilute (osmolality <100 mOsm/kg) with a relatively high rate of urine flow (up to 18 L/day).

In the presence of vasopressin, V_2 receptors are activated and cAMP is generated in the principal cells. This stimulates phosphorylation by cAMP-dependent protein kinase A, which subsequently results in remodeling of cytoskeletal components and the exocytic insertion of preformed subapical vesicular water channels, aquaporin-2, into the apical membrane [45]. The insertion of these water channels results in a large increase in water permeability of the luminal epithelial membrane (up to 100-fold), allowing diffusion of water along its osmotic gradient from the lumen of the tubule into the hypertonic inner medullary interstitium. This net movement of water in excess of solute allows return of free water to the systemic circulation, reduction in urine volume and excretion of concentrated urine.

The water channels themselves belong to a family of related proteins, the aquaporins, which differ in their sites of expression and pattern of regulation. The aquaporins consist of a single polypeptide chain with six membrane-spanning domains thought to function as homotetramers in the plasma membrane [46]. Aquaporin-2 (AQP-2) comprises the specifically vasopressin-

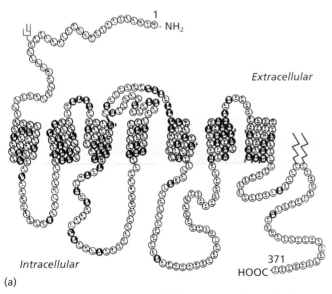

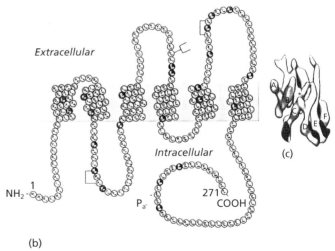

Figure 15.7 The arginine vasopressin (AVP) V_2 receptor and aquaporin-2 (AQP-2). (a) Schematic representation of the seven transmembrane V_2 receptor. The locations of known missense or nonsense mutations are indicated by solid circles. A number accompanying a solid circle indicates that there is more then one known mutation in that codon. (b) Schematic representation of the AQP-2 protein. A monomer has six transmembrane helices. The location of the protein kinase A phosphorylation site (Pa) is indicated. Solid symbols indicate the location of known mutations. (c) Three-dimensional representation of the six-helix barrel of aquaporin-2, viewed parallel to the bilayer. (From Bonnardeaux & Bichet [104] with permission.)

regulated water channel in the kidney, its predominant site of expression. At this site, V_2 receptor-mediated protein kinase A activation results in phosphorylation of serine 256 in AQP-2, an event required for trafficking to the apical membrane [47]. More prolonged stimulation by vasopressin increases the production of aquaporin-2 which, over the course of several hours, further enhances urinary concentrating capacity [48]. The gene that encodes AQP-2 in humans has been localized to chromosome 12q13 and has been found to be mutated in patients with autosomal recessive NDI (Fig. 15.7b,c) [49].

Aquaporins-1, -3 and -4 are also expressed in the kidney but have a less prominent and vasopressin-independent role in water balance. Aquaporins-3 and -4 are expressed on the basolateral, rather than the apical, surface of the collecting duct epithelium. In genetically altered animal models, mutations of aquaporin-3 or -4 result in mild defects in urinary concentrating ability [50,51]. Aquaporin-1 is expressed in the proximal tubule. Defects in aquaporin-1 function result in increased delivery of free water to the distal nephron and impaired urine-concentrating ability in mice [52] but humans missing this protein are normal [53].

The dose–response analyses of vasopressin and urine concentration, while variable in adult subjects, have shown that an increase in plasma vasopressin of 0.5 pg/mL (0.45 pmol/L) raises urine osmolality by approximately 150–250 mOsm/kg [19]. Maximum urinary concentration results when plasma vasopressin concentration reaches 5 pg/mL (4.5 pmol/L). Vasopressin may also have a role in limiting insensible water loss from the skin and lungs but this effect is small and easily overcome by changes in environmental conditions such as temperature and humidity, as well as exercise.

Thirst and regulation of water intake

Thirst, the conscious sensation of the need to drink, is the essential mechanism by which water losses are replaced. Thirst is regulated by many of the same physiological factors that regulate vasopressin release, of which plasma osmolality is the most potent [54]. Osmotic regulation of thirst occurs by osmosensors in the anterior hypothalamus and includes modulatory activity by neurons in the ventromedial nucleus of the hypothalamus [55]. Stimulation of thirst is also mediated by angiotensin II sensed in the subformical organ, outside of the blood–brain barrier [56]. While lesion studies of the anteroventral third ventricle suggest anatomic proximity of osmosensors controlling thirst and vasopressin release, the sensors controlling vasopressin release and thirst are not likely to be identical [57].

The set point for thirst is at a plasma osmolality that is 10 mOsm/kg higher than the threshold for secretion of vasopressin. This difference allows physiologic regulation of plasma osmolality between these two thresholds. If the plasma osmolality drops below the lower threshold, vasopressin will not be released and free water will be excreted to raise plasma osmolality. If the plasma osmolality rises above the upper threshold, thirst will be activated and drinking will decrease the plasma osmolality. The graded release of vasopressin between the two thresholds (progressively decreasing urine output as osmolality rises from the vasopressin threshold to the thirst threshold) allows for regulation of osmolality without constant access to water.

If the set points for vasopressin release and thirst were identical or offset in the opposite direction, thirst would be activated before significant vasopressin release, the ingested fluid would not be retained and a sustained polyuric and polydipsic state would ensue. Even before plasma osmolality changes significantly, drinking water causes vasopressin secretion to diminish and thirst to abate. This negative feedback protects against excessive ingestion and overhydration and is thought to arise from chemoreceptors that respond to both the volume and the temperature of the fluid ingested [58]. Humans, rats and rabbits meter drinking to replace half of their water deficit and then drink again 20 min later. Camels, dogs and sheep meter drinking to replace their entire water deficit at once.

Hypovolemia and hypotension increase thirst. The magnitude of intravascular depletion or hypotension needed to stimulate thirst has not been defined in humans but is probably larger than that associated with vasopressin release. Similar to the consequences for vasopressin secretion, volume and blood pressure changes alter the threshold set point and gain for thirst [59].

Fluid intake often occurs for reasons other than thirst. These include social cues of others drinking, pleasurable taste or other effects of an ingested beverage, hunger or dry mouth resulting from factors independent of hydration such as anxiety or medication. When water intake exceeds homeostatic requirements, plasma vasopressin decreases to undetectable concentrations, allowing excretion of the extra water. Thirst and vasopressin efficiently maintain plasma tonicity in the appropriate range under normal circumstances.

With defects in either thirst or urine concentrating ability, plasma tonicity can still be maintained within the normal range. Thus, a patient with inability to concentrate their urine because of a deficiency in vasopressin release or action usually has a normal random plasma osmolality if the patient has adequate access to water because an intact thirst mechanism stimulates water ingestion up to 10 L/m^2/day. Similarly, normal vasopressin regulation can mask mild to moderate impairment of thirst, preventing dehydration by avidly retaining water but, when centers controlling both thirst and vasopressin secretion are disrupted simultaneously, the occurrence of potentially life-threatening dysregulation of plasma osmolality and intravascular volume is high.

Volume and pressure sensors and effector pathways
Renin-angiotensin-aldosterone system

The renin-angiotensin system is the primary system to regulate intravascular volume to maintain euvolemia [60]. Renin, a proteolytic enzyme that catalyzes the cleavage of circulating angiotensinogen from the liver, is synthesized in the renal juxtaglomerular cells and released into the circulation in response to a number of stimuli associated with hypovolemia. These include decreased renal arteriolar pressure, decreased intratubular fluid sodium concentration and increased renal sympathetic nerve activation.

The proteolytic action of renin releases the decapeptide angiotensin I from angiotensinogen. Inactive angiotensin I serves as a substrate for angiotensin-converting enzyme in the lungs and other peripheral sites to generate the biologically active octapeptide angiotensin II that can be further metabolized to angiotensin III. The effects of angiotensin II include vascular smooth muscle contraction and blood pressure elevation and both angiotensin II and III stimulate aldosterone release from the zona glomerulosa of the adrenal.

Aldosterone increases sodium reabsorption and potassium excretion in the distal renal tubule by augmenting the production of sodium channels trafficked to the apical plasma membrane, mitochondrial ATP synthesis and production of subunits of the Na^+, K^+-ATPase [61]. In addition to stimulating aldosterone-mediated sodium reabsorption, angiotensin II stimulates sodium–hydrogen exchange and bicarbonate reabsorption in the proximal tubule. Both these increases in active sodium transport increase water absorption, thereby supporting intravascular volume expansion.

In addition to intravascular volume status, aldosterone release from the adrenal zona glomerulosa is stimulated directly by elevated plasma potassium concentration [60]. Acute increases in plasma levels of ACTH or vasopressin have the capacity transiently to stimulate aldosterone secretion but chronic administration of either does not result in sustained increases. Aldosterone release is inhibited by atrial natriuretic peptide, somatostatin and dopamine [62,63].

Angiotensin II is also sensed in the subfornical organ in the brain and stimulates drinking and salt-seeking, providing another avenue for the renin-angiotensin system to augment intravascular volume [64].

The natriuretic peptide system

The natriuretic peptides [atrial natriuretic peptide (ANP), brain natriuretic peptide (BNP) and C-type natriuretic peptide (CNP)] contribute to salt and water balance by promoting renal salt excretion and altering vasopressin secretion from the hypothalamus [65]. These structurally related peptides of 28, 22 and 32 amino acids, respectively, each contain a 17-member ring formed by an intramolecular disulfide bond and are produced from much larger precursor peptides(Fig. 15.8). The natriuretic peptides interact with different receptors [66]. Two of them, NPR-A and NPR-B, possess guanyl cyclase activity. NPR-A binds both ANP and BNP with high affinity, while NPR-B binds CNP with much higher affinity than either ANP or BNP. The third receptor, NPR-C, is membrane-bound but is not a guanyl cyclase and clears all three ligands from the circulation [67].

The natriuretic effects of ANP were the first to be elucidated [68]. ANP synthesis occurs in both the left and the right atria in response to increasing wall pressure and increased heart rate. Secretion into the circulation is modulated in a volume-

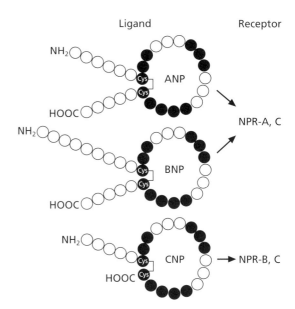

Figure 15.8 Structure of the natriuretic peptides and their receptor specificity. Atrial natriuretic peptide (ANP), brain natriuretic peptide (BNP) and C-type natriuretic peptide (CNP) each consist of a 17-member ring structure closed by a disulfide bond between cysteine residues, along with amino- and carboxy-terminal tails of variable length. Conserved amino acids are indicated by the filled circles. Each family member binds the NPR-C clearance receptor, while ANP and BNP exert their effects through binding NPR-A and CNP activates NPR-B.

dependent manner. ANP released into the peripheral circulation produces sodium excretion and some diuresis. It inhibits sodium reabsorption in the medullary collecting duct, impairs the salt-retaining actions of angiotensin II on the proximal tubule and partially antagonizes the water retention effects of vasopressin [69]. In addition, ANP inhibits aldosterone synthesis by inhibiting actions of aldosterone secretagogues, particularly the action of angiotensin II. ANP reduces plasma renin activity, which reduces the generation of angiotensin II, further diminishing aldosterone secretion and renal salt reabsorption. ANP is also produced within the brain at sites with potential for neuroendocrine regulation in the periventricular, arcuate, anteroventral preoptic and lateral hypothalamic nuclei [70].

BNP was first isolated from porcine brain [71] but it is secreted from both atria and ventricles, with production augmented in congestive heart failure and hypertension; it causes renal and adrenal effects similar to ANP [69]. The brain is the primary site of CNP production and CNP expression overlaps with ANP expression in the hypothalamus [72]. Little CNP is present in plasma normally or in response to volume overload.

Disorders of water balance
Vasopressin deficiency
Deficiencies in vasopressin secretion or action result in polyuria, characterized by chronic excretion of abnormally large volumes of dilute urine (exceeding 2 L/m^2/day) and consequent polydipsia. Vasopressin-deficient or -resistant polyuria and polydipsia

are known as diabetes insipidus. The signs and symptoms of DI are primarily urinary frequency with high urine output, nocturia in older children and adults and persistent enuresis or delayed toilet training in younger children. These symptoms are accompanied by thirst and increased fluid intake throughout the day and night. Children with untreated DI typically crave cold fluids, especially water.

Polyuria and polydipsia caused by pathological reduction of vasopressin secretion (central DI) or action (nephrogenic DI) can result in hypernatremia if access to water is restricted or the thirst mechanism is impaired. DI should be differentiated from other causes of urinary frequency. These include a reduced bladder capacity or bladder irritation, in which fluid intake and the 24-h urine volume are normal, and diabetes mellitus (DM) or other forms of solute diuresis, in which fluid intake and urine output is increased, or conditions of increased water intake (dipsogenic polydipsia or psychogenic polydipsia).

Diagnostic approach to DI

Patients presenting with polyuria and polydipsia should have urine tested for glycosuria to exclude DM. When the possibility of DI is being considered, fluid intake and output should be established to determine whether polyuria (urine output >2 L/ m^2/day) is indeed present. If possible, an intake–output record should be kept at home to determine the volume of urine in 24 h. If the child is not toilet trained or has a condition that makes it difficult to collect urine, the measurement of fluid intake or weighing diapers are possible alternatives. After an overnight fast, the first morning urine is ordinarily concentrated because of insensible fluid loss and urine production overnight. A morning urine with specific gravity <1.005 suggests the possibility of DI and >1.010 makes it unlikely.

The answers to specific questions can be helpful:
• Does the need to drink and urinate interfere with normal activities?
• Is nocturia or enuresis present?
• Does the patient need to drink at night?
• Is there a psychological or psychiatric component to the need to drink?
• What is the preferred drink?
• What is the color of the patient's urine?
• Does the history (including longitudinal growth) suggest other deficient or excessive pituitary hormone secretion?
• Was the onset sudden or gradual?
• Are there symptoms suggestive of a CNS mass?
• Is there bone pain or skin rash?
• Is the child taking medication that could result in vasopressin resistance?

If pathological polyuria or polydipsia appears to be present, serum osmolality and concentrations of sodium, potassium, glucose, calcium and urea and urinary osmolality, specific gravity and glucose should be measured, either as an outpatient or as the first step in a water deprivation test. A urine osmolality >600 mOsm/kg excludes DI and DI is also unlikely if the serum osmolality and sodium are low or low-normal. Serum sodium >145 mmol/L or serum osmolality >300 mOsm/kg with urine osmolality <600 mOsm/kg confirms the diagnosis of DI and a water deprivation test is not necessary and potentially dangerous.

Because measurement of serum osmolality is often not as accurate as that of serum sodium, interpretation of a single elevated serum osmolality should be made with caution if it is not accompanied by a concordant change in serum sodium. As intact thirst results in compensatory fluid intake, the majority of patients with DI have serum sodium and osmolality in the normal range. Therefore, most patients with dilute urine and intake–output records at home suggesting significant polyuria and polydipsia need a formal water deprivation test to establish a diagnosis of DI and then to differentiate central from nephrogenic causes.

A water deprivation test is used to determine if excessive urine output will allow the serum sodium and osmolality to rise to abnormally high values in the absence of drinking. The test should be performed either at an outpatient site appropriate for 8–10 h of close observation and assessment or as an inpatient. Because patients with DI can become dehydrated in a few hours, it is not appropriate to begin fluid restriction before the patient arrives for the test unless the clinical history suggests that the child can comfortably go for an extended period of time without drinking. In that case, the child can be fluid restricted for that length of time before the test begins.

During the test, the environment must be controlled to avoid surreptitious water intake because the intense drive to drink can lead to fluid intake from unusual sources including the toilet. Physical signs and biochemical parameters are measured hourly (Fig. 15.9). As measurement of serum osmolality is relatively imprecise, serum sodium is often more reliable than osmolality during water deprivation. The laboratory should be aware of the need for prompt assessment of the specimens.

A common recommendation is to stop the test when a 5% loss of body weight is recorded, but this may result in the test being stopped before a diagnosis can be made. Unless vital signs or other symptoms suggest hypovolemia, the patient should be monitored and the test can proceed until diagnostic results are obtained.

Diagnosis of DI is made only when the serum osmolality has risen to an abnormally high value (>300 mOsm/kg, sodium >145 mmol/L) and the urine is not appropriately concentrated (<600 mOsm/kg). If possible, the test should be continued for an additional hour to perform a confirmatory set of measurements to avoid making a diagnosis based on a single set of laboratory values. If the serum osmolality plateaus at a normal value (<300 mOsm/kg), with an increasing urine osmolality (>600 mOsm/kg) and decreasing hourly urine volume, the patient does not have DI but may have dipsogenic or psychogenic polydipsia.

Once a diagnosis of DI is made, differentiation of central from nephrogenic DI requires measurement of plasma vasopressin and the renal response to exogenous vasopressin. In the hyperna-

Time	Serum	Urine			BP	Weight
(min)	Sodium (Osm)	Sodium Osm	Volume/hr			
−30						
0						
60						
120						
180						
240						
300						
360						
420						
480						
Aqueous AVP administration						
0						
30						
60						

If serum osm <300 (Na <145 and urine osm <600) continue the test unless vital signs suggest hyovolemia

If urine osm >1000 or >600 and stable over two time points, stop test. Normal

If serum osm >300 and urine osm <600 and stable over two time points, stop test. DI. Give vasopressin 1 unit/m² sub cu and measure response over following hour. OK to drink modestly.

Figure 15.9 Flow sheet for water deprivation testing for diagnosis of diabetes insipidus.

tremic state at the end of a water deprivation test, vasopressin concentration will be appropriately elevated in nephrogenic DI but the kidneys will not be able to respond. In central DI (CDI), vasopressin will be inappropriately low [73].

The response to exogenous vasopressin can also be tested to determine whether the urine output decreases appropriately (CDI) or whether the dilute urine production continues (nephrogenic DI). This is frequently carried out immediately following the water deprivation test but can be performed independently. Aqueous vasopressin (5 unit/m²) is administered subcutaneously and fluid restriction should be stopped because continued restriction in a child with NDI will result in progressive dehydration.

dDAVP (1 µg/m² subcutaneously) can also be used for this test but is potent and long lasting, so giving dDAVP to a patient who actually has psychogenic or primary polydipsia or giving a large dose of dDAVP to an infant taking liquid nutrition can lead to water intoxication [74].

No rise in urine osmolality in the subsequent hour is consistent with complete nephrogenic DI. A doubling of urine osmolality and a decrease in urine volume in the hour following vasopressin administration suggests CDI with a normal renal response to vasopressin. The rise in osmolality will be intermediate in partial central and partial nephrogenic DI. If partial nephrogenic DI is suspected, a standard dose of dDAVP may not decrease urine output but a subsequent larger subcutaneous test dose of 10 µg/m² may be sufficient to activate a V₂ receptor with decreased activity or affinity for vasopressin. A positive response could suggest an unconventional treatment of this form of nephrogenic DI with high dose dDAVP. Patients with long-standing primary polydipsia may appear to have mild nephrogenic DI as of dilution of their renal medullary interstitium.

An alternative to a water deprivation test that is rarely used in children is to induce hypernatremia with a 3% saline infusion at 0.1 mL/kg/min for up to 2 h, measuring urine and serum sodium and osmolality every 30 min until serum osmolality is >290 mOsm/kg and sodium >145 mmol/L which should induce vasopressin release and urinary concentration. If not, this diagnoses DI and the vasopressin level and response to vasopressin or dDAVP can be assessed.

Central diabetes insipidus
The most common form of DI results from deficiency of vasopressin secretion. CDI (neurogenic, pituitary, hypothalamic, neurohypophyseal, cranial or vasopressin-responsive) results when pituitary vasopressin production is reduced. Losses up to 90% of

normal vasopressin secretion can occur without overt clinical manifestations in otherwise well individuals. Further loss of vasopressin secretion results in onset of polyuria and polydipsia so the onset of symptoms is generally perceived to be sudden and patients or their families often identify a discrete time. Once symptoms develop, the degree of polyuria and polydipsia depends on the severity of vasopressin deficiency and on other factors, such as the integrity of thirst, renal function, dietary salt load and normality of other endocrine systems. Urinary losses up to 400 mL/m^2/h can occur. CDI responds well to vasopressin replacement therapy with vasopressin or more typically its longer-acting analog, dDAVP.

Causes of central diabetes insipidus

Genetic causes

The inherited forms of CDI account for less than 10% of cases of DI (Table 15.2).

Autosomal dominant neurohypophyseal DI. The most frequent inherited form of DI, is caused by mutations in the vasopressin-NPII gene and more than 40 mutations have been described. The majority are in the neurophysin coding region or in the signal peptide and are presumed to impair processing, folding or dimerization. Symptoms appear at several years of age. Vasopressin secretion is normal initially and declines gradually until DI of variable severity supervenes [75].

Cell culture and animal studies have shown that the mutant proteins are trapped in the endoplasmic reticulum (ER) and high-level expression of mutant protein results in abnormal ER morphology and increased cell death [76]. Autopsy studies reveal a markedly subnormal number of vasopressin-producing magnocellular neurons in the supraoptic and paraventricular nuclei of the hypothalamus, associated with moderate gliosis [77]. These findings are consistent with degeneration of these neurons and suggest that accumulation of the abnormal vasopressin prohormone in the ER causes neuronal degeneration and cell death. Neurotoxicity with degeneration of the magnocellular neurons due to accumulation of abnormal prohormone would explain both the autosomal dominant inheritance and the delayed onset of DI.

A single mutation in the *AVP-NPII* gene produces *autosomal-recessive neurohypophyseal DI* [78]. A missense mutation at nucleotide 301 changes the proline at position 7 of vasopressin to a leucine. The mutant hormone is a weak agonist for the V$_2$ receptor, with approximately 30-fold reduced binding affinity. Affected sibs were asymptomatic for the first 1–2 years of life, presumably as increased secretion of the mutant hormone is able to compensate for its decreased activity in early life. There is evidence that the mutation does not alter ER handling of the precursor but may impair final processing and limit the amount that can be secreted [79].

Vasopressin deficiency is part of Wolfram syndrome, a rare progressive neurodegenerative condition also known as DIDMOAD (*d*iabetes *i*nsipidus, *d*iabetes *m*ellitus, *o*ptic *a*trophy and *d*eafness) [80]. The minimal features required for diagnosis

Table 15.2 Causes of central diabetes insipidus.

Genetic
AVP-NPII gene:
  Autosomal dominant
  Autosomal recessive
Wolfram syndrome

Congenital
Septo-optic dysplasia
Midline craniofacial defects
Holoprosencephalic syndromes
Agenesis of the pituitary

Acquired
Neoplasms:
  Craniopharyngioma
  Germinoma
  Pinealoma
  Leukemia/lymphoma
Inflammatory/infiltrative:
  Langerhans cell histiocytosis
  Systemic lupus erythematosus
  Neurosarcoidosis
  Lymphocytic neurohypophysitis
Infectious:
  Meningitis
  Encephalitis
  Congenital infection
Traumatic injury:
  CNS surgery
  Head trauma
  Hypoxic injury

Idiopathic

are juvenile-onset insulin-dependent diabetes and optic atrophy. CDI, sensorineural deafness, urinary tract atony, ataxia, peripheral neuropathy, mental retardation and psychiatric illness develop in the majority of patients. Onset of DI is usually in the second decade. The condition is probably genetically heterogeneous because it is associated with autosomal recessive mutations in the *WFS1* gene on chromosome 4p16.1 [81], autosomal recessive mutations in the *CIDS2* gene on 4q22-24 (82) and deletions in mitochondrial DNA [83].

There is some evidence that *WFS1* mutations may cause the mitochondrial deletions [84]. *WFS1* codes for an 890 amino acid transmembrane protein, wolframin, that is ubiquitously expressed and predominantly localized to the ER. *CIDS2* encodes ERIS (endoplasmic reticulum intermembrane small protein) that also localizes to the ER [82]. Dominant mutations in *WFS1* cause low-frequency hearing loss and have been associated with isolated diabetes mellitus and isolated psychiatric disease.

Congenital intracranial midline anatomic defects are associated with CDI and estimated to account for 5–10% of pediatric cases.

DI may become apparent in the first weeks of life but diagnosis may be delayed. The most frequent defect is septo-optic dysplasia (SOD, de Morsier syndrome) characterized by hypoplasia of the optic nerves with other midline cerebral anomalies (agenesis of the corpus callosum), schizencephaly and pituitary hormone deficiencies. Mutations in the homeobox gene *Hesx1* have been associated with SOD in less than 1% of cases [85,86].

Other anomalies associated with CDI include nasal encephalocele, porencephaly, holoprosencephaly, hydrocephalus and hydranencephaly. MRI evaluation generally reveals an absent posterior pituitary bright spot, in addition to the accompanying CNS lesions. Visible midline craniofacial defects associated with congenital CDI include single central incisor, cleft lip or palate, high arch palate, micrognathia, synophrys, hypoteleorism, flat nasal bridge or other midface hypoplasia but many children with congenital CDI have no external evidence of midline abnormalities. Deficiencies of anterior pituitary hormones and defects in thirst perception are not uncommon. In patients who have cortisol deficiency, symptoms of DI may be masked as cortisol deficiency impairs renal free water clearance. In such cases, glucocorticoid therapy may unmask vasopressin deficiency and precipitate polyuria.

Acquired CDI
Non-familial acquired DI accounts for the majority of CDI.

Tumor. Brain tumours and those who develop DI following surgery account for up to 50% of acquired DI. Tumors account for 10–15% of acquired DI in children and include germinoma, astrocytoma, pinealoma, CNS lymphoma, glioma and craniopharyngioma. Although craniopharyngioma infrequently causes DI before surgery, the majority of children develop DI following resection and craniopharyngiomas ultimately account for the majority of tumor-associated CDI in children.

Because hypothalamic vasopressin neurons are distributed over a large area within the hypothalamus, tumors that cause DI must be large, infiltrative or located at the point of convergence of the hypothalamo-neurohypophyseal axonal tract in the infundibulum. As germinomas and pinealomas typically arise near the base of the hypothalamus, where vasopressin axons converge as they enter the posterior pituitary, they are the tumors most commonly associated with DI at diagnosis. Germinomas can be small and undetectable by MRI for several years following the onset of DI [87]. The β-subunit of human chorionic gonadotropin and alpha-fetoprotein are often secreted by germinomas and pinealomas and repeated measurements and MRI scans should be performed in children with idiopathic or unexplained DI. Tumor-associated DI is rare before 5 years of age [88].

Neurosurgical intervention. Surgery is one of the most common causes of CDI. In the postoperative period, it is important to be aware of the risk of DI and to distinguish polyuria associated with DI from polyuria due to the normal diuresis of fluids given during surgery and polyuria associated with cerebral salt-wasting. In both DI and normal diuresis, the urine may be very dilute and of high volume but, with postoperative diuresis, serum sodium and osmolality will be normal, whereas they will be high in DI if the patient does not have free access to water.

In cerebral salt-wasting, urine volumes are also high but urinary sodium concentrations are high and serum osmolality and sodium are low. Postoperative DI is characterized by an abrupt onset of polyuria, usually within the first 12–24 h. This phase is often transient, resolving spontaneously in 1–2 days, and thought to be caused either by acute injury to the neurohypophysis with inhibition of vasopressin secretion or release of biologically inactive vasopressin-like peptide hormones from the damaged hypothalamo-neurohypophyseal system that interfere with the binding of vasopressin to the V_2 receptor [89].

Not infrequently, a "triple-phase" response is seen. Following the initial DI, the syndrome of inappropriate ADH secretion (SIADH) is seen, typically starting in 4–5 days and lasting for 10 days resulting from the unregulated release of vasopressin from dying neurons. A third phase of permanent DI follows if sufficient numbers of vasopressin-producing cells were destroyed. Although cranial irradiation is associated with the development of anterior pituitary hormone deficiencies, it is not associated with DI.

Infections. Infections involving the base of the brain, such as meningococcus, group B streptococci, *Haemophilus influenzae*, *Streptococcus pneumoniae*, cryptococcal and listeria meningitides, congenital cytomegalovirus, tuberculoma or toxoplasmosis can cause CDI, which may be transient or permanent. When permanent, DI is often combined with anterior pituitary endocrinopathies.

Langerhans cell histiocytosis (LCH). The most common infiltrative disorder causing CDI, this may be responsible for up to 10% of acquired cases. LCH is generally considered a disease of childhood, although the diagnosis is also made in adults. It is characterized by a clonal proliferation of abnormal dendritic histiocytes (Langerhans cells) with an accompanying infiltration of lymphocytes, eosinophils and neutrophils. It can involve many body organ systems or tissues and often targets the posterior hypothalamo-pituitary region.

Ten percent of patients with LCH have DI at presentation and another 10% develop DI over time [90,91]. A minority has concurrent anterior hormone deficiencies, which can develop many years after the onset of DI but rarely without it. DI associated with LCH is almost always a multisystem disease, with lesions in bone (68%), skin (57%), lung (39%) and lymph nodes (18%) [92]. X-ray evaluation for skeletal lesions and clinical symptoms of multisystem disease should be sought when LCH is considered in a differential diagnosis. Thickening of the pituitary stalk may be seen on cranial MRI but the pituitary stalk can also appear normal. DI can also be associated with sarcoid but neurological manifestations of sarcoid are rare in children [93].

Trauma. Trauma to the base of the brain can cause swelling around or severance of the magnocellular neurons, resulting in transient or permanent DI, even after seemingly minor trauma. As in CNS surgery, the DI associated with trauma may develop rapidly after the injury and can be transient or permanent. Occasionally, onset can be delayed as the magnocellular neurons degenerate.

Autoimmune DI. Autoantibodies to vasopressin-secreting cells are present in more than half of adults less than 30 years of age presenting with idiopathic DI and are much more common in individuals with a history of prior autoimmune disease or pituitary stalk thickening [94]. Based on the presence of these antibodies, it has been suggested that autoimmune lymphocytic neurohypophysitis may account for a significant proportion of patients with idiopathic DI but 16% of patients with non-idiopathic CDI also have antibodies. It is possible that antibodies directed against vasopressin-containing cells are not pathogenic but are markers of previous neuronal cell destruction. Patients with other autoimmune diseases may have vasopressin-secreting cell antibodies without evidence of DI [95]. Biopsy-proven lymphatic hypophysitis or infundibulo-neurohypophysitis with associated DI has been reported infrequently in children, so the magnitude of its contribution to acquired childhood DI is unknown.

Hypoxic injury. Brain damage caused by carbon monoxide poisoning, smoke inhalation, respiratory failure, cardiopulmonary arrest, septic shock and sudden infant death syndrome may cause CDI. The interval between the insult and development of DI ranges from a few hours to many days. As the neurohypophyseal system has a bilateral blood supply and is relatively resistant to hypoxic injury, the appearance of DI following hypoxic injury is ominous and generally indicative of widespread neurological damage. DI is present in approximately 40% of children with brain death and CDI should be considered in the differential diagnosis of polyuria occurring in any patient who has suffered hypoxic injury.

Idiopathic DI. The remaining 12–20% of cases of DI are idiopathic. MRI may be normal or the pituitary stalk may be thickened. Thickening is observed in approximately one-third of children with CDI. Some of these have a cause for their DI at presentation, most often LCH but the majority have idiopathic DI. Patients with idiopathic DI and thickening of the pituitary stalk appear to be more likely to have or to develop anterior pituitary hormone deficiencies but all patients should have anterior pituitary function tests at presentation and during follow-up. Patients with or without thickening of the pituitary stalk should be followed with repeated MRI, as DI is the most common initial presentation of germinoma and may occur before radiographic evidence of the tumor is present. Evidence of a tumor is usually within 2.5 years after diagnosis and 1.3 years after thickening of the pituitary stalk is noted on MRI.

Concomitant gonadotropin deficiency is a marker for a structural lesion underlying DI [96].

Treatment of central DI

Once CDI has been diagnosed, management requires a search for a cause. In 80–90% of healthy children and adults, the posterior pituitary emits a hyperintense signal ("bright spot") on T1-weighted non-infused mid-sagittal images (Fig. 15.10). The posterior pituitary bright spot is absent in more than 90% of children with CDI at the time of diagnosis. This is not diagnostic of CDI as the bright spot is also absent in NDI, presumably because of increased release of vasopressin. The bright spot is notably normal in primary polydipsia. If initial studies do not reveal the etiology, repeat MRI at 6-month intervals is recommended for 2 years. Imaging frequency can then be decreased to yearly if the pituitary is stable or stalk thickening is present but improving. Anterior pituitary function should also be evaluated. In some cases, a lumbar puncture may be needed to identify a germinoma as cerebrospinal fluid (CSF), α-fetoprotein or human chorionic gonadotropin concentrations may be elevated in the absence of an elevation in serum levels.

Treatment of CDI is usually lifelong as recovery from a deficiency lasting more than a week is uncommon, even if the underlying cause is eliminated. With intact thirst and free access to water, an individual with DI will drink sufficiently to maintain normal serum osmolality and high-normal serum sodium. To relieve symptoms, the treatment of choice is administration of dDAVP (desmopressin) (Fig. 15.2). dDAVP (4 μg/mL) is available for subcutaneous injection in doses from 0.1 to 1 μg once or twice per day. dDAVP as a nasal solution (10 μg/0.1 mL) can be delivered in increments of 2.5 μg by tube or by 10-μg increments as spray in the same concentration. It is approximately 10-fold less potent than the injected form. Oral dDAVP is available as 0.1 or 0.2 mg tablets and is slower in onset of action and approximately 20-fold less potent than when given via the intranasal route (200-fold less potent than injection).

Treatment should begin with the lowest amount that gives the desired antidiuretic effect. Dosing can be once or twice per day and patients with intact thirst should be allowed to escape from the antidiuretic effect briefly at least once a day to allow excessive water to be excreted and reduce the risk of water intoxication. The antidiuretic effect of dDAVP is rapid with subcutaneous or intranasal forms, with a somewhat slower onset of 30–60 min with the oral form. The maximum effect may not be achieved until 24–48 h after the first dose because of the blunting of concentrating capacity caused by chronic water diuresis. Antidiuresis is followed promptly by a 1–2% increase in body water and a similar decrease in plasma osmolality and sodium, which relieves thirst and results in a reduction in fluid intake.

dDAVP does not typically reduce urine free water output below the level of free water intake in a standard diet, so hyponatremia is unlikely to occur in the absence of excess fluid intake but, as dDAVP reduces free water excretion, hyponatremia will occur if fluid intake is excessive. Patients and parents should be

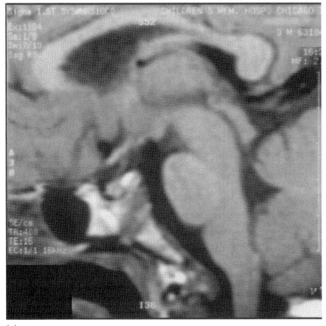

(a)

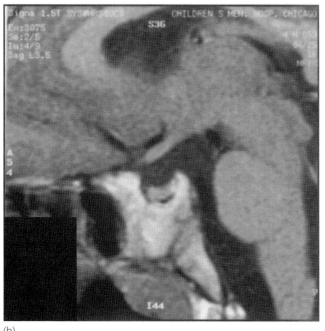

(b)

Figure 15.10 Magnetic resonance imaging of the hypothalamus and pituitary in central diabetes insipidus (CDI). Both images are T$_1$ weighted and obtained before the infusion of gadolinium. (a) This sagittal image is from a healthy 4-year-old boy and shows the hyperintense signal normally emitted by the posterior pituitary. (b) This comparable image from a boy with autosomal dominant neurohypophyseal diabetes insipidus lacks the posterior pituitary bright spot.

educated about the risk of excessive fluid intake and the signs and symptoms of water intoxication. Patients and families should be advised that intake should be guided solely by thirst and patients should avoid incidental or social drinking. It may be helpful to

suggest limiting the intake of juice, soda, alcoholic beverages and other non-nutrient drinks and offering plain water to prevent taste-induced drinking.

Treatment of CDI associated with hypodipsia or adipsia. The osmoregulation of thirst is normal in more than 90% of patients with CDI but a few have hypodipsia or adipsia, mostly those with a history of congenital midline CNS malformations or hypothalamic surgery or, to a lesser extent in children, head trauma, ruptured anterior communicating artery aneurysms or suprasellar malignancy. As thirst adjusts water intake to compensate for changes in urine output and insensible losses, intact thirst protects against dehydration and hypernatremia or overhydration and hyponatremia during treatment of DI. When hypodipsia or adipsia are present, this greatly complicates management, as changing urine output is no longer compensated by spontaneous adjustment in fluid intake. The situation is complicated by the fact that many adipsic DI patients have significant associated neurologic and cognitive dysfunctions.

Management of DI in this situation requires a fixed dose of dDAVP and a daily water intake to meet fluid needs under usual conditions of treatment, diet, temperature and activity. In the absence of periods of significant diuresis, the required free water intake will be approximately 1 L/m^2/day. Patients and their families can be taught to adjust the intake from the fixed target amount based on situational changes, which include changes in urine output due to variation in dDAVP effectiveness or dietary solute load and increased insensible losses secondary to changes in ambient temperature, illness or physical activity. Daily weight can be helpful in determining the need to make interval adjustments in the daily fluid intake but target weights need to be recalibrated periodically to compensate for growth. Periodic monitoring of serum sodium is essential, usually weekly, with additional tests for unexpected weight loss or gain. This requires frequent trips to the laboratory but, with the availability of small analyzers designed for point-of-care monitoring, families can be taught to carry out sodium monitoring in the home [97].

Treatment of CDI in infants. Neonates and young infants need large fluid intakes to deliver adequate calories. Combining this high fluid intake with conventional dosing of dDAVP can result in hyponatremia. There are several approaches to this situation.

Most infants with CDI cannot concentrate urine to reach an osmolality greater than the renal solute concentration of the feed and therefore excessive urine output and hypernatremia results. Large volumes of supplemental free water with daily weight and periodic sodium assessment is standard therapy but the large volume of water intake may result in inadequate calorie intake and poor growth. Decreasing the solute load with low-solute formula or breast milk can reduce the obligate urine output, allowing fluid balance to be achieved with modest free water supplementation in infants who can concentrate their urine to 70–100 mOsm/L. If DI is severe and urine cannot be spontaneously concentrated to 70 mOsm/L, addition of a thiazide diuretic (chlorothiazide 5 mg/kg every 12 h) with low solute formula is helpful in increasing urine osmolality and reducing urine output [98].

Another successful approach is to give small frequent doses of dDAVP orally to concentrate urine to 100–150 mOsm/L and thereby decrease urine output to approximately normal volume. A surprisingly small amount of dDAVP is required, approximately 0.5–5 µg orally every 6 h for a neonate. The intranasal solution is 10 µg/100 µL or 100 µg/1 mL and the dDAVP can be dosed with an insulin syringe (1 unit volume is 1 µg) or diluted and dispensed in a larger volume. Close follow-up with daily weights and periodic serum sodium is essential with all therapies.

Treatment of postoperative CDI. In the acute postoperative management of DI, vasopressin should be used with caution because hyponatremia can occur with intravenous fluid intake not regulated by thirst. A continuous vasopressin infusion allows modulation of the urine output and can be titrated rapidly to meet changing conditions. This is not possible with dDAVP, which is generally inadvisable immediately postoperatively. Fluid therapy alone can be used to treat postoperative DI but the large volumes of urine output and intravenous fluid infusion can lead to rapid undesirable changes in osmolality.

When intravenous fluid therapy is used alone, input is matched with hourly output, with an initial limit of 3–5 L/m^2/day. A basal infusion rate of 1 L/m^2/day (40 mL/m^2/h) should be given as 5% dextrose in 0.22% saline to replace baseline sodium loss. No additional fluid should be administered for hourly urine volumes under 40 mL/m^2/h. For hourly urine volumes above 40 mL/m^2/h, the additional volume should be replaced with 5% dextrose–water to a maximum of 120–200 mL/m^2/h (3–5 L/m^2/day). For urine outputs above 120 mL/m^2/h, the initial total infusion rate should be 120 mL/m^2/h and may be adjusted up to 200 mL/m^2/h. In the presence of DI, this will result in serum sodium in the 150 mmol/L range. This mildly volume-contracted state should produce a prerenal reduction in urine output, generally avoiding the need to give larger volumes of fluid, and will also allow the assessment of thirst and the return of normal vasopressin function or the emergence of SIADH.

Patients may become mildly hyperglycemic with this regimen, particularly if they are also receiving postoperative glucocorticoids. Frequent assessment of fluid balance, urine specific gravity and serum electrolytes to determine appropriate adjustments in therapy are essential to avoid fluctuations in volume status, particularly in cases where the triple-phase response develops. If the child is awake and able to drink, free access to water based on thirst should be allowed, with advice to avoid non-thirst-mediated fluid intake. If there is concern about impaired thirst, oral intake should be matched to urine output. Patients with post-neurosurgical DI should be switched from intravenous to oral fluid intake at the earliest opportunity because thirst sensation, if intact, will help regulate blood osmolality and minimize the risk of significant hypernatremia or hyponatremia.

Intravenous vasopressin infused at 1.5–2.5 mU/kg/h concentrates urine within 1–6 h [99]. A loading dose of 1–2 mU/kg accelerates control. Occasionally, following hypothalamic surgery, higher concentrations of vasopressin are required initially to treat acute DI, which may be attributable to the release of biologically inactive vasopressin-like peptides acting as antagonists to normal vasopressin activity [89]. When fluid requirements are no longer fluctuating, the patient can be changed to dDAVP if required.

Nephrogenic DI

Nephrogenic (vasopressin-resistant) diabetes insipidus (NDI) is characterized by impaired urinary concentrating ability despite normal or elevated plasma concentrations of vasopressin: it can be genetic or acquired. Genetic etiologies are diagnosed during childhood and are generally more severe than acquired causes. Acquired NDI can occur as a component of acquired kidney disease, in a number of metabolic abnormalities or in response to drugs.

Causes of NDI

Genetic NDI

In contrast to familial CDI, polyuria and polydipsia are present from birth with NDI but the average age at which the diagnosis is recognized is 9 months (Table 15.3). Pregnancies involving affected infants can be complicated by hydramnios. Unless the disease is recognized, affected children have repeated episodes of dehydration, sometimes complicated by convulsions and death. Affected infants are irritable and present with vomiting, anorexia, failure-to-thrive, fever and constipation. Serum sodium is generally elevated because babies cannot increase free water intake.

Table 15.3 Causes of nephrogenic diabetes insipidus.

Genetic
X-linked recessive (AVP-V$_2$ receptor)
Autosomal recessive (aquaporin-2)
Autosomal dominant (aquaporin-2)

Acquired
Drugs:
  Lithium
  Foscarnet
  Demeclocycline
  Many others
Metabolic:
  Hyperglycemia
  Hypercalcemia
  Hypokalemia
  Protein malnutrition
Renal:
  Chronic renal failure
  Ischemic injury
  Impaired medullary function
  Outflow obstruction

Growth failure may be secondary to the ingestion of large amounts of water, which the child may prefer over other higher calorie substances, and/or because of general poor health resulting from dehydration and hypernatremia. Mental retardation of variable severity has been reported [100] but it is probable that this results from prolonged episodes of dehydration or frequent swings in osmolality which can be prevented by earlier recognition and appropriate management [101,102].

Even with early institution of therapy, short stature remains common in children with congenital NDI. Some patients develop severe dilatation of the urinary tract, which may predispose to rupture after minor trauma. Intracranial calcification has been described.

Congenital X-linked NDI. This accounts for >90% of cases and has an estimated prevalence of eight per million males, although the frequency is higher in some populations. It is caused by loss-of-function mutations in the vasopressin V_2 receptor gene, which is located at Xq28. Although it is X-linked, heterozygous females may be affected, presumably as a result of X chromosome inactivation of the wild-type locus in a significant number of the cells of the renal collecting ducts in one or both kidneys [103].

More than 180 mutations in the V_2 receptor have been identified (Fig. 15.7a) [104]. They are mostly single base mutations that result in amino acid substitutions (50%), translational frame-shifts (27%) or termination of peptide synthesis (11%). Most result in abnormal misfolded proteins that are trapped in the endoplasmic reticulum as a result of failed processing through the N-linked glycosylation pathway. A few have been demonstrated to result in proteins with normal abundance on the cell surface but impaired vasopressin binding or G-protein coupling. Almost all mutations in the V_2 receptor gene result in severe NDI but there are a few exceptions associated with a milder phenotype and later presentation [105].

Autosomal recessive NDI. Autosomal recessive NDI, caused by mutations in the aquaporin-2 gene, located in the 12q13 chromosome region, constitutes <10% of cases. More than 30 mutations have been identified (Fig. 15.7b,c) [104] that impair the ability of the luminal membrane to undergo an increase in water permeability following signaling through the V_2 receptor. Most mutations in AQP-2 result in autosomal recessive disease. The mutations result in misfolding and misrouting of AQP-2 mutant proteins, with retention of the protein within the ER.

Autosomal dominant NDI. This is also caused by a mutation in the *AQP-2* gene and has been described in a few families. Oocyte expression studies have shown that the autosomal dominant protein behaves in a dominant-negative way by forming hetero-oligomers with wild-type AQP-2 and impairing routing of both wild-type and mutant proteins out of the Golgi apparatus to the plasma membrane [106].

AQP-2 mutations can be distinguished from the V_2 receptor mutation forms by genetic or functional studies demonstrating the presence of extrarenal V_2-mediated responses to dDAVP. Patients with autosomal NDI show normal increases in von Willebrand factor, factor VIII and tissue-type plasminogen activator levels in response to dDAVP, while these responses are absent in X-linked NDI. These tests are difficult to perform in infants and have been replaced by molecular identification of the mutations in AQP-2 or the V_2 receptor. If the family history is suggestive of familial DI, genetic characterization of the defect is appropriate. Patients with a family history can be evaluated for the disorder in the prenatal or perinatal period by DNA sequence analysis, allowing therapy to be initiated without delay [107].

Acquired NDI

Drug-induced NDI. This is not common but 50% of patients receiving lithium have impaired urinary concentrating ability and 10–20% develop symptomatic NDI on long-term therapy. Lithium appears to act by decreasing AQP-2 protein targeting to the apical membrane [108]. The risk of symptomatic DI increases with duration of lithium therapy and NDI may be slow to recover or persist following discontinuation of lithium therapy.

Other drugs associated with NDI include foscarnet, cidofovir, clozapine, fluvoxamine, amphotericin B, gentamicin, demeclocycline, cyclophosphamide, isophosphamide, cisplatin, rifampicin, methicillin, methotrexate, cimetidine, verapamil, methoxyflurane, colchicine and glyburide. Most cause NDI in the setting of severe illness. Foscarnet, the second most common drug associated with NDI, appears to interfere with the transduction of the vasopressin signal proximal to cAMP and its effect can be blocked by non-steroidal anti-inflammatory drugs (NSAIDs), suggesting that it may be mediated via prostaglandins. How other agents cause NDI is not known.

Metabolic causes. Hyperglycemia, hypokalemia and hypercalcemia are associated with vasopressin-resistant polyuria and polydipsia. Hyperglycemia causes an osmotic diuresis, preventing normal water reabsorption in the face of intact signaling with increased urine osmolality. The DI in hypokalemia is not as severe as that seen with familial or lithium-induced NDI but does appear to result from a true reduction in vasopressin responsiveness, probably by a reduction in total AQP-2. Hypercalcemia-associated polyuria and polydipsia is associated with AQP-2 downregulation and diminished trafficking of AQP-2 to the collecting duct apical membrane [109].

Kidney disease. Impaired urinary concentrating capacity and unresponsiveness to vasopressin occurs in acute and chronic renal failure when impairment of the counter-current concentrating mechanism probably contributes to reduced concentrating ability. Defective medullary counter-current function resulting in a vasopressin-resistant concentrating defect is seen in other diseases that cause medullary damage, such as sickle cell disease, Sjögren syndrome, amyloidosis, sarcoid and cystinosis. Protein malnutrition or low sodium intake can also lead to diminished tonicity of the renal medullary interstitium and diminish the driving force for water reabsorption. Urinary tract obstruction produces polyuria, which appears to be multifactorial but includes decreased AQP-2 [110].

Treatment of NDI

Once the diagnosis and cause of acquired NDI has been established, treatment focuses first on elimination of the underlying disorder or drug. In congenital NDI, the main goals are to ensure adequate intake of calories for growth and avoid dehydration. Therapies for congenital NDI do not completely eliminate polyuria but reduction to 3–4 L/m^2/day is often achievable.

Foods with the highest ratio of calorie content to osmotic load should be used to maximize growth and minimize the urine volume required to excrete solute. Thiazide diuretics (hydrochlorothiazide 2–4 mg/kg/day divided two or three times daily) with low sodium intake and amiloride or indometacin are the most useful treatments. Thiazides inhibit the NaCl co-transporter in the distal convoluted tubule and the resultant increased sodium excretion coupled with dietary sodium restriction results in extracellular volume contraction, decreased glomerular filtration rate (GFR) and increased proximal tubule sodium and water reabsorption. This results in decreased delivery of water and sodium to the collecting tubules and therefore decreased urine output. Thiazides may also directly increase water resorption in the collecting duct [111].

Indometacin enhances proximal tubular sodium and water absorption but is associated with nephrotoxicity and gastrointestinal side effects. Amiloride, in a regimen of 0.3 mg/kg/day divided three times per day, prevents thiazide-induced hypokalemia, which can itself cause vasopressin-resistant polyuria, avoids the toxicity associated with indometacin and is well tolerated, even with prolonged treatment [112].

In cases of X-linked NDI with V_2 receptors that are expressed on the cell surface but have a decreased affinity for vasopressin, dDAVP at higher than typical doses can sometimes be used [113]. Some patients with lithium-induced NDI are effectively treated with thiazides and amiloride because the latter inhibits lithium uptake by collecting duct epithelial cells [114].

Synthetic membrane-permeable vasopressin antagonists can act as chemical chaperones, increasing the successful processing of mutant V_2 receptors and allowing increased movement to the plasma membrane. Once there, some of the mutant proteins are capable of generating vasopressin-mediated cAMP production and presumably vasopressin-mediated water uptake [115,116]. These antagonists offer hope of more effective therapy for some forms of X-linked NDI.

Primary polydipsia

Polyuria and polydipsia with low vasopressin levels can result from excessive intake of water and is often mistaken for DI but, in contrast to DI, hypernatremia is never seen, even with fluid restriction. Excessive intake of water slightly lowers serum osmolality and inhibits the secretion of vasopressin allowing water diuresis to compensate for the increased intake. This condition,

primary polydipsia, must be distinguished from DI because dDAVP therapy is contraindicated in most cases. In a water deprivation test, the polyuria will be interrupted and the urine will become concentrated and decrease in volume. Therapy with dDAVP in the face of continued drinking may cause water intoxication to develop rapidly, usually within 24–48 h with development of hyponatremia and central nervous symptoms and signs. dDAVP should not be used to treat a polyuric patient with a normal water deprivation test.

Psychogenic polydipsia

Primary polydipsia, which can occur as part of a general cognitive defect associated with schizophrenia or other psychiatric disorders, is usually called psychogenic polydipsia or compulsive water drinking. Rare in children, it may occur in adolescents. Patients do not complain of thirst and usually attribute polydipsia to disordered beliefs. Water intake is often in excess of that necessary to maintain fluid balance, even in DI, and may occasionally exceed the renal capacity to excrete free water, predisposing individuals with this form of primary polydipsia to hyponatremia. Treatment focuses on the underlying psychiatric disorder. If water intake has been sufficient to cause hyponatremia in the absence of dDAVP, the patient may need supervised care to control access to water.

Dipsogenic polydipsia

In dipsogenic polydipsia, increased water consumption is caused by an increase in thirst [117]. This can be seen in diseases involving the hypothalamus, although it is most often idiopathic. Management should include a search for the cause and for the presence of associated defects in hypothalamic and anterior pituitary function. Some cases appear to result from resetting the osmotic threshold for thirst below the threshold for vasopressin release. Because vasopressin secretion is suppressed at the thirst osmotic threshold, ingested water is rapidly excreted and thirst persists. dDAVP may be beneficial when thirst and vasopressin osmotic threshold are reversed because it allows the serum osmolality to fall below the threshold for thirst, thereby suppressing water ingestion [118]. If the thirst threshold is reset too low, significant hyponatremia may result with the removal of the protective renal diuresis mechanism.

Iatrogenic polydipsia

Primary polydipsia can also be prompted by overzealous adoption or incorrect understanding of advice to increase fluid intake offered by physicians, nurses, complementary medicine practitioners or the lay media. It is usually mild and rarely results in urine outputs of more than 5 L/day. It can be corrected if those involved are amenable to adopting more moderate fluid intake practices.

Hypernatremia

Hypernatremia (serum sodium concentration >145 mmol/L) is caused by loss of water or gain of sodium. Because the increased serum osmolality induces intense thirst, even a modest rise in serum sodium stimulates water ingestion, preventing progression of hypernatremia, so hypernatremia rarely occurs in a normal ambulatory individual with intact thirst and access to water, even with DI.

Adipsic hypernatremia

Primary adipsia is usually caused by lesions in the anterior hypothalamus and the resulting hypernatremia can be exacerbated by concomitant DI with impaired vasopressin release in response to increasing serum osmolality. The water intake associated with a normal diet is insufficient to match obligate renal, bowel and insensible water losses and periodic supplemental drinking is required to prevent hypernatremia. If thirst is absent, drinking does not occur and hypernatremic dehydration results.

Hypernatremia develops slowly and even moderate to severe elevations in plasma sodium may be well tolerated and cause no obvious clinical abnormalities. The development of hypernatremia can be accelerated by an increase in urinary or stool water loss or an increase in insensible losses associated with exercise, increase in environmental temperature or fever. If hypernatremic dehydration develops rapidly or is particularly severe, it usually results in overt clinical signs of hypovolemia and damage to the brain and other organs can occur.

As with DI, adipsia requires cranial MRI to evaluate the hypothalamus. The long-term management should prevent or minimize recurrences of hypertonic dehydration by minimizing urinary water losses using dDAVP if DI is present and ensuring that fluid intake is sufficient to replace total water output. Even in the absence of dDAVP, caution should be taken to avoid excessive fluid intake as some individuals also have an impaired ability to downregulate vasopressin secretion and may be at risk of water intoxication with increased fluid intake.

Physical obstacles to drinking

Adipsic hypernatremia should be distinguished from the presence of physical obstacles to drinking, such as occur in patients who are debilitated by acute or chronic illness, have neurological impairment or are at the extremes of age. Immobilized patients who can communicate are less likely to develop hypernatremia because they can indicate their desire to drink but very young children or those with significant developmental delay are at risk of dehydration if obligate fluid losses are not anticipated and replaced.

Excessive free water losses (not due to DI)

When acute illness results in inadequate fluid intake or excessive free water losses, which cannot be compensated by increased fluid intake due to the ongoing disease process, hypernatremia can result. Gastroenteritis with prolonged vomiting and diarrhea is the most common example. In severely ill patients, hypernatremia can also be caused by inadequate replacement of increased insensible water loss, which may occur in patients with burns or high fever or by failure to adequately replace increased losses from other sources.

Excessive sodium intake

Increased sodium intake can be caused by accidental ingestion of large quantities of salt or intravenous administration of hypertonic solutions. Increased water intake corrects the hyperosmolality and excess sodium is rapidly excreted as long as thirst and renal function are intact and there are no physical limitations preventing access to water. In infants, severely ill or debilitated patients, excessive sodium administration can result in persistent hypernatremia until adequate free water is provided to allow salt diuresis.

Correction of hypernatremia

The initial treatment of hypernatremia should replace the water deficiency and minimize further losses by treating DI, diabetes mellitus or other underlying pathology. Free water should be given orally if possible but can also be infused intravenously either as 0.45% saline, 5% dextrose in 0.22% saline or as 5% dextrose–water (if hyperglycemia is not present). 0.45% saline provides equal volumes of normal saline and free water whereas 0.22% saline is equivalent to one part normal saline and three parts free water. The net increase in body water that must be achieved to correct the deficit can be estimated by the formula:

$$\Delta H_2O = [(P_{Na} - 140)/140] \times 0.6 \times BW$$

where ΔH_2O is the estimated water deficit in liters, P_{Na} is the plasma sodium concentration expressed in mmol/L and BW is the body weight in kilograms.

Non-acute hypernatremic dehydration or hypernatremic dehydration of uncertain duration should be corrected gradually. Hypernatremia results in an efflux of fluid from the intracellular space to maintain osmotic equilibrium which leads to transient intracellular dehydration. The brain significantly increases its content of sodium, potassium, amino acids (taurine and glutamine) and other osmotically active substances, such as myoinositol and betaine [119] and regains 98% of its water content within 1 week, despite persistent hypernatremia [120]. Although protective during hypernatremia, these compensatory increases in intracellular osmoles will result in cellular swelling if hypernatremia is corrected too rapidly. Swelling of cells in the brain after the closure of the fontanelles increases intracranial pressure rapidly leading to seizures, coma and death.

Therefore, when hypernatremia has been present for more then 12 h or the duration is uncertain, the target should be to replace the free water deficit over a minimum of 48 h and to avoid changes in sodium concentration exceeding 0.5–1 mmol/L/h. The rate of fluid administration will be determined by the free water deficit divided by the desired time over which the deficit is to be replaced added to fluid administration sufficient to replace estimated or measured renal and gastrointestinal output and estimated insensible losses. During the correction of hypernatremia, fluid intake, output and plasma sodium (and glucose if hyperglycemia is present) should be monitored frequently and the treatment plan adjusted as necessary.

Hyponatremia

The primary defense against hyponatremia is the ability to generate dilute urine and excrete free water which excess vasopressin or primary renal disease can interrupt. If dilute urine cannot be produced and water intake not reduced sufficiently to match the reduction in urine output, free water accumulates and dilutes body fluids, resulting in hypotonic hyponatremia. Clinical manifestations result from the effects of hyponatremia on the CNS: both alterations in electrolyte concentrations and direct effects of cellular swelling. Slow development of hyponatremia may result in mild symptoms but rapid development causes anorexia, headache, nausea, lethargy, psychosis, convulsions, intracranial hypertension and coma or death from herniation. The severity of neurological effects depends on the degree of hyponatremia, the rate of decline and the age of the patient. Children are more susceptible to symptomatic hyponatremia after closure of the fontanelles, which leaves less room for brain expansion [121]. Females after menarche and before menopause are at increased risk of developing symptomatic hyponatremia probably because estrogen inhibits compensatory changes in intracellular osmolality and may increase the risk of consequent hypoxic damage by promoting cerebral vasoconstriction [122]. If hyponatremia develops rapidly (over less than 24–48 h) and/or is exceptionally severe (<120 mmol/L), it usually results in symptoms and signs.

Determining the etiology is critical because it affects management [123]. The duration and degree of hyponatremia and the presence or absence of symptoms are important: acute (<24–48 h) hyponatremia can be corrected quickly but chronic asymptomatic hyponatremia should be corrected slowly because rapid correction is associated with CNS injury, including central pontine myelinolysis [124]. Symptomatic chronic hyponatremia requires a phase of rapid correction until symptoms remit, followed by further gradual correction.

Diagnostic approach to hyponatremia

Hyponatremia typically occurs with hypotonicity but can also be found with a normal or elevated serum osmolality. The first step in evaluation is confirmation that it is associated with hypotonicity by measuring serum osmolality (Fig. 15.11). The most common cause of hypertonic hyponatremia is hyperglycemia. Glucose-induced hyperosmolality causes an osmotic shift of fluid from the intracellular into the extracellular space, resulting in a dilutional decrease in sodium. If hyperglycemia is present, the observed plasma sodium (PNa) should be corrected for dilution to determine the plasma sodium that would be present in the absence of hyperglycemia using the formula:

$$P\text{-}Na_{Cor} = P_{Na} + [(Glu - 100) \times 1.6]/100$$

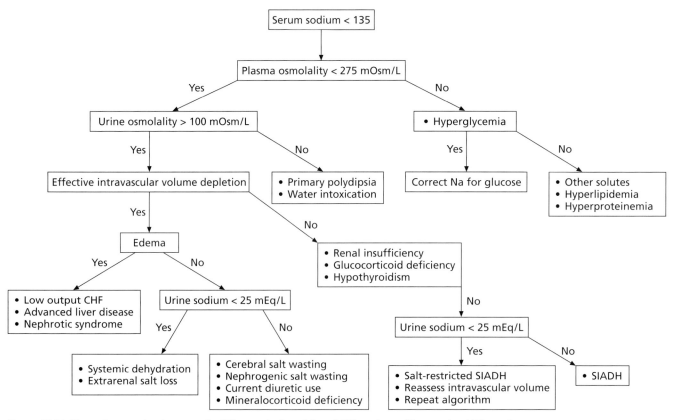

Figure 15.11 Diagnostic approach to hyponatremia. CHF, congestive heart failure; SIADH, syndrome of inappropriate ADH secretion.

where P-Na$_{Cor}$ is the corrected plasma sodium in mmol/L and Glu is the plasma glucose in mg/dL (mmol/L × 18). Other solutes, such as mannitol, sorbitol, maltose and radiocontrast, can also produce hypertonic hyponatremia.

Normotonic hyponatremia can be seen in severe hyperproteinemia or hyperlipidemia, which cause a displacement of plasma water. When sodium is measured by methods that involve dilution of the specimen before measurement, sodium concentration appears to be low, although if measured by an ion selective electrode in the aqueous phase of undiluted serum, the sodium is normal. Hyponatremia in this situation is thus a laboratory artifact, pseudohyponatremia.

Hypotonic hyponatremia results either from sodium loss or free water gain. A dilute urine osmolality (<100 mOsm/L) suggests excess free water gain from primary polydipsia. Sodium loss or diminished water excretion result in concentrated urine, generally with osmolality >300 mOsm/kg. A clinical and laboratory assessment of whether the patient is hypovolemic, suggesting sodium loss, or euvolemic or hypervolemic, suggesting diminished water excretion, is required. Information on recent intake and output, weight changes, medication and underlying medical illnesses may be useful in making the distinction. Weight loss, decreased skin turgor, decreased perfusion and elevated heart rate suggest hypovolemia, as do elevated blood urea nitrogen (BUN), renin, aldosterone and uric acid.

Urine sodium also distinguishes hypovolemia from hypervolemia. In hypovolemia, sodium will be avidly retained and the urinary sodium will be less than 10 mmol/L, except when the hypovolemia is brought about by cerebral salt-wasting, ongoing diuretic use or renal salt-wasting. In hypervolemia, the urine sodium is generally >40 mmol/L.

Euvolemic or hypervolemic hyponatremia can be caused by inappropriately elevated vasopressin or by vasopressin "appropriately" elevated as the result of effectively decreased plasma volume, such as in congestive heart failure, diuretic use or cirrhosis. Because many forms of hyponatremia have associated increases in vasopressin levels, it is important to determine whether the increased vasopressin reflects a physiologically appropriate process or is due to inappropriate increases in vasopressin secretion (Fig. 15.12) [125].

Inappropriate vasopressin secretion

Osmotically inappropriate vasopressin secretion that cannot be explained by a non-osmotic stimulus implies a primary abnormality in the regulation of vasopressin secretion, SIADH [126]. Patients with SIADH fail to suppress vasopressin secretion, even

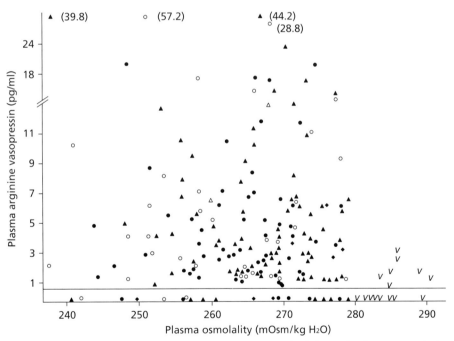

Figure 15.12 Plasma vasopressin concentration in hyponatremia. It is generally not helpful to measure vasopressin levels during the evaluation of hyponatremia as most patients with hyponatremia have vasopressin levels that are inappropriately elevated for their serum osmolality. Fifteen healthy volunteers (v) who drank 1 L water per hour for 8–10 h suppressed their vasopressin levels as their plasma osmolality declined and did not develop hyponatremia. In contrast, in 51 patients with congestive heart failure (CHF) associated hyponatremia (△), 35 patients with cirrhosis-associated hyponatremia (▲) and 55 patients with volume depletion-associated hyponatremia (■), the majority have elevated vasopressin levels despite their hyponatremia. This is presumed to be due to intravascular volume depletion-mediated vasopressin release and these vasopressin levels are indistinguishable from those seen in 36 individuals with SIADH (○). Nine patients without a known etiology of their hyponatremia are also included (◆). The line at 0.75 pg/mL indicates the minimum detectable vasopressin level in the assay used. The numbers in parentheses at the top indicate the value of plasma vasopressin measurements that are beyond the scale of this diagram. (From Gross *et al.* [152] with permission.)

when plasma osmolality falls below the normal osmotic threshold for stimulated vasopressin release. This causes impaired renal free water clearance and results in total body free water excess and hyponatremia if free water intake is not limited. SIADH is the most common etiology of severe hyponatremia but the mechanism is not fully understood.

Mechanism of hyponatremia with euvolemia in SIADH

Even maximal antidiuresis by vasopressin causes little or no decrease in plasma sodium unless fluid intake is maintained at a level greater than total urinary and insensible output. Excessive fluid intake in patients can be caused by inappropriate administration of intravenous or nasogastric fluids, non-thirst-mediated drinking or an abnormality in the osmoregulation of thirst. Under these conditions, excess water accumulates, expanding and diluting body fluids. When the expansion of body water exceeds 5–6%, plasma renin activity and aldosterone are suppressed, atrial natriuretic peptide levels increase and urine sodium excretion begins to rise. These compensatory mechanisms interrupt further increase in the extracellular volume expansion, preventing extreme volume expansion, but aggravate the hyponatremia.

Because of these compensatory changes, individuals with SIADH are clinically euvolemic and, once they have reached this phase of SIADH, urine free water and sodium excretion rates parallel the rates of water and sodium intake. The increase in urine sodium mediated by the vasopressin-induced volume expansion helps to distinguish SIADH from other forms of hypotonic hyponatremia. In the absence of diuretic use or renal disease, hyponatremia with low urine output and increased urine sodium (>20–30 mmol/L) is consistent with SIADH but SIADH should not be diagnosed if there is clinical evidence of hypovolemia or peripheral edema. Low normal BUN, creatinine and low uric acid can provide additional laboratory evidence of the mild volume expansion expected with SIADH.

Causes of SIADH

Tumors. SIADH was first described with bronchogenic carcinoma and has since been recognized in patients with several other types of tumors, particularly of neuroendocrine origin. Small-cell lung carcinomas are capable of ectopic synthesis and release of vasopressin. A small percentage of other lung tumors also produce and release vasopressin. Head and neck tumors have also been associated with SIADH. Although many SIADH-associated tumors produce vasopressin, a number have not. In those cases, it is presumed that the tumor produces a substance that promotes vasopressin secretion. Most SIADH-associated tumors are not seen in children.

Drugs. Drugs can cause impaired free water clearance (Table 15.4) resulting from alteration in vasopressin release, enhanced vasopressin effect at the same plasma vasopressin concentration or vasopressin-independent changes in distal collecting tubule water permeability. Carbamazepine [127], chlorpropamide [128],

Table 15.4 Drugs associated with impaired water clearance.

Class	Common drugs
Angiotensin-converting enzyme inhibitors	Lisinopril
Anticonvulsants	Carbamazepine
	Oxacarbazepine
	Valproic acid
Anitneoplastics	Cis-platinum
	Cyclophosphamide
	Vinblastine
	Vincristine
Antiparkinsonian	Amantadine
	Trihexyphenidyl
Antipsychotics	Haloperidol
	Thioridazine
Antipyretics	Acetaminophen
Hypolipidemics	Clofibrate
Oral hypoglycemics	Chlorpropamide
	Tolbutamide
Selective serotonin uptake inhibitors	Fluoxetine
	Sertraline
Tricyclic antidepressants	Imipramine
	Amitriptyline
Other	Ecstasy

vinblastine [129], vincristine [130], tricyclic antidepressants [131] and 3,4-methylenedioxymethamphetamine (ecstasy) [132] increase antidiuretic hormone (ADH) secretion and result in hyponatremia.

CNS disorders. These include inflammatory processes, such as systemic lupus, sarcoid and Guillain–Barré syndrome, and infectious causes, such as meningitis and encephalitis. Tuberculous meningitis has an unusually high association with SIADH, with 70% of tuberculous meningitis cases in children affected [133]. SIADH has also been seen with tumors or brain abscesses, following cerebrovascular accident and following CNS surgery or traumatic injury. In CNS injury, care must be taken to distinguish SIADH from cerebral salt-wasting, which also causes hyponatremia but requires markedly different management.

Non-malignant pulmonary disorders. These, including hypoxia and hypercapnia, elevate plasma vasopressin levels. SIADH has been seen in advanced chronic obstructive pulmonary disease and several other pulmonary disorders, including tuberculosis, severe asthma, respiratory syncytial virus (RSV) bronchiolitis, cystic fibrosis (CF) exacerbation and pneumonia. SIADH generally occurs with acute respiratory failure but is limited to the period of respiratory failure. Mechanical ventilation, particularly positive pressure ventilation, has been associated with increased vasopressin release and SIADH probably because decreased vascular return to the heart results in decreased cardiac output and decreased stretch on the baroreceptors.

SINGLETON HOSPITAL
STAFF LIBRARY

Postoperative hyponatremia. It has long been recognized that the use of hypotonic saline for hydration during acute postoperative management puts patients at risk of hyponatremia and, for this reason, isotonic saline solutions are widely used for fluid support following surgery. Unfortunately, children are still sustaining neurological morbidity and mortality associated with hospital-acquired hyponatremia associated with receiving hypotonic fluids postoperatively [134]. The etiology of postoperative hyponatremia is multifactorial but generally associated with a self-limited increase in vasopressin. Nausea, a common postoperative symptom, is a stimulus for vasopressin secretion, as are pain, stress, anxiety and fever. Whether brought about by intravascular volume depletion or other stimuli, vasopressin levels are high in the immediate postoperative period so hypotonic fluids should be used cautiously.

Adrenal insufficiency/hypothyroidism. An SIADH-like syndrome occurs in patients with adrenal insufficiency [30], which impairs free water excretion. Cortisol-deficient states are associated with increased vasopressin levels and also cause antidiuresis in patients with CDI, suggesting that cortisol may also have an effect on urine concentration independent of vasopressin. As in true SIADH, the development of hyponatremia is dependent upon excessive water intake. Patients with hyponatremia resulting from isolated glucocorticoid deficiency do not have hyperkalemia or signs of hypovolemia and can be reliably differentiated from patients with SIADH only by testing the hypothalamic-pituitary-adrenal axis. Severe hypothyroidism can also produce an SIADH-like hyponatremia, the etiology of which is unknown [135]. SIADH should not be diagnosed until hypothyroidism and adrenal insufficiency have been excluded.

Exercise-induced SIADH. Marathon runners are susceptible to development of hyponatremia during a race. Fluid intake is encouraged while nausea, pain, exercise itself and release of IL-6 from low grade rhabdomyolysis all promote vasopressin secretion and can lead to fatal hyponatremia from SIADH [136]. NSAIDs may enhance the renal activity of inappropriately secreted vasopressin and may potentiate development of SIADH.

Inherited. A constitutively activating mutation in the gene encoding the V_2 receptor causes a congenital SIADH-like syndrome in the absence of elevated vasopressin levels. This condition has been named nephrogenic syndrome of inappropriate antidiuresis [137].

Management of SIADH
The primary management of SIADH is fluid restriction while the underlying cause is identified and treated. Fortunately, SIADH is generally temporary and fluid restriction will be necessary only until it remits spontaneously. In cases when excess hormone is made ectopically, given exogenously, results from a deficiency in glucocorticoid or thyroid hormone or is released from the posterior pituitary in response to a medication, the cause can be addressed specifically. Symptomatic SIADH is less common but requires urgent therapy.

Asymptomatic hyponatremia
When hyponatremia is not severe (serum sodium >120 mmol/L) and is asymptomatic, fluid restriction is the optimal therapy. The goal is to promote a gradual increase in sodium, followed by stabilization in the normal range. Rapid correction of hyponatremia has been associated with central pontine myelinolysis, a rare and sometimes fatal neurological disorder characterized by demyelination that involves the central portion of the base of the pons and causes spastic quadriparesis, pseudobulbar paralysis with dysphagia and dysarthria. Myelinolysis lesions may also be extrapontine and then the syndrome has been called osmotic demyelinating syndrome. It may result from disruption of the blood–brain barrier that allows complement to damage oligodendrocytes and produce a pathological pattern resembling fulminate multiple sclerosis [138].

Patients in whom hyponatremia has been present for more than 48 h may have fewer symptoms but are more likely to have serious complications from rapid correction of hyponatremia. The target is to increase the sodium at not more than 0.5 mmol/h or 8–12 mmol/day. To promote an increase in serum sodium, fluid restriction to amounts below obligate urine and insensible losses is required, generally 600–800 mL/m²/day. The expected rate of increase in sodium with such a fluid restriction in place is well below the maximum target of 10–12 mmol/day. Once the sodium has risen into the desired range, maintenance of it in that range can generally be achieved with a fluid restriction of 0.8–1 L/m²/day. Fluid restriction can be difficult in infants and young children because the water content of formula or baby food is relatively high and fluid restriction may result in unintentional calorie deficit. Fluid restriction can also become burdensome to older children when SIADH is prolonged and additional measures may be needed.

The children with nephrogenic syndrome of inappropriate antidiuresis have a persistent form of antidiuresis and are treated with fluid restriction and oral urea to eliminate free water by induction of an osmotic diuresis [137].

Inhibiting the vasopressin effect. Body water can be reduced by treatments that inhibit the antidiuretic effects of vasopressin. Demeclocycline, a tetracycline derivative, at conventional doses of up to 1.2 g/day in adults, causes a reversible form of NDI in almost all patients with SIADH in a week or more [139]. Its potential renal toxicity may cause a rise in plasma urea which is reversible when the drug is stopped. Its efficacy and safety in treating infants and children with SIADH is unknown but it is incorporated into tooth and bone and therefore its use should be restricted to patients with chronic SIADH not amenable to fluid restriction.

Lithium carbonate causes a form of NDI but, at conventional doses, this effect is inconsistent and, with its narrow therapeutic window, it is prone to produce undesirable side effects. For these reasons, lithium should not be used for treatment of SIADH in children [140]. Oral urea in a 30% solution at 0.1 g/kg/day divided into four doses rapidly establishes an osmotic diuresis and eliminates free water safely and effectively [141].

A potent intravenous non-peptide V_1/V_2 receptor antagonist, conivaptan, that blocks the antidiuretic effect of vasopressin has been approved for use in humans. Oral V_2-specific vasopressin antagonists (tolvaptan, lixivaptan, satavaptan) capable of blocking the antidiuretic effect of vasopressin have been developed and tested in humans. They appear to be safe and effective in promoting a gradual water diuresis and raising the plasma sodium in adults with SIADH [103,126,127] but they have not been studied in children.

Severe or symptomatic hyponatremia

Brain edema can result in decreased cerebral blood flow, hypoxic brain injury, herniation and cardiopulmonary arrest. Symptomatic hyponatremia is a medical emergency, requiring prompt treatment to prevent permanent brain damage or death. Fluid restriction should be instituted but hypertonic saline should also be used to begin an immediate rise in serum sodium, because of the risk of central pontine myelinolysis, hypertonic saline (3% saline at a rate of 1–2 mL/kg/h) should be used only to the extent necessary to raise plasma sodium until acute symptoms resolve and then at only 1–2 mmol/L/h. Some [142] but not all [143] advocate concomitant furosemide therapy. If hyponatremia is of long-standing, hypertonic saline treatment must be undertaken with particular caution and correction rates of 0.5–1 mmol/L/h may be more appropriate. Urine output as well as plasma sodium should be monitored at least every 2 h during hypertonic saline infusion and every 2–4 h during subsequent fluid restriction.

Once symptoms associated with hyponatremia have remitted, hypertonic saline should be stopped and further correction achieved with fluid restriction alone, with fluid rates sufficient to produce sodium increases no greater than 0.5 mmol/L/h and limited to 10–12 mmol in any 24-h period. Following the rapid correction phase, this may mean that no further increase in sodium is attempted during the first 24 h of care. Normal saline alone is not appropriate for the treatment of severe hyponatremia in SIADH because the sodium infused will be excreted rapidly while water is retained, potentially worsening the hyponatremia.

Overtreatment. During treatment of severe chronic hyponatremia, overtreatment leading to an increase in sodium above 10–12 mmol/L/24 h may occur despite careful monitoring. If overcorrection is associated with a change in mental state, suggesting possible brain injury or is greater than 15 mmol/L/24 h, it may be appropriate to lower the sodium again to levels at which the patient's symptoms improve or the daily increase in sodium remains below 10 mmol/L/24 h. This can be accomplished with infusion of 5% dextrose or 5% dextrose following administration of dDAVP if the SIADH has resolved. Once the patient has stabilized at the lower sodium, the process of correction can be restarted at a slower rate.

Appropriately increased secretion of vasopressin
Hypovolemic hyponatremia

Osmotically inappropriate but physiologically appropriate thirst and vasopressin secretion occur during large reductions in extracellular volume or blood pressure. The syndrome of hypovolemic hyponatremia can result from a number of salt- and water-depleting diseases, such as severe gastroenteritis, renal tubular acidosis, salt-wasting nephropathy, chronic pyelonephritis, deficiency of aldosterone or aldosterone action and during diuretic therapy.

Primary water depletion

Diseases such as gastroenteritis cause a fall in renal GFR that results in an increase in proximal tubular sodium and water reabsorption with a concomitant decrease in distal tubular water excretion. This, with the associated stimulation of the renin-angiotensin-aldosterone system and suppression of atrial natriuretic peptide secretion by decreased vascular volume, results in the excretion of concentrated urine very low in sodium. As dehydration progresses, hypovolemia and/or hypotension become major stimuli for vasopressin release, even in the presence of hypotonicity.

These responses, although they preserve volume, can cause hyponatremia, especially if water replacement in excess of salt replacement is given. Hyponatremia may be evident from increased heart rate and decreased skin turgor and laboratory studies will show hemoconcentration and elevated BUN but the diagnosis may be subtle and urine sodium concentration can be very helpful. It should be low in dehydration- or salt loss-associated hyponatremia (<10–20 mmol/L) in the absence of diuretic use or renal disease.

In contrast to the hyponatremia associated with SIADH, patients with systemic dehydration should be rehydrated with isotonic salt-containing fluids, such as normal saline or lactated Ringer's solution. As of activation of the renin–angiotensin–aldosterone system, the administered sodium will be avidly conserved and a water diuresis will ensue as volume is restored and vasopressin concentrations fall. Hypernatremic fluid administration should not be needed in this situation. As in SIADH, care must be taken to prevent too rapid correction of hyponatremia to avoid central pontine myelinolysis by controlling the rate of fluid administration if the hyponatremia has been prolonged.

Primary sodium deficiency

When salt loss exceeds intake, sodium deficiency can result in hyponatremia. Salt loss from the kidney can result from primary renal diseases, such as congenital polycystic kidney disease, acute interstitial nephritis, chronic renal failure, deficient mineralocorticoid secretion or action and diuretic use. Primary salt loss can occur from the skin in patients with burns or cystic fibrosis. An imbalance between sodium intake and output can also occur as a result of insufficient nutritional sodium intake, although this is less common.

Early in salt deficiency, hyponatremia is countered by suppression of vasopressin release, which results in increased water excretion. With continuing salt loss, hypovolemia develops, resulting in non-osmotic stimulation of vasopressin. Hypovolemia leads to increased thirst and the ingestion of fluids with low solute content contributes to the hyponatremia.

Dehydration is often evident, as is the cause of sodium-wasting but, if thirst is intact and fluid intake is not interrupted oral intake may partially correct the volume deficit and evidence of hypovolemia may be subtle. If the kidney is the site of salt loss, hyponatremia may be accompanied by high urine sodium content, which would otherwise be unexpected in hypovolemic hyponatremia, so assessment of renal function is a vital component of the evaluation of hyponatremia.

Aldosterone deficiency or pseudohypoaldosteronism present special cases of hypovolemic hyponatremia with hyperkalemia. In addition to congenital pseudohypoaldosteronism, aldosterone resistance can be seen in urinary tract obstruction or infection. As in other forms of renal salt-wasting, urinary sodium excretion is inappropriately high.

Patients with hyponatremia due to salt loss require isotonic saline replacement and ongoing supplementation with sodium chloride and fluids. Intravenous fluids can be followed by oral salt supplementation and oral hydration when the patient is clinically stable. If salt loss is significant and ongoing and the hyponatremia is severe, hypertonic saline may be used to raise the sodium more quickly. As with SIADH, hypertonic therapy should be used only until symptoms resolve.

Hypervolemic hyponatremia

Severe low output congestive heart failure, advanced liver cirrhosis with ascites and nephrotic syndrome are all characterized by increased total body sodium and water, resulting in peripheral edema. They decrease "effective" intravascular volume due to decreased cardiac output and/or reduction in blood volume caused by a shift of salt and water from plasma to the interstitial space. As with systemic dehydration, the renin-angiotensin-aldosterone system is stimulated and water and salt excretion by the kidney is reduced. As the disease progresses, decreases in baroreceptor stimulation result in a compensatory increase in vasopressin secretion, leading to a further reduction in water clearance. If water intake is not restricted, hyponatremia can develop and hyponatremia in these clinical situations is common, although severe hyponatremia is rare.

In patients with impaired cardiac output and elevated atrial or ventricular volume (e.g. congestive heart failure or lung disease), atrial and/or brain natriuretic peptide concentrations are elevated, which can contribute to hyponatremia by promoting natriuresis. On evaluation of hypervolemic hyponatremia, urinary sodium is usually low and urea, creatinine and urate are increased, because of the reduction in effective blood volume and GFR. The presence of a predisposing disease and edema distinguishes this form of hyponatremia from that associated with systemic hypovolemia.

This type of hyponatremia is often mild, may be asymptomatic and may not need treatment but it is associated with a poor prognosis in patients with cirrhosis and congestive heart failure (CHF). Although this may reflect the fact that patients with the most severe disease are at greatest risk of hyponatremia, it also raises the possibility that hyponatremia may itself contribute to a poor outcome. This is particularly true in CHF, where hyponatremia can have direct effects on myocardial contractility. This has resulted in an increased interest in identifying effective ways of treating hypervolemic hyponatremia, which can be difficult to reverse.

When possible the underlying disease should be treated, but often this is not possible. Fluid and salt restriction and diuretics are commonly used but can worsen hyponatremia. Fluid restriction can be very difficult to maintain because the intravascular volume depletion contributes to increased thirst. Use of twice-daily hypertonic saline infusion with high-dose loop diuretic and fluid restriction to 1 L/day has been shown to increase serum sodium and improve outcome in refractory CHF [144].

Vasopressin V_2 receptor antagonists have been studied in the treatment of CHF and cirrhosis-induced hyponatremia. In animal models, the antagonists produce a water diuresis and increase serum sodium. When studied over short periods in humans, they are effective in increasing urine output and plasma sodium in both CHF [145] and cirrhosis [146] and do so at doses that do not produce hypernatremia or a clinically significant worsening of intravascular volume depletion but, during therapy for hypervolemic hyponatremia with these antagonists, endogenous vasopressin levels become further elevated and additional study is needed to determine whether this leads to increased stimulation of the V_1 receptor, which could be counterproductive in CHF.

dDAVP stimulates von Willebrand factor, factor VIIIa and tissue plasminogen activator through vasopressin V_2R, so it is possible that use of the vasopressin V_2R antagonists might increase the risk of bleeding in individuals with hepatic disease already at risk as of portal hypertension and/or impaired hepatic protein synthesis.

As with SIADH, acute treatment of symptomatic hyponatremia can be accomplished with hypertonic saline but the underlying disorder makes it difficult to maintain the administered fluid within the intravascular space. Furthermore, patients with cardiac disease administered hypertonic saline may require concomitant treatment with a diuretic such as furosemide to prevent worsening of heart failure and already have increased natriuretic peptide levels. Both of these increase natriuresis and make correction more difficult. Frequent monitoring of sodium and fluid balance is critical and, once symptoms have been controlled, therapy should be adjusted so that the hyponatremia is corrected slowly to avoid the risk of neurological injury associated with rapid correction.

Other causes of hyponatremia
Water intoxication

Water intoxication in the absence of disease is rare and seen primarily in psychogenic polydipsia, as adults with normal solute

Table 15.5 Comparison of findings in syndrome of inappropriate ADH secretion (SIADH), cerebral salt-wasting (CSW) and central diabetes insipidus (CDI).

	SIADH	CSW	CDI
Plasma volume	↑	↓	↓
Clinical evidence of volume depletion	–	+	+
Serum sodium/osmolality	↓	↓	↑
Urine sodium/osmolality	↑	↑↑	↓
Urine flow rate	↓	↑↑	↑
Plasma renin activity	↓	↓	↑
Plasma aldosterone concentration	↓ or →	↓	↑
Plasma AVP concentration	↑	↑ or →	↓
BUN/creatinine	↓/↓	↑/↑	↓/↑
Hematocrit	↓	↑	↑
Albumin concentration	↓	↑	↑
Serum uric acid concentration	↓	↓ or ›	↑
Plasma ANP or BNP concentration	↑	↑	↓
Treatment	Fluid restriction	Salt and fluid replacement	Salt-poor fluid replacement

ANP, atrial natriuretic peptide; AVP, arginine vasopressin; BNP, brain natriuretic peptide; BUN, blood urea nitrogen.

intake and the ability to produce a maximally dilute urine can theoretically ingest up to 20 L/day without becoming hyponatremic. Infants are at increased risk of water intoxication, as they have a decreased ability to produce a dilute urine. As infants take their nutrition in liquid form and hunger can overcome hypotonic inhibition of drinking, hungry infants will accept low-solute fluids even in the face of falling serum osmolality. As a result, infants fed overly dilute formula or water in place of formula are at risk of water intoxication.

Cerebral salt-wasting

Following CNS injury, a syndrome of hyponatremia associated with increased urine sodium concentration, increased urine volume and volume depletion known as cerebral salt-wasting (CSW) can develop. This is associated with primary renal salt losses in the absence of primary renal disease. It is critical to distinguish CSW from the two other major disturbances of water metabolism that can occur associated with CNS injury: DI and SIADH. Each of these shares some clinical features (Table 15.5), yet the distinction between them is of considerable clinical importance, given the wholly divergent nature of the treatments. Fluid restriction is the treatment of choice for SIADH, whereas the treatment of CSW involves vigorous sodium and volume replacement and DI requires volume replacement with fluids of low salt content. DI and CSW can be distinguished easily by measuring serum sodium. Determination of volume status is the key to distinguishing SIADH from CSW.

CSW follows subarachnoid hemorrhage and numerous other CNS perturbations. In children, these include CNS tumor resection, severe closed head injury, craniofacial surgery, hydrocephalus and stroke. There is now considerable evidence that the hyponatremia associated with CSW is related to hypersecretion of atrial and/or brain natriuretic peptide, which is presumed to drive the inappropriate natriuresis [147]. Apparently inconsistent with the clinical evidence of hypovolemia, renin and aldosterone levels are frequently low, presumably because of natriuretic peptide inhibition. Low aldosterone levels further promote salt loss but renin and aldosterone suppression are also present in SIADH as a result of volume expansion and are therefore not useful in distinguishing these entities, even if measurements were available immediately.

Clinical differentiation of the syndromes requires careful attention to urine output and volume status. Findings that support a diagnosis of CSW include orthostatic changes in blood pressure and pulse, dry mucous membranes, weight loss and negative fluid balance with urinary sodium >150 meq/L. Useful laboratory findings are hemoconcentration, with increased hematocrit or albumin and increased BUN/creatinine.

CSW is transient but appropriate management while it persists involves vigorous administration of intravenous isotonic saline solutions. As this therapy would be expected to worsen hyponatremia in SIADH and worsen hypernatremia in DI, the diagnosis and clinical and laboratory markers of volume status and serum osmolality should be reassessed frequently during therapy. As might be expected with inappropriately low aldosterone, the efficacy of hypervolemic therapy appears to be improved by administration of fludrocortisone to inhibit natriuresis [148].

References

1 Friis-Hansen B. Water distribution in the foetus and newborn infant. *Acta Paediatr Scand Suppl* 1983; **305**: 7–11.

2 Fomon SJ, Nelson SE. Body composition of the male and female reference infants. *Annu Rev Nutr* 2002; **22**: 1–17.

3 Aperia A, Zetterstrom R. Renal control of fluid homeostasis in the newborn infant. *Clin Perinatol* 1982; **9**: 523–533.

4 Lolait SJ, O'Carroll AM, McBride OW, Konig M, Morel A, Brownstein MJ. Cloning and characterization of a vasopressin V2 receptor and possible link to nephrogenic diabetes insipidus. *Nature* 1992; **357**: 336–339.

5 Summar ML, Phillips JA 3rd, Battey J, Castiglione CM, Kidd KK, Maness KJ, *et al*. Linkage relationships of human arginine vasopressin-neurophysin-II and oxytocin-neurophysin-I to prodynorphin and other loci on chromosome 20. *Mol Endocrinol* 1990; **4**: 947–950.

6 Sausville E, Carney D, Battey J. The human vasopressin gene is linked to the oxytocin gene and is selectively expressed in a cultured lung cancer cell line. *J Biol Chem* 1985; **260**: 10236–10241.

7 Mohr E, Bahnsen U, Kiessling C, Richter D. Expression of the vasopressin and oxytocin genes in rats occurs in mutually exclusive sets of hypothalamic neurons. *FEBS Lett* 1988; **242**: 144–148.

8 Arvan P, Castle D. Sorting and storage during secretory granule biogenesis: looking backward and looking forward. *Biochem J* 1998; **332** (Pt 3): 593–610.

9 Eubanks S, Nguyen TL, Deeb R, Villafania A, Alfadhli A, Breslow E. Effects of diabetes insipidus mutations on neurophysin folding and function. *J Biol Chem* 2001; **276**: 29671–29680.

10 Deeb R, Breslow E. Thermodynamic role of the pro region of the neurophysin precursor in neurophysin folding: evidence from the effects of ligand peptides on folding. *Biochemistry* 1996; **35**: 864–873.

11 Breslow E, Mombouyran V, Deeb R, Zheng C, Rose JP, Wang BC, *et al*. Structural basis of neurophysin hormone specificity: geometry, polarity and polarizability in aromatic ring interactions. *Protein Sci* 1999; **8**: 820–831.

12 Moses AM, Miller M. Accumulation and release of pituitary vasopressin in rats heterozygous for hypothalamic diabetes insipidus. *Endocrinology* 1970; **86**: 34–41.

13 Vavra I, Machova A, Holecek V, Cort JH, Zaoral M, Sorm F. Effect of a synthetic analogue of vasopressin in animals and in patients with diabetes insipidus. *Lancet* 1968; **1**: 948–952.

14 Lang J, Schafer K. [The origin and ramifications of the intracavernous section of the internal carotid artery]. *Gegenbaurs Morphol Jahrb* 1976; **122**: 182–202.

15 Antoni FA. Vasopressinergic control of pituitary adrenocorticotropin secretion comes of age. *Front Neuroendocrinol* 1993; **14**: 76–122.

16 Thrasher TN, Keil LC, Ramsay DJ. Lesions of the organum vasculosum of the lamina terminalis (OVLT) attenuate osmotically-induced drinking and vasopressin secretion in the dog. *Endocrinology* 1982; **110**: 1837–1839.

17 Iovino M, Steardo L. Vasopressin release to central and peripheral angiotensin II in rats with lesions of the subfornical organ. *Brain Res* 1984; **322**: 365–368.

18 Zerbe RL, Miller JZ, Robertson GL. The reproducibility and heritability of individual differences in osmoregulatory function in normal human subjects. *J Lab Clin Med* 1991; **117**: 51–59.

19 Robertson GL. The regulation of vasopressin function in health and disease. *Recent Prog Horm Res* 1976; **33**: 333–385.

20 Robertson GL, Shelton RL, Athar S. The osmoregulation of vasopressin. *Kidney Int* 1976; **10**: 25–37.

21 Hammer M, Ladefoged J, Olgaard K. Relationship between plasma osmolality and plasma vasopressin in human subjects. *Am J Physiol* 1980; **238**: E313–317.

22 Zerbe RL, Robertson GL. Osmoregulation of thirst and vasopressin secretion in human subjects: effect of various solutes. *Am J Physiol* 1983; **244**: E607–614.

23 Vokes TP, Aycinena PR, Robertson GL. Effect of insulin on osmoregulation of vasopressin. *Am J Physiol* 1987; **252** (4 Pt 1): E538–548.

24 Thrasher TN. Baroreceptor regulation of vasopressin and renin secretion: low-pressure versus high-pressure receptors. *Front Neuroendocrinol* 1994; **15**: 157–196.

25 Robertson GL, Athar S. The interaction of blood osmolality and blood volume in regulating plasma vasopressin in man. *J Clin Endocrinol Metab* 1976; **42**: 613–620.

26 Robertson GL, Athar S. Osmotic control of vasopressin function. In: Andreoli TE, Grantham JJ, Rector FC, eds. *Disturbances in Body Fluid Osmolality*. Bethesda: American Physiological Society; distributed by Williams & Wilkins, 1977: 125.

27 Koch KL, Summy-Long J, Bingaman S, Sperry N, Stern RM. Vasopressin and oxytocin responses to illusory self-motion and nausea in man. *J Clin Endocrinol Metab* 1990; **71**: 1269–1275.

28 Seckl JR, Johnson M, Shakespear C, Lightman SL. Endogenous opioids inhibit oxytocin release during nicotine-stimulated secretion of vasopressin in man. *Clin Endocrinol (Oxf)* 1988; **28**: 509–514.

29 Wolff K, Tsapakis EM, Winstock AR, Hartley D, Holt D, Forsling ML, *et al*. Vasopressin and oxytocin secretion in response to the consumption of ecstasy in a clubbing population. *J Psychopharmacol* 2006; **20**: 400–410.

30 Oelkers W. Hyponatremia and inappropriate secretion of vasopressin (antidiuretic hormone) in patients with hypopituitarism. *N Engl J Med* 1989; **321**: 492–496.

31 Green HH, Harrington AR, Valtin H. On the role of antidiuretic hormone in the inhibition of acute water diuresis in adrenal insufficiency and the effects of gluco- and mineralocorticoids in reversing the inhibition. *J Clin Invest* 1970; **49**: 1724–1736.

32 Viinamaki O, Erkkola R, Kanto J. Plasma vasopressin concentrations and serum vasopressinase activity in pregnant and nonpregnant women. *Biol Res Pregnancy Perinatol* 1986; **7**: 17–19.

33 Iwasaki Y, Oiso Y, Kondo K, Takagi S, Takatsuki K, Hasegawa H, *et al*. Aggravation of subclinical diabetes insipidus during pregnancy. *N Engl J Med* 1991; **324**: 522–526.

34 Kennedy S, Hall PM, Seymour AE, Hague WM. Transient diabetes insipidus and acute fatty liver of pregnancy. *Br J Obstet Gynaecol* 1994; **101**: 387–391.

35 Katz VL, Bowes WA Jr. Transient diabetes insipidus and preeclampsia. *South Med J* 1987; **80**: 524–525.

36 Durr JA, Hoggard JG, Hunt JM, Schrier RW. Diabetes insipidus in pregnancy associated with abnormally high circulating vasopressinase activity. *N Engl J Med* 1987; **316**: 1070–1074.

37 Jard S. Vasopressin receptors: a historical survey. *Adv Exp Med Biol* 1998; **449**: 1–13.

38 Lolait SJ, O'Carroll AM, Brownstein MJ. Molecular biology of vasopressin receptors. *Ann N Y Acad Sci* 1995; **771**: 273–292.

39 Frattini A, Zucchi I, Villa A, Patrosso C, Repetto M, Susani L, *et al*. Type 2 vasopressin receptor gene, the gene responsible nephrogenic diabetes insipidus, maps to Xq28 close to the LICAM gene. *Biochem Biophys Res Commun* 1993; **193**: 864–871.

40 Ostrowski NL, Lolait SJ, Bradley DJ, O'Carroll AM, Brownstein MJ, Young WS 3rd. Distribution of V1a and V2 vasopressin receptor

messenger ribonucleic acids in rat liver, kidney, pituitary and brain. *Endocrinology* 1992; **131**: 533–535.

41 Hirsch AT, Dzau VJ, Majzoub JA, Creager MA. Vasopressin-mediated forearm vasodilation in normal humans: evidence for a vascular vasopressin V2 receptor. *J Clin Invest* 1989; **84**: 418–426.

42 Johnson EM, Theler JM, Capponi AM, Vallotton MB. Characterization of oscillations in cytosolic free Ca^{2+} concentration and measurement of cytosolic Na^+ concentration changes evoked by angiotensin II and vasopressin in individual rat aortic smooth muscle cells: use of microfluorometry and digital imaging. *J Biol Chem* 1991; **266**: 12618–12626.

43 Aguilera G. Regulation of pituitary ACTH secretion during chronic stress. *Front Neuroendocrinol* 1994; **15**: 321–350.

44 Wersinger SR, Ginns EI, O'Carroll AM, Lolait SJ, Young WS 3rd. Vasopressin V1b receptor knockout reduces aggressive behavior in male mice. *Mol Psychiatry* 2002; **7**: 975–984.

45 Harris HW Jr, Strange K, Zeidel ML. Current understanding of the cellular biology and molecular structure of the antidiuretic hormone-stimulated water transport pathway. *J Clin Invest* 1991; **88**: 1–8.

46 Harris HW, Paredes A, Zeidel ML. The molecular structure of the antidiuretic hormone elicited water channel. *Pediatr Nephrol* 1993; **7**: 680–684.

47 Fushimi K, Sasaki S, Marumo F. Phosphorylation of serine 256 is required for cAMP-dependent regulatory exocytosis of the aquaporin-2 water channel. *J Biol Chem* 1997; **272**: 14800–14804.

48 Knepper MA. Molecular physiology of urinary concentrating mechanism: regulation of aquaporin water channels by vasopressin. *Am J Physiol* 1997; **272** (1 Pt 2): F3–12.

49 Oksche A, Rosenthal W. The molecular basis of nephrogenic diabetes insipidus. *J Mol Med* 1998; **76**: 326–337.

50 Ma T, Song Y, Yang B, Gillespie A, Carlson EJ, Epstein CJ, *et al.* Nephrogenic diabetes insipidus in mice lacking aquaporin-3 water channels. *Proc Natl Acad Sci U S A* 2000; **97**: 4386–4391.

51 Ma T, Yang B, Gillespie A, Carlson EJ, Epstein CJ, Verkman AS. Generation and phenotype of a transgenic knockout mouse lacking the mercurial-insensitive water channel aquaporin-4. *J Clin Invest* 1997; **100**: 957–962.

52 Schnermann J, Chou CL, Ma T, Traynor T, Knepper MA, Verkman AS. Defective proximal tubular fluid reabsorption in transgenic aquaporin-1 null mice. *Proc Natl Acad Sci U S A* 1998; **95**: 9660–9664.

53 Preston GM, Smith BL, Zeidel ML, Moulds JJ, Agre P. Mutations in aquaporin-1 in phenotypically normal humans without functional CHIP water channels. *Science* 1994; **265**: 1585–1587.

54 Robertson GL. Thirst and vasopressin function in normal and disordered states of water balance. *J Lab Clin Med* 1983; **101**: 351–371.

55 Kucharczyk J, Mogenson GJ. Separate lateral hypothalamic pathways for extracellular and intracellular thirst. *Am J Physiol* 1975; **228**: 295–301.

56 Phillips MI. Functions of angiotensin in the central nervous system. *Annu Rev Physiol* 1987; **49**: 413–435.

57 Gruber KA, Wilkin LD, Johnson AK. Neurohypophyseal hormone release and biosynthesis in rats with lesions of the anteroventral third ventricle (AV3V) region. *Brain Res* 1986; **378**: 115–119.

58 Salata RA, Verbalis JG, Robinson AG. Cold water stimulation of oropharyngeal receptors in man inhibits release of vasopressin. *J Clin Endocrinol Metab* 1987; **65**: 561–567.

59 Thrasher TN. Volume receptors and the stimulation of water intake. In: Ramsay DJ, Booth DA, eds. *Thirst: Physiological and Psychological Aspects.* London, New York: Springer-Verlag; 1991: 93–107.

60 Quinn SJ, Williams GH. Regulation of aldosterone secretion. *Annu Rev Physiol* 1988; **50**: 409–426.

61 Morris DJ. The metabolism and mechanism of action of aldosterone. *Endocr Rev* 1981; **2**: 234–247.

62 Chartier L, Schiffrin EL. Atrial natriuretic peptide inhibits the effect of endogenous angiotensin II on plasma aldosterone in conscious sodium-depleted rats. *Clin Sci (Lond)* 1987; **72**: 31–5.

63 Rebuffat P, Mazzocchi G, Gottardo G, Nussdorfer GG. Further studies on the involvement of dopamine and somatostatin in the inhibitory control of the growth and steroidogenic capacity of rat adrenal zona glomerulosa. *Exp Clin Endocrinol* 1989; **93**: 73–81.

64 Simpson JB. The circumventricular organs and the central actions of angiotensin. *Neuroendocrinology* 1981; **32**: 248–256.

65 Saavedra JM. Brain and pituitary angiotensin. *Endocr Rev* 1992; **13**: 329–380.

66 Garbers DL, Koesling D, Schultz G. Guanylyl cyclase receptors. *Mol Biol Cell* 1994; **5**: 1–5.

67 Maack T, Suzuki M, Almeida FA, Nussenzveig D, Scarborough RM, McEnroe GA, *et al.* Physiological role of silent receptors of atrial natriuretic factor. *Science* 1987; **238**: 675–678.

68 de Bold AJ, Borenstein HB, Veress AT, Sonnenberg H. A rapid and potent natriuretic response to intravenous injection of atrial myocardial extract in rats. *Life Sci* 1981; **28**: 89–94.

69 Espiner EA. Physiology of natriuretic peptides. *J Intern Med* 1994; **235**: 527–541.

70 Gundlach AL, Knobe KE. Distribution of preproatrial natriuretic peptide mRNA in rat brain detected by *in situ* hybridization of DNA oligonucleotides: enrichment in hypothalamic and limbic regions. *J Neurochem* 1992; **59**: 758–761.

71 Sudoh T, Kangawa K, Minamino N, Matsuo H. A new natriuretic peptide in porcine brain. *Nature* 1988; **332**: 78–81.

72 Herman JP, Langub MC Jr, Watson RE Jr. Localization of C-type natriuretic peptide mRNA in rat hypothalamus. *Endocrinology* 1993; **133**: 1903–1906.

73 Zerbe RL, Robertson GL. A comparison of plasma vasopressin measurements with a standard indirect test in the differential diagnosis of polyuria. *N Engl J Med* 1981; **305**: 1539–1546.

74 Koskimies O, Pylkkanen J, Vilska J. Water intoxication in infants caused by the urine concentration test with vasopressin analogue (dDAVP). *Acta Paediatr Scand* 1984; **73**: 131–132.

75 Elias PC, Elias LL, Torres N, Moreira AC, Antunes-Rodrigues J, Castro M. Progressive decline of vasopressin secretion in familial autosomal dominant neurohypophyseal diabetes insipidus presenting a novel mutation in the vasopressin-neurophysin II gene. *Clin Endocrinol (Oxf)* 2003; **59**: 511–518.

76 Nijenhuis M, Zalm R, Burbach JP. Mutations in the vasopressin prohormone involved in diabetes insipidus impair endoplasmic reticulum export but not sorting. *J Biol Chem* 1999; **274**: 21200–21208.

77 Green JR, Buchan GC, Alvord EC Jr, Swanson AG. Hereditary and idiopathic types of diabetes insipidus. *Brain* 1967; **90**: 707–714.

78 Willcutts MD, Felner E, White PC. Autosomal recessive familial neurohypophyseal diabetes insipidus with continued secretion of mutant weakly active vasopressin. *Hum Mol Genet* 1999; **8**: 1303–1307.

79 Christensen JH, Siggaard C, Corydon TJ, Robertson GL, Gregersen N, Bolund L, et al. Differential cellular handling of defective arginine vasopressin (AVP) prohormones in cells expressing mutations of the AVP gene associated with autosomal dominant and recessive familial neurohypophyseal diabetes insipidus. *J Clin Endocrinol Metab* 2004; **89**: 4521–4531.

80 Minton JA, Rainbow LA, Ricketts C, Barrett TG. Wolfram syndrome. *Rev Endocr Metab Disord* 2003; **4**: 53–59.

81 Strom TM, Hortnagel K, Hofmann S, Gekeler F, Scharfe C, Rabl W, et al. Diabetes insipidus, diabetes mellitus, optic atrophy and deafness (DIDMOAD) caused by mutations in a novel gene (wolframin) coding for a predicted transmembrane protein. *Hum Mol Genet* 1998; **7**: 2021–2028.

82 Amr S, Heisey C, Zhang M, Xia XJ, Shows KH, Ajlouni K, et al. A homozygous mutation in a novel zinc-finger protein, ERIS, is responsible for Wolfram syndrome 2. *Am J Hum Genet* 2007; **81**: 673–683.

83 Rotig A, Cormier V, Chatelain P, Francois R, Saudubray JM, Rustin P, et al. Deletion of mitochondrial DNA in a case of early-onset diabetes mellitus, optic atrophy and deafness (Wolfram syndrome, MIM 222300). *J Clin Invest* 1993; **91**: 1095–1098.

84 Barrientos A, Volpini V, Casademont J, Genis D, Manzanares JM, Ferrer I, et al. A nuclear defect in the 4p16 region predisposes to multiple mitochondrial DNA deletions in families with Wolfram syndrome. *J Clin Invest* 1996; **97**: 1570–1576.

85 Dattani MT, Martinez-Barbera JP, Thomas PQ, Brickman JM, Gupta R, Martensson IL, et al. Mutations in the homeobox gene HESX1/Hesx1 associated with septo-optic dysplasia in human and mouse. *Nat Genet* 1998; **19**: 125–133.

86 McNay DE, Turton JP, Kelberman D, Woods KS, Brauner R, Papadimitriou A, et al. HESX1 mutations are an uncommon cause of septooptic dysplasia and hypopituitarism. *J Clin Endocrinol Metab* 2007; **92**: 691–697.

87 Appignani B, Landy H, Barnes P. MR in idiopathic central diabetes insipidus of childhood. *AJNR Am J Neuroradiol* 1993; **14**: 1407–1410.

88 Alter CA, Bilaniuk LT. Utility of magnetic resonance imaging in the evaluation of the child with central diabetes insipidus. *J Pediatr Endocrinol Metab* 2002; **15** (Suppl 2): 681–687.

89 Seckl JR, Dunger DB, Bevan JS, Nakasu Y, Chowdrey C, Burke CW, et al. Vasopressin antagonist in early postoperative diabetes insipidus. *Lancet* 1990; **335**: 1353–1356.

90 Broadbent V, Pritchard J. Diabetes insipidus associated with Langerhans cell histiocytosis: is it reversible? *Med Pediatr Oncol* 1997; **28**: 289–293.

91 Dunger DB, Broadbent V, Yeoman E, Seckl JR, Lightman SL, Grant DB, et al. The frequency and natural history of diabetes insipidus in children with Langerhans-cell histiocytosis. *N Engl J Med* 1989; **321**: 1157–1562.

92 Howarth DM, Gilchrist GS, Mullan BP, Wiseman GA, Edmonson JH, Schomberg PJ. Langerhans cell histiocytosis: diagnosis, natural history, management and outcome. *Cancer* 1999; **85**: 2278–2290.

93 Konrad D, Gartenmann M, Martin E, Schoenle EJ. Central diabetes insipidus as the first manifestation of neurosarcoidosis in a 10-year-old girl. *Horm Res* 2000; **54**: 98–100.

94 Pivonello R, De Bellis A, Faggiano A, Di Salle F, Petretta M, Di Somma C, et al. Central diabetes insipidus and autoimmunity: relationship between the occurrence of antibodies to arginine vasopressin-secreting cells and clinical, immunological and radiological features in a large cohort of patients with central diabetes insipidus of known and unknown etiology. *J Clin Endocrinol Metab* 2003; **88**: 1629–1636.

95 De Bellis A, Bizzarro A, Amoresano Paglionico V, Di Martino S, Criscuolo T, Sinisi AA, et al. Detection of vasopressin cell antibodies in some patients with autoimmune endocrine diseases without overt diabetes insipidus. *Clin Endocrinol (Oxf)* 1994; **40**: 173–177.

96 Charmandari E, Brook CG. 20 years of experience in idiopathic central diabetes insipidus. *Lancet* 1999; **353**: 2212–2213.

97 Green RP, Landt M. Home sodium monitoring in patients with diabetes insipidus. *J Pediatr* 2002; **141**: 618–624.

98 Pogacar PR, Mahnke S, Rivkees SA. Management of central diabetes insipidus in infancy with low renal solute load formula and chlorothiazide. *Curr Opin Pediatr* 2000; **12**: 405–411.

99 Lee YJ, Shen EY, Huang FY, Kao HA, Shyur SD. Continuous infusion of vasopressin in comatose children with neurogenic diabetes insipidus. *J Pediatr Endocrinol Metab* 1995; **8**: 257–262.

100 Niaudet P, Dechaux M, Leroy D, Broyer M. Nephrogenic diabetes insipidus in children. *Front Horm Res* 1985; **13**: 224–231.

101 Hoekstra JA, van Lieburg AF, Monnens LA, Hulstijn-Dirkmaat GM, Knoers VV. Cognitive and psychosocial functioning of patients with congenital nephrogenic diabetes insipidus. *Am J Med Genet* 1996; **61**: 81–88.

102 van Lieburg AF, Knoers NV, Monnens LA. Clinical presentation and follow-up of 30 patients with congenital nephrogenic diabetes insipidus. *J Am Soc Nephrol* 1999; **10**: 1958–1964.

103 Moses AM, Sangani G, Miller JL. Proposed cause of marked vasopressin resistance in a female with an X-linked recessive V2 receptor abnormality. *J Clin Endocrinol Metab* 1995; **80**: 1184–1186.

104 Bonnardeaux A, Bichet DG. Inherited disorders of the renal tubule. In: Brenner BM, Rector FC, eds. *Brenner & Rector's The Kidney*, 7th edn. Philadelphia, PA: Saunders, 2004: 1697–1741.

105 Faerch M, Christensen JH, Corydon TJ, Kamperis K, de Zegher F, Gregersen N, et al. Partial nephrogenic diabetes insipidus caused by a novel mutation in the AVPR2 gene. *Clin Endocrinol (Oxf)* 2008; **68**: 395–403.

106 Marr N, Bichet DG, Lonergan M, Arthus MF, Jeck N, Seyberth HW, et al. Heteroligomerization of an Aquaporin-2 mutant with wild-type Aquaporin-2 and their misrouting to late endosomes/lysosomes explains dominant nephrogenic diabetes insipidus. *Hum Mol Genet* 2002; **11**: 779–789.

107 Bichet DG. Molecular and cellular biology of vasopressin and oxytocin receptors and action in the kidney. *Curr Opin Nephrol Hypertens* 1994; **3**: 46–53.

108 Robben JH, Knoers NV, Deen PM. Cell biological aspects of the vasopressin type-2 receptor and aquaporin 2 water channel in nephrogenic diabetes insipidus. *Am J Physiol Renal Physiol* 2006; **291**: F257–270.

109 Earm JH, Christensen BM, Frokiaer J, Marples D, Han JS, Knepper MA, et al. Decreased aquaporin-2 expression and apical plasma membrane delivery in kidney collecting ducts of polyuric hypercalcemic rats. *J Am Soc Nephrol* 1998; **9**: 2181–2193.

110 Schrier RW, Cadnapaphornchai MA. Renal aquaporin water channels: from molecules to human disease. *Prog Biophys Mol Biol* 2003; **81**: 117–131.

111 Cesar KR, Magaldi AJ. Thiazide induces water absorption in the inner medullary collecting duct of normal and Brattleboro rats. *Am J Physiol* 1999; **277** (5 Part 2): F756–760.

112 Kirchlechner V, Koller DY, Seidl R, Waldhauser F. Treatment of nephrogenic diabetes insipidus with hydrochlorothiazide and amiloride. *Arch Dis Child* 1999; **80**: 548–552.

113 Ala Y, Morin D, Mouillac B, Sabatier N, Vargas R, Cotte N, et al. Functional studies of twelve mutant V2 vasopressin receptors related to nephrogenic diabetes insipidus: molecular basis of a mild clinical phenotype. *J Am Soc Nephrol* 1998; **9**: 1861–1872.

114 Batlle DC, von Riotte AB, Gaviria M, Grupp M. Amelioration of polyuria by amiloride in patients receiving long-term lithium therapy. *N Engl J Med* 1985; **312**: 408–414.

115 Morello JP, Salahpour A, Laperriere A, Bernier V, Arthus MF, Lonergan M, et al. Pharmacological chaperones rescue cell-surface expression and function of misfolded V2 vasopressin receptor mutants. *J Clin Invest* 2000; **105**: 887–895.

116 Bernier V, Lagace M, Lonergan M, Arthus MF, Bichet DG, Bouvier M. Functional rescue of the constitutively internalized V2 vasopressin receptor mutant R137H by the pharmacological chaperone action of SR49059. *Mol Endocrinol* 2004; **18**: 2074–2084.

117 Robertson GL. Dipsogenic diabetes insipidus: a newly recognized syndrome caused by a selective defect in the osmoregulation of thirst. *Trans Assoc Am Physicians* 1987; **100**: 241–249.

118 Perkins RM, Yuan CM, Welch PG. Dipsogenic diabetes insipidus: report of a novel treatment strategy and literature review. *Clin Exp Nephrol* 2006; **10**: 63–67.

119 Trachtman H. Cell volume regulation: a review of cerebral adaptive mechanisms and implications for clinical treatment of osmolal disturbances: II. *Pediatr Nephrol* 1992; **6**: 104–112.

120 De Petris L, Luchetti A, Emma F. Cell volume regulation and transport mechanisms across the blood–brain barrier: implications for the management of hypernatraemic states. *Eur J Pediatr* 2001; **160**: 71–77.

121 Arieff AI, Ayus JC, Fraser CL. Hyponatraemia and death or permanent brain damage in healthy children. *Br Med J* 1992; **304**: 1218–1222.

122 Arieff AI. Influence of hypoxia and sex on hyponatremic encephalopathy. *Am J Med* 2006; **119** (7 Suppl 1): S59–564.

123 Janicic N, Verbalis JG. Evaluation and management of hypo-osmolality in hospitalized patients. *Endocrinol Metab Clin North Am* 2003; **32**: 459–481, vii.

124 Kleinschmidt-DeMasters BK, Norenberg MD. Rapid correction of hyponatremia causes demyelination: relation to central pontine myelinolysis. *Science* 1981; **211**: 1068–1070.

125 Gross P, Reimann D, Neidel J, Doke C, Prospert F, Decaux G, et al. The treatment of severe hyponatremia. *Kidney Int Suppl* 1998; **64**: S6–11.

126 Ellison DH, Berl T. Clinical practice: the syndrome of inappropriate antidiuresis. *N Engl J Med* 2007; **356**: 2064–2072.

127 Van Amelsvoort T, Bakshi R, Devaux CB, Schwabe S. Hyponatremia associated with carbamazepine and oxcarbazepine therapy: a review. *Epilepsia* 1994; **35**: 181–188.

128 Weissman PN, Shenkman L, Gregerman RI. Chlorpropamide hyponatremia: drug-induced inappropriate antidiuretic-hormone activity. *N Engl J Med* 1971; **284**: 65–71.

129 Zavagli G, Ricci G, Tataranni G, Mapelli G, Abbasciano V. Life-threatening hyponatremia caused by vinblastine. *Med Oncol Tumor Pharmacother* 1988; **5**: 67–69.

130 Escuro RS, Adelstein DJ, Carter SG. Syndrome of inappropriate secretion of antidiuretic hormone after infusional vincristine. *Cleve Clin J Med* 1992; **59**: 643–644.

131 Liskin B, Walsh BT, Roose SP, Jackson W. Imipramine-induced inappropriate ADH secretion. *J Clin Psychopharmacol* 1984; **4**: 146–147.

132 Fallon JK, Shah D, Kicman AT, Hutt AJ, Henry JA, Cowan DA, et al. Action of MDMA (ecstasy) and its metabolites on arginine vasopressin release. *Ann N Y Acad Sci* 2002; **965**: 399–409.

133 Cotton MF, Donald PR, Schoeman JF, Aalbers C, Van Zyl LE, Lombard C. Plasma arginine vasopressin and the syndrome of inappropriate antidiuretic hormone secretion in tuberculous meningitis. *Pediatr Infect Dis J* 1991; **10**: 837–842.

134 Moritz ML, Ayus JC. Prevention of hospital-acquired hyponatremia: a case for using isotonic saline. *Pediatrics* 2003; **111**: 227–230.

135. Nakano M, Higa M, Ishikawa R, Yamazaki T, Yamamuro W. Hyponatremia with increased plasma antidiuretic hormone in a case of hypothyroidism. *Intern Med* 2000; **39**: 1075–1078.

136 Siegel AJ, Verbalis JG, Clement S, Mendelson JH, Mello NK, Adner M, et al. Hyponatremia in marathon runners due to inappropriate arginine vasopressin secretion. *Am J Med* 2007; **120**: 461, e11–117.

137 Feldman BJ, Rosenthal SM, Vargas GA, Fenwick RG, Huang EA, Matsuda-Abedini M, et al. Nephrogenic syndrome of inappropriate antidiuresis. *N Engl J Med* 2005; **352**: 1884–1890.

138 Baker EA, Tian Y, Adler S, Verbalis JG. Blood–brain barrier disruption and complement activation in the brain following rapid correction of chronic hyponatremia. *Exp Neurol* 2000; **165**: 221–230.

139 Anmuth CJ, Ross BW, Alexander MA, Reeves GD. Chronic syndrome of inappropriate secretion of antidiuretic hormone in a pediatric patient after traumatic brain injury. *Arch Phys Med Rehabil* 1993; **74**: 1219–1221.

140 Forrest JN, Jr., Cox M, Hong C, Morrison G, Bia M, Singer I. Superiority of demeclocycline over lithium in the treatment of chronic syndrome of inappropriate secretion of antidiuretic hormone. *N Engl J Med* 1978; **298**: 173–177.

141 Huang EA, Feldman BJ, Schwartz ID, Geller DH, Rosenthal SM, Gitelman SE. Oral urea for the treatment of chronic syndrome of inappropriate antidiuresis in children. *J Pediatr* 2006; **148**: 128–131.

142 Adrogue HJ, Madias NE. Hyponatremia. *N Engl J Med* 2000; **342**: 1581–1589.

143 Smith DM, McKenna K, Thompson CJ. Hyponatraemia. *Clin Endocrinol (Oxf)* 2000; **52**: 667–678.

144 Licata G, Di Pasquale P, Parrinello G, Cardinale A, Scandurra A, Follone G, et al. Effects of high-dose furosemide and small-volume hypertonic saline solution infusion in comparison with a high dose of furosemide as bolus in refractory congestive heart failure: long-term effects. *Am Heart J* 2003; **145**: 459–466.

145 LeJemtel TH, Serrano C. Vasopressin dysregulation: hyponatremia, fluid retention and congestive heart failure. *Int J Cardiol* 2007; **120**: 1–9.

146. Ferguson JW, Therapondos G, Newby DE, Hayes PC. Therapeutic role of vasopressin receptor antagonism in patients with liver cirrhosis. *Clin Sci (Lond)* 2003; **105**: 1–8.

147 Betjes MG. Hyponatremia in acute brain disease: the cerebral salt wasting syndrome. *Eur J Intern Med* 2002; **13**: 9–14.

148 Mori T, Katayama Y, Kawamata T, Hirayama T. Improved efficiency of hypervolemic therapy with inhibition of natriuresis by fludrocortisone in patients with aneurysmal subarachnoid hemorrhage. *J Neurosurg* 1999; **91**: 947–952.

149 Muglia LJ, Majzoub JA. Disorders of the posterior pituitary. In: Sperling M, ed. *Pediatric Endocrinology*, 2nd edn. Philadelphia: Saunders, 2002: 289–322.

150 Dunn FL, Brennan TJ, Nelson AE, Robertson GL. The role of blood osmolality and volume in regulating vasopressin secretion in the rat. *J Clin Invest* 1973; **52**: 3212–3219.

151 Robertson GL. Regulation of vasopressin secretion. In: Seldin DW, Giebisch GH, eds. *The Kidney: Physiology and Pathophysiology*. New York: Raven Press, 1985: 869–884.

152 Gross P, Ketteler M, Hausmann C, Reinhard C, Schomig A, Hackenthal E, *et al.* Role of diuretics, hormonal derangements and clinical setting of hyponatremia in medical patients. *Klin Wochenschr* 1988; **66**: 662–669.

16 The Parathyroid and Disorders of Calcium and Bone Metabolism

Jeremy Allgrove

Royal London Hospital and Great Ormond Street Hospital for Children, London, UK

Calcium and phosphate not only have a role in maintaining normal neuromuscular and cellular function but they also have a structural role as components of bone. Their physiology is complex and the mechanisms of homeostasis can be disrupted in many ways.

Many causes of mineral and bone disorders have a genetic basis. Many of the genetic conditions are rare but have value in shedding light on physiology. All the conditions and the genes that determine them are referred to by their Online Mendelian Inheritance in Man (OMIM) numbers so that further details and references can be obtained directly from http://www.ncbi.nlm.nih.gov/sites/entrez?db=OMIM.

Physiology of calcium metabolism

Cations and anions

Calcium

About 1200 g of calcium are present in a fully grown adult, of which 99% is in bone, the remainder circulating in three fractions. The ionized fraction, which constitutes about 50% of the total and is at a concentration of 1.1–1.3 mmol/L (4.4 and 5.2 mg/dL), determines neuromuscular function and is maintained by various endocrine factors. Approximately 40% circulates bound to albumin and conditions associated with hypoalbuminemia may reduce the total circulating concentration without affecting the ionized calcium. The remainder circulates as complexes with other molecules such as citrate and sulfate. The control of ionized calcium in plasma is mainly under the influence of parathyroid hormone (PTH) and 1,25-dihydroxyvitamin D [1,25(OH)$_2$D], both of which raise concentrations. Calcitonin (CT) and parathyroid hormone related peptide (PTHrP) have a lesser influence. Fibroblast growth factor 23 (FGF23) has a significant effect on phosphate metabolism.

Brook's Clinical Pediatric Endocrinology, 6th edition. Edited by C. Brook, P. Clayton, R. Brown. © 2009 Blackwell Publishing, ISBN: 978-1-4051-8080-1.

It is possible to measure ionized calcium directly, although this is not routinely available in most laboratories, which usually measure total calcium and albumin, often making an adjustment to allow for the albumin concentration. In practice, these adjustments usually have little clinical relevance unless severe hypoalbuminemia is present. A suitable estimate can be obtained from the formula:

$$Ca_{CORR} = Ca_{TOTAL} + (41 - [Alb]) * 0.017$$

where Ca_{TOTAL} is the observed total calcium (in mmol/L) and [Alb] is the plasma albumin in g/L (for calcium measured in mg/dL the albumin correction factor is 0.068).

Intestinal absorption, renal tubular reabsorption and equilibration with bone stores regulate plasma calcium by transport across intestinal and renal epithelial cells by paracellular and transcellular processes [1]. The paracellular mechanisms occur by the tight junctions, which are made up of a combination of proteins including, amongst others, the claudins: the most important, claudin 16 (*603959), also known as paracellin 1, facilitates the passive transport of calcium and magnesium across intestinal and renal tubular cells.

Active transcellular transport occurs by separate processes at the luminal surface, cytosolic transport and baso-lateral extrusion all influenced by different proteins. At the luminal surface, two members of the transient receptor potential (TRP) channel protein family, TRPV5 (*606679) and TRPV6 (*606680), act as "gatekeepers" facilitating the ingress of calcium into cells. They are inwardly rectifying calcium channels that have a greater affinity for calcium than magnesium. TRPV6 is probably the most important in the intestine and is stimulated by 1,25(OH)$_2$D. Cytosolic diffusion is facilitated by calbindin$_{28K}$ (*114050) and calbindin$_{9K}$ (*302020) which bind calcium and transport it across the cell cytoplasm. Extrusion of calcium at the baso-lateral surface is facilitated by an ATP-dependent Ca$^+$-ATPase (PMCA1b) (*108731) and a Na$^+$/Ca$^+$ exchanger (NCX1) (*182305). The former is more important in the small intestine and is under the influence of 1,25(OH)$_2$D. Absorption of calcium may be reduced by large quantities of calcium-binding agents such as phytate or oxalate.

Excretion is mainly by the kidney and increased by dietary factors including sodium, protein and acid load [2]. Most reabsorption occurs in the proximal tubule (70%) as a passive process in conjunction with sodium. Twenty percent is absorbed in the thick ascending loop of Henle by the same paracellular mechanism as in the intestine. Passive reabsorption occurs only where claudin 16 is present. The 5–10% reabsorbed in the distal tubule is under hormonal control [3] similar to that in the intestine but TRPV5 is more important at the luminal surface. Cytosolic diffusion is also facilitated by calbindins but, at the baso-lateral surface, NCX1 is more important and is under the influence of PTH (Fig. 16.1).

The highest proportion of ingested calcium is absorbed during the phases of rapid growth in infancy and adolescence when calcium absorption exceeds excretion sufficiently to allow for bone mineralization.

Urinary calcium excretion is measured by assessing the ratio of calcium to creatinine (Ca:Cr) in a mid-morning urine specimen and this should not normally exceed 0.7 mmol/mmol (0.25 mg/mg) [4]. Excess calcium excretion occurs in hypercalcemic conditions associated with hyperparathyroidism and vitamin D excess, as well as in those not associated with hypercalcemia such as activating mutations of the calcium-sensing receptor and distal renal tubular acidosis, all of which can cause nephrocalcinosis. Primary renal tubular disorders are also frequently associated with hypercalciuria and nephrocalcinosis or nephrolithiasis.

In contrast, hypercalcemia associated with inactivating mutations of the calcium-sensing receptor or hypocalcemia caused by hypoparathyroidism results in low urinary calcium excretion.

Magnesium

Magnesium circulates in plasma in a concentration of 0.7–1.2 mmol/L (1.7–2.9 mg/dL) and is necessary because adequate magnesium is required for normal PTH secretion. It is absorbed in the small intestine by paracellular and transcellular mechanisms similar to those of calcium but less well understood. Active transport across luminal cells is similar but transport across the luminal surface is probably facilitated by TRP proteins TRPM6 (*607009) and TRPM7 (*605692) which are different from those of calcium. One form of autosomal recessive hypomagnesemia with secondary hypocalciuria (HOMG1) (#602014) is probably caused by mutations in TRPM6 which has been mapped to chromosome 9p22. Passive absorption is not affected in this condition and calcium excretion is low.

Renal tubular transport also occurs by both paracellular and transcellular mechanisms. Following filtration by the glomerulus, passive reabsorption occurs along the ascending loop of Henle at the same sites as calcium. Mutations in the claudin 16 (paracellin 1) gene (*603959) result in impaired magnesium and calcium reabsorption and is a cause of hypomagnesemia, hypercalciuria and nephrocalcinosis (HOMG3) syndrome (#248250). In the collecting ducts, a similar tight junction protein, claudin 19 (*610036), permits transport of calcium and magnesium and

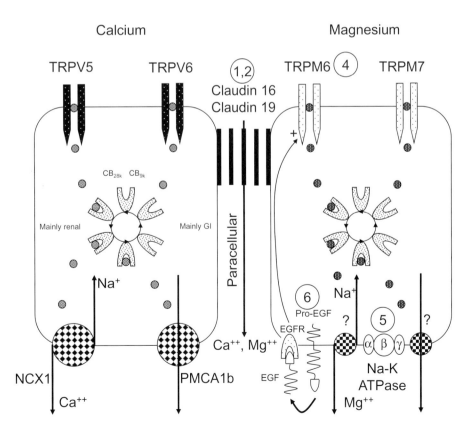

Figure 16.1 Divalent cation transport across gastrointestinal and renal cells. Calcium is shown on the left and magnesium on the right. The luminal surface is at the top and the baso-lateral surface at the bottom. EGF, epidermal growth factor; EGFR, EGF receptor; GI, gastrointestinal.

mutations cause renal hypomagnesemia with ocular involvement (#248190).

Active transcellular absorption occurs mainly in the distal tubule: TRPM6 is probably the most specific of the proteins responsible for transport across the luminal surface and renal reabsorption is also affected in hypomagnesemia with secondary hypocalcemia (HOMG) (#602014). The activity of TRPM6 is influenced by epidermal growth factor (EGF) (*131530), a soluble protein derived from pro-EGF which is membrane-bound on the baso-lateral membrane of the renal tubules. Once EGF has been cleaved from pro-EGF, it interacts with the EGF receptor (*131550), which stimulates magnesium absorption by TRPM6 on the luminal surface. Mutations in the EGF gene disrupt the baso-lateral sorting of pro-EGF resulting in understimulation of TRPM6 and impaired magnesium reabsorption (isolated recessive renal hypomagnesemia) [5].

Cytoplasmic transfer is probably effected by intracellular proteins such as calbindin$_{28K}$ but the mechanisms are not well understood. At the baso-lateral membrane, active transport occurs by means of the Na^+,K^+-ATPase pump. The mechanism is not understood but mutations in the FXYD2 (*601814) gene that codes for the γ-subunit of this protein cause autosomal dominant renal hypomagnesemia associated with hypocalciuria (HOMG2) (#154020) and sometimes causes severe symptomatic hypomagnesemia. The thiazide-sensitive sodium chloride co-transporter (NCC) is also involved in magnesium transport and mutations in the coding gene, SLC12A3 (*600968), cause Gitelman syndrome (#263800) of which hypermagnesuria is a feature. Raised urinary magnesium excretion is also present in some cases of Bartter syndrome which is caused by mutations affecting chloride and sodium reabsorption in the loop of Henle. Renal tubular transport of magnesium can be increased by several non-genetic causes, such as diuretics, diabetic ketoacidosis, gentamicin, mercury-containing laxatives, transplanted kidney, urinary tract obstruction, the diuretic phase of acute renal failure and cisplatin.

Phosphate

A fully grown adult contains approximately 700 g phosphate, about 80% of which is contained in bone. Of the remainder, 45% (9% of the total) is present in skeletal muscle, 54.5% in the viscera and only 0.5% in extracellular fluid. Most is present in inorganic form but plays a crucial part in many intracellular processes. Phosphate circulates as phospholipids, phosphate esters and free inorganic phosphate (P_i). Plasma P_i concentrations are not as tightly controlled as those of calcium and reflect the fluxes of phosphate entering and leaving the extracellular pool. In contrast to calcium, phosphate concentrations in plasma vary considerably during life, being highest during phases of rapid growth. Thus, phosphate concentrations in premature infants are normally above 2.0 mmol/L (6.4 mg/dL), falling to 1.3–2.0 mmol/L (4.2–6.4 mg/dL) during infancy and childhood and to 0.7–1.3 mmol/L (2.2–4.3 mg/dL) in young adults.

Phosphate transport across membranes is controlled by sodium-dependent active transport mechanisms (Na/Pi co-transporters). Type 1 is present in renal tubular brush borders but is not thought to have a major role. The three subtypes of Type 2 (a–c) are probably the most important in regulating phosphate absorption and reabsorption. Type 3 is present in many tissues but is thought to have more of a "gatekeeping" role. Phosphate is readily absorbed throughout the small bowel by passive and active mechanisms. Approximately 70% is absorbed by Type 2b Na/Pi co-transporter, the remainder being by passive absorption. The active transport is stimulated by 1,25(OH)$_2$D and indirectly by hypocalcemia and PTH. Because hypophosphatemia is a powerful stimulant of 25-hydroxyvitamin D-1-alfahydroxylase (1α-hydroxylase), phosphate deficiency itself stimulates increased absorption but the total amount absorbed is dependent on the dietary phosphate load and may be inhibited by phosphate-binding agents such as calcium acetate (Phosex®), carbonate (Tetralac®) or sevelamer (Renagel®), which are of value in hyperphosphatemic states when phosphate absorption needs to be limited, such as chronic renal failure.

Regulation of plasma phosphate occurs principally in the renal tubule by the Type 2a and 2c Na/Pi co-transporters. Type 2c (*609826) is probably the most important in humans and its activity is dependent on the activity of FGF23, a major phosphotonin, which stimulates phosphate excretion. Excess FGF23 results in hypophosphatemia and low concentrations are associated with hyperphosphatemia, which has significant clinical implications. Of filtered phosphate 85–98% is reabsorbed, mainly by the proximal renal tubule, which represents about 10 times the amount absorbed by the intestine. Tubular reabsorption of phosphate (TRP) is saturable and determined both by the filtered load, itself determined by glomerular filtration rate (GFR) and plasma concentration, and by hormonal factors, particularly PTH and FGF23, both of which increase phosphate excretion.

Assessment of phosphate excretion is crucial to diagnosing some conditions, particularly hypophosphatemic rickets. It is most easily assessed by measuring the fractional excretion of phosphate (FE$_{PO_4}$), the ratio of the clearance of phosphate to the clearance of creatinine, which requires estimation of plasma and urine phosphate and creatinine on single samples taken simultaneously. It makes the assumption that creatinine clearance approximates to GFR but does not require any timed urine samples. FE$_{PO4}$ is calculated according to the formula:

$$FE_{PO_4} = [U_{PO_4}]/[P_{PO_4}] \times [P_{Creat}]/[U_{Creat}]$$

where all the results for phosphate and creatinine are expressed in the same units.

TRP is 1-FE$_{PO_4}$ and is usually expressed as a percentage. Values are normally in excess of 85% and frequently approach 98% in children. In hyperphosphaturic conditions, the value may be below 50% but this parameter is dependent on the filtered load: the lower the plasma concentration, the greater the proportion that can be reabsorbed. A more precise measure of renal tubular phosphate handling, which eliminates any effect of plasma phosphate, can be obtained by calculating the theoretical tubular maximal phosphate threshold as a function of GFR (Tm_{PO_4}/GFR). This is most easily obtained by a nomogram from the plasma phosphate concentration and the FE_{PO_4} [6]. Tm_{PO_4}/GFR is reduced in hyperparathyroidism and phosphate-losing conditions and increased in hypoparathyroidism. It is higher in children and adolescents than in adults [7].

Hormones and other calciotropic agents
Alkaline phosphatase
This is present in several tissues in three main isoforms: intestinal (IAP) (*171740), placental (PLAP) (*171810) and tissue non-specific (TNAP) (*171760). A gene on chromosome 2q34-37 codes for the first two and a gene on chromosome 1p36.1-p34 codes for the last [8]. Different post-translational modifications of TNAP enzyme result in three tissue-specific forms found in bone, liver and kidney that can be distinguished by their different isoelectric points and heat lability, the bone-specific form (bTNAP) being the least stable.

bTNAP is present in osteoblasts and promotes bone mineralization. Circulating TNAP is largely derived from liver and bone. Concentrations in plasma during childhood reflect growth rate [9] and are raised in the presence of rickets, in juvenile Paget disease (#239000) and in fibrous dysplasia. Low concentrations are seen in hypophosphatasia, which results from mutations in the TNAP gene. A database that keeps track of these mutations (currently 194) can be accessed at http://www.sesep.uvsq.fr/Database.html.

Parathyroid hormone
Parathyroid hormone (*168450) is a single-chain 84-amino-acid polypeptide hormone encoded by a gene on chromosome 11 from prepro-PTH, which has an additional 31 amino acids. Synthesis occurs in the ribosomes, where the initial 25 amino acid pre sequence acts as a signal peptide to aid transport through the rough endoplasmic reticulum. The pre sequence is cleaved and pro-PTH then travels to the Golgi apparatus where the 6 amino acid pro sequence is cleaved to yield the mature hormone, which is stored in secretory vesicles that fuse with the plasma membrane before secretion of the hormone [10]. Little PTH is stored within the glands and most of the secreted hormone is newly synthesized. Mutations in the PTH gene have been described.

Only the first 34 N-terminal amino acids are required for full activity and the function of the remainder of the molecule is not understood. The half-life of PTH in the circulation is 1–2 min [10]. The molecule is cleaved at various sites, which results in a number of fragments that can be identified in the circulation. The best modern assays of PTH measure intact PTH, are able to measure physiological concentrations of PTH, correlate with bioactivity and ignore the inactive fragments. Normal concentrations are about 1–6 pmol/L (10–60 pg/mL) but vary depending on the assay.

Control of PTH secretion
The calcium-sensing receptor
PTH is secreted in response to changes in ionized calcium. A calcium-sensing receptor (CaSR) (+601199) is present in many tissues, particularly the parathyroid glands and renal tubule, and in bone, cartilage and other tissues [11]. Its gene is located on chromosome 3q13-21 and the CaSR is a large molecule consisting of 1078 amino acid residues of which 610 form the extracellular calcium-binding domain, 250 comprise the seven-transmembrane domain and another 210 the intracellular cytosolic component. Ca^{2+} binds to the extracellular domain and influences PTH secretion by both phospholipase Cb and G-protein second messengers. As a consequence, PTH secretion changes in a sigmoidal fashion in response to acute changes in plasma calcium (Fig. 16.2) and there is a continuous tonic secretion of PTH, which maintains plasma-ionized calcium at whatever concentration is set by the CaSR [12]. Magnesium also binds to the CaSR and influences PTH secretion in a fashion similar to that of calcium. Magnesium deficiency inhibits PTH secretion, probably because the adenylate cyclase coupled to the G-protein is itself magnesium dependent.

Two other loci on chromosomes 19p and 19q13 have been identified by family linkage studies. The precise nature of the gene products of these loci remains uncertain but mutations within them result in syndromes similar to those resulting from inactivating mutations of the CaSR itself.

Mutations within the CaSR gene result in either inactivation or activation of the receptor, which result in hypercalcemia and hypocalcemia, respectively. Inactivating mutations cause insensitivity to calcium, which shifts the curve of PTH secretion in response to plasma calcium to the right (Fig. 16.2). As a consequence, PTH secretion is switched off at a higher concentration than normal and hypercalcemia results [11]. The receptors are also present in the renal tubule and renal calcium excretion is thereby reduced. The resulting condition is known as familial benign hypercalcemia (FBH) or familial hypocalciuric hypercalcemia (FHH) (#145980). In contrast, activating mutations of the receptor shift the PTH secretion curve to the left (Fig. 16.2), causing chronic hypocalcemia and hypercalciuria, a condition known as autosomal dominant hypocalcemia (ADH).

Many of the mutations found in FBH are clustered around the aspartate- and glutamate-rich regions of the extracellular domain of the molecule and it has been postulated that this region contains low-affinity binding sites for calcium. Many of the FBH kindreds have been found to have unique mutations. Mutations have also been detected within the transmembrane domain but only rarely within the intracellular domain. Most activating mutations that cause ADH are present within the extracellular calcium-binding domain. One hundred and twenty-eight mutations, three of which are polymorphisms, have been described (http://www.casrdb.mcgill.ca).

Not all families with FBH have mutations within the CaSR gene and it has been suggested that there may be abnormalities either within the CaSR gene promoter or within one of the two loci found on chromosome 19. The three variants of FBH linked to chromosome 3q, 19p and 19q, have therefore been referred to as FBH types 1–3.

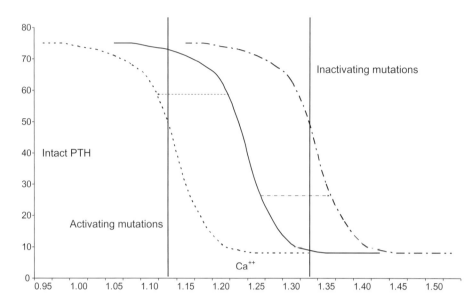

Figure 16.2 The sigmoidal relationship between ionized Ca (Ca^{2+}) and intact parathyroid hormone (PTH) secretion. The vertical lines represent the normal range of Ca^{2+}. Also shown is the effect of inactivating mutations (right shift) and activating (left shift) of the CaSR. The degree to which these shifts occur is dependent on the mutation involved. (After original data of Conlin *et al.* [12].)

Parathyroid glands

The parathyroid (PT) glands, usually four in number, are derived embryologically from the third (lower glands) and fourth (upper glands) branchial arches. Several transcription factors are involved in their development [13]. Some, such as Hoxa3 (thyroid and thymus) (*142954) and GATA3 (sensorineural deafness, renal anomalies, chromosome 10p13-14) (*131320), are involved in the development of other structures. Several genes, including Tbx1 (thymus, cardiac outflow tract and the face, chromosome 22q11) (*602054) and UDF1L, are located on the long arm of chromosome 22. Mutations within the genes responsible for these factors result in congenital hypoparathyroidism, which may be either isolated or associated with other conditions such as the hypoparathyroidism, deafness, renal anomalies (HDR) (#146255) syndrome and the CATCH 22 complex, of which the DiGeorge syndrome (DGS) (#188400) is part.

The homolog of Drosophila glial cells missing 2 (GCM2) (*603716) is a highly conserved gene necessary for PT gland development that has no other function in humans. Mutations cause autosomal recessive familial isolated hypoparathyroidism (FIH) (#146200). The SRY-related HMG-box gene 3 (SOX3) (*313430), located on the X chromosome, is also thought to be involved in PT gland development and mutations may be responsible for X-linked recessive FIH (%307700).

Actions of PTH

PTH has two principal target organs: bone and kidney. In bone, it promotes bone mineralization by an action on osteoblasts when present in physiological concentrations. During phases of hypocalcemia, when PTH concentrations rise, its main effect is on the osteoclast, where it stimulates bone resorption within the bone remodeling unit (BMU) by the RANKL/RANK system. The two processes do not occur independently and increases in bone resorption are accompanied by stimulation of osteoblast activity by a series of paracrine and autocrine mechanisms that result in an increase in bone turnover.

In the nephron, most filtered calcium is reabsorbed passively in the proximal tubule by a paracellular mechanism. In the convoluted and straight parts of the proximal renal tubule, PTH also acts to stimulate 1α-hydroxylase, the enzyme that converts vitamin D to its active metabolite, 1,25(OH)$_2$D. PTH actively promotes calcium and magnesium transcellular reabsorption in the distal nephron. Phosphate excretion increases in response to PTH, which, following PTH-stimulated bone resorption, allows any excess phosphate that has been removed from bone with calcium to be excreted. PTH also stimulates renal excretion of bicarbonate and amino acids. Thus, hyperparathyroidism results in a mild acquired form of the Fanconi syndrome.

Mechanisms of action of PTH

The PTH receptor

PTH acts by two receptors. The first and principal is PTH1R (also called PTH/PTHrP) receptor (*168468), which has equal affinity for both PTH and PTHrP. It consists of 593 amino acids coded by a gene on the long arm of chromosome 3 [14]. It has an extracellular binding domain of 190 residues, a seven-transmembrane domain and a cytosolic component of 134 residues. Both inactivating and activating mutations of the PTH1R have been described. These result in Blomstrand lethal chondrodysplasia (#215045) and Jansen disease (#156400), respectively. A second PTH2 receptor (PTH2R) is present in the central nervous system. PTHrP is not a ligand for it.

Intracellular signaling

Intracellular signaling occurs principally by coupling of the cytosolic component of the PTH1R to G-protein second messengers, Gs and Gq [15]. These are heterotrimeric, consisting of α, β and γ subunits. In the resting state, they are associated and the Gsα subunit is bound to GDP (Fig. 16.3a) which results in guanosine diphosphate (GDP) being exchanged for guanosine triphosphate (GTP) and dissociation of the Gsα subunit from the β,γ complex. The Gsα subunit is then free to stimulate adenylate cyclase, which results in an increase in intracellular cAMP, which activates the various actions of PTH by specific protein kinases (Fig. 16.3b). Intrinsic GTPase activity associated with the Gsα subunit hydrolyzes GTP to GDP, which causes reassociation of the components of the G-protein. At the same time, phosphodiesterases inactivate cAMP to AMP and the cell reverts to its resting state (Fig. 16.3c). This mechanism is common to thyroid-stimulating hormone (TSH), gonadotropins and growth hormone-releasing hormone (GHRH) [15].

The Gsα subunit is coded by a gene, *GNAS1*, (+139320) located on chromosome 20q13.3. This complex gene contains 13 exons that code for the Gsα subunit itself plus several other exons which, by alternative promoter use and splicing, results in at least four different mRNA transcripts. In most tissues, these show biallelic expression but some of the transcripts are derived either from the maternal or paternal alleles. The Gqα subunit activates phospholipase Cb to generate inositol triphosphate (IP$_3$), although this is a lesser effect than cAMP generation.

Several factors modify responsiveness to PTH. Mutations within the *GNAS1* gene for the Gsα subunit of the G-protein second messenger cause resistance by preventing activation of adenylate cyclase, which results in some of the forms of pseudo-hypoparathyroidism. PTH can also modify responsiveness to itself. Acute infusions cause desensitization by uncoupling the receptor from the G-protein and, in the presence of chronic hyperparathyroidism, downregulation of the receptors occurs as a result of reduction in the number of receptors.

Resistance to PTH has been assessed traditionally by examining the effects of PTH on phosphate excretion (the Ellsworth–Howard test) or on cAMP production in either urine or plasma. It has not been possible recently to undertake such stimulation tests since PTH has not been available. The development of synthetic PTH (teriparatide) for use in involutional osteoporosis should allow it to be used for such purposes again, although the manufacturers have not made it available in suitably small quantities. Since understanding of the genetic mechanisms underlying many of the conditions has advanced, the need for stimulation tests has declined.

Vitamin D

Vitamin D is a secosteroid that exists in two forms. Cholecalciferol is synthesized as a result of the action of ultraviolet (UV) light breaking the B ring of 7-dehydrocholesterol to produce previtamin D, which is then converted to native vitamin D (cholecalciferol) by the action of body heat. Ergocalciferol is synthesized by plants and differs slightly in structure in having an extra double bond in the side-chain but it is equipotent with cholecalciferol and metabolized similarly. Vitamin D includes both compounds.

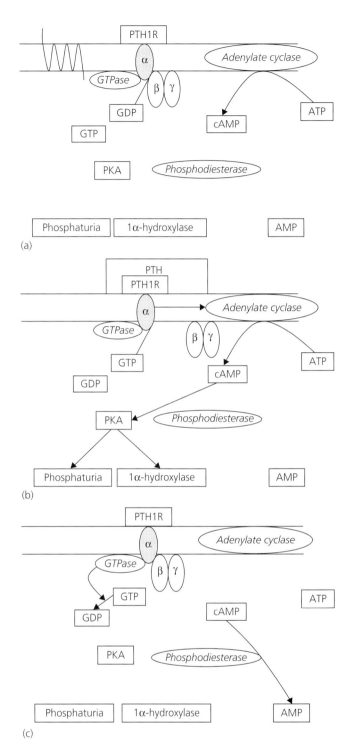

Figure 16.3 Simplified representation of mechanism of action of parathyroid hormone (PTH) in relation to the G-protein second messenger. (a) In the resting state, the Gsα subunit is bound to GDP and associated with the β,γ subunit. (b) When PTH binds to the receptor, GDP is exchanged for GTP which causes dissociation of the Gsα subunit from the β,γ subunit. The Gsα subunit is then free to stimulate membrane bound adenylate cyclase, which increases intracellular cAMP, which has its effects by protein kinases. (c) The intrinsic GTPase activity associated with the Gsα subunit then hydrolyses GTP back to GDP, which causes reaggregation of the G-protein. At the same time, phosphodiesterases inactivate the cAMP to AMP and the situation reverts to the quiescent state (a). In this diagram, the less important Gq second messenger, which acts by inositol triphosphate (IP$_3$), is not shown.

Under normal circumstances, 80% of vitamin D consists of cholecalciferol synthesized in skin, the remainder being acquired from dietary sources as both cholecalciferol and ergocalciferols but the amount of vitamin D synthesized in skin is dependent upon skin color and exposure. Following synthesis, it becomes bound to a specific vitamin D-binding protein (DBP) and passes to adipose tissue and the liver for storage and further metabolism. Vitamin D does not have significant biological activity. Its activity requires two hydroxylation steps, at the 25 and 1 positions (Fig. 16.4) [16].

All of the steps in vitamin D metabolism are catalyzed by cytochrome P450 enzymes (Fig. 16.4). The first step is catalyzed by at least four different vitamin D 25 hydroxylases distinguishable by their different affinities and capacities and intracellular localization. The first, a low-affinity high-capacity enzyme (CYP27A1) (*606530), is located in mitochondria. There are no reports of rickets resulting from mutations in this gene but they do cause cerebrotendinous xanthomatosis (#213700). A second high-affinity low-capacity enzyme (CYP2R1) (*608713), which may be of greater physiological significance, is located within hepatic microsomes. Although they have not yet been fully characterized, cases of rickets are described associated with mutations (#600081). Two other enzymes, CYP3A4 (*124010) and CYP2J2 (*601258), probably also have some effect on 25-hydroxylase but are mainly involved in drug metabolism.

25-hydroxyvitamin D (25OHD), circulates in plasma bound to the DBP and is the most abundant vitamin D metabolite, circulating in nanomolar concentrations. Assay gives a measure of vitamin D status, the concentration depending on the supply of vitamin D with considerable annual variation, peaking about 6 weeks after maximal exposure to sunlight. It has some weak activity which is not normally of clinical significance but may become so in the presence of vitamin D excess. Vitamin D 25 hydroxylase also catalyzes the conversion of 1α-hydroxy-cholecalciferol (alfacalcidol) and 1α-hydroxy-ergocalciferol (doxercalciferol), to $1,25(OH)_2D$.

25OHD is metabolized to its active hormone, $1,25(OH)_2D$, by 25-hydroxyvitamin D 1α-hydroxylase, which is active only against metabolites that are already hydroxylated at position 25 [17]. A single enzyme located in convoluted and straight portions of the proximal renal tubule has been identified. Activity is also present in osteoblasts, keratinocytes and lymphohematopoietic cells, where 1,25(OH)2D may have an autocrine or paracrine role. During fetal life, 1α-hydroxylase activity is found in the placenta. In pathological states, it is present in the macrophages of sarcoid tissue and subcutaneous fat necrosis. It is a mitochondrial enzyme (CYP27B1) (*609506) consisting of 508 amino acids with considerable homology to other P450 enzymes encoded by a single gene on chromosome 12q13.1-q13.3. Mutations are responsible for the condition known variously as pseudo-vitamin D deficiency rickets (PDDR), vitamin D-dependent rickets type I (VDDR-I) or 1α-hydroxylase deficiency (#264700).

Activity of 1α-hydroxylase is stimulated by PTH by its cAMP– protein kinase actions. Hypocalcemia stimulates 1α-hydroxylase activity but this effect is mediated by PTH and not directly. Plasma phosphate has a direct effect on 1α-hydroxylase activity, although there is some evidence to suggest that this may be modulated by growth hormone (GH) and calcitonin. Its activity is inhibited by FGF23.

$1,25(OH)_2D$ is a potent compound circulating in picomolar concentrations. Its synthesis is tightly controlled by the plasma calcium concentration. In order to enable changes in $1,25(OH)_2D$

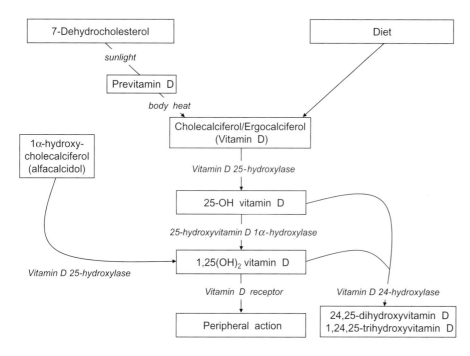

Figure 16.4 The principal steps involved in vitamin D metabolism.

to occur rapidly, 25-hydroxyvitamin D 24-hydroxylase (25OHD 24-OHase) (*126065), another cytochrome P450 enzyme, exists that can use both 25OHD and 1,25(OH)₂D as substrates to form 24,25-dihydroxyvitamin D (24,25(OH)₂D) and 1α,24,25-trihydroxyvitamin D (1,24,25(OH)₃D), respectively. The role of this enzyme is probably to divert metabolism of 25OHD away from 1,25(OH)₂D synthesis when this is not needed and to participate in the degradation of existing 1,25(OH)₂D. It is inhibited by PTH and stimulated by 1,25(OH)₂D and FGF23.

1,24,25(OH)₃D has limited potency (about 10% of 1,25(OH)₂D) and is probably an intermediate degradation metabolite of 1,25(OH)₂D. Its role, if any, is uncertain but people of South Asian origin possess higher 25OHD 24-OHase activity than those of European origin [18] and this seems to contribute to their susceptibility to vitamin D deficiency rickets.

1,25(OH)₂D acts by a specific vitamin D receptor [19] (*601769). It is a member of the steroid-thyroid-retinoid superfamily of nuclear receptors and, in many respects, is typical of this group with ligand binding, DNA binding, dimerization and transcriptional activation domains. It is encoded by a gene on chromosome 12 near the 1α-hydroxylase gene. The receptors are widely distributed in gut, parathyroid glands, chondrocytes, osteoblasts and osteoclast precursors. 1,25(OH)₂D has a critical role in promoting calcium absorption in the small intestine, suppresses PTH secretion from the parathyroids, influences growth plate mineralization and stimulates differentiation of osteoclasts. In addition, there are receptors present in many tissues that are not directly related to calcium homeostasis, such as skin, breast, prostate and colon, and it has been postulated that it may play a part in preventing cancers of these tissues.

Mutations in the vitamin D receptor occur throughout the molecule but particularly in either the ligand-binding (ligand-binding negative) or the DNA-binding (ligand-binding positive) domains. These mutations cause severe rickets and many individuals, especially those with defects in DNA binding, also have alopecia. Originally referred to as vitamin D-dependent rickets type II (VDRR-II), it is now more properly called hereditary 1,25(OH)₂D-resistant rickets (HVDRR) (#277440). In another form of HVDRR, no mutations of the receptor have been identified but is thought to be caused by overexpression of a nuclear ribonucleoprotein that binds with the hormone receptor complex to attenuate its action (*600785).

Fibroblast growth factor 23

FGF23 (*605380) is mainly secreted by osteoblasts and osteocytes. It circulates in plasma and is one of a number of fibroblast growth factors that function by fibroblast growth factor receptors (FGFRs) in a variety of tissues as a classic hormone (Fig. 16.5). FGF23 is the principal "phosphotonin" that acts by FGFR1c (*136350) to stimulate phosphate excretion by the Type 2c Na/Pi co-transporter. It also inhibits 1α-hydroxylase so that hyperphosphaturic conditions caused by raised FGF23 are not accompanied by the expected increase in 1,25(OH)₂D.

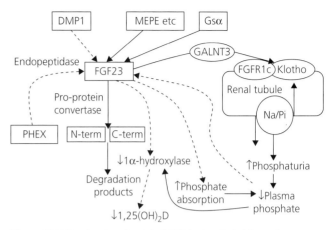

Figure 16.5 The phosphate fountain. FGF23 is the principal factor that controls phosphate metabolism and is influenced by a host of other factors that either alter its metabolism or affect its secretion. Inhibitory effects are represented by dotted arrows and stimulation by solid arrows.

The FGF23 gene is located on chromosome 12p13 and encodes a 251-amino-acid peptide that is further processed to amino- and carboxy-terminal fragments. Mutations prevent this processing, resulting in raised FGF23 in plasma which is responsible for the excess phosphate wasting seen in autosomal dominant hypophosphatemic rickets (ADHR) (#193100). Excess FGF23 is also responsible for the hyperphosphaturia seen in X-linked dominant hypophosphatemic vitamin D resistant rickets (VDRR) (#307800), autosomal recessive hypophosphatemic rickets (ARHP) (#241520), some cases of tumor-induced hypophosphatemic osteomalacia (TIO) and McCune–Albright syndrome (MAS) (#174800). Inactivating mutations result in low concentrations of FGF23 which causes hyperphosphatemia and tumoral calcinosis. In addition, post-translational modification of FGF23 includes glycosylation before full activity is obtained. This is effected by UDP-polypeptide N-acetylgalactosaminyl transferase 3 (GALNT3) (*601756). Mutations in the GALNT3 gene cause familial tumoral calcinosis (#211900).

Several other factors have a direct or indirect effect on FGF23. For the active receptor to be generated, another protein, Klotho (KL) (*611135), is required which combines with the receptor and allows it to be responsive to FGF23. The KL gene is located on chromosome 13q12 and codes for a 1014 amino acid protein that contains two internal repeats. The precise mechanism by which it activates FGF23 is still uncertain but it is thought to confer specificity of action to FGF23 within certain tissues, mainly kidney, parathyroid and pituitary. Inactivating mutations of KL also cause hyperphosphatemia and tumoral calcinosis with high circulating concentrations of FGF23 [20].

The *PHEX* gene (phosphate-regulating gene with homology to endopeptidases on the X chromosome) (*300550) encodes a 749 amino acid, seven trans-membrane glycoprotein and is present in several tissues but not kidney [21]. It is probably responsible, by its endopeptidase activity, for the processing and cleavage of FGF23 to prevent hyperphosphaturia. The gene is located on the X chromosome and mutations cause classical X-linked dominant hypophosphatemic rickets (VDRR) (#307800) (http://phexdb.mcgill.ca). It is not clear how it causes excess phosphaturia but mutations are associated with raised concentrations of circulating FGF23 probably caused by reduced inactivation of FGF23.

Secretion of FGF23 is controlled by dentin matrix protein 1 (DMP1) (*600980), one of a number of small integrin-binding ligand, N-linked glycoproteins (SIBLING) that promote mineralization. It is a factor secreted mainly by osteocytes. It probably acts as a mechanostat to influence bone mineralization directly but also inhibits FGF23 secretion. Mutations in the DMP1 gene cause an autosomal recessive form of hypophosphatemic rickets (ARHP) (#241520) because FGF23 secretion is unrestrained. Other SIBLING proteins include bone sialoprotein (BSP) (*166490), osteopontin (OPN) (*166490), dentin sialophosphoprotein (DSPP) (*125485) and matrix extracellular phosphoglycoprotein (MEPE) (*605912). Some of these are upregulated in certain forms of cancer and may be responsible for alterations in FGF23 secretion that causes tumor-induced hypophosphatemic osteomalacia. Some individuals with McCune–Albright polyostotic fibrous dysplasia, caused by somatic mutations in the α-subunit of the stimulatory G-protein (Gsα), have an associated excess phosphate excretion secondary to increased FGF23 by an, as yet, ill understood mechanism.

Hypophosphatemia and rickets are seen in several primary renal tubular abnormalities, such as the Fanconi syndrome (whatever the cause) and in hereditary hypophosphatemia with hypercalciuria (HHRH) (#241530) which results from a mutation in the Type 2c Na/Pi co-transporter. In these conditions, FGF23 is not raised and the expected increase in 1,25(OH)2D with consequent hypercalciuria may occur and cause nephrocalcinosis.

Parathyroid hormone-related peptide

Following the observation that some cancers are associated with hypercalcemia with undetectable PTH, it became apparent that another factor sharing many of the properties of PTH was the cause of the hypercalcemia. It is now known that PTHrP (+168470) is secreted by many of these tumors [22]. PTHrP is a polypeptide with considerable homology to PTH, particularly at the N-terminal end. It is secreted as a prohormone, which is cleaved into several fragments. The N-terminal fragment binds with the PTH1R in a way similar to PTH and has similar actions.

PTHrP does not circulate in amounts detectable in plasma and has no significant classic hormonal actions in postnatal life but it does have paracrine effects, particularly in bone. It is of importance as the factor that promotes and maintains the positive gradient of calcium across the placenta in fetal life [23]. It is also secreted by the lactating breast and may play a part in calcium homeostasis during lactation. Women with primary hypoparathyroidism may become hypercalcemic while breast feeding and

require a reduction in their dosage of vitamin D analog. This effect is thought to be caused by PTHrP.

Calcitonin

Calcitonin (CT) is a polypeptide hormone secreted by the C-cells of the thyroid derived from the ultimobranchial bodies that become incorporated into the thyroid. It is secreted in response to hypercalcemia and acts by specific receptors mainly to counteract the effects of PTH in osteoclasts. It therefore has a calcium-lowering effect, which wanes in the presence of sustained CT secretion. Secretion also occurs in response to a specific tetrapeptide sequence present on, among other molecules, glucagon. CT acts by a receptor, the gene for which is located on chromosome 7q21.

The physiological role of CT has been difficult to establish but it may play a part in moderating bone turnover and may be of greater importance to the developing skeleton than to the mature one. In practice, CT appears to have little clinical significance except as a therapeutic agent for acute hypercalcemia and as a tumor marker for medullary carcinoma of the thyroid (MCT) (#171400).

Physiology of bone metabolism

Bone consists of matrix, mineral and cells, which are present in different proportions in the various parts of bone. Matrix provides the protein scaffolding on which mineral is laid down. Both of these components are synthesized and removed by the various bone cells. Most bones are formed from cartilage and are called endochondral bones. Intramembranous bones, the flat bones of the skull, the scapulae and the pelvis, do not have a cartilage template and develop from differentiation of mesenchymal cells into bone forming cells.

Endochondral bones consist of an epiphysis at each end of the bone, the diaphysis or shaft and metaphyses between them. Bone consists of a tubular outer section of densely calcified bone, the cortex and an inner more loosely packed trabecular area in which the bone is constructed from a latticework of cross-struts in between which the bone marrow lies. Trabecular bone is particularly prominent in the epiphyses and metaphyses as in the vertebral bodies. In children, a fourth component, the cartilage growth plate, is present situated between the epiphysis and metaphysis. Once growth ceases, this area calcifies and disappears.

In endochondral bone, growth occurs by increase in length as a result of proliferation and subsequent ossification of the growth plates and in size by a combination of bone accretion on the outer aspect of the cortex and bone resorption on the inner (modeling). Intramembranous bones grow as a result of proliferation of preosteoblasts and calcification. Where the bones meet, they form sutures which interdigitate with one another. In certain conditions, including osteogenesis imperfecta, the calcification process is defective and gives rise to the characteristic appearance of Wormian bones, seen radiologically as multiple areas of calcification surrounded by undermineralized bone.

The cartilaginous growth plate contains four layers within which the predominant cell type is the chondrocyte. Furthest from the metaphysis is the resting layer beneath which is the proliferative layer. The chondrocytes differentiate, increase in size and their division rate decreases as they enter the prehypertrophic layer. Under the influence of Indian hedgehog (IHH) (*600726), one of a family of highly conserved genes related to *Drosophila* "hedgehog" genes, further differentiation occurs as they finally enter the hypertrophic layer, which is non-mitotic. This is regulated by PTHrP through its receptor, PTH1R, before becoming apoptotic and being invaded by blood vessels and replaced with osteoblasts.

Development of the chondrocytes is influenced by the actions of a series of bone morphometric proteins (BMPs) that are controlled in turn by another protein called Noggin (*602991). Together they are responsible for joint development. Noggin is an inhibitor of BMPs and a number of chondrodysplasias, such as symphalangism and brachydactyly are caused by mutations in their genes.

Bone matrix
Collagen
The collagens are widely distributed in connective tissue and consist of heterotrimers or homotrimers of fibrils cross-linked and wound into triple helices. One or other type of collagen comprises 80% of the protein content of bone, the most abundant form of collagen being Type I, a heterotrimer of two strands of Type 1A1 and one of Type 1A2. Each strand is synthesized as a proprotein and, during the course of post-translational modification, the proprotein peptides, procollagen Type 1 C-terminal (P1CP) and procollagen Type 1 N-terminal (P1NP) peptides, are cleaved and circulate in plasma. Measurement of procollagen peptides is sometimes used as a measure of bone formation during bone turnover studies. Similarly, during bone resorption, the N-terminal cross-links between fibrils (NTX) are released and can be measured, usually in urine, as an indicator of bone resorption.

Mutations in the COL1A1 (+120150) and COL1A2 (*120160) genes, resulting in either qualitative or quantitative abnormalities in the respective proteins, cause the majority of cases of osteogenesis imperfecta (OI). The process of cross-linking of the collagen fibers is complex and consists of a combination of hydroxylation of lysine and proline molecules within the fibrils, aldehyde formation and glycosylation. Cartilage associated protein (CRTAP) (*605497), a cofactor in the post-translational modification of collage, combines with prolyl 3-hydroxylase-1 (P3H1) (*610339) and cyclophylin B involved in the coiling of the collagen protein. Mutations in CRTAP cause both OI Types IIB and VII while mutations in LEPRE1 gene that codes for P3H1 cause OI Type VIII. No mutations in cyclophylin B have yet been identified in humans. The other more minor form of collagen

that occurs in bone is Type V, which co-localizes with Type 1. It is a heterotrimer of Type 5A1 (*120215) and Type 5A2 (*120190) collagen and mutations in one or other of these genes cause some forms of Ehlers–Danlos syndrome.

Four different forms of collagen are secreted by cartilage with different ones being produced at different stage of growth plate development. During the proliferative phase, the principal form is Type II with smaller amounts of Types IX and XI. Type II collagen is also found in the vitreous of the eye and many of the conditions involving mutations of this gene are accompanied by ocular abnormalities. Once the prehypertrophic and hypertrophic phases are entered, Type X becomes the prominent form of collagen, which is only present in this tissue. Mutations in the genes for all these proteins can give rise to a variety of osteo and chondrodysplasias (Table 16.1).

Non-collagenous matrix proteins
Non-collagenous matrix proteins, proteoglycans, glycoproteins and g-carboxylated proteins (gla proteins), constitute the 15% of bone matrix not occupied by collagen. Proteoglycans are present either as macromolecules that fill the spaces between the collagen fibrils or as smaller proteins with more specific functions. Mutations in the gene for one of them, aggrecan, leads to spondyloepiphyseal dysplasia (#608361). Glycoproteins are components of bone and cartilage matrix because they bind to macromolecules and to cell surface receptors and maintain cell–cell interactions. One of the most significant of these in cartilage is cartilage oligomeric matrix protein (COMP), mutations in the gene for which cause pseudoachondroplasia (#177170) and multiple epiphyseal dysplasia (#132400). The gla proteins are vitamin K-dependent proteins for matrix calcification and maturation. Matrix-gla protein (MGP) seems to be important in cartilage calcification and mutations in its gene cause Keutel syndrome (#245150), in which cartilage calcification is defective. Bone-gla protein, otherwise known as osteocalcin, is secreted by osteoblasts in proportion to their activity and is involved in bone mineral formation. Some osteocalcin escapes into the circulation and can be used to measure osteoblast activity in bone turnover studies. The relationship with vitamin K is demonstrated by the development of chondrodysplasia punctata in infants of mothers treated with warfarin during pregnancy.

Bone mineral
Bone mineral consists mainly of hydroxyapatite, 10 carbon atoms combined with three pyrophosphate molecules, each of which contains two phosphate atoms. It is laid down on the matrix scaffolding by osteoblasts under the influence of the many factors secreted by them. Pyrophosphate molecules have the structural formula:

$$PO_3 - O - PO_3$$

The bisphosphonates, which are increasingly used as treatment for osteoporotic conditions, have a similar structure.

Table 16.1 Disorders of collagen found in bone and cartilage.

Collagen type	Principal location	Hetero-/homotrimer	Genes	Gene location	Pathological conditions	Inheritance	OMIM
Type I	Bone	Heterotrimer	COL1A1	17q21.31-q22	Osteogenesis imperfecta Type I	AD	#166200
					Osteogenesis imperfecta Type IIA	AD	#166210
					Osteogenesis imperfecta Type III	AD	#259420
					Osteogenesis imperfecta Type IV	AD	#166220
					Ehlers–Danlos Type I	AD	#130000
					Ehlers–Danlos Type VII	AD	#130060
					Caffey disease	AD/Sporadic	#114000
			COL1A2	7q22.1	Osteogenesis imperfecta Type I	AD	#166200
					Osteogenesis imperfecta Type IIA	AD	#166210
					Osteogenesis imperfecta Type III	AD	#259420
					Ehlers–Danlos Type VII	AD	#130060
Type II	Cartilage (Proliferative)	Homotrimer	COL2A1	12q13.11-q13.2	Stickler Type 1	AD	#108300
					Achondrogenesis Type II	AD	#200610
					Spondyloepimetaphyseal dysplasia (Strudwick)	AD	#184250
					Spondyloepiphyseal dyplasia congenital Kneist dysplasia	?AD	#183900
					Multiple epiphyseal dysplasia, myopia, deafness	AD	#156550
Type V	Bone	Hetero- or homo-	COL5A1	9q34.2-q34.3	Multiple epiphyseal dysplasia	AD	#130000
						AD	#130010
			COL5A2	2q31	Ehlers–Danlos Type I	AD	#130000
					Ehlers–Danlos Type II	AD	#130010
			COL5A3	19p13.2			
Type IX	Cartilage (Proliferative)	Hetero-	COL9A1	6q13	Multiple epiphyseal dysplasia Type I	AD	120210.0001
					Stickler syndrome	AR	120210.0002
			COL9A2	1p33-p32.2	Multiple epiphyseal dysplasia Type II	AD	#600204
			COL9A3	20q13.3	Multiple epiphyseal dysplasia Type III	AD	#600969
Type X	Cartilage (Prehypertrophic and hypertrophic)	Homo-	COL10A1	6q21-q22.3	Schmid type metaphyseal chondrodysplasia	AD	#156500
Type XI	Cartilage (Proliferative)	Hetero-	COL11A1	1p21	Stickler Type 2	AD	#604841
					Marshall syndrome	AD	#154780
			COL11A2	6p21.3	Stickler Type 3	AD	#184840
					Otospondylomegaepiphyseal dysplasia	AR	#215150
					Weissenbacher–Zweymuller syndrome	AD	#277610

Disorders of collagens that are present in bone and cartilage. The OMIM numbers relate to the disorders caused by mutations in the various collagens and refer to the Online Mendelian Inheritance in Man code numbers (http://www.ncbi.nlm.nih.gov/sites/entrez?db=OMIM).

Bone cells

Osteoblasts, osteoclasts and osteocytes exist in bone and chondrocytes in cartilage. The main function of osteoblasts is to lay down new bone, both matrix and mineral. In doing so, they secrete alkaline phosphatase and osteocalcin, both of which, together with P1CP or P1NP, can be used as markers of bone turnover. They also control the activity of osteoclasts by secreting the osteoclast-transforming factors RANKL and osteoprotegerin and are themselves controlled by osteocytes which secrete sclerostin.

Osteoblasts are derived from mesenchymal stem cells and, under the influence of activators and inhibitors, transformed by the Wnt signaling system into mature osteoblasts. The Wnt protein (*164820) binds with Frizzled protein (*603408) coupled to low density lipoprotein receptor protein 5 (LRP5) (*603506) on the cell surface of the osteoblast precursors to activate the canonical pathway mediated by β-catenin [24]. This induces gene transcription by the Tcf/Lef family of transcription factors and is essential for differentiation of osteoblasts from precursors. Inactivating and activating mutations of LRP5 cause a variety of bone fragility conditions [25]. Factors controlling osteoblast differentiation and function include bone morphogenic proteins (BMPs), Runx2 (*600211), which has been described as a master switch for bone formation by modifying genes within the osteoblast [26] and Type 1 activin A receptor (ACVR1) (*102576). Sclerostin (*605740), which is derived from osteocytes, inhibits BMPs and mutations in the gene (SOST) for sclerostin cause the bone sclerosing conditions van Buchem disease (#239100) and sclerosteosis (#269500) (Fig. 16.6). ACVR1 is a BMP type 1 receptor and mutations in this gene are responsible for fibrodysplasia ossifi-

cans progressiva (FOP) (#135100). Mutations in Runx2 cause cleidocranial dysostosis (#119600).

Osteoclasts are the principal bone resorbing cells. When they occur on the same surface of bone as osteoblasts, they act in tandem to resorb bone which is then replaced by the associated osteoblasts (remodeling) and the combination of the two types of cell is called a bone remodeling unit (BMU). Osteoclasts are derived from macrophage precursors and are under considerable influence by osteoblasts. Macrophages secrete macrophage colony-stimulating factor (M-CSF) which acts on receptors (c-fms) on the osteoclast progenitors to begin the maturation process (Fig. 16.7) but M-CSF is unable by itself to complete the process which requires activation of the RANK (NF-κB) receptors on the cell surface. These are stimulated by tissue necrosis factors (TNFs) and RANK-ligand (RANKL). Activation of RANKL results in fusion of several cells so that the mature osteoclasts are multinucleated. RANKL is secreted by osteoblasts in response to PTH, 1,25(OH)₂D, PTHrP and various cytokines. There are abundant PTH receptors on osteoblasts but few on osteoclasts, so bone resorption has to be mediated indirectly by osteoblasts. Osteoblasts also produce osteoprotegerin (OPG), a decoy receptor for RANKL. By binding to it, OPG acts as a restraining factor to prevent overactivity of RANK causing excessive bone resorption. Mutations in the RANKL gene cause a mild form of autosomal recessive osteopetrosis (#259710) while OPG mutations cause juvenile Paget disease (#239000).

In order to resorb bone, the osteoclast attaches itself to an area of bone by the ruffled border on its base where it forms a depression, known as a resorption lacuna. The ruffled border is bounded by a skirt which is tightly attached to the bone and limits the area of resorption to the base of the osteoclast. The cells are respon-

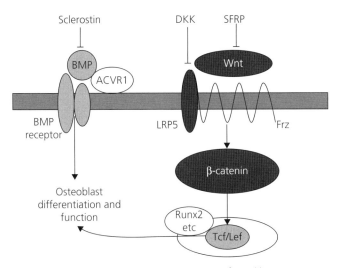

Figure 16.6 Simplified diagrammatic representation of osteoblast differentiation. ACVR1, type 1 activin A receptor; BMP, bone morphogenic protein; DKK, Dickkopf; Frz, Frizzled protein; Lef, lymphoid enhancer-binding factor; LRP5, low density lipoprotein receptor protein 5; Runx2, Runt related transcription factor 2; SFRP, soluble Frizzled related protein; Tcf, transcription factor; Wnt, Wingless-type MMTV integration site family member.

Figure 16.7 Osteoclast differentiation and function. The upper part of the diagram shows the factors synthesized by osteoblasts that control osteoclast transformation together with the factors that stimulte osteoblasts to induce this transformation. The lower half shows an osteoclast with the various factors that they produce to maintain the acid environment that allows bone resorption. ANKH, homology of mouse ANK; CAII, carbonic anhydrase II; ClCN7, chloride channel 7; CTSK, cathepsin K; M-CSF, macrophage colony-stimulating factor; OPG, osteoprotegerin; OSTM1, osteopetrosis-associated transmembrane protein 1; PLEKHM1, Pleckstrin homology domain-containing protein, family M, member 1; Ppi, inorganic phosphate; PTH, parathyroid hormone; PTHrP, parathyroid hormone related peptide; RANK, tumor necrosis factor ligand superfamily, member 11; RANKL, RANK ligand; SOST, sclerostin; TCIRG1, T cell immune regulator 1; TGFβ1: transforming growth factor, beta-1.

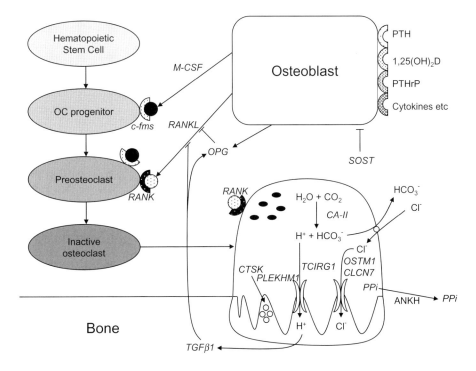

sible for removal of mineral and matrix, the former effected by the creation of hydrochloric acid (HCl) which dissolves the mineral. The H^+ ions are produced by carbonic anhydrase and the Cl^- ions by exchange of HCO_3^- (formed by carbonic anhydrase) for Cl^-. The protons are externalized into the resorption lacunae by an ATP-dependent vacuolar pump (TCIRG1) (*604592) while the Cl^- ions are transported by a specific chloride channel (CLCN7) (*602727). CLCN7 has a β-subunit, OSTM1 (*607649) while the vacuolar transport also requires plekstrin (PLEKHM1). Mutations in one or other of these processes impair osteoclast function and result in the various forms of osteoclast-rich osteopetrosis. Matrix removal requires the activity of cathepsin K and mutations in the gene for this protein (CTSK) (*601105) cause pycnodysostosis (#265800) in which a high bone density is also present.

Osteocytes

Osteocytes, the most abundant of the bone cells, are derived from mature osteoblasts and incorporated into bone where they are responsible for maintaining bone health. They lie in small spaces within the bone known as lacunae, connected to one another by processes contained within canaliculae that connect the lacunae. These lacunae and their accompanying canaliculae are arranged in concentric circles in cortical bone and a group of them makes an Haversian system.

Interactions between calciotropic agents

The primary aim of interactions between the various influences on calcium metabolism is to maintain plasma ionized calcium concentration within narrow limits, an aim that is normally successful (Fig. 16.8). At the same time, bone metabolism must be allowed to proceed satisfactorily so that calcium and phosphate accumulation and bone remodeling can occur during growth.

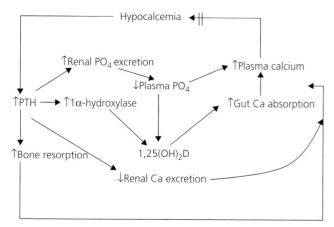

Figure 16.8 The principal responses to a hypocalcemic stimulus. (After Allgrove J. The parathyroid and disorders of calcium metabolism. In: Brook CGD, Clayton PH, Brown R, eds. *Clinical Pediatric Endocrinology*, 5th edn. Oxford: Blackwell, 2003.)

Fetal and neonatal calcium metabolism

Parathyroid glands are active in the human fetus from about 12 weeks' gestation, maintaining a positive gradient of calcium of 0.25–0.5 mmol/L (1–2 mg/dL) across the placenta. Little PTH is detectable in fetal plasma using immunoassays but bioassays showed significant bioactivity [23] because the principal factor is PTHrP rather than PTH itself. A term infant contains approximately 27 g calcium, most of it acquired during the last trimester and the net transfer of calcium across the placenta is 300–400 mg/day at term. Fetal bone is active and turnover of calcium at birth is more than 1% per day of total body calcium, compared with about 1/50th of this rate in adults.

After birth, the maternal supply of calcium is terminated which results in a rapid fall in plasma calcium to a nadir of 1.8–2.0 mmol/L (7.2–8 mg/dL) by 48 h. The normal concentration of 2.2–2.6 mmol/L (8.8–10.4 mg/dL) is achieved toward the end of the first week as the supply of calcium is resumed in milk and physiological mechanisms are established.

Postneonatal calcium, phosphate and magnesium metabolism and the calcium cascade

Following the establishment of physiological concentrations of calcium in plasma, there is little variation throughout life, despite a 50-fold increase in bone mineral to about 1200 g by adulthood. By contrast, concentrations of phosphate vary, being highest during periods of greatest demand for bone mineral, particularly during the neonatal period and adolescence (Fig. 16.9). Concentrations of magnesium are maintained within a narrow range of 0.6–1.2 mmol/L (1.4–2.8 mg/dL). Of the four factors that maintain calcium homeostasis, PTH, vitamin D and its metabolites, PTHrP and calcitonin, the first two are the most relevant outside fetal life. Magnesium has a part to play because deficiency interferes with PTH secretion. Calcium concentration is detected by a calcium-sensing receptor located on the surface of the parathyroid glands linked to secretion of PTH by an adenylate cyclase system. PTH acts by receptors on the various target organs through adenylate cyclase, to which it is linked by G-proteins. Defects in any part of this cascade can give rise to hypercalcemia or hypocalcemia.

Investigation of calcium and bone disorders

Calcium disorders
Clinical assessment of hypocalcemia
Symptoms of hypocalcemia do not usually occur until total calcium falls below 1.8 mmol/L (7.2 mg/dL) and some patients remain asymptomatic with a plasma calcium as low as 1.2 mmol/L (4.8 mg/dL). Symptoms include muscle twitching

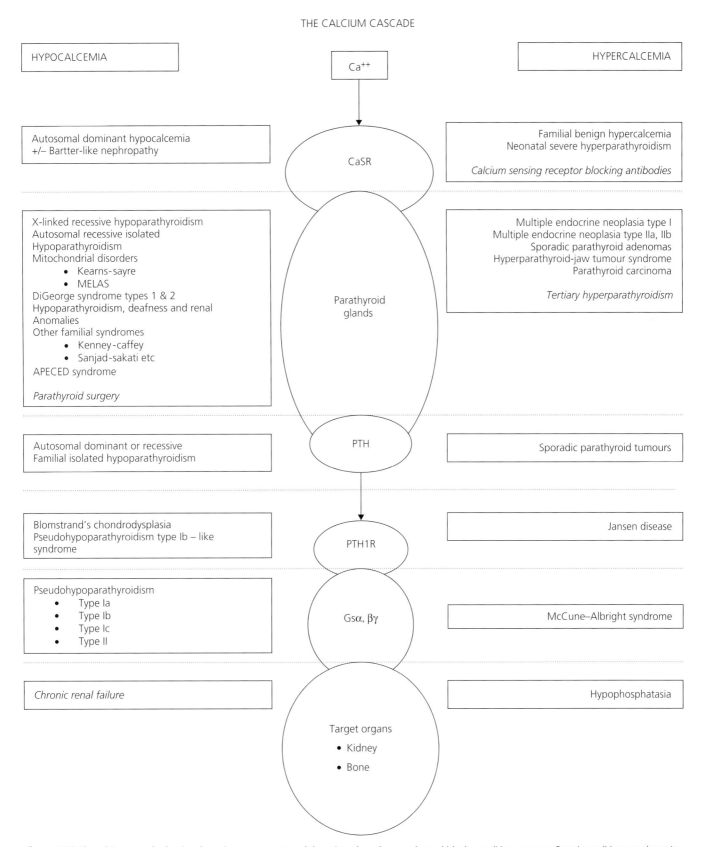

Figure 16.9 The calcium cascade showing the various components and the points along the cascade at which abnormalities can occur. Genetic conditions are shown in normal type and acquired conditions in italics. (From Allgrove J. The parathyroid and disorders of calcium metabolism. In: Brook CGD, Clayton PH, Brown R, eds. *Clinical Pediatric Endocrinology*, 5th edn. Oxford: Blackwell, 2003 with permission.) APECED, autoimmune polyendocrinopathy-candidiasis-ectodermal dystrophy; MELAS, **M**itochondrial myopathy, **E**ncephalopathy, **L**actic **A**cidosis and **S**troke.

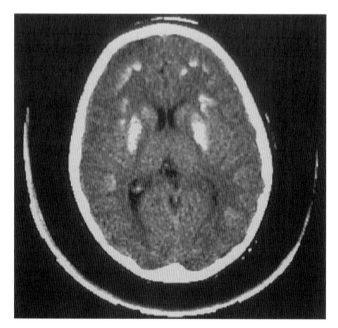

Figure 16.10 Computed tomography image of basal ganglion and frontal lobe calcification in pseudohypoparathyroidism Type Ia. Extensive calcification is seen in the basal ganglia and frontal lobes.

and spasms, which can be painful, apnea, stridor, carpopedal spasms and focal or generalized seizures. Measurement of plasma calcium should always be part of the investigation of unexplained fits to avoid confusion with epilepsy, even if fever is present and febrile convulsions are suspected. Clinical examination may reveal positive Chvostek or Trousseau signs and chronic hypocalcemia may cause calcification of the lens of the eye. In infants whose hypocalcemia is secondary to vitamin D deficiency, a form of dilated cardiomyopathy may develop. This does not occur with other causes of hypocalcemia (e.g. hypoparathyroidism) and is probably the result of a direct effect of the vitamin D deficiency on cardiac muscle. If cardiorespiratory support is effective, the prognosis for the cardiomyopathy is good, although it may take several months to recover. Some syndromes are associated with specific dysmorphic features. Rickets may be present in some instances. Soft tissue calcification is sometimes present in pseudohypoparathyroidism and computed tomographic (CT) scanning of the brain may reveal the presence of basal ganglion and frontal lobe calcification in both hypoparathyroidism and pseudohypoparathyroidism (Fig. 16.10).

Clinical assessment of hypercalcemia

The symptoms of hypercalcemia in childhood are age-dependent. Mild hypercalcemia may be asymptomatic but, as the calcium concentration rises above 3.0 mmol/L, symptoms become more common. Infants present with failure to thrive, vomiting and constipation. Muscle hypotonia, lethargy, anorexia, abdominal pain and constipation may be present in older children. Polyuria and polydipsia result from a concentrating defect in the renal tubule and long-standing hypercalciuria can lead to nephrocalcinosis, kidney stones and renal failure. Occasionally, psychiatric disturbance accompanies hypercalcemia and reverses when calcium returns to normal. Although not as common as the disorders causing hypocalcemia, many of those causing hypercalcemia are also genetic in origin.

Laboratory and radiological investigation

First line investigations should include measurement of total (and, if available, ionized) calcium, phosphate, albumin, magnesium, alkaline phosphatase, creatinine, PTH and 25OHD in blood, a sample of which should also be stored for future measurement of $1,25(OH)_2D$ if this is relevant, particularly if rickets is also present (Table 16.2). Urine should be taken for measurement of calcium, phosphate and creatinine. Fasting phosphate concentrations are of value if hypophosphatemic rickets is suspected. X-rays will reveal the presence of rickets, skeletal dysplasias (e.g. in pseudohypoparathyroidism), hyperparathyroid bone disease or soft tissue calcification. They are insensitive in detecting intracranial calcification, for which CT scanning is most appropriate. Early nephrocalcinosis can best be detected by ultrasound. Where a genetic cause for a disorder of calcium metabolism is suspected, blood should be taken and DNA extracted for analysis.

Metabolic bone disorders

Clinical assessment

The diagnosis of osteoporosis in children is primarily clinical, supported as necessary by radiological, bone density and genetic data. When a child presents with multiple fractures, particularly if they originate from mild trauma, a careful history, including family history, is taken. Biochemical investigation includes measurement of a bone profile with PTH and 25OHD as a measure of vitamin D status. All these parameters are usually normal, although urinary excretion of calcium may be elevated, particularly in idiopathic juvenile osteoporosis (IJO) and those forms of osteogenesis imperfecta where growth is poor. Blood may also be taken for DNA analysis [27]. Conditions associated with high bone density may also present with fractures; X-rays will usually give a clue to the diagnosis which can then be confirmed with biochemical and genetic tests as appropriate.

Radiology

Bone density rises gradually during childhood, increases sharply during adolescence and continues to rise more slowly in the late teenage years before reaching a peak in the early twenties. Routine X-rays give a poor indication of osteoporosis because 30–50% of bone mineral has to be lost before it becomes radiologically apparent. They are useful at demonstrating fractures, fracture healing and vertebral morphology and will often give an indication of the presence of increased bone density.

Several methods of bone density measurements are available but the most widely used is dual energy X-ray absorptiometry (DEXA) [28] which has a particular advantage in that it delivers

Table 16.2 Investigation of disorders of calcium and bone metabolism.

Blood – initial investigations

Calcium

Phosphate

Albumin

Alkaline phosphatase

Creatinine

25OHD

Intact PTH

Save serum for $1\alpha,25(OH)_2D$

Subsequent investigations as necessary

Blood gases

$1\alpha,25(OH)_2D$

DNA analysis for genetic abnormalities

PTHrP

Bone turnover markers

Radiology and nuclear medicine

Hand and knee for rickets

Skeletal survey for bone abnormalities

Renal ultrasound for nephrocalcinosis

Parathyroid ultrasound for parathyroid tumors

CT scan for intracranial calcification

SestaMIBI scan for PT gland localization

DEXA scan

Urine – initial investigations

Calcium

Phosphate

Creatinine

Calculate

Ca : creatine ratio

FE_{PO4} and TRP

T_mPO_4/GFR

Subsequent investigations as necessary

Glucose and amino acids

Bone turnover markers

Bone biopsy

Table of investigations that are indicated when a patient presents with a disorder of calcium or bone metabolism. Not all investigations are indicated in all patients.

---

a low radiation dose so repeat measurements can be undertaken with safety. In principle, it uses X-rays of two different energies to determine the amount of bone mineral by differential absorption but, while DEXA is a potentially useful in children because of the rapidly changing density during the phases of growth and adolescence, there are considerable pitfalls in interpretation. Several methods have been developed to take into account the fact that DEXA gives a two-dimensional measurement and to allow for variations in height, age, gender and pubertal status, although the best method has yet to be determined [28]. It is particularly important that the use of the T score, which relates bone density to the peak bone density achieved in adults, is avoided. Bone densities are usually reported as an age-related Z score and serial DEXA measurements on the same child are often useful. Lateral DEXA is also sometimes used to assess vertebral morphology at a lower radiation dose than lateral X-rays of the spine but its value has yet to be evaluated.

Other methods used to assess bone density include peripheral quantitative computerized tomography (pQCT) and various ultrasound techniques. QCT of the spine gives more precise measurements, particularly as it provides a three-dimensional measurement but it delivers too high a radiation dose for routine use. Whatever method is used, bone density does not necessarily relate to bone strength, particularly in children, in whom the definitions of osteopenia and osteoporosis, as defined in adults, do not necessarily apply.

Bone biopsy

Biopsy of bone can be useful where there is doubt about a diagnosis [29]. It is usually performed by taking a full-thickness biopsy through the iliac crest which includes both inner and outer cortices as well as the intervening trabecular bone. Most value is gained if the patient has had tetracycline labeling during the 3 weeks before biopsy. Tetracycline is laid down on mineralization fronts and, when viewed under ultraviolet light, can give useful quantitative information concerning bone activity. The biopsies can also be viewed under polarizing light to give information about the lamellar pattern and may provide a definitive diagnosis (e.g. in OI Type VI).

Bone turnover markers

Two types of marker are used, those that reflect bone formation and those that result from bone resorption [30]. Bone resorption markers derived from osteoblast activity are present as Type 1 collagen propeptide (P1CP), bone specific alkaline phosphatase (bALP) or osteocalcin (bone gla-protein). P1CP is derived from cleavage of the propeptide sequence of Type 1 collagen as it is laid down to form bone matrix. Measurement of bALP relies on its greater heat lability than other forms of ALP and osteocalcin is derived solely from bone but escapes into the circulation at the time of matrix formation.

Bone resorption markers are derived from the products of matrix removal. The most commonly used are urinary N- or C-terminal telopeptides of collagen (NTX-1, CTX-1) which are related to creatinine to allow for variations in urine concentration. Tartrate-resistant acid phosphatase (TRAP) is specifically secreted by osteoclasts and may give a measure of osteoclast activity. It is particularly useful in determining the effectiveness of bone marrow transplantation in osteopetrosis. Urinary pyridinoline, deoxypyridinoline and hydroxyproline are rarely used.

Markers of bone turnover may be used for a diagnosis or for monitoring treatment. Thus, OI is usually accompanied by high and IJO by low bone turnover. Bisphosphonates gradually reduce the rate of bone turnover.

Pathology of hypocalcemia

Neonatal hypocalcemia

Hypocalcemia may occur within the first 2–3 days of life or toward the end of the first week. In the former, the physiological fall in plasma calcium is exaggerated, especially in the preterm infant, following birth asphyxia, in sick infants and in those born to diabetic mothers. The mechanisms are unclear but may represent a delayed response to the rise of PTH following hypocalcemia. There may be an exaggerated response of calcitonin, especially where hypoglycemia is present because of the secretagog effect of glucagons but this is unlikely to be the explanation in the infant of a diabetic mother in whom glucagon responses to hypoglycemia are known to be impaired, presumably because of chronic hyperglycemia in utero. Magnesium deficiency may be a factor, particularly if the mother's diabetes has been poorly controlled, and measurement of magnesium should be included in the investigation of neonatal hypocalcemia and corrected if necessary. Early-onset hypocalcemia usually corrects itself spontaneously but additional calcium supplements may be required if symptoms persist. Relative hypophosphatemia is frequently present in preterm infants and may contribute to the development of bone disease of prematurity.

Late neonatal hypocalcemia is usually symptomatic. It can be the first manifestation of hypoparathyroidism but vitamin D deficiency or primary hyperparathyroidism in the mother must be considered. In the former, hypocalcemia can present at any time after birth depending on the severity of the deficiency and is not necessarily associated with radiological evidence of rickets, particularly if the presentation is soon after birth. It is almost confined to infants of mothers from ethnic minority groups and routine vitamin D supplementation of 400 IU/day, even from birth, may not be sufficient to prevent hypocalcemia in these infants. Hyperparathyroid mothers may be asymptomatic and the presence of hypocalcemia in the infant may be a clue to maternal disease. Measurement of vitamin D in mother and infant and of bone profile in the mother should form part of the investigation of late neonatal hypocalcemia. Excess phosphate in the diet may also cause hypocalcemia. In the past this has usually been because of the introduction of unsuitable milk preparations too soon after birth; this is not seen in breast fed infants and, with the increasing sophistication of formula feeds, is rarely a problem.

Symptomatic neonatal hypocalcemia requires intravenous 10% calcium gluconate (0.225 mmol/mL–0.9 mg/mL) given as a slow infusion of 1–3 mL/kg. This can be continued as an infusion of 1–2 mmol/kg/day (40–80 mg/kg/day) or as oral supplements. It is important to ensure a secure intravenous site because extravasation causes unsightly burns. In the event of vitamin D deficiency, additional vitamin D supplements of 1000–1500 IU/day are required. If hypocalcemia persists, and particularly if hypoparathyroidism is suspected, active metabolites of vitamin D may be required.

Bone disease of prematurity

Most calcium and phosphorus is accumulated during the last trimester. Thus, if an infant is born prematurely, there has been insufficient time for bone mineralization and extremely premature infants are at risk of developing bone disease of prematurity (BDP) [31]. It is difficult to maintain mineral accretion at the same rate as occurs in utero, even if the infant has few neonatal problems but if, in addition, nutritional, respiratory or cardiac problems requiring diuretic therapy supervene, the difficulties are compounded.

BDP has its origin in mineral deficiency, particularly phosphate but physical inactivity may also be a risk factor. Infants at risk need to be monitored and additional supplements given as necessary to maintain plasma phosphate >2 mmol/L (6.4 mg/dL): a rise in alkaline phosphatase above 1000 IU/L is usually indicative of active bone disease. Vitamin D supplements are usually given as a matter of routine and vitamin D deficiency is not usually a problem but, if neonatal hepatitis supervenes, it may be necessary to use a small dose of calcitriol in addition to the other supplements if bone healing is not achieved. Other aspects of nutrition, such as protein and calorie intake, should be optimized.

Postneonatal hypocalcemia

Disorders related to PTH

Hypocalcemia in childhood can result from defects in any part of the calcium metabolic cascade, many of them genetic in origin (Fig. 16.9; Table 16.3). Causes that affect the early part of the cascade are generally associated with low and those affecting the latter part with high PTH. The reverse is true of hypercalcemic conditions.

Disorders of the calcium-sensing receptor
Autosomal dominant hypocalcemia
Autosomal dominant hypocalcemia (ADH) is one form of familial isolated hypoparathyroidism (FIH) (#146200) caused by an activating mutation of the CaSR gene [11] (+601199). Calcium is sensed as being normal at subphysiological concentrations and PTH secretion is therefore switched off inappropriately, causing hypoparathyroidism. The extent of the resulting hypoparathyroidism is determined by how much the mutation shifts the calcium response curve to the left (Fig. 16.2). Patients may or may not be asymptomatic. Several mutations have been described and, although there is no genotype–phenotype correlation, symptoms are related to the degree of hypocalcemia, which remains fairly constant within individuals. Inheritance is usually autosomal dominant but sporadic cases have been described.

It can be difficult to distinguish ADH from other forms of FIH in the absence of a family history; germline mosaicism in an apparently unaffected parent can confuse the issue further and make prediction of recurrence difficult. Diagnosis depends on demonstrating hypocalcemia with normal PTH concentrations. In contrast to primary hypoparathyroidism, urinary calcium excretion is high and these patients are susceptible to nephrocalcinosis, especially if treated to prevent symptoms.

Continued on p. 392

Table 16.3 Hypocalcemic disorders associated with genetic abnormalities.

Location in calcium cascade	Metabolic abnormality	OMIM	Location	Gene	Gene product	OMIM	Inheritance	Principal clinical features
Calcium sensing receptor								
	Autosomal dominant hypocalcemia	#146200	3q13.3-q21	CaSR	Calcium sensing receptor	+601199	AD	(Symptomatic) hypocalcemia, hypercalciuria, nephrocalcinosis
	Autosomal dominant hypocalcemia with Bartter-like features		3q13-1	CaSR	Calcium sensing receptor	+601199	AD	
Parathyroid glands								
	X-linked recessive hypoparathyroidism	%307700	Xq26-7	?SOX3	SRY-related homeobox	*313430	XLR	Infantile onset hypoparathyroidism
	Autosomal recessive isolated hypoparathyroidism	#146200	6p24.2	GCM2	Homolog of Drosophila glial cells missing	*603716	AR	Isolated hypoparathyroidism
	Mitochondrial disorders							
	Kearns–Sayre	#530000	Mitochondrial gene deletion	Various mitochondrial			Maternal	Hypoparathyroidism, progressive ophthalmoplegia, pigmentary retinopathy, heart block or cardiomyopathy, short stature, primary gonadal failure, sensorineural deafness, proximal myopathy, diabetes mellitus
	MELAS	#540000	Mitochondrial gene point mutation	Various mitochondrial			Maternal	Hypoparathyroidism, mitochondrial encephalopathy, lactic acidosis, stroke-like episodes, proximal myopathy, diabetes mellitus
	DiGeorge syndrome Type I	#188400	22q11.2	TBX1 (and others)	Transcription factors	*602054	Sporadic or AD or Unbalanced translocation	Neonatal hypoparathyroidism, thymic aplasia, ear, nose and mouth deformities, aortic arch abnormalities – truncus arteriosus, right-sided aortic arch, etc.

Table 16.3 *Continued*

Location in calcium cascade	Metabolic abnormality	OMIM	Location	Gene	Gene product	OMIM	Inheritance	Principal clinical features
	DiGeorge syndrome Type II	#188400	10p13-4	?	?		Sporadic	Neonatal hypoparathyroidism, immune deficiency
	Hypoparathyroidism, deafness, renal anomalies	#146255	10p14-0pter	GATA3	T-cell antigen receptor enhancer binding protein	*131320	AD	Hypoparathyroidism, sensorineural deafness, cystic renal changes
Other familial syndromes								
	Autosomal dominant Kenny–Caffey	%127000	?	?	?		AD	Similar to AR Kenny–Caffey
	Autosomal recessive Kenny–Caffey	#244460	1q43-4	TBCE	Tubulin-specific Chaperone E	*604934	AR	Hypoparathyroidism, extreme short stature, cortical thickening and medullary stenosis of tubular bones, normal bone age, absent diploic space, delayed closure of anterior fontanelle, normal intelligence
	Sanjad-Sakati and Richardson & Kirk	#241410	1q43-4	TBCE	Tubulin-specific Chaperone E	*604934	AR	Hypoparathyroidism, deep-set eyes, microcephaly, thin lips, long philtrum, beaked nose, external ear anomalies, micrognathia, depressed nasal bridge, mental retardation
	Dahlborg & Borer		?	?	?		AR or XLR	Hypoparathyroidism, congenital lymphedema, nephropathy, mitral valve prolapse, brachytelophalangy
	Pluriglandular autoimmune hypoparathyroidism (APECED)	#240300	21q22.3	AIRE-1	Autoimmune regulator	*607358	AR	Mucocutaneous candidiasis, hypoparathyroidism, adrenal insufficiency, hypogonadism, diabetes mellitus, nail pitting, keratopathy, alopecia, hepatitis, intestinal malabsorption

PTH

Familial isolated hypoparathyroidism	#146200	11p15	PTH	Parathyroid hormone	*168450	AD	Hypoparathyroidism
Familial isolated hypoparathyroidism	#146200	11p15	PTH	Parathyroid hormone	*168450	AR	Hypoparathyroidism

PTH/PTHrP receptor

Blomstrand chondrodysplasia	#215045	3p21.1-p22	PTH1R	Parathyroid hormone receptor	*168468	AR	Advanced bone maturation, accelerated chondrocyte maturation, increased bone density, poor bone modeling, rapidly lethal
Eiken skeletal dysplasia	#600002	3p21.1-p22	PTH1R	Parathyroid hormone receptor	*168468	?AR	Retarded ossification. Abnormal bone modeling
Pseudohypoparathyroidism Type Ib-like syndrome		3p21.1-p22	PTH1R	Parathyroid hormone receptor	*168468	?AR	Hypoparathyroidism with raised PTH

Post-receptor events

Pseudohypoparathyroidism Type Ia	#103580	20q13.2-3.3	GSαAD paternally imprinted	Gsα subunit	+139320	AD paternally imprinted	Hypoparathyroidism with raised PTH, short stature, round facies, short metacarpals and metatarsals (Albright hereditary osteodystrophy), mild hypothyroidism, disturbance of ovarian function, mild developmental delay
Pseudopseudohypoparathyroidism		20q13.2-3.3	GSαAD maternally imprinted	Gsα subunit	+139320	AD maternally imprinted	As above but with no hypoparathyroidism
Pseudohypoparathyroidism with testotoxicosis		20q13.2-3.3	Gsα – differential heat sensitivity	Gsα subunit	+139320	AD paternally imprinted	As for PHP-Ia but with testotoxicosis
Pseudohypoparathyroidism Type Ib	#603233	20q13	STX16	Syntaxin 16	*603666	AD ?paternally imprinted	Hypoparathyroidism with raised PTH but no features of AHO. May retain bone sensitivity
Pseudohypoparathyroidism Type Ic	?	?	?	?		?AD	Multiple hormone resistance with AHO

Continued on p. 394

Table 16.3 *Continued*

Location in calcium cascade	Metabolic abnormality	OMIM	Location	Gene	Gene product	OMIM	Inheritance	Principal clinical features
	Pseudohypoparathyroidism Type II	%203330	?	?	?	?	?	Hypoparathyroidism with normal cAMP but impaired phosphaturic response
Magnesium deficiency								
	Familial primary hypomagnesemia	#602014	9q12-2.2	TRPM6	Transient receptor potential cation channel M6	*607009	AR	Isolated defect of magnesium transport in gut, hypocalciuria
	Isolated renal magnesium wasting	#154020	11q23	FXYD2	Na,K-ATPase γ	*601814	AD	Hypermagnesuria with hypomagnesemia. Hypocalciuria
	Isolated recessive renal hypomagnesemia	#611718	4q25	EGF	Epidermal growth factor	*131530	AR	Isolated hypomagnesemia, normal plasma and urine calcium, psychomotor retardation, seizures, brisk reflexes
	Gitelman syndrome	#263800	16q13	SLC12A3	Thiazide sensitive Na-Cl co-tranporter	*600968	AR	Hypermagnesuria, hypokalemic alkalosis, hypocalciuria, chronic dermatitis
	Familial hypomagnesemia with hypercalciuria and nephrocalcinosis	#248250	3q	CLDN16 (PCLN-1)	Paracellin-1	*603959	AR	Hypermagnesuria, hypercalciuria, hypomagnesemia, nephrocalcinosis, renal failure
	Renal hypomagnesemia with ocular involvement	#248190	1p34.2	CLDN 19	Claudin 19	*610036	AR	Hypermagnesuria, hypercalciuria, hypomagnesemia, nephrocalcinosis, renal failure, ocular abnormalities

Genetic conditions that cause hypocalcemia. The conditions are classified according to which part of the calcium cascade they affect and, where known, the gene location, gene product, inheritance and principal clinical features are shown. OMIM numbers in columns 3 and 7 relate to the disorders and the genes respectively and refer to the Online Mendelian Inheritance in Man code numbers (http://www.ncbi.nlm.nih.gov/sites/entrez?db=OMIM). AHO, Albright hereditary osteodystrophy.

In patients whose plasma calcium is >1.95 mmol/L (7.8 mg/dL), treatment is unnecessary and, in those with a lower concentration of calcium, treatment is required only if symptoms are present. An active vitamin D metabolite (alfacalcidol or calcitriol) should be used cautiously and in the smallest dosage required and it is not necessary to restore plasma calcium to normal. Urinary calcium excretion should be monitored to avoid nephrocalcinosis and regular renal ultrasonography can be helpful in detecting early changes. If it proves difficult to prevent symptomatic hypocalcemia without causing nephrocalcinosis, thiazide diuretics may also be used. Selective CaSR blocking agents may become available in the future: there is one report of the successful short-term use of synthetic PTH, teriparatide (Forsteo⁻), in the treatment of this condition [32].

Another phenotype associated with activating mutations of the CaSR has been described and probably represents a more extreme example of the same condition [33]. These patients presented with apparent neonatal hypoparathyroidism and were treated with calcium and vitamin D or calcitriol. They subsequently presented in late childhood, adolescence or early adulthood with a Bartter-like syndrome of impaired renal function, hypercalciuria, nephrocalcinosis, hyperreninemia, hypokalemia and hyperaldosteronism in various degrees. In all cases, activating mutations of the CaSR were identified resulting in a marked left shift of the dose–response curve for extracellular calcium signaling.

The mechanism of these biochemical changes is not clear but it has been suggested that the CaSR defect prevents calcium and magnesium reabsorption, which normally takes place in conjunction with sodium. This leads to sodium wasting and a concentrating defect that stimulates hyperreninemia and hyperaldosteronism and leads to increased potassium losses. At the same time, the distal convoluted tubule (DCT) then has to compensate for the sodium losses, which leads to further calcium excretion and hypokalemic alkalosis. Caution is therefore urged in the use of thiazide diuretics, which might theoretically worsen the calcium excretion.

Disorders of the parathyroid glands

X-linked recessive familial isolated hypoparathyroidism

In X-linked recessive familial isolated hypoparathyroidism (HYPX) (%307700), a mutant gene on chromosome Xq26-q27 has been described in two apparently unrelated families [34]. Mitochondrial DNA studies have shown them to be related. The nature of the gene product is not known for certain but it is likely that SOX3 (*313430) is involved in parathyroid development and that genes that influence SOX3 may be involved in the development of HYPX. Affected males have infantile onset of hypoparathyroidism and histological studies have suggested that the cause is parathyroid agenesis.

Autosomal recessive isolated hypoparathyroidism

Autosomal recessive isolated hypoparathyroidism presents at an early age [34]. In one family, apparently unrelated, a homozygous

mutation was found in the GCM2 (*603716) gene [35] located on chromosome 6p24.2, while in an extended Pakistani family where consanguinity was present, a different mutation was found [36]. These two mutations have been shown to result in reduced transcriptional activity of the gene which is expressed only in PT glands and appears to have a role in PT gland development. In addition, there appears to be a group of patients with isolated hypoparathyroidism, sometimes familial, in whom heterozygous mutations within the GCM2 gene have been demonstrated but these have also been found in unaffected family members and do not appear to reduce transcriptional activity [37]. The precise role of GCM2 in PTG development has therefore yet to be elucidated.

Kearns–Sayre syndrome

The Kearns–Sayre syndrome (KSS) (#530000) comprises hypoparathyroidism with progressive external ophthalmoplegia, pigmentary retinopathy, heart block or cardiomyopathy and proximal myopathy. It may also be associated with diabetes mellitus. It overlaps with the MELAS syndrome (#540000) in which hypoparathyroidism is associated with a childhood onset of mitochondrial encephalopathy, lactic acidosis and stroke-like episodes [34]. Proximal myopathy and diabetes mellitus have also been described with this condition. Several different mutations in the mitochondrial genome have been reported in some of these patients, although the role of these mutations is not understood.

DiGeorge syndrome

The DiGeorge syndrome (DGS) (#188400) is the most common gene deletion syndrome with an incidence of 1 in 4–5000 live births. It consists of parathyroid gland hypoplasia, thymic immunodeficiency, congenital heart disease and facial anomalies, structures all derived from the third and fourth branchial pouches [38]. It is related to velocardiofacial (VCFS) (#192430) and conotruncal anomaly facial (CTAFS) (#217095) syndromes and a number of non-syndromic cardiac conditions, such as pulmonary atresia with ventricular septal defect, Fallot tetralogy, truncus arteriosus and interrupted aortic arch. Only DGS includes hypoparathyroidism.

They are linked under the umbrella of the CATCH22 syndrome (cardiac anomalies, abnormal facies, thymic hypoplasia, cleft palate and hypocalcemia associated with microdeletions in the long arm of chromosome 22).

Most cases of DGS are associated with de novo deletions of variable size in chromosome 22q11.2. Autosomal dominant transmission has been described in association with an unbalanced translocation and deletion involving the same chromosomal area [39]. The TBX1 gene (*602054), which is in the center of the DiGeorge region of chromosome 22q11.1, seems to have a crucial role in the early development of the pharyngeal pouches and otic vesicles. The precise role of the gene products is not understood but they are probably DNA-binding proteins [40]. Another gene, UDF1L, is also located within the 22q11 region and deletions have been found in all patients with the CATCH22 syndrome [41]. Not all patients with DGS have been shown to have mutations in the 22q region. Those who have are designated as DGS1. Mutations in a second locus on chromosome 10p13-14 have also been seen with hypoparathyroidism and immune deficiency, which has been designated DGS2 (%601362). The gene involved in this syndrome is not known for certain. Some features of DGS may also be seen in the fetal alcohol syndrome [42].

In DGS, the emphasis is on the PT and thymus glands and the cardiac anomalies. The severity of the condition varies but most infants present with cardiac abnormalities and often hypocalcemia is overlooked. Thymus gland aplasia is suspected by the absence of a thymic shadow on chest X-ray and can be confirmed by a low T-cell count, although the total lymphocyte count may be normal.

Late-onset DGS has also been described. These patients present with hypocalcemia in late childhood or adolescence and have only minor dysmorphic features. Microdeletions of the 22q11 chromosome have also been identified [43]. If hypocalcemia does not become symptomatic during infancy it may remain dormant until adolescence when the increased demand for calcium during the adolescent growth spurt precipitates hypocalcemic convulsions. The use of loop diuretics for cardiac failure may precipitate hypocalcemia because of their hypercalciuric effects.

Autosomal dominant hypoparathyroidism, deafness and renal anomalies

Autosomal dominant hypoparathyroidism, deafness and renal anomalies (HDR) (#146255) was first described in 1992 [34]. The hypoparathyroidism is associated with low or inappropriately normal concentrations of PTH with normal responsiveness to PTH, the deafness is sensorineural and the renal anomalies consist of cystic changes that lead to renal impairment in some patients. Cytogenetic abnormalities of chromosome 10p14-10pter have been identified in these patients. This region does not overlap the DGS2 region and contains a gene, GATA3, (*131320) that is involved in the developing kidney, otic vesicles and parathyroid glands. Thirteen different mutations have been demonstrated, mostly causing a loss of DNA binding [44] and it is probably the same syndrome as described by Barakat et al. [45] and by Shaw et al. [46].

Hypoparathyroidism retardation dysmorphism

The autosomal recessive Kenny–Caffey (#244460) [34] and Sanjad–Sakati [34] syndromes and that described by Richardson and Kirk [47] are probably all phenotypic variants of the hypoparathyroidism retardation dysmorphism (HRD) syndrome (#241410) caused by mutations in the tubulin specific chaperone E (TBCE) gene (*604934). Hypoparathyroidism is associated with extreme short stature and developmental delay. They have been described mainly in consanguineous families from Saudi Arabia and Kuwait and mutations have been mapped to chromosome 1q42-43. Other familial syndromes are also described, although the chromosomal locations and gene defects have not been identified (Table 16.3 [34]).

Autoimmune polyendocrinopathy-candidiasis-ectodermal dystrophy (APECED)

The APECED syndrome (#240300), also known as the polyglandular autoimmune type 1 syndrome, is an evolving association between mucocutaneous candidiasis and hypoparathyroidism that usually develops in mid-childhood [48]. About 70% of patients develop adrenal insufficiency and other endocrinopathies, such as hypogonadism and hypothyroidism; diabetes mellitus may develop in later life. Other associated features include nail pitting, keratopathy, alopecia, hepatitis and intestinal malabsorption, all of which are autoimmune mediated.

Several mutations in the autoimmune regulator (AIRE-1) gene (*607358) on chromosome 21q22.3 have been recognized. The condition is particularly prominent in Finnish families, in which a mutation at codon 257 (Arg257Ter) has been identified in 82% of subjects. It has also been identified in Iranian Jews.

Patients usually present with mucocutaneous candidiasis and later develop hypoparathyroidism followed by other features. Adrenal insufficiency should be suspected if hypercalcemia supervenes in a previously stable patient. This is probably because of changes in renal calcium reabsorption following the hypovolemia associated with mineralocorticoid deficiency. These patients require careful follow-up in order to identify adrenal insufficiency.

Disorders of PTH
Autosomal dominant familial isolated hypoparathyroidism

Autosomal dominant familial isolated hypoparathyroidism (FIH) has been described in a patient in whom a single base substitution in exon 2 of the PTH gene results in a single amino acid substitution (arginine for cysteine) that impedes processing of the mutant prepro sequence [49]. Different mutations, also involving the prepro sequence, have been found to cause autosomal recessive FIH [50,51].

Disorders of the PTH/PTHrP receptor
Blomstrand chondrodysplasia

Blomstrand chondrodysplasia (BOCD) (#215045) is an autosomal recessive condition that results in advanced bone maturation, accelerated chondrocyte maturation, increased density of the skeleton, increased ossification and poor bone modeling, particularly of the long bones [52]. It is rapidly lethal. Mutations of the PTH/PTHrP receptor (*168468) have consisted of nucleotide exchanges in the maternal allele (the paternal allele not being expressed), single nucleotide insertions or deletions resulting in frameshifts or nonsense mutations resulting in a truncated protein.

Eiken skeletal dysplasia

Another syndrome caused by mutations in the PTHR1 receptor is Eiken skeletal dysplasia (#600002) [53]. Many of the features are the opposite of those of BOCD in that delayed ossification, particularly of the epiphyses, pelvis, hands and feet, was noted along with abnormal bone modeling. The subjects appeared normal at birth and hypocalcemia does not seem to be a problem.

Three siblings in one family have been described who presented with features similar to those of pseudohypoparathyroid-

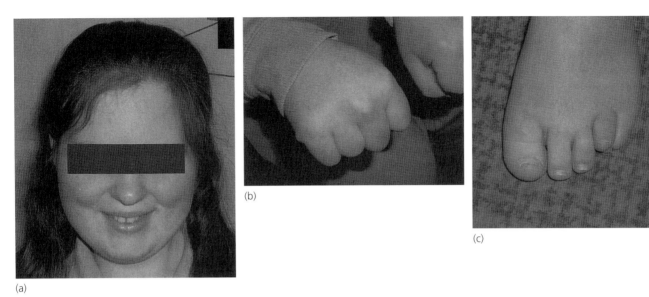

(b)

(c)

(a)

Figure 16.11 The face (a) showing the typical rounded facies and of the right hand (b) and left foot (c) of a patient with pseudohypoparathyroidism Type Ia showing the typical shortening of the metacarpals and metatarsals seen as part of Albright hereditary osteodystrophy (AHO). The patient had presented with short stature. A mutation in the GNAS1 gene has been demonstrated in this patient. (Reproduced with the kind permission of the patient.)

ism Type Ib and were found to have a single amino acid deletion (del382Ile) in the C-terminal end of the PTH/PTHrP receptor [51]. This mutation appears to uncouple the PTH/PTHrP receptor from the Gsα while not affecting other hormones.

Parathyroid hormone resistance

This group of conditions, which occurs as a result of defects toward the end of the calcium cascade, is characterized by hypocalcemia, usually but not always accompanied by hyperphosphatemia and raised PTH. The two most important are pseudohypoparathyroidism and deficiencies in the supply or metabolism of vitamin D.

Pseudohypoparathyroidism Type Ia

Pseudohypoparathyroidism Type Ia (PHP-Ia) (#103580) is an autosomal dominant condition characterized by hypoparathyroidism (hypocalcemia and hyperphosphatemia) with raised concentrations of PTH. Resistance to the action of PTH can be confirmed by demonstrating lack of cAMP or phosphaturic responses to PTH infusion. A characteristic set of features includes short stature, round facies, shortening of the metacarpals and metatarsals, particularly the fourth and fifth, and obesity, collectively termed Albright hereditary osteodystrophy (AHO) (Fig. 16.11). Other features include intracranial calcification (Fig. 16.10), sensorineural deafness and a poor sense of smell and many subjects have developmental delay. Resistance to other cAMP-dependent hormones, especially TSH and gonadotropins, may be present, leading to mild hypothyroidism and menstrual irregularity. This syndrome is referred to as PHP1a. Following the discovery of the Gsα subunit of the G-protein (+139320), it was recognized that inactivating mutations within the gene are responsible for the PTH resistance [54].

Ten years after the original description of PHP1a, a second syndrome was described in which AHO was present without an abnormality of calcium metabolism. This was termed pseudopseudohypoparathyroidism (PPHP). It subsequently became apparent that both conditions can occur within the same family but not within the same sibship. While both conditions are associated with the skeletal manifestations, it emerged that, when hypocalcemia was present, the gene had been inherited from an affected mother and paternal transmission of the gene did not result in PTH resistance, despite the fact that identical mutations could be demonstrated within families. Gene imprinting was suspected [54] and subsequently confirmed by detailed genetic studies.

The GNAS1 gene has 13 exons that code for the Gsα subunit plus at least five additional exons including those that code for transcripts known as A/B, XL, Nesp55 and Nespas. By a complex arrangement of splicing, four different mRNA transcripts are known to result (Fig. 16.12). All have the products of codons 2–13 in common.

Native Gsα also contains exon 1 and this mRNA is expressed in most tissues in a biallelic manner but the transcripts containing A/B, XL and Nespas are expressed only by the paternal allele, because the maternal allele is methylated, resulting in inactivation; the Nesp55 allele is expressed only in the maternal allele, the paternal allele being methylated [55]. In the kidney only the maternal allele is expressed in the proximal tubule (where most calcium reabsorption occurs) although it is expressed biallelically in the thick ascending loop of Henle and collecting ducts. This causes hypocalcemia although, in contrast to hypoparathyroidism, hypercalciuria is not usually a problem during treatment because of the presence of an active paternal allele lower down the tubule. It is proposed that it is this that distinguishes the phenotypes. Thus, if a mutation occurs within the maternal allele,

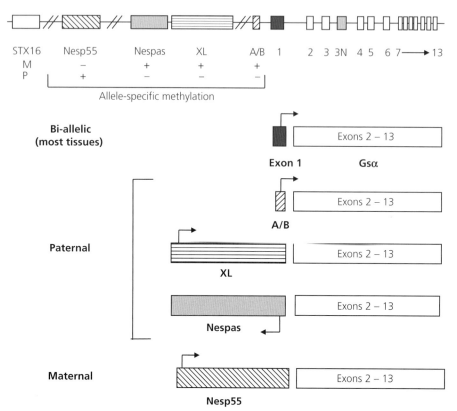

Figure 16.12 The intron–exon organization of the GNAS1 gene showing the different mRNAs that are derived as a result of alternative splicing. Native Gsα is thought to be expressed in most tissues and to be biallelic. Mutations result in AHO. The A/B, XL and Nespas alternative transcripts are principally expressed in the paternal allele while the Nesp55 transcript, which is mainly found in the kidney, is expressed from the maternal allele. Therefore paternally acquired mutations result in pseudopseudohypoparathyroidism while pseudohypoparathyroidism results from maternally acquired mutations. (Adapted and reprinted from Bastepe *et al.* [59] with permission from Elsevier.)

PTH resistance and hypocalcemia are present while hypocalcemia is absent if the paternal allele is mutated.

Several mutations have been described throughout the GNAS1 gene but most frequently in exon 7. There is no obvious phenotype–genotype correlation, apart from a missense mutation at codon 366 consisting of an Ala122Ser substitution, which results in a temperature-sensitive Gsα mutant. At 37°C, it is inactivated, resulting in PHP; at 34°C, it is activated and results in testotoxicosis [56].

Pseudohypoparathyroidism Type Ib

In pseudohypoparathyroidism Type Ib (PHPIb) (#603233), features of AHO are absent but PTH resistance is present. Renal resistance to PTH can be demonstrated by impaired cAMP and phosphaturic responses. Some patients exhibit hyperparathyroid bone disease, indicating that some measure of bone sensitivity to PTH is retained. These patients have been variously referred to as pseudohypohyperparathyroidism or pseudohypoparathyroidism with raised alkaline phosphatase [57]. The term PHP1b is preferred. The precise mechanism by which the PHP develops has not been fully elucidated. No mutations in the GNAS1 gene have been detected but linkage studies have suggested that the gene responsible is located on chromosome 20q13 near to or in the same position as the GNAS1 gene. PHP1b appears to be paternally imprinted in the same way as PHP-1a [58]. It is possible that tissue- or cell-specific promoters or enhancers of GNAS1 may be responsible. A microdeletion in the STX16 gene (*603666), which lies about 280 kb downstream from the GNAS

gene, may be the crucial factor that results in differential loss of methylation of the A/B exon of the GNAS gene, thus resulting in renal resistance but without causing AHO [59].

Pseudohypoparathyroidism Type Ic

Pseudohypoparathyroidism Type Ic (PHP-Ic) is characterized by multiple hormone resistance, including PTH, together with features of AHO. No defect in Gsα has been demonstrated and the genetic defect is not known, although it is presumed to reside within the adenylate cyclase receptor system.

Pseudohypoparathyroidism type II

Pseudohypoparathyroidism type II (PHPII) (%203330) is reserved for a small group of patients who have PTH resistance without features of AHO. The PTH resistance is confined to the phosphaturic response, whereas cAMP responses are normal. The defect, which has not been identified, presumably lies beyond the adenylate cyclase system.

Treatment of hypoparathyroidism and pseudohypoparathyroidism

Treatment is aimed at maintaining plasma calcium concentrations within the lower part of the normal range without causing hypercalciuria. The mainstay of treatment is vitamin D, either in its active form, 1,25(OH)2D (calcitriol) or the analog 1α-hydroxycholecalciferol (alfacalcidol). The dose of calcitriol is usually 15–30 ng/kg/day to maintain normocalcemia but requires twice or thrice daily dosage. Alfacalcidol usually requires about twice the dose but, because it has to be metabolized first, it has a longer half-life and needs to be given only once daily. Calcium supplements are usually required, which may enable the dose of alfacalcidol to be reduced. This is a particular advantage in hypoparathyroid disorders in which the renal tubular reabsorptive effects of PTH are lacking and hypercalciuria may supervene. In patients in whom cardiac failure is present (e.g. DiGeorge syndrome), loop diuretics such as furosemide should be used with caution because the hypercalciuric effects of these agents may precipitate symptomatic hypocalcemia. Regular renal ultrasound may detect early nephrocalcinosis. Synthetic PTH (1–34) and PTH analogs may be useful in the future.

The principles of treatment of PHP are similar to those of hypoparathyroidism. Alfacalcidol (1–3 µg/day) is usually sufficient to maintain normocalcemia. Hypercalciuria is less likely to occur and the plasma calcium concentration can usually be kept within the normal range. Patients with PHP1a or PHP1c, and occasionally PHP1b, may have resistance to other hormones. TSH is frequently slightly raised and thyroxine is required to suppress this and allow optimum thyroid function. Menstrual irregularities may require estrogen therapy. The role of growth hormone for short stature is controversial but has been used in some patients with variable effect. If resistance to GRF can be demonstrated, there is some logic to this therapy. No treatment has a significant effect on the AHO.

Disorders related to magnesium deficiency

Hypomagnesemia usually arises as a result of impaired intestinal absorption or increased urinary losses, which can be distinguished by measuring the urinary magnesium : creatinine ratio. In some of these conditions there is hypercalciuria but low urinary calcium excretion is present in others.

Magnesium is a ligand for the CaSR and, if plasma magnesium concentrations fall, PTH secretion is stimulated in a manner similar to that of hypocalcemia. More severe hypomagnesemia (<0.5 mmol/L) inhibits PTH secretion in response to hypocalcemia. Initially, this inhibition is incomplete and PTH remains elevated but not as high as would be expected from the degree of hypocalcemia. As concentrations fall to 0.2–0.3 mmol/L, PTH secretion is inhibited completely and a state of hypoparathyroidism then exists [60]. During the initial phase of mild hypomagnesemia, when PTH concentrations are still elevated, resistance to the action of PTH, caused by either desensitization or downregulation, worsens the hypocalcemia. Thus, hypocalcemia secondary to hypomagnesemia is resistant to treatment until magnesium concentrations have been restored to normal.

Hypomagnesemia with hypocalciuria
Hypomagnesemia with secondary hypocalciuria
Hypomagnesemia with secondary hypocalciuria (HOMG1) (#602014) was initially thought to be an X-linked recessive condition because this condition has a preponderance of males but it is now known to be autosomal recessive and is caused by a primary defect in magnesium absorption as a result of mutations in the TRPM6 gene (*607009) involved in active transport of magnesium in the gut (Fig. 16.1). Chronic hypomagnesemia leads to impaired PTH secretion and responsiveness with consequent hypocalcemia early in the neonatal period. If patients survive, treatment is best undertaken using magnesium supplements in large quantity, often as much as 20 times normal requirements, although this may be difficult because of secondary diarrhea. Acquired malabsorption of magnesium can also occur as a result of Crohn or Whipple diseases.

Hypomagnesemia with associated hypocalciuria
In hypomagnesemia with associated hypocalciuria (HOMG2) (#154020), misrouting of the γ-subunit of the Na^+/K^+-ATPase on the inner membrane of the renal tubule causes magnesium wasting (Fig. 16.1). Mutations of the FXYD2 gene (*601814), which codes for this protein, cause autosomal dominant hypomagnesemia with reduced urinary calcium excretion.

Isolated recessive renal hypomagnesemia
Isolated recessive renal hypomagnesemia (IRH, HOMG4) (#611718) is an autosomal recessive condition caused by a mutation in the EGF gene (*131530) which controls magnesium reabsorption by TRPM6 (Fig. 16.1). Isolated hypomagnesemia is associated with normal plasma and urine calcium but the patients have psychomotor retardation and seizures with brisk reflexes, presumably as a result of other effects of EGF.

Gitelman syndrome
Gitelman syndrome (#263800), sometimes referred to as a benign form of Bartter syndrome, is a separate entity, although there is some overlap. Mutations in the thiazide-sensitive sodium chloride transporter (SLC12A3) (*600968) result in hypokalemic alkalosis with salt-wasting, hypomagnesemia and hypocalciuria. Patients usually present after the age of 5 years with episodes of muscle weakness, lethargy, tetany and muscle cramps. Dermatitis may be present and, although the syndrome is described as benign, a prolonged cardiac Q-T interval may give rise to arrhythmias and syncopal attacks. Chondrocalcinosis is a feature which these patients share with others with chronic hypomagnesemia. Urinary calcium excretion is low. Treatment consists of correcting the biochemical abnormalities, particularly the potassium and magnesium deficiencies, with oral supplementation.

Hypomagnesemia with hypercalciuria
Claudin 16 (paracellin 1), located in the tight junctions of the epithelium of ascending loop of Henle, is mutated in hypermagnesuria with hypercalciuria and nephrocalcinosis (HOMG3) (#248250). It allows excessive excretion of both magnesium and calcium. Several different homozygous or compound heterozygous mutations have been described and the severity of the condition varies according to genotype. In some cases the problem is self-limiting while in others renal failure may ensue. Hypocalcemia is occasionally present.

Renal hypomagnesemia with ocular involvement

Renal hypomagnesemia with ocular involvement (#248190) is also autosomal recessive and is similar to HOMG3 but also includes ocular abnormalities such as coloboma, myopia and horizontal nystagmus. No mutations are found in the claudin 16 gene but they are found in the similar claudin 19 gene (*610036). This is located mainly in the collecting ducts of the renal tubule.

Acquired tubulopathies leading to hypermagnesuria may occur in diabetic ketoacidosis, chronic alcoholism or following the chronic use of various drugs, such as loop diuretics, ciclosporin, aminoglycoside antibiotics, cisplatin and cetuximab. Treatment of hypomagnesemia is aimed at restoring plasma magnesium concentrations to normal to prevent inhibition of PTH secretion.

Rickets and other disorders with abnormal supply or metabolism of vitamin D

Vitamin D deficiency

The definition of vitamin D deficiency is controversial but a consensus is emerging that suggests that true deficiency should be considered in children when 25OHD concentrations are <30–35 nmol/L (12–14 ng/mL) and that insufficiency is present when concentrations are above this but <50 nmol/L (20 ng/mL). Some physicians regard 70–80 nmol/L (28–32 ng/mL) to be the lower limit of normal on the grounds that some adults show increases in PTH below this concentration but not everyone who has vitamin D deficiency as defined above presents with symptoms and it is likely that calcium intake plays a part in determining whether or not problems arise [61].

Calcium deficiency rickets is also described, particularly from West and South Africa and parts of tropical Asia, in patients in whom vitamin D deficiency was unimportant but who had low calcium intakes [62]. These patients tend to present later than those with vitamin D deficiency and respond better to treatment with calcium supplementation than to vitamin D.

Vitamin D deficiency and nutritional rickets remain significant causes of abnormalities of calcium metabolism. Following the recognition of the importance of vitamin D, rickets was virtually eliminated in Western societies with fortification of foods and administration of vitamin D supplements to children. A resurgence of vitamin D deficiency was seen following the increase in immigration to the UK, particularly from the Caribbean and Indian subcontinent in the 1950s and 1960s. Various campaigns, such as the Glasgow Stop Rickets campaign during the 1970s, reduced the incidence of rickets and vitamin D deficiency but, recently, there has been a third wave seen in both the UK and the USA. Vitamin D deficiency remains the single most common cause of rickets in the UK and in many other countries worldwide. Vitamin D deficiency can also arise as a result of impaired absorption of vitamin D in gastrointestinal disorders, such as celiac disease, especially if the supply of vitamin D from sunlight is restricted.

Disorders associated with vitamin D deficiency

Three particular conditions have been described in association with vitamin D deficiency. Young infants and adolescents may present with hypocalcemic convulsions and other symptoms. Radiological evidence of rickets is often not present, particularly in teenagers. The muscle spasm that accompanies the hypocalcemia can be painful but is rapidly relieved by intravenous infusion of calcium. This situation arises early during the development of vitamin D deficiency and occurs in children who are growing rapidly before rickets has a chance to develop [63]. The biochemical abnormalities are rapidly corrected by high dose vitamin D with calcium supplements.

Classic rickets develops in older infants and toddlers but may also be seen later in childhood. The more typical biochemical findings of mild hypocalcemia, hypophosphatemia and greatly elevated alkaline phosphatase are usually seen. As rickets worsens, hypocalcemia ensues and may become symptomatic. Patients present with walking difficulties caused by muscle weakness and bowing of the legs. Genu valgum, genu varum or a combination of the two, giving the so-called windswept appearance, are more common in older children. Swelling of the wrists and knees and a rickety rosary are apparent (Fig. 16.13). Developmental delay of motor milestones is often seen. The classic radiological features are widening and splaying of the epiphyses with a motheaten appearance to the epiphyses, the so-called champagne glass appearance (Fig. 16.14). The bones have an osteopenic appearance and evidence of secondary hyperparathyroidism, including microcysts along the borders of the phalanges and periosteal reaction, can be seen. Fractures may also be present [64]. Treatment consists of high dose vitamin D, which usually corrects the biochemical abnormalities within a few weeks, although the rickets takes longer to heal. Bowing of the legs and other skeletal deformities may take several months to correct and referral for orthopedic procedures, particularly in young children, should be delayed until it is clear that further remodeling is not going to occur.

A third, potentially fatal, complication of vitamin D deficiency, dilated cardiomyopathy, may occur in infants under the age of 6 months [65]. They present with feeding difficulties and respiratory distress and on examination are found to have heart failure associated with dilated cardiomyopathy. The combination of hypocalcemia and heart failure should strongly suggest this diagnosis. Urgent treatment with vitamin D and supportive therapy for the heart failure, which may include extracorporeal membrane oxygenation, is required. The prognosis is good, unlike that of almost all other kinds of cardiomyopathy in infancy, although, while the biochemical abnormalities are usually correctable within a few days, cardiac function may take months to return to normal. These infants are most frequently born to mothers of South Asian or Afro-Caribbean origin who are themselves vitamin D deficient and the infants are born vitamin D deficient. Breast feeding increases the likelihood of vitamin D deficiency because there is little vitamin D in breast milk.

In addition to the clearly defined syndromes of vitamin D deficiency, many children with vitamin D insufficiency complain

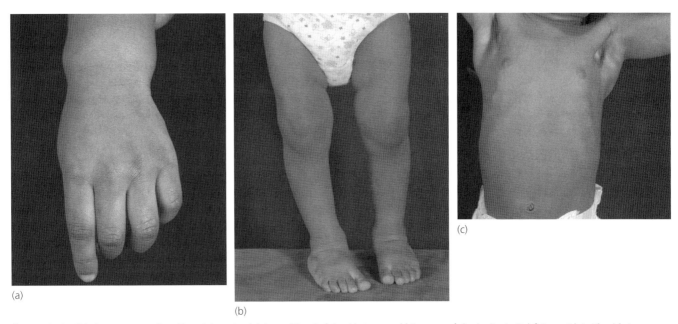

Figure 16.13 Clinical appearances of swelling of the wrists (a), knees (b) and of the rickety rosary (c) in a case of classic vitamin D deficiency rickets. The rickety rosary is seen lateral and parallel to the costal margins. (Reproduced with kind permission of the patient's family.)

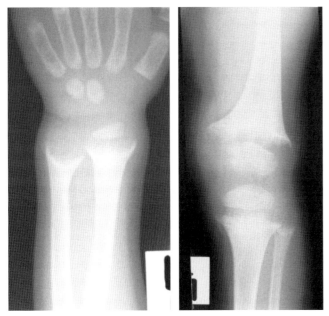

Figure 16.14 X-ray appearances of wrists (a) and knees (b) in classic vitamin D deficiency rickets. Both show the typical champagne glass appearances of the epiphyses with concave margins and a ragged appearance.

of aches and pains and backache without overt evidence of rickets or hypocalcemia. They respond to treatment with vitamin D and calcium supplements.

Biochemical abnormalities may not be seen, even in the presence of undetectable vitamin D concentrations, but when present they develop in three stages, although these are not clearly demarcated and may overlap (Fig. 16.15) [66].

In stage 1, hypocalcemia and hyperphosphatemia are present, bone turnover is increased and alkaline phosphatase is usually moderately raised. PTH is raised secondary to hypocalcemia and these patients can present with severe hypocalcemic symptoms. The presence of hypocalcemia and hyperphosphatemia with raised PTH resembles an acquired PHP-like state and, indeed, PTH resistance, as demonstrated by cAMP responses to PTH, is present. Because of this, it is not possible to define a cause for hypocalcemia until vitamin D deficiency has been excluded or corrected. In some parts of the UK, vitamin D deficiency remains the most common cause of hypocalcemia outside the neonatal period.

In stage 2, PTH rises further and seems to overcome the resistance seen in stage 1. Consequently, plasma calcium is only slightly low and hypophosphatemia supervenes in response to hyperparathyroidism. Alkaline phosphatase increases as the rickets develops.

In stage 3, hypocalcemia worsens and may again become symptomatic, whereas the hypophosphatemia persists. Rickets becomes worse and alkaline phosphatase rises further. At this stage, the radiological appearances become more obvious.

In vitamin D deficiency, 25OHD concentrations are usually low but a normal concentration does not exclude the diagnosis, especially if vitamin D has been administered or sunlight exposure obtained before presentation. 1,25(OH)$_2$D concentrations (if measured) are usually low but may be normal or even elevated if vitamin D treatment has already begun because 1,25(OH)$_2$D rises

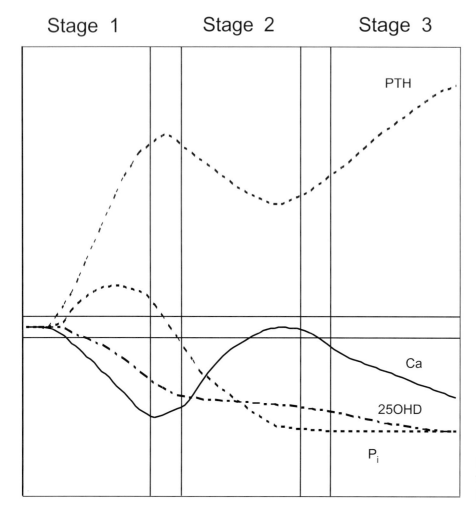

Figure 16.15 Stages in the development of vitamin D deficiency. (After Arnaud *et al.* [66] with permission from de Gruyter.)

to supraphysiological concentrations in response to the high PTH following administration of vitamin D and falls to physiological concentrations only as the rickets heal [67].

Treatment of vitamin D deficiency is best undertaken with vitamin D and not one of its analogs. A dose of 1500 IU/day in infants and 3000 IU/day for 3 months in older children and 6000 IU/day in adolescents is usually sufficient to correct the biochemistry and restore vitamin D stores [67]. Acute symptomatic hypocalcemia may require calcium infusions until symptoms subside. It is advisable to give oral calcium supplements as well as vitamin D. Alfacalcidol should be avoided because it does not correct vitamin D deficiency and may be ineffective in healing the rickets because supraphysiological concentrations are required for adequate healing.

Disorders of vitamin D metabolism

The biochemical changes seen in rickets associated with abnormalities of vitamin D metabolism are the same as those seen in vitamin D deficiency, with the exception of the vitamin D metabolites (Table 16.4). Chronic liver disease may affect 25-hydroxylation of vitamin D but this is not usually of clinical sig-

nificance because patients with chronic liver disease are usually given vitamin D supplements. In low birthweight infants (23–25 weeks' gestation), who often develop a degree of hepatitis, poor 25-hydroxylation may be significant and these infants sometimes require treatment with calcitriol rather than alfacalcidol to overcome this defect. In selective 25-hydroxy vitamin D_3 deficiency (#600081), caused by mutations in one of the vitamin D 25-hydroxylases, (CYP2R1) (*608713) [68], patients require treatment with high dose vitamin D or calcitriol.

Vitamin D-dependent rickets Type 1

Patients with vitamin D-dependent rickets Type 1 (VDDR-I, 1a-hydroxylase deficiency) (#264700), caused by mutations in the vitamin D 1α-hydroxylase gene (CYP27B1) (*609506), usually present with rachitic features during the toddler age. $1,25(OH)_2D$ concentrations are low or only just within the normal range despite adequate concentrations of 25OHD and high PTH. Alfacalcidol (or calcitriol) is the treatment of choice in large doses (150–200 ng/kg/day) until the rickets heal. This mimics the supraphysiological concentrations of $1,25(OH)_2D$ that occur during the initial phase of treatment of vitamin D deficiency. Patients

Table 16.4 Vitamin D metabolism and pathology.

Enzyme	Gene	Location	OMIM	Clinical condition	OMIM	Principal features
Vitamin D 25-hydroxylase	CYP27A1	2q33-qter	*606530	Cerebrotendinous xanthomatosis	#213700	Cerebellar ataxia, pseudobulbar palsy, premature atherosclerosis, cataracts. Rickets *not* a feature
	CYP2R1	11p15.2	*608713	25-hydroxyvitamin D deficiency	#600081	Rickets appearing in early childhood. Responds to high dose vitamin D or calcitriol
	CYP3A4	7q22.1	*124010	nil		Drug metabolism
	CYP2J2	1p31.3-p31.2	*601258	nil		Drug metabolism
25OHD-1α hydroxylase	CYP27B1	12q13.1-q13.3	*609506	Vitamin D dependent rickets Type 1	#264700	Classic rickets appearing in toddler age range. Responds to 1α-hydroxylated vitamin D metabolites
25OHD-24 hydroxylase	CYP24A1	20q13.2-q13.3	*126065	nil		May be upregulated in some ethnic groups
Vitamin D receptor	VDR	12q12-q14	*601769	1α,25(OH)$_2$D-resistant rickets, ligand binding positive	#277440	Severe rickets usually unresponsive to vitamin D metabolites. Alopecia usual
Vitamin D receptor	VDR	12q12-q14	*601769	1α,25(OH)$_2$D-resistant rickets, ligand binding negative	#277440	Severe rickets usually unresponsive to vitamin D metabolites. Alopecia usually absent
Vitamin D receptor	VDR	?		Vitamin D dependent rickets Type II with normal vitamin D receptor	%600785	Rickets with lower limb deformities. Good physical condition. Muscle weakness, alopecia, etc. *not* present

Vitamin D enzymes and the disorders that arise from their mutations. The OMIM numbers in column 4 relate to the enzymes themselves and those in column 6 to the disorders caused by mutations in the various enzymes and refer to the Online Mendelian Inheritance in Man code numbers (http://www.ncbi.nlm.nih.gov/sites/entrez?db=OMIM).

need to be monitored and the dose reduced to prevent hypercalciuria or hypercalcemia as the bones heal.

Vitamin D-dependent rickets Type 2

Vitamin D-dependent rickets Type 2, more properly known as hereditary 1α,25(OH)$_2$D-resistant rickets (HVDRR) (#277440), is caused by mutations in the vitamin D receptor (VDR) (*601769) either within the ligand-binding domain (ligand-binding negative) or the DNA binding domain (ligand-binding positive). A wide variety of mutations has been demonstrated and those that are ligand-binding positive generally have alopecia while those that are ligand-binding negative have normal hair. Infants present with severe rickets and failure to thrive. Hypocalcemia, hypophosphatemia and raised alkaline phosphatase are present with radiological signs of rickets. 1,25(OH)$_2$D concentrations are usually raised, regardless of whether or not treatment has been begun, because of impaired 24-hydroxylase activity. Treatment with vitamin D analogs raises concentrations further.

Treatment of HVDRR can prove difficult. Some patients respond to large doses of calcitriol whereas others prove almost completely resistant. The most successful treatment has been with infusions of large doses of calcium which allows mineralization to take place. Once this has been established, it may be possible to maintain satisfactory calcium balance, although this may become more difficult during puberty.

Vitamin D-dependent rickets with normal vitamin D receptor

In one other form of HVDRR, vitamin D-dependent rickets with normal vitamin D receptor (%600785), patients present with lower limb deformities, normal muscle power and none of the other features normally associated with rickets. Plasma calcium concentrations are low or low-normal and 1,25(OH)$_2$D and alkaline phosphatase elevated. No abnormalities have been demonstrated in the VDR and post-translation defects leading to failure of normal protein binding are thought to be the cause.

Distal renal tubular acidosis

Renal tubular acidosis (RTA) can result from defects either in the proximal or distal tubule (Table 16.5). In proximal RTA, the defect results from failure to excrete bicarbonate ions and is usually associated with other proximal tubular abnormalities (e.g.

Table 16.5 Distal renal tubular acidosis and miscellaneous renal tubular disorders associated with hypercalciuria, hyperphosphatemia and hypermagnesuria.

Clinical condition	OMIM	Location	Gene	Gene product	OMIM	Inheritance	Features
Distal renal tubular acidosis							
Autosomal dominant distal renal tubular acidosis	#179800	17q21-q22	SLC4A1	Band 3 glycoprotein	+109270	AD	Nephrocalcinosis, nephrolithiasis, rickets
Distal renal tubular acidosis with progressive nerve deafness	#267300	2cen-q13	ATP6V1B1	Vacuolar ATPase	*192132	AR	Nephrocalcinosis, rickets, sensorineural deafness
Autosomal recessive distal renal tubular acidosis	#602722	7q33-q34	ATP6N1B	Multisubunit H(+)-ATPase pump	*605239	AR	Nephrocalcinosis, nephrolithiasis, rickets
Autosomal recessive distal renal tubular acidosis	#602722	17q21-q22	SLC4A1	Band 3 glycoprotein	109270	AR	Nephrocalcinosis, nephrolithiasis, rickets. Elliptocytosis in some patients
Renal tubular acidosis III	267200	?	?	?	?	?AR, ?XL	Rickets, nephrolithiasis, nephrocalcinosis
Other renal tubular disorders causing proximal renal tubular acidosis, hypercalciuria, etc.							
Absorptive hypercalciuria 2	#143870	1q24	SAC	Soluble adenylyl cyclase	*605205	AD	Hypercalciuria, recurrent calcium oxalate stones
Absorptive hypercalciuria 1	%607258	4q33-qter	?	?		?	Hypercalciuria, nephrocalcinosis, dysmorphic features
Dent disease 1	#300009	Xp11.22	CLCN5	Chloride channel 5	*300008	XLR	Rickets, hypercalciuria, hyperphosphaturia, aminoaciduria, nephrolithiasis, renal failure
X-linked recessive nephrolithiasis	#310468	Xp11.22	CLCN5	Chloride channel 5	*300008	XLR	Nephrolithiasis, renal failure
Low molecular weight proteinuria with hypercalciuria and nephrocalcinosis	#308990	Xp11.22	CLCN5	Chloride channel 5	*300008	XLR	Low molecular weight proteinuria, hypercalciuria, nephrocalcinosis
X-linked recessive hypophosphatemic rickets*	#300554	Xp11.22	CLCN5	Chloride channel 5	*300008	XLR	Hypophosphatemic rickets +/– nephrocalcinosis

Disorder	OMIM	Location	Gene	Protein	OMIM	Inheritance	Clinical features
Dent disease 2	#300555	Xq26.1	OCRL1	Phosphatidylinositol 4,5-bisphosphate-5-phosphatase	*300535	XLR	Similar to Dent 1
Lowe oculocerebrorenal syndrome	#309000	Xq26.1	OCRL1	Phosphatidylinositol 4,5-bisphosphate-5-phosphatase	*300535	XLR	Vitamin D resistant rickets, ocular abnormalities, mental retardation
Wilson disease	#277900	13q14.3-q21.1	ATP7B	Copper transporting ATPase Beta polypeptide	*606882	AR	Liver cirrhosis, neurological manifestations, low caeruloplasmin, hypercalciuria, nephrocalcinosis
IMAGE	300290	Chr.X	?	?		XLR	Hypercalciuria, hypercalcemia, IUGR, adrenal insufficiency, mild dysmorphism, hypogonadotrophic-hypogonadism
Fanconi–Bickel syndrome	#227810	3q26.1-q26.3	GLUT2	Glucose transporter 2	*138160	AR	Hypophosphatemic rickets, hepatorenal glycogenosis, proximal renal tubulopathy
Fanconi renotubular syndrome	%134600	15q15.3	?	?		AD	Fanconi syndrome, mild rickets
Cystinosis	#219800	17p13	CTNS	Cystinosin	*606272	AR	Hypophosphatemic rickets, metabolic acidosis, photophobia, short stature, hypothyroidism, renal failure
Antenatal Bartter syndrome, Type 1	#601678	15q15-q21.1	SLC12A1	Sodium-potassium-chloride cotransporter-2	*600839	AR	Hypokalemic hypochloremic alkalosis, salt-wasting, hypercalciuria, nephrocalcinosis, osteopenia
Antenatal Bartter syndrome, Type 2	#241200	11q24	KCNJ1	Inward-rectifying apical potassium channel	*600359	AR	Hypokalemic hypochloremic alkalosis, salt-wasting, hypercalciuria, nephrocalcinosis, osteopenia
Bartter syndrome, Type 3	#607364	1p36	CLCNKB	Kidney chloride channel B	*602023	AR	Hypokalemic hypochloremic alkalosis, salt-wasting, hypercalciuria, nephrocalcinosis, osteopenia, occasional hypomagnesemia
Infantile Bartter syndrome with sensorineural deafness, Type 4	#602522	1p31	BSND	Barttin	*606412	AR	Hypokalemic hypochloremic alkalosis, salt-wasting, hypercalciuria, nephrocalcinosis, osteopenia
Gitelman syndrome*	#263800	16q13	SLC12A3	Thiazide sensitive Na-Cl cotransporter	600968	AR	Hypochloremic, hypokalemic alkalosis, hypocalciuria, renal magnesium wasting

Table of renal tubular disorders including distal renal tubular acidosis (DRTA) and a number of miscellaneous disorders related to abnormalities of renal tubular dysfunction. Most of these are not described in detail in the text apart from DRTA and those marked with (*) which also appear in other tables and are described in detail in the text. OMIM numbers in columns 2 and 6 relate to the disorders and the genes respectively and refer to the Online Mendelian Inheritance in Man code numbers (http://www.ncbi.nlm.nih.gov/sites/entrez?db=OMIM).

in Fanconi syndrome). Rickets may result but is usually associated with hyperphosphaturia. In distal RTA (DRTA), the defect resides in one or other of the mechanisms that promote hydrogen ion excretion through the luminal surface of the tubule. A specific H^+-ATPase pump on the luminal surface contains both A1 and B1 subunits as well as several others. Chloride and bicarbonate are exchanged across the baso-lateral surface through an anion exchanger (SLC4A1). Mutations within the genes coding for these proteins are responsible for DRTA. It is usually accompanied by hypercalciuria and a tendency to nephrocalcinosis. The diagnosis needs to be distinguished from vitamin D-related rickets because treatment with vitamin D or its analogs worsens the hypercalciuria whereas treatment with oral bicarbonate corrects the metabolic acidosis, heals the rickets and diminishes hypercalciuria.

Patients present at any age with failure to thrive, rickets and metabolic acidosis; unlike proximal RTA, there is no threshold for acidification of the urine. Vitamin D metabolites are usually normal but hypercalciuria is present and nephrocalcinosis may be seen on renal ultrasound. Alkaline phosphatase is raised and hypokalemia with recurrent episodes of hypokalemic flaccid paralysis may be a feature.

There are several causes of DRTA [69]. Autosomal recessive DRTA with progressive nerve deafness (#267300) is caused by mutations in the ATP6B1 gene (*192132) which codes for the B-subunit of the apical proton pump mediating distal nephron acid secretion. This is also present in the cochlea and accounts for the progressive deafness.

Autosomal recessive DRTA without progressive deafness (RTADR) (*192132) is a separate entity caused by abnormalities of the ATP6V0A4 gene that codes for the A-subunit of the proton pump. Hearing loss is not usually a feature although it may become so later in life. The acidosis can become apparent as early as 3 weeks of age.

Autosomal recessive (#611590) and dominant (#179800) forms of DRTA have been described in association with mutations in the anion exchanger SLC4A1 gene (+109270). This is also present in the red cell membrane where it is known as Band 3 protein. A wide variety of mutations in the gene has been identified, as a result of which some patients have predominantly DRTA while others mainly have elliptocytosis and hemolytic anemia. Mutations are found mostly in South-East Asian populations and may confer resistance to malaria.

Patients with carbonic anhydrase II (CAII) mutations, which cause autosomal recessive osteopetrosis Type 3 (OPTB3), have a degree of distal RTA.

Systemic conditions associated with hypocalcemia

Tumor-lysis syndrome occurs in 30% of children during the initial phases of treatment of some hematological tumors. The release of large quantities of phosphate, potassium and uric acid results in a syndrome characterized biochemically by hyperphosphatemia, hyperuricemia, hyperkalemia, uremia and hypocalcemia. The hypocalcemia is consequent upon the hyper-

phosphatemia, which itself occurs secondarily to the acute renal failure of hyperuricemia. The condition can be prevented by a combination of forced alkaline diuresis and the use of the recombinant urate oxidase inhibitor, rasburicase (Fasturtec®), which, although more expensive that allopurinol, has been found to be useful and cost-effective [70].

Chronic renal failure (CRF) has a serious impact on calcium metabolism. Reduced GFR results in retention of phosphate, plasma concentrations which begin to rise once GFR falls below 30 mL/min/1.73 m². As the kidney is the only site of 1a-hydroxylase activity, concentrations of $1,25(OH)_2D$ fall, particularly when GFR falls below 50–60 mL/min/1.73 m². Metabolic acidosis, either directly as a result of the CRF or caused by renal tubular disorders that may have led to the CRF, is often a factor. Hypocalcemia results, which induces secondary hyperparathyroidism. Renal osteodystrophy therefore consists of a spectrum of both high turnover resulting from the hyperparathyroidism and low turnover secondary to osteomalacia [71]. Additional factors influencing renal osteodystrophy include calcium, phosphorus, vitamin D analogs and aluminum.

The principles of minimizing renal osteodystrophy depend upon preventing hyperphosphatemia, reversing the effects of the reduced 1a-hydroxylase activity and preventing hyperparathyroidism. Oral phosphate-binding agents are used for the former and selevamer (Renagel®) is most commonly used. It is an orally active phosphate binding agent that is not absorbed and which has the advantage over calcium carbonate of not causing adynamic bone while being as effective. Alfacalcidol or calcitriol is used to maintain $1,25(OH)_2D$ concentrations but must be monitored to prevent hypercalciuria or hypercalcemia, which might worsen the renal failure. The vitamin D analog, 19-nor-1α,25(OH)$_2$D2, paricalcitol (Zemplar®) has been used because this has a preferential effect on reducing PTH without increasing renal calcium excretion [72].

Hypercalcemia

Disorders related to PTH
Disorders of the calcium-sensing receptor
Familial benign hypercalcemia
Familial benign hypercalcemia (FBH) or familial hypocalciuric hypercalcemia (FHH) (#145980) is caused in most cases by inactivating mutations of the CaSR gene (Table 16.6) [11]. There are a few families in whom mutations in the CaSR have not been demonstrated. In one, the a locus was identified on chromosome 19p while in another linkage to 19q [73] has been found. These two variants have been designated FHH2 (%145981) and FHH3 (Oklahoma) (%600740). All cases are autosomal dominant and most of the patients are heterozygous. It is often identified incidentally or as a result of investigation of FBH kindreds. In some families, there is a history of parathyroidectomy for presumed hyperparathyroidism. Plasma calcium usually remains elevated throughout life. There is a high degree of penetrance and hyper-

Table 16.6 Hypercalcemic disorders associated with genetic abnormalities.

Location in calcium cascade	Metabolic abnormality	OMIM	Location	Gene	Gene product	OMIM	Inheritance	Principal clinical features
Calcium sensing receptor	Familial benign hypercalcemia Type 1	#145980	3q13.3-q21	CaSR	Calcium sensing receptor	+601199	AD	Asymptomatic hypercalcemia with hypocalciuria. Occasional pancreatitis
	Familial benign hypercalcemia Type 2	%145981	19p13.3	?			AD	As above
	Familial benign hypercalcemia Type 3	%600740	19q13	?			AD	Oklahoma variant
	Neonatal severe primary hyperparathyroidism	#239200	3q13.3-q21	CaSR	Calcium sensing receptor	+601199	AD – homozygous	Severe neonatal hyperparathyroidism with grossly elevated calcium and PTH
Parathyroid glands	Multiple endocrine neoplasia Type 1	+131100	11q13	MEN1	MENIN		AD	Parathyroid adenomas with hyperparathyroidism, pancreatic tumors, anterior pituitary tumors
	Multiple endocrine neoplasia Type 2a	#171400	10q11.2	c-ret protooncogene	RET receptor tyrosine kinase	*164761	AD	Parathyroid tumors, medullary carcinoma of the thyroid, phaeochromocytomas
	Multiple endocrine neoplasia Type 2b	#162300	10q11.2	c-ret protooncogene	RET receptor tyrosine kinase	*164761	AD	Medullary carcinoma of the thyroid, mucosal neurofibromas, intestinal autonomic ganglion dysfunction
	Medullary carcinoma only	#155240	10q11.2	c-ret protooncogene	RET receptor tyrosine kinase	*164761	AD	Medullary carcinoma of the thyroid
			1q21-q22	NRK1	Neurotrophic receptor tyrosine kinase	*191315	AD	
	Multiple endocrine neoplasia Type 4	#610755	12p13	CDKN1B	Cyclin-dependent kinase	*600778	AD	Primary hyperparathyroidism, pituitary adenomas
	Sporadic parathyroid adenomas		1p32-ter		?Tumor suppressor		Sporadic	Isolated hyperparathyroidism

Continued on p. 408

Table 16.6 *Continued*

Location in calcium cascade	Metabolic abnormality	OMIM	Location	Gene	Gene product	OMIM	Inheritance	Principal clinical features
	Hyperparathyroid-jaw tumor syndrome	#145001	1q25-q31	HRPT2	Parafibromin complex	*607393	AD	Parathyroid adenomas and carcinomas, mandibular and maxillary jaw tumors
	Familial isolated primary hyperparathyroidism		Various		Various		AD	Isolated hyperparathyroidism (occasionally carcinoma)
	Parathyroid carcinomas	#608266	1q25-q31 13q14.1-q14.2		Parafibromin complex Retinoblastoma			May be part of hyperparathyroid-jaw tumor syndrome
PTH	Sporadic parathyroid adenomas	#156400	11q13	PRAD1	Cyclin D1	*168461	Sporadic	Primary hyperparathyroidism
PTH/PTHrP receptor	Jansen disease	#156400	3p22-p21.1	PTH1R	Parathyroid hormone receptor 1	*168468	AD	Neonatal hyperparathyroidism with low PTH, short stauture, abnormal chondrocyte proliferation
Target organs	Hypophosphatasia – infantile	#241500	1p36.1-p34	TNAP	Tissue non-specific alkaline phosphatase	*171760	AR	Hypercalcemia, hyperphosphatemia, severe undermineralization of bone, variable severity depending on age of presentation
	Hypophosphatasia – childhood	#241510	1p36.1-p34					
	Hypophosphatasia – adult type	#146300	1p36.1-p34					
Abnormal Vitamin D metabolism	Williams–Beuren syndrome	#194050	7q11.2 7q11.23	ELN LIMK1	Elastin LIM-kinase	*130160 *601329	AD but usually sporadic	Failure to thrive, poor feeding, irritability, "elfin" facies, radioulnar synostosis, "cocktail party" conversation

Genetic conditions that cause hypercalcemia. The conditions are classified according to which part of the calcium cascade they affect and, where known, the gene location, gene product, inheritance and principal clinical features are shown. OMIM numbers in columns 3 and 7 relate to the disorders and the genes respectively and refer to the Online Mendelian Inheritance in Man code numbers (http://www.ncbi.nlm.nih.gov/sites/entrez?db=OMIM).

calcemia has usually developed before 10 years of age but often much earlier. Most patients remain asymptomatic, although some infants may develop mild symptoms during the first year. In FHH3 PTH concentrations may become elevated later in life which can make it difficult to distinguish from primary hyperparathyroidism [74]. Pancreatitis has been described as a rare complication. It is not clear whether this is a true association or whether the hypercalcemia may be the cause. Some mutations may confer susceptibility to pancreatitis in a subgroup of patients.

FBH must be distinguished from primary hyperparathyroidism. Although plasma calcium is elevated, sometimes >3.0 mmol/L (12 mg/dL), PTH remains normal unless attempts have been made to reduce the plasma calcium with low-calcium diets, etc. The PTH has normal biological activity but, in contrast to hyperparathyroidism, plasma magnesium is usually slightly elevated, urinary calcium excretion is inappropriately low for the degree of hypercalcemia and nephrocalcinosis does not develop. Treatment of FBH is usually unnecessary and, when the condition is diagnosed in a child of a kindred known to carry the gene, reassurance is all that is required.

Neonatal severe primary hyperparathyroidism

Neonatal severe primary hyperparathyroidism (NSPHT) (#239200) is usually caused by a homozygous inactivating mutation in the CaSR gene and occurs mostly in consanguineous families [11]. Newborns fail to thrive, feed poorly and suffer constipation and atonia shortly after birth. Gross hypercalcemia and hypophosphatemia are present. PTH is markedly elevated and hyperparathyroid bone disease develops such that respiratory distress necessitating assisted ventilation may result from poor rib compliance. The bones become thin and develop a motheaten appearance because of the severe hyperparathyroidism, which can be identified by the presence of microcysts in the subperiosteal areas. Multiple fractures may occur and be mistaken for rickets. Once the diagnosis has been established, total parathyroidectomy is required to eliminate the hypercalcemia. As sometimes happens with primary hyperparathyroidism following surgery, a hungry bone condition develops, which requires infusion of large quantities of intravenous calcium to prevent hypocalcemia until the bones recover. Bisphosphonates may be useful before surgery to restore normocalcemia.

NSPHT may also develop in infants who have a heterozygous mutation of the CaSR gene from an affected father, the mother being normocalcemic. The fetus senses the maternal calcium as low and develops a degree of secondary hyperparathyroidism that settles progressively, usually by 6 months of age [75]. Alternatively, the degree of set point abnormality or bone responsiveness to PTH may be responsible. In these cases, conservative management may be sufficient until the hypercalcemia settles spontaneously to a concentration at which it becomes asymptomatic and identifying the mutation in the father but not the mother may be helpful in determining whether or not an expectant attitude can be taken.

Another phenotype similar to FBH is associated with the presence of CaSR blocking antibodies that lead to secondary hyperparathyroidism [33]. Mutational analysis of the CaSR was negative in all cases, most of whom had other autoimmune conditions such as hypothyroidism or celiac disease. The principal difference between this and primary hyperparathyroidism was the absence of hypercalciuria, the raised plasma magnesium and the normal PTH concentrations. The natural history of this condition is not known but there is a likelihood that it may remit spontaneously as the antibody concentrations decline.

Disorders of the parathyroid glands

Primary hyperparathyroidism can result from generalized PT gland hyperplasia or from single or multiple adenomas which may be isolated and sporadic or form part of one of the inherited tumor syndromes.

Familial isolated primary hyperparathyroidism

Familial isolated primary hyperparathyroidism (FIHP) (#145000) may be caused by mutations in either the HRPT2 gene that causes hyperparathyroid jaw tumor syndrome or in the MEN1 gene responsible for multiple endocrine neoplasia Type 1a. A third locus mapped to chromosome 2p14-p13.3 has also been described, although the function of the gene is not known. Familial hyperparathyroidism may be seen in MEN2A and in MEN4. Sporadic hyperparathyroidism has been seen in connection with mutations in the PTH gene or in PRAD1, genes thought to be oncogenes or tumor suppressor genes. In sporadic cases, a single hit mutation affects a proto-oncogene such as PRAD1 resulting in preferential growth of a single cell line. In the familial syndromes, a germline first hit mutation affects a tumor suppressor gene and makes the parathyroid (and other) glands susceptible to a second hit [59]. Tumors that arise in familial hyperparathyroidism are usually the result of hyperplasia while those occurring in sporadic cases are adenomas but these can be multiple and it is sometimes difficult to distinguish the two.

Multiple endocrine neoplasias

Multiple endocrine neoplasia Type I (MEN1) (+131100) is characterized by parathyroid (90% of patients), endocrine pancreatic (40%) and anterior pituitary (30%) tumors. Adrenocortical and carcinoid tumors such as lipomas, angiofibromas and collagenomas may also occur [76]. The etiology is probably an inactivating mutation of the MEN1 gene (131100.0020), located on chromosome 11q13, which normally codes for a tumor suppressor protein, MENIN. Nonsense mutations, deletions, insertions, donor-splice site mutations and missense mutations have all been described. Parathyroid tumors are usually the first to present, generally in late adolescence or the twenties or thirties.

Three variants of MEN2 are described. In the most common, MEN2A (#171400), parathyroid tumors (20%) are associated with medullary carcinoma of the thyroid (MCT) and pheochromocytomas [77]. MEN2B (#162300) is not usually associated with parathyroid tumors but has an association with pheochromocytomas, mucosal neurofibromas and intestinal autonomic ganglion dysfunction. In the third variant, MCT-only (#155240), no tumors other than MCT occur.

All three are linked by mutations in a gene that maps to chromosome 10cen-10q11.2 which contains the *c-ret* proto-oncogene (*164761) but different mutations have been found in all three variants and identification of them is useful in the diagnosis and management of family members at risk. Mutations in a second gene, NTRK1 (*191315) have also been shown to cause isolated MCT.

MEN4 (#610755) is caused by mutations in the CDKN1B gene (*600778). Pituitary, parathyroid and other tumors feature in this condition, although usually only in adulthood. The gene product is thought to be a suppressor of cell proliferation which acts by cyclin-dependent kinases.

Allelic loss of chromosome 1p32-pter has been found in a number of cases of isolated sporadic parathyroid adenomas [78]. This region contains a putative tumor suppressor gene but the gene product is unidentified.

Hyperparathyroid-jaw tumor syndrome

Hyperparathyroid-jaw tumor syndrome (HYP-JT) (#145001) is an autosomal dominant syndrome. Parathyroid adenomas and carcinomas are associated with mandibular and maxillary jaw tumors that are fibro-osseous in nature. Renal tumors are also seen on occasions. Different tumors may occur in different members of the same family. Inactivating mutations of the HRPT2 gene (*607393), located on chromosome 1q21-q31, are thought to be responsible [79]. The parafibromin gene, together with three other genes, forms a parafibromin complex that associates with RNA polymerase and acts as a tumor suppressor.

Parathyroid carcinoma

Parathyroid carcinoma (#608266) can be difficult to distinguish histologically from parathyroid adenoma, unless metastases are present. It is an important diagnosis to make as it may cause aggressive hyperparathyroidism which can be difficult to treat especially once it has metastasized. It may be a feature of HPT-JT syndrome and many patients with sporadic PT carcinoma have deletions in the HRPT2 gene [80]. PT carcinoma has also been shown to be associated with allelic deletions of the retinoblastoma (Rb) gene, which has three polymorphic markers, located on chromosome 13q14. Loss of heterozygosity of at least one of the markers at the Rb locus of the gene occurs in all cases of carcinoma but also occurs in some cases of parathyroid adenoma but all parathyroid adenomas show some positivity for the retinoblastoma protein (pRb), whereas this is lacking in all carcinomas [81]. Lack of translation of the pRb seems to be the distinguishing feature. Treatment is surgical.

Disorders of the PTH gene

Sporadic parathyroid tumors may result from mutations within the PTH gene itself. The PRAD1 gene (*168461) is derived from a rearrangement of exon 1 of the PTH gene, which is not trans-

lated, with new non-PTH DNA located on chromosome 11q13. It encodes a 295 amino acid protein, cyclin D1 [82]. Mutations resulting in overexpression of this gene cause parathyroid cell proliferation and hyperparathyroidism. The mutations appear to be somatic and are not inherited.

A 22-bp deletion within exon 2 of the PTH gene has been described [83]. It is possible that silencing of the PTH gene leads to overexpression of the PRAD1/cyclin D1 gene, thus causing the parathyroid tumors seen in this condition which may cause confusion when assaying PTH because it may not react in all immunoassays.

Disorders of the PTH1R

Metaphyseal chondrodysplasia, Jansen type

Metaphyseal chondrodysplasia, Jansen type (#156400) is an autosomal dominant condition that presents in the neonatal period with apparent hyperparathyroidism but without detectable PTH or PTHrP. It is characterized by short-limbed short stature caused by abnormal regulation of chondrocyte proliferation and differentiation in the metaphyseal growth plate as a result of mutations of the PTH/PTHrP receptor, which autoactivate in the absence of either hormone [84]. Treatment is difficult but the condition is said to respond to calcitonin and, theoretically, bisphosphonates should be of value to reduce osteoclast activity and bone turnover.

Diagnosis and treatment of hyperparathyroidism

Hypercalcemia and hypophosphatemia are associated with raised PTH concentrations. Urinary calcium excretion is also raised and a partial Fanconi syndrome (generalized aminoaciduria and mild metabolic acidosis) is usually present. Plasma magnesium is often slightly low, in contrast to FHB. Radiological examination may reveal the presence of subperiosteal microcysts and severe hyperparathyroidism can be confused with rickets.

Localization of parathyroid tumors is best undertaken with the aid of radionuclide scanning with ^{99m}Tc-MIBI (methoxyisobutyl isonitrile) (Fig. 16.16) or ^{99m}Tc-tetrofosmin. These methods are more sensitive than either ultrasonography or magnetic resonance imaging (MRI) scanning and have proved invaluable in locating persistent tumors, especially after primary surgery has failed to eradicate the problem. They are sometimes combined with thyroid subtraction scintigraphy and, if performed shortly before surgery, can be combined with the use of a handheld gamma camera to pinpoint the tumor at operation. Perioperative measurement of PTH has also proved useful in determining whether or not a tumor (or tumors) has been fully resected because it disappears rapidly from the circulation.

Surgical removal of the tumors should be undertaken only by those experienced in the procedure. It may be necessary to control hypercalcemia before surgery by forced diuresis and furosemide. Failing this, bisphosphonates (e.g. pamidronate 0.5 mg/kg/day for 2–3 days) is usually sufficient to restore plasma calcium to normal. Plasma calcium usually declines postoperatively within a few hours and the patient may become hypocalcemic and remain so

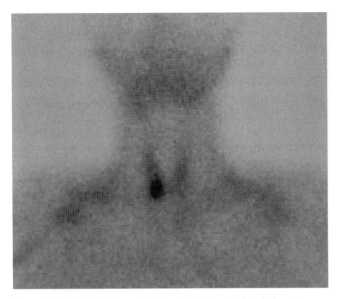

Figure 16.16 SestaMIBI scan taken in a child with a single right lower parathyroid adenoma. She presented with hypercalcemia. A single adenoma was removed at operation and she remains normocalcemic. No mutations of the MEN1 or HYP-JT genes have been demonstrated.

for some time if hyperparathyroidism has been long-standing. In this case, a hungry bone syndrome develops that requires infusion of calcium in large quantities.

Hypercalcemia associated with abnormal vitamin D metabolism

Subcutaneous fat necrosis

Subcutaneous fat necrosis usually occurs in term infants who have suffered a mild degree of birth asphyxia. Firm lumps appear in the subcutaneous tissues and may be multiple. Hypercalcemia develops within the first few weeks after birth accompanied by hypercalciuria and nephrocalcinosis [85]. The skin lesions are invaded by macrophages and the etiology of the hypercalcemia is thought to be inappropriate activation of 1α-hydroxylase within them, which results in high concentrations of circulating $1,25(OH)_2D$ and vitamin D intoxication. The condition is self-limiting but steps may need to be taken to reduce the plasma calcium concentration. Calcium and vitamin D restriction, steroids and bisphosphonates may be of value.

Sarcoidosis

A similar process is thought to occur in sarcoidosis and other granulomatous diseases. Some 30–50% of children with sarcoidosis develop hypercalcemia, which may be precipitated by sunlight. Others have hypercalciuria without hypercalcemia. Tuberculosis and cat-scratch disease may also cause hypercalcemia by a similar mechanism [86]. The hypercalcemia usually resolves with treatment of the underlying condition.

In large doses, vitamin D may cause hypercalcemia, mainly because of the high concentrations of 25OHD that result from

this consequent upon the uncontrolled metabolism of vitamin D by 25-hydroxylase. Although 25OHD has limited activity, high concentrations cause increased bone resorption. A more common cause is seen in patients treated with excess doses of either alfacalcidol or calcitriol. Symptoms are typical of hypercalcemia from other causes and complications of prolonged hypercalcemia are ectopic calcification, nephrocalcinosis and impaired renal function. Hypercalcemia following excess vitamin D is usually more prolonged than that caused by the vitamin D metabolites because vitamin D itself is stored in fat, whereas the metabolites have a much shorter half-life. Treatment is directed toward restricting the source of excess vitamin D. If acute symptoms are present, steroids or bisphosphonates may be of value.

Williams–Beuren syndrome

Williams–Beuren syndrome (#194050) may be autosomal dominant but is usually sporadic [87]. During infancy, patients have a characteristic phenotype consisting of elfin facies caused by periorbital fullness, a long philtrum, malar hypoplasia and an open-mouthed appearance caused by an arched upper lip and full lower lip. As they get older, features change, become coarsened and radioulnar synostosis may develop. Many patients develop hypercalcemia during infancy, which rarely lasts beyond the first year. Subsequently, cardiac anomalies, subvalvar aortic stenosis or peripheral pulmonary stenosis, manifest themselves. Developmental delay is a feature and patients develop a tendency to cocktail party conversation as children and young adults, in which it appears that they are conducting an intelligent conversation which, on reflection, is largely meaningless.

The etiology of the hypercalcemia is not clear. Some patients have been thought to have abnormalities of vitamin D metabolism or CT deficiency while hypercalcemic, whereas others have been found to have no identifiable defect in any of the parameters of calcium metabolism after the hypercalcemia resolves. Most cases have a microdeletion of chromosome 7q11.23, which encompasses the elastin gene [88] (*130160). A number of other genes including LIM-kinase (*601329), RFC2 (*600404), GTF21RD1 (*604318) and GTF21 (*601679), all of which are located near the elastin gene on the long arm of chromosome 7, have also been implicated. Some of these are expressed in the central nervous system and variations in the extent of the microdeletion presumably account for the variable nature of the condition. Mutations of the CT receptor gene (7q21) are not thought to be responsible.

Infant patients present with failure to thrive, poor feeding and irritability. Treatment consists of a low-calcium diet. Where patients live in hard water areas, there may be sufficient calcium in the water to negate the effect of diet. If symptoms are severe, a short course of prednisolone, 1 mg/kg/day, is useful and can usually be stopped after a few weeks. Correcting the hypercalcemia has no effect on the progress of the other features of the disease, which may evolve without hypercalcemia ever having been present.

Idiopathic infantile hypercalcemia

Idiopathic infantile hypercalcemia (IIH) (143880) was originally described in infants born to mothers who had been ingesting large quantities of vitamin D and the incidence declined with a general reduction in vitamin D supplementation but some cases continued to occur with no evidence of excess vitamin D intake. Familial cases have been described. Some features of this condition resemble Williams syndrome and can include hypertension, strabismus and radioulnar synostosis with failure to thrive. The dysmorphic features are usually absent and correction of the hypercalcemia allows normal development, although the tendency to hypercalcemia may last beyond the first year. Lack of mutations in the elastin gene allows this condition to be distinguished from Williams syndrome [89].

The etiology of this condition is uncertain. It has been suggested that an intrinsic hypersensitivity to vitamin D is present and elevated concentrations of N-terminal PTHrP were demonstrated during hypercalcemia in one series. Treatment consists of lowering the plasma calcium with a calcium- and vitamin D-restricted diet, steroids and bisphosphonates if necessary. Cellulose phosphate has been used to limit calcium absorption.

Other causes of hypercalcemia in childhood

Immobilization

Hypercalcemia occurs in a small proportion of patients, especially adolescents, who are immobilized following quadriplegia or other neurological insults [90]. Symptoms consist of lethargy, mood changes, nausea, vomiting and anorexia but may be overlooked in the context of other problems. They usually arise within a few days or weeks of the original insult when bone turnover is rapid.

Hypercalcemia and hypercalciuria are present and nephrocalcinosis can result. Bone biopsy shows loss of trabecular volume, increased osteoclast and decreased osteoblast activity with an overall increase in bone turnover as demonstrated by raised bone turnover markers. The etiology is probably multifactorial, including lack of mechanical stress, poor vascularity, metabolic changes in bone and denervation [90]. If remobilization is not possible and conventional treatment with intravenous fluids and loop diuretics (which may increase urinary calcium excretion) are ineffective in controlling hypercalcemia, pamidronate 0.5 mg/kg/day for 2–3 days is usually effective for several weeks but may need to be repeated. The effect of calcitonin is not so rapid and it has to be given in divided daily doses for prolonged periods. The hypercalcemia is self-limiting as bone turnover slows.

Hypercalcemia of malignancy

Hypercalcemia is a rare complication of malignancy in childhood and has been reported to occur in about 0.4% of cases [91]. It may be a presenting feature of leukemia but also occurs in Hodgkin disease, non-Hodgkin lymphoma and a variety of solid tumors, such as rhabdomyosarcoma, hepatoblastoma, neuroblastoma and angiosarcoma.

As with other conditions complicated by hypercalcemia, the symptoms may be overlooked. The cause is usually related to excess secretion of PTHrP and PTH concentrations are low. Bone turnover is increased and, if the hypercalcemia does not remit on treatment of the underlying malignancy, it usually responds to bisphosphonate therapy as for immobilization.

Hypophosphatasia

This condition is caused by mutations in the tissue non-specific alkaline phosphatase (TNAP) gene (171760). Six different conditions are described depending on the age of presentation and severity [92,93]. Hypercalcemia and hyperphosphatemia occur in the more severe forms. In perinatal hypophosphatasia, infants are born with undermineralized rachitic bones, a high-pitched cry and unexplained fevers and seizures. They usually die shortly after birth, probably with the homozygous form of the condition.

In infantile hypophosphatasia (#241500), hypercalcemia and its attendant symptoms together with bone abnormalities develop during the first 6 months after birth. Initial development may be normal until the onset of symptoms and, if they survive, there tends to be a gradual improvement with time and the prognosis is good. Raised intracranial pressure may result from premature fusion of the cranial sutures.

Childhood hypophosphatasia (#241510) presents later and is variable in its manifestations. It is often accompanied by premature tooth loss which is distinguished from normal loss of deciduous teeth by minimal tooth root resorption. Short stature is often a feature and apparent rachitic changes are seen on X-ray. Characteristic tongues of demineralized bone are seen at the metaphyses. A dolichocephalic shape to the skull may be caused by premature fusion of the sutures. The condition tends to improve at adolescence, although osteomalacia may reappear later in life.

Adult hypophosphatasia (#146300) is mild but there may be a history of tooth loss and rickets during early life. Diagnosis is made by a combination of a low alkaline phosphatase and the characteristic radiological and clinical features. Raised concentrations of phosphoethanolamine and pyridoxal phosphate are found as both of these are substrates for alkaline phosphatase.

In odontohypophosphatasia premature tooth loss is the only feature and pseudohypophosphatasia is characterized by infants who appear to have the clinical features of hypophosphatasia but with normal alkaline phosphatase. This is thought to be caused by abnormally inactive enzyme.

Treatment is symptomatic. Raised intracranial pressure may require neurosurgical intervention and orthopedic surgery, physiotherapy and dental care may be needed. Infusions of plasma containing high concentrations of alkaline phosphatase have been tried with generally disappointing results. Bisphosphonates have been tried in the infantile form without success, presumably because these drugs target the osteoclasts rather than the osteoblasts.

Tertiary hyperparathyroidism

This occasionally occurs in children after chronic hyperstimulation of the PT glands, particularly in CRF. It may also result from chronic vitamin D deficiency. PTH concentrations are usually elevated and the hyperplastic glands become susceptible to developing autonomous nodules. It is not clear whether or not this adenomatous formation is polyclonal or monoclonal in origin but the latter may be present in a majority of cases. Treatment consists of parathyroidectomy.

Disorders of bone metabolism

Disorders that affect bone can be divided between those that affect bone matrix and those that result from poor bone mineralization. Most conditions result in changes in bone density but those that demonstrate uniform changes are referred to as the osteoporoses while those in which mineralization defects are paramount are known as the osteomalacias. In children, osteomalacia is most obviously apparent in the growth plates and gives rise to rickets, which cannot occur in adults once the growth plates have fused. In addition, there are several conditions in which changes in bone density occur in specific areas while leaving the remainder of the bone intact.

Disorders of bone matrix accompanied by low bone density

Osteoporosis

Osteoporoses in children can result from:
- Failure to achieve normal bone density during growth and development;
- Increased bone resorption;
- Failure to replace bone during remodeling [94].

In practice, many osteoporoses result from a combination of these processes. The primary osteoporoses result from intrinsic defects in matrix formation, with subsequent failure of normal mineral deposition or from abnormalities in one or other of the cell types within bone. In the secondary osteoporoses there is no intrinsic defect in bone function but outside influences (e.g. excessive steroid therapy) affect bone density in otherwise normal bone.

Primary osteoporosis

The most common cause of primary osteoporosis is osteogenesis imperfecta (OI), a group of conditions resulting from intrinsic defects in bone matrix caused by abnormalities, either quantitative or qualitative, in bone collagen. The original classification of OI [95] divided it into four types based on clinical differences related to collagen defects. Other causes of bone matrix abnormality have been described and are now included in the classification (Table 16.7).

Osteogenesis imperfecta Type I

Osteogenesis imperfecta Type I (#166200), the mildest form of OI, results from a quantitative defect in either COL1A1 or COL1A2. It is sometimes associated with dentinogenesis imperfecta (DI) (Type 1a) and sometimes not (Type Ib). Blue sclerae are frequently present and can be assessed objectively [96]. Fractures, which are uncommon in infancy, occur in childhood with minimal trauma but they do not usually result in bone deformity if treated adequately. The frequency tends to increase during phases of rapid growth such as puberty when patients are particularly prone to vertebral compression fractures that may need treatment with bisphosphonates. Fracture frequency increases after the menopause and later in men. Hearing difficulties, usually conductive, may develop during adolescence and progress to profound deafness. Patients may bruise easily and have hypermobile joints. Excessive sweating is characteristic. Growth is usually normal. Radiological evidence of Wormian bones is usually present at birth.

Osteogenesis imperfecta Types IIA and IIB

Osteogenesis imperfecta Types IIA and IIB are the most severe forms of OI and usually fatal. If the infants are born live, they have multiple fractures and poorly mineralized bones. Respiratory problems usually supervene rapidly because of the poor rib compliance. Heterozygous mutations in COL1A1 or COL1A2 are responsible in most cases. This is designated Type IIA (#166210), and an autosomal recessive condition. Type IIB (#610854), which is clinically similar, is caused by a mutation in the CRTAP gene.

Osteogenesis imperfecta Type III

Osteogenesis imperfecta Type III (#259420), caused by a qualitative defect in COL1A1 or COL1A2, is the most severe form of OI compatible with life. Affected infants suffer multiple fractures *in utero* and are born small for gestational age. They continue to have multiple fractures with mild trauma. Blue sclerae at birth may whiten with age. The bones become progressively deformed and multiple orthopedic procedures are frequently needed. Growth is often poor and raised urinary calcium excretion may cause nephrocalcinosis. A characteristic radiological feature is the development of "popcorn" bones [97]. These are not present at birth, increase in number and severity during childhood but disappear as growth ceases. They occur within the epiphyses and metaphyses always in close proximity to the growth plate and appear to be detached fragments of growth plate probably in response to trauma. They mostly occur in the lower extremities, particularly the lower femur and upper tibia and less frequently in the upper limbs.

Osteogenesis imperfecta Type IV

Osteogenesis imperfecta Type IV (#166220) is an intermediate form of OI with variable degrees of bone deformity. The sclerae are typically white but may have a bluish tinge. Fracture rates are variable and may not be particularly troublesome but growth is often impaired and it may be this rather than fractures that the patients are more concerned about. It is caused by qualitative defects in either COL1A1 or COL1A2.

Table 16.7 Primary osteoporoses.

Condition	OMIM	Gene location	Gene	Gene product	OMIM	Inheritance	Severity, clinical features	Sclerae
Osteogenesis imperfecta								
Type I	#166200	17q21.31-q22	COL1A1	Type 1A1 collagen	+120150	AD	Mild to moderate. May have dentinogenesis imperfecta (Type IA) or not (Type IB)	Usually blue
	#166200	7q22.1	COL1A2	Type 1A2 collagen	+120140	AD		
Type IIA	#166210	17q21.31-q22	COL1A1	Type 1A1 collagen	+120150	AD	Severe, usually lethal	
	#166210	7q22.1	COL1A2	Type 1A2 collagen	+120140	AD		
Type IIB	#610854	3p22	CRTAP	Cartilage associated protein	*605497	AR	Severe, usually lethal	
Type III	#259420	17q21.31-q22	COL1A1	Type 1A1 collagen	+120150	AD	Severe, multiple fractures and deformities at birth	Blue
	#259420	7q22.1	COL1A2	Type 1A2 collagen	+120140	AD		
Type IV	#166220	17q21.31-q22	COL1A1	Type 1A1 collagen	+120150	AD	Mild to moderate, often associated with short stature	White or pale blue
	#166220	7q22.1	COL1A2	Type 1A2 collagen	+120140	AD		
Type V	%610967	N/K	N/K			AD	Moderate, radioulnar membrane with impaired supination, exuberant callus formation	White
Type VI	%610968	?AR	N/K			AD	Moderate, bone deforming, characteristic "fish-scale" appearance on bone biopsy	White or pale blue
Type VII	#610682	3p22, 3p24.1-p22	CRTAP	Cartilage associated protein	*605497	AR	Variable, usually mild to moderate. Rhizomelia, coax vara	White
Type VIII	#610915	1p34	LEPRE1	Prolyl 3 Hydroxylase 1	*610339	AR	Severe growth deficiency, extreme skeletal undermineralization, bulbous metaphyses	White
Bruck 1	%259450	17p12	N/K	N/K	?	AR	Contractures. Mild DI. Moderately-severe bone disease	White
Bruck 2	#609220	3q23-q24	PLOD2	Bone-specific telopeptide lysyl hydroxylase	*601865	AR	Clinical phenotype as for Bruck 1	White
Cole–Carpenter	112240	N/K	N/K	N/K	?	N/K	Normal at birth; develop craniosynostosis, ocular proptosis, hydrocephalus and diaphyseal fractures	White
Other primary osteoporoses								
OPS	#259770	11q13.4	LRP5	Low density lipoprotein receptor-related peptide 5	*603506	AR	Moderate, associated with "optic pseudoglioma" and impaired vision	White
IJO	259750	N/K	N/K			?AR	↓Bone density with fractures. No other features of OI	White
Juvenile Paget disease	#239000	8q24	TNFRSF11B	Osteoprotegerin	*602643	AR	Large head, expanded bowed extremities, markedly raised alkaline phosphatase	White

Disorders causing primary osteoporosis. The various forms of osteogenesis imperfecta are shown at the beginning, followed by the other causes of primary osteoporosis. OMIM numbers in columns 2 and 6 relate to the disorders and the genes respectively and refer to the Online Mendelian Inheritance in Man code numbers (http://www.ncbi.nlm.nih.gov/sites/entrez?db=OMIM). IJO, idiopathic juvenile osteoporosis; OI, osteogenesis imperfecta; OPG, osteoporosis-pseudoglioma syndrome.

Osteogenesis imperfecta Type V

Osteogenesis imperfecta Type V (%610967) differs from other forms of OI in that no mutations in either COL1A1 or COL1A2 have been demonstrated and the etiology is unknown [98]. Moderately deforming, patients have limited supination of the radius and ulna caused by the presence of a calcified interosseous membrane between the two bones. They also have exuberant callus formation at the site of fractures and elsewhere and this can present as hard lumps which can be confused with osteosarcoma. The callus progresses initially but may eventually disappear [99]. A third feature is the presence of a radio-opaque metaphyseal band adjacent to the growth plate.

Osteogenesis imperfecta Type VI

The few patients described with osteogenesis imperfecta Type VI (%610968) presented with fractures between 4 and 18 months and fractured more frequently than in Type IV [100]. Although none of the patients had radiological evidence of rickets, bone biopsy showed a characteristic fish scale pattern and there was evidence of increased osteoid suggestive of a mineralization defect. Alkaline phosphatase was raised more than in Type IV. No evidence of COL1A1 or COL1A2 defects has been identified and the etiology remains unknown.

Osteogenesis imperfecta Type VII

Osteogenesis imperfecta Type VII (#610682) is another rare form of OI [101]. Unlike most of the other forms of OI, Type VII is autosomal recessive. Fractures occur throughout childhood and seem to diminish in frequency during adolescence. Short stature is common as a result of bone deformity. Rhizomelia and coxa vara are characteristic radiological features. Hearing loss, diabetes insipidus and ligamentous laxity are not seen. Homozygous mutations in the CRTAP gene (*605497) have been shown to be the cause.

Osteogenesis imperfecta Type VIII

Osteogenesis imperfecta Type VIII (#610915) is a severe, often lethal, form of OI which overlaps the clinical features of Types II and III. It is caused by homozygous mutations in the LEPRE1 gene that codes for prolyl-3 hydroxylase-1 (P3H1) (*610339) which catalyzes proline hydroxylation in the crosslinks of Type 1 collagen fibrils [102]. Affected individuals have radiological evidence of fractures *in utero*. The survivors develop bulbous metaphyses and vertebral compression fractures and have extremely low bone density. The hands are large compared to the forearms. The sclerae are white.

Bruck syndrome

Two forms of this condition are described. Both have a similar phenotype consisting of moderately severe bone disease similar to OI Type 4 but with additional joint contractures which fre-quently limit mobility more than the bone disease would warrant. Bruck 1 (%259450) has no known underlying etiology but Bruck 2 (#609220) is caused by mutations in the *PLOD2* gene (*601865) that is involved in maturation of Type 1 collagen crosslinks.

Cole–Carpenter syndrome (112240)

This is of unknown etiology but is characterized by diaphyseal fractures, craniosynostosis and proptosis. The infants are normal at birth.

Osteoporosis-pseudoglioma syndrome

Osteoporosis-pseudoglioma syndrome (OPG) (#259770) shares many of the clinical features of mild to moderate deforming OI. It is not classified amongst the OIs because it is not primarily a disorder of bone matrix, the principal defect lying within the osteoblast. It is an autosomal recessive condition caused by mutations in the LRP5 gene (*603506). LRP5 is the factor that is present in the cell surfaces of osteoblast precursors which forms a receptor complex with frizzled-related protein for which Wnt (the homolog of the *Drosophila* wingless gene) is the ligand. This results in transformation of preosteoblasts into osteoblasts (Fig. 16.6). LRP5 is present in many other tissues, notably retinal vessels, and OPG is associated with severely reduced vision caused by the presence of pseudoglioma of the retina that results from disordered retinal development. The term pseudoglioma is a non-specific expression used to describe any lesion that resembles retinoblastoma. When bilateral, it must be distinguished from Norrie disease (#310600), which is X-linked and not associated with low bone density. Patients present with early onset low trauma fractures which are often deforming but of variable severity. Vision is severely impaired and most patients are registered blind. Treatment is undertaken along similar lines to that of OI and responds to bisphosphonates.

Heterozygous carriers of LRP5 mutations have low bone density and some cases of IJO have been associated with this. Carriers do not have ophthalmic abnormalities but may develop osteoporosis later in life. Some mutations in the LRP5 gene are associated with increased bone density.

Idiopathic juvenile osteoporosis

Idiopathic juvenile osteoporosis (IJO) (259750) is, as the name implies, of unknown etiology, presenting with low trauma fractures during mid to late childhood. These are not usually deforming if treated but include vertebral collapse which may be associated with a marked kyphosis and long bone fractures, particularly around the metaphyses [103–105]. It can be sufficiently debilitating to render the patients wheelchair-bound. It improves after puberty but may require treatment with bisphosphonates to allow increased mobility before its natural improvement.

It is distinguished from OI by the absence of other features, either clinical or genetic, and appears to be a condition primarily of failure of adequate bone formation. Bone biopsy, using double

415

tetracycline labeling, has shown diminished cancellous bone volume but bone resorption is normal. Thus, in contrast to OI, bone turnover is low rather than increased.

Juvenile Paget disease

Juvenile Paget disease (JPD) (#239000), in contrast to IJO, is an autosomal recessive condition of increased bone resorption caused by abnormal osteoclast function usually caused by mutations in the TNFRSF11B gene that codes for osteoprotegerin (*602643). This normally exercises an inhibitory effect on RANKL to prevent overstimulation of osteoclasts by the RANK receptors on osteoclast precursors (Fig. 16.7). Bone turnover is high and markers of bone turnover, such as alkaline phosphatase, NTX and hydroxyproline are increased.

Patients present in early life with a large head. The long bones are bowed and greatly expanded and show coarse trabeculation on X-ray. The calvaria show marked thickening with isolated areas of increased density. Treatment with bisphosphonates should be of value but the most logical treatment is with recombinant osteoprotegerin, which has been used in adults with success [106]. There are no reports of its use in children.

Secondary osteoporoses

Secondary osteoporosis is more common that primary disease and may arise either because of an underlying condition or because of treatment of that condition. Diseases such as celiac disease, juvenile chronic arthritis and β-thalassemia often cause reduced bone mass, partly because the inflammatory processes occurring in association with those diseases have an adverse effect on bone through inflammatory markers and partly because steroids and other drugs detrimental to bone are used. Immobilization is another cause of osteoporosis that may result in a tendency to spontaneous or low trauma fractures.

Treatment of the osteoporoses

For the more severe forms, a multidisciplinary approach is required from a team including a pediatrician, pediatric endocrinologist, physiotherapist, occupational therapist orthopedic surgeon, dentist, specialist nurse and social worker [107]. Access to a geneticist is advisable. Specialist ophthalmology and audiology may also be required.

Apart from the routine treatment of fractures, surgery is often required to correct bone deformity. This may involve surgical fracture of bones with insertion of rods to maintain the integrity of the bones. Physiotherapy and other measures to increase mobility are essential because immobility has a detrimental effect which can be reversed by mobilization. The mainstay of medical treatment is intravenous or, more rarely, oral bisphosphonates which have a dramatic effect on diminishing bone pain, improving bone density, decreasing fracture rates and enabling mobilization of previously immobile patients.

Secondary osteoporosis is best treated by removing the cause. If the patient can be weaned off steroids or adequately mobilized, bone density may improve. If this proves impossible (e.g. in paraplegic patients), the use of bone-sparing drugs such as the bisphosphonates may be of value.

Diseases characterized by increased bone density

Conditions associated with increased bone density occur as a result of a mismatch between osteoblast and osteoclast function that favors the former (Table 16.8). The osteoclasts may either be poorly formed (osteoclast-poor) or they may be poorly functioning (osteoclast-rich). This group of conditions includes the osteopetroses, pyknodysostosis, van Buchem disease and sclerosteosis.

Osteopetrosis

Eight kinds of osteopetrosis (OPT) are described of which six are autosomal recessive and two autosomal dominant. They vary in their severity and are described as being malignant, benign or intermediate. The malignant forms present with early onset symptoms and can be diagnosed radiologically during the antenatal period. Bone overgrowth results in apparent macrocephaly, progressive blindness and deafness and anemia because of encroachment on the bone marrow. Hepatosplenomegaly from extramedullary hematopoiesis is present. Despite the increased bone density, the bones are more fragile than normal and fractures may occur. Hypocalcemia may be present, particularly in the malignant forms, and rickets may also be present despite the osteosclerosis.

Several treatments have been tried. Bone marrow transplantation is the most effective but must be undertaken as early as possible before excessive bone overgrowth has occurred [108]. High dose calcitriol [109] and recombinant human interferon γ1b [110] have been tried with some success.

Autosomal recessive osteopetrosis Type 1

Autosomal recessive osteopetrosis Type 1 (OPTB1) (#259700), an osteoclast-rich infantile malignant form of OPT, is caused by mutations in the T-cell immune regulator subunit of the vacuolar proton pump (TCIRG1 subunit) (*604592). This results in failure to generate a suitably acid environment by the osteoclast ruffled border for bone resorption to occur because the protons cannot be transported to the extracellular space (Fig. 16.7).

Autosomal recessive osteopetrosis Type 2

Autosomal recessive osteopetrosis Type 2 (OPTB2) (#259710) is mild and characterized by prognathism, genu valgum and an increased fracture tendency. Anemia and hepatosplenomegaly are present in some cases. The underlying cause is mutations in the TNFS11 gene (*602642) otherwise known as RANKL (Fig. 16.7). Osteoclasts are not transformed in normal numbers and bone resorption is therefore defective.

Autosomal recessive osteopetrosis Type 3

Autosomal recessive osteopetrosis Type 3 (OPTB3) (#259730) is a benign form of OPT caused by mutations in the carbonic anhydrase II (CA2) gene (*611492). Like the vacuolar proton pump, it contributes to the development of the bone resorbing acid envi-

Table 16.8 Osteopetrotic conditions.

Condition	OMIM	Location	Gene	Gene product	Inheritance	Osteoclasts	Severity	Cause
Osteopetroses								
Autosomal recessive 1	#259700	11q13-4q13.5	TCIRG1 subunit	T-cell immune regulator subunit of the vacuolar proton pump	AR	Osteoclast rich	Malignant	Failure of acidification
Autosomal recessive 2	#259710	13q14	TNFSF11 RANK L	Tumor necrosis factor superfamily 11 RANK ligand	AR	Osteoclast poor	Benign	Failure of osteoclast transformation
Autosomal recessive 3	#259730	8q22	CA2	Carbonic anhydrase II	AR	Osteoclast rich	Intermediate	Failure of acidification; RTA
Autosomal recessive 4	#611490	16p13	CLCN7	Chloride channel-7 protein	AR	Osteoclast rich	Malignant	Failure of acidification
Autosomal recessive 5	#259720	6q21	OSTM1	Osteopetrosis-associated transmembrane protein-1	AR	Osteoclast rich	Malignant	Failure of acidification
Autosomal recessive 6	#611497	17q21.3	PLEKHM1	Plekstrin homology domain-containing protein, family M member 1	AR	Osteoclast rich	Intermediate	Abnormal vesicular transport
Autosomal recessive	#612301	18q22.1	RANK	Tumor necrosis factor superfamily member 11a	AR	Osteoclast poor	Benign	Failure of osteoclast transformation
Autosomal dominant 1*	#607634	11q13.4	LRP5	Low density lipoprotein receptor protein 5	AD	Osteoclast rich	Benign	Increased osteoblast signaling
Autosomal dominant 2	#166600	16p13	CLCN7	Chloride channel-7 protein	AD	Osteoclast rich	Benign	Failure of acidification
Other bone sclerosing conditions								
Pyknodysostosis	#265800	1q21	CTSK	Cathepsin K	AR	Osteoclast rich		Failure of bone matrix resorption
Hyperostosis corticalis generalisata (van Buchem disease)	#239100	17q12-q21	SOST	Sclerostin	AR	Osteoclast rich		Increased osteoblast signaling
Sclerosteosis	#269500	17q12-q21	SOST	Sclerostin	AR	Osteoclast rich		Increased osteoblast signaling

Disorders of primary bone sclerosis. The various forms of osteopetrosis are shown at the beginning followed by the other causes of bone sclerosis. Note that this does not include those conditions that are characterized by soft tissue calcification. OMIM numbers in columns 2 and 6 relate to the disorders and the genes respectively and refer to the Online Mendelian Inheritance in Man code numbers (http://www.ncbi.nlm.nih.gov/sites/entrez?db=OMIM). RTA, renal tubular acidosis. *No longer strictly an osteopetrosis as there is no defect of osteoclast formation or function.

ronment of the osteoclast ruffled border. It is therefore an osteo-clast-rich form of the condition. It is associated with mild nerve compression, particularly of the optic nerve, dental malocclusion, short stature and a degree of mental retardation. Mild anemia may also be present but tends to resolve with time. The CA2 deficiency also gives rise to a degree of renal tubular acidosis.

Autosomal recessive osteopetrosis Type 4
Autosomal recessive osteopetrosis Type 4 (OPTB4) (#611490) is a malignant infantile form of OPT caused by mutations in chloride channel 7 (CLCN7) gene (*602727) responsible for transporting the chloride ions that provide the hydrochloric acid that dissolves bone mineral. The clinical features are similar to those of OPTB1.

Autosomal recessive osteopetrosis Type 5
Autosomal recessive osteopetrosis Type 5 (OPTB5) (#259720), similar to OPTB4, is another infantile malignant form of OPT. Mutations in OSTM1 (*607649) result in an abnormal β-subunit of CLCN7 which also results in failure of osteoclast acidification.

Autosomal recessive osteopetrosis Type 6
Autosomal recessive osteopetrosis Type 6 (OPTB6) (#611497) is a mild form of OPT which presents with walking difficulties and leg pains. Initially the patients have dense metaphyseal bands on X-ray but later develop an Erlenmeyer flask appearance of the distal femora. Mutations in the plekstrin gene (PLEKHM1) (*611466) involved in vacuolar transport in osteoclasts are responsible.

Autosomal dominant osteopetrosis Type 1
Autosomal dominant osteopetrosis Type 1 (OPTA1) (#607634) is an osteoclast-poor form of OPT caused by mutations in the *LRP5* gene. In contrast to OPPG, these mutations result in an abnormal protein that cannot bind to, and therefore be inhibited by, Dickkopf (Fig. 16.6). As a result, LRP5 binds avidly to Frizzled protein and overstimulates osteoblast activity. The osteosclerosis is mainly seen in the skull vault while the spine is almost completely spared with no evidence of a bone within bone appearance (Table 16.8).

Autosomal dominant osteopetrosis Type 2
Autosomal dominant osteopetrosis Type 2 (OPTA2) (#166600) is another milder form of OPT caused by heterozygous mutations in the CLCN7 gene (see OPTB4). As chloride channels exist as dimers, it seems that a dominant negative effect is present to account for the abnormality. The condition can be differentiated from OPTA1 by the distribution of the osteosclerosis which mainly affects the skull base, spine and pelvis. A bone within bone appearance is seen in the vertebrae. Increased bone fragility and dental abscesses are prominent.

Other miscellaneous conditions
Pycnodysostosis
Pycnodysostosis (#265800) is caused by mutations in the gene coding for cathepsin K (CTSK) (*601105) which is synthesized

by the osteoclasts and responsible for resorption of bone matrix once the mineral has been removed. Extreme short stature, abnormalities of the skull vault, with delayed fusion of the sutures and acroosteolysis of the maxilla and phalanges are prominent features. Increased bone fragility is present and stress fractures of the tibia and femur and of the lumbar and cervical vertebrae may occur. Bone overgrowth can sometimes lead to extramedullary hematopoiesis similar to the more severe forms of OPT.

Sclerosteosis and van Buchem disease
Sclerosteosis (SOST) (#269500) and van Buchem Disease (VBCH) (#239100) are both caused by mutations in the sclerostin (SOST) gene (*605740). Sclerostin, normally produced by osteocytes, inhibits the action of bone matrix proteins (BMPs) which stimulate osteoblast differentiation. Bone overgrowth results because osteoblast transformation is unrestrained. SOST is the more severe disease with tall stature, increased body weight and overgrowth of the long bones and skull, the latter resulting in cranial nerve compression which is often multiple. It is particularly common in the Afrikaner population of South Africa.

VBCH is less severe and may result from mutations downstream of the SOST gene itself within a proposed SOST gene regulator. It usually presents in late childhood or adolescence with osteosclerosis of the skull, which may be up to four times normal weight, mandible, long bones and ribs. Cranial nerve compression, particularly of the optic and auditory nerves may occur.

Craniometaphyseal dysplasia
Craniometaphyseal dysplasia (CMDD) (#123000), caused by mutations in the ANKH gene (*605145) which is responsible for transporting pyrophosphate from the intracellular to extracellular space in osteoclasts, is a condition that particularly affects the craniofacial bones. Widening of the bridge of the nose (with the development of leonine facies) may result in cranial nerve compression. Increases in pyrophosphate concentrations inhibit bone resorption leading to bone overgrowth.

Several other conditions associated with mutations within the TNFRSF11B (RANKL) gene or of the genes which regulate RANKL, such as sequestosome 1 (*601530) and TGFβ1 (*190180) have been shown to be responsible for other rare conditions such as familial expansile osteolysis (FEO) (#174810), expansile skeletal hyperphosphatasia, Paget disease of bone (PDB) (#602080) and Camurati–Engelmann disease (CED) (#131300) [111].

Disorders of phosphate metabolism
It has become clear over the past few years that the key to the control of phosphate metabolism is FGF23 and much work has been done to elucidate the mechanisms by which the conditions associated with altered phosphate metabolism arise (Table 16.9). They can be divided into those in which FGF23 is raised and those in which it is too low. Plasma phosphate is usually low in those with raised FGF23 and vice versa. There is also a group of condi-

Table 16.9 Conditions associated with disorders of phosphate metabolism and soft tissue calcification.

Condition	OMIM	Location	Gene	Gene product	OMIM	Inheritance	Clinical features
Hypophosphatemia							
X-linked dominant hypophosphatemic rickets	#307800	Xp22.2-p22.1	PHEX	Phosphate regulating gene with homologies to endopeptidases	*300550	XLD	Hypophosphatemic, vitamin D resistant rickets
Autosomal dominant hypophosphatemic rickets	#193100	12p13.3	FGF23	Fibroblast growth factor 23	*605380	AD	Hypophosphatemic, vitamin D resistant rickets
Autosomal recessive hypophosphatemic rickets	#241520	4q21	DMP1	Dentin matrix protein 1	*600980	AR	Hypophosphatemic, vitamin D resistant rickets
Hereditary hypophosphatemic rickets with hypercalciuria	#241530	9q34	SLC34A3	Sodium/phosphate co-transporter	*609826	AR	Hypophosphatemic, vitamin D resistant rickets with hypercalciuria
X-linked recessive hypophosphatemic rickets	#300554	Xp11.22	CLCN5	Chloride channel 5	*300008	XLR	Hypophosphatemic rickets +/- nephrocalcinosis
McCune–Albright syndrome	#174800	20q13.2	GNAS1	G-protein α subunit	+139320	Somatic mutation	Polyostotic fibrous dysplasia
Tumor induced osteomalacia		4q21.1 / 12p13.3	MEPE / FGF23	Matrix extracellular phosphoprotein / Fibroblast growth factor 23	*605912 / *605380	Sporadic / Sporadic	Tumor induced osteomalacia / Tumor induced osteomalacia
Hyperphosphatemia							
Hyperphosphatemic familial tumoral calcinosis	#211900	2q24-q31	GALNT3	UDP-n-acetyl-α-d-galactosamine: polypeptide n-acetylgalactosaminyltransferase 3	*601756	AR	Progressive deposition of basic calcium crystals in periarticular spaces and soft tissues
	#211900 / #211900	12p13.3 / 13q12	FGF23 / KL	Fibroblast growth factor 23 / Klotho	*605380 / +604824	AR / AR	
Hyperostosis–hyperphosphatemia syndrome	#610233	2q24-q31	GALNT3	UDP-n-acetyl-α-d-galactosamine: polypeptide n-acetylgalactosaminyltransferase 3	*601756	AR	Recurrent, transient, painful swellings of the long bones, periosteal reaction, cortical hyperostosis. Bone but not skin involvement
Other soft tissue calcification disorders							
Normophosphatemic familial tumoral calcinosis	#610455	7q21	SAMD9	Sterile alfa motif domain-containing protein 9	*610456	AR	As above but with normal plasma phosphate
Progressive osseous heteroplasia	#166350	20q13.2	GNAS1	Gsα subunit	+139320	AD	Osteoma cutis. Variable severity. May be a feature of Albright hereditary osteodytrophy
Fibrodysplasia ossificans progressiva	#135100	2q23-q24	ACVR1	Activin A receptor 1	*102576	AD	Progressive life-threatening ectopic ossification. Uniphalangic great toes. Mild mental retardation
Generalized arterial calcification of infancy	#208000	6q22-q23	ENPP1	Ectonucleotide pyrophosphatase/ phosphodiesterase 1	*173335	AR	Progressive arterial calcification. Often early death from coronary artery occlusion
Williams–Beuren syndrome	#194050	7q11.23, 7q11.23	ELN / LIMK1	Elastin / LIM-kinase	*130160	AD/sporadic	Infantile hypercalcemia, failure to thrive, subvalvar aortic stenosis, peripheral pulmonary stenosis, aortic calcification

Table of disorders associated with abnormalities of phosphate metabolism. The table also includes those conditions characterized by soft tissue calcification in which plasma phosphate is normal. OMIM numbers in columns 2 and 6 relate to the disorders and the genes respectively and refer to the Online Mendelian Inheritance in Man code numbers (http://www.ncbi.nlm.nih.gov/sites/entrez?db=OMIM).

tions in which plasma phosphate is normal but which cause soft tissue calcification.

Hypophosphatemic rickets

X-linked dominant hypophosphatemic rickets

X-linked dominant hypophosphatemic (vitamin D resistant) rickets (XLH) (#307800), caused by mutations in the phosphate-regulating endopeptidase gene (PHEX) (*300550) located on the X chromosome, is the most common form of hypophosphatemic rickets. Affected individuals usually present within the first or second year of life with bowed legs and clinical signs of rickets. There may be a family history. Boys are more severely affected than girls because of the absence of a normal allele on the second X chromosome. The phenotype in females is variable and not necessarily consistent within families so that maternal carriers may be unaware that they have it until tested following diagnosis in a child.

The signs of rickets are similar to those of vitamin D-related rickets although often without the muscle weakness and pain. Radiological signs of rickets differ from those of vitamin D-related rickets in showing rather coarser trabeculation which may suggest the diagnosis. Growth may also be impaired. Diagnosis is made by demonstrating a raised urinary phosphate excretion and low plasma phosphate. Plasma calcium is normal in the untreated state and alkaline phosphatase and FGF23 are raised.

Treatment consists of a combination of oral phosphate supplements together with alfacalcidol or calcitriol to counteract the suppressive effect of FGF23 on 1α-hydroxylase activity and to prevent hypocalcemia. Unfortunately, because urinary excretion is so rapid, the phosphate supplements need to be given four or five times a day if adequate concentrations are to be maintained. The dose of phosphate is often limited by diarrhea. Getting the balance right between these two treatments and preventing hypocalcemia while healing the rickets can be difficult. Growth hormone has also been used with some effect to try to improve growth and it may have a temporary beneficial effect on phosphate excretion [112,113]. Monitoring of treatment requires regular measurements of calcium, phosphate and alkaline phosphatase in plasma. Measurements of FGF23 have yet to be fully evaluated. Repeat X-rays may help to show healing of the rickets but it is important to understand that, unlike vitamin D-related rickets, the bone never returns to normal and biopsy evidence of osteomalacia persists, however effective the treatment. Orthopedic intervention may be required.

Autosomal dominant hypophosphatemic rickets

Autosomal dominant hypophosphatemic rickets (ADHR) (#193100) caused by mutations in the FGF23 gene (#241520) is clinically and biochemically similar to that of XLH, although the onset may not be until a later age. The mutations are thought to prevent the natural cleavage of the molecule which thus maintains higher than normal concentrations of FGF23. It is rarer than

XLH but treatment is similar. The hypophosphatemia occasionally resolves with age.

Autosomal recessive hypophosphatemic rickets

Autosomal recessive hypophosphatemic rickets (ARHR) (#241520) is clinically and biochemically similar to XLH and ADHR but caused by mutations in the DMP1 gene (*600980). DMP1 is secreted by osteocytes and normally provides a restraining influence on FGF23 secretion. FGF23 is therefore elevated in this condition. Treatment is the same as that for XLH and ADHR.

Hereditary hypophosphatemia with hypercalciuria

Hereditary hypophosphatemia with hypercalciuria (HHRH) (#241530), unlike XLH, ADHR and ARHR, is not related to abnormalities in FGF23. It is an autosomal recessive condition caused by a defect in the sodium–phosphate co-transporter of the renal tubule (*609826) which results directly in increased phosphate excretion, although heterozygous carriers show some intermediate effects on calcium and phosphate transport between homozygotes and normal individuals. As a consequence, FGF23 concentrations are low and $1,25(OH)_2D$ concentrations are appropriately raised as a result of the hypophosphatemia and the lack of inhibition by FGF23. Urinary calcium excretion is therefore elevated with the subsequent risk of nephrocalcinosis. Treatment consists of phosphate supplements alone. These usually correct the biochemical abnormalities, apart from the low renal phosphate threshold. Vitamin D analogs should not be used because of the tendency to increase urinary calcium excretion.

Fanconi syndrome

Fanconi syndrome, a generic term for a number of proximal renal tubular disorders that, in its full manifestation, consists of bicarbonaturia, glycosuria, aminoaciduria and phosphaturia [114], has a wide variety of acquired and genetic causes, the most common of which is cystinosis. Rickets may be the first manifestation but chronic renal failure may supervene without appropriate treatment. Specific treatment of the rickets consists of correcting the acidosis (which may require large quantities of bicarbonate) and reversing the hypophosphatemia.

Polyostotic fibrous dysplasia and McCune–Albright syndrome

Polyostotic fibrous dysplasia (PFD) and McCune–Albright syndrome (MAS) (#174800) are caused by mosaicism for activating somatic mutations in the GNAS1 gene (+139320). Fibrous dysplastic lesions can occur in any bone and may be limited or widespread. Apart from the fact that fractures may occur through the dysplastic lesions, they may also cause hypophosphatemic rickets and osteomalacia because of increased concentrations of FGF23. The mechanism by which this occurs is not understood but is probably dependent on how widespread the lesions are and it is likely that a humoral factor is responsible.

Bisphosphonates are sometimes used as specific treatment for PFD, particularly for the accompanying bone pain [115]. The bone lesions do not return to normal but pain relief is sometimes considerable. Because there is no specific abnormality of the otherwise normal bone, treatment is aimed at symptom relief rather than being given regularly. If hypophosphatemia is present before treatment, oral phosphate supplements should be given to prevent worsening hypophosphatemia causing acute cardiovascular disturbances.

Tumor-induced osteomalacia

Occasionally, tumors are associated with rickets and osteomalacia that is hypophosphatemic in nature. The tumors are usually of mesenchymal origin. The precise mechanism is not clear but probably results from the production of humoral factors such as MEPE by the tumor. The condition is best treated by tumor removal.

Phakomatosis pigmentokeratotica and Schimmelpenning–Feuerstein–Mims syndrome

Several epidermal nevus syndromes, such as phakomatosis pigmentokeratotica and Schimmelpenning–Feuerstein–Mims syndrome (%163200), have been reported to be associated with hypophosphatemic rickets [116–118]. The mechanism is uncertain but thought to be similar to that of TIO and FGF23 concentrations are raised. Effective removal of the nevi is sufficient to cure the osteomalacia.

Soft tissue calcification disorders

Hyperphosphatemic familial tumoral calcinosis

Hyperphosphatemic familial tumoral calcinosis (HFTC) (#211900) is an autosomal recessive condition characterized by progressive deposition of painful calcific nodules in periarticular spaces and soft tissues, including the skin. The nodules consist of calcium phosphate and should be distinguished from extraskeletal ossification. The underlying biochemical defect is hyperphosphatemia secondary to inactive or ineffective FGF23 and can be caused by inactivating mutations of the FGF23 gene itself (*605380), by mutations in the GALNT3 gene (*601756), which prevents FGF23 from being processed properly, or by mutations in the Klotho gene (+604824) which prevent FGFR1 from being able to act as a suitable receptor for FGF23 (Fig. 16.5). As a consequence, tubular reabsorption of phosphate is increased and calcium phosphate deposition occurs. Angioid streaks in the retina, similar to those of pseudoxanthoma elasticum (#264800), are also usually present.

Treatment is difficult but some success has been achieved with a low phosphate diet and phosphate binding agents such as aluminum hydroxide. The newer phosphate binding agent, sevelamer, should also be effective without running the risk of aluminum toxicity.

Hyperostosis-hyperphosphatemia syndrome

Hyperostosis-hyperphosphatemia syndrome (HHS) (#610233) overlaps HFTC and is also caused by mutations in the GALNT3 gene but it is characterized by recurrent transient episodes of swelling and pain in long bones which are accompanied by radiological evidence of periosteal reactions. Skin and other soft tissues are not involved in the same way as in HFTC.

Other causes of soft tissue calcification

Normophosphatemic familial tumoral calcinosis

Normophosphatemic familial tumoral calcinosis (NFTC) (#610455) is similar to HFTC but not accompanied by hyperphosphatemia. It is caused by inactivating mutations in the SAMD9 gene (*610456) that is involved in fibromatous tumor suppression.

Progressive osseous heteroplasia

Progressive osseous heteroplasia (POF) (#166350) is caused by heterozygous paternally inherited inactivating mutations of the GNAS1 gene (+139320). In contrast to HFTC and HHS, the lesions in this condition consist of bony spicules that contain normal membranous bone structures. Osteoma cutis (hard swellings in the skin) occur initially, often in young children and later become ossified and visualized radiologically. There is clearly some overlap between this condition and Albright hereditary osteodystrophy (#103580) in which heterotopic ossification can also occur and which is caused by similar mutations.

Fibrodysplasia ossificans progressiva

Fibrodysplasia ossificans progressiva (FOP) (#135100) is an autosomal dominant condition in which progressive extraskeletal ossification begins at a variable age from childhood to late adulthood but on average by 5 years. It is caused by mutations in the Type 1 activin A receptor gene (ACVR1) (*102576). The activins are mainly involved in the control of gonadotropin secretion but, being part of the TGFβ superfamily, also have an influence on ossification by osteoblasts. Progressive ossification occurs in a characteristic way from head to foot, back to front, trunk to limbs and proximal to distal and results in increasing disability. It is associated with abnormalities of the great toes, which may be uniphalangeal.

Drugs used in the treatment of disorders of calcium and bone metabolism

Vitamin D

The normal requirement for vitamin D in individuals not exposed to adequate sunshine is 200–400 units/day (5–10 μg/day). Vitamin D is the treatment of choice for vitamin D deficiency given either as cholecalciferol or ergocalciferol. The former is probably more effective but there is little to choose between them. In the presence of deficiency, it can be given as a daily supplement (1500–10 000 units/day depending on age) for a total of 3 months in the first instance. If there are concerns about compliance or if there is a problem of malabsorption, larger single doses can be given, a regimen known as stosstherapy [119], in divided doses orally during one day or as a single intramuscular dose (150 000–600 000 units) every 3 months, depending on age. Many preparations containing either vitamin D in combination with calcium or as a multivitamin formula are available.

Vitamin D metabolites

1,25-dihydroxycolecalciferol (calcitriol)

1,25-dihydroxycolecalciferol (calcitriol) is the fully active metabolite of vitamin D. Because it does not need to be metabolized before becoming active, it has a half-life of only 5–6 h and therefore needs to be given at least twice and preferably three times daily. Its principal value is in situations where 25-hydroxylation of vitamin D is impaired, such as in chronic liver disease and in bone disease of prematurity, especially where there is coexistent hepatitis. In countries where alfacalcidol is not available, calcitriol 15–30 ng/kg/day is usually used.

1α-hydroxycolecalciferol (alfacalcidol)

1α-hydroxycolecalciferol (alfacalcidol) is vitamin D_3 that has been hydroxylated in the 1-position but not in the 25-position. It is active orally but, once absorbed, has to be converted to $1,25(OH)_2D_3$ in the liver. It has a half-life of around 30–35 h which make it ideal to be given daily. It is the treatment of choice in hypoparathyroidism, hypophosphatemic rickets, 1α-hydroxylase deficiency rickets and chronic renal failure, although vitamin D deficiency as a cause of raised PTH in the latter must be excluded and treated first [72]. The usual dose requirement is 30–50 ng/kg/day and treatment must be monitored regularly to make sure that hypercalcemia and/or hypercalciuria do not supervene. Higher doses may be needed initially until plasma calcium concentrations are stabilized. In hypoparathyroidism plasma calcium concentrations may need to be maintained at the lower end of the normal range or even lower, as long as the patient remains asymptomatic, particularly when activating mutations of the CaSR (ADH) are responsible, in order to prevent hypercalciuria.

Unfortunately, alfacalcidol is not available in some countries, including the USA, and calcitriol is usually used instead. 1α-hydroxyergocalciferol (Hectorol®) is available in the USA and licensed for use in chronic renal failure. It has half to two-thirds of the potency of alfacalcidol.

Paricalcitol (Zemplar®)

This is 19-nor calcitriol and has a preferential effect on the VDR in the kidney and less effect in the gut. It is sometimes used instead of alfacalcidol or calcitriol in chronic renal disease for this reason.

Teriparatide (Forsteo®)

This is synthetic PTH 1–34 available for the treatment of post-menopausal osteoporosis and hypoparathyroidism in adults. It is not licensed for treatment in children and there are few short-term studies of its use in pediatric patients with hypoparathyroid-

ism. It is effective in raising plasma calcium concentrations and may have a specific benefit in patients in whom hypercalciuria and nephrocalcinosis is a particular problem, such as in ADH [32]. There are no long-term safety studies in children and the manufacturers have raised concerns about the possibility of developing osteosarcomas with long-term treatment because of similar problems in rats given high doses.

The bisphosphonates

These are analogs of pyrophosphate in which the central oxygen atom is replaced with carbon, the tetravalent nature of which allows the addition of extra residues on the spare side-chains, designated R1 and R2. In most bisphosphonates, R1 is an hydroxyl group that allows it to bind with pyrophosphate. The variety of the R2 residues determines the properties of the bisphosphonates and much work has been devoted to developing products that have a differential effect on bone accretion and resorption. The first generation of bisphosphonates (e.g. etidronate and clodronate) showed some of this differential but care has to be exercised in ensuring that they do not cause a mineralization defect and the later generations of drugs are not only much more potent (zoledronate is 10 000 times more potent than etidronate) but also have a greater effect on osteoclasts than on osteoblasts.

First generation bisphosphonates act by forming acyclic analogs of ATP which are cytotoxic and lead to cell apoptosis [120,121]. The second to fourth generation bisphosphonates contain an amino group and act by inhibiting farnesyl diphosphate synthase which inhibits protein prenylation (transfer of fatty acid chains) into intracellular proteins that are unable to be incorporated normally into cell membranes by the mevalonic acid pathway [122]. This disrupts cell function and leads to apoptosis. The effect is temporary and, after a few weeks, the osteoclasts recover and resume their functions. Each episode of treatment can be identified radiologically by the presence of a dense band across the metaphyses and, as growth slows, these bands become closer together until eventually they fuse.

The most frequently used bisphosphonate in children is pamidronate which reduces bone pain and fracture frequency and increases bone strength and density [123]. Pamidronate has become standard for children with moderate to severe OI. It is usually given by intravenous infusion in a regimen of 1 mg/kg/day for 3 days every 3–4 months. Trials of the newer bisphosphonate zoledronate have been undertaken and the results are awaited. Bisphosphonates can be given orally but are poorly absorbed because of their highly polar nature. They should be given at least 2 h before or after food. Trials of oral alendronate or olpadronate have proved disappointing and the most potent, risedronate, is still under investigation.

The indications for the use of bisphosphonates in children are:
• Generalized osteoporotic conditions, such as OI and OPG, as well as the secondary osteoporoses if symptomatic (e.g. back pain, crush fractures).

- Hypercalcemic conditions such as that caused by immobilization, malignancy or hyperparathyroidism. These patients are usually sensitive to treatment and may respond successfully to as little as a single dose of 0.5 mg/kg.
- Soft tissue calcification. There are no large series reporting the effects of bisphosphonates in these conditions but several case reports have demonstrated their value in a variety of conditions including dermatomyositis, fibrodysplasia ossificans progressiva, scleroderma and infantile arterial calcification.
- Miscellaneous conditions, particularly polyostotic fibrous dysplasia. The effects here are principally to reduce pain and the treatment has little effect on the bone lesions. Because the aim is not principally to increase bone density, treatment is usually given when the patient's symptoms demand it rather than on a regular basis.

Bisphosphonates are accompanied by a number of side effects:
- Acute phase reaction. This effect only occurs with the amino-bisphosphonates and is accompanied by fever, aches and pains and sometimes vomiting. They respond to simple analgesics and antipyretics. These usually only occur during the first cycle of treatment and subsequent cycles do not usually cause problems.
- Hypocalcemia and hypophosphatemia occur to a certain extent but do not usually cause problems unless exaggerated by the presence of vitamin D deficiency. Patients should always be screened for this and, if necessary, treated before initiation of bisphosphonates.
- Increased risk of fractures. If treatment of conditions such as OI is commenced, it should continue at least until growth has ceased since there appears to be an increase in fracture risk at the junction of treated and untreated bone [124].
- Esophagitis. Some of the oral bisphosphonates, particularly alendronate and olpadronate, are reported to cause some esophagitis. This seems to be less of a problem in children than in adults and less so with risedronate.
- Osteonecrosis of the jaw has been reported in adults but there are no reports of its occurrence in children.
- Osteopetrosis and undertubulation. There is one report of a child treated for non-specific bone pain with pamidronate at monthly intervals [125]. He developed dense bones, similar to those seen in osteopetrosis and undertubulation which results from failure of remodeling of the long bones. All known causes of osteopetrosis were excluded. The bone abnormalities persisted even after treatment had been stopped for 18 months.
- Iritis has been reported following treatment with both oral risedronate and intravenous pamidronate. This appears to be less of a problem in children than in adults but, in the event of eye problems developing, early referral to an ophthalmologist is advised.

Treatment with bisphosphonates should be undertaken only in centers where there is expertise in their use.

Calcitonin

This is occasionally used for its hypocalcemic effects when severe hypocalcemia has not responded to forced diuresis, etc. Its use has now been largely supplanted by bisphosphonates.

Phosphate supplements

These form part of the treatment of hypophosphatemic conditions, especially hypophosphatemic rickets. Phosphate is rapidly absorbed from the gastrointestinal tract and is also rapidly excreted, especially when TRP is low. Unfortunately, there are no slow-release preparations of phosphate available so it has to be given up to four or five times daily to maintain adequate concentrations. It is often difficult to achieve this because of problems of compliance both because of the taste and frequency of administration. Diarrhea may limit the total dose that can be given.

Phosphate binders

These are most useful in chronic kidney disease (CKD) when a reduced GFR limits phosphate excretion. Aluminum hydroxide has now been largely supplanted by calcium carbonate (Tetralac®) and sevelamer (Renagel®). While calcium carbonate is effective at reducing plasma phosphate, it has been associated with the development of adynamic bone. Sevelamer is not absorbed by the gut and does not have this problem. Sevelamer may also be useful in situations where soft tissue calcification arises as a result of hyperphosphatemia but there are no reports of its use in this situation.

Cinacalcet (Mimpara®)

Cinacalcet acts by increasing the sensitivity of the parathyroids to plasma calcium. It thus shifts the CaSR–PTH curve to the left (Fig. 16.2). It has been developed principally for the treatment of secondary hyperparathyroidism in CKD but there are also reports of its successful use in familial benign hypercalcemia (FBH) [126,127]. It is not clear if it is effective in homozygous forms of this condition. It is effective orally but requires twice daily administration.

Magnesium supplements

These may be required in large quantities in hypomagnesemic states, particularly where the hypomagnesemia causes secondary hypoparathyroidism. Magnesium sulfate is likely to cause diarrhea if used in large quantities. Magnesium glycerophosphate causes fewer such side effects. Magnesium sulfate can be given intramuscularly. A 50% solution contains 2 mmol/mL (46 mg/mL) and the dose may be repeated as required to maintain concentrations >0.7 mmol/L (1.6 mg/dL). It may also be given intravenously but must be given with caution as it causes intense vasodilatation if given too quickly.

Acknowledgments

I am grateful to Drs Moira Cheung and Caroline Brain for their helpful comments.

References

1 Hoenderop JG, Nilius B, Bindels RJ. Calcium absorption across epithelia. *Physiol Rev* 2005; **85**: 373–422.

2 Heaney RP. Nutrition and risk of osteoporosis. In: Marcus R, Feldman D, Kelsey J, eds. *Osteoporosis*. San Diego: Academic Press, 2001.

3 Friedman PA, Gesek FA. Cellular calcium transport in renal epithelia: measurement, mechanisms and regulation. *Physiol Rev* 1995; **75**: 429–471.

4 Kruse K, Kracht U, Kruse U. Reference values for urinary calcium excretion and screening for hypercalciuria in children and adolescents. *Eur J Pediatr* 1984; **143**: 25–31.

5 Groenestege WM, Thebault S, van der WJ, van den BD, Janssen R, Tejpar S, *et al.* Impaired basolateral sorting of pro-EGF causes isolated recessive renal hypomagnesemia. *J Clin Invest* 2007; **117**: 2260–2267.

6 Walton RJ, Bijvoet OL. Nomogram for derivation of renal threshold phosphate concentration. *Lancet* 1975; **2**: 309–310.

7 Kruse K, Kracht U, Gopfert G. Renal threshold phosphate concentration (TmPO4/GFR). *Arch Dis Child* 1982; **57**: 217–223.

8 Smith M, Weiss MJ, Griffin CA, Murray JC, Buetow KH, Emanuel BS, *et al.* Regional assignment of the gene for human liver/bone/kidney alkaline phosphatase to chromosome 1p36.1-p34. *Genomics* 1988; **2**: 139–143.

9 Round JM, Butcher S, Steele R. Changes in plasma inorganic phosphorus and alkaline phosphatase activity during the adolescent growth spurt. *Ann Hum Biol* 1979; **6**: 129.

10 Kronenberg HM, Bringhurst FR, Segre GV, Potts JT. Parathyroid hormone biosynthesis and metabolism. In: Bilezikian JP, Marcus R, Levine MA, eds. *The Parathyroids: Basic and Clinical Concepts*. San Diego: Academic Press, 2001, pp. 17–30.

11 Brown EM, MacLeod RJ. Extracellular calcium sensing and extracellular calcium signaling. *Physiol Rev* 2001; **81**: 239–297.

12 Conlin PR, Fajtova VT, Mortensen RM, LeBoff MS, Brown EM. Hysteresis in the relationship between serum ionized calcium and intact parathyroid hormone during recovery from induced hyper- and hypocalcemia in normal humans. *J Clin Endocrinol Metab* 1989; **69**: 593–599.

13 Parfitt AM. Parathyroid growth: normal and abnormal. In: Bilezikian JP, Marcus R, Levine MA, eds. *The Parathyroids: Basic and Clinical Concepts*. San Diego: Academic Press, 2001, pp. 293–330.

14 Nissensen RA. Receptors for parathyroid hormone and parathyroid hormone-related protein: signaling and regulation. In: Bilezikian JP, Marcus R, Levine MA, eds. *The Parathyroids: Basic and Clinical Concepts*. San Diego: Academic Press, 2001, pp. 93–104.

15 Farfel Z, Bourne HR, Iiri T. The expanding spectrum of G protein diseases. *N Engl J Med* 1999; **340**: 1012–1020.

16 Okuda K, Usui E, Ohyama Y. Recent progress in enzymology and molecular biology of enzymes involved in vitamin D metabolism. *J Lipid Res* 1995; **36**: 1641–1652.

17 St Arnaud R, Messerlian S, Moir JM, Omdahl JL, Glorieux FH. The 25-hydroxyvitamin D 1-alpha-hydroxylase gene maps to the pseudovitamin D-deficiency rickets (PDDR) disease locus. *J Bone Miner Res* 1997; **12**: 1552–1559.

18 Awumey EM, Mitra DA, Hollis BW, Kumar R, Bell NH. Vitamin D metabolism is altered in Asian Indians in the southern United States: a clinical research center study. *J Clin Endocrinol Metab* 1998; **83**: 169–173.

19 Haussler MR, Whitfield GK, Haussler CA, Hsieh JC, Thompson PD, Selznick SH, *et al.* The nuclear vitamin D receptor: biological and molecular regulatory properties revealed. *J Bone Miner Res* 1998; **13**: 325–349.

20 Ichikawa S, Imel EA, Kreiter ML, Yu X, Mackenzie DS, Sorenson AH, *et al.* A homozygous missense mutation in human KLOTHO causes severe tumoral calcinosis. *J Clin Invest* 2007; **117**: 2684–2691.

21 Francis F, Strom TM, Hennig S, Boddrich A, Lorenz B, Brandau O, *et al.* Genomic organization of the human PEX gene mutated in X-linked dominant hypophosphatemic rickets. *Genome Res* 1997; **7**: 573–585.

22 Martin TJ, Moseley JM, Williams ED. Parathyroid hormone-related protein: hormone and cytokine. *J Endocrinol* 1997; **154** (Suppl): S23–S37.

23 Allgrove J, Adami S, Manning RM, O'Riordan JL. Cytochemical bioassay of parathyroid hormone in maternal and cord blood. *Arch Dis Child* 1985; **60**: 110–115.

24 Bodine PV, Komm BS. Wnt signaling and osteoblastogenesis. *Rev Endocr Metab Disord* 2006; **7**: 33–39.

25 Johnson ML, Rajamannan N. Diseases of Wnt signaling. *Rev Endocr Metab Disord* 2006; **7**: 41–49.

26 Stein GS, Lian JB, van Wijnen AJ, Stein JL, Montecino M, Javed A, *et al.* Runx2 control of organization, assembly and activity of the regulatory machinery for skeletal gene expression. *Oncogene* 2004; **23**: 4315–4329.

27 Byers PH, Krakow D, Nunes ME, Pepin M. Genetic evaluation of suspected osteogenesis imperfecta (OI). *Genet Med* 2006; **8**: 383–388.

28 Fewtrell MS. Bone densitometry in children assessed by dual X-ray absorptiometry: uses and pitfalls. *Arch Dis Child* 2003; **88**: 795–798.

29 Rauch F. Watching bone cells at work: what we can see from bone biopsies. *Pediatr Nephrol* 2006; **21**: 457–462.

30 Szulc P, Seeman E, Delmas PD. Biochemical measurements of bone turnover in children and adolescents. *Osteoporos Int* 2000; **11**: 281–294.

31 Sharp M. Bone disease of prematurity. *Early Hum Dev* 2007; **83**: 653–658.

32 Shiohara M, Shiozawa R, Kurata K, Matsuura H, Arai F, Yasuda T, *et al.* Effect of parathyroid hormone administration in a patient with severe hypoparathyroidism caused by gain-of-function mutation of calcium-sensing receptor. *Endocr J* 2006; **53**: 797–802.

33 Sayer JA, Pearce SH. Extracellular calcium-sensing receptor dysfunction is associated with two new phenotypes. *Clin Endocrinol (Oxf)* 2003; **59**: 419–421.

34 Bassett JH, Thakker RV. Molecular genetics of disorders of calcium homeostasis. *Baillieres Clin Endocrinol Metab* 1995; **9**: 581–608.

35 Ding C, Buckingham B, Levine MA. Familial isolated hypoparathyroidism caused by a mutation in the gene for the transcription factor GCMB. *J Clin Invest* 2001; **108**: 1215–1220.

36 Baumber L, Tufarelli C, Patel S, King P, Johnson CA, Maher ER, *et al.* Identification of a novel mutation disrupting the DNA binding activity of GCM2 in autosomal recessive familial isolated hypoparathyroidism. *J Med Genet* 2005; **42**: 443–448.

37 Maret A, Ding C, Kornfield SL, Levine MA. Analysis of the GCM2 gene in isolated hypoparathyroidism: a molecular and biochemical study. *J Clin Endocrinol Metab* 2008; **93**: 1426–1432.

38 Gong W, Emanuel BS, Collins J, Kim DH, Wang Z, Chen F, *et al.* A transcription map of the DiGeorge and velo-cardio-facial syndrome minimal critical region on 22q11. *Hum Mol Genet* 1996; **5**: 789–800.

39 Scambler PJ, Carey AH, Wyse RK, Roach S, Dumanski JP, Nordenskjold M, *et al.* Microdeletions within 22q11 associated with sporadic and familial DiGeorge syndrome. *Genomics* 1991; **10**: 201–206.

40 Augusseau S, Jouk S, Jalbert P, Prieur M. DiGeorge syndrome and 22q11 rearrangements. *Hum Genet* 1986; **74**: 206.

41 Yamagishi H, Garg V, Matsuoka R, Thomas T, Srivastava D. A molecular pathway revealing a genetic basis for human cardiac and craniofacial defects. *Science* 1999; **283**: 1158–1161.

42 Ammann AJ, Wara DW, Cowan MJ, Barrett DJ, Stiehm ER. The DiGeorge syndrome and the fetal alcohol syndrome. *Am J Dis Child* 1982; **136**: 906–908.

43 Scire G, Dallapiccola B, Iannetti P, Bonaiuto F, Galasso C, Mingarelli R, *et al.* Hypoparathyroidism as the major manifestation in two patients with 22q11 deletions. *Am J Med Genet* 1994; **52**: 478–482.

44 Ali A, Christie PT, Grigorieva IV, Harding B, Van Esch H, Ahmed SF, *et al.* Functional characterization of GATA3 mutations causing the hypoparathyroidism-deafness-renal (HDR) dysplasia syndrome: insight into mechanisms of DNA binding by the GATA3 transcription actor. *Hum Mol Genet* 2007; **16**: 265–275.

45 Barakat AY, D'Albora JB, Martin MM, Jose PA. Familial nephrosis, nerve deafness and hypoparathyroidism. *J Pediatr* 1977; **91**: 61–64.

46 Shaw NJ, Haigh D, Lealmann GT, Karbani G, Brocklebank JT, Dillon MJ. Autosomal recessive hypoparathyroidism with renal insufficiency and developmental delay. *Arch Dis Child* 1991; **66**: 1191–1194.

47 Richardson RJ, Kirk JM. Short stature, mental retardation and hypoparathyroidism: a new syndrome. *Arch Dis Child* 1990; **65**: 1113–1117.

48 Ahonen P, Myllarniemi S, Sipila I, Perheentupa J. Clinical variation of autoimmune polyendocrinopathy-candidiasis-ectodermal dystrophy (APECED) in a series of 68 patients. *N Engl J Med* 1990; **322**: 1829–1836.

49 Arnold A, Horst SA, Gardella TJ, Baba H, Levine MA, Kronenberg HM. Mutation of the signal peptide-encoding region of the preproparathyroid hormone gene in familial isolated hypoparathyroidism. *J Clin Invest* 1990; **86**: 1084–1087.

50 Parkinson DB, Thakker RV. A donor splice site mutation in the parathyroid hormone gene is associated with autosomal recessive hypoparathyroidism. *Nat Genet* 1992; **1**: 149–152.

51 Sunthornthepvarakul T, Churesigaew S, Ngowngarmratana S. A novel mutation of the signal peptide of the preproparathyroid hormone gene associated with autosomal recessive familial isolated hypoparathyroidism. *J Clin Endocrinol Metab* 1999; **84**: 3792–3796.

52 Blomstrand S, Claesson I, Save-Soderbergh J. A case of lethal congenital dwarfism with accelerated skeletal maturation. *Pediatr Radiol* 1985; **15**: 141–143.

53 Eiken M, Prag J, Petersen KE, Kaufmann HJ. A new familial skeletal dysplasia with severely retarded ossification and abnormal modeling of bones especially of the epiphyses, the hands and feet. *Eur J Pediatr* 1984; **141**: 231–235.

54 Weinstein LS, Yu S, Warner DR, Liu J. Endocrine manifestations of stimulatory G protein alpha-subunit mutations and the role of genomic imprinting. *Endocr Rev* 2001; **22**: 675–705.

55 Hayward BE, Kamiya M, Strain L, Moran V, Campbell R, Hayashizaki Y, *et al.* The human GNAS1 gene is imprinted and encodes distinct paternally and biallelically expressed G proteins. *Proc Natl Acad Sci U S A* 1998; **95**: 10038–10043.

56 Nakamoto JM, Zimmerman D, Jones EA, Loke KY, Siddiq K, Donlan MA, *et al.* Concurrent hormone resistance (pseudohypoparathyroidism type Ia) and hormone independence (testotoxicosis) caused by a unique mutation in the G alpha s gene. *Biochem Mol Med* 1996; **58**: 18–24.

57 Farfel Z. Pseudohypohyperparathyroidism-pseudohypoparathyroidism type Ib. *J Bone Miner Res* 1999; **14**: 1016.

58 Zheng H, Radeva G, McCann JA, Hendy GN, Goodyer CG. Gαs transcripts are biallelically expressed in the human kidney cortex: implications for pseudohypoparathyroidism type 1b. *J Clin Endocrinol Metab* 2001; **86**: 4627–4629.

59 Bastepe M, Jüppner H, Thakker RV. Parathroid disorders. In: Glorieux FH, Pettifor JM, Jüppner H, eds. *Pediatric Bone: Biology & Diseases*. San Diego: Academic Press, 2003, pp. 485–508.

60 Allgrove J, Adami S, Fraher L, Reuben A, O'Riordan JL. Hypomagnesaemia: studies of parathyroid hormone secretion and function. *Clin Endocrinol (Oxf)* 1984; **21**: 435–449.

61 Khadilkar A, Das G, Sayyad M, Sanwalka N, Bhandari D, Khadilkar V, *et al.* Low calcium intake and hypovitaminosis D in adolescent girls. *Arch Dis Child* 2007; **92**: 1045.

62 Thacher TD, Fischer PR, Strand MA, Pettifor JM. Nutritional rickets around the world: causes and future directions. *Ann Trop Paediatr* 2006; **26**: 1–16.

63 Ladhani S, Srinivasan L, Buchanan C, Allgrove J. Presentation of vitamin D deficiency. *Arch Dis Child* 2004; **89**: 781–784.

64 Mughal Z. Rickets in childhood. *Semin Musculoskelet Radiol* 2002; **6**: 183–190.

65 Maiya S, Sullivan I, Allgrove J, Archer N, Tulloh R, Daubeney P, *et al.* Hypocalcaemia and Vitamin D deficiency: an but preventable cause of life threatening infant heart failure. *Heart* 2007; **94**: 581–584.

66 Arnaud SB, Arnaud CD, Bordier PJ. The interrelationships between vitamin D and parathyroid hormone in disorders of mineral metabolism in man. In: Norman AW, ed. *Vitamin D and Problems of Uremic Bone Disease*. de Gruyter, 1975, pp. 397–416.

67 Papapoulos SE, Clemens TL, Fraher LJ, Gleed J, O'Riordan JL. Metabolites of vitamin D in human vitamin-D deficiency: effect of vitamin D3 or 1,25-dihydroxycholecalciferol. *Lancet* 1980; **2**: 612–615.

68 Casella SJ, Reiner BJ, Chen TC, Holick MF, Harrison HE. A possible genetic defect in 25-hydroxylation as a cause of rickets. *J Pediatr* 1994; **124**: 929–932.

69 Fry AC, Karet FE. Inherited renal acidoses. *Physiology (Bethesda)* 2007; **22**: 202–211.

70 Annemans L, Moeremans K, Lamotte M, Garcia CJ, van den BH, Myint H, *et al.* Pan-European multicentre economic evaluation of recombinant urate oxidase (rasburicase) in prevention and treatment of hyperuricaemia and tumour lysis syndrome in haematological cancer patients. *Support Care Cancer* 2003; **11**: 249–257.

71 Salusky IB, Goodman WG. Growth hormone and calcitriol as modifiers of bone formation in renal osteodystrophy. *Kidney Int* 1995; **48**: 657–665.

72 KDOQI NKF. K/DOQI clinical practice guidelines for bone metabolism and disease in children with chronic kidney disease. *Am J Kidney Dis* 2005; **46**: S1–121.

73 Lloyd SE, Pannett AA, Dixon PH, Whyte MP, Thakker RV. Localization of familial benign hypercalcemia, Oklahoma variant

(FBHOk), to chromosome 19q13. *Am J Hum Genet* 1999; **64**: 189–195.

74 McMurtry CT, Schranck FW, Walkenhorst DA, Murphy WA, Kocher DB, Teitelbaum SL, *et al*. Significant developmental elevation in serum parathyroid hormone concentrations in a large kindred with familial benign (hypocalciuric) hypercalcemia. *Am J Med* 1992; **93**: 247–258.

75 Pearce S, Steinmann B. Casting new light on the clinical spectrum of neonatal severe hyperparathyroidism. *Clin Endocrinol (Oxf)* 1999; **50**: 691–693.

76 Pannett AA, Thakker RV. Multiple endocrine neoplasia type 1. *Endocr Relat Cancer* 1999; **6**: 449–473.

77 Thakker RV. Multiple endocrine neoplasia: syndromes of the twentieth century. *J Clin Endocrinol Metab* 1998; **83**: 2617–2620.

78 Williamson C, Pannett AA, Pang JT, Wooding C, McCarthy M, Sheppard MN, *et al*. Localisation of a gene causing endocrine neoplasia to a 4 cM region on chromosome 1p35-p36. *J Med Genet* 1997; **34**: 617–619.

79 Szabo J, Heath B, Hill VM, Jackson CE, Zarbo RJ, Mallette LE, *et al*. Hereditary hyperparathyroidism-jaw tumor syndrome: the endocrine tumor gene HRPT2 maps to chromosome 1q21-q31. *Am J Hum Genet* 1995; **56**: 944–950.

80 Weinstein LS, Simonds WF. HRPT2, a marker of parathyroid cancer. *N Engl J Med* 2003; **349**: 1691–1692.

81 Cetani F, Pardi E, Bycava P, Pollina GD, Fanelli G, Picone A, *et al*. A reappraisal of the Rb1 gene abnormalities in the diagnosis of parathyroid cancer. *Clin Endocrinol (Oxf)* 2004; **60**: 99–106.

82 Motokura T, Bloom T, Kim HG, Juppner H, Ruderman JV, Kronenberg HM, *et al*. A novel cyclin encoded by a bcl1-linked candidate oncogene. *Nature* 1991; **350**: 512–515.

83 Odell WD, Hobbs MR, Benowitz B. An immunologically anomolous parathyroid hormone variant causing hyperparathyroidism. *Clin Endocrinol (Oxf)* 2001; **55**: 417–420.

84 Schipani E, Langman C, Hunzelman J, Le Merrer M, Loke KY, Dillon MJ, *et al*. A novel parathyroid hormone (PTH)/PTH-related peptide receptor mutation in Jansen's metaphyseal chondrodysplasia. *J Clin Endocrinol Metab* 1999; **84**: 3052–3057.

85 Burden AD, Krafchik BR. Subcutaneous fat necrosis of the newborn: a review of 11 cases. *Pediatr Dermatol* 1999; **16**: 384–387.

86 Chesney RW, Hamstra AJ, DeLuca HF, Horowitz S, Gilbert EF, Hong R, *et al*. Elevated serum 1,25-dihydroxyvitamin D concentrations in the hypercalcemia of sarcoidosis: correction by glucocorticoid therapy. *J Pediatr* 1981; **98**: 919–922.

87 American Academy of Pediatrics. Health care supervision for children with Williams syndrome. *Pediatrics* 2001; **107**: 1192–1204.

88 Perez Jurado LA, Peoples R, Kaplan P, Hamel BC, Francke U. Molecular definition of the chromosome 7 deletion in Williams syndrome and parent-of-origin effects on growth. *Am J Hum Genet* 1996; **59**: 781–792.

89 McTaggart SJ, Craig J, MacMillan J, Burke JR. Familial occurrence of idiopathic infantile hypercalcemia. *Pediatr Nephrol* 1999; **13**: 668–671.

90 Kaul S, Sockalosky JJ. Human synthetic calcitonin therapy for hypercalcemia of immobilization. *J Pediatr* 1995; **126**: 825–827.

91 McKay C, Furman WL. Hypercalcemia complicating childhood malignancies. *Cancer* 1993; **72**: 256–260.

92 Cole DE. Hypophosphatasia update: recent advances in diagnosis and treatment. *Clin Genet* 2008; **73**: 232–235.

93 Whyte MP. Hypophosphatasia and the role of alkaline phosphatase in skeletal mineralization. *Endocr Rev* 1994; **15**: 439–461.

94 Raisz LG. Pathogenesis of osteoporosis: concepts, conflicts and prospects. *J Clin Invest* 2005; **115**: 3318–3325.

95 Sillence DO, Senn A, Danks DM. Genetic heterogeneity in osteogenesis imperfecta. *J Med Genet* 1979; **16**: 101–116.

96 Zack P, Zack LR, Surtees R, Neville BG. A standardized tool to measure and describe scleral colour in osteogenesis imperfecta. *Ophthalmic Physiol Opt* 2007; **27**: 174–178.

97 Goldman AB, Davidson D, Pavlov H, Bullough PG. Popcorn calcifications: a prognostic sign in osteogenesis imperfecta. *Radiology* 1980; **136**: 351–358.

98 Glorieux FH, Rauch F, Plotkin H, Ward L, Travers R, Roughley P, *et al*. Type V osteogenesis imperfecta: a new form of brittle bone disease. *J Bone Miner Res* 2000; **15**: 1650–1658.

99 Cheung MS, Glorieux FH, Rauch F. Natural history of hyperplastic callus formation in osteogenesis imperfecta type V. *J Bone Miner Res* 2007; **22**: 1181–1186.

100 Glorieux FH, Ward LM, Rauch F, Lalic L, Roughley PJ, Travers R. Osteogenesis imperfecta type VI: a form of brittle bone disease with a mineralization defect. *J Bone Miner Res* 2002; **17**: 30–38.

101 Ward LM, Rauch F, Travers R, Chabot G, Azouz EM, Lalic L, *et al*. Osteogenesis imperfecta type VII: an autosomal recessive form of brittle bone disease. *Bone* 2002; **31**: 12–18.

102 Cabral WA, Chang W, Barnes AM, Weis M, Scott MA, Leikin S, *et al*. Prolyl 3-hydroxylase 1 deficiency causes a recessive metabolic bone disorder resembling lethal/severe osteogenesis imperfecta. *Nat Genet* 2007; **39**: 359–365.

103 Rauch F, Travers R, Norman ME, Taylor A, Parfitt AM, Glorieux FH. Deficient bone formation in idiopathic juvenile osteoporosis: a histomorphometric study of cancellous iliac bone. *J Bone Miner Res* 2000; **15**: 957–963.

104 Smith R. Idiopathic juvenile osteoporosis: experience of twenty-one patients. *Br J Rheumatol* 1995; **34**: 68–77.

105 Smith R. Idiopathic osteoporosis in the young. *J Bone Joint Surg Br* 1980; **62-B**: 417–427.

106 Cundy T, Davidson J, Rutland MD, Stewart C, DePaoli AM. Recombinant osteoprotegerin for juvenile Paget's disease. *N Engl J Med* 2005; **353**: 918–923.

107 Rauch F, Glorieux FH. Osteogenesis imperfecta, current and future medical treatment. *Am J Med Genet C Semin Med Genet* 2005; **139**: 31–37.

108 Fischer A, Griscelli C, Friedrich W, Kubanek B, Levinsky R, Morgan G, *et al*. Bone-marrow transplantation for immunodeficiencies and osteopetrosis: European survey, 1968–1985. *Lancet* 1986; **2**: 1080–1084.

109 Key L, Carnes D, Cole S, Holtrop M, Bar-Shavit Z, Shapiro F, *et al*. Treatment of congenital osteopetrosis with high-dose calcitriol. *N Engl J Med* 1984; **310**: 409–415.

110 Key LL Jr, Rodriguiz RM, Willi SM, Wright NM, Hatcher HC, Eyre DR, *et al*. Long-term treatment of osteopetrosis with recombinant human interferon gamma. *N Engl J Med* 1995; **332**: 1594–1599.

111 Janssens K, Van Hul W. Molecular genetics of too much bone. *Hum Mol Genet* 2002; **11**: 2385–2393.

112 Ariceta G, Langman CB. Growth in X-linked hypophosphatemic rickets. *Eur J Pediatr* 2007; **166**: 303–309.

113 Borghi MM, Coates V, Omar HA. Evaluation of stature development during childhood and adolescence in individuals with familial hypophosphatemic rickets. *Sci World J* 2005; **5**: 868–873.

114 Quigley R. Proximal renal tubular acidosis. *J Nephrol* 2006; **19** (Suppl 9): S41–45.

115 Plotkin H, Rauch F, Zeitlin L, Munns C, Travers R, Glorieux FH. Effect of pamidronate treatment in children with polyostotic fibrous dysplasia of bone. *J Clin Endocrinol Metab* 2003; **88**: 4569–4575.

116 Bouthors J, Vantyghem MC, Manouvrier-Hanu S, Soudan B, Proust E, Happle R, *et al.* Phacomatosis pigmentokeratotica associated with hypophosphataemic rickets, pheochromocytoma and multiple basal cell carcinomas. *Br J Dermatol* 2006; **155**: 225–226.

117 Hoffman WH, Jueppner HW, Deyoung BR, O'dorisio MS, Given KS. Elevated fibroblast growth factor-23 in hypophosphatemic linear nevus sebaceous syndrome. *Am J Med Genet A* 2005; **134**: 233–236.

118 Saraswat A, Dogra S, Bansali A, Kumar B. Phakomatosis pigmentokeratotica associated with hypophosphataemic vitamin D-resistant rickets: improvement in phosphate homeostasis after partial laser ablation. *Br J Dermatol* 2003; **148**: 1074–1076.

119 Shah BR, Finberg L. Single-day therapy for nutritional vitamin D-deficiency rickets: a preferred method. *J Pediatr* 1994; **125**: 487–490.

120 Shaw NJ, Bishop NJ. Bisphosphonate treatment of bone disease. *Arch Dis Child* 2005; **90**: 494–499.

121 Russell RG. Bisphosphonates: mode of action and pharmacology. *Pediatrics* 2007; **119** (Suppl 2): S150–S162.

122 Roelofs AJ, Thompson K, Gordon S, Rogers MJ. Molecular mechanisms of action of bisphosphonates: current status. *Clin Cancer Res* 2006; **12**: 6222s–6230s.

123 Glorieux FH, Bishop NJ, Plotkin H, Chabot G, Lanoue G, Travers R. Cyclic administration of pamidronate in children with severe osteogenesis imperfecta. *N Engl J Med* 1998; **339**: 947–952.

124 Rauch F, Cornibert S, Cheung M, Glorieux FH. Long-bone changes after pamidronate discontinuation in children and adolescents with osteogenesis imperfecta. *Bone* 2007; **40**: 821–827.

125 Whyte MP, Wenkert D, Clements KL, McAlister WH, Mumm S. Bisphosphonate-induced osteopetrosis. *N Engl J Med* 2003; **349**: 457–463.

126 Festen-Spanjer B, Haring CM, Koster JB, Mudde AH. Correction of hypercalcaemia by cinacalcet in familial hypocalciuric hypercalcaemia. *Clin Endocrinol (Oxf)* 2008; **68**: 324–325.

127 Timmers HJ, Karperien M, Hamdy NA, de Boer H, Hermus AR. Normalization of serum calcium by cinacalcet in a patient with hypercalcaemia due to a *de novo* inactivating mutation of the calcium-sensing receptor. *J Intern Med* 2006; **260**: 177–182.

17 Endocrine Neoplasia in Childhood

Joanne C. Blair

Alder Hey Children's NHS Foundation Trust, Liverpool, UK

Endocrine neoplasia is rare in childhood and its management is challenging. Children typically present with clinical features of hormone excess or enlargement of an endocrine gland but optimal management often requires collaboration between a large number of professionals, including oncologists, specialist surgeons, geneticists, clinical biochemists, pathologists, radiotherapists and anesthetists.

Endocrine tumors present more commonly in adult life and collaboration with adult endocrinologists can be invaluable. Many children require lifelong endocrine therapies or surveillance for recurrent or associated disease and from diagnosis close collaboration with specialists in adult practice facilitates seamless transition into adult medical services.

The rarity of these tumors is reflected in a lack of knowledge of the natural history of some of these conditions and a paucity of evidence informing the management of children with advanced or relapsed disease. National and international collaborations seek to address these deficiencies by establishing disease registries and delivering rigorous clinical trials.

Endocrine neoplasia often occurs in the context of constitutional genetic abnormalities, which may be associated with an increased lifetime risk of malignant disease of a number of endocrine or non-endocrine organs. Cross-sectional and prospective studies of large cohorts of patients have informed surveillance programs and prophylactic therapy. Such advances in the care of patients and families with inherited endocrine neoplasia have improved the morbidity and mortality in some of these conditions.

Tumors of the adrenal gland

Adrenocortical tumors

Adrenocortical tumors (ACT) occur with a worldwide incidence of 0.2–0.3 cases per million with a marked geographical variation:

Brook's Clinical Pediatric Endocrinology, 6th edition. Edited by C. Brook, P. Clayton, R. Brown. © 2009 Blackwell Publishing, ISBN: 978-1-4051-8080-1.

children in Brazil are affected 10–15 times more commonly that those in North America. Approximately 90% of ACT are malignant and they account for 0.2% of all pediatric solid malignancies. There is a bimodal age distribution in the first and fourth decades of life and most children present before the age of 5 years. Girls are affected more commonly than boys and female predominance increases from early childhood, when the female : male ratio is 1.5 : 1, to 6 : 1 during adolescence [1].

Childhood ACT is usually associated with constitutional genetic abnormalities. Fifty percent of children have Li–Fraumeni syndrome, a dominantly inherited condition that results from mutations of the p53 gene. A number of other malignancies occur with increased frequency in early adult life, including sarcomas, brain tumors, breast and lung cancers. Childhood ACT may be the first presentation of Li–Fraumeni syndrome in a family.

The p53 gene is a tumor suppressor gene located on chromosome 17p13.1. It encodes a 53-kDa transcription factor which responds to diverse cellular stresses to regulate cell cycle arrest, apoptosis, senescence, DNA repair or changes in metabolism. Regulation of apoptosis by p53 is also induced through non-transcriptional cytoplasmic processes. In unstressed cells, p53 is kept inactive. Loss of heterozygosity of p53 has been widely documented in ACT tumor cells with deletion of the wild-type allele and accumulation of the mutant p53 protein within the cell nuclei.

Atypical p53 germline mutations are found in 80% of children with sporadic ACT. The cancer family history of these patients may be unremarkable because p53 mutations have low penetrance and are likely to be tissue-specific. Nevertheless, the cancer risk for carriers of p53 mutations is increased and the presence of a p53 mutation of any type greatly increases the risk of childhood ACT. Genetic counseling and testing should be considered for all families of children with ACT. Germline mutations of p53 do not appear to be associated with ACT in older children and young adults.

The prevalence of ACT is increased in a number of other genetic conditions. Beckwith–Wiedemann syndrome occurs with a prevalence of 1 in 13 700. The mode of inheritance is complex.

Possible patterns include autosomal dominant inheritance with variable expressivity, genomic imprinting resulting from a defective or absent copy of the maternally derived gene and contiguous gene duplication at 11p15. The cardinal features are exomphalos, midline abdominal wall defects, macroglossia, neonatal hyperinsulinemia and macrosomia. Ear pits and ear creases are also commonly observed. Patients are at increased risk of malignant and benign tumors including Wilms tumor, ACT, hepatoblastoma, neuroblastoma and rhabdomyosarcoma. Patients with apparently dominantly inherited disease have genetic alternations in the region 11p15.5 and duplication of this region may confer an increased risk of ACT.

Isolated hemihypertrophy is a term applied to patients with asymmetric overgrowth of single or multiple organs or regions of the body. Approximately 1 in 86 000 live born infants are affected and a female preponderance is observed. A number of tumors occur with increased frequency, including ACT, hepatoblastoma, Wilms tumor and neuroblastoma. In one study of nine affected children, two developed ACT [2].

Carney complex is a dominantly inherited condition characterized by pigmented lesions of the skin and mucosae and cardiac, endocrine, cutaneous and neural myxomatous tumors. At least two genetic loci have been associated with Carney complex: type 1 is caused by mutation in the protein kinase A regulatory subunit-1α gene on chromosome 17q and type 2 has been mapped to chromosome 2p16. Twenty five percent of patients with Carney complex develop Cushing syndrome due to primary pigmented nodular adrenocortical disease. Papillary and follicular thyroid carcinomas, benign thyroid adenomas and large-cell calcifying Sertoli cell tumor have also been reported to occur with increased frequency.

ACT are described in patients with congenital adrenal hyperplasia. Adrenal carcinomas, adenomas, myelolipomas and hemangioma have all been reported. The reasons for this association are unknown but tumorigenesis is likely to be related to chronic stimulation of the adrenal gland by elevated concentrations of ACTH.

Multiple endocrine neoplasia type 1 (MEN1) is discussed in detail below. Approximately 35% of adult patients have adrenal nodules of which the majority are benign and nonfunctional. Benign cortisol secreting tumors, pheochromocytoma and adrenocortical carcinomas have also been reported.

Diagnosis
Clinical features
Ninety percent of ACT affecting young children are functional and the majority of children present with clinical features of androgen excess: accelerated growth and skeletal maturity, acne, pubic hair growth, growth of the penis in boys and cliteromegaly in girls. Estrogen secretion occurs very rarely and induces accelerated growth and skeletal maturity, breast development and, in girls, vaginal bleeding. Approximately 40% of patients are hypertensive at diagnosis because of glucocorticoid or mineralocorticoid excess or compression of the renal artery [1]. A minority of patients present with hypertensive seizures. Glucocorticoid excess results in the clinical characteristics of Cushing syndrome in a minority of patients. Older patients are more likely to have nonfunctioning tumors and present more commonly with abdominal pain and weight loss.

Biochemical evaluation
The endocrine profile of the tumor should be defined at diagnosis by measurement of serum cortisol, dihydroepiandrosterone sulfate (DHEAS), testosterone androstendione, 17 hydroxyprogesterone, estradiol, renin, aldosterone and 11 deoxycortisol. Congenital adrenal hyperplasia and exaggerated adrenarche can be excluded on 24-h urinary steroid profile. Non-functioning ACT can be distinguished from pheochromocytoma and neuroblastoma by analysis of 24-h urinary catecholamines or metanephrines.

Blood glucose and electrolytes should also be monitored as hyperglycemia and hypokalemia are found commonly in children with functional tumors.

Diagnostic imaging
The use of radiation should be used sparingly for the diagnosis and surveillance of children with ACT given the high prevalence of p53 gene mutations and known risk of secondary malignancies.

Ultrasound is the examination of first choice for the definition of tumor location, dimensions and characteristics. Large tumors often have a stellate appearance due to hemorrhage, necrosis and fibrosis. Calcification is common. Tumor thrombus occurs in 20% of patients and can be visualized in the inferior vena cava on ultrasound examination. Extension into the right atrium is not uncommon.

Detailed scanning by magnetic resonance imaging (MRI) or computerized tomography (CT) is essential for surgical planning, in particular to gain further information regarding tumor invasion of adjacent structures. The MRI appearances of ACT are illustrated in Fig. 17.1. The liver should also be examined for evidence of metastatic spread. Tumors should never be biopsied because of the risk of tumor spillage.

The presence of lung metastases should be investigated by CT of the chest. Metastases to bone and brain are also common and require specific imaging.

Imaging with fluorine[18]-labeled fluorodeoxyglucose positron emission tomography (FDG-PET) is being used increasingly for the diagnosis and staging of a number of malignancies. FDG is a glucose analog that enters cells in the same manner as glucose but is trapped within the cell after phosphorylation and is not metabolized further, so intracellular FDG reflects intracellular glucose metabolism and is markedly increased in a variety of tumor cells. The identification of local recurrence can be difficult by conventional CT and MRI and in this scenario FDG-PET is a particularly valuable investigation that also identifies distant metastases.

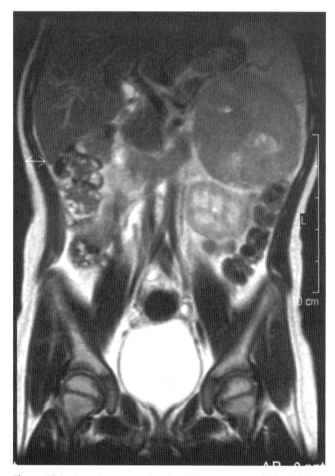

Figure 17.1 Magnetic resonance imaging (MRI) appearances of a left-sided adrenocortical carcinoma.

Pathology

The distinction between cortical adenomas (benign) and carcinomas (malignant) can be very difficult. Tumor size and weight offer a rough indication of malignant potential in that tumor nodules less than 5 cm in diameter and less than 200 g are likely to be adenomas (Plates 17.1 & 17.2).

A large number of parameters to distinguish benign and malignant disease have been studied. The presence of necrosis (greater than two high-power fields in diameter) and broad fibrous bands/septae were useful discriminatory features, in addition to a diffuse pattern of growth, nuclear polychromasia and vascular invasion [3].

Tumors with high nuclear grade (>5 mitoses/50 high power field), atypical mitoses, diffuse growth pattern, invasion of venous, sinusoidal and capsular structures, clear cells comprising <25% of the tumors were likely to pursue a malignant course. Tumors with less than two of these features never metastasized, whereas those with more than four almost invariably recurred or metastasized [4].

Benign cortical tumors in children were significantly more likely to have higher mitotic activity, necrosis, broad fibrous bands and nuclear polymorphism than adenomas in adults [5].

These observations warn us that the set of criteria established for differentiation of adult ACT tumors cannot be directly applied to the pediatric population. Although early DNA studies suggested that cytofluorometric analysis of DNA content could be an effective predictor of clinical outcome when histomorphological features are ambiguous, cortical adenomas may be aneuploid and carcinomas diploid, indicating that ploidy is not a reliable discriminatory feature between adenomas and carcinomas.

Management

Preoperative medical management

Hypertension is common at diagnosis and may be difficult to treat. Specific therapies that block one or more enzymatic steps of steroid biosynthesis may be more successful than conventional therapies. Such medications include metyrapone, ketoconazole or mitotane but all have a delayed onset of action. Spironolactone, an aldosterone antagonist, has a more rapid effect and may be required in large doses in children with severe or refractory hypertension. Hyperglycemia and electrolyte abnormalities should also be corrected.

Surgery

Surgery should aim for complete en bloc tumor resection and this may include adjacent kidney, portions of the pancreas and liver and other adjacent structures. Patients in whom there is residual disease have a much poorer prognosis than those in whom surgical resection is complete.

In 20% of patients, the inferior vena cava is infiltrated with tumor thrombus making radical surgery difficult. For this reason, the inferior vena cava should be palpated and thrombus removed before tumor resection is attempted. In extensive disease, a combined thoracic and abdominal approach may be required.

Large tumors often show local recurrence and modified lymph node dissection of the ipsilateral nodes is recommended from the renal vein to the bifurcation of the common iliac vessel. If the contralateral nodes are enlarged, these should also be dissected.

Postoperative medical management

All patients with glucocorticoid secreting tumors experience adrenal insufficiency in the postoperative period because of adrenocorticotropic hormone (ACTH) suppression. Replacement therapy with hydrocortisone at stress concentrations is required and gradually weaned until there is recovery of the hypothalamo-adrenal-pituitary axis which may take many months or even years. Patients with bilateral disease have a life-long need for glucocorticoid and mineralocorticoid replacement therapy. Patients who were hypertensive in the preoperative period are at risk of profound hypotension following surgery and pressor support may be required.

The urinary steroid profile should be checked during the first postoperative week in patients with functional tumors. Hormones typically return to normal within 7 days of complete tumor resection. The use of hydrocortisone as a glucocorticoid replacement will render urinary cortisol meaningless and, if it is anticipated that urinary cortisol will be used as a tumor marker, replacement therapy should be with dexamethasone. Serum cortisol measured 12 h following an oral dose of hydrocortisone can be used to assess endogenous cortisol production.

Management of advanced and metastatic disease
Second look surgery
Recurrent or metastatic disease should be surgically resected wherever possible.

Mitotane therapy
The place of mitotane in the management of ACT is uncertain. Up to 30% of patients with advanced disease have an objective response; however, this is usually transient and the overall effect on survival is unknown [6]. Complete responses have been reported in children with advanced or metastatic disease but appear to be unusual.

Mitotane in low doses inhibits glucocorticoid biosynthesis and, in high doses, it induces cell death in the zona fasciculata. The zona glomerulosa is also affected but less severely so. Mitotane accelerates the metabolic clearance of glucocorticoids, thyroid and parathyroid hormones so glucocorticoid and mineralocorticoid replacement therapy is required in all patients and many also require thyroid hormone supplementation.

The antitumor effect of mitotane relies on the maintenance of high serum concentrations for prolonged periods of time. This is only achieved in 50–60% of patients using standard protocols because severe side effects limit patient compliance [7]. Gastrointestinal side effects include nausea, vomiting and abdominal pain but somnolence, lethargy, depression, ataxia and vertigo are the most profound effects. Improved tolerability and favorable therapeutic results have been reported using low dose mitotane regimens and therapeutic concentrations can be achieved with gradual increments over 3–5 months [8]. Mitotane in lower doses also has a place in palliation of symptoms related to hormone excess in the management of children with advanced disease.

Chemotherapy
The effect of chemotherapy on ACT in childhood has been less extensively studied. The use of cisplatin alone can induce remission in up to 25% of patients with advanced disease [9]. Combination therapy of cisplatin with doxorubicin and cyclophosphamide or 5-fluorouracil increases remission rates to 20–40% [10,11].

The use of mitotane in combination with etoposide-based chemotherapy is attractive to reduce the occurrence of multidrug resistance and improved remission rates of 63% have been reported when mitotane is combined with cisplatin, etoposide and doxorubicin [12].

Radiotherapy
In general, ACT are considered radio-resistant. The high prevalence of p53 gene mutations in these patients and associated risk of secondary malignancies also makes it an unattractive therapy. A number of children treated with radiotherapy have been reported, in whom secondary sarcoma in the radiation field proved fatal.

Staging and prognosis
The staging guidelines for ACT are given in Table 17.1. Prognosis is closely related to the stage of the tumor at diagnosis, event-free survival at 5 years being 91% for children presenting with stage I disease and 53% for those with stage III disease [1]. Very few children present with stage II or IV disease but the prognosis is extremely poor for these patients.

Data from the International Pediatric Adrenocortical Tumor Registry reported that 44.1% of children had stage I disease at diagnosis and 31.5% had stage II disease and the mean duration of symptoms prior to diagnosis was 5 months [1]. It is important to note that 79.5% of children on this registry were from southern Brazil, where the high prevalence of the disease is likely to prompt early investigation of children presenting with the clinical characteristics of ACT, particularly those from previously affected families. In contrast, the mean duration of symptoms before diagnosis in a small British cohort was 31 months [13].

Prognosis is more favorable in children who present below the age of 3 years, those with tumor weighing less than 200 g and isolated virilization at presentation.

Surveillance
Stage I disease
Patients in whom tumor resection is complete and tumor size is less than 100 g in weight or 200 mL in volume should enter a tumor surveillance program for 5 years.

Stage II–IV disease
Children in whom tumor resection is incomplete, tumor size exceeds 100 g in weight or 200 mL in volume and those with evidence of metastatic disease should be considered for either mitotane or chemotherapy. Those with complete resection of large tumors and no biochemical evidence of residual disease may be followed closely clinically, with biochemical profiles and abdominal imaging for evidence of recurrent or residual disease. There are currently no robust clinical trials to inform the selection of adjuvant therapy.

Table 17.1 Staging of adrenocortical tumors.

Stage I	Total excision of tumor; tumor volume <200 cm³ (100 g)
	Absence of metastases and normal hormone concentrations after surgery
Stage II	Microscopic residual tumor, tumor volume >200 cm³ (100 g)
	Persistently elevated adrenocortical hormone concentrations after surgery
IIA	Resected tumors (>200 cm³/100 g) 50% surgically cured
IIB	Microscopic residual disease or persistant hormone excess – 100% progression
Stage III	Gross residual or inoperable tumor
Stage IV	Distant metastases

Surveillance and transitional care

Once the child has entered remission they should enter a program of tumor surveillance with periodic clinical review, evaluation of urinary steroid excretion and imaging.

Patients who have completed 5 years of tumor surveillance should continue under the care of the endocrinologist until adult life to ensure that growth and puberty progresses normally. Virilized girls with cliteromegaly may be best seen in a multidisciplinary service for children with disorders of sex development to enable their psychological, surgical and medical needs to be met.

Patients with any of the genetic syndromes discussed above require lifelong tumor surveillance to facilitate early tumor diagnosis and treatment of associated neoplasms. Planned transition from pediatric to adult services is critical if patients are to comply with complex and sometimes demanding surveillance programs. This is most likely to succeed in a service designed specifically to meet the needs of families with genetic conditions associated with neoplasia. Such services may be complex, drawing on the expertise of health care professionals of many disciplines and delivering a range of surveillance programs. Adult oncologists are best placed to lead such a service and expert nurses should have a central role in family education and coordination of the surveillance program.

Palliative care

A significant number of children with ACT have inoperable disease or recurrent disease resistant to current treatment modalities. These children require the care of a pediatric palliative care team. Palliation of the symptoms of hormone excess and replacement of hormone deficiencies is best achieved when the endocrinologist works alongside the palliative care team.

Pheochromocytoma and paraganglioma

Pheochromocytoma and paraganglioma are tumors of the sympathetic and parasympathetic paraganglia. Both originate from chromaffin cells derived from the neural crest and are highly vascularized, slowly growing tumors. Parasympathetic paraganglia are found in the head and neck and are generally non-functioning. Sympathetic paraganglia arise from the adrenal medulla or the sympathetic ganglia and generally secrete catecholamines.

The term pheochromocytoma is applied to catecholamine secreting paraganglia located within the abdomen or thorax.

The incidence is 1.55–2 per million and 10–20% of tumors occur in children and adolescents. Pheochromocytoma are rarely malignant in childhood. Anecdotally, pheochromocytoma was known as the "10% tumor": 10% were believed to be malignant, 10% were extra-adrenal, 10% were bilateral and 10% were believed to be hereditary. In fact, about 40% of cases are associated with a germline mutation in one of five major susceptibility genes (Table 17.2) and this figure is likely to be higher in childhood.

Genotype–phenotype studies have informed surveillance programs for those at risk of inherited disease. The need to screen asymptomatic patients has prompted re-evaluation of established diagnostic tests and the development of new biochemical tests better suited to surveillance than conventional investigations. Such programs should enable the early identification of active disease, facilitating safer surgical intervention.

The prognosis for elective surgical management of pheochromocytoma is excellent and the perioperative mortality is 0–3% for all age groups. In contrast, undiagnosed or ill-prepared patients experience a perioperative mortality as high as 50%.

Inherited pheochromocytoma and paraganglioma syndromes

Chronic hypoxia is associated with the development of paraganglioma of the carotid body and this observation led to speculation that genes involved in oxygen sensing and signaling may be important in the etiology of this condition.

Succinate dehydrogenase (SDH) was an attractive candidate gene in the search for the genetic cause of hereditary pheochromocytoma. Loss of function of this complex may result in the constant signaling of hypoxia within the cell and upregulation of hypoxic angiogenic response genes has been associated with mutations of the genes encoding SDH [14].

Table 17.2 Genetic syndromes associated with pheochromocytoma.

Syndrome	Gene	Frequency of pheochromocytoma (%)	Frequency of head and neck paraganglia (%)	Youngest age at presentation (years)
MEN2	RET oncogene	30–50	0	5
von Hippel–Lindau	von Hippel–Lindau suppressor gene	15–20	0	5
Neurofibromatosis-1	Neurofibromatosis type 1	1–5	0	
Paraganglioma syndrome type 1	SDHD	58	79	5
Paraganglioma syndrome type 3	SDHC	0	100	13
Paraganglioma syndrome type 4	SDHB	87	15	5

MEN2, multiple endocrine neoplasia type 2; SDH, succinate dehydrogenase (subunits B, C & D).

SDH is also known as complex II of the electron transport chain. This pathway includes four protein complexes that link the Krebs cycle and oxidative phosphorylation, the process by which mitochondria generate adenosine triphopshate (ATP). SDH generates a proton gradient by catalyzing the oxidation of succinate to fumarate and thereby transferring its reducing equivalent to ubiquinone.

SDH is composed of four subunits: two catalytic subunits A and B that are anchored in the inner mitochondrial membrane by subunits C and D. Mutations of SDHB, -C and -D have been reported in patients and cause paraganglioma syndrome types 4, 3 and 1, respectively. Mutations of SDHA are associated with Leigh syndrome, a necrotizing encephalomyopathy in which cerebrospinal fluid (CSF) glucose is reduced and lactic acidosis occurs intermittently, and a syndrome of optic atrophy, ataxia and myopathy.

Patients with mutations of SDHB usually present in early adult life. The mean age at diagnosis is 35 years, although children as young as 5 years of age have been affected. Eighty-seven percent of patients develop a pheochromocytoma, which is most commonly extra-adrenal in location. Multiple tumors are common and occur in 28% of patients, of which 35% are malignant [15]. There are case reports of renal and thyroid carcinoma occurring in patients with SDHB mutations but the data are inadequate to determine whether this is a true association.

Mutations of the gene encoding SDHC are less common than those affecting either SDHB or SDHD. Pheochromocytoma have not yet been reported in association with SDHC gene mutations and paraganglia appear to be restricted to the head and neck. The carotid body is the most common site of disease. The mean age at diagnosis is 46 years; the youngest affected patient reported was 13 years. Multiple lesions occur in 10% of patients but malignant disease has not yet been described [16].

Patients carrying mutations of the SDHD gene present at a mean age of 40 years and the youngest affected patient was 5 years of age [15]. Seventy-nine percent of patients develop paraganglia of the head and neck and approximately 50% develop pheochromocytoma, most commonly affecting the adrenal gland. Malignant disease has not yet been reported, although a number of cases of thyroid carcinoma have reported in patients with SDHD gene mutations.

Von Hippel–Lindau disease

Von Hippel–Lindau (VHL) disease is inherited in an autosomal dominant manner. It occurs with an incidence of 1 in 36 000 and has a penetrance of 97% by the age of 60 years. Approximately 20% of patients develop pheochromocytoma and its absence or presence classifies patients as having type 1 or 2, respectively. Other features of the disease include retinal angiomas, hemangioblastomas of the central nervous system, renal cysts and clear cell carcinomas, pancreatic cysts, neuroendocrine pancreatic tumors, tumors of the endolymphatic sac and epididymal cystadenoma. The classification of VHL can be further refined into 2A or 2B, the former unaffected by renal cell carcinoma and the latter affected.

Mean age at diagnosis of pheochromocytoma in patients with VHL is 28 years but children as young as 5 years of age have been affected. Patients are more likely to present with multifocal disease than those with sporadic pheochromocytoma but patients are generally asymptomatic and malignancy is less common.

The VHL gene is located on chromosome position 3p25 and consists of three exons. More than 200 different mutations have been reported, including large deletions, frameshift mutations and insertions which result in truncated proteins, nonsense and missense mutations. Genotype–phenotype studies report that only missense mutations occur in families with pheochromocytoma. Two alternative transcripts result from the presence or absence of exon 2, resulting in two proteins of 213 and 160 amino acids, respectively. The function of these proteins appears to be very similar. Like SDH, the VHL protein has an important role in the regulation of hypoxia-inducible gene expression. Loss of VHL protein function results in upregulation of these genes. The VHL protein has also been implicated in the cell cycle regulation and mRNA stability.

The VHL gene is a tumor repressor gene and genes on both alleles must be inactive before the syndrome manifests. The first mutation is inherited but the second is a somatic event that usually involves partial or complete gene deletion.

Neurofibromatosis

Neurofibromatosis type 1 (NF-1) is the most common inherited disease associated with central nervous system tumors and has an incidence of 1 in 3000. The estimated prevalence of pheochromocytoma is 0.1–5.7%, although autopsy reports place this figure at 3–13%. Examination findings that should alert the physician to the diagnosis include cutaneous, nodular or plexiform neurofibromas, café-au-lait lesions of more than 1.5 cm in diameter, Leisch nodules of the iris, auxiliary freckling and macrocephaly. Other manifestations include intestinal tumors, malignant gliomas and juvenile chronic myeloid leukemia.

The mean age at diagnosis of pheochromocytoma in patients with NF-1 is approximately 40 years, although presentation in childhood has been reported. In a cohort of 148 individuals with NF-1 and pheochromocytoma, 84% of patients had unilateral disease, 9.6% bilateral disease and 6.1% ectopic disease. Eleven percent of patients had malignant disease [17].

The NF-1 gene is located on chromosome 17q11.2. It spans 300 kb of genomic DNA and contains 60 exons which encode neurofibrimin, a protein that has been shown to regulate the Ras and cyclic adenosine monophosphate (cAMP) signaling pathways. Mutational analysis of the gene is difficult because of the gene size, lack of mutational hot spots and high rate of new mutations. For these reasons, extensive mutational analysis of NF-1 in large cohorts of patients has seldom been undertaken and mutations have been described in only about 15% of patients.

Diagnosis

Clinical features

Pheochromocytoma secrete large amounts of catecholamines, including epinephrine, norepinephrine, dopamine and various peptides, and ectopic hormones, including encephalins, somatostatin, calcitonin, oxytocin, vasopressin, insulin and adrenocorticotropic hormones. The clinical manifestations of the disease reflect hormone excess, e.g. headache, sweating, weight loss and diarrhea, or mass effects such as abdominal pain. Hypertension and tachycardia are usual but may be episodic. Blood glucose may be elevated and hypokalemia is common in children.

Biochemical evaluation

The diagnosis of pheochromocytoma has traditionally depended on the demonstration of catecholamine excess by analysis of urinary excretion of catecholamines or their metabolites. Analysis of two 24-h urine collections for catecholamines (norepinephrine, epinephrine and dopamine) and metanephrines (normetanephrine or metanephrine) identifies 95% of patients with a pheochromocytoma.

The differential diagnosis of a retroperitoneal mass in childhood includes neuroblastoma and, if this diagnosis is suspected, urinary vanillylmandelic acid (VMA) and 4-hydroxy-3-methoxymandelic acid (HMMA) should also be measured.

Catecholamine secretion may be intermittent in patients with pheochromocytoma and concentrations may be normal between episodes. A minimum of two negative samples are required to exclude the diagnosis. Elevated concentrations may result from conditions other than pheochromocytoma and some medications, including some antihypertensives, affect catecholamine excretion and may need to be discontinued before investigation.

Analysis of plasma free metanephrines (o-methylated metabolites of catecholamines) circumvents many of these problems and may be a more useful diagnostic test. In adult practice, the sensitivity and specificity of fractionated plasma metanephrines for the diagnosis of pheochromocytoma is reported to be as high as 99% and 89%, respectively, in contrast to plasma catecholamines (85% and 80%) and urinary catecholamines (83% and 88%) [18].

Diagnostic imaging

The localization of pheochromocytoma and paraganglia and assessment for metastatic disease relies on anatomical imaging and assessment of tumor function using radioisotopes.

On CT, pheochromocytoma are seen as rounded or oval lesions of density similar to surrounding tissues. Scattered calcification is seen in approximately 10% of lesions. Most lesions enhance rapidly with contrast medium but the use of ionic contrast media can precipitate a hypertensive crisis. If these media are to be used, the patient should receive α-adrenergic blockade.

MRI provides excellent anatomical detail without the use of ionizing radiation. Rapid scanning techniques enable whole body assessment and avoid the potentially dangerous use of contrast required for CT. The MRI appearances of an extra-adrenal pheochromocytoma are illustrated in Fig. 17.2.

The radionuclide imaging technique of choice is ^{123}I-MIBG scintigraphy, which detects a wide range of neural crest tumors. It is similar in structure and uptake to norepinephrine and uptake is observed normally in the heart, salivary glands, liver, spleen and urinary tract. A number of medications interfere with MIBG uptake, including calcium antagonists and labetalol, which should be withdrawn 48–72 h before imaging. If necessary, hypertension can be treated with phenoxybenzamine and propranolol.

Because of the mechanism of uptake, MIBG is a highly specific investigation but 5–10% of lesions do not take it up. Anatomical resolution is also limited and it may be most appropriately employed in patients in whom biochemical investigations are inconclusive or for the localization of paraganglia not identified on MRI. Appearances of an extra-adrenal pheochromocytoma are shown in Fig. 17.3.

Positron emission tomography (PET) with fluorine-18-labeled dopamine (^{18}F-DOPA) is based on the capacity of neurendocrine tumors to take up, decarboxylate and store amino acids such as dopamine. Normal uptake is observed in the striatum, gallbladder, urinary tract, pancreas and occasionally colon.

This imaging modality has a number of advantages over MIBG and in time may replace it as the radionuclide investigation of first choice. PET scanning enables superior anatomical resolution compared to gamma camera, resulting in better image quality and greater sensitivity for small lesions compared to either MIBG or somatostatin analogs. The low background uptake enables identification of paraganglia and pheochromocytoma with a greater degree of certainty. Finally, interference of ^{18}F-DOPA uptake with medications has not yet been reported.

FDG-PET employs a fluorine-18-labeled glucose analog to identify areas of increased glucose uptake and metabolism.

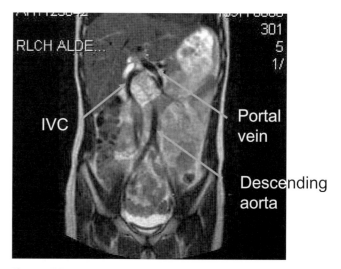

Figure 17.2 Magnetic resonance imaging (MRI) appearances of a left-sided extra-adrenal pheochromocytoma illustrating displacement of the inferior vena cava (IVC), portal vein and descending aorta.

Because most tumors are metabolically active, tumors that do not take up MIBG can generally be visualized using FDG. Specificity is less acceptable because FDG uptake simply reflects intracellular metabolism and the scan cannot differentiate pheochromocytoma or paraganglioma from a number of other tumors.

Management

Preoperative medical management

Once the diagnosis of pheochromocytoma is made, medical therapy should commence with the aim of achieving complete blockade of α-adrenergic receptors and correcting the metabolic consequences of catecholamine excess.

Patients are stabilized with an α-adrenergic antagonist, most commonly phenoxybenzamine, although doxazosin is an acceptable alternative. Successful α-blockade results in postural hypotension due to vasodilatation so it is important to maintain

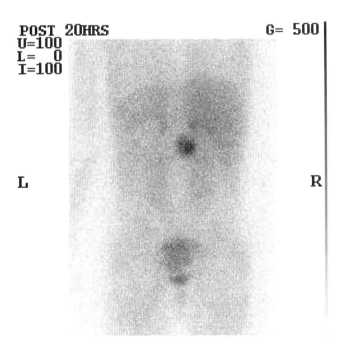

Figure 17.3 MIBG images of a right-sided extra-adrenal pheochromocytoma.

adequate hydration to expand the intravascular space during α-blockade. This can usually be achieved using oral fluids during phenoxybenzamine therapy. Blood hematocrit can be measured at the start of therapy and subsequently to monitor volume expansion and hemodilution.

Blockade of β-adrenergic receptors may be necessary to control symptoms of tachycardia and hypoglycemia using propranolol. It is critical that α-blockade is complete before β-blockade because unopposed stimulation of α-adrenergic receptors can precipitate a hypertensive crisis. Medical therapy should be maintained for a minimum of 4 weeks preoperatively to enable full α-blockade to minimize the risk of profound hypertension during surgery and enable re-expansion of the intravascular compartment to minimize the risk of hypotension during the postoperative period.

If the tumor is located in the left adrenal, consideration should be given to pneumococcal vaccination in case of splenic trauma.

Intra-operative management

Resection of pheochromocytoma should be undertaken by experienced endocrine and pediatric surgeons and anesthetists often working together.

The tumors may be approached either laparoscopically or through an open operation. When the tumor is handled, catecholamine release may precipitate hypertensive episodes. Sodium nitroprusside is a potent arterio-venodilator with a rapid onset and offset of action ideally suited to the management of intra-operative hypertension. After tumor removal or on venous clamping, the anesthetist should be warned of the risk of sudden and profound hypotension. Sodium nitroprusside should be stopped and intravenous fluid expansion with or without pressor agents may be needed to maintain adequate perfusion. The anesthetic charts of a patient undergoing resection of a pheochromocytoma are illustrated in Fig. 17.4.

Postoperative medical management

In the postoperative period, the child should be nursed in an intensive care unit and monitored closely for cardiovascular

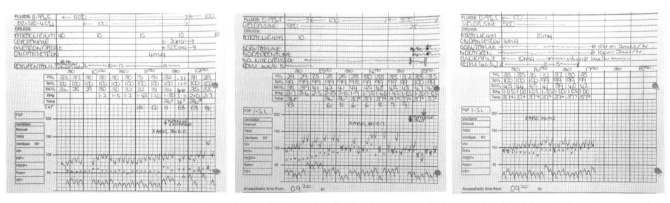

Figure 17.4 Anesthetic charts illustrating hemodynamic changes during resection of a pheochromocytoma. As the tumor is mobilized the patient experiences surges in blood pressure which are controlled with sodium nitroprusside. When the tumor is clamped dobutamine is commenced to maintain blood pressure.

instability. Postoperative hypoglycemia can be profound, especially in the first 24 h because inhibition of pancreatic β-cell secretion is removed resulting in increased insulin secretion while lipolysis and glycogenolysis are inhibited by residual α-blockade.

Management of malignant disease

Malignant pheochromocytoma is rare in children and the evidence base informing the management of these patients is drawn primarily from the adult literature. In adults, 5-year survival is approximately 50%.

Nearly all pheochromocytoma occurring in patients with MEN2, more than 90% of those with VHL and 90% of those with NF-1 appear to be benign. The prevalence of malignancy is much higher in patients with mutations of SDHB.

A number of biochemical, morphological and molecular markers have been investigated as potential markers of malignant disease but none has reliably identified the presence of malignant tissue. The only criterion currently accepted for the diagnosis of malignant disease is the presence of metastatic disease.

Surgery to debulk the tumor is widely regarded as the mainstay of treatment. Reduction of tumor size reduces exposure of target organs to high concentrations of catecholamine and, in those treated with ^{131}I-MIBG, improves the delivery of radiotherapy to residual tumor tissue.

Chemotherapy with cyclophosphamide, vincristine and dacarbazine has induced a complete response in a significant number of patients (14–50%), although in the majority of patients the disease stabilizes or progresses [19].

Radiotherapy with ^{131}I-MIBG was introduced in 1983. Since that time outcome data report tumor responses, which are generally partial, in 24–45% of patients and disease progression after 2 years is common. In the pediatric population, the use of ^{131}I-MIBG in the treatment of neuroblastoma has been associated with myeloid leukemia as a secondary malignancy in 1.7% of patients [20]. Chemotherapy and ^{131}I-MIBG combination therapy has been used with some success; however, the toxicity is considerable and the benefits of combination therapy over either chemotherapy or radiotherapy alone are unclear.

Surveillance and transitional care

All patients with pheochromocytoma require lifelong follow-up because of the risk of contralateral tumors. In addition, approximately 40% of patients who present with a pheochromocytoma in childhood harbor a germline mutation of one of the five genes described in Table 17.2. They and their families are best cared for in a clearly structured multidisciplinary team (MDT). A comprehensive service focused on delivering care to families rather than independent pediatric and adult services delivering services to individuals is more likely to succeed in maintaining patients in surveillance programs from the point of diagnosis in childhood through adolescence and into adult life.

The core MDT should include clinical geneticists, pediatric and adult endocrinologists, endocrine surgeons and specialist endo-

crine nurses. Close collaboration with an extended team of clinical biochemists, radiologists, ophthalmologists and neurosurgeons is necessary to meet the complex needs of these patients.

The primary purpose of the MDT should be to identify and treat tumors associated with these syndromes at an early stage of development thereby minimizing the impact of these syndromes on patients' morbidity, mortality and quality of life. The MDT also has an important role in educating patients of the value of predictive testing for family members at risk of inheriting a germline mutation.

Surveillance programs for the early diagnosis of tumors associated with these conditions have been published [21,22] and these are summarized in Table 17.3.

Thyroid neoplasia

Thyroid cancer is the most common pediatric endocrine malignancy and the third most common pediatric solid tumor, accounting for 1–1.5% of all childhood cancers with an incidence of 0.5 per million per year. Five to ten percent of all thyroid cancers occur in children. Females are more commonly affected than males, the female : male ratio increasing steadily with age from 1.5 : 1 in those aged less than 15 years, to 3 : 1 in those aged 15–20 years to 4 : 1 in the adult population.

Where the diagnosis is confirmed patient management should be undertaken in consultation with a pediatric oncologist, a clinical oncologist or nuclear medicine physician and an experienced thyroid surgeon.

Thyroid neoplasia can be broadly subdivided into those tumors arising from the follicular epithelium and those of non-follicular origin. Well-differentiated thyroid cancers account for 60–90% of childhood thyroid cancers. Histological classification of papillary, follicular or papillary-follicular does not affect treatment, although children with papillary or papillary-follicular tumors are more likely to relapse than those with follicular disease.

Papillary-follicular thyroid carcinoma

Thyroid malignancies in childhood are most commonly well-differentiated papillary or follicular carcinomas that arise from follicular epithelium, although all histological subtypes have been observed.

Papillary carcinomas (75% of malignant tumors in childhood) are irregular, solid or cystic. On histological examination they show a variety of patterns, ranging from properly formed papillary to frond-like structures covered by distinct uniform tumor cells showing occasional mitoses. Both papillary and follicular components are often seen within the same tumor. The most important histological diagnostic criteria of papillary carcinoma are the typical nuclear features of the cells and not the histological pattern or organization of the tumor.

Table 17.3 Recommended surveillance schedule for patients with syndromes associated with hereditary pheochromocytoma.

Syndrome	Tumor	Age to begin (years)	Biochemical tests	Imaging tests
MEN2	Pheochromocytoma	15	Annual plasma metanephrines	Every 3–5 years
	Hyperparathyroidism		Every 3–5 years: Plasma calcium and PTH	MRI or CT adrenals
VHL	Pheochromocytoma	5	Annual plasma metanephrines	Annually: US of the adrenal
				Every 3 years: MRI of the adrenals
	Retinal hemangioblastoma	5		Annually: fluroscein angiography
	CNS hemangioblastoma	10		Every 3 years: MRI brain and spinal cord
	Renal carcinoma	5		Annually: US kidneys
				Every 3 years: MRI kidneys
Paraganglioma syndrome type 1	Pheochromocytoma Paraganglioma	10	Annual plasma metanephrines	Annual MRI of neck, thorax, chest and abdomen
Paraganglioma syndrome type 3	Paraganglioma	10		Annual MRI of neck, thorax, chest and abdomen
Paraganglioma syndrome type 4	Pheochromocytoma Paraganglioma	10	Annual plasma metanephrines	Annual MRI of neck, thorax, chest and abdomen

CNS, central nervous system; CT, computed tomography; MEN2, multiple endocrine neoplasia type 2; MRI, magnetic resonance imaging; PTH, parathyroid hormone; US, ultrasound; VHL, von Hippel–Lindau disease.

Tumor cell nuclei of papillary carcinoma are uniformly round and pale, an appearance described as clear, washed out or ground glass. Within cell nuclei, fine grooves are observed. The presence of psammoma bodies is helpful. The histological appearances of papillary thyroid carcinoma are demonstrated in Plate 17.3. Papillary carcinomas metastasize via the lymphatic route, resulting in multiple tumor deposits in regional or distant lymph nodes.

Follicular carcinoma (18% of thyroid malignancies) are generally encapsulated tumors with highly cellular follicles and microfollicles. Nuclei are of fairly uniform size, usually centrally located, compact in appearance and dark. The distinction between follicular carcinoma and adenoma is often difficult and is not based on cellular and nuclear features of malignancy but depends on identification of tumor cell invasion into the capsule and angioinvasion (into the lumen of a medium-sized vein). Plate 17.4 illustrates the histological appearances of follicular carcinoma with angioinvasion. Unless these features are identified, the tumor should be regarded as benign, regardless of its size and other features. Angioinvasion of follicular carcinoma results in hematogenous spread with frequent and early metastasis into the lungs, brain and bone.

The behavior of both these tumors is more aggressive in childhood than in adult life. Local lymph node metastases are palpable at presentation in 60–80% of patients and distant metastases are found in 10%. Extracapsular extension of the tumor is observed in 30–50% of patients.

There appear to be two common genetic events that trigger malignant transformation of thyroid cells. Mutations of two genes integral to the regulation of the mitogen-activated protein kinase (MAPK) signaling pathway, RET and BRAF, have been reported in adult and pediatric patients. The MAPK signaling pathway is a crucial intracellular cascade that regulates cell growth, differentiation and death in response to growth factors, hormones and cytokines.

Activation of RET occurs following inversion or translocation, known as RET/PTC rearrangement, which breaks the RET gene and results in fusion of its 3′ end to the 5′ end of several unrelated genes. Sixteen different types of RET/PTC have been described, of which RET/PTC1 (fusion of RET with the gene CCDC6) and RET/PTC3 (fusion of RET with the gene NcoA4) occur most commonly. Both these genes are constitutively expressed in thyroid cells. Because the mechanisms by which these genes are activated continue to operate transcription of the fusion gene is also activated. The MAPK cascade is triggered and the expression of proliferation genes is increased. Overexpression of RET by the generation of fusion genes is only the initiating event in the malignant transformation of thyroid cells and much less is understood about subsequent events.

The frequency with which RET/PTC rearrangements are manifest in papillary thyroid carcinoma varies with the populations studied, probably reflecting ethnic diversity and methodological differences between study groups. However, it is now clear that rearrangements of RET/PTC occur much more commonly in young people and children than in older patients and are encountered in 40–70% of sporadic papillary carcinomas described in this population [23]. The highest prevalence of RET/PTC rearrangements is reported in papillary thyroid carcinoma in children exposed to ^{131}I following the Chernobyl disaster and 87% of these patients are found to harbour a RET/PTC rearrangement [24].

The RET/PTC3 rearrangement appears to be associated with a shorter latency period and is reported most commonly in the youngest children while carcinomas associated with RET/PTC1 appear to have a longer latency period and are also reported to occur commonly in patients exposed to external irradiation.

The MAPK signaling cascade can also be activated by mutations in the gene encoding BRAF kinase. Activating mutations in this gene result in constitutive activation of BRAF kinase and therefore of the MAPK signaling cascade. Mutations of BRAF occur much more commonly in adults than in children and are reported in 40–60% of adult patients but only 0–12% of children [25].

Medullary thyroid carcinoma

Medullary thyroid carcinoma (MTC) arises from the parafollicular C cells of the thyroid gland. At least 50% of cases are dominantly inherited as often part of a constellation of endocrine malignancies and tumors of neuroectodermal origin that are collectively described as the multiple endocrine neoplasia (MEN) syndrome type 2 (Plate 17.5). This figure is likely to be higher in children and young people.

Nodular hyperplasia and follicular adenomas

The distinction between hyperplastic non-neoplastic nodules from follicular adenomas (FA) may be difficult. Hyperplastic nodules are polyclonal in origin, whereas FA are monoclonal and therefore true neoplasms. Follicular adenomas are considered to be benign in nature but some subtypes may have malignant potential, e.g. FA of Hürtle cell origin or atypical FA. These lesions should be considered as suspicious if there is:

1 Partial infiltration of the capsule;

2 The presence of abnormal thyrocytes within the capsule or neighboring lymph nodes;

3 The growth of an oxyphilic tumor into the thickened capsule without crossing its border; or

4 The presence of a neoplastic lesion within the capsule.

Tumors demonstrating any of these "borderline" features should be described as "a well-differentiated tumor of uncertain malignant potential" (WDT-UMP) if they demonstrate questionable papillary type nuclear changes, or as a "follicular tumor of uncertain malignant potential" (FT-UMP) if they show questionable capsular penetration without nuclear changes. Tumors that display these characteristics can present in childhood and the long-term prognosis is uncertain. These tumors should be treated as benign by surgery with thyroxine supplementation to maintain thyroid stimulating hormone (TSH) in the normal range, with surveillance for evidence of malignant change [26].

Etiology

Radiation and thyroid cancer

Radiation exposure, either internal or external, is a well-recognized risk factor for the development of thyroid cancer. The risk of developing thyroid cancer is strongly related to the radiation dose. External irradiation is a valuable treatment for a number of childhood conditions including Hodgkin lymphoma and preparation for bone marrow transplantation. Such children are at increased risk of developing thyroid cancer and should remain under lifelong observation with periodic ultrasound examination of the thyroid. The latent period between exposure and the appearance of thyroid cancer may be up to 40 years. Those developing thyroid nodules of more than a few millimetres in size should be thoroughly investigated.

The incidence of thyroid cancer increased up to 100-fold in populations across Eastern Europe exposed to ^{131}I following the Chernobyl disaster in 1987. An increase in the incidence of thyroid cancer, predominantly papillary carcinoma, was observed first in Belarus and the Ukraine. Children living in iodine deficient areas and those aged under 2 years at the time of exposure were particularly vulnerable. There are also a number of reports of thyroid cancer in children who were fetuses at the time of exposure, while the disease was rare in children aged more than 5 years. Those at a greater distance from Chernobyl accumulated lower doses of radioiodine and suffered later. After an initial peak in patients presenting with papillary thyroid carcinoma, a second peak of follicular carcinoma was observed, indicating the longer latency period of this malignancy.

Congenital abnormalities of the thyroid and thyroid cancer

Some causes of congenital hypothyroidism are associated with an increased risk of thyroid nodules and possibly thyroid cancer. Neoplastic transformation is reported in children with dyshormonogenesis or defects of iodine transport in whom thyroxine replacement therapy is inadequate and thyrotropin concentrations are elevated for prolonged periods of time. These lesions are generally benign but malignant lesions most commonly follicular in nature have been reported.

Thyroglossal cysts are the most common developmental abnormality of the thyroid and occur in up to 7% of the normal population. They are most commonly located in the midline between the base of the tongue and the hyoid bone and are usually clinically silent. There is debate regarding the additional risk these lesions represent for the development of thyroid cancer. If there is an additional risk, it appears to be small and thyroid cancer has been reported in association with a thyroglossal cyst in only eight children.

Autoimmune thyroid disease and thyroid cancer

Papillary thyroid cancer has been reported in children with both Graves disease and autoimmune hypothyroidism but the number of cases is small and this association remains controversial.

Diagnosis

Thyroid nodules in children are not common but data pooled from 16 cohort studies of thyroid nodules in childhood reported malignant disease in 299 out of 1134 (26%) nodules [26]. For this reason all should be carefully investigated.

Clinical features

Presentation of thyroid cancer is with a painless mass that is frequently an incidental finding on routine examination or is identified by the child or parent. The appearance of a thyroid tumor at presentation in a 12-year-old boy is illustrated in Plate 17.6.

Characteristics that are associated with malignant disease include firm texture, rapid growth, tethering to adjacent tissues, cervical lymphadenopathy and lack of movement on swallowing. Many malignant tumors do not demonstrate these characteristics and the classic features of adult thyroid malignancy (pain, tenderness, upper airway obstruction, vocal cord paralysis and difficulty swallowing) are rarely present in children. Size is not predictive of malignancy, although most malignant tumors are more than 1.5 cm in diameter but the rate of tumor growth is more closely related to risk of malignancy.

Eighty to ninety percent of patients are euthyroid at presentation and the clinical state (euthyroid, hypothyroid or thyrotoxic) is not predictive of malignancy.

Biochemical evaluation

Thyroid hormones should be measured in all children at presentation. The presence of hypothyroidism or thyrotoxicosis does not inform the differential diagnosis but abnormalities of thyroid hormones should be corrected preoperatively. Serum thyroglobulin (Tg) is a glycoprotein that is synthesized only by normal or neoplastic thyroid follicular cells. Elevated concentrations are highly suggestive of malignancy. Measurement of Tg is also of value in the long-term surveillance of patients treated with total thyroidectomy and radioiodine remnant ablation. Concentrations may be falsely elevated in the presence of heterophile or anti-Tg antibodies.

Calcitonin is secreted in excessive amounts in MTC and can be used as a marker of disease activity, although basal concentrations may be normal at early stages of tumor development. Some tumors also secrete chorionic embryonic antigen (CEA), although this may become undetectable in advanced disease.

Diagnostic imaging

Thyroid ultrasound is the examination of first choice for assessment of thyroid nodules. Although ultrasound is not sufficiently sensitive or specific for the diagnosis of thyroid malignancy for it to be considered a diagnostic test, it does have a place in the selection of patients requiring more detailed investigation.

Ultrasound examination allows assessment of the number of follicles, their size and location and ultrasound appearances may also contribute significantly to the differential diagnosis of benign versus malignant disease, although this is an area of some controversy. Appearances suggestive of the presence of malignancy are outlined in Table 17.4. Multiple, solid isoechogenic or hypoechogenic lesions and those with a peripheral halo are likely to be benign. Lesions with a thick or irregular halo are more likely to be malignant. The use of color Doppler can lend further information, and high intranodular blood flow in the presence of a

Table 17.4 Ultrasound appearances of a thyroid nodule suggestive of malignancy.

Solitary solid lesion
Hypoechogenic
Subcapsular localization
Irregular margins
Invasive growth
Heterogeneous appearances
Multifocal lesions within an otherwise solitary module
Microcalcification
High intranodular flow on Doppler with normal TSH
Suspicious regional lymph nodes

TSH, thyroid stimulating hormone.

normal TSH is suggestive of malignant disease. MRI gives further anatomical detail to aid surgical planning in the child with extensive local disease.

Thyroid scintigraphy gives information on iodine uptake. It is of limited value in the further assessment of thyroid nodules. Most lesions show reduced uptake, while hyperfunctioning or "hot" nodules are occasionally malignant. Scintigraphy is relatively insensitive, failing to identify up to 20% of nodules visualized on ultrasound. Thus, the appearance of a thyroid nodule on scintigraphy does not inform the differential diagnosis nor aid the selection of patients for thyroidectomy: its use should be restricted to the assessment of the thyrotoxic patient with thyroid nodules. By contrast, whole body scanning may be useful in the identification of metastatic disease, especially of the lungs, which may not be easily visualized on X-ray or CT.

Fine needle aspiration

Fine needle aspiration (FNA) is being used increasingly in children and adolescents for preoperative diagnosis and selection of patients for thyroidectomy. The diagnostic accuracy of FNA in childhood varies from 77 to 90.4% and sensitivity and specificity 89–100% and 63–83%, respectively [26]. Success requires experienced aspirationists and histopathologists in specialized centers.

The procedure is well-tolerated in children with the use of transdermal and infiltrative local anesthesia. Recognized complications include papillary endothelial cell hyperplasia, hemorrhage, vascular proliferation, vascular thrombosis, fibrosis, cystic change, infarction and abscess formation.

Selection of patients for FNA should be based on clinical features and ultrasound appearances. Children too young to cooperate with FNA should undergo excisional biopsy under general anesthetic.

Thyroid hormone concentrations should be measured before FNA because high concentrations of serum TSH induce morphological changes in epithelial follicular cells which may lead to a false diagnosis of papillary thyroid carcinoma. If serum TSH were elevated in a patient with a multinodular goiter, thyroxine should be started and follow-up with reassessment of thyroid hormone concentrations should be arranged 4–6 weeks later. Ultrasound should be repeated after 3 months and only if TSH is in the normal range and concern persists regarding the nature of the thyroid mass should the patient proceed to FNA.

Molecular analysis of FNA biopsies

The diagnostic accuracy of FNA may be improved by the use of reverse transcriptase polymerase chain reaction (RT-PCR) to identify genetic markers of malignancy. A number of markers have been identified, including telomerase, Hector Battifora mesothelial cell (HBME-1), galectin -3, CD44v6 and cytokeratin-19. None of these alone is sufficiently specific for diagnostic purposes (e.g. galectin-3 is expressed in both benign multinodular goiter and Hashimoto thyroiditis). The expression of genes in tandom (e.g. HBME-1 and galectin-3) significantly increases the specificity of testing. Expression of the gene encoding calcitonin is supportive of a diagnosis of MTC. Up to 60% of children with papillary thyroid carcinoma harbor a RET/PTC rearrangement and BRAF gene mutations may be identified in a further 10% of patients.

The use of microarrays has enabled the identification of thousands of genes expressed in papillary thyroid carcinoma that are not expressed in normal thyroid tissue, many of which are related to an immune response. These gene patterns are not yet of routine diagnostic value but they offer the prospect of accurate and rapid molecular diagnosis in the future.

Staging and prognosis

The American Joint Committee on Cancer (AJCC) TNM staging system for thyroid carcinoma is given in Table 17.5. Clinical features that adversely affect prognosis include male gender, age less than 10 years, large tumor size, extrathyroidal expansion, palpable lymph nodes and distant metastases [27].

The progression-free survival for children with differentiated thyroid cancer is 76–80% at 5 years, 61–83% at 10 years and 46–66% at 20 years. Despite this the long-term survival of differentiated thyroid cancer diagnosed in childhood is excellent: 99.5–100% at 5 years, 90–100% at 10 years and 90–99% at 20 years, indicating effective salvage of relapsed patients [27].

Management
Surgery

The majority of children with thyroid cancer present with extrathyroidal invasion of tumor tissue or cervical lymph node spread which is a significant negative predictor of progression-free survival. Children have a high risk of local tumor recurrence, either in the thyroid bed or in cervical lymph nodes. In light of these observations, excision of as much tumor tissue as possible is logical and the operations of choice are total or near-total thyroidectomy and cervical lymph node dissection. Multivariate analysis has demonstrated that radical surgery is the strongest predictor of event-free survival in childhood [28]. Radical surgery is associated with an increased risk of permanent hypoparathyroidism, recurrent laryngeal paralysis and Horner syndrome compared to hemithyroidectomy; a surgical team skilled in

Table 17.5 Tumor Node Metastases (TNM) staging system for thyroid cancer according to the American Joint Committee on Cancer.

Primary tumor

pT0	No evidence of primary tumor
pT1	Intrathyroidal tumor <1 cm in greatest dimension
pT2	Intrathyroidal tumor 1–4 cm in greatest dimension
pT3	Intrathyroidal tumor >4 cm in greatest dimension and limited to the thyroid
pT4	Tumor of any size extending beyond the thyroid capsule
pTX	Tumor cannot be assessed

Regional lymph nodes (cervical and upper mediastinal)

NX	Regional nodes cannot be assessed
N0	No lymph node metastasis
N1	Regional lymph node metastasis
N1a	Metastasis in ipsilateral cervical nodes
N1b	Metastasis in bilateral, midline or contralateral cervical or superior mediastinal nodes

Distant metastasis

MX	Distant metastases cannot be assessed
M0	No distant metastases
M1	Distant metastases

Stage grouping

Papillary or follicular

Stage I	Any T, any N, M0
Stage II	Any T, any N, M1

Medullary

Stage I	T1, N0, M0
Stage II	T2, N0, M0
	T3, N0, M0
	T4, N0, M0
Stage III	Any T, N1, M0
Stage IV	Any T, any N, M1

thyroid cancer surgery is mandatory, and collaboration with surgeons with adult thyroid patients maybe necessary.

Radioiodine remnant ablation

All patients should undergo radioiodine remnant ablation (RRA) 4–6 weeks after thyroidectomy with the aim of destroying any residual normal thyroid and microscopic tumor deposits. Ablation of all thyroid tissue facilitates interpretation of whole body scintigraphy and serum Tg concentrations as markers of tumor recurrence and metastatic disease. Pregnancy should be excluded in adolescent girls before administration of ^{131}I and avoided for at least 6 and preferably 12 months following treatment. Cryopreservation of sperm should be considered in peripubertal and adolescent boys.

The use of RRA has been associated with a reduction in relapse and disease-related mortality in a large cohort of 1510 adults and children with tumors of more than 1.5 cm at presentation with no distant metastases [29]. A smaller study of 60 children and adolescents in whom the dose of ^{131}I was modified according to the presence of distant metastases reported a reduction in regional relapse of from 42% to 6.3% in those treated with RRA compared with those untreated [30].

Exposure to iodine should be limited before RRA to facilitate uptake of [131]I. Iodinated radiographic contrasts and antiseptics should be avoided for 12 weeks before RRA and foods high in iodine (sea salt, seafood and vitamin preparations containing iodine) for 2 weeks.

In the postoperative period, tri-iodothyronine should be used for replacement. This should be stopped 2 weeks before RRA to enable TSH to rise to above 30 mU/L. Immediately before RRA, an uptake scan using 2 mCi ^{123}I is recommended to visualize the size of the local remnant, assess local invasion and calculate absolute uptake value of radioactive iodine.

There is some evidence that the dose of ^{131}I should be stratified according to risk [27]. Patients who are aged less than 10 years with tumors more than 1.5 cm in size, capsular invasion, residual disease or lymph node involvement are at high risk and should be treated with a 100 miC dose. Lower risk patients should receive a dose modified for body surface area of 100 miC/1.73 m^2.

Thyroid hormone replacement therapy

Thyroxine replacement should start 3 days following ^{131}I administration. Most differentiated thyroid carcinomas express TSH receptors and the growth of follicular cells is dependent on TSH stimulation. It is anticipated that suppression of serum TSH using supraphysiological doses of thyroxine will minimize the risk of TSH stimulated tumor regrowth and a reduction in disease recurrence has been reported in children with thyroid cancer treated in this way [31]. The aim of thyroid hormone replacement therapy should be to maintain the child in a clinically euthyroid state with serum T4 and T3 in the near normal range, while suppressing TSH to <0.1 μU/mL in most cases and to undetectable concentrations in children with extensive disease.

Management of recurrent disease

Recurrence is diagnosed when there are clinical features of disease such as a palpable mass or bone pain, when a biopsy sample is positive in a patient considered disease-free for more than 6 months, if stimulated Tg is greater than 10 ng/mL (10 μg/L) or stimulated Tg is greater than 2 ng/mL (2 μg/L) and there is a trend of rising Tg or if there is ^{131}I uptake in an area that previously showed no uptake. Persistent disease is defined as positive ^{131}I uptake persisting more than 6 months after treatment or Tg greater than 10 ng/mL (10 μg/L) persisting for more than 2 years after therapy [27].

Surgical excision is the treatment of choice for palpable lesions and bulky lesions affecting bone and some mediastinal lesions. If lesions are not amenable to surgery, ^{131}I in a dose of 100–270 mCi should be administered 6-monthly.

Dosing regimens are complicated in children. Tumor burden is often higher in children than in adults but ^{131}I uptake is greater and radioactive iodine treatment maybe more effective at a similar dose. Repeated dosing may be required and excessive doses should be avoided to minimize the risk of the complications of chronic radioiodine, pulmonary fibrosis, lymphadenitis pulmonis, chronic sialadenitis, bone marrow suppression, leukemia and ovarian damage.

Surveillance and transitional care

Surveillance should enable identification and treatment of tumor recurrence as well as identification and management the complications of supraphysiological doses of thyroxine. Clinical examination for thyroid masses and cervical lymphadenopathy is supported by the use of serum Tg, neck ultrasound and [131/123]I diagnostic whole body scan (DWBS). No single investigation is sufficiently sensitive for the identification of recurrent disease.

The sensitivity of serum Tg and DWBS can be improved by TSH stimulation and the avoidance of iodine-rich foods. TSH stimulation can be achieved in two ways: either by withdrawal of thyroxine or by administration of recombinant human TSH (rhTSH). The latter avoids the unpleasant symptoms of hypothyroidism.

TSH stimulation by the induction of hypothyroidism has traditionally been achieved by the substitution of T4 with T3 5 weeks before DWBS followed by the withdrawal of T3 2 weeks before scanning, but withdrawal of T4 2–3 weeks prior to DWBS is equally effective with improved quality of life [32]. Using this regime, a dose of 2–5 mCi ^{131}I should be used for DWBS.

A recommended protocol for the use of rhTSH includes withdrawal of T4 on day 1, subcutaneous administration of rhTSH days 2 and 3, radioactive iodine dose on day 4 and DWBS on day 6. A higher dose of 4 mCi ^{131}I is used for DWBS in using this regimen than in hypothyroid patients, allowing for the reduced renal clearance of iodine in the hypothyroid state. Serum Tg concentrations should be measured on day 3.

Using either regimen, a stimulated Tg greater than 10 ng/ml (10 μg/L) should be considered indicative of residual or recurrent disease [27].

Neck ultrasound is valuable for the identification of recurrent disease and may be more sensitive than either stimulated Tg or DWBS for the identification of positive lymph nodes. The appearance of lesions of more than 4 mm in diameter, rounded in shape and/or containing areas of microcalcification or cystic components should be considered suspicious. A hypervascular appearance on color Doppler is also suggestive of malignant disease.

Patients are at lifelong risk of recurrence but it usually occurs in the first 10 years following surgery with a range of 8 months to 44 years. Lifelong surveillance for recurrence, relapse and the complications of prolonged exposure to supraphysiological doses of thyroxine is indicated in all patients. Close collaboration with thyroid surgeons and nuclear medicine physicians at the point of diagnosis should facilitate communication and transition into the adult services. Specialists from both services deliver thyroid cancer services and the direction of referral will reflect local practice. Whatever the favored route of referral, optimal care requires careful planning, excellent communication between clinicians and patients and, wherever possible, a period of joint consultation during adolescence.

Multiple endocrine neoplasia syndromes

The multiple endocrine neoplasia (MEN) syndromes 1 and 2 are dominantly inherited cancer syndromes that may present in childhood. Neoplasms that develop in the context of these inherited cancer syndromes are characterized by a preneoplastic phase of benign glandular hyperplasia, presentation at an earlier age than sporadic disease and a high prevalence of multifocal disease affecting a number of different organs. Identification of the genetic causes of the MEN syndromes has enabled the diagnosis of asymptomatic carriers, informing the selection and timing of prophylactic surgery in patients with MEN2 and early diagnosis and treatment of clinically silent tumors in patients with MEN1 and MEN2. In order to improve the prognosis for carriers of MEN gene mutations, the target organ must be expendable or its function must be amenable to replacement therapy and its removal must pose minimal risk for the patient.

Medullary thyroid carcinoma associated with MEN2 meets these criteria and early thyroidectomy has improved morbidity and mortality [33]. The benefit of early diagnosis and surveillance of asymptomatic carriers of MEN1 gene mutations is less certain.

Families affected by MEN1 or MEN2 require the expertise of a multidisciplinary team, including adult and pediatric endocrinologists, pediatric and adult endocrine surgeons and clinical geneticists. Such a team should enable seamless transition of the affected child from pediatric to adult services.

The identification of a potentially lethal genetic disease is associated with considerable stress, anxiety and guilt, particularly in the parents of an affected child. The support of clinical psychology may be invaluable in supporting these families through many years of disease surveillance and intervention.

Multiple endocrine neoplasia Type 1

MEN1 is a dominantly inherited condition affecting 1–10 per 100 000 individuals. More than 20 benign and malignant endocrine and non-endocrine tumors are recognized (Table 17.6) but parathyroid adenomas, pituitary and enteropancreatic tumors are most common. The age-related penetrance for MEN1 is near zero below the age of 5 years, 50% by 20 years and above 95% at 40 years of age.

Genetic testing

Mutations in the MEN1 gene are identified in 80–90% of clinically diagnosed patients. The gene is located on chromosome 11q13 and consists of 10 exons. It encodes a 610 amino acid protein known as menin. Genetic linkage studies suggest that all familial MEN1 traits arise from the same chromosomal locus and therefore the same gene. Failure to identify a mutation in 10–20% of cases is likely to occur when mutations are located in regions of the gene not routinely studied or in the presence of large gene deletions that are not detected by routine PCR amplification methods.

Table 17.6 Endocrine and non-endocrine manifestations of multiple endocrine neoplasia type 1 (MEN1).

Endocrine features	Non-endocrine features
Parathyroid adenoma	Lipomas
Enteropancreatic tumor	Facial angiomas
Gastrinoma	Collagenomas
Insulinomas	
VIPoma	
Somatostatinoma	
Non-functioning	
Foregut carcinoid	
Thymic carcinoid	
Bronchial carcinoid	
Gastric enterochromaffin-like tumor	
Anterior pituitary	
Prolactinoma	
GH + prolactinoma	
GH	
Non-functioning	
ACTH	
TSH	
Adrenal cortex, non-functioning	
Pheochromocytoma	

ACTH, adrenocorticotropic hormone; GH, growth hormone; TSH, thyroid stimulating hormone.

Mutations of the MEN1 gene are scattered in and around the open reading frame and most commonly result in truncation of the menin protein. Nonsense mutations are reported in 25% of patients, 45% have small deletions, 15% small insertions, 10% missense mutations and fewer than 5% donor-splice mutations. At present there appears to be no correlation between specific mutations, the type of tumor, behavior of specific tumors or clinical presentation (age and tumor site). The phenotypic presentation of an MEN1 mutation may vary significantly between and within families.

The MEN1 gene is a tumor suppressor that is recessive at the tumor level, i.e. both alleles must be inactivated for neoplastic clonal expansion, but a heterozygous germline mutation combined with the frequent occurrence of somatic mutations leads to a dominant pattern of inheritance. Somatic mutations frequently result in the loss of large regions of the gene and whole gene deletion is not uncommon. This phenomenon is described as loss of heterozygosity. Biallelic inactivation is observed in approximately one-quarter of sporadic MEN1 type tumors when both MEN1 alleles are inactivated within the same somatic cell line.

Menin is located in the cell nucleus where it interacts with a number of transcription factors, such as JunD, to inhibit JunD activated cell proliferation. Menin also has a role in the inhibition of transforming growth factor B mediated cell growth and inhibition of SMAD3 activity by inhibition of SMAD3/DNA binding at specific transcriptional regulatory sites.

Whether to test potential MEN1 carriers during childhood is debatable. Presentation in early childhood is extremely rare and a positive test in childhood will not lead to a major therapeutic intervention. It will, however, deny the patient an independent choice about genetic testing.

Current recommendations for starting surveillance for MEN1-related tumors reflect the youngest age at which MEN1-related tumors have been reported and surveillance therefore starts in early childhood. The issue of whether or not surveillance programs should be based upon single case reports of young patients is also a matter of some debate because these data give little insight into an individual's risk of developing a tumor during childhood.

Major endocrine tumors of MEN1

Parathyroid hyperplasia

Hyperparathyroidism occurs in nearly all patients by the age of 50 years, the typical age of the onset of symptoms being 20–25 years, approximately 30 years earlier than sporadic hyperparathyroidism. Longitudinal studies of asymptomatic carriers of MEN1 gene mutations indicate that serum calcium starts to rise sharply from the age of 10 years and the bone mineral density of women with MEN1 and hyperparathyroidism is significantly reduced by the age of 35 years, probably indicating long-standing disease.

Hyperparathyroidism is associated not only with impaired bone mineral density but also with nephrocalcinosis, nephrolithiasis and hypertension. Treatment is by total parathyroidectomy with autograft of a small remnant in the forearm or near-total parathyroidectomy, in which a small (approximately 50 mg) volume of parathyroid tissue is left *in situ* and tagged to enable easy identification. Ninety to 95% of patients should be euparathyroid postoperatively and 5–10% hypoparathyroid but the residual parathyroid tissue has a slow progression to hyperparathyroidism and further surgery is necessary 8–12 years after apparent cure in 50% of patients.

Entero-pancreatic islet tumors

Entero-pancreatic islet cell tumors occur in 30–75% of patients and are found in 80% at postmortem. The onset of symptoms occurs most commonly from the age of 40 years. Insulinomas have been reported in children as young as 13 years of age and biochemical screening of asymptomatic carriers of a MEN1 gene mutation has identified affected patients as young as 15 years of age.

Lesions are generally multifocal and vary from microadenomas to macroadenomas to invasive and metastatic disease. The majority of gastrinomas are found in the duodenum, while pancreatic lesions are found to contain chromogranin A and B, pancreatic polypeptide, glucagon, insulin, proinsulin, somatostatin, gastrin, vasoactive intestinal polypeptide (VIP), serotonin, calcitonin, growth hormone releasing hormone (GHRH) and neurotensin. Malignant disease is rare before the age of 30 years but by middle age approximately 50% of patients are affected and metastatic malignant disease is the leading cause of MEN1-related death.

Approximately 40% of patients develop gastrinomas. Lesions are frequently multiple and metastatic spread is present in 50% of patients at diagnosis. For these reasons surgery is seldom curative. The presence of a primary lesion located in the pancreas, metastatic disease and ectopic Cushing syndrome are features associated with a poor prognosis. Prognosis is also related to the concentration of serum gastrin at diagnosis.

The role and timing of surgery in the management of gastrinomas is controversial. Because the primary aim is to prevent cancer, some advocate surgical intervention as soon as the biochemical diagnosis is unequivocal. Others recommend surgery in patients with tumors of more than 1 cm in diameter and a more conservative approach, operating only on patients with tumors of more than 3 cm in diameter, is also advocated. A large case series reporting patients with sporadic and MEN1-related gastrinoma of 3 cm or more in size reported cure rates of 16% and 5 years following surgery only 6% of patients remained free of disease [34]. Whether outcomes are significantly improved by earlier intervention is uncertain.

With the exception of insulinomas, hormone excess from MEN1-related entero-pancreatic islet cell tumors can be well controlled medically. Proton pump inhibitors control symptoms relating to gastrinomas, and somatostatin analogs effectively treat symptoms relating to oversecretion of other hormones.

Pituitary tumors

Up to 25% of patients with sporadic disease present first with an anterior pituitary tumor, usually a microadenoma. For patients with familial disease diagnosed prospectively, this figure is 10%. The reported prevalence of pituitary tumors ranges from 10% to 60%. Pituitary tumors of all types occur, with the exception of gonadotropinomas. Prolactinomas are most common in all age groups and can be effectively treated with dopamine antagonists, such as bromocriptine or cabergoline. Large prolactinomas sometimes require trans-sphenoidal resection to relieve compression of adjacent structures. The youngest reported case to date is of a 5-year-old who presented with rapid growth, acromegalic features and hyperprolactinemia. Immunohistochemical examination of the tumor cells was positive for both growth hormone and prolactin [35].

Other expressions of MEN1

Adrenal cortical lesions are often observed on imaging. Adenomas, diffuse hyperplasia, nodular hyperplasia and malignancy have all been described in adults. Carcinoid tumors arise in 10% of adult patients and show a predilection for the thymus in males and the bronchi in females. The foregut may also be affected.

Multiple endocrine neoplasia Type 2

Multiple endocrine neoplasia type 2 (MEN2) is a dominantly inherited condition that affects tissues of neuroectodermal origin. Approximately 1 in 50 000 people are affected. Three clinically distinct forms are recognized: MEN2A, MEN2B and familial medullary thyroid carcinoma (MTC). MTC is a common feature of all three MEN2 subtypes. Pheochromocytoma is observed in patients with MEN2A and MEN2B and hyperparathyroidism occurs in association with MEN2A. Historically patients succumbed to undiagnosed pheochromocytoma and progressive MTC. The introduction of predictive gene testing, enabling prophylactic thyroidectomy and early diagnosis of pheochromocytoma, has reduced the mortality from hereditary MTC from 15–20% [36] to less than 5% [33] and deaths from pheochromocytoma have been virtually eliminated.

Genetic testing

MEN2 is caused by mutations of the RET proto-oncogene, a 21 exon gene which encodes for a transmembrane tyrosine kinase receptor. The gene is located on chromosome 10q11.2. Activating mutations of RET result in a constitutively active receptor in patients with MEN2. Mutations affecting the extracellular domain induce homodimerization of the receptor and those in the intracellular domain induce RET kinase enzymatic activity. Mutations of RET are found in more than 98% of patients with MEN2. Rearrangements of RET are found in papillary thyroid carcinoma and inactivating mutations in Hirschsprung disease.

Mutations in exons 10 and 11, which encode the extracellular domain of the receptor, occur most commonly in patients with MEN2A. Mutations of exons 13 and 14, which encode the intracellular tyrosine kinase 1 domain, occur less frequently. Ninety five percent of patients with MEN2B harbor mutations in codon 918 located in exon 16, which encodes the intracellular tyrosine kinase 2 domain. Mutations in codon 883 of exon 15, which also encodes the intracellular tyrosine kinase 2 domain, are found in 2–3% of patients with MEN2B. A cartoon of the RET proto-oncogene illustrating mutation sites and related phenotype is given in Fig. 17.5.

A strong genotype–phenotype relationship exists for mutations of MEN2 which has enabled stratification of risk according to genotype. The recommendations of the International Working Party on Multiple Endocrine Neoplasia on risk allocation are outlined in Table 17.7 [21].

Total thyroidectomy should be performed within the first 6 months of life in those classified as having level 3 disease. Those with level 2 disease should proceed to total thyroidectomy before the age of 5 years. The management of those in level 1 is debated. Some authors favor prophylactic thyroidectomy by the age of 5 years, others by the age of 10 years, while others propose a periodic pentagastrin stimulation test and total thyroidectomy at the first abnormal result.

MEN2A

Ninety to 95% of patients with MEN2 have MEN2A. Almost all affected patients develop MTC. Hyperparathyroidism develops as a result of multigland parathyroid hyperplasia in 20–30% of patients with MEN2A. Patients with mutations in codon 634 are most susceptible, while those with mutations affecting codons 768 and 891 and those with the V804M mutation are rarely affected. Mutations in codons 609, 611, 618, 620, 790 and 791 confer an intermediate risk. Hyperparathyoidism in patients with

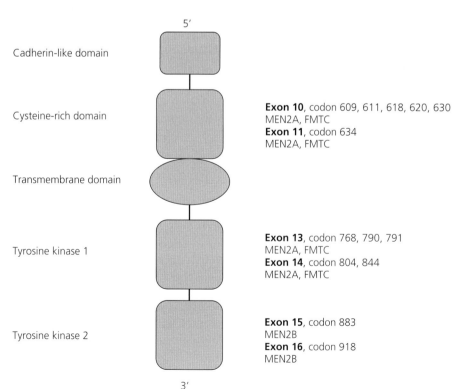

5′

Cadherin-like domain

Cysteine-rich domain

Exon 10, codon 609, 611, 618, 620, 630
MEN2A, FMTC
Exon 11, codon 634
MEN2A, FMTC

Transmembrane domain

Tyrosine kinase 1

Exon 13, codon 768, 790, 791
MEN2A, FMTC
Exon 14, codon 804, 844
MEN2A, FMTC

Tyrosine kinase 2

Exon 15, codon 883
MEN2B
Exon 16, codon 918
MEN2B

3′

Figure 17.5 Cartoon of the RET proto-oncogene illustrating the location of mutations associated with the MEN2 syndrome.

Table 17.7 Stratification of risk for medullary thyroid carcinoma (MTC) and primary treatment of patients with mutations of RET proto-oncogene.

RET germline mutations	Risk of MCT	Primary treatment
883, 918, 922	Level 3 The highest risk of MTC	Total thyroidectomy + bilateral central neck dissection within the first 6 months (preferably first month) of life or at diagnosis
611, 618, 620, 634	Level 2 A high risk of MTC	Total thyroidectomy by age 5 years or when mutation identified
609, 768, 790, 791, 804, 891	Level 1 The least high risk of MTC	Total thyroidectomy by age 10 years or when mutation identified

MEN2A is a less aggressive disease than in MEN1, with an indolent course that seldom requires treatment in childhood.

Pheochromocytoma is reported in patients with mutations of RET affecting all codons identified in patients with MEN2 to date, other than 609, 768, 891 and the V804M mutation. Mutations in the codon 634 are associated with an early onset of disease and pheochromocytoma has been reported in children as young as 5 years of age. More than 50% of patients are affected.

Associated pathologies include paraneoplastic syndromes such as lichen amyloidosis of the skin. Some patients present during early childhood with the clinical features of Hirschprung disease. In contrast to MEN2, Hirschprung disease is usually associated with inactivating mutations of RET which result in complete loss of receptor function. The mechanism by which Hirschprung disease develops in children with MEN2A is not known.

MEN2B

MEN2B is the most aggressive from of MEN2. It is characterized by an earlier age at onset of disease and a number of developmental abnormalities including a marfanoid body habitus, mucosal neuromas, ganglioneuromatosis of the intestinal tract and myelinated corneal nerves. MTC develops very early in MEN2B, often during infancy, and behaves in an aggressive manner. Pheochromocytoma occurs in 40–50% of patients.

There is an age-related pattern of non-endocrine manifestations, including lip and mucosal neuromas, corneal fibres, conjunctivitis sicca and conjunctival neuromas. Joint hypermobility and muscle weakness may be present in childhood and scoliosis and hip epiphysiolysis occur in later life.

Like MEN2A, MEN2B can present with gastrointestinal symptoms which result from colonic dysfunction caused by ganglioneuromatosis. Constipation may be severe in childhood and surgical intervention is required in up to one-quarter of patients to relieve symptoms of intestinal obstruction. In adult life diarrhea is reported more commonly.

Medullary thyroid carcinoma

Medullary thyroid carcinoma occurs in all patients with MEN2. It derives from the parafollicular c cells that are part of the amine precursor uptake and decarboxylase system (APUD) and a spectrum of c cell abnormality is observed. Early disease is indicated by the presence of c cell hyperplasia that develops into intrathyroidal MTC. Regional and distant metastases occur as the disease progresses.

Diagnosis
Clinical features

MTC presents as a painless thyroid mass with or without cervical lymphadenopathy.

Biochemical evaluation

Calcitonin is secreted only by c cells and elevated serum calcitonin is a highly specific tumor marker. Calcitonin concentrations in excess of 100 pg/mL (10 ng/L) can be considered diagnostic of MTC and a direct relationship exists between serum calcitonin and tumor size and prognosis. Patients in whom serum calcitonin is 20–100 pg/mL (20–100 ng/L) should undergo stimulation testing with pentagastrin to clarify the diagnosis. It is important to note that calcitonin concentrations may be normal or low in the presence of poorly differentiated MTC. In these patients carcinoembryonic antigen (CEA) concentrations are often high and both markers should be measured preoperatively.

Diagnostic imaging

Ultrasound examination of the thyroid is the most commonly used investigation to identify the presence and extent of local disease. In older patients, FNA will give a histological diagnosis, although this is seldom necessary in patients with a RET gene mutation or a positive family history. More detailed anatomical information can be obtained by CT or MRI to inform surgical planning.

Metastatic disease affecting the neck and chest is most readily identified by technetium-99-m-sestamibi scans and distant metastases are more easily visualized on MRI or CT. ^{131}I-anti-CEA monoclonal antibodies have been successfully used for the identification of occult disease.

Tumor staging

The AJCC staging system for thyroid cancer is given in Table 17.5.

Management

It is essential that pheochromocytoma is excluded preoperatively in those with MEN2A or MEN2B.

Surgery

Total thyroidectomy with lymphadenectomy of the cervicocentral compartment offers the only prospect of cure in those with MTC and success is mainly dependent on the adequacy of the initial operation [36]. Ipsilateral modified radical lymph node dissection should be undertaken if the primary tumor is more than 1 cm in diameter in those with MEN2A or more than 0.5 cm in diameter in those with MEN2B and for those with central node metastases. More advanced disease requires a more extensive operation which may involve resection of involved neck structures. Patients undergoing prophylactic thyroidectomy do not require central node dissection if preoperative basal and stimulated calcitonin are normal and there are no areas of abnormality on ultrasound examination of the thyroid.

Patients in whom hyperparathroidism is diagnosed preoperatively should undergo parathyroidectomy at the time of thyroid exploration.

Postoperative medical care

Hypocalcemia occurs commonly following total thyroidectomy with lymph node dissection. Serum calcium should be measured 4 h postoperatively and 12-hourly thereafter. Slow intravenous infusions of calcium or oral calcium with vitamin D supplementation may be required. All patients require physiological thyroxine replacement.

The prognosis of patients with MTC is influenced by stage of disease at diagnosis and fall in calcitonin during the postoperative period. Serum calcitonin and CEA should be measured 3–7 days following surgery and 2–3 months later. Patients in whom calcitonin and CEA concentrations return to normal can be monitored by periodic measurements of serum markers and imaging examinations. Persistent elevation of calcitonin following surgery is indicative of recurrent, persistent or generalized disease.

Management of persistent or recurrent disease

Patients with recurrent disease can experience a good quality of life but diarrhea can be debilitating and bone metastases can give rise to pain. Distant metastases, which occur in patients with large tumors at diagnosis and those with extrathyroidal growth and lymph node involvement, are the main cause of death. Distant metastases often affect multiple organs, including the lungs, bones and liver and, more rarely, brain, skin and breast. Survival rates of approximately 25% 5 years following the identification of distant metastases and 10% at 10 years are reported [37].

If calcitonin concentrations remain elevated in the postoperative period or rise during surveillance it is important to define the location and extent of tumor tissue. Reoperation is indicated if residual disease is identified in the neck or upper mediastinum and there is no evidence of distant metastatic disease. Cure is possible at reoperation if lymph nodes in all compartments of the neck and upper mediastinum are dissected.

The only place for surgery in patients with distant metastases is to palliate symptoms related to tumor mass and to relieve the symptoms of diarrhea which results from the humoral factors produced by MTC.

Standard chemotherapy regimes have not been successful in the treatment of MTC and the tumors are not very sensitive to X-ray or thermal radiation therapy. Imatinib, a tyrosine kinase inhibitor, was thought to be an attractive agent for the treatment of metastatic MTC. Early clinical trials showed promising results but observation over 12 months found no evidence of objective response. Furthermore, mucosal swelling of the larynx during therapy required emergency tracheotomy in some patients [38].

The role of radiotherapy using radioiodine-labeled bispecific antibodies directed to CEA and diethylenetriamine penta-acetic acid monoclonal antibodies is under investigation. Early clinical trials indicate that the overall survival of patients with extensive disease is significantly improved with this therapy while toxic effects appear to be tolerable [39]. In the assessment of new therapies it is important to note that patients can survive long-term and symptom-free even with substantial tumor burdens.

Surveillance and transitional care of patients with MEN

The standards of care for patients and families with MEN1 and MEN2 are very similar to those for families with inherited endocrine neoplasia. Services should be designed to meet the needs of families rather than individuals to facilitate seamless transition from pediatric to adult services. It is necessary to draw on the expertise of specialists from a number of disciplines including clinical geneticists, pediatric and adult endocrinologists, endocrine surgeons and specialist endocrine nurses who should work together in a well-structured team to deliver tumor surveillance according to the best available evidence. Close collaboration should exist with clinical biochemists, radiologists and neurosurgeons, and patients with MEN1 also require the care of gastroenterologists.

In 2001, a consensus statement from the Seventh International Working Party on Multiple Endocrine Neoplasia was published [21]. This included recommendations for surveillance of carriers of MEN1 gene mutation (Table 17.8).

Of particular relevance to children are the following:

1 Prophylactic intervention is not possible to prevent the leading cause of death in this syndrome;

2 The effectiveness of early detection and intervention has not yet been demonstrated; and

3 There is potential for genetic discrimination in employment. Expression of MEN1 in the pediatric population is very rare and the course of the disease is generally indolent. For these reasons, some advocate genetic testing in early adolescence allowing the patient an opportunity to give assent.

Predictive testing of children for the diagnosis of MEN2 is more easily justified. The International Working Party on Multiple Endocrine Neoplasia has recommended that screening for pheochromocytoma should start at the age of 15 years and comprise annual assessment of plasma metanephrines with MRI or CT imaging of the adrenal glands every 3–5 years. Patients in whom there is a family history of hyperparathyroidism should be screened annually by the measurement of serum calcium and parathyroid hormone from early adult life.

Table 17.8 Recommended surveillance for carriers of multiple endocrine neoplasia type 1 (MEN1) gene mutations.

Tumor	Age to begin (years)	Biochemical tests annually	Imaging tests every 3 years
Parathyroid adenoma	8	Calcium, PTH	None
Gastrinoma	20	Gastrin, gastric acid output, secretin-stimulated gastrin	None
Insulinoma	5	Fasting glucose: insulin	
Other enteropancreatic	20	Chromogranin-A, glucagon, proinsulin	^{111}In-DPTA octreotide scan; CAT or MRI
Anterior pituitary	5	Prolactin, IGF-I	MRI
Foregut carcinoid	20	None	CT

CT, computed tomography; IGF, insulin-like growth factor; MRI, magnetic resonance imaging; PTH, parathyroid hormone.

Tumors of the ovary

Ovarian tumors occur in 2.6 per 100 000 girls per year. The majority of ovarian tumors in children are benign and ovarian malignancies account for less than 1% of all childhood cancers.

Tumors may arise from sex cord stromal, germ and epithelial cells. Gonadoblastomas are unusual mixed germ cell–sex cord tumors arising most commonly in intra-abdominal dysgenetic gonads. Ovaries may be involved in girls with leukemia or lymphoma or may be a site of metastatic spread in girls with other malignant disease. A classification of adapted from the World Health Organization (WHO) Histological Classification of Ovarian Tumors is given in Table 17.9.

Sex cord stromal tumors

Ovarian tumors presenting in early childhood most commonly arise from the stromal component of the ovary, such as granulosa, Sertoli or Leydig cells. Histological techniques have enabled more accurate description of tumor types which are now considered to comprise granulosa cell tumors, Sertoli–Leydig cell tumors (SLCT), sclerosing stromal tumor (SST), sex cord tumor with annular tubules, stromal tumor and thecoma.

Sex cord stromal cell tumors (SCST) are associated with Peutz–Jeghers syndrome, a dominantly inherited condition which results from genomic mutations of the serine-threonine kinase 1 (STK11) tumor suppressor gene. Affected individuals develop melanocytic maculas on the lips, labial mucosa and fingers and multiple hamartomatous intestinal polyps. Patients with Peutz–Jeghers syndrome develop SCST at an earlier age than unaffected girls. Bilateral disease occurs more commonly but malignant disease is less frequent. The prognosis is better than for those in whom the tumor is sporadic.

Juvenile granulosa cell tumors

Juvenile granulosa cell tumors are the most common ovarian tumor occurring during infancy and early childhood; 80% occurring in children aged less than 10 years. The histological characteristics and clinical behavior of granulosa cell tumors differ from adult patients and the tumor is referred to as a juvenile granulosa cell tumor (JGCT). Almost all JGCT are confined to the ovary at

Table 17.9 Classification of ovarian tumors.

Germ cell tumors
Undifferentiated
Dysgerminoma

Embryonic
Teratoma
Embryonal carcinoma

Extra-embryonal
Endodermal sinus tumor
Choriocarcinoma

Sex cord stromal tumors
Juvenile granulosa cell
Sertoli–Leydig cell

Epithelial cell
Mucinous cystadenoma/cystadenoma

diagnosis and have an excellent prognosis, even when malignant characteristics are present on histological examination. In 83 of 125 patients with follow-up data, 80 patients presented with stage 1 disease of whom two succumbed to their disease. Only three patients presented with stage 2 disease or more and it was fatal in all [40].

Surgery alone should be curative for patients presenting with disease stage 1B or less. The outcome for patients with stage 1C disease is dictated by the presence of preoperative tumor rupture or malignant ascites. The prognosis for patients in whom the tumor is ruptured during surgery is currently indistinguishable from those with stage 1B disease or less.

The management of patients with advanced disease is controversial. In a current trial, cisplatin-based chemotherapy is used for girls presenting with tumor stage 1C due to spontaneous tumor rupture and those with stage 2 disease or more.

Sertoli cell tumors of the ovary

Sertoli cell tumors affect young women. Secretion of estrogen and androgens is common and presentation in childhood is with precocious puberty, amenorrhea or virilization. Tumor growth may be rapid and patients also present with increasing abdominal girth and symptoms resulting from tumor compression of intra-abdominal structures.

Sertoli cell tumors have been subclassified into pure Sertoli cell tumor of the ovary, which arises from the multipotential stromal ovarian cell, sex cord stromal tumors, with annular tubules and histological features intermediate between SLT and JGCT, mixed Sertoli–Leydig cell tumors and Sertoli–Leydig tumors with retiform pattern with histological features of the rete ovarii, analogous to the rete testis in the male. This last subgroup presents at an earlier age than other Sertoli cell tumors and carries a worse prognosis, with a 25% chance of malignancy.

Gonadoblastoma

Gonadoblastoma is a tumor in which germ cells and immature Sertoli/granulosa cells are intimately mixed. They are not malignant *per se* but 30% demonstrate overgrowth of the germinal component, in which case the tumor is no longer considered benign and is reclassified as a dysgerminoma. Ten percent of gonadoblastomas develop different types of germ cell neoplasia, such as yolk sac tumor, immature teratoma, embryonal carcinoma or choriocarcinoma.

Eighty percent of patients are phenotypic females with intra-abdominal dysgenetic gonads and the presence of Y chromosome material. The risk of developing a gonadoblastoma is reported to be in excess of 30% in girls with a 45X, 46XY karyotype although there is some evidence that this is an overestimate. Up to 40% of girls with Turner syndrome and no Y material on karyotype have molecular evidence of Y chromosome material on polymerase chain reaction. In these patients, the risk of developing a gonadoblastoma is 7–10% and the risk of contralateral disease is approximately 40%.

Girls with androgen insensitivity syndrome are also at increased risk of gonadoblastoma, with 30–60% of girls being affected. In light of these observations it is recommended that girls with these syndromes undergo prophylactic gonadectomy, although the timing of this procedure is controversial. Gonadoblastomas are reported in infancy and early childhood but the majority present at a later stage and are indolent in nature, prompting some to argue for a delay in gonadectomy.

Molecular studies have localized the gonadoblastoma locus on the Y chromosome (GBY) near its centromere. This locus contains a number of known genes including testis-specific protein Y. This gene is expressed at high concentrations in gonadoblastoma tissues and evidence from *in vitro* and animal studies suggest that it has an important role in the regulation of cell proliferation and tumorigenesis.

Other benign sex cord tumors

Fewer than 10% of fibromas are found in patients below the age of 30 years. If they are large (more than 10 cm in diameter) they may be associated with Meigs syndrome, the triad of a fibrous ovarian tumor, ascites and pleural effusion. They also occur in association with the basal cell nevus syndrome, where fibromas tend to be bilateral, calcified and multinodular.

Approximately 3% of thecomas present in patients aged less than 20 years. Estrogen and androgen secretion are common and patients present with menstrual disturbance or virilization.

Germ cell tumors

Germ cell tumors arise from the primitive germ cells and may occur in any part of the reproductive tract. Ectopic germ cell tumors occur as a result of aberrant patterns of primordial germ cell migration. Germ cell proliferation as a pure germ cell tumor results in dysgerminoma of the ovary, seminoma of the testes or germinoma in ectopic sites. The totipotential primitive germ cell may also develop as a benign mature teratoma, an immature teratoma of uncertain malignant potential, or a malignant tumor (embryonal carcinoma or if extra-embryonic tissue is present, yolk sac tumor or choriocarcinoma). The term "mixed germ cell tumor" describes tumors composed of more than one histological type of germ cell. Each tumor type expresses different tumor markers and has different malignant potential.

Germ cell tumors account for 75–80% of all neoplastic ovarian lesions in childhood. The incidence of the tumor increases with age and 70% of cases are diagnosed in girls aged 10–14 years.

Teratomas

Teratomas are derived from all three embryonic layers, ectoderm, endoderm and mesoderm, and are the most common ovarian tumor of childhood. They are classified as mature if they are characterized by differentiated tissues, immature if some immature non-malignant tissue is present or malignant if there are features of yolk sac tumor, choriocarcinoma or embryonal carcinoma. The appearances of a mature teratoma are illustrated in Plate 17.7. Seventy percent of teratomas are mature and are frequently asymptomatic until they reach a large size. Immature lesions are graded histologically from 1 to 3 based on the number of immature regions visualized per low power field. Fewer that 10% of microscopic foci contain immature tissue in grade 1 disease, which rises to 10–50% in grade 2 and more than 50% in grade 3.

In adult patients, the least mature lesions demonstrate the greatest risk of recurrence and malignant change. For this reason, high grade tumors in children have historically been treated with chemotherapy. However, the findings of a recent intergroup study between the Children's Oncology Group and the Pediatric Oncology Group indicate that surgical treatment alone, together with close observation for recurrence, is a safe and adequate treatment in children and adolescents [41,42].

Thirty percent of ovarian teratomas are malignant, of which one-third are pure endodermal sinus tumors and one-third contain mixed elements. Detailed examination of any solid component of a teratoma is mandatory to ensure that no immature neural elements or occult foci of malignancy are present. Metastatic spread may be local to peritoneum or distant, most commonly to lung, liver, brain and bone. Surgery alone is curative for tumors limited to the ovary.

If tumor markers are elevated at presentation they can be monitored in the postoperative period as an indicator of residual disease. Serum alfa fetoprotein (AFP) has a half-life of 5 days and serum human chorionic gonadotropin (β-hCG) a half-life of 16 h. Failure of these tumor markers to fall indicates persisting active tumor and the patient should proceed to chemotherapy. Patients in whom tumor markers are not elevated should be followed closely with MRI or ultrasound.

Dysgerminomas

Dysgerminomas arise from germ cell lines with suppressed differentiation. They are malignant but are associated with a good prognosis because they tend to present at an early stage and are highly sensitivity to radiation and chemotherapy. Bilateral disease is found in 10–15% of patients. Serum lactic dehydrongenase (LDH) may be elevated in the presence of dysgerminoma and can be a useful tumor marker. Other tumor markers reported to be positive in dysgerminoma include neuron-specific enolase, β-hCG and CA-125.

Embryonal carcinoma and choriocarcinoma are rarely seen in isolation and are most commonly observed together with elements of endodermal sinus tumor in mixed malignant tumors. Such mixed tumors comprise 30% of malignant ovarian germ cell tumors. Patients may have elevated concentrations of β-hCG or AFP or both.

Epithelial cell tumors

Epithelial cell tumors are the second most common ovarian neoplasia affecting adolescents but they are not seen before puberty.

Only one subtype of epithelial cell tumor is seen in childhood, the cystadenoma. This tumor type can be further classified as serous, the most common form, or mucinous. The majority of cystadenomas presenting in childhood are benign and can be treated successfully by cystectomy or unilateral oophorectomy alone.

Adenocarcinomas are fortunately extremely rare in childhood. Serum CA-125 tumor antigen, AFP or CEA may be elevated and can be a useful indicator of residual tumor burden following surgery and response to chemotherapy.

Borderline ovarian epithelial cell tumors are indolent tumors which are frequently bilateral and locally invasive. They are defined as epithelial cell tumors with varying concentrations of nuclear atypia and they lack stromal invasion of the ovary. Tumors generally present early and the prognosis in these patients is excellent following surgery so fertility-sparing procedures should be attempted. However, the tumor is highly heterogeneous and some patients will have extensive disease at diagnosis requiring radical surgery and chemotherapy. Death in childhood has been reported.

Diagnosis
Clinical features

Young girls with functional tumors present at an early stage with the clinical features of precocious puberty or virilization. In older girls, hormone production from functional tumors may induce galactorrhea, virilization and menstrual irregularity. Patients with non-functioning tumors present with abdominal pain, an abdominal mass or urinary symptoms and, in the presence of malignancy, ascites or pleural effusion.

Diagnostic imaging

Ovarian lesions can be well visualized on ultrasound assessment. Sonolucent lesions with very thin walls and no solid component are very unlikely to be malignant. Lesions with thick irregular walls and septa, papillary projections and solid components are likely to be malignant and laparotomy and intra-operative staging is indicated. Further anatomical detail may be obtained from MRI or CT.

Staging of ovarian tumors

The staging of malignant disease in both childhood and adult life has been standardized by the International Federation of Gynecology and Obstetrics (FIGO) and details of this staging system are given in Table 17.10. Tumor stage, the level of mitotic activity within the tumor on histological examination, the presence or absence of endocrine features and age are important prognostic indicators.

A separate staging system for ovarian germ cell tumors has been devised by the Pediatric Oncology Group (Table 17.11).

Treatment
Surgery

The surgical management of ovarian tumors in childhood presents a particular challenge. Benign lesions occur much more commonly than malignant lesions and conservative surgical techniques should be employed to preserve ovarian tissue and minimize adhesion formation. However, some malignant lesions are associated with a high mortality rate and careful preoperative assessment is essential to inform surgical planning. The place for laparoscopic cystectomy in the treatment of ovarian lesions is controversial and the question of whether the risk of overlooking malignancy outweighs the benefit of this less invasive approach remains unanswered. The Germ Cell Committee and the Children's Oncology Group specifically discourage this approach because the risk of tumor rupture can result in upgrading of undiagnosed malignant lesions.

The prognosis of ovarian tumors is closely related to the extent of disease as defined by the FIGO system and tumor staging at the time of surgery has an important role in determining the need for postoperative chemotherapy. This should include collection of ascites for cytology, sampling of lymph nodes, omentectomy, peritoneal biopsies and assessment of the contralateral ovary. Such extensive examination may not be necessary in girls with germ cell tumors in the absence of gross disease.

Table 17.10 FIGO staging system for primary carcinoma of the ovary.

Stage I	Growth limited to the ovaries
IA	Growth limited to one ovary, no tumor on the external surface; capsule intact
IB	Growth limited to both ovaries, no tumor on the external surface; capsule intact
IC	Tumor stage either IA or IB but with ascites or peritoneal washings containing malignant cells; tumor on the surface or capsule ruptured
Stage II	Growth involving one or both ovaries with pelvic extension
IIA	Extension to the uterus or tubes
IIB	Extension to other pelvic structures
IIC	Tumor either IIA or IIB but with ascites or peritoneal washings containing malignant cells; tumor on the surface or capsule ruptured
Stage III	Tumor involving one or both ovaries with peritoneal implants outside the pelvis or positive retroperitoneal or inguinal lymph nodes; superficial liver metastasis equals stage III; tumor is limited to the true pelvis but with histologically proven malignant extension to small bowel or omentum
IIIA	Tumor grossly limited to the true pelvis with negative nodes but histologically proven microscopic seeding of the peritoneal surfaces
IIIB	Tumor of one or both ovaries with histologically confirmed implants of abdominal peritoneal surfaces, none exceeding 2 cm in diameter, nodes are negative
IIIC	Abdominal implants are greater than 2 cm in diameter or positive retroperitoneal or inguinal lymph nodes
Stage IV	Growth involving one or both ovaries with distant metastases; if pleural effusion present, there must be positive cytology to allot a case to stage IV; parenchymal liver metastases equals stage IV

Table 17.11 Staging of pediatric ovarian germ cell tumors according to the American Pediatric Oncology Group and Children's Cancer Group.

Stage I	Limited to ovary (ovaries) peritoneal washings negative for malignant cells; no clinical, radiographic or histological evidence of disease beyond the ovary; tumor markers normal after appropriate half-life decline (AFP, 5 days; β-hCG, 16 h)
Stage II	Microscopic residual disease or disease in lymph nodes <2 cm; peritoneal washings negative for malignant cells; tumor markers positive or negative
Stage III	Gross residual disease or biopsy only; lymph nodes >2 cm; contiguous spread to other organs (omentum, intestine, bladder); peritoneal washings positive for malignant cells
Stage IV	Metastatic disease, which may include liver

The risk of recurrence of borderline epithelial tumors is related to the primary surgical procedure. Recurrence is reported in 5.7% of patients undergoing radical surgery (hysterectomy and bilateral salpingo-oophorectomy) while recurrence in those treated by adnexectomy and cystectomy is 15.5% and 36.3%, respectively. Recurrent disease can be reliably detected by ultrasound and pelvic examination and successfully treated surgically and conservative surgery probably does not affect the overall survival if patients are able to comply with a program of tumor surveillance [42].

The treatment of adenocarcinomas is with surgical debulking followed by chemotherapy.

Chemotherapy

Chemotherapy is indicated for any ovarian germ cell tumor that has spread outside the confines of the ovary. Overall, the treatment of germ cell tumors with chemotherapy is extremely successful, even in advanced cases. The combination of bleomycin, etoposide and cisplatin has been associated with an event-free survival in excess of 95% [43] for patients at all stages of disease.

Following surgery girls with adenocarcinomas are treated with platinum-based chemotherapy based on adult protocols. Unlike other pediatric ovarian malignancies, the prognosis for girls with malignant adenocarcinoma is poor. A recent publication of 463 women treated for this malignancy reported 21% survival at 5 years, 13.5% survival at 10 years and 12% survival at 15 years [44].

Tumors of the testes

Testicular tumors account for 1% of all pediatric solid tumors and occur with an incidence of 0.5–2.0 per 100 000 boys. Two peaks in presentation are observed, the first during the first 2 years of life and the second after the age of 10 years.

Testicular tumors affecting the prepubertal boy differ markedly from those seen in older boys and adult men, both in terms of tumor type and tumor behavior. Germ cell tumors account for 60–70% of tumors in children, while 95% of testicular tumors are of germ cell origin in adults. Seminomas and embryonal carcinomas are not observed in prepubertal boys, while teratomas, which are uniformly benign in prepubertal boys, are often malignant in adults. Sex cord stromal tumors account for 7–8% of childhood tumors. Prepubertal testicular tumors are classified according to the cell line of origin and a modified version of the WHO classification of prepubertal testicular tumors is given in Table 17.12.

Germ cell tumors

Germ cell tumors arise from the primitive germ cells and may occur in any part of the reproductive tract. Pure germ cell proliferation results in seminoma of the testis. The totipotential primitive germ cell may also develop as a benign mature teratoma, an

Table 17.12 Classification of prepubertal testicular tumors.

Germ cell tumors
Yolk sac
Teratoma
Seminoma
Mixed germ cell

Gonadal stromal tumors
Leydig cell
Sertoli cell
Granulosa cell
Mixed gonadal stromal cell

Gonadoblastoma

Tumors of supporting tissue
Fibroma
Fibrosarcoma
Leiomyoma
Hemangioma

Lymphomas and leukemias

Tumor-like lesions
Epidermid cyst
Testicular adrenal rest tumors (TART)

Secondary tumors

Tumors of the adnexa
Rhabdomyosarcoma, fibroma, fibrosarcoma, leiomyoma, leiomyosarcoma,
   hemangioma, lipoma

immature teratoma of uncertain malignant potential or a malignant tumor (embryonal carcinoma or, if extra-embryonic tissue is present, yolk sac tumor or choriocarcinoma). The term "mixed germ cell tumor" describes tumors composed of more than one histological type of germ cell.

Three entities of testicular tumors can be defined on the basis of epidemiological, clinical and histological characteristics. These three entities have a different pathogenesis. The first group includes the yolk sac teratomas. These tumors usually present before the age of 4 years and always before puberty and are likely to have their origin during fetal life. The second group, referred to as testicular germ cell tumors (TGCT), is found in pubertal and adult males and comprises seminomas and teratomas. Tumorigenesis in this group is likely to be related to spermatogenesis during puberty and beyond. The final group, spermatocytic seminomas, are diagnosed in elderly men.

Yolk sac tumors

Yolk sac tumors have a prevalence of 0.1 per 100 000 in prepubertal boys with more than 75% of cases presenting in the first 2 years of life. The youngest affected patients are diagnosed in the neonatal period. Early reports related the age at diagnosis to metastatic disease and outcome but data from the Prepubertal Testis Tumor Registry, established by the Section of Urology in the American Academy of Pediatrics, suggest this is not true.

The vast majority of tumors present early at stage I and surgery alone should be curative. More than 99% of all patients with yolk sac tumors are expected to survive.

Testicular tumors in childhood demonstrate hematogenous spread to lungs, liver and brain.

Teratomas of childhood

Testicular teratomas are the second most common testicular tumor in prepubertal boys. They are generally mature and derived from embryonic tissue from all three germ layers. Ultrasound examination reveals a cystic septated appearance with intervening solid components including calcification.

Mixed germ cell tumor

Tumors comprising more than one type of germ cell neoplasm are found in the testes, ovary, mediastinum and brain. The most common combinations include teratoma with yolk sac, teratoma with embryonal carcinoma and choriocarcinoma and teratoma with embryonal carcinoma. The presence of choriocarcinoma significantly decreases survival. Treatment is dictated by the most malignant component of the tumor.

Testicular germ cell tumors of adolescence

The worldwide incidence of TGCTs in this age group has doubled in the last 40 years, an increase that follows a birth cohort effect. As the genetic composition of a population cannot change in one or two generations, environmental influences must be important in the etiology of the disease.

There is speculation that prenatal exposure to high concentrations of estrogen may be important in the etiology of infertility, cryptorchidism and sperm quality and TGCT. This hypothesis can be explored through twin studies that compare the prevalence of TGCT in male twins to that of singletons because maternal estrogen concentrations are higher during twin pregnancies than singleton pregnancies and higher in dizygotic twin pregnancies than monozygotic pregnancies. Genetic influences can be studied by comparing the rate of concordance (both twins affected) in monozygotic and dizygotic twins. Males from twin pregnancies are at increased risk of TGCT compared to singletons and those from dizygotic pregnancies are at increased risk compared to those from monozygotic pregnancies (odds ratio 1.5) [45].

More research is required to investigate the pathogenetic mechanisms that lead to the increased risk of TGCT in dizygotic twins. Twinning itself is, to some extent, genetically determined and it is possible that coinherited genetic factors could contribute to the increased risk of TGCT rather than the increase in maternal estrogen.

To date only one study has compared the rate of concordance in males from monozygotic pregnancies with that in dizygotic pregnancies [46]. In this study, which included six pairs of concordant twins, monozygotic twins were most commonly affected.

Gonadal stromal tumors

Gonadal stromal tumors are benign tumors in childhood arising from Leydig and Sertoli cells.

Leydig cell tumor

Testicular Leydig cell tumors can occur at any age but are seen most commonly in prepubertal boys aged 5–10 years and in adult males aged 30–60 years. They are always benign in childhood but behave as malignant tumors in 10% of adult patients. Leydig cell tumors secrete androgens and sometimes estrogen. Boys may present with pseudo-precocious puberty, in which growth and skeletal maturity are advanced together with pubic and axillary hair growth and genital development in the absence of pubertal testicular growth. Breast tenderness and gynecomastia may result from estrogen secretion by the tumor, although this is rare in childhood, or from peripheral aromatization of testosterone to estrogen.

Ultrasound appearances are of a homogeneous hypoechoic lesion and Doppler examination often shows a hypervascular tumor with prominent peripheral and circumferential blood flow. Tumor markers (AFP, β-hCG and placental alkaline phosphatase) should be within the normal range.

Sertoli cell tumor

Sertoli cell tumors (SCT) account for only 1.3% of tumors recorded on the American Academy of Pediatrics Section on Urology Prepubertal Testicular Tumor Registry. There are no case reports to date of Sertoli cell tumors presenting in the neonatal period and only three case reports of boys being affected in the first decade of life. In the pediatric population they are most commonly diagnosed in infancy when they present as painless testicular masses. Occasionally, infants present with gynecomastia but virilization is unusual. To date, there are no reported cases of malignancy in boys aged less than 5 years and surgical treatment should be considered curative. In older boys, malignant behavior is observed in 10% of tumors and is related to tumor size and mitotic activity. Tumor necrosis and vascular infiltration are also suggestive of malignant disease.

Large cell calcifying Sertoli cell tumor (LCCSCT) is seen predominantly in children and adolescents and it is the most common form of SCT seen in childhood. Ultrasound examination reveals the presence of multiple hyperechoic lesions within the tumor representing areas of calcification. Tumors are generally benign and are associated with Peutz–Jeghers syndrome and Carney complex. Malignancy is more likely in tumors more than 4 cm in diameter.

Sertoli cell hyperplasia and adenoma are often observed in patients with androgen insensitivity syndrome.

Juvenile granulosa cell tumors

Testicular juvenile granulosa cell tumors are diagnosed only in the first year of life and most commonly before the age of 6 months. They are non-functioning benign tumors which are cured by surgical resection. These testicular lesions are reported to occur more commonly in boys with anomalies of the Y chromosome, mosaicism and ambiguous genitalia.

Lymphoma and leukemia

Lymphoma and leukemia account for 2–5% of all testicular tumors and the majority of bilateral tumors.

The reported incidence of testicular involvement in boys with acute lymphoblastic leukemia (ALL) ranges 8–25% but most studies report a figure of less than 10%. As survival from ALL improves, the incidence of testicular leukemia has increased. The testes may be the site of residual tumor after chemotherapy and the testes are the most common site of relapse. These observations have prompted speculation that the blood–testis barrier may protect the intratesticular cells from chemotherapy, although animal studies do not support this hypothesis.

The clinical presentation is with a painless testicular mass but only a minority of tumors are clinically apparent. Diagnosis is confirmed by wedge biopsy and treatment is with chemotherapy and bilateral testicular irradiation.

Lymphomatous involvement of the testes has been reported in all ages, although 80% of cases occur in men over 50 years of age. It is usually limited to non-Hodgkin lymphoma, although occasionally other histological types are reported.

Tumor-like lesions
Epidermoid cysts

Epidermoid cysts are benign lesions of epithelial cell origin that account for fewer than 2% of all childhood testicular tumors. On ultrasound examination they are found to be cystic with a hyperechoic centre indicating the presence of central keratinized debris and a hyperechoic rim, representing squamous and fibrous elements. The lesions are universally benign and surgery is curative.

Testicular adrenal rest tumors in patients with congenital adrenal hyperplasia

Testicular adrenal rest tumors (TART) occur in association with congenital adrenal hyperplasia (CAH) when glucocorticoid replacement therapy is insufficient to suppress serum ACTH. Most tumors are bilateral and develop synchronously. They are ACTH dependent and shrink in response to adequate glucocorticoid therapy. Should they persist, it is important to consider the possibility that they have developed autonomy and are true neoplasms, in which case enucleation is indicated.

A recent study investigated the prevalence of TART on high resolution ultrasound examination in prepubertal boys with CAH and compared testicular function with controls of the same age. Inhibin B and anti-Müllerian hormone were used as markers of Sertoli cell function. Leydig cell function was assessed from the increment in serum testosterone from baseline to 72 h following stimulation with β-hCG 5000 units/m². Twenty-one percent of boys with CAH had TART. Inihibin B, anti-Müllerian hormone and the increment in serum testosterone were lower in boys with CAH than in controls. As expected, those with inadequate control were most severely affected [47].

Tumors of the adnexa

Tumors arising from the adnexa are most commonly rhabdomyosarcomas. Very rarely, paratesticular mesotheliomas arise in the epididymus, tunica vaginalis or spermatic cord, almost always in patients over the age of 18 years. In contrast to adult patients, the clinical course of these tumors appears to be benign in children, although data describing the natural history of the disease are limited. Paratesticular leiomyomas and leiomyosarcomas have been described in childhood.

Rhabdomyosarcomas

Rhabdomyosarcomas are soft tissue malignant tumors of skeletal muscle origin. They have a bimodal distribution and occur in boys aged 3–4 months and in teenagers. Tumors present as painless testicular masses or hydroceles and ultrasound examination reveals a mass located within the spermatic cord. As many as 70% of patients have involvement of the retroperitoneal lymph nodes at presentation. These tumors are highly aggressive and 20% of patients have disease in the lymphatics or direct extension to the lungs, the cortical bone or to the bone marrow at the time of diagnosis. Radical inguinal orchiectomy followed by retroperitoneal lymph node dissection is recommended for all children older than 10 years and in those younger than 10 years with retroperitoneal disease. Those with positive lymph nodes are treated with multimodal therapy (chemotherapy and radiation).

Diagnosis

Clinical features

The most common mode of presentation is with a painless testicular mass that does not transilluminate. Patients may also complain of testicular pain and presentation following trauma, which presumably prompts testicular examination and identification of a testicular mass, is also common. In 10–25% of cases malignant tumors present with a hydrocele. Functional tumors that secrete androgens present with features of virilization in the prepubertal boy and those that secrete estrogen present with chest tenderness and gynecomastia. The time between onset of symptoms and treatment varies from 3 to 6 months in boys with germ cell tumors but is delayed for up to 24 months in those with tumors of non-germ cell origin.

Biochemical evaluation

Serum AFP is elevated in 60–90% of boys with yolk sac tumors. It is a valuable marker of the patient's response to treatment and the presence of residual and recurrent disease. Patients in whom serum AFP is greater than 10000 ng/mL at diagnosis have a significantly poorer prognosis than those in whom serum AFP is lower. The half-life of AFP is about 5 days and concentrations should return to normal (<20 ng/mL) within a month after complete surgical resection. Failure of AFP to fall is highly suggestive of residual or metastatic disease. It is important to note that high concentrations of serum AFP are physiological during the first 6–12 months of life and may not be of diagnostic value in this age group. However, preoperative and postoperative concentrations are still of value to monitor response to treatment and identify relapsed disease. The mean serum AFP concentrations according to age are given in Table 17.13 [48].

Serum testosterone or estradiol may be elevated in boys with Leydig cell tumors and serum hCG may be elevated in gonadoblastomas. Like AFP, these markers of tumor activity can be helpful in the assessment of response to treatment.

Serum AFP and hCG should be measured in all adolescent boys at diagnosis of a testicular germ cell tumor. Concentrations of these tumor markers are used along with imaging techniques to allocate a prognostic group for the patient (Table 17.16).

Diagnostic imaging

Preoperative assessment should include ultrasound of the testes to define the location and size of the tumor and to assess its characteristics. Tumors located entirely within the testis may be amenable to testes-preserving surgery. The presence of liver metastasis and involvement of the retroperitoneal lymph nodes should be assessed by MRI and lung metastases by chest X-ray or chest CT. Metastatic spread to brain, bone or other parenchymal organs may be suspected but diagnostic tests can be safely deferred until a histological diagnosis is made at surgery. Imaging of the chest, abdomen and pelvis is essential for staging with adolescent boys testicular germ cell tumors.

Staging

A staging system designed for the evaluation of testicular tumors in prepubertal boys has been devised by Committee on Tumors, Section of Urology, Academy of Pediatrics. This staging system is detailed in Table 17.14. The staging system for pediatric testicular germ cell tumors is given in Table 17.15 and for adolescent tumors the TNMS system according to the AJCC is given in Table 17.16.

Table 17.13 Reference values of serum alfa fetoprotein (AFP) [48].

Patient age	AFP (µg/L or ng/mL)
Premature	80 000–220 000
Newborn	2000–130 000
0–2 weeks	8000–130 000
2 weeks–1 month	300–70 000
1 month	90–10 000
2 months	40–1000
3 months	20–300
4 months	0–300
5 months	0–100
6 months	0–40
7 months	0–40
8 months	0–20
9 months–adult	0–10

Table 17.14 Staging of childhood testicular tumors according to the Committee on Tumors, Section of Urology in the American Academy of Pediatrics.

Group 1	Tumor confined to the testes, AFP normal within 1 month following orchidectomy, imaging of the retroperitoneum and chest normal
Group 2	Similar to group 1 but retroperitoneal lymph node dissection reveals unsuspected nodal metastases
Group 3	Retroperitoneal lymph node metastases on imaging studies, serum AFP concentrations persistently elevated
Group 4	Demonstrable metastases beyond the retroperitoneum

AFP, alfa fetoprotein.

Table 17.15 Staging of pediatric testicular germ cell tumors according to the American Pediatric Oncology Group and Children's Cancer Group.

Stage I	Limited to testis, completely resected by high inguinal orchiectomy; no clinical, radiographic or histological evidence of disease beyond the testis; tumor markers normal after appropriate half-life decline (AFP, 5 days; β-hCG, 16 h)
Stage II	Transcrotal orchiectomy; microscopic disease in scrotum or high in spermatic chord (<5 cm from proximal end); retroperitoneal lymph node involvement (<2 cm) and/or increased tumor markers after appropriate decline
Stage III	Tumor positive retroperitoneal lymph nodes >2 cm in diameter: no visceral or extra-abdominal involvement
Stage IV	Metastatic disease, which may include liver

AFP, alfa fetoprotein; hCH, human chorionic gonadotropin.

Treatment

Surgery

The operation of choice for boys with malignant disease, including yolk sac tumors, is radical inguinal orchidectomy with high ligation of the spermatic chord. Retroperitoneal lymph node dissection is now considered unnecessary because tumor spread in childhood is most commonly hematogenous to lung, liver and brain. Furthermore, retroperitoneal lymph node dissection is associated with a risk of adhesions, intra-operative injury and ejaculatory dysfunction and there is no evidence that retroperitoneal lymph node dissection improves survival.

Patients with yolk sac tumors and evidence of metastatic disease and those with persistently elevated AFP should be treated with combination chemotherapy with cisplatin, etoposide and bleomycin. This therapy has significantly improved the prognosis of those with advanced disease and event-free survival in excess of 90% at 6 years has been reported [41]. If AFP concentrations remain elevated following chemotherapy, dissection of the retroperitoneal lymph nodes may be required.

Table 17.16 The American Joint Committee on Cancer TNMS staging system for testicular tumors in pubertal and adult males.

Primary tumor (T)

pTX	Primary tumor cannot be assessed*
pT0	No evidence of primary tumor (e.g. histologic scar in testis)
pTis	Intratubular germ cell neoplasia (carcinoma *in situ*)
pT1	Tumor limited to the testis and epididymis without lymphatic/vascular invasion; tumor may invade into the tunica albuginea but not the tunica vaginalis
pT2	Tumor limited to the testis and epididymis with vascular/lymphatic invasion or tumor extending through the tunica albuginea with involvement of the tunica vaginalis
pT3	Tumor invades the spermatic cord with or without vascular/lymphatic invasion
pT4	Tumor invades the scrotum with or without vascular/lymphatic invasion

Regional lymph nodes (N)

NX	Regional lymph nodes cannot be assessed
N0	No regional lymph node metastasis
N1	Metastasis with a single lymph node mass 2 cm or less in greatest dimension; or multiple lymph nodes, none more than 2 cm in greatest dimension
N2	Metastasis with a single lymph node mass more than 2 cm but not more than 5 cm in greatest dimension; or multiple lymph nodes, none more than 5 cm in greatest dimension
N3	Metastasis with a lymph node mass more than 5 cm in greatest dimension

Distant metastasis (M)

MX	Presence of distant metastasis cannot be assessed
M0	No distant metastasis
M1	Distant metastasis
M1a	Non-regional nodal or pulmonary metastasis
M1b	Distant metastasis other than to non-regional lymph nodes and lungs

Serum tumor markers (S)

SX	Marker studies not available or not performed
S0	Marker study concentrations within normal limits
S1	LDH <1.5 × N* *and* hCG (mIu/mL) <5000 *and* AFP (ng/ml) <1000
S2	LDH 1.5–10 × N* *or* hCG (mIu/mL) 5000–50 000 *or* AFP (ng/mL) 1000–10 000
S3	LDH >10 × N* *or* hCG (mIu/mL) >50 000 *or* AFP (ng/mL) >10 000

*If no radical orchidectomy has been performed. AFP, serum alfa fetoprotein; hCG, human chorionic gonadotropin; LDH, lactic dehydrogenase; N, upper limit of normal for LDH assay.

Prepubertal teratomas, Leydig and Sertoli cell tumors are benign and patients should expect to be cured by surgery alone. Traditionally, this comprised orchidectomy with high ligation of the spermatic chord but this approach is being modified as data reported from a number of registries emphasize the benign behavior of most testicular tumors in prepubertal boys. Furthermore, in this age group testicular tumors generally present at an early stage and those with more extensive disease respond well to chemotherapy.

Table 17.16 The AJCC staging system for testicular tumors in pubertal and adult males (*cont*).

Stage grouping

Stage 0
pTis, N0, M0, S0

Stage I
pT1–4, N0, M0, SX

Stage IA
pT1, N0, M0, S0

Stage IB
pT2, N0, M0, S0
pT3, N0, M0, S0
pT4, N0, M0, S0

Stage IS
Any pT/Tx, N0, M0, S1–3

Stage II
Any pT/Tx, N1–3, M0, SX

Stage IIA
Any pT/Tx, N1, M0, S0
Any pT/Tx, N1, M0, S1

Stage IIB
Any pT/Tx, N2, M0, S0
Any pT/Tx, N2, M0, S1

Stage IIC
Any pT/Tx, N3, M0, S0
Any pT/Tx, N3, M0, S1

Stage III
Any pT/Tx, any N, M1, SX

Stage IIIA
Any pT/Tx, any N, M1a, S0
Any pT/Tx, any N, M1a, S1

Stage IIIB
Any pT/Tx, N1–3, M0, S2
Any pT/Tx, any N, M1a, S2

Stage IIIC
Any pT/Tx, N1–3, M0, S3
Any pT/Tx, any N, M1a, S3
Any pT/Tx, any N, M1b, any S

Testis-sparing surgery has potential cosmetic, psychological and functional advantages over orchidectomy and long-term outcome data indicate that it is both adequate and appropriate in selected cases. Long-term observational studies from boys with teratoma treated in this way report no recurrences and no cases of testicular atrophy [49] and it is recommended that this procedure be offered to prepubertal boys in whom there is viable testicular tissue on ultrasound and serum AFP is normal. Frozen section biopsies are obtained after temporary occlusion of the spermatic cord at the inguinal canal. If the frozen section confirms the presence of a benign tumor, the testis is closed and left *in situ*. In the presence of malignant disease, orchidectomy is performed. In peripubertal boys with a frozen section diagnosis of teratoma, intra-operative assessment should also include a biopsy of surrounding normal testicular tissue. If testicular tissue appearances are pubertal, orchidectomy is performed because testicular teratomas may behave in a malignant manner in this age group.

Patients should remain under long-term surveillance to facilitate early identification and treatment of recurrent or persistent disease. During the first year following diagnosis, serum AFP is measured monthly. A chest X-ray should be performed every 2 months for 2 years and MRI of the retroperitoneum should be performed every 3 months for the first year and biannually thereafter.

Ten percent of pubertal boys with Sertoli cell tumors have malignant disease at diagnosis and treatment is with radiotherapy, chemotherapy and retroperitoneal lymph node dissection.

All germ cell tumors in pubertal boys are treated by inguinal orchidectomy. Consideration should be given to semen analysis and sperm banking in adolescent boys. Boys should also be offered insertion of a testicular prosthesis at the time of primary surgery.

The contralateral testes should be biopsied once sperm has been banked and those with evidence of carcinoma *in situ* should be offered irradiation of the testes.

It is now a widely held belief that there is no place for observation of pubertal and adult males with seminomas and adjuvant radiotherapy is recommended for all patients with stage I disease. Those without risk factors for pelvic node disease are treated with prophylactic irradiation of the para-aortic glands alone. The field is extended to include the ipsilateral pelvic nodes in patients with risk factors for pelvic nodal disease. If there is evidence of invasion of lymphatic or blood vessels, the patient should be treated with chemotherapy. Patients with metastatic disease are treated with para-aortic and ipsilateral pelvic lymph node radiotherapy and cisplatin-based chemotherapy.

Pubertal boys with stage I teratoma and no high risk features can be managed by surveillance following orchidectomy. The chest and abdomen should be routinely imaged as part of the surveillance program. Metastatic disease is treated with bleomycin, etoposide and cisplatin.

References

1 Michalkiewicz E, Sandrini R, Figueiredo B, Miranda EC, Caran E, Oliveira-Filho AG, *et al*. Clinical and outcome characteristics of children with adrenocortical tumors: a report from the International Pediatric Adrenocortical Tumor Registry. *J Clin Oncol* 2004; **22**: 838–845.

2 Hoyme HE, Seaver LH, Jones KL, Procopio F, Crooks W, Feingold M. Isolated hemihyperplasia (hemihypertrophy): report of a prospective multicenter study of the incidence of neoplasia and review. *Am J Med Genet* 1998; **79**: 274–278.

3 Hough AJ, Hollifield JW, Page DL, Hartman WH. Prognostic factors in adrenal cortical tumours: a mathematical analysis of clinical and morphologic data. *Am J Clin Pathol* 1979; **72**: 390–399.

4 Weiss LM. Comparative histological study of 43 metastasizing and non-metastasizing adrenocortical tumors. *Am J Surg Pathol* 1984; **8**: 163–169.

5 Cagle PT, Hough AJ, Pyeher J, Page DL, Johnson EH, Kirkland RT, et al. Comparison of adreno cortical tumors in children and adults. *Cancer* 1986; **57**: 2235–2237.

6 Mayer SK, Oligny LL, Deal C, Yazbeck S, Gagné N, Blanchard H. Childhood adrenocortical tumors: case series and reevaluation of prognosis – a 24-year experience. *J Pediatr Surg* 1997; **32**: 911–915.

7 Baudin E, Pellegriti G, Bonnay M, Penfornis A, Laplanche A, Vassal G, et al. Impact of monitoring plasma 1,1-dichlorodiphenildichloroethane (o,p'DDD) concentrations on the treatment of patients with adrenocortical carcinoma. *Cancer* 2001; **15**: 1385–1392.

8 Dickstein G, Shechner C, Arad E, Best LA, Nativ O. Is there a role for low doses of mitotane (o,p'-DDD) as adjuvant therapy in adrenocortical carcinoma? *J Clin Endocrinol Metab* 1998; **83**: 3100–3103.

9 Chun HG, Yagoda A, Kemeny N, Watson RC. Cisplatin for adrenal cortical carcinoma. *Cancer Treat Rep* 1983; **67**: 513–514.

10 van Slooten H, van Oosterom AT. CAP (cyclophosphamide, doxorubicin and cisplatin) regimen in adrenal cortical carcinoma. *Cancer Treat Rep* 1983; **67**: 377–379.

11 Schlumberger M, Brugieres L, Gicquel C, Travagli JP, Droz JP, Parmentier C. 5-Fluorouracil, doxorubicin and cisplatin as treatment for adrenal cortical carcinoma. *Cancer* 1991; **67**: 2997–3000.

12 Zancanella P, Pianovski MA, Oliveira BH, Ferman S, Piovezan GC, Lichtvan LL, et al. Mitotane associated with cisplatin, etoposide and doxorubicin in advanced childhood adrenocortical carcinoma: mitotane monitoring and tumor regression. *J Pediatr Hematol Oncol* 2006; **28**: 513–524.

13 Patil KK, Ransley PG, McCullagh M, Malone M, Spitz L. Functioning adrenocortical neoplasms in children. *BJU Int* 2002; **89**: 562–565.

14 Gimenez-Roqueplo AP, Favier J, Rustin P, Rieubland C, Kerlan V, Plouin PF, et al. Functional consequences of a SDHB gene mutation in an apparently sporadic pheochromocytoma. *J Clin Endocrinol Metab* 2002; **87**: 4771–4774.

15 Neumann HP, Pawlu C, Peczkowska M, Bausch B, McWhinney SR, Muresan M, et al. European-American Paraganglioma Study Group. Distinct clinical features of paraganglioma syndromes associated with SDHB and SDHD gene mutations. *JAMA* 2004; **25**: 943–951.

16 Schiavi F, Boedeker CC, Bausch B, Peçzkowska M, Gomez CF, Strassburg T, et al. European-American Paraganglioma Study Group. Predictors and prevalence of paraganglioma syndrome associated with mutations of the SDHC gene. *JAMA* 2005; **26**: 2057–2063.

17 Walther MM, Reiter R, Keiser HR, Choyke PL, Venzon D, Hurley K, et al. Clinical and genetic characterization of pheochromocytoma in von Hippel–Lindau families: comparison with sporadic pheochromocytoma gives insight into natural history of pheochromocytoma. *J Urol* 1999; **162**: 659–664.

18 Pacak K, Linehan WM, Eisenhofer G, Walther MM, Goldstein DS. Recent advances in genetics, diagnosis, localization and treatment of pheochromocytoma. *Ann Intern Med* 2001; **134**: 315–329.

19 Scholz T, Eisenhofer G, Pacak K, Dralle H, Lehnert H. Clinical review: current treatment of malignant pheochromocytoma. *J Clin Endocrinol Metab* 2007; **92**: 1217–1225.

20 Garaventa A, Gambini C, Villavecchia G, Di Cataldo A, Bertolazzi L, Pizzitola MR, et al. Second malignancies in children with neuroblastoma after combined treatment with 131I-metaiodobenzylguanidine. *Cancer* 2003; **97**: 1332–1338.

21 Brandi ML, Gagel RF, Angeli A, Bilezikian JP, Beck-Peccoz P, Bordi C, et al. Guidelines for diagnosis and therapy of MEN type 1 and type 2. *J Clin Endocrinol Metab* 2001; **86**: 5658–5671.

22 Johnston LB, Chew SL, Trainer PJ, Reznek R, Grossman AB, Besser GM, et al. Screening children at risk of developing inherited endocrine neoplasia syndromes. *Clin Endocrinol* 2000; **52**: 127–136.

23 Jarzab B, Handkiewicz-Junak D. Differentiated thyroid cancer in children and adults: same or distinct disease? *Hormones (Athens)* 2007; **6**: 200–209.

24 Nikiforov YE, Rowland JM, Bove KE, Monforte-Munoz H, Fagin JA. Distinct pattern of ret oncogene rearrangements in morphological variants of radiation-induced and sporadic thyroid papillary carcinomas in children. *Cancer Res* 1997; **57**: 1690–1694.

25 Rosenbaum E, Hosler G, Zahurak M, Cohen Y, Sidransky D, Westra WH. Mutational activation of BRAF is not a major event in sporadic childhood papillary thyroid carcinoma. *Mod Pathol* 2005; **18**: 898–902.

26 Niedziela M. Pathogenesis, diagnosis and management of thyroid nodules in children. *Endocr Relat Cancer* 2006; **13**: 427–453.

27 Rachmiel M, Charron M, Gupta A, Hamilton J, Wherrett D, Forte V, et al. Evidence-based review of treatment and follow-up of pediatric patients with differentiated thyroid carcinoma. *J Pediatr Endocrinol Metab* 2006; **19**: 1377–1393.

28 Jarzab B, Handkiewicz Junak D, Włoch J, Kalemba B, Roskosz J, Kukulska A, et al. Multivariate analysis of prognostic factors for differentiated thyroid carcinoma in children. *Eur J Nucl Med* 2000; **27**: 833–841.

29 Mazzaferri EL, Kloos RT. Clinical review 128: current approaches to primary therapy for papillary and follicular thyroid cancer. *J Clin Endocrinol Metab* 2001; **86**: 1447–1463.

30 Chow SM, Law SC, Mendenhall WM, Au SK, Yau S, Mang O, et al. Differentiated thyroid carcinoma in childhood and adolescence: clinical course and role of radioiodine. *Pediatr Blood Cancer* 2004; **42**: 176–183.

31 Landau D, Vini L, A'Hern R, Harmer C. Thyroid cancer in children: the Royal Marsden Hospital experience. *Eur J Cancer* 2000; **36**: 214–220.

32 Kuijt WJ, Huang SA. Children with differentiated thyroid cancer achieve adequate hyperthyrotropinemia within 14 days of levothyroxine withdrawal. *J Clin Endocrinol Metab* 2005; **90**: 6123–6125.

33 Gagel RF, Tashjian AH Jr, Cummings T, Papathanasopoulos N, Kaplan MM, DeLellis RA, et al. The clinical outcome of prospective screening for multiple endocrine neoplasia type 2a: an 18-year experience. *N Engl J Med* 1988; **318**: 478–484.

34 Norton JA, Fraker DL, Alexander HR, Venzon DJ, Doppman JL, Serrano J, et al. Surgery to cure the Zollinger–Ellison syndrome. *N Engl J Med* 1999; **341**: 635–644.

35 Stratakis CA, Schussheim DH, Freedman SM, Keil MF, Pack SD, Agarwal SK, et al. Pituitary macroadenoma in a 5-year-old: an early expression of multiple endocrine neoplasia type 1. *J Clin Endocrinol Metab* 2000; **85**: 4776–4780.

36 Kakudo K, Carney JA, Sizemore GW. Medullary carcinoma of thyroid: biologic behavior of the sporadic and familial neoplasm. *Cancer* 1985; **55**: 2818–2821.

37 Bergholm U, Bergström R, Ekbom A. Long-term follow-up of patients with medullary carcinoma of the thyroid. *Cancer* 1997; **79**: 132–138.

38 de Groot JW, Zonnenberg BA, van Ufford-Mannesse PQ, de Vries MM, Links TP, Lips CJ, *et al.* A phase II trial of imatinib therapy for metastatic medullary thyroid carcinoma. *J Clin Endocrinol Metab* 2007; **92**: 3466–3469.

39 Chatal JF, Campion L, Kraeber-Bodéré F, Bardet S, Vuillez JP, Charbonnel B, *et al.* French Endocrine Tumor Group. Survival improvement in patients with medullary thyroid carcinoma who undergo pretargeted anti-carcinoembryonic-antigen radioimmuno-therapy: a collaborative study with the French Endocrine Tumor Group. *J Clin Oncol* 2006; **24**: 1705–1711.

40 Young RH, Dickersin GR, Scully RE. Juvenile granulosa cell tumor of the ovary: a clinicopathological analysis of 125 cases. *Am J Surg Pathol* 1984; **8**: 575–596.

41 Cushing B, Giller R, Ablin A, Cohen L, Cullen J, Hawkins E, *et al.* Surgical resection alone is effective treatment for ovarian immature teratoma in children and adolescents: a report of the Pediatric Oncology Group and the Children's Cancer Group. *Am J Obstet Gynecol* 1999; **181**: 353–358.

42 Morice P, Wicart-Poque F, Rey A, El-Hassan J, Pautier P, Lhommé C, *et al.* Results of conservative treatment in epithelial ovarian carcinoma. *Cancer* 2001; **92**: 2412–2418.

43 Rogers PC, Olson TA, Cullen JW, Billmire DF, Marina N, Rescorla F, *et al.* Pediatric Oncology Group 9048; Children's Cancer Group 8891. Treatment of children and adolescents with stage II testicular and stages I and II ovarian malignant germ cell tumors: A Pediatric Intergroup Study–Pediatric Oncology Group 9048 and Children's Cancer Group 8891. *J Clin Oncol* 2004; **22**: 3563–3569.

44 Lambert HE, Gregory WM, Nelstrop AE, Rustin GJ. Long-term survival in 463 women treated with platinum analogs for advanced epithelial carcinoma of the ovary: life expectancy compared to women of an age-matched normal population. *Int J Gynecol Cancer* 2004; **14**: 772–778.

45 Pettersson A, Richiardi L, Nordenskjold A, Kaijser M, Akre O. Age at surgery for undescended testis and risk of testicular cancer. *N Engl J Med* 2007; **356**: 1835–1841.

46 Swerdlow AJ, De Stavola BL, Swanwick MA, Maconochie NE. Risks of breast and testicular cancers in young adult twins in England and Wales: evidence on prenatal and genetic aetiology. *Lancet* 1997; **350**: 1723–1728.

47 Martinez-Aguayo A, Rocha A, Rojas N, García C, Parra R, Lagos M, *et al.* Chilean Collaborative Testicular Adrenal Rest Tumor Study Group. Testicular adrenal rest tumors and Leydig and Sertoli cell function in boys with classical congenital adrenal hyperplasia. *J Clin Endocrinol Metab* 2007; **92**: 4583–4589.

48 Wu JT, Book L, Sudar K. Serum alpha fetoprotein (AFP) concentrations in normal infants. *Pediatr Res* 1981; **15**: 50–52.

49 Sugita Y, Clamette TD, Cooke-Yarborough C, *et al.* Testicular and paratesticular tumours in children: 30 years experience. *Aust N Z J Surg* 1999; **69**: 505–508.

18 Diabetes Mellitus

Andrew W. Norris[1] & Joseph I. Wolfsdorf[2]

[1] Division of Endocrinology and Diabetes, University of Iowa Children's Hospital, Iowa City, IA, USA
[2] Division of Endocrinology, Children's Hospital, Boston, MA, USA

Diabetes mellitus is characterized by persistent hyperglycemia resulting from defects in insulin secretion, insulin action or both. Chronic hyperglycemia is associated with long-term damage, dysfunction and failure of various organs, especially the eyes, kidneys, nerves, blood vessels and heart [1]. Most children and adolescents have type 1 diabetes mellitus caused by deficiency of insulin secretion or type 2 diabetes caused by a combination of resistance to insulin action and an inadequate compensatory insulin secretory response. Abnormalities in carbohydrate, fat and protein metabolism characteristic of diabetes are attributable to deficiency of insulin action on target tissues.

There is no biological marker that separates people with diabetes mellitus from non-diabetic individuals. The lack of a marker has led to reliance on hyperglycemia as measured by fasting plasma glucose (FPG) or 2-h post-prandial venous plasma glucose (PG) concentration to make the diagnosis. The diagnostic concentrations of FPG and 2-h post-prandial PG are based on their association with the risk of having or developing retinopathy (Table 18.1). The same disease process may not have progressed sufficiently to cause sustained hyperglycemia necessary to fulfill the criteria for the diagnosis of diabetes mellitus but can cause lesser degrees of impaired glucose regulation, such as impaired fasting glucose (IFG) and/or impaired glucose tolerance (IGT). IGT and IFG are considered to be states of pre-diabetes associated with increased risk for cardiovascular morbidity [1].

Definition and diagnosis of diabetes in children

Diabetes mellitus is diagnosed by:
1 Classic symptoms of diabetes plus casual (defined as any time of day without regard to time since last meal) PG concentration ≥11.1 mmol/L (200 mg/dL);
2 Fasting (for at least 8 h) PG ≥7.0 mmol/L (126 mg/dL);

Brook's Clinical Pediatric Endocrinology, 6th edition. Edited by C. Brook, P. Clayton, R. Brown. © 2009 Blackwell Publishing, ISBN: 978-1-4051-8080-1.

3 2-h post load PG ≥11.1 mmol/L (200 mg/dL) during an oral glucose tolerance test (OGTT).

In the absence of unequivocal hyperglycemia with acute metabolic decompensation, these criteria should be confirmed by repeat testing on a different day. The OGTT is not recommended for routine clinical use [1] but, when indicated, the test should be performed after at least 3 days of adequate (≥150 g/1.73 m²) carbohydrate consumption and using a glucose load containing the equivalent of 75 g anhydrous glucose dissolved in water for individuals weighing >43 kg and 1.75 g/kg for individuals weighing ≤43 kg.

Symptoms of hyperglycemia include polyuria, polydipsia, weight loss, sometimes polyphagia and blurred vision. Chronic hyperglycemia in girls and infants and toddlers of both genders, commonly leads to perineal candidiasis. The diagnosis of type 1 diabetes is usually obvious because most children present with classic symptoms which have been present for a few days to a few weeks accompanied by marked hyperglycemia or with diabetic ketoacidosis (DKA).

These definitions are based on venous plasma glucose concentrations. Although portable glucose meters are useful for screening purposes in clinics and physicians' offices, the diagnosis of diabetes mellitus should be confirmed by measurement of venous plasma glucose on an analytic instrument in a clinical chemistry laboratory. Precautions should be taken to process the blood sample properly and deliver it to the laboratory without delay to prevent glucose utilization by leukocytes that could lead to spuriously low PG concentrations.

Classification

Table 18.2 shows an etiologic classification of diabetes mellitus and Table 18.3 the major clinical characteristics. Genetic studies have led to changes in the classification of diabetes and better understanding of its many causes. They have reinforced the polygenic multifactorial nature of type 1 and 2 diabetes while identifying numerous monogenic causes accounting for a large proportion of neonatal or youth-onset diabetes that is neither type 1 nor type 2.

Table 18.1 Biochemical criteria for diabetes mellitus and lesser degrees of impaired glucose regulation [1].

Test	Normal	Impaired fasting glucose	Impaired glucose tolerance	Diabetes mellitus
FPG mmol/L (mg/dL)	<5.6 (<100)	5.6–6.9 (100–125)		≥7.0 (126)
2-h PG mmol/L (mg/dL)	<7.8 (<140)		7.8–11.0 (140–199)	≥11.1 (200)
Casual PG mmol/L (mg/dL)	<11.1 (200)			≥11.1 (200)

FPG, fasting plasma glucose; PG, plasma glucose.

Table 18.2 Etiologic classification of diabetes mellitus [1].

I. Type 1 diabetes
A. Immune-mediated
B. Idiopathic

II. Type 2 diabetes

III. Other specific types
A. Genetic defects of β-cell function
  MODY
  Mitochondrial DNA
  Monogenic neonatal diabetes

B. Genetic defects in insulin action
  Type A insulin resistance
  Leprechaunism
  Rabson–Mendenhall syndrome
  Lipoatrophic diabetes

C. Diseases of the exocrine pancreas
  Cystic fibrosis
  Hemochromatosis
  Pancreatectomy

D. Endocrinopathies
  Cushing syndrome
  Pheochromocytoma
  Hyperthyroidism

E. Drug- or chemical-induced
  Glucocorticoids
  Diazoxide
  β-Adrenergic agonists
  Pentamidine
  Nicotinic acid
  α-Interferon
  Tacrolimus

F. Infections
  Congenital rubella
  Cytomegalovirus

G. Uncommon forms of immune-mediated diabetes
  "Stiff-man" syndrome
  Anti-insulin receptor antibodies

H. Other genetic syndromes sometimes associated with diabetes
  Down syndrome
  Turner syndrome
  Klinefelter syndrome
  Wolfram syndrome
  Friedreich ataxia
  Prader–Willi syndrome
  Bardet–Biedl syndrome
  Myotonic dystrophy

IV. Gestational diabetes mellitus

MODY, maturity onset diabetes of the young.

Type 1 diabetes mellitus

Type 1A diabetes results from chronic progressive T-cell mediated autoimmune destruction of the β cells of the pancreas leading to severe insulin deficiency and manifested by low or undetectable plasma concentrations of C-peptide. Markers of the process of immune-mediated destruction of β cells include autoantibodies to insulin (IAA), autoantibodies to glutamic acid decarboxylase (GAD$_{65}$) and autoantibodies to the tyrosine phosphatases IA-2 and IA-2β. At least one of these is present in 85–98% of newly diagnosed children. The disease has strong human leukocyte antigen (HLA) associations, with linkage to the major histocompatibility complex (MHC) class II genes DQA, DQB and DRB. Specific HLA-DR/DQ alleles can either predispose to type 1A diabetes or be protective. High-risk alleles include DQA1*0301/

DQB1*0302 or DQA1*0501/DQB1*0201, whereas HLA-DQB1*0602 confers protection [2].

The rate of β-cell destruction is variable, being rapid in some individuals, especially infants and young children, and slower in adolescents and adults, some of whom may retain the ability to secrete insulin for several years (Fig. 18.1) [3]. The disease occurs throughout childhood and adolescence in genetically predisposed individuals but is also related to poorly understood environmental factors. Type 1A diabetes predominantly affects Europoid Caucasians, is somewhat less frequent in African-Americans and is much less common in Asians and Native North Americans.

The classic phenotype used to be that of a thin child with a history of polyuria, polydipsia and weight loss but, with increasing prevalence of obesity in childhood, 20–25% of newly diag-

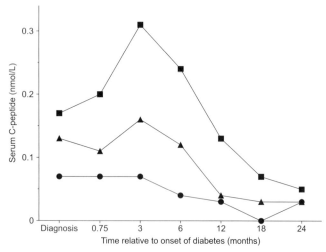

Figure 18.1 Younger children more rapidly lose endogenous insulin production, as evidenced by plasma C-peptide concentrations from the time of diagnosis of type 1 diabetes. Data are stratified by age of onset: 5–14.9 years old (squares), 2–4.9 years old (triangles) and <2 years old (circles). Toddlers have the lowest plasma C-peptide concentrations at diagnosis. The temporary partial remission experienced by older children is readily apparent and is notably absent in toddlers. Copyright 2002 American Diabetes Association, from [3], adapted with permission.

nosed type 1 patients are obese. Patients with type 1A diabetes are prone to other autoimmune disorders.

Type 1 diabetes with no known etiology, so-called type 1B diabetes, is strongly inherited but there is no HLA association nor evidence of β-cell autoimmunity.

Atypical diabetes mellitus

Atypical forms of diabetes mellitus have been described in various populations and have been referred to as Flatbush diabetes, atypical diabetes mellitus, idiopathic type 1 diabetes, ketosis-prone diabetes and type 1.5 diabetes. The hallmark is a propensity to hyperglycemic ketosis or ketoacidosis without key features of type 1 diabetes such as evidence of autoimmunity or sustained insulin dependence. These forms of diabetes have been described primarily in individuals of African or Asian ancestry and there is often a strong family history. Homozygous mutations in Pax4 may contribute to a small number of cases but the genetic defects remain to be determined in the majority of cases. Treatment of atypical diabetes should be based on individual clinical characteristics.

Characteristics distinguishing the common forms of diabetes are shown in Table 18.3.

Genetic defects of insulin secretion
Maturity onset diabetes of the young

Maturity onset diabetes of the young (MODY) was originally described as a form of non-insulin-dependent or "maturity-onset" type diabetes with onset before age 25 and inherited in an autosomal dominant pattern. MODY, which may account for 1–

5% of all cases of diabetes in industrialized countries, is a heterogeneous group of disorders caused by a variety of monogenic mutations (Table 18.4). Hyperglycemia in MODY is the result of varying degrees of insulin deficiency with minimal or no defect in insulin action. Onset is typically in the pubertal or young adult years with mild to moderate hyperglycemia. Other features include a family history of diabetes in successive generations, no evidence of insulin resistance, absent pancreatic autoantibodies, no propensity to ketosis and no predisposition to obesity beyond that of the general population. Confirmation of the diagnosis and of the specific type of MODY requires molecular genetic testing.

Treatment of MODY

The type of MODY predicts the therapeutic response and some variants exhibit excellent clinical response to sulfonylureas (Table 18.4) [4]. Patients with MODY require monitoring to ensure glycemic control to avoid complications. Exercise and medical nutrition therapy to maintain normal weight and insulin sensitivity should be emphasized and pharmacologic treatment, when necessary, is tailored to the patient's specific MODY type and level of hyperglycemia.

Mitochondrial diabetes

Diabetes may be the presenting manifestation of syndromes caused by mutations in mitochondrial DNA [5]. **Maternally inherited diabetes and deafness syndrome** (MIDD; MIM 520000) may present in children. The most common mutation occurs at position 3243 in the tRNA leucine gene, leading to an A-to-G transition. This and other mutations in related tRNA mitochondrial genes can also be associated with multiple other features including myopathy, encephalopathy, lactic acidosis and myoclonic epilepsy. **Kearns–Sayre syndrome** (MIM 530000) is also caused by mitocondrial gene mutations and is characterized by ophthalmoplegia, retinal pigmentary degeneration and cardiomyopathy and may include several hormone deficiencies including diabetes in approximately 13% of cases. Diabetes can be treated with diet and sulfonylureas but may require insulin. Patients with impaired mitochondrial function are prone to develop lactic acidosis and therefore metformin should not be used.

Other molecular disorders

Thiamine-responsive megaloblastic anemia syndrome (MIM 249270) is caused by mutations in a thiamine transport gene (SLC19A2) and is often accompanied by diabetes mellitus and/or sensorineural deafness. Treatment with thiamine corrects the anemia and sometimes improves the diabetes but insulin is often required.

Rare defects in prohormone convertase activity inherited in an autosomal dominant pattern leads to impaired processing of proinsulin and mild glucose intolerance. A few families have been identified who secrete mutant insulins with impaired ability to bind to the insulin receptor. Glucose metabolism may be normal or only mildly impaired in these individuals.

Table 18.3 Characteristics of prevalent forms of primary diabetes mellitus in children and adolescents.

	Type 1A	Type 2	MODY	ADM*
Prevalence	Common	Increasing	≤5% in Caucasians	≥10% in African-American
Age at onset	Throughout childhood	Pubertal	Pubertal	Pubertal
Onset	Acute severe	Insidious to severe	Gradual	Acute severe
Ketosis at onset	Common	~1/3	Rare	Common
Affected relative	5–10%	60–90%	90%	>75%
Female:male	1:1	1.1–1.7:1	1:1	Variable
Inheritance	Polygenic	Polygenic	Autosomal dominant	Autosomal dominant
HLA-DR3/4	↑ Association	No association	No association	No association
Ethnicity	All, Caucasian at highest risk	All†	Caucasian	African-American/Asian
Insulin secretion	Decreased/absent	Variable	Decreased	Variably decreased
Insulin sensitivity	Normal when controlled	Decreased	Normal	Normal
Insulin dependence	Permanent	Variable	Variable	Episodic
Obesity	No‡	>90%	Uncommon	Varies with population
Acanthosis nigricans	No	Common	No‡	No‡
Pancreatic autoantibodies	Yes§	No	No	No

ADM, atypical diabetes mellitus; HLA, human leukocyte antigen; MODY, maturity onset diabetes of the young.

*ADM, also referred to as Flatbush diabetes, type 1.5 diabetes, ketosis-prone diabetes and idiopathic type 1 diabetes mellitus.

†In North America, type 2 diabetes predominates in African-American, Mexican-American, Native American, Canadian First Nation children and adolescents and is also more common in Asians and South Asians than in Caucasians.

‡Mirrors rate in general population.

§Autoantibodies to insulin (IAA), islet cell cytoplasm (ICA), glutamic acid decarboxylase (GAD) or tyrosine phosphatase (insulinoma associated) antibody (IA-2 and IA-2 β) at diagnosis in 85–98%.

Table 18.4 Classification of maturity onset diabetes of the young (MODY).

Type(MIM)*	Gene	Frequency	Associated features	Common treatments
MODY1 (125850)	HNF-4α	Uncommon	Glucosuria; reduced serum lipids; macrosomia and hyperinsulinemic hypoglycemia in infancy	Sulfonylurea
MODY2 (125851)	Glucokinase	Common	Stable mild hyperglycemia	Diet and exercise
MODY3 (600496)	HNF-1α	Common		Sulfonylurea
MODY4 (606392)	IPF-1	Rare		Oral hypoglycemic agent, insulin
MODY5 (137920)	HNF-1 β	Rare	Renal dysplasia, renal cysts	Insulin
MODY6 (606394)	NeuroD1	Rare		Insulin
MODY7 (610508)	KLF11	Rare		Oral hypoglycemic agent and/or insulin
MODY8 (609812)	CEL	Rare	Pancreatic exocrine dysfunction	Oral hypoglycemic agent and/or insulin
MODY9 (612225)	PAX4	Rare		Diet, oral hypoglycemic agent
INS-related†	Insulin	Rare		Insulin

*MIM, Mendelian Inheritance in Man. †As yet unnamed.

Impaired insulin sensitivity

Genetic defects of insulin signaling

Several rare insulin resistance syndromes are caused by genetic defects in the insulin receptor or its cellular signaling apparatus. **Leprechaunism** (MIM 246200) is the most severe presenting at birth with low birthweight, characteristic facial features, near total lack of adipose tissue, acanthosis nigricans and extreme insulin resistance. It is usually fatal in infancy. **Rabson–Mendenhall syn**drome (MIM 262190) is characterized by extreme insulin resistance with acanthosis nigricans, abnormalities of the skeleton, teeth and nails, growth retardation, genitomegaly and pineal gland hyperplasia. **Type A insulin resistance syndrome** (MIM 610549) typically presents in thin young women with extreme hyperinsulinism, acanthosis nigricans, glycosuria, hyperandrogenism with virilization and polycystic ovarian syndrome (PCOS).

Inherited lipoatrophic diabetes

Lipoatrophic diabetes is associated with widespread loss of adipose tissue and severe insulin resistance. Hyperlipemia, hepatomegaly, acanthosis nigricans and elevated basal metabolic rate are common findings. Several forms of lipoatrophic diabetes are caused by gene defects. **Seip–Berardinelli syndrome** (MIM 269700) is inherited as an autosomal recessive and usually presents in the first year of life with lack of subcutaneous adipose tissue. Insulin resistance, acanthosis nigricans and diabetes mellitus develop before adolescence. **Familial partial lipodystrophy, Dunnigan syndrome** (MIM 151660), is caused by an autosomal dominant mutation in the lamin A/C gene or peroxisome proliferator-activated receptor gamma gene. It presents in adolescence with loss of subcutaneous adipose tissue from the trunk and extremities but with excess adipose tissue on the face and neck.

Acquired insulin resistance

Severe generalized acquired lipoatrophy may present during childhood. Diabetes ensues within a few years of the loss of adipose tissue. Some forms of acquired lipoatrophic diabetes are caused by immune-mediated destruction of adipocytes and are frequently associated with other autoimmune diseases. Some patients with **HIV disease treated with protease inhibitors** develop partial lipodystrophy. **Type B insulin resistance syndrome** is a rare cause of diabetes caused by circulating antibodies directed against the insulin receptor.

Diabetes as a component of specific genetic syndromes

In **Wolfram syndrome** (MIM 222300), also known as DIDMOAD (diabetes insipidus, diabetes mellitus, optic atrophy and deafness), insulin-deficient diabetes mellitus is often the presenting characteristic, with a median age at onset of 6 years. Most cases have an identifiable mutation of the Wolframin gene inherited in an autosomal recessive fashion.

Many other syndromes are associated with an increased risk of diabetes (Table 18.2). **Alstrom, Prader–Willi** and **Bardet–Biedl** syndromes combine severe obesity with insulin-resistant diabetes mellitus.

Neonatal diabetes mellitus

A monogenic defect (Table 18.5) can now be determined in most cases of diabetes with onset within the first 6 months of life and, occasionally, when diabetes has its onset between 6 and 12 months of life. Many of the monogenic etiologies are associated with congenital defects, conditions or syndromes (Table 18.5). Approximately half of cases are transient, resolving within months

Table 18.5 Classification of neonatal diabetes mellitus.

Region	Gene	Genetics	Associated features	Outcome/treatment	Familial diabetes	OMIM
Transient						
6q24	Probably ZAC	pUPD or pDUP	Macroglossia, anterior wall defects	Diabetes often recurs in adolescence	Often	601410
Transient or permanent						
11p15.1	KCNJ11	AD	Dysmorphology; neurological features possible	Typically responds to sulfonylureas; transient cases often relapse	Often	610582
11p15.1	ABCC8	AD,AR	Neurological features possible	Typically responds to sulfonylureas; transient cases often relapse	Often	610374
17cen-q21.3	HNF1B	AD	Renal cysts; pancreatic atrophy	Lifelong treatment	Often	137920
Permanent						
Xp11.23-q13.3	FOXP3	XR	IPEX	Poor prognosis	No	304790
2p12	EIF2AK3	AR	Wolcott–Rallison sydrome	Early death	No	226980
11p15.5	INS	AD	Possibly acanthosis nigricans	Lifelong diabetes treatment	Often	–
13q12.1	IPF1	AR	Pancreatic agenesis	Lifelong treatment; exocrine pancreas replacement therapy	Often	260370
10p12.3	PTF1A	AR	Cerebellar and pancreatic hypogenesis	Early mortality	No	609069
9p24.3-p23	GLIS3	AR	Severe congenital hypothyroidism, facial anomalies, congenital glaucoma, hepatic fibrosis and polycystic kidneys	Early mortality	No	610199
7p15-p13	GK	AR	Growth retardation	Lifelong diabetes treatment	Often	138079

AD, autosomal dominant; AR, autosomal recessive; IPEX, immune dysregulation, polyendocrinopathy, enteropathy, X-linked; pDUP, paternal duplication; pUPD, paternal uniparental disomy; XR, X-linked recessive.

but mild non-insulin-dependent diabetes recurs in adolescence or early adulthood in a substantial proportion of patients. Imprinting defects in chromosome region 6q24 are the most common etiology of transient neonatal diabetes. Activating mutations in the Kir6.2 inwardly rectifying ATP-sensitive potassium channel (KCNJ11) or the sulfonylurea receptor (ABCC8) genes account for a majority of the remaining cases [6] and are associated with later onset and less microsomia than 6q24 defects and can often be treated with high doses of sulfonylureas. Sulfonylurea treatment may improve some of the peripheral nerve abnormalities that can accompany neonatal diabetes mellitus caused by KCNJ11 mutations [6].

Mutations in KCNJ11 and ABCC8 are common causes of permanent neonatal diabetes, as are specific defects in the insulin (INS) gene. Homozygous mutations in the genes for MODY2 and MODY4 or heterozygous mutation in the gene for MODY5 are uncommon causes of permanent neonatal diabetes mellitus.

The IPEX (immunodysregulation, polyendocrinopathy, enteropathy, X-linked) syndrome is characterized by intractable diarrhea, diabetes and autoimmunity and is often fatal. The Wolcott–Rallison syndrome is characterized by multiple epiphyseal dysplasia and early-onset diabetes.

The initial treatment of neonatal diabetes consists of administration of insulin to control hyperglycemia. Once replacement therapy has been initiated, catch-up growth is usually rapid. A trial of therapy with a high dose (0.5–1.0 mg/kg/day) of glibenclamide (glyburide) should be attempted in cases with mutations of KCNJ11 or ABCC8.

Secondary causes of diabetes
Cystic fibrosis related diabetes

Because of the increasing life expectancy of patients with cystic fibrosis, cystic fibrosis related diabetes (CFRD) has become more common. Insulinopenia is caused by pancreatic destruction and amyloid deposition in the islets. Insulin resistance may be a prominent feature during exacerbations of pulmonary disease and causes deterioration in glycemia. First-phase insulin release is particularly affected but ketoacidosis is rare. CFRD can present in the first decade but is usually seen in the second and third decades of life. The development of CFRD is associated with progressive clinical deterioration and increased mortality. Screening for glucose intolerance should begin at age 14 years and hyperglycemia should be treated aggressively [7].

Insulin is the only treatment for CFRD. It prevents protein catabolism, promotes weight gain and improves pulmonary function. Ideally, a basal-bolus regimen using insulin glargine and rapid-acting insulin is used and diet should not be restricted. Patients should be taught carbohydrate counting and how to use rapid-acting insulin with meals. Destruction of the pancreatic α-cells results in glucagon deficiency and chronic use of glucocorticoids can cause adrenocortical insufficiency. Patients with CFRD are thereby at increased risk for severe hypoglycemia owing to malabsorption and impaired counter-regulatory responses.

Hemosiderosis

Frequent blood transfusions and chelation therapy has improved the prognosis of thalassemia major. However, adolescents and young adult patients are at increased risk of developing diabetes mellitus as a result of the effects of iron overload on β-cell function and insulin sensitivity. Insulin is required for treatment.

Drug-induced diabetes

Various pharmacological agents can cause hyperglycemia [8]. **Glucocorticoids** induce severe hepatic and peripheral insulin resistance and are potent hyperglycemic agents. Glucocorticoid-induced diabetes is relatively common in children who receive massive doses of glucocorticoids after organ transplantation, as a component of chemotherapy for malignancy and in other circumstances in which glucocorticoids are used as anti-inflammatory or immunosuppressive agents. **Growth hormone** is an occasional cause of glucose intolerance or diabetes. Atypical **antipsychotic agents** increase the risk of diabetes mellitus probably by inducing insulin resistance, sometimes but not always, associated with weight gain. **Antiretroviral protease inhibitors** increase the risk of diabetes mellitus associated with features of the metabolic syndrome and lipoatrophic changes. **Beta-adrenergic agents** used for treatment of acute asthma are common causes of transient hyperglycemia. **Diazoxide** decreases insulin secretion by direct action on the K_{ATP}/Kir6.2 potassium channel involved in the regulation of insulin secretion. Pediatric transplant recipients are especially prone to insulin-requiring diabetes when treated with the calcineurin inhibitor **tacrolimus** (FK506). **Ciclosporin** has also been reported to have toxic effects on the β cell. L-Asparaginase often causes transient insulin-requiring diabetes.

Type 1 diabetes mellitus

Epidemiology of type 1 diabetes mellitus

The incidence of type 1 diabetes varies 400-fold between geographic regions, with age-adjusted rates of 40.9/100 000 per year in Finland and 0.1/100 000 per year in areas of China and Venezuela (Fig. 18.2) [9] but the incidence of childhood diabetes is climbing worldwide at a rate of 2.8% per year, with increases documented in six continents [9]. A significant proportion of this variation is attributable to differences in the prevalence of protective HLA-DQ alleles among populations. The incidence of type 1 diabetes in children ≤14 years of age is similar in UK and USA, 15–26 and 15–18 per 100 000 per year, respectively [9]. Incidence also varies among ethnic subgroups within a given geographical area. Some migrant populations retain their original risk of type 1 diabetes, whereas others show a trend toward acquiring the diabetes risk of their new location. Secular increases in the incidence of pediatric type 1 diabetes during the mid-late 20th century have been documented in North America and Western Europe at rates higher than can be explained by genetic shifts (Fig. 18.3) [10].

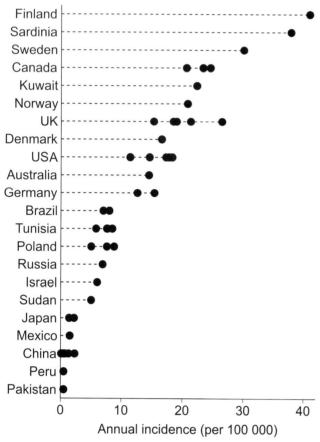

Figure 18.2 Variations in the incidence of type 1 diabetes in children ≤14 year of age among regions of selected countries from six continents. Rates were measured throughout the 1990s. Multiple symbols indicate rates measured in different regions or ethnic populations within that country. Data from the DiaMond study [9].

There has also been an alarming trend towards younger age of onset. Diabetes is no longer uncommon in toddlers and pre-school-aged children (Fig. 18.4) [9,10]. These temporal and age-related shifts in diabetes incidence all underscore the increasing need for expert pediatric diabetes care.

Etiology, genetics and family risk of type 1A diabetes

Type 1A diabetes mellitus occurs in genetically susceptible individuals as a consequence of chronic T-cell-mediated destruction of insulin-secreting β cells of the islets of Langerhans [11]. Auto-antibodies are detected in 85–98% of newly diagnosed children. Insulitis, characterized by lymphocytic infiltration of the islets of Langerhans, is observed in children who died soon after the onset of type 1 diabetes. There is strong linkage to the MHC locus.

Variation in the MHC locus accounts for about half of the genetic risk for type 1A diabetes. Increased susceptibility to type 1A diabetes is conferred by certain MHC alleles such as DRB1*0401/2/5-DQA1*0301-DQB1*0302 (HLA-DR4-DQ8) and DRB1*0301-DQA1*0501-DQB1*0201 (HLA-DR3-DQ2) [12]. Numerous non-MHC genetic loci contribute weakly to type 1A diabetes risk. Decreased susceptibility to type 1A diabetes is conferred by several MHC alleles including DRB1*1501-DQA1*0102-DQB1*0602 (HLA-DR2-DQ6) [12].

Most (85%) new cases of type 1A diabetes occur in persons without an affected first-degree relative [12]. The risk to siblings of an affected child is approximately 6%. The risk to the child of a parent with type 1A diabetes is 1.3–4% or 6–9%, respectively, depending on whether the mother or the father has diabetes. Concordance rates for monozygotic twins are 21–70% and 0–13% for dizygotic twins. These data indicate that both genetic and environmental factors contribute to the pathogenesis of type 1A diabetes. The environmental factor(s) that contribute to the

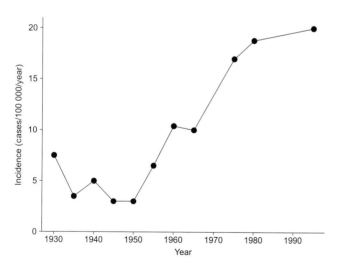

Figure 18.3 Secular increases in the incidence of childhood type 1 diabetes, as measured among Norwegian children less than 10 years old. Similar trends have been documented in the USA and in many countries in Europe. Copyright 2002 American Diabetes Association, from Gale [160], adapted with permission.

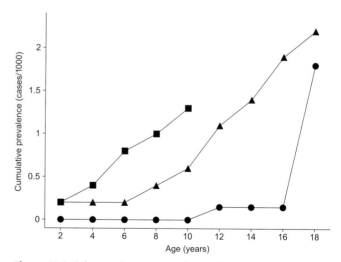

Figure 18.4 Shifts towards younger age of onset of type 1 diabetes in three UK birth cohorts born in 1946 (circles), 1958 (triangles) and 1970 (squares). Copyright 2002 American Diabetes Association, from Gale (160), adapted with permission.

pathogenesis of type 1A diabetes are not known with certainty and there are no proven environmental interventions that reduce the risk of type 1 diabetes. Possible environmental factors include viral infections, diet, hygiene and toxins [13]. It is likely that environmental induction of type 1 diabetes relates to the chronology of exposure and on interactions with genetic susceptibility.

Prediction and prevention of type 1 diabetes

The onset of overt diabetes represents the endpoint of a progressive selective immunologically mediated attack on β cells [14]. Clinical diabetes occurs when 90% have been damaged or destroyed in genetically susceptible individuals. It is a cellular-mediated process, presumably a specific reaction to one or more β-cell proteins (autoantigens), although probably initiated by some environmental factor(s). There is consequent progressive impairment of β-cell function and decline in β-cell mass.

A secondary humoral immune response is characterized by the appearance of autoantibodies that serve as markers of the immune damage to β cells [15]. This insidious process may evolve over a period of years [16]. The decline in β-cell function and mass is evidenced by loss of the first-phase insulin response to an intravenous glucose challenge [17] and later by impaired glucose tolerance or, less often, by impaired fasting glucose concentration [18].

Prediction of diabetes in relatives of a person with type 1 diabetes and in the general population can be determined by a risk assessment that includes HLA genotyping and measurement of immunologic markers (autoantibodies directed against islet constituents – insulin, glutamic acid decarboxylase, IA-2) combined with tests of β-cell function [16]. Autoantibodies restricted to a single antigen have little prognostic value but an immune response that has spread to multiple antigens and is stable over time is highly predictive. Individuals who have multiple islet autoantibodies are destined to develop immune-mediated diabetes.

The latency period between the detection of antibodies and the clinical onset of disease may extend over several years and offers an opportunity to intervene [14]. Interventions, including parenteral insulin [16], oral insulin [19] and nicotinamide [20], have failed to arrest or retard the diabetes disease process. We can predict the development of type 1 diabetes but do not yet have a safe and effective preventive therapy so whether screening should be performed outside the context of clinical studies is controversial.

At the onset of symptoms, about 10% of β cells are viable and there is good evidence that residual β-cell function has clinical benefit. The Diabetes Control and Complications Trial (DCCT) identified a "virtuous circle" whereby residual insulin secretion resulted in better glucose control with less hypoglycemia and slower progression to vascular complications and better control, in turn, prolonged β-cell function [21]. Much investigation has been directed at arresting the type 1 diabetes disease process, both during the evolution of the disease and at the time of presentation [14]. The goal is to halt destruction of remaining β cells, perhaps allowing them to recover function, thereby lessening the severity of clinical manifestations and disease progression. Success is measured by preservation of C-peptide.

Trials of immune intervention with ciclosporin and azathioprine at the time of diagnosis have demonstrated prolonged β-cell function and provided the proof of principle but the effect was modest and not sustained when treatment was stopped and the side effects, especially of ciclosporin, could not justify long-term use. Short-term interventions in recent-onset type 1 diabetes designed to alter the immune response in a manner that might result in sustained beneficial effects without continuous exposure to the intervention have included an immunomodulatory peptide from heat-shock protein-60 (p277 peptide) [22], a GAD vaccine [23] and infusion of anti-CD3 monoclonal antibodies [24,25], all of which have suggested preservation of β-cell function. It is not known whether the effect will be sustained beyond the initial period for which the results have been reported.

A primary prevention study, the Trial to Reduce IDDM in the Genetically at Risk (TRIGR), is in progress directed at high-risk children with genetic risk factors but prior to expression of measurable β-cell autoimmunity. Its goal is to determine if removal of cow's milk proteins (substituting casein hydrolysate) during early life will decrease the frequency of type 1 diabetes [26].

Type 1A diabetes mellitus and other autoimmune diseases (see also Chapter 14)

Individuals with type 1A diabetes are at increased risk for several other autoimmune diseases. There are also several autoimmune syndromes whose phenotype includes type 1 diabetes.

Autoimmune thyroid disorders are common [27], approximately 22% of patients having thyroid autoantibodies, but the prevalence of thyroid dysfunction varies widely and hypothyroidism can be expected to develop in 6–14% of pediatric patients. Even subclinical hypothyroidism may increase the risk of hypoglycemia. Asymptomatic individuals should be screened annually for thyroid dysfunction.

In Western Europe, North America and Australia, the prevalence of **celiac disease** (gluten-induced enteropathy) is 4.1% (0–10.4%). Screening shows that 3.7–9.9% (mean 7.4%) of children with type 1 diabetes have anti-endomysial or tissue transglutaminase antibodies and the majority of these have a positive biopsy. Most cases detected by serologic screening with biopsy confirmation have silent disease with villous atrophy only or a subclinical form of the disease with subtle manifestations that may be recognized only in retrospect. It has been suggested that all children with type 1 diabetes should be screened for celiac disease but the potential benefits and risks of screening children with diabetes for celiac disease have not been systematically assessed [28]. If screening is not performed routinely, clinicians should consider the possibility of celiac disease in patients with unexplained poor growth, poor glycemic control, diarrhea, abdominal pain or recurrent hypoglycemia. Measurement of anti-endomysial or tissue transglutaminase antibodies should be combined with measurement of the serum IgA concentration to rule out IgA deficiency, which can cause a false-negative serologic result.

Anti-21-hydroxylase antibodies occur in 1.6–2.3% of individuals with type 1 diabetes but only 1 in 200–300 progress to develop clinical adrenocortical insufficiency [29]. The risk increases to 1 in 30 in patients with two autoimmune processes (e.g. diabetes and thyroiditis). The development of adrenocortical insufficiency in type 1 diabetes is characterized by recurrent unexplained hypoglycemia and decreasing insulin requirements.

Polyautoimmune disorders associated with type 1 diabetes

Autoiummune polyendocrine syndrome type 1 (APS-1, MIM 240300)

APS-1, also known as autoimmune polyendocrinopathy-candidiasis-ectodermal dystrophy (APECED) syndrome, is a rare autosomal recessive disorder caused by mutation of the autoimmune regulator gene (AIRE-1). At least two of three major criteria are required for the diagnosis: primary hypoparathyroidism, Addison disease and chronic mucocutaneous candidiasis. Additional autoimmune features may appear over the course of a patient's life, including autoimmune thyroiditis, type 1A diabetes, vitiligo, autoimmune hepatitis, alopecia, ovarian failure and hypophysitis.

Immune dysregulation, polyendocrinopathy, enteropathy, X-linked syndrome (IPEX, MIM 304790)

IPEX syndrome, caused by mutations in FOXP3, is a rare X-linked recessive disorder characterized by early-onset type 1A diabetes and severe atopy, chronic immune-mediated diarrhea, failure to thrive, thyroiditis, eosinophilia and hemolytic anemia.

Autoiummune polyendocrine syndrome type 2 (APS-2)

Like type 1A diabetes, genetic susceptibility to APS-2 appears to be conferred by high-risk HLA alleles. Unlike APS-1, it is not a monogenic disorder. Diagnosis of APS-2 requires at least two of three major criteria: Addison disease, autoimmune thyroid disease and type 1A diabetes. Associated findings may include celiac disease, autoimmune hepatitis, gonadal failure, vitiligo, alopecia, pernicious anemia and myasthenia gravis.

Type 2 diabetes mellitus

Type 2 diabetes results from a combination of insulin resistance and inadequate compensatory insulin secretion (relative insulin deficiency). The relative contributions of these two pathophysiological components range from predominantly insulin resistance to predominantly β-cell failure. The β-cell failure is not autoimmune mediated and there are no reliable biomarkers for type 2 diabetes. Owing to insulin resistance, circulating insulin concentrations may be elevated but may be abnormally low if β-cell dysfunction is severe. Most youths with type 2 diabetes are overweight or obese, which exacerbates insulin resistance. The pathophysiology is complex and incompletely understood but clearly involves both genetic and lifestyle factors.

Type 2 diabetes, which currently affects 7% of the US population and 4% of Britons, is a leading cause of morbidity and mortality. Youth-onset of type 2 diabetes was rarely reported before the mid-1990s. Since then, rising prevalence and/or incidence rates of youth-onset type 2 diabetes have been documented in many populations, ethnic groups and geographical locations. Some characteristics of youth-onset type 2 diabetes differ substantially from those of adult-onset type 2 diabetes but, as in adults, the disease is closely linked to obesity and family history. There have been very few longitudinal studies of youth-onset type 2 diabetes. Thus, the natural history, optimal therapy and long-term prognosis remain to be determined.

Epidemiology

Table 18.6 shows rates of youth-onset type 2 diabetes in various populations throughout the world over the past several decades. Although these studies cannot strictly be compared owing to differences in methodology and diabetes classification, several consistent features are apparent. Type 2 diabetes is uncommon before puberty and studies conducted in multi-ethnic populations clearly show that ethnicity has a strong impact. The highest rates are in the Pima American Indian population. Other high-risk groups include Canadian First Nation, Hispanic, African, Asian, Pacific Islander and indigenous Australian (Aboriginal) youths, whereas Europoid-Caucasians tend to have relatively lower rates. Studies spanning several decades have documented increasing rates of type 2 diabetes among young persons, which have been attributed to rising rates of pediatric obesity and environmental factors such as sedentary lifestyle and excessive consumption of calorie- and sugar-dense foods. As these characteristics of Western affluence spread to the economically developing regions of the world with their predominance of high-risk ethnicities, global rates of youth-onset type 2 diabetes are expected to continue to rise.

Genetic and environmental risk factors

Type 2 diabetes is highly heritable, as evidenced by concordance rates of 50–92% in monozygotic compared to 37–42% in dizygotic twins. The inheritance pattern is polygenic. Recent genome-wide association studies involving large numbers of individuals with type 2 diabetes show that no single gene strongly contributes to type 2 diabetes risk. Rather, common variants at a small number of genetic loci weakly contribute to the development of type 2 diabetes with a relative risk of 1.10–1.37 [30]. Because the vast majority of subjects in these studies have adult-onset type 2 diabetes, the importance of these genetic variants to the risk of youth-onset type 2 diabetes is unknown. Furthermore, these association studies were conducted on homogeneous Northern European populations. Thus, it is not yet clear which genes contribute to the vast majority of youth-onset type 2 diabetes worldwide.

Multiple risk factors have been identified for the development of youth-onset type 2 diabetes (Table 18.7) but few longitudinal studies have been conducted to determine which of these factors

Table 18.6 Rates of type 2 diabetes mellitus in youth.

Country	Method	Classification	Ethnicity	Year	Ages	Rate
Incidence*						
Japan	UA	Strict	–	1974–1979	6–15	1.7
			–	1982–2002		2.8
Libya	MR	Strict	–	1981–1990	15–19	5.9
USA	MR	Strict	–	1982	0–19	0.7
				1994		7.2
USA	MR	Broad	H, AA	1985–1989	0–17	2.6
				1990–1994		3.8
Taiwan	UA	Strict	–	1992–1999	6–18	6.5
Austria	MR	Strict	–	1999–2001	0–15	0.25
USA	MR,SR	Broad	–	2002–2003	0–4	0
					5–9	0.8
					10–14	8.1
					15–19	11.8
Australia	MR	Broad	I	2002	<17	16
			Non-I			1
UK	MR	Strict	White	2004–2005	0–16	0.5
			Black			3.9
			Asian			1.3
Prevalence (%)						
USA	OGTT	NR	Pima	1967–1976	15–19	2.6
				1987–1996		4.6
Canada	MR	Broad	I	1978–1992	0–15	0.25
Tanzania	FG,OGTT	Screen	–	1982–1983	0–19	0.15
Togo	OGTT	Screen	–	1987	<20	0[†]
USA	FG	Screen	–	1988–1994	12–19	0.13
Canada	MR	Strict	I	1990	5–14	0.05
USA	MR	Broad	I	1990	15–19	0.32
				1998		0.54
Bangladesh	OGTT	Screen	–	1995	15–19	0.06
Saudi Arabia	OGTT	Screen	–	~1999	<14	0.12
USA	FG	Screen	–	1999–2002	12–19	0.15
USA	MR,SR	Broad	NHW	2001	10–19	0.02
			AA			0.11
			H			0.05
			API			0.05
			I			0.17
Israel	MR	Broad	–	~2002	17	0.03
USA	FG,OGTT	Strict	–	~2003	~10–19	0.12
Turkey	FG	Screen	–	~2003	12–18	0[†]
India	FG	Strict	–	~2005	12–19	0.04

Data tabulated from 24 studies of various populations based on cross-sectional sampling, prospective registries, health systems with defined broad catchment, school systems or mandatory conscription. Classifications used in each study were defined as:

Strict – requiring negative islet-related antibodies, documented hyperinsulinism and/or glycemic control without insulin;

Screen – study assumes that asymptomatic cases identified by screening are type 2 diabetes;

Broad – other approaches including diagnostic codes or less stringent criteria.

FG, fasting glucose; OGTT, oral glucose tolerance test; MR, medical record review; SR, self-report; UA, urinalysis screening for glycosuria; AA, African-American; API, Asian/Pacific Islander; H, Hispanic; I, Indigenous such as American Indian; NHW, non-Hispanic White; NR, not reported.

*Per 100 000 per year.

†Studies reporting rates of zero screened at least 800 youth.

Table 18.7 Risk factors for the development of youth-onset type 2 diabetes mellitus.

Well established or widely accepted
Obesity
Impaired glucose tolerance
Impaired fasting glucose
Elevated fasting insulin
Family history of type 2 diabetes
In utero exposure to maternal diabetes
Low or high birthweight for gestational age
Dyslipidemia
Hypertension
PCOS
Acanthosis nigricans
Ethnicity

Modifiable factors contributing to childhood obesity
Sugar-sweetened beverages
Sedentary lifestyle
Protective effect of having been breastfed

Suspected
Binge eating disorder

PCOS, polycystic ovarian syndrome.

predict who will actually develop diabetes. Among Pima Indians aged 5–19 years, the best predictors of youth-onset type 2 diabetes were fasting and 2-h plasma glucose concentrations during an OGTT, a low HDL-cholesterol concentration and body mass index [31] but overall prediction was imperfect with the optimized multivariate model based on 10 diabetes-associated factors accounting for a relative risk of only 3.4.

Prevention

Progression from IGT to type 2 diabetes over 3–6 years in overweight adults can be reduced by 31–58% by intensive lifestyle modification. Successful interventions have incorporated weight reduction goals, low-fat diets and regular moderate exercise, supported by frequent individualized dietary and exercise counseling. The efficacy of these approaches in preventing type 2 diabetes in the young have yet to be determined but studies have demonstrated the potential usefulness of a variety of programs based on principles of behavioral therapy, to improve lifestyle choices and/or type 2 risk factors among the young at risk in schools, community, camp and family.

Metformin and thiazolidinediones (insulin sensitizing agents), acarbose (carbohydrate absorption blocker) and orlistat (lipid absorption blocker) reduce the progression to type 2 diabetes in high-risk adults by 9–89% over 3–4 years of intervention. Thiazolidinediones, which reduce risk by 50–89%, are accompanied by significant side effects, including weight gain, osteoporosis, fluid retention and risk of heart failure.

Metformin reduces risk of progression to type 2 diabetes without major side effects by 31%. There are no data on type 2 diabetes as a clinical endpoint in the young but metformin has been shown to improve hyperinsulinemia in obese children with IGT. The American Diabetes Association currently recommends that, in addition to lifestyle counseling, primary prevention with metformin may be considered in those who are at high risk as defined by the combination of obesity, IGT and IFG. Enthusiasm for application of this recommendation to children is currently hampered by lack of evidence of efficacy on clinical endpoints, lack of data to allow identification of a high probability of progressing to type 2 diabetes and lack of data regarding the benefit:risk ratio of long-term use of these medications.

Presentation

Type 1 diabetes mellitus

Most children with newly diagnosed type 1 diabetes present with polyuria, polydipsia and weight loss for a few days to several weeks. Other presentations include recent onset of enuresis in a previously toilet-trained child, failure to gain weight appropriately in a growing child, vaginal candidiasis, especially in a prepubertal child, recurrent skin infections, irritability and deteriorating school performance [32].

The frequency of DKA at diabetes onset varies widely by geographic location, ranging from 15 to 67% in Europe and North America and more in developing countries [33,34]. There is an inverse relation between the frequency of DKA and the incidence of type 1 diabetes in different populations. DKA at initial presentation is more frequent in infants, toddlers and preschool-age children, in children who do not have a first-degree relative with type 1 diabetes and in children whose families are of lower socio-economic status [33].

Prospective follow-up of high-risk subjects shows that the diagnosis can be made in the majority of asymptomatic individuals when metabolic abnormalities are still relatively mild [16,35]. The progression of type 1 diabetes tends to follow a clinical course that includes an abrupt onset of classic symptoms that rapidly disappear after starting insulin replacement. This is often followed by a temporary remission ("honeymoon phase") with partial recovery of endogenous insulin secretion, demonstrable by plasma C-peptide concentrations (Fig. 18.1), and characterized by stable near-normal blood glucose concentrations and decreasing insulin requirements [32]. Severe DKA and young age at presentation reduce the likelihood of a remission phase. Recurrence or persistence of the autoimmune attack on β cells, however, leads invariably to further β-cell destruction and progressive decline in insulin production until it eventually ceases completely.

Type 2 diabetes mellitus

A major difficulty in analyzing and interpreting the many studies that have examined the characteristics at onset of type 2 diabetes in various populations of children is the wide range of definitions used to classify type 2 diabetes. The studies that employ strict criteria for the diagnosis show several common characteristics (Table 18.8), including obesity, frequent family history, acanthosis nigricans, female preponderance and average age in mid-puberty. The presentation can range from insidious to severe and DKA is not uncommon, which contrasts with adult-onset type 2 diabetes, in which DKA is rare. The characteristics shown in Table 18.8 are recapitulated in numerous additional studies of youth-onset type 2 diabetes that employ less stringent definitions (Table 18.9). Many young people with type 2 diabetes present with classic symptoms including weight loss. Diagnosis in asymptomatic individuals is common, either as a consequence of the incidental finding of glycosuria or hyperglycemia or as a result of screening individuals at risk. It is probable that many individuals with youth-onset type 2 diabetes experience a prolonged period of mild hyperglycemia with minimal or no symptoms.

Distinguishing type 1 from type 2 diabetes

The increasing incidence in children of type 2 diabetes and the current high prevalence of overweight and obesity have presented clinicians with a diagnostic challenge when evaluating a patient with new-onset diabetes mellitus. Distinguishing diabetes type 1 from type 2 may be difficult because there may be considerable overlap in presentation (Table 18.3) and there are clearly patients who have clinical and biochemical features of both types. The overall frequency of obesity at diagnosis of type 1 diabetes has tripled in the past decade, irrespective of race, gender and age at onset, and a recent report indicates that 25% of patients with type 1 diabetes are obese [36].

In contrast to type 2 diabetes in adults, in which ketonuria is unusual, a substantial fraction of adolescents with type 2 diabetes will have ketonuria or even DKA at presentation (Tables 18.8 & 18.9). Insulin requirements typically decrease after several weeks of treatment of type 2 diabetes, which may resemble the remission or "honeymoon" period of type 1 diabetes. Measuring pancreatic autoantibodies and markers of insulin secretion (fasting C-peptide concentrations) at the time of diagnosis helps distinguish type 1 from type 2 in obese patients. A fasting plasma C-peptide level >0.85 ng/mL (300 pmol/l) suggests type 2 diabetes [37]. Plasma C-peptide concentrations, however, may be temporarily low in type 2 diabetes initially owing to glucotoxicity and lipotoxicity; rechecking the level after several weeks or even months of therapy will sometime demonstrate hyperinsulinism, helping to establish a diagnosis of type 2 diabetes.

Table 18.9 Characteristics at diagnosis of youth with type 2 diabetes mellitus.

Characteristic	Average* (range)
Measurement	
BMI (kg/m^2)	31.8 (25.5–37.7)
Glucose (mg/dL); mmol/L	446 (344–549); 24.8 (19.1–30.5)
HbA1c	10% (10–11)
Prevalence at presentation†	
Symptoms of diabetes	56% (19–96)
Ketonuria	36% (24–63)
DKA	14% (5–46)
Weight loss	55% (47–62)
Screening or incidental	48% (32–57)
Candidal vulvovaginitis	24% (24–24)
Prevalence of ethnicity‡	
African	36% (9–76)
Asian/Pacific	15% (3–46)
Indigenous	23% (3–53)
Hispanic	25% (10–63)
White	26% (3–57)

Data from 17 studies (each included at least 40 subjects) representing 2916 youth from four continents.

BMI, body mass index; DKA, diabetic ketoacidosis.

*Mean of the averages reported by each study, with the range of reported averages shown in parentheses.

†Among studies not based on primary screening.

‡Among studies reporting mixed ethnic composition.

Table 18.8 Clinical characteristics of youth at diagnosis of strictly defined type 2 diabetes mellitus.

Region	N	Method	FHx (%)	M : F	↑ BMI (%)	Age	AN (%)	DKA (%)	Ketosis (%)
New South Wales, Australia	128	Registry	75	1 : 1.1	90	15	NR	NR	NR
Cincinnati, USA	54	Chart review	85	1 : 1.7	92	14	60	~	~
Tokyo, Japan	232	Urinalysis	57	1 : 1.2	84	14	NR	~	~
UK	67	Registry	84	1 : 1.3	95	14	57	7	28
Toronto, Canada	44	Chart review	95	1 : 1.7	80	14	69	8	30
Taiwan	137	Urinalysis	21	1 : 1.7	48	13	NR	~	~

Data tabulated from studies employing strict definitions of type 2 diabetes: including either negative islet-cell antibodies, sustained glycemic control without insulin and/or confirmed insulin hypersecretion.

AN, acanthosis nigricans; ↑ BMI, obese or overweight; DKA, diabetic ketoacidosis; FHx, family history of type 2 diabetes; M : F, male : female ratio; NR, not reported; ~ not pertinent because of method of ascertainment or case definition.

Fasting insulin-like growth factor binding protein-1 (IGFBP-1) level, whose secretion is acutely inhibited by insulin, is a marker of insulinization and another useful biochemical parameter. A very low IGFBP-1 concentration is highly suggestive of type 2 diabetes [37].

There have been several reports of autoantibody positivity in children with clinical features of type 2 diabetes and latent autoimmune diabetes in youth (LADY) has been proposed to describe this subgroup. It is not always possible to categorize patients at the time of diagnosis but, irrespective of the type of diabetes, the choice of initial therapy must be made on the basis of the metabolic state, as determined by clinical assessment. Subsequent therapy should be guided by the individual patient's response to treatment and modified if necessary.

Differential diagnosis

Other causes of glycosuria

Diabetes mellitus is occasionally diagnosed in an asymptomatic individual because glycosuria is discovered incidentally. The diagnosis must always be confirmed by at least two independent measurements of plasma glucose concentration. Glycosuria can occur without hyperglycemia as a result of renal tubular dysfunction, e.g. Fanconi–Bickel syndrome, Fanconi syndrome, or because of an isolated reduction of the renal tubular threshold for glucose reabsoprtion (benign glycosuria). This disorder is diagnosed by performing an OGTT with simultaneous measurements of plasma and urine glucose concentrations. Glycosuria will be evident with plasma glucose concentrations in the normal range. Hepatic glycogen synthase deficiency (glycogen storage disease type 0) is an uncommon cause of intermittent post-prandial hyperglycemia and glycosuria in children.

Transient hyperglycemia

The incidence of transient hyperglycemia is estimated to be approximately 1 per 8000 pediatric office visits and 1 per 200 emergency department or hospital visits [38]. A minority of children with transient hyperglycemia develop diabetes mellitus. When transient hyperglycemia is detected in a child who does not have a severe illness, the risk of developing diabetes is much higher than if a severe illness were present. The presence of pancreatic autoantibodies and/or a low first-phase insulin response during an intravenous glucose tolerance test strongly predicts progression to diabetes.

Management

Initial management of newly diagnosed type 1 diabetes mellitus

Whenever possible, the child with DKA should be cared for by nursing staff trained in DKA management and access to a clinical chemistry laboratory that can provide frequent and timely measurement of serum chemistry. Children with severe DKA (long duration of symptoms, compromised circulation, depressed level of consciousness) and those at increased risk for cerebral edema (<5 years of age, new-onset diabetes) should be treated in a pediatric intensive care unit or in a children's ward that specializes in diabetes care and can provide comparable resources and supervision of care [39].

The goals of initial management depend on the clinical presentation and are to restore fluid and electrolyte balance, to stabilize the metabolic state with insulin and to provide basic diabetes education and self-care training for the child (if age and developmentally appropriate) and other caregivers (parents, grandparents, older siblings, daycare providers and babysitters).

The diagnosis of diabetes in a child is a crisis for the family, which requires considerable emotional support and time for adjustment and healing. Shocked, grieving and overwhelmed parents typically require at least 2–3 days to acquire basic "survival" skills while they are coping with the emotional upheaval that typically follows the diagnosis. Even if they are not acutely ill, children with newly diagnosed type 1 diabetes are usually admitted to hospital for stabilization, diabetes education and self-management training but outpatient or home-based management is preferred at some centers that have appropriate resources. The results comparing initial hospitalization with home-based and/or outpatient management of children who are not acutely ill with newly diagnosed type 1 diabetes are inconclusive but the data suggest that outpatient and/or home initial management of type 1 diabetes in children does not lead to any disadvantages in terms of metabolic control, acute complications, hospitalizations, psychosocial or behavioral variables. The decision whether a child with newly diagnosed diabetes should be admitted to hospital depends on several factors, including the severity of the metabolic derangements, a psychosocial assessment of the family and the resources available at the treatment center. Outpatient management in a comprehensive day center staffed by a multidisciplinary diabetes team is an appropriate alternative to hospitalization for many newly diagnosed children.

Psychosocial issues

The diagnosis of diabetes in a child or adolescent hurls the parent from a secure and known reality into a frightening and foreign world [40]. At diagnosis, they grieve the loss of their healthy child and cope with normal distress reactions such as shock, disbelief and denial, fear, anxiety, anger and blame or guilt. However, while grieving, parents are expected to acquire an understanding of the disease and behavioral skills to manage the illness at home and to assist the child to achieve acceptable blood glucose control. Parents should receive the support required to begin coping with the emotional distress and not be overwhelmed by unrealistic expectations from a well-meaning diabetes treatment team.

Diabetes presents family members with the task of being sensitive to the balance between the child's need for a sense of autonomy and mastery of self-care activities and the need for ongoing family support and involvement. The struggle to balance independence and dependence in relationships between the child and family members presents a long-term challenge and raises different issues for families at different stages of child and adolescent development. Focusing on normal developmental tasks at each stage of the child's growth and development provides the most effective structure with which to address this concern [40].

A medical social worker should perform an initial psychosocial assessment of all newly diagnosed patients to identify high-risk families who need additional services. Thereafter, patients are referred to the mental health specialist when emotional, social, environmental or financial concerns are suspected or identified that interfere with the ability to maintain acceptable diabetes control [40]. Some of the more common problems in families include parental guilt resulting in poor adherence to the treatment regimen, difficulty coping with the child's rebellion against treatment, anxiety, depression, fear of hypoglycemia, missed appointments, financial hardship, loss of health insurance affecting the ability to attend scheduled clinic appointments and/or purchase of supplies. Recurrent ketoacidosis is the most extreme indicator of psychosocial stress and management of such patients is incomplete without a comprehensive psychosocial assessment.

The treatment of pediatric diabetes is complicated by many factors inherent to childhood. Because childhood is characterized by cognitive and emotional immaturity, the involvement of responsible adults is essential to the treatment of diabetes which takes place within a family dynamic: treatment-related conflicts are not uncommon, arising in part from natural discord in goals between caretakers and/or the child.

Each phase of childhood has characteristics that complicate treatment, such as the unpredictable eating of toddlers and the unscheduled intense physical play of school-age children that can hinge on unpredictable factors such as the weather. Adolescence is characterized by multiple physiologic and psychosocial factors that make glycemic control more difficult. Optimal diabetes treatment has to be tailored to each child and family, based on factors including age, gender, family resources, cognitive faculties, the schedule and activities and the goals and desires of the child and family.

Current rates of psychological ill-health in diabetic youth are disturbingly high and longitudinal data indicate that mental health issues are likely to persist into early adulthood and possibly beyond. Such mental health issues appear to be prognostic of maladaptive lifestyle practices and of long-term problems with diabetes control and earlier-than-expected onset of complications. Based on these considerations, mental health should be given equivalence to and perhaps even precedence over the screening of other complications undertaken in diabetes clinics. Routine screening for behavioral disturbance should begin at the time of diagnosis, with further assessment of parental mental health and family functioning for those children identified as "at risk." Interventions can then be targeted based on the specific needs of individual children and families [41].

Outpatient diabetes care

The diabetes team

Optimal care of children with type 1 diabetes is complex and time-consuming. Few primary care practitioners or pediatricians have the resources and expertise, nor can they devote the time required to provide all of the components of an optimal treatment program for children with diabetes. Children with diabetes should be managed by a multidisciplinary diabetes team that provides diabetes education and care in collaboration with the child's primary care physician [42]. The team should consist of a pediatric endocrinologist or pediatrician with training in diabetes, a pediatric diabetes nurse educator, a dietitian and a mental health professional, either a clinical psychologist or social worker. A member of the diabetes team should always be available by telephone to respond to metabolic crises that require immediate intervention and to provide guidance and support to parents and patients.

Initial diabetes education

The diabetes education curriculum should be adapted to the individual child and family. Parents and children with newly diagnosed diabetes are anxious and overwhelmed and cannot assimilate a large amount of abstract information. Therefore, the education program should be staged: initial goals should be limited to "survival" skills so that the child can be safely cared for at home and return to his/her daily routine. Initial education should include understanding what causes diabetes, how it is treated, how to administer insulin, basic meal planning, self-monitoring of blood glucose and ketones, recognition and treatment of hypoglycemia and how and when to contact a member of the diabetes team.

Continuing diabetes education and long-term supervision of diabetes care

When the child is medically stable and parents and other care providers have mastered "survival" skills, the child is discharged from the hospital or ambulatory treatment center. In the first few weeks after diagnosis, frequent telephone contact provides emotional support, helps parents to interpret the results of blood glucose monitoring and adjust insulin doses if necessary.

Within a few weeks of diagnosis, many children enter a partial remission, evidenced by normal or near-normal blood glucose concentrations on a low dose (<0.25 units/kg/day) of insulin. By this time, most patients and parents are less anxious and have mastered basic diabetes management skills through experience and repetition and are now more prepared to begin to learn the details of intensive management.

At this stage, the diabetes team should begin to provide patients and parents with the knowledge and skills they need to maintain optimal glycemic control while coping with the challenges imposed by exercise, fickle appetite and varying food intake, intercurrent illnesses and the other variations that normally occur in a child's daily life. In addition to teaching facts and practical skills, the education program should promote desirable health beliefs and attitudes in the young person who has a chronic incurable disease. For some children, this may best be accomplished in a non-traditional educational setting such as summer camp. The educational curriculum must be concordant with the child's level of cognitive development and has to be adapted to the learning style and intellectual ability of the individual child and family. Parents, grandparents, older siblings, school nurse and other important people in the child's life are encouraged to participate in the diabetes education program so they can share in the diabetes care and help the child to live a normal life.

In the first month after diagnosis, the patient is seen frequently by the diabetes team to review and consolidate the diabetes education and practical skills acquired in the first few days and to extend the scope of self-care training. Thereafter, follow-up visits with members of the diabetes team should occur at least every 3 months. Regular clinic visits are to ensure that the child's diabetes is being appropriately managed at home and the goals of therapy are being met. A focused history should obtain information about self-care behaviors, the child's daily routines, the frequency, severity and circumstances surrounding hypoglycemic events and blood glucose monitoring data should be reviewed.

At each visit, height and weight are measured and plotted on a growth chart. The weight curve is especially helpful in assessing adequacy of therapy. Significant weight loss usually indicates that the prescribed dose is insufficient or the patient is not receiving all the prescribed doses of insulin.

A more complete physical examination should be performed at least twice each year focusing on blood pressure, stage of puberty, evidence of thyroid disease, mobility of the joints in the hands, scarring of the fingertips from frequent lancing and injection sites for lipohypertrophy or lipoatrophy.

Regular clinic visits also provide an opportunity to review, reinforce and expand upon the diabetes self-care training begun at the time of diagnosis. The goal at each visit is to reinforce the goals of treatment while increasing the patient's and family's understanding of diabetes management, the interplay of insulin, food and exercise and their impact on blood glucose concentrations. As cognitive development progresses, the child should become more involved in management and assume increasing age-appropriate responsibility for daily self-care. Parents are encouraged to call for advice if the pattern of blood glucose concentrations changes between routine visits suggesting the need to adjust the insulin dose or change the regimen. Eventually, when parents and patients have sufficient knowledge and experience, they are encouraged to adjust the insulin dose(s) independently.

Goals of therapy

The DCCT [43,44], and a similar smaller study in Sweden [45], ended the debate about whether the microvascular complications of diabetes are caused by hyperglycemia and can be prevented or ameliorated. Additional evidence for the importance of glycemic control was provided by the UK Prospective Diabetes Study (UKPDS) in adults with type 2 diabetes [46,47]. These clinical trials and the long-term follow-up observations of the DCCT cohort demonstrate unequivocally the importance of lowering glycated hemoglobin (HbA1c) values to reduce the risk of development and progression of retinopathy, nephropathy, neuropathy and macrovascular disease. Treatment regimens that reduce average HbA1c to approximately 7% (about 1% above the upper limit of normal) are associated with fewer long-term micro- and macrovascular complications [48] and improved glycemic control is associated with a sustained decreased rate of development of diabetic complications [49,50].

The aim of diabetes management is to achieve recommended glycemic targets known to reduce the risk of long-term complications but there is no consensus on the targets appropriate for children of different ages. The recommendations of a sample of national diabetes organizations are shown in Table 18.10.

Management of young children with diabetes, especially those younger than 5 years old, must balance opposing risks of hypoglycemia and future vascular complications. The relative contribution of the prepubertal years to the development of microvascular complications has been uncertain but longer prepubertal duration of diabetes increases the risk of retinopathy and possibly microalbuminuria in adolescence and young adulthood but at a slower rate than the postpubertal years [51].

Biochemical goals of treatment for children and adolescents have recently been published by the International Society for Pediatric and Adolescent Diabetes (ISPAD): ideal HbA1c is <6.05%, optimal <7.5%, suboptimal 7.5–9.0% and action is required when the value exceeds 9.0% [52]. The ISPAD guidelines are accompanied by the statement: "Each child should have their targets determined individually with the goal of achieving a value as close to normal as possible while avoiding severe hypoglycemia as well as frequent mild to moderate hypoglycemia."

The risk for microalbuminuria increases steeply with HbA1c >8% [53]. Based on these considerations, an HbA1c of ≤8.0% is a reasonable general goal for children with diabetes but biochemical goals should be individualized taking into account both medical and psychosocial considerations. Less stringent treatment goals are appropriate for preschool-age children, those with developmental handicaps, psychosocial challenges, lack of appropriate family support, children who have experienced severe hypoglycemia or those with hypoglycemia unawareness.

Insulin therapy

Most children with type 1 diabetes are severely insulin-deficient and depend on insulin replacement for survival. Ideally, the insulin regimen should mimic physiologic insulin secretory patterns but physiologic replacement of insulin remains elusive. Insulin pump therapy or multiple daily insulin injections are the methods that most closely mimic insulin secretion.

The first step in choosing an insulin regimen is to establish glycemic goals. For most patients, this means that more than half of PG values should fall within the following ranges: preprandial 90–130 mg/dL (5–7.2 mmol/L), bedtime 100–140 mg/dL (5.6–7.8 mmol/L), 1–2 h post-prandial <180 mg/dL (10 mmol/L)

Table 18.10 Recommended glycemic targets.

	Blood glucose goal range (mmol/L)		A1c

American Diabetes Association

	Preprandial	Bedtime	
Toddlers and preschool age children (<6 years)	5.6–10	6.1–11.1	<8.5 (but >7.5%)
School-age children (6–12 years)	5–10	5.6–10	<8%
Adolescents and young adults	5–7.2	5–8.3	<7.5%*

Australasian Paediatric Endocrine Group

	Preprandial	Post-prandial	
Children and adolescents[a]	4–8	<10	<7.5%

Canadian Diabetes Association

	Preprandial	
Age < 5 years	6–12	≤9%[b]
Age 5–12 years	4–10	≤8%[c]
Age 13–18 years	4–7	≤7%[d]
	4–6	≤6%[e]

Diabetes UK (National Institute for Clinical Excellence)

	Preprandial	Post-prandial	
Children and young people	4–8	<10	≤7.5%[f]

International Society for Pediatric and Adolescent Diabetes[g]

	Preprandial	Post-prandial	
Ideal	3.6–5.6	4.5–7	<6.05
Optimal	5–8	5–10	<7.5
Suboptimal (action suggested)	>8	10–14	7.5–9
High risk (action required)	>9	>14	>9

*A lower goal (<7%) is reasonable if it can be achieved without excessive hypoglycemia.

[a]"In very young children, . . . glycemic targets need to be at the upper part of these ranges or a little higher."

[b]Extreme caution is required to avoid severe hypoglycemia.

[c]Targets should be graduated to the child's age.

[d]Appropriate for most patients.

[e]Consider for patients in whom these targets can be achieved safely.

[f]". . . without frequent disabling hypoglycemia."

[g]These targets are intended as guidelines and each child should have their targets individually determined with the goal of achieving a value as close to normal as possible while avoiding severe hypoglycemia as well as frequent mild to moderate hypoglycemia [52].

(Table 18.10). It is very important to individualize blood glucose goals.

In children with severe insulin deficiency, practical considerations, including socio-economic circumstances, age, supervision of care, ability and willingness to self-administer insulin several times each day and difficulty maintaining long-term adherence, make physiologic replacement of insulin challenging. There is no insulin regimen that can be used for all children with type 1 diabetes. The diabetes team has to design an insulin regimen that meets the needs of the individual patient and is acceptable to the patient and/or family member(s) responsible for administering insulin to the child or supervising its administration.

The route of insulin administration is determined by the severity of the child's condition at presentation. Insulin is preferably given intravenously for treatment of DKA. Children who are metabolically stable without vomiting or significant ketosis may be started with subcutaneous (SC) insulin administration. SC insulin treatment in the newly diagnosed child should be started with at least three injections per day or a basal-bolus regimen (Table 18.11). Some clinicians start insulin pump therapy at the time of diagnosis regardless of the severity of presentation or age of the child.

In addition to severity of metabolic decompensation, the child's age, weight and pubertal status guide the initial insulin dose selection. When diabetes has been diagnosed early, before significant metabolic decompensation, 0.25–0.5 unit/kg/day usually is an adequate starting dose. When metabolic decompensation is more severe (e.g. ketosis without acidosis or dehydration) the initial dose is typically at least 0.5 unit/kg/day. After recovery from DKA, prepubertal children usually require at least 0.75 unit/kg/day, whereas adolescents require at least 1 unit/kg/day.

In the first few days of insulin therapy, while the focus of care is on diabetes education and emotional support, it is reasonable to aim for pre-meal blood glucose concentrations in the range 4.5–11 mmol/L (80–200 mg/dL) and to supplement, if necessary, with 0.05–0.1 unit/kg of rapid- or short-acting insulin SC at 3–4 h intervals.

Three major categories of insulin preparations classified according to their time course of action are available (Table 18.12). Various regimens consisting of a mixture of short- or rapid-acting insulin with an intermediate- or long-acting insulin used in children and adolescents (Table 18.11), typically given two to four (or more) times daily. Clear superiority of any one regimen in children and adolescents in terms of metabolic outcomes has not been demonstrated [54,55].

All insulin regimens have the same general goal to provide basal insulin throughout the day and night with additional insulin to cover meals and snacks. When a two-dose regimen is used, the total daily dose is usually divided so that two-thirds is given before breakfast and one-third is given in the evening. With a three-dose regimen, short- or rapid-acting insulin is administered before supper and the second dose of intermediate-acting insulin is given at bedtime rather than before the evening meal.

Table 18.11 Insulin regimens used to treat children and adolescents.

Number of daily doses	Breakfast	Lunch	Dinner	Bedtime
2	S/R + N*		S/R + N	
3	S/R + N		S/R	S/R + N
	S/R + N	S/R	S/R + N	
	S/R + N	S/R	S/R+ Glarg/Det†	
	S/R + N		S/R	Glarg/Det
4	S/R	S/R	S/R	S/R + N
	S/R + N	S/R	S/R	S/R + N
	S/R	S/R	S/R	S/R + Glarg/Det
	S/R + Glarg/Det	S/R	S/R	S/R
	S/R + Det	S/R	S/R	S/R + Det
	S/R	S/R	S/R + Glarg/Det	S/R
CSII‡	S/R	S/R	S/R	S/R

CSII, continuous subcutaneous insulin infusion; Det, insulin detemir; Glarg, insulin glargine; N, neutral protamine Hagedorn (isophane); R, regular (soluble) insulin; S, short-acting insulin (insulin lispro, insulin aspart, insulin glulisine).
*Premixed combinations such as, either 70% NPH and 30% regular or 70% protamine-crystallized aspart (PA) and 30% soluble insulin aspart or 75% neutral protamine lispro (NPL) and 25% insulin lispro are usually used in twice daily fixed dose insulin regimens.
†Insulin glargine is almost always given once daily, either with breakfast or in the evening with dinner or at bedtime. According to the manufacturers, both glargine and detemir should be given as a separate injection and cannot be mixed with another insulin in the same syringe. However, recent studies suggest that rapid-acting insulin analogs can be mixed with glargine in the same syringe with no detrimental effect on insulin action provided they are injected immediately [154,155].
Insulin detemir may be used once (typically with dinner or at bedtime) or twice daily (with breakfast and a second dose either with dinner or at bedtime).
‡CSII (pump) boluses are given with meals and snacks together with basal insulin throughout the day and night.
Intensified insulin therapy is defined as the use of at least three daily doses of insulin or CSII.

The initial ratio of rapid- to intermediate-acting insulin at both times is approximately 1:2. Toddlers and young children typically require a smaller fraction of short- or rapid-acting insulin (10–20% of the total dose) and proportionately more intermediate-acting insulin. Rapid-acting insulin (lispro, aspart, glulisine) insulin is given 5–15 min before eating.

The optimal ratio of rapid- or short-acting to intermediate-acting insulin is determined empirically for each patient, guided by the results of frequent blood glucose measurements. At least five daily measurements are required to determine the effects of each component of the insulin regimen. The blood glucose concentration is measured before each meal, before the bedtime snack and once between midnight and 4 a.m. Parents are taught to look for patterns of hyperglycemia or hypoglycemia that indicate the need for an adjustment in the dose.

Table 18.12 Insulin preparations classified according to their pharmacodynamic profiles.

	Onset of action (h)	Peak action (h)	Effective duration of action (h)
Rapid-acting			
Insulin lispro*	0.25–0.5	0.5–2.5	≤5
Insulin aspart*	<0.25	1–3	3–5
Insulin glulisine	<0.25	1–1.5	3–5
Short-acting			
Regular (soluble)	0.5–1	2–3	5–8
Intermediate-acting			
NPH (isophane)	1–2	4–10	10–16
Long-acting			
Insulin glargine*	2–4	Relatively peakless	20–24
Insulin detemir*	0.8–2	Relatively peakless	12–24†
Premixed combinations			
50% NPH, 50% regular	0.5–1	Dual	10–16
50% NPL, 50% lispro	<0.25	Dual	10–16
70% NPH, 30% regular	0.5–1	Dual	10–16
70% PA, 30% aspart*	<0.25	Dual	15–18
75% NPL, 25% lispro*	<0.25	Dual	10–16

Pharmacodynamic effects of lispro insulin and insulin aspart appear to be equivalent [156].
NPL, neutral protamine lispro suspension; PA, protamine-crystallized insulin aspart suspension. Both PA + soluble aspart and NPL + lispro are stable premixed combinations of intermediate- and rapid-acting insulins.
The human insulins and insulin analogs are available in vials, prefilled disposable pen injectors and cartridges for non-disposable pen injectors.
These data are for human insulins and are approximations from studies in adult test subjects. Time action profiles are estimates only. The kinetics of NPH insulin may be more rapid in children [157]. The times of onset, peak and effective duration of action vary within and between patients and are affected by numerous factors, including size of dose, site and depth of injection, dilution, exercise, temperature, regional blood flow, local tissue reactions.
*Insulin analog developed by modifying the amino acid sequence and/or chemical adducts of the human insulin molecule.
†Dose-dependent; 12 h for 0.2 U/kg; 20–24 h for ≥0.4 U/kg.

Adjustments to individual components of the insulin regimen are usually made in 5–10% increments or decrements in response to patterns of consistently elevated (above the target range for several consecutive days) or unexplained low blood glucose concentrations. This is referred to as pattern adjustment. The insulin dosage is adjusted until satisfactory blood glucose control is achieved with >50% of blood glucose values in or close to the individual child's target range.

At the time of diagnosis, most children have some residual β cells and often enter a period of partial remission ("honeymoon") within several days to a few weeks, during which normal or near-normal glycemic control is relatively easily achieved with a low dose of insulin. At this stage, the dose of insulin should be reduced to prevent hypoglycemia but should not be discontinued. As destruction of the remaining β cells occurs, the insulin dose increases ("intensification phase"), eventually reaching a full replacement dose. The average daily insulin dose in prepubertal children with long-standing diabetes is approximately 0.8 unit/kg/day and in adolescents about 1–1.5 unit/kg/day.

Insulin therapy in young children

Caring for young children with diabetes is challenging for many reasons, one of which is the need accurately and reproducibly to measure and inject tiny doses of insulin that is supplied in a concentration of 100 units/mL (U100 insulin). To administer a dose of 1 unit requires the ability accurately to measure 10 μL (1/100 mL) of insulin. When the dose is less than 2 U of U100 insulin, neither parents of children with diabetes nor skilled pediatric nurses are able to measure the dose accurately. Furthermore, a dose change of 0.25 U translates into a volume difference of 2.5 μL in a 300 μL (30 unit) syringe. When parents attempt to measure insulin doses in increments of 0.25 U insulin (e.g. 3.0, 3.25, 3.5 U) using a standard commercial 30 unit (300 μL) syringe, they consistently measure more than the prescribed amount.

To enhance accuracy and reproducibility of small doses, insulin should be diluted to U10 (10 units/mL) with diluent available from the manufacturer. Using U10 insulin, each line ("unit") on a syringe is actually 0.1 U insulin.

To avoid intramuscular injections in infants and children with little subcutaneous fat, syringes with 31 gauge (5 mm) needles should be used.

Intensified insulin therapy in children

There is little evidence to guide clinical decisions concerning the risk–benefit ratio of strict control in the pre-adolescent patient. Clinical trials comparable to the DCCT have not been conducted in prepubertal children but many experts believe that it is reasonable to extrapolate that prepubertal children will also benefit from strict control of their diabetes.

Limitations of twice daily split-and-mixed insulin regimens

Beyond the remission period, it is not generally possible to achieve near-normal glycemia with two injections per day without incurring a greater risk of hypoglycemia, especially during the night. A major problem with the two dose "split-and-mixed" regimens (rapid- or short-acting insulin combined with intermediate-acting insulin administered before breakfast and before the evening meal; Table 18.11) is that the peak effect of the pre-dinner intermediate-acting insulin tends to occur at the time of lowest insulin requirement (midnight to 4 a.m.), increasing the risk of nocturnal hypoglycemia. Thereafter, insulin action declines

from 4 to 8 a.m., when the basal insulin requirement normally increases. Consequently, the tendency for blood glucose concentrations to rise before breakfast (dawn phenomenon) may be aggravated by waning insulin effect before breakfast and/or by counter-regulatory hormones secreted in response to a fall in blood glucose concentrations during sleep, post-hypoglycemic hyperglycemia (Somogyi phenomenon).

A three-dose insulin regimen with mixed short- or rapid- and intermediate-acting insulins before breakfast, short- or rapid-acting insulin before dinner and intermediate-acting insulin at bedtime may significantly reduce these problems (Table 18.11; Fig. 18.6) [56]. Intensive insulin regimens that employ intermediate-acting insulin (Fig. 18.5) demand consistency in the daily meal schedule, in the amounts of food consumed at each meal and in the timing of insulin injections.

Basal-bolus regimens and continuous subcutaneous insulin infusion

Insulin therapy with at least three injections each day or with continuous subcutaneous insulin infusion (CSII) using an insulin pump can more closely simulate normal insulin profiles, can overcome many of the limitations inherent in a two-dose regimen and permit greater flexibility with respect to timing and content of meals. Doses of rapid-acting insulin are adjusted meal-to-meal based on preprandial glucose values, anticipated carbohydrate intake and activity. A peakless long-acting insulin, insulin glargine or detemir, can be used to provide basal insulin (typically 40–60% of the total daily dose) and is used together with short- or rapid-acting insulin injected before each meal (basal-bolus regimen; Fig. 18.6b).

Insulin glargine is an insulin analog, produced by recombinant DNA technology, with an approximately 24-h duration of action. It has little peak activity and is typically administered once daily,

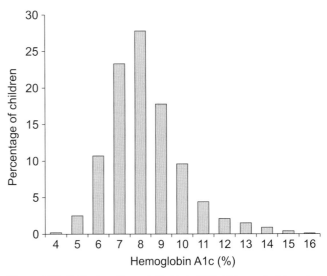

Figure 18.5 Distribution of hemoglobin A1c in 2873 children and adolescents with type 1 diabetes from 18 countries. Data from Mortensen [161].

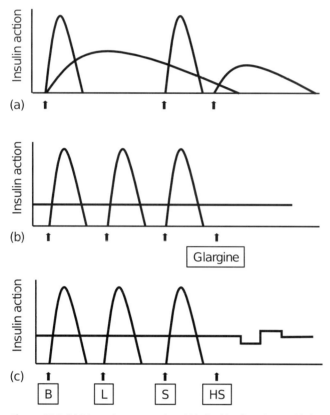

Figure 18.6 (a) Schematic representation of idealized insulin action provided by a regimen consisting of a mixture of rapid-acting insulin (lispro or aspart) and intermediate-acting insulin (NPH) before breakfast, rapid-acting insulin (lispro or aspart) before supper and intermediate-acting insulin (NPH or Lente) at bedtime. (b) Schematic representation of idealized insulin action provided by an insulin regimen consisting of four daily injections: rapid-acting insulin (lispro or aspart) before each meal (B, L, S) and a separate injection of insulin glargine, either at bedtime (as shown here) or at dinner or breakfast. (c) Schematic representation of idealized insulin effect provided by continuous subcutaneous insulin infusion via an insulin pump with insulin aspart or lispro. In this figure, alternative basal rates are illustrated; insulin delivery is shown to decrease from midnight to 3 a.m. and to increase before breakfast. B, breakfast; L, lunch; S, supper; HS, bedtime. Arrows indicate times of insulin injection or boluses before meals.

either before breakfast or in the evening with dinner or at bedtime. It should be injected at about the same time each day; whereas short- or rapid-acting insulin is injected separately before each meal, whenever it is eaten. Insulin glargine has been used safely in children and adolescents [57] and, because it does not have the peak of activity characteristic of NPH [58], can reduce nocturnal hypoglycemic episodes without jeopardizing glycemic control [59,60].

Insulin detemir has become available as an alternative long-acting, peakless basal insulin [61]. Detemir has effects similar to those of glargine during the first 12-h after administration but thereafter its effect wanes and, accordingly, it usually has to be administered twice daily in patients with severe insulin deficiency [62].

In 1996, less than 5% of patients starting pump therapy were under 20 years of age. Over the past several years, there has been a worldwide marked increase in the number of children and adolescents using CSII (pump) therapy [63] and a current estimate is that more than 80 000 children and adolescents worldwide are using a pump. An insulin pump has the advantage over insulin injections in the ability to program changes in basal dosage to meet an anticipated increase or decrease in need (Fig. 18.6c). This feature can help combat the dawn phenomenon or hypoglycemia during or after exercise. In addition to programing various basal rates, the use of dual wave and square wave bolus delivery significantly lowers 4-h post-prandial blood glucose concentrations. Also, the infusion set typically only has to be replaced every 2–3 days. A meta-analysis of randomized controlled clinical trials concluded that CSII resulted in a small (approximately 0.5%) improvement in HbA1c [64].

Although an insulin pump is a complex and medical device that requires extensive training in its use, many children can manage the added responsibility of using a pump and, with appropriate education and training and with support from parents and a school nurse, benefit from its advantages [65]. Only short- or rapid-acting insulin is used with CSII so any interruption in the delivery of insulin leads rapidly to metabolic decompensation. To reduce this risk, meticulous care must be devoted to the infusion system and blood glucose concentrations must be measured frequently. Increased lifestyle flexibility, reduced blood glucose variability, improved glycemic control and reduced frequency of severe hypoglycemia are all documented advantages of CSII [63]. Success requires motivation to achieve normal blood glucose concentrations, frequent blood glucose monitoring, record keeping, carbohydrate counting and frequent contact with the diabetes team. Patients must understand that to be successful, CSII therapy requires more time, effort and active involvement in diabetes care by patients and parents and considerable education and support from the diabetes team. The individual who is unable to master a multiple dose injection regimen is not likely to be successful with CSII.

Despite concerns that it might have adverse psychosocial consequences owing to the added burden of treatment, especially in adolescents, the opposite effect has been observed. Short-term studies have shown that more aggressive and successful management of their diabetes by teenagers can be accompanied by enhanced psychosocial well-being. In teenagers, CSII offers a treatment option that can lead to improved control and lower the risk of severe hypoglycemia.

Puberty

Owing to physiologic peripheral insulin resistance of puberty [66], adolescents require large doses of rapid- or short-acting insulin to control post-prandial blood glucose excursions. However, a large increase in the dose of regular insulin markedly delays its peak effect (to 3–4 h) and prolongs its total duration of action to 6–8 h. Puberty does not cause hepatic insulin resistance and hyperinsulinemia therefore suppresses hepatic glucose production for several hours and increases the risk of post-prandial hypoglycemia, especially at night between 10 p.m. and 2 a.m. This is an important reason to use rapid-acting insulin analogs (insulin lispro, aspart or glulisine) in preference to regular (soluble) insulin in treating adolescents, especially before the evening meal to reduce the risk of nocturnal hypoglycemia.

Technological innovations have provided patients with insulin preparations whose pharmacokinetic properties make it possible crudely to simulate physiologic insulin kinetics. It is now possible for children to safely achieve unprecedented levels of glycemic control without excessive severe hypoglycemia. The diabetes care provider should frankly discuss treatment options with parents and child and explain the advantages and disadvantages of each in attempting to meet the overall goals of treatment. The most suitable regimen for a given child and family should be determined by mutual consent.

Biochemical outcomes in type 1 diabetes mellitus

Studies performed in the post-DCCT era show that metabolic control of type 1 diabetes in children and adolescents continues to be unsatisfactory. For example, the mean HbA1c of 2873 children from 22 pediatric diabetes centers in 18 countries was 8.6 ± 1.7 (SD)% (equivalent to a mean of 8.3% using the DCCT method) [67] and did not change significantly when re-examined 3 years later, despite significant increases in insulin dose and number of daily insulin injections (Fig. 18.5) [68]. In a nationwide cross-sectional study of 2579 French children with type 1 diabetes, mean HbA1c was 8.97 ± 1.98 (SD)%, of whom 33% had an HbA1c of ≤8% [69]. Likewise, a nationwide study of 1755 Scottish children with type 1 diabetes found an average HbA1c of 9.1% [70]. Despite many changes in diabetes management in the past decade, glycemic control has not improved at many pediatric diabetes centers and major differences in metabolic outcome persist [55].

The differences are not explained by demography, ethnic issues or insulin regimens. Poorly understood differences in the implementation of insulin treatment are thought to account for the variation in metabolic outcomes. In a large cohort (26 687 patients) of children and adolescents (mean age 13.6 years, mean duration of diabetes 5.4 years) treated for type 1 diabetes in 152 hospitals and clinics in Germany and Austria from 1995 to 2005, 73% were treated with ≥4 daily injections (intensified conventional therapy), 14% with CSII and 13% with 1–3 injections per day (i.e. 87% of patients were treated with ICT or CSII). While this percentage increased over the observation period, mean HbA1c was almost constant [71]. Thus, the therapeutic goal of achieving optimal glycemic control has still not been achieved in the majority of patients, which may indicate a need to improve glucose monitoring and patient education in order to exploit the full potential of intensified therapeutic options [71].

By contrast, a population-based cohort (1335 children) from Western Australia showed that the overall average HbA1c significantly decreased (by 0.2% per year from 10.9 ± 1.7 in 1992 to $8.1 \pm 1.5\%$ in 2002), suggesting that recent approaches to therapy

may allow a degree of improved control without the expected increased risk of severe hypoglycemia [72]. The reason(s) for the differences in biochemical outcome between centers are still not well understood.

Management of type 2 diabetes mellitus

Data are sparse regarding the treatment of type 2 diabetes in young people and approaches have generally been adopted from the care of adults with type 2 diabetes informed by the treatment of children with type 1 diabetes. Lifestyle changes, oral hypoglycemic agents and insulin are the mainstays of treatment.

Lifestyle changes directed at reducing obesity, optimizing dietary choices and increasing physical activity should be recommended for all young persons with type 2 diabetes. Such changes are sufficient by themselves for the treatment of motivated youngsters with mild hyperglycemia. Oral hypoglycemic agents are an effective adjuvant to lifestyle changes and metformin, an insulin-sensitizing agent, is the agent of choice.

At the onset of diabetes, insulin is required if there is ketosis and/or marked symptomatic hyperglycemia. Metformin can be added once ketosis has resolved. It is not uncommon for the hyperglycemia to improve significantly in the first few weeks after diagnosis, allowing reductions in the dose and even cessation of insulin treatment.

After an initial period of improvement, many children with type 2 diabetes experience progressive worsening of glycemia, despite use of an oral hypoglycemic agent. There are no data regarding whether the best escalation of therapy is to add a second oral hypoglycemic agent or initiate insulin treatment but many patients eventually require insulin to maintain glycemic targets.

Lifestyle interventions

Even modest reductions in weight can produce significant improvements in glycemia. Lifestyle education and counseling should aim to produce incremental progressive improvements in lifestyle choices. Families should be involved in this process and encouraged to provide positive reinforcement for any improvements the child makes. Realistic weight reduction goals should be tailored to each child and be accompanied by nutritional and physical activity counseling to provide the knowledge and motivation necessary to accomplish this difficult task. An appropriate exercise plan should be prescribed with the goal of at least 30–60 min/day physical exercise and less than 1–2 h/day of video, TV or computer "screen time."

The daily calorie consumption should be reduced to induce gradual weight loss and reduce dietary glycemic exposure. Patients should be advised to stop drinking sugar-sweetened beverages. This one step can produce significant improvements in hyperglycemia in the child who has been consuming large quantities. The daily fat intake should be reduced to 25–35% of total daily calories. The child and family should be counseled on portion control, limiting the amounts of high-calorie foods and the importance of eating meals on a regular schedule. In contrast to type 1 diabetes, snacks should not be prescribed for the child with type 2 diabetes unless needed to avoid hypoglycemia. Low glycemic index diets may have therapeutic benefit for the motivated family but are untested in the child with type 2 diabetes.

Many children with type 2 diabetes have great difficulty implementing lifestyle changes. Other family members may have unhealthy dietary habits and sedentary behaviors, creating a *de facto* barrier to the child's adoption of a healthy lifestyle.

Oral hypoglycemic agents

Oral hypoglycemic agents typically produce moderate improvements of hyperglycemia. Metformin is an insulin-sensitizing agent that improves glycemia without promoting weight gain and is considered the oral hypoglycemic agent of choice for type 2 diabetes. A 16-week double-blind randomized clinical trial demonstrated the efficacy and safety of metformin compared with a placebo, with an improvement in HbA1c of slightly more than 1% [73]. A large longitudinal study in adults demonstrated favorable effects of metformin compared with other therapeutic approaches on clinical endpoints, including reductions in diabetes-related complications, all-cause mortality and stroke. These effects were achieved with less weight gain and fewer episodes of hypoglycemia [74].

Metformin is generally safe but should not be used by patients with renal insufficiency because of the risk of severe lactic acidosis and renal function should be assessed before initiating therapy and the serum creatinine concentration measured at least annually thereafter. Other contraindications include metabolic acidosis. Metformin should not be prescribed for young people with recurrent DKA. A small number of patients develop vitamin B_{12} deficiency and red blood cell counts and measurement of vitamin B_{12} concentrations should be performed annually. Patients should be counseled about the most common side effects, which include diarrhea, nausea, dyspepsia, flatulence and abdominal pain, which are not usually sufficient to warrant stopping the medication and usually lessen with time. They are milder if the dosage is slowly titrated upward. The starting dosage is 500 mg/day, usually taken with the evening meal. Dosage increments of 500 mg can be made weekly (or 850 mg every 2 weeks) as tolerated, up to a maximum of 2000 mg/day for patients <16 years given in divided doses or 2550 mg/day for patients aged ≥16 years divided into 2–3 doses given with meals.

The sulfonylureas are insulin secretagogues. Glimepiride was as effective as metformin in improving hyperglycemia in a 26-week randomized comparison study but young patients treated with glimepiride experienced a relative increase in BMI Z score compared to a decrease in those treated with metformin. Drawbacks of sulfonylurea therapy include weight gain, increased risk of hypoglycemia (compared to metformin) and rare side effects of nausea, vomiting, rashes, leukopenia and hemolytic anemia. Second- and third-generation sulfonylureas have favorable side effect profiles compared to first-generation agents. Sulfonylureas offer an alternative for patients who cannot tolerate metformin.

Other classes of oral hypoglycemic agents have been used to treat type 2 diabetes in children but there are no data on their efficacy or safety. In adults, none of the medications has been found to be superior to metformin in efficacy, although the hypoglycemic effects of the thiazolidinediones may be more durable compared to metformin. Until data become available, we do not advocate the use of these agents in the pediatric patient with type 2 diabetes.

Insulin therapy for type 2 diabetes mellitus

Insulin is often required to achieve optimal glycemic control. A recommended starting dose is 0.5–1.0 U/kg/day, which should be adjusted until blood glucose concentrations reach target levels (Table 18.10). For some, a daily long-acting insulin or intermediate-acting insulin at bedtime or twice daily may be sufficient to bring blood glucose concentrations into the target range but the addition of short- or rapid-acting insulin at meal times to achieve target glycemia is often required using the principles outlined for insulin therapy of type 1 diabetes. Because poor adherence is common, simple insulin regimens are preferable for most children with type 2 diabetes and premixed insulin preparations may be attractive.

Biochemical outcomes in type 2 diabetes mellitus

Metabolic control is often unsatisfactory. In a study of 331 youth with type 2 diabetes from 11 countries in the Western Pacific, the median HbA1c was 7% and 60% achieved a level <7.5% [75]. One-quarter were treated with lifestyle alone, half with an oral hypoglycemic agent and one-quarter received insulin. More frequent blood glucose monitoring predicted improved outcome. The prevalence of hypertension and microalbuminuria were 24% and 8%, respectively, but only 4% received antihypertensive medication.

Among 72 patients in Milwaukee, USA followed longitudinally from diagnosis, the mean HbA1c improved from 10.1% at diagnosis to 9.1% after 1 year of treatment. It should be noted, however, that 20% of the patients were lost to follow-up. Poorer outcomes were predicted by higher initial HbA1c and by nonadherence to medical therapy [76]. Several smaller studies from three other cities in North America have likewise found poor metabolic outcomes with mean HbA1c values in the range 8.1–9.8% after at least 1 year's treatment.

Medical nutrition therapy

Nutritional management is one of the cornerstones of the management of all types of diabetes mellitus and nutrition education is an essential component of education for patients and their families [77,78]. Medical nutrition therapy (MNT) should be individualized, with consideration given to the patient's usual eating habits and other lifestyle factors. Monitoring clinical and metabolic parameters including blood glucose, HbA1c, lipids, blood pressure and body weight, as well as quality of life, is crucial to ensure successful outcomes. Modern diabetes management, combining frequent self-monitoring of blood glucose with intensive insulin therapy and mastery of carbohydrate counting, enables children and adolescents to enjoy dietary flexibility while maintaining glycemic control.

Patients with both types of diabetes have the same goals to achieve and maintain target blood glucose and glycated hemoglobin concentrations (Table 18.13). The initial focus of MNT, however, differs between the two major types of diabetes. Children with type 2 diabetes are typically obese at presentation and there is great emphasis on weight loss, limiting calorie intake and distributing meals evenly throughout the day. In type 2 diabetes, even modest weight reduction alone increases sensitivity to insulin and improves fasting and post-prandial plasma glucose concentrations. Similarly, moderate calorie reduction decreases plasma glucose concentrations.

In adults, structured intensive lifestyle programs involving participant education, individualized counseling, reduced energy and fat intake (30% of total energy), regular physical activity and frequent participant contact are necessary to produce long-term weight loss of 5–7% of starting weight [79]. Accordingly, lifestyle changes that lead to weight loss are the cornerstone of therapy in adult patients with type 2 diabetes. In the child with type 1 diabetes, the primary goal is to match insulin delivery and carbohydrate consumption to achieve blood glucose concentrations in the age-specific target range.

There is no evidence that the nutritional needs of children with diabetes differ from those of other children. The total intake of energy must be sufficient to balance the daily expenditure and has to be adjusted periodically to achieve an ideal body weight and maintain a normal rate of growth and development.

Carbohydrate

A total of 60–70% of total energy should be from carbohydrate and monounsaturated fat [80]. Dietary dogma, based on the assumption that simple sugars are more rapidly digested and absorbed than starches and would aggravate hyperglycemia to a greater degree, has been to avoid simple sugars and replace them with complex carbohydrates.

The glycemic index (GI), proposed in 1981 as an alternative system for classifying carbohydrate-containing foods, measures the glycemic response after ingestion of carbohydrate. GI is defined as the incremental area under the plasma glucose response curve after consumption of a standard amount of carbohydrate from a test food relative to that of a control food, either white bread or glucose. The glycemic and hormonal responses to a large number of carbohydrates have been systematically examined and their GIs defined. There is a wide spectrum of biologic responses to different complex and simple carbohydrates with so much overlap that they cannot be simply classified into distinct groups. Even a single food produces a substantially different glycemic response when prepared in different ways. The physical structure and form of a carbohydrate-containing food, in addition to its chemical composition, influences post-prandial glycemia by altering its rate of digestion and absorption. Fruits and milk cause a lower glycemic response than most starches and sucrose causes a glycemic response similar to that of bread, rice and potatoes. In general, most refined starchy foods have a high GI, whereas nonstarchy vegetables, fruits and legumes tend to have a low GI.

The usefulness of low GI diets in individuals with type 1 diabetes continues to be controversial and the data in children are few. A meta-analysis of randomized controlled clinical trials, some of which have included children, shows that low GI diets have a modest long-term beneficial effect on blood glucose and lipid concentrations [81].

The glycemic load of meals and snacks is more important than the source or type of carbohydrate. The glycemic load, defined as the weighted average of the GI of individual foods multiplied by the percentage of dietary energy as carbohydrate, has been proposed as a method to characterize the impact of foods and dietary

Table 18.13 Goals of medical nutrition therapy of children and adolescents with diabetes mellitus. After [158,159].

Goals that apply to all persons with diabetes	1. Attain and maintain optimal metabolic outcomes including:
	  a. Blood glucose concentrations in the normal range or as close to normal as is safely attainable
	  b. A lipid and lipoprotein profile that reduces the risk for vascular disease
	  c. Blood pressure concentrations in the normal range or as close to normal as is safely possible
	2. To prevent or at least slow, the rate of development of the chronic complications of diabetes by modifying nutrient intake and lifestyle
	3. To address individual nutrition needs, taking into account personal and cultural preferences, economic circumstances and willingness to change
	4. To maintain the pleasure of eating by only limiting food choices when indicated by scientific evidence

Goals specific to type 1 diabetes	To provide adequate energy to ensure normal growth and development, integrate insulin regimens into usual eating and physical activity habits
Goals specific to type 2 diabetes	To facilitate changes in eating and physical activity habits that reduce insulin resistance and improve metabolic control
Goals specific to patients on insulin or insulin secretagogues	To provide self-management education for treatment and prevention of hypoglycemia, acute illnesses and exercise-related blood glucose problems

patterns with different macronutrient composition on glycemic responses. For example, a carrot has a high GI but a low glycemic load, whereas a potato has both a high GI and a high glycemic load. Individuals who use intensive insulin therapy select their pre-meal insulin doses based on the carbohydrate content of their meals, whereas individuals who receive fixed daily insulin doses should attempt to maintain day-to-day consistency with respect to the carbohydrate content of their meals and snacks. Although the use of low GI foods may reduce post-prandial glycemic excursions and may have long-term benefit on HbA1c concentrations, emphasis should be on the total amount of carbohydrate consumed and its source should be a secondary consideration [77].

Sucrose

Sucrose as part of the meal plan does not adversely affect blood glucose control in individuals with either type of diabetes. Sucrose and sucrose-containing foods may be substituted (gram for gram) for other carbohydrates. The nutrient content of sucrose-containing foods, as well as the presence of other nutrients frequently ingested with sucrose, such as fat, must be taken into consideration.

Fructose

Fructose is present as the free monosaccharide in many fruits, vegetables and honey. About one-third of dietary fructose comes from fruits, vegetables and other natural sources in the diet and about two-thirds comes from food and beverages to which fructose has been added. Fructose is absorbed more slowly from the intestinal tract than glucose, sucrose or maltose and is converted to glucose and glycogen in the liver. Post-prandial plasma glucose concentrations are reduced when an isocaloric amount of fructose replaces sucrose or starch in the diets of people with diabetes. Fructose has been used in children in amounts up to 0.5 g/kg/day but the potential benefit is tempered by concern that fructose may have adverse effects on serum lipids, especially low density lipoprotein (LDL) cholesterol. Consumption of large amounts of fructose [15–20% of daily energy intake (90th centile of usual intake)] increases fasting total and LDL cholesterol in subjects with diabetes and fasting total and LDL cholesterol and triglycerides in non-diabetic subjects. Because of the potential adverse effect of large amounts of fructose on serum lipids, fructose may have no overall advantage over other nutritive sweeteners. There is no reason to avoid naturally occurring sources of fructose.

Carbohydrate counting and exchange lists

Carbohydrate counting is a meal planning method in which the amount of carbohydrate or number of carbohydrate servings eaten at each meal and snack are counted. Carbohydrate is the main nutrient in starches, fruits, milk and sugar-containing foods and has the greatest effect on blood glucose concentrations. Therefore, it is the most important macronutrient to control in order to maintain optimal glycemic control. Using exchange lists, one starch choice is considered to be equivalent to either one fruit or milk choice; each contains approximately 15 g carbohydrate and is equal to one "carbohydrate choice" (Table 18.14).

The "nutrition facts" on food labels list the portion size and total amount of carbohydrate measured in grams per serving. Carbohydrate counting allows flexibility in food choices and minimizes "cheating" as all foods can be included in the meal

Groups/lists	Carbohydrate (g)	Protein (g)	Fat (g)	Calories
Carbohydrate choices				
Starch	15	3	0–1	80
Fruit	15	0	0	60
Milk				90–150
Fat-free, low fat	12	8	0–3	90
Reduced fat	12	8	5	120
Whole	12	8	8	150
Other carbohydrates	15	Varies	Varies	Varies
Non-starchy vegetable				
(when using carbohydrate choices, a single serving is "free"; 3 servings = 1 carbohydrate choice)	5	2	0	25
Meat and meat substitutes				
Very lean	0	7	0–1	35
Lean	0	7	3	55
Medium fat	0	7	5	75
High fat	0	7	8	100
Fat group	0	0	5	45

Table 18.14 Calorie and macronutrient content of exchange lists.

Table 18.15 An example of a patient's daily food allowance distributed among the food groups.

Group	Exchanges	Carbohydrate (g)	Protein (g)	Fat (g)
Starch	8	120	16	
Fruit	4	60		
Milk	3 low fat (1%)	36	24	9
Vegetables	1	5	2	
Meat	6 medium fat		42	30
Fat	4			20
Grams		221	84	59
Calories (%)		884 (50.5)	336 (19.2)	531 (30.3)

plan. Table 18.15 shows an example of a patient's daily meal plan incorporating both the exchange servings and grams of carbohydrate.

Fiber, which refers to the indigestible portion of a plant, influences the digestion, absorption and metabolism of many nutrients. Inclusion of plant fiber in the diet may benefit patients with diabetes by diminishing post-prandial glycemia and certain soluble plant fibers significantly reduce serum cholesterol and fasting serum triglyceride concentrations in patients with diabetes who have hypertriglyceridemia. Dietary fiber guidelines for children with diabetes are the same as for non-diabetic children and can be readily achieved by increasing the consumption of minimally processed foods, such as grains, legumes, fruits and vegetables. In diabetic adolescents using intensive insulin treatment methods, optimal blood glucose control is more common in those who have a higher intake of fiber, fruits and vegetables [82].

Protein

Protein requirements are not increased when diabetes is well controlled with insulin and children with diabetes should follow the recommended daily allowance guidelines. Physiologic requirements are determined by the amount of protein necessary to sustain normal growth, which is based on ideal weight-for-height and varies with age, being highest in infancy and early childhood. Protein intake should be 0.9–2.2 g/kg body weight/day and constitutes 15–20% of the total daily intake of energy, the same as for non-diabetic children and adolescents. The consumption of saturated fat can be reduced by eating less red meat, whole milk and high-fat dairy foods and by eating more poultry, fish and vegetable proteins and drinking more low-fat milk.

Fat

A carbohydrate meal that also has a high content of saturated fat significantly increases and prolongs the glycemic effect of the meal and requires anticipatory adjustment of the dose of insulin to combat the effect. Excessive saturated fat, cholesterol and total energy lead to increased blood concentrations of cholesterol and triglycerides. Because hyperlipidemia is a major determinant of atherosclerosis and patients with type 1 diabetes eventually develop atherosclerosis and its sequelae, the meal plan should attempt to mitigate this risk factor.

Children and adolescents with well-controlled type 1 diabetes are not at high risk for dyslipidemia but should be screened and monitored according to recommended guidelines (see below). If the child or adolescent is growing and developing normally and has normal plasma lipid concentrations, <10% of energy should come from saturated fat, the daily intake of cholesterol should be <300 mg/day and consumption of transunsaturated fatty acids should be minimized. Total dietary fat should be reduced in the obese child to reduce total energy consumption. The National Cholesterol Education Program (NCEP) Step II diet guidelines should be implemented in the patient with elevated LDL cholesterol [>2.6 mmol/L (100 mg/dL)]. Total fat should constitute ≤30% of total calories, <7% of calories from saturated fat and dietary cholesterol is limited to 200 mg/day [83,84].

MNT education and formulation of the meal plan

Newly diagnosed children usually present with weight loss. Therefore, the initial meal plan includes an estimation of energy requirements to restore and then maintain an appropriate body weight and allow normal growth and development. Energy requirements vary with age, height, weight, stage of puberty and level of physical activity. Because the energy needs of growing children change continuously, the meal plan should be re-evaluated every 6 months in young children and annually in adolescents.

MNT begins with an assessment by a dietitian, heeding the ethnic, religious and economic factors pertaining to the individual patient and family. The meal plan must take account of the child's school schedule, early or late lunches, physical education classes, after-school physical activity and differences in a child's activities on weekdays compared with weekends and holidays. Young children typically have three meals and two or three snacks daily, depending on the interval between meals, age of the child and level of physical activity.

Although their daily energy intake is relatively constant over time, young children adjust their energy intake at successive meals. The highly variable food consumption from meal to meal typical of normal children is especially challenging when the child has type 1 diabetes. Rapid-acting insulin based on estimation of the actual amount of carbohydrate consumed may be administered immediately after the meal and diminishes parental anxiety.

The purpose of snacks is to prevent hypoglycemia and hunger between meals. If the basal insulin component is adjusted appropriately, patients who use a basal-bolus insulin regimen or insulin pump therapy may not require snacks. Data from pre- and postprandial blood glucose monitoring and individualized insulin : carbohydrate ratios are used to select insulin doses to match anticipated carbohydrate intake.

The dietitian's role is to evaluate the patient's and family's knowledge and understanding of nutrition and to formulate an individualized meal plan. Even intensive insulin replacement regimens are not successful without careful attention to meal planning. Nutrition education, like all aspects of diabetes education, has to be an ongoing process with periodic review and revision of the meal plan and assessment of the child's and parents' levels of comprehension, ability to analyze and solve problems and adherence to the nutrition goals. The patient with newly diagnosed diabetes and his/her parents should consult with a dietitian several times during the first few days after diagnosis. Within a few weeks of the child resuming his/her usual schedule and activities, the patient and family should review the meal plan with a dietitian, who should also be available to patients for telephone consultation. If the patient's glycemic control is poor, if growth is failing, if weight gain is excessive or if other problems arise related to MNT, the dietitian should be reconsulted.

The meal plan

The individualized meal plan must be simple, practical, easy to modify and offer interesting, tasty and inexpensive foods. Dietary strategies principally are determined by the patient's insulin replacement regimen (Table 18.16). We advocate meal planning adapted to the ethnic, religious and economic circumstances of each family and based on a combination of carbohydrate counting and the exchange system. Each list in the exchange system for meal planning indicates the appropriate size or volume of each food exchange. Each portion of food within a group is exchangeable because it contains approximately the same nutritional value in terms of calories, carbohydrate, protein and fat. By prescribing the meal plan in terms of a number of exchanges for each meal, consistency of total calories and the proportions of nutrients can be maintained, while allowing the patient to choose among numerous foods. Accurate measurement of portion sizes has to be learned, and weighing and measuring foods help to achieve familiarity with the sizes of food portions specified in the exchange list. Weighing and measuring food should be viewed as an edu-

cational exercise to train the eye and need not be continued indefinitely but, if blood glucose control appears inexplicably to deteriorate, it is useful to resume weighing and measuring food portions to ensure that amounts are accurate. The exchange system should not be used in isolation; rather, it should be one component of a nutritional program directed by a trained dietitian.

An example of how this system can be applied to a hypothetical patient is as follows. An 11-year-old girl's height is 144 cm (50th percentile on the Centers for Disease Control and Prevention growth chart) and weight is 37.4 kg (50th percentile). Her daily energy requirement to support growth in the 50th percentile is 1756 calories. An appropriate distribution of macronutrients is 50% of total calories from carbohydrate, 20% as protein and 30% as fat (Table 18.15).

Exercise

Children with diabetes should be encouraged to participate in sports and include regular exercise in their lives. Participation in physical exercise normalizes the child's life, enhances self-esteem, improves physical fitness, helps to control weight and may improve glycemic control. Regular exercise increases insulin sensitivity, cardiovascular fitness and lean body mass, improves blood lipid profiles and lowers blood pressure.

Although physical exercise is complicated for the child with type 1 diabetes, especially by the need to prevent hypoglycemia, with proper guidance and planning, exercise can be a safe and enjoyable experience [85]. Blood glucose responses to prolonged moderate-intensity exercise are reliable and repeatable when pre-exercise meal, exercise and insulin regimens are kept constant [86]. Exercise acutely lowers the blood glucose concentration by increasing utilization of glucose to a variable degree depending on the intensity and duration of physical activity and the concurrent level of insulin in the blood. Note, however, that in type 1 diabetes increased concentrations of epinephrine and glucagon

Table 18.16 General approaches to meal management.

Type 1 diabetes	Split-mixed insulin regimen	3 meals and 2 or 3 snacks daily
		Meals and snacks spaced 2–3 h apart
		Consistent carbohydrate intake
		Snack before bed to decrease risk of overnight hypoglycemia
		Meal times consistent from day-to-day
		Continued education and assessment of readiness to change lifestyle to achieve Heart Healthy diet
	Basal-bolus or insulin pump therapy	Carbohydrate content can vary
		Must accurately count carbohydrate and match insulin dose to pre-determined insulin:carbohydrate ratio
		Should eat at least 3 meals daily
		Should not eat less than a predetermined amount of carbohydrate per day
		Continued education and assessment of readiness to change lifestyle to achieve Heart Healthy diet
Type 2 diabetes		Meal plan to assist with evenly spaced carbohydrate intake and increased emphasis on reducing calories to promote weight loss

Age-related issues: children's activities often differ on weekdays compared to weekends and holidays and appropriate allowance must be made for these differences. The meal plan must take into account the child's school schedule, early or late lunches, gym classes and after-school physical activity.

in response to acute strenuous anaerobic exercise may cause transient hyperglycemia for 30–60 min.

Hypoglycemia can usually be prevented by a combination of anticipatory reduction in the pre-exercise insulin dose or a temporary interruption or reduction of basal insulin infusion (with CSII) and supplemental snacks before, during and after physical activity, depending on its duration and intensity. Nearly all forms of activity lasting more than 30 min require some adjustment to food and/or insulin. Continuous moderate intensity exercise tends to cause a lesser decline in blood glucose concentrations than intermittent high-intensity exercise of short duration [87]. The optimal strategy depends on timing of the exercise relative to the child's meal plan and on the insulin regimen.

Consideration is given to several factors when selecting the content and size of the snack. Among these are the current blood glucose level, the action of insulin most active during and after the period of anticipated exercise, the interval since the last meal and the duration and intensity of physical activity. The appropriate amount is learned by trial and error but a useful initial guide is to provide up to 1 g carbohydrate per kilogram of body mass per hour of strenuous exercise.

Prolonged and strenuous exercise in the afternoon or evening should be followed by a 10–30% reduction in the pre-supper or bedtime dose of intermediate- or long-acting insulin or an equivalent reduction in overnight basal insulin delivery in patients using CSII. In addition, to reduce the risk of nocturnal or early morning hypoglycemia caused by the lag effect of exercise, the bedtime snack should be larger than usual and contain carbohydrate, protein and fat. Parents should be encouraged to monitor the blood glucose concentration in the middle of the night until they are experienced, modifying the evening dose of insulin after exercise.

Blood glucose monitoring is essential for the active child with diabetes because it allows identification of trends in glycemic responses. Records should include blood glucose concentrations, timing, duration and intensity of exercise as well the strategies used to maintain glucose concentrations in the target range. Blood glucose concentrations should be measured before, during and after exercise and, to prevent nocturnal hypoglycemia, before bed (Table 18.17).

Exercising the limb into which insulin has been injected accelerates the rate of insulin absorption. If possible, the insulin injection preceding exercise should be given in a site least likely to be affected by exercise. Because physical training increases tissue sensitivity to insulin, children who participate in organized sports are advised to reduce the dose of the insulin preparation predominantly active during the period of sustained physical activity (Table 18.17). The size of such reductions is determined by measuring blood glucose concentrations before and after exercise and is generally in the order of 10–30% of the usual dose.

In the child with poorly controlled diabetes, vigorous exercise can aggravate hyperglycemia and ketoacid production; accordingly, a child with ketonuria should not exercise until satisfactory biochemical control has been restored (Table 18.17).

Table 18.17 Practical guidelines for exercise. After Riddell and Iscoe [85].

1 Consider the timing, mode, duration and intensity of exercise
2 Eat a carbohydrate-containing meal 1–3 h before exercise
3 Measure blood glucose level
  (a) If BG <90 mg/dL (5 mmol/L) and concentrations are decreasing, extra calories needed
  (b) If BG 90–270 mg/dL (5–15 mmol/L), extra calories may not be needed, depending on duration of exercise and individual's response to exercise
  (c) If BG >270 mg/dL (>15 mmol/L) and urine or blood ketones are increased, delay exercise until concentrations are restored to normal with supplemental insulin
4 If the exercise is aerobic, determine whether insulin or additional carbohydrate will be needed based on the peak insulin activity
  (a) If insulin dose is to be changed for long duration moderate–high intensity activity, reduce premeal insulin dose by 50% 1 h before exercise. On subsequent days, adjust dose based on measured individual response
  (b) Inject insulin in a site that will not be affected by exercising muscles
  (c) If additional carbohydrate is required, start with 1 g/kg/h of moderate–high intensity exercise performed during peak insulin activity; less carbohydrate is required as time elapsed since last injection increases
  (d) Alter the amount of carbohydrate on subsequent days based on measured individual response

BG, blood glucose.

Monitoring diabetes control
Self-monitoring of blood glucose

Self-monitoring of blood glucose (SMBG) is the cornerstone of modern diabetes care. Most glucose meters now display plasma values, which are about 10–15% higher than those for whole blood. Patients and parents must be taught how to use the data to assess the efficacy of therapy and to adjust the components of their treatment regimen to achieve individual blood glucose goals. Most glucose meters have an electronic memory but it is valuable for patients and parents to keep written records of their results and to analyze the data for patterns and trends and to make adjustments when necessary.

For most patients with type 1 diabetes, SMBG should be performed at least four times daily: before each meal and at bedtime. To minimize the risk of nocturnal hypoglycemia, blood glucose (BG) should be measured between midnight and 4 a.m. once each week or every other week and whenever the evening dose of insulin is adjusted. If HbA1c targets are not being met, patients should be encouraged to measure BG concentrations more frequently, including 90–120 min after meals. Frequency of BG monitoring is a predictor of glycemic control in children with type 1 diabetes [88,89]. The optimal frequency of SMBG for patients with type 2 diabetes is not known but should be sufficient to guide adjustments in medication and facilitate attainment of the individual patient's glycemic goals. Children who are able to perform SMBG independently must be properly supervised because it is not unusual for children to fabricate data with disastrous consequences. Common reasons for deterioration of metabolic control are shown in Table 18.18.

Table 18.18 Causes of deterioration of metabolic control in children and adolescents with diabetes mellitus.

Increased insulin requirement
Progressive loss of residual β-cell function
Failure to increase dose with growth
Failure to increase dose during puberty
Increased calorie intake
Illness or significant psychological stress
Diminished physical activity (often seasonal)
Medications that cause insulin resistance (e.g. glucocorticoids)

Insulin omission (inadvertent or deliberate)

"Failure" of administered insulin
Inappropriate timing of insulin in relation to food consumption
Failure to completely suspend intermediate-acting insulin suspension
Lipohypertrophy at site of insulin injection
Loss of insulin potency (frozen, heated or expired)
Improper injection technique (intramuscular or intra-epidermal injection)

Miscellaneous causes
Fabricated blood glucose data
Glucose meter malfunction
Celiac disease
Hyperthyroidism
High titer insulin antibodies

Continuous glucose monitoring

The technology of continuous glucose monitoring (CGM) has evolved rapidly. Current CGM devices measure glucose in the interstitial fluid by means of a short thin subcutaneous probe that can be used for 3–7 days. The accuracy of CGM devices is improving but not yet considered sufficient to substitute for SMBG by portable glucose meters. Furthermore, each newly placed CGM probe must be calibrated during a period of stable glycemia over several hours by performing simultaneous capillary blood glucose measurements. Importantly, there is a several minute lag between actual plasma glucose and interstitial glucose concentrations. Thus, current CGM devices cannot substitute for SMBG; they are used as an adjunct to provide BG information between SMBG measurements.

The latest generation of continuous glucose devices report the estimated plasma glucose values in real time (RT-CGM) every 1–5 min via a user interface. Several such RT-CGM devices are commercially available and approved for use in the USA and Europe. Information from RT-CGM allows the user to detect the early phases of a hyperglycemic or hypoglycemic episode, thereby enabling corrective action to be taken after confirmatory SMBG. Short-term (3 month) uncontrolled trials of current-generation RT-CGM have demonstrated improved HbA1c concentrations and a high level of patient satisfaction [90]. Whether RT-CGM will lead to durable improvements of glycemia and/or reduction in risk of acute diabetic complications is unknown.

Urine ketone testing

Urine should be tested for ketones during acute illness or stress, when blood glucose concentrations are persistently elevated (e.g. two consecutive blood glucose values >300 mg/dL, 16.7 mmol/L) or when the patient feels unwell, especially with abdominal pain, nausea or vomiting. False-negative readings may occur when the strips have been exposed to air (e.g. improperly stored) or when urine is highly acidic (e.g. after consumption of large doses of ascorbic acid). Urine ketone tests using nitroprusside-containing reagents can give false-positive results in patients who take valproic acid or any sulfhydryl-containing drug, including captopril.

Blood ketone testing

Meters available for home use that measure blood β-hydroxybutyric acid (βOHB) concentrations are expensive and not widely used. Quantification of blood βOHB, the predominant ketone body, is preferred over urine ketone testing for diagnosing and monitoring metabolic decompensation as may occur with intercurrent illness, pump failure and in ketoacidosis [91]. Blood ketone determination is helpful in avoiding emergency room visits [92] and offers the advantage of accurately assessing improvement after starting treatment [91].

Glycated hemoglobin (HbA1c)

HbA1c is a minor fraction of adult hemoglobin, which is formed slowly and non-enzymatically from hemoglobin and glucose. Because erythrocytes are freely permeable to glucose, HbA1c is formed throughout the lifespan of the erythrocyte; its rate of formation is directly proportional to the ambient glucose concentration. The concentration of HbA1c, therefore, provides a "glycemic history" of the previous 120 days, the average lifespan of erythrocytes. Although HbA1c reflects glycemia over the preceding 12 weeks, it is weighted toward the most recent 4 weeks. Blood glucose and blood or urine ketone testing provide useful information for day-to-day management of diabetes, whereas HbA1c provides important information about recent average glycemic control. It is an integral component of the management of patients with diabetes and is used to monitor long-term glycemic control and as a measure of the risk for the development of diabetes complications.

More than 30 different methods are used to measure HbA1c which has led to different non-diabetic reference ranges because different glycated hemoglobin fractions are measured [93]. The International Federation of Clinical Chemistry has developed a new reference method that precisely measures the concentration of glycated hemoglobin (betaN1-deoxyfructosyl-hemoglobin) [94] and a recently completed international study has determined the relationship between mean blood glucose over many weeks and the glycated hemoglobin concentration. It is anticipated that the new assay will be reported as "estimated average blood glucose" or "A1C-derived average glucose" and the units will be mmol/L or mg/dL [95].

HbA1c should be measured approximately every 3 months to determine whether a patient's metabolic control has reached or has been maintained within a target range. The HbA1c is primarily used to monitor the effectiveness of glycemic therapy and as an indicator for when therapy needs to be modified.

Average glucose concentrations are underestimated by HbA1c in conditions that shorten the average circulating red blood cell lifespan, such as hemolysis, sickle cell disease, transfusion and iron deficiency anemia. When accurate HbA1c measurement is not possible, as in the above conditions, alternative measures of chronic glycemia such as fructosamine or glycated serum albumin should be used. These measure the glycation of serum proteins rather than hemoglobin, and reflect glycemia over the preceding 2–4 weeks.

Acute complications of diabetes

Diabetic ketoacidosis
In Canada, the USA and Europe, annual rates of hospitalization for DKA in established and new patients with type 1 diabetes have remained stable at about 8–10 per 100 000 children over the past 20 years [96]. The risk of DKA in patients with established type 1 diabetes is 1–10% per patient per year [39]. It is increased in children with poor metabolic control or previous episodes of DKA, peripubertal and adolescent girls, children with psychiatric disorders, including those with eating disorders, and those with difficult family circumstances, including lower socioeconomic status and lack of health insurance. In the era of CSII, interruption of insulin delivery, irrespective of the reason, is an important cause of DKA. Children rarely have DKA when insulin administration is closely supervised or performed by a responsible adult. In established patients, most instances of DKA are probably associated with insulin omission or treatment error, while the remainder are caused by inadequate insulin therapy during intercurrent illness.

The biochemical criteria for the diagnosis of DKA include hyperglycemia (blood glucose >11 mmol/L (approximately 200 mg/dL)) with acidosis (venous blood pH <7.3 and/or serum bicarbonate ≤15 mmol/L), ketonemia with total serum ketones (β-hydroxybutyrate and acetoacetate) >3 mmol/L and ketonuria. DKA is generally categorized as mild (venous pH <7.30, bicarbonate <15 mmol/L), moderate (pH <7.2, bicarbonate <10 mmol/L) or severe (pH <7.1, bicarbonate <5 mmol/L).

Pathophysiology
DKA is the result of absolute or relative deficiency of circulating insulin and the combined effects of increased concentrations of the counter-regulatory hormones, catecholamines, glucagon, cortisol and growth hormone. Absolute insulin deficiency occurs in previously undiagnosed type 1 diabetes and when patients on treatment deliberately or inadvertently do not take insulin. Relative insulin deficiency occurs when the concentrations of counter-regulatory hormones increase under conditions of stress such as

sepsis, trauma or gastrointestinal illness with diarrhea and vomiting. Low serum concentrations of insulin and high concentrations of the counter-regulatory hormones results in an accelerated catabolic state whose effects are: increased glucose production by the liver and kidney (via glycogenolysis and gluconeogenesis), impaired peripheral glucose utilization resulting in hyperglycemia and hyperosmolality and increased lipolysis and ketogenesis, causing ketonemia and metabolic acidosis. Hyperglycemia and hyperketonemia cause osmotic diuresis, dehydration and obligatory loss of electrolytes often exacerbated by vomiting (Table 18.19).

DKA may be aggravated by lactic acidosis from poor tissue perfusion and/or sepsis and is characterized by severe depletion of water and electrolytes (Table 18.20). Despite dehydration, patients continue to have considerable urine output unless they are extremely volume depleted. The magnitude of specific deficits in an individual patient at the time of presentation depends on the duration of illness, the extent to which the patient was able to maintain intake of fluid and electrolytes, as well as the content of food and fluids consumed before presentation.

Management of DKA
Initial evaluation
• Perform a clinical evaluation to establish the diagnosis and determine its cause (especially any evidence of infection).
• Weigh the patient and measure height or length to determine body surface area.
• Assess the patient's degree of dehydration.
• Determine the blood glucose concentration with a glucose meter and the blood or urine ketone concentration.

Table 18.19 Clinical manifestations of diabetic ketoacidosis (DKA).

Dehydration
Rapid, deep, sighing (Kussmaul) respiration
Nausea, vomiting, abdominal pain that may mimic an acute abdomen
Increased leukocyte count with left shift
Non-specific elevation of serum amylase
Fever when there is infection
Progressive obtundation and loss of consciousness

Table 18.20 Usual losses of fluids and electrolytes in diabetic ketoacidosis and normal maintenance requirements. These data are from measurements in only a few children and adolescents [39].

	Average losses per kg (range)	Maintenance requirements per meter^2
Water	70 mL (30–100)	1500 mL
Sodium	6 mmol (5–13)	45 mmol
Potassium	5 mmol (3–6)	35 mmol
Chloride	4 mmol (3–9)	30 mmol
Phosphate	(0.5–2.5) mmol	10 mmol

- Obtain a blood sample for laboratory measurement of glucose, electrolytes and TCO_2, blood urea nitrogen, creatinine, serum osmolality, venous (or arterial in critically ill patient) pH, pCO_2, pO_2, hemoglobin, hematocrit, total and differential white blood cell count, calcium, phosphorus and magnesium concentrations.
- Perform a urinalysis and obtain appropriate specimens for culture (blood, urine, throat).
- Perform an electrocardiogram for baseline evaluation of potassium status.

Supportive measures

- Secure the airway and empty the stomach by continuous nasogastric suction to prevent pulmonary aspiration in the unconscious or severely obtunded patient.
- Give antibiotics to febrile patients after obtaining appropriate cultures of body fluids.
- Give supplementary oxygen to patients with severe circulatory impairment or shock.
- Catheterization of the bladder is usually not necessary but if the child is unconscious or unable to void on demand (e.g. infants and very ill young children), the bladder should be catheterized.
- A flow chart is essential to record the patient's clinical and laboratory data, including vital signs [heart rate, respiratory rate, blood pressure, level of consciousness (Glasgow coma scale)], details of fluid and electrolyte therapy, amount of administered insulin and urine output. One key to successful management of diabetic ketoacidosis is meticulous monitoring of the patient's clinical and biochemical response to treatment so that timely adjustments in the treatment regimen can be made when indicated by the patient's clinical or laboratory data. Frequent re-examination of laboratory parameters is required to prevent serious electrolyte imbalance and administration of either insufficient or excessive fluid.
- A heparin-locked intravenous catheter should be placed for convenient and painless repetitive blood sampling.
- A cardiac monitor should be used for continuous electrocardiographic monitoring.

Fluid and electrolyte therapy

All patients with DKA are dehydrated and suffer total body depletion of sodium, potassium, chloride, phosphate and magnesium (Table 18.20). The high effective osmolality of the extracellular fluid (ECF) compartment results in a shift of water from the intracellular fluid compartment (ICF) to the ECF and decreases the serum sodium concentration approximately 1.6 mmol/L per 5.6 mmol/L (100 mg/dL) of blood glucose above normal. The presence of hyperlipidemia may also lower the measured serum sodium concentration (depending on the methodology used to measure serum sodium concentration) so the serum sodium concentration may give a misleading estimate of the degree of sodium loss. The effective osmolality (see formula below) at the time of presentation is frequently in the range 300–350 mOsm/L. Increased serum urea nitrogen and hematocrit are useful markers

of severe ECF contraction. At the time of presentation, patients are ECF contracted and clinical estimates of the deficit in patients with severe DKA are usually in the range of 7–10%. In mild to moderately severe DKA, fluid deficits are more modest, in the range 30–50 mL/kg. Shock with hemodynamic compromise is uncommon in childhood.

The onset of dehydration is associated with a reduced glomerular filtration rate (GFR), which results in decreased glucose and ketone clearance. Intravenous fluid administration expands the intravascular volume and increases glomerular filtration, which increases renal excretion of glucose and ketones and results in a prompt decrease in blood glucose concentration.

The goals of fluid and salt replacement therapy in DKA are to restore circulating volume, replace sodium and the ECF and ICF water to restore GFR (with enhanced clearance of glucose and ketones from the blood) and avoid cerebral edema (Table 18.21). In both animals and humans, intracranial pressure rises as intravenous fluids are given. Although there is no compelling evidence showing superiority of any fluid regimen over another, there are data that suggest that rapid fluid replacement with hypotonic fluid in the first several hours of treatment is associated with an increased risk of cerebral edema; slower fluid deficit correction with isotonic or near-isotonic solutions results in earlier reversal of acidosis. Large amounts of 0.9% saline have also been associated with the development of hyperchloremic metabolic acidosis (Table 18.22).

Initial intravenous fluid administration and, when necessary, volume expansion, should begin immediately with an isotonic solution (0.9% saline or balanced salt solution such as Ringer's lactate). The volume and rate of administration depends on the patient's circulatory status. When volume expansion is clinically indicated, 10–20 mL/kg is given over 1–2 h and may be repeated if necessary. Continue to use 0.9% saline for at least 4–6 h. Thereafter, use a solution with a tonicity ≥0.45% saline [0.9% saline or balanced salt solution (Ringer's lactate) or 0.45% saline with added potassium]. The rate of intravenous fluid administration should be calculated to rehydrate the patient at an even rate over 48 h.

Table 18.21 Goals of therapy.

Correct dehydration
Restore blood glucose to near normal concentrations
Correct acidosis and reverse ketosis
Avoid complications of treatment

Table 18.22 Complications of therapy.

Inadequate rehydration
Hypoglycemia
Hypokalemia
Hyperchloremic acidosis
Cerebral edema

Because the severity of dehydration may be difficult to determine and is often overestimated, the daily volume of fluid should not usually exceed 1.5–2 times the usual daily requirement based on age, weight or body surface area (Table 18.20). Urinary losses should not be added to the calculation of replacement fluids. The development of hyponatremia or failure to observe a progressive rise in serum sodium concentration with a concomitant decrease of blood glucose concentration during treatment is a risk factor for cerebral edema (Table 18.23). Monitor the effective serum osmolality and allow it to decrease gradually. If the effective osmolality starts low or does not increase appropriately as the plasma glucose concentration falls, increase the sodium concentration.

When the blood glucose concentration reaches approximately 17 mmol/L (300 mg/dL), 5% dextrose is added to the infusion fluid. Adjust the dextrose concentration to avoid hypoglycemia. It may be necessary to use ≥10% dextrose. Administration of intravenous fluids should be continued until acidosis is corrected (venous pH ≥7.30 and anion gap near to normal) and the patient can tolerate fluids and food. Inadequate fluid administration should be evident from examination of the cumulative fluid balance and persistent tachycardia in the absence of a fever.

Insulin

Hydration decreases the plasma glucose concentration but insulin is essential to restore blood glucose to normal, to suppress lipolysis and ketogenesis and reverse ketoacidosis. Several routes (subcutaneous, intramuscular and intravenous) of insulin administration and doses have been used but "low dose" intravenous insulin administration is the standard of care. Intravenous regular (soluble) insulin at a dose of 0.1 unit/kg/h achieves steady state serum insulin concentrations of 50–200 μU/mL within 60 min, which are adequate to offset the insulin resistance characteristic of DKA. They suppress glucose production, significantly increase peripheral glucose uptake and inhibit lipolysis and ketogenesis. The dose of insulin should remain at 0.1 unit/kg/h until resolution of ketoacidosis (pH >7.30 and bicarbonate >15 mmol/L and/or closure of the anion gap).

It may be necessary to reduce the dose to 0.05–0.075 unit/kg/h in more insulin sensitive patients, especially young children and patients with mild to moderate DKA, provided acidosis continues to resolve. It should be noted, however, that resolution of keto-acidemia takes longer than restoration of blood glucose concentrations to normal. Therefore, intravenous insulin therapy must

Table 18.23 Factors associated with increased risk of cerebral edema.

An attenuated rise in measured serum sodium concentration during treatment
More severe acidosis
Administration of bicarbonate to correct acidosis
More profound hypocapnia at presentation
Increased serum urea nitrogen at presentation reflecting more severe dehydration

not be discontinued until ketoacidosis has resolved, even if the blood glucose concentration is normal or near normal. To prevent an unduly rapid fall in blood glucose concentration and development of hypoglycemia, dextrose should be added to the intravenous fluid when the plasma glucose has fallen to approximately 17 mmol/L (300 mg/dL).

Continuous intravenous insulin should be administered via an infusion pump. Regular insulin is diluted in normal saline (50 units regular insulin in 50 mL saline) and is given at a rate of 0.1 unit/kg/h. The insulin infusion should commence after initial volume expansion, 1–2 h after starting fluid therapy. An intravenous priming dose is both unnecessary and may increase the risk of cerebral edema [97]. This rate of insulin infusion is sufficient to reverse ketoacidosis in most patients but if the response is inadequate, especially if blood glucose level is falling but acidosis is not improving owing to severe insulin resistance, the rate of insulin infusion should be increased until a satisfactory response is achieved.

It is essential to monitor the blood glucose, venous (or arterial) pH and anion gap response to insulin therapy and, very occasionally, patients with severe insulin resistance do not respond satisfactorily to low-dose insulin infusion and require two or three times the usual dose. Other possible explanations for failure to respond to insulin and especially an error in insulin preparation should be considered.

When intravenous administration is not possible, the intramuscular or subcutaneous route of insulin administration may be used and hourly or 2-hourly rapid-acting insulin (lispro or aspart) may be preferable to regular insulin in these circumstances. Poor tissue perfusion in a severely dehydrated patient will impair SC absorption of insulin and, initially, insulin should be given intramuscularly.

The serum half-life of insulin is 5 min so that if the insulin infusion is stopped, insulin concentration decreases rapidly. If the infusion were to infiltrate and this was not recognized promptly, inadequate serum insulin concentrations would ensue rapidly. Therefore, low-dose intravenous insulin therapy must be carefully supervised.

When ketoacidosis has resolved and the change to subcutaneous insulin is planned, the first subcutaneous injection should be given before stopping the infusion to allow sufficient time for the subcutaneously injected insulin to begin to be absorbed.

Potassium

Potassium is predominantly lost from the intracellular pool as a result of hypertonicity, insulin deficiency and buffering of hydrogen ions within the cell. During acidosis, intracellular potassium enters the extracellular compartment and is lost in urine and vomit. At the time of presentation, serum potassium concentrations may be normal, increased or, infrequently, decreased. Hypokalemia at presentation is related to prolonged duration of disease and persistent vomiting, whereas hyperkalemia results primarily from impaired renal function. Adults with DKA have total body potassium deficits of the order of 4–6 mmol/kg and, although data in children are few, similar deficits have been described.

Insulin promotes uptake of glucose and potassium by cells and correction of acidosis promotes the return of potassium to the intracellular compartment. The serum potassium concentration may decrease abruptly, predisposing the patient to cardiac arrhythmias. In the unusual patient who presents with hypokalemia, insulin administration should be deferred and potassium replacement should be started immediately. Otherwise, it should be started after initial volume expansion and concurrent with commencing insulin therapy. If the patient presents with hyperkalemia, potassium administration should be deferred until urine output has been documented and the potassium concentration has decreased to a normal level.

The amount of potassium administered should be sufficient to maintain serum potassium concentrations in the normal range. The usual starting potassium concentration in the infusate should be 40 mmol/L and potassium administration should continue throughout the period of intravenous fluid therapy. The usual maximum rate of intravenous potassium administration is 0.5 mmol/kg/h. Careful monitoring of the serum level and provision of adequate potassium is essential to prevent hypokalemia and life-threatening arrhythmias.

Electrocardiography (ECG) can be used as a guide to therapy and is especially valuable while waiting for the serum potassium concentration to be measured. Flattening of the T wave, widening of the QT interval and the appearance of U waves indicate hypokalemia. Tall peaked symmetrical T waves and shortening of the QT interval are signs of hyperkalemia.

The plasma potassium concentration should be checked every hour if the plasma concentration is outside the normal range. Potassium may be given as chloride, acetate or phosphate. Use of potassium acetate and potassium phosphate reduces the total amount of chloride administered and partially corrects the phosphate deficit.

Phosphate

Depletion of intracellular phosphate occurs in DKA as a result of osmotic diuresis. In adults, deficits are in the range 0.5–2.5 mmol/kg but comparable data in children are few. After starting therapy, plasma phosphate concentrations decrease rapidly as a result of urinary excretion and because insulin causes phosphate to re-enter cells. Low serum phosphate concentrations have been associated with a variety of metabolic disturbances but the effect of hypophosphatemia on 2,3-diphosphoglycerate concentrations and on tissue oxygenation are especially relevant to DKA management. Although phosphate depletion persists for several days after resolution of DKA, prospective studies have not shown any significant clinical benefit from phosphate replacement. Nevertheless, serum phosphate should be monitored and severe hypophosphatemia treated with potassium phosphate while serum calcium is carefully monitored to avoid phosphate-induced hypocalcemia.

Acidosis and bicarbonate

Even severe acidosis is reversible by fluid and insulin replacement by stopping synthesis of ketoacids and promoting ketone utilization because the metabolism of ketones results in regeneration of bicarbonate and correction of acidemia. Treatment of hypovolemia improves tissue perfusion and restores renal function, thus increasing the excretion of organic acids, and reverses lactic acidosis, which may account for up to 25% of the acidemia.

In DKA, the anion gap is increased primarily because of a marked increase in the concentrations of β-OHB and acetoacetate. Acetone is formed by spontaneous decarboxylation of acetoacetate. Acetoacetate and acetone, but not β-OHB, are measured by the commonly used clinical reagent strip or tablet methods that employ the sodium nitroprusside reaction. At initial presentation with DKA, the concentration of β OHB is 4 to 10 fold higher than that of acetoacetic acid. With insulin therapy and correction of the acidosis, the β-OHB is re-oxidized to acetoacetate, which is eventually metabolized. Blood ketone meters measure only β-OHB.

The indications for bicarbonate therapy in DKA are unclear. Controlled trials have not shown clinical benefit nor any important difference in the rate of rise of plasma bicarbonate concentration. There are physiologic reasons not to use bicarbonate. Its use may cause paradoxical CNS acidosis. Bicarbonate combines with H^+ and then dissociates to CO_2 and H_2O. The HCO_3^- diffuses poorly across the blood–brain barrier, whereas CO_2 freely diffuses into the cerebrospinal fluid. Hence, the use of bicarbonate may worsen acidosis within the central nervous system while serum acidosis improves. Rapid correction of acidosis causes hypokalemia, may aggravate sodium load and contributes to serum hypertonicity. It may also impair tissue oxygenation by increasing the affinity of hemoglobin for oxygen (i.e. shift the hemoglobin–oxygen dissociation curve to the left). Alkali therapy may increase hepatic ketone production and thus slow the rate of recovery from ketosis [39]. The use of bicarbonate in children with DKA is associated with an increased risk for cerebral edema [98].

However, there may be patients who benefit from cautious alkali therapy, including patients with severe acidemia (arterial pH <6.9) in whom decreased cardiac contractility and peripheral vasodilatation can further impair tissue perfusion and patients with life-threatening hyperkalemia. Administration of bicarbonate is indicated when acidosis is severe (arterial pH ≤6.9) and when hypotension, shock or an arrhythmia is present. In these circumstances, 1–2 mmol/kg sodium bicarbonate may be infused over 2 h and the plasma bicarbonate concentration rechecked. Bicarbonate should not be given as a bolus because this may precipitate acute cardiac arrhythmia.

Clinical and biochemical monitoring

Initially, plasma glucose should be measured hourly. Thereafter, plasma glucose, serum electrolytes (and corrected sodium), pH, pCO_2, TCO_2, anion gap, calcium and phosphorus should be measured every 2–4 h for the first 8 h and then every 4 h until they are normal. The data must be carefully recorded on a flow sheet.

Investigating the cause of ketoacidosis

The management of DKA is not complete until its cause has been identified and treated. An intercurrent infection is not the usual cause when the patient is properly educated in diabetes management, is receiving regular follow-up care and has access to a diabetes treatment team. In previously diagnosed patients on treatment with insulin, omission of insulin, either inadvertently or deliberately, is the most common cause. In users of CSII, the most common cause of DKA is failure to take extra insulin with a pen or syringe when hyperglycemia and hyperketonemia or ketonuria occur.

There is often an important psychosocial reason for insulin omission. This can be an attempt to lose weight (e.g. in an adolescent girl with an eating disorder), a means of escaping an intolerable or abusive home situation, clinical depression or other reason for the inability of the patient to manage his/her own diabetes unassisted [39]. A psychiatric social worker or clinical psychologist should be consulted to help to identify the psychosocial reason(s) underlying the development of DKA.

Useful calculations for managing DKA

1 Effective osmolality $= 2[Na^+ + K^+] +$ glucose (mmol/L)
2 Corrected sodium $= [Na^+] + (1.6 \times [\text{plasma glucose mmol/L} -5.6] \div 5.6)$
3 Anion gap $= [Na^+] - [Cl^- + HCO_3^-]$
4 Evaluation for pure metabolic acidosis: $pCO_2 =$ last two numbers of the pH

$$pCO_2 = 1.5 [\text{serum } HCO_3^-] + 8 \pm 2$$

Effective serum osmolality correlates with mental status abnormalities. Blood or serum urea nitrogen freely diffuses into cells and does not contribute to effective osmolality. Corrected serum sodium assists in estimation of free water deficits. A decreasing anion gap indicates successful therapy of metabolic acidosis. A lower than predicted pCO_2 indicates respiratory alkalosis and may be a clue to sepsis.

Morbidity and mortality from DKA in children

DKA is the leading cause of acute morbidity and mortality in children with type 1 diabetes [39]. Reported mortality rates from DKA in national population-based studies are reasonably constant in the range of 0.15–0.31%. In areas with sparse medical facilities, the risk of dying from DKA is greater and children may die before receiving treatment. Cerebral edema accounts for 57–87% of all deaths from DKA. The incidence of cerebral edema has been fairly consistent between national population-based studies; 0.46% in Canada to 0.87% in the USA. Mortality rates from cerebral edema in population-based studies are 21–25%. Significant morbidity occurs in 10–26% of survivors. Other causes of DKA-related morbidity and mortality include hypokalemia, hyperkalemia, hypoglycemia, sepsis and other CNS complications such as thrombosis [39].

Cerebral edema

This typically occurs 4–12 h after commencement of treatment but can occur before treatment has begun or at any time during treatment. Symptoms and signs are variable and include onset of headache, change in neurological status (restlessness, irritability, drowsiness, deterioration in level of consciousness), inappropriate slowing of the heart rate and an increase in blood pressure [99]. Cerebral edema is more common in children with severe DKA, new-onset type 1 diabetes, younger age and longer duration of symptoms [98]. The cause remains poorly understood [100].

Treatment of cerebral edema

Treatment should be initiated as soon as the condition is suspected [39]. The rate of fluid administration should be reduced by one-third. Intravenous mannitol (0.5–1 g/kg) should be given over 20 min and repeated if there is no response in 30 min. Hypertonic saline (3%), 5–10 mL/kg over 30 min has been used as an alternative to mannitol and is recommended if there is no response to mannitol. Intubation may be necessary for the patient with impending respiratory failure but aggressive hyperventilation [to a pCO_2 <22 mmHg (2.9 kPa)] has been associated with poor outcome and is not recommended [101].

After treatment for cerebral edema has been started, a cranial computed tomography (CT) scan should be obtained to rule out other possible intracerebral causes of neurologic deterioration (10% of cases), especially thrombosis or hemorrhage, which may benefit from specific therapy.

Management of sick days: prevention of DKA

Even a relatively minor illness in a child with type 1 diabetes can cause rapid deterioration of metabolic control. The stress of infection, surgery, injury or emotional upset increases counter-regulatory hormone concentrations, which cause hyperglycemia and stimulate lipolysis and ketogenesis. Even when carbohydrate consumption is reduced by illness, blood glucose concentrations usually increase and these metabolic disturbances can rapidly progress to DKA. The aim of sick day management is to minimize deterioration of metabolic control and prevent DKA (Tables 18.24 & 18.25).

Failure to administer the child's usual basal doses of insulin can have disastrous consequences. Supplemental injections of rapid- or short-acting insulin are often required to prevent or

Table 18.24 Principles of sick day management.

Treat the underlying illness
Never omit intermediate- or long-acting insulin injections or basal insulin infusion
Maintain hydration
Frequently measure blood glucose and blood or urine ketone concentrations
Administer supplemental rapid- or short-acting insulin every 2–4 h when indicated (refer to guidelines in Table 18.25)
Treat the underlying illness
Monitor for signs and symptoms that demand urgent medical attention

Table 18.25 Guidelines for supplemental insulin when the child is ill. After [103].

Ketones		Blood glucose				
Blood ketones (mmol/L)	Urine ketones	<5.5 mmol/L (<100 mg/dL)	5.5–10 mmol/L (100–180)	10–14 mmol/L 180–250 mg/dL	14–22 mmol/L 250–400 mg/dL	>22 mmol/L >400 mg/dL
<0.6	Negative or trace	No extra insulin; if <4 mmol/L consider mini dose glucagon*	No extra insulin	Increase dose of insulin for next meal if BG is still elevated	Give extra 5% of TDD† or 0.05 U/kg	Give extra 10% of TDD or 0.1 U/kg
0.6–0.9	Trace or small	Starvation ketosis; extra carbohydrate and fluid	Starvation ketosis; extra carbohydrate and fluid	Give extra 5% of TDD or 0.05 U/kg	Give extra 5–10% of TDD or 0.05–0.1 U/kg	Give extra 10% of TDD or 0.1 U/kg
1–1.4	Small or moderate	Starvation ketosis; extra carbohydrate and fluid	Starvation ketosis; extra carbohydrate and fluid	Extra carbohydrate and fluid. Give extra 5–10% of TDD or 0.05–0.1 U/kg	Give extra 10% of TDD or 0.1 U/kg	Give extra 10% of TDD or 0.1 U/kg
1.5–2.9	Moderate or large	Starvation ketosis; extra carbohydrate and fluid. Recheck BG and ketones in 1–2 h	Starvation ketosis; extra carbohydrate and fluid. Give extra 5% of TDD or 0.05 U/kg	Extra carbohydrate and fluid. Give 10% of TDD or 0.1 U/kg	Give extra 10–20% of TDD or 0.1 U/kg	Give extra 10–20% of TDD or 0.1 U/kg
≥3	Large	Starvation ketosis; extra carbohydrate and fluid. Recheck BG and ketones in 1–2 h	Starvation ketosis; extra carbohydrate and fluid. Give extra 5% of TDD or 0.05 U/kg	Extra carbohydrate and fluid. Give 10% of TDD or 0.1 U/kg	Give extra 10–20% of TDD or 0.1 U/kg	Give extra 10–20% of TDD or 0.1 U/kg

*Mini dose glucagon SC: ≤2 years of age, 20 μg; 2–15 years, 10 μg/year of age; >15, 150 μg [102].
†TDD, total daily dose. To calculate TDD, add up all the insulin given on a usual day (rapid- or short-acting insulin + intermediate- or long-acting insulin) or the sum of basal rate and boluses delivered by pump.
Supplemental insulin may be either rapid-acting insulin analogs (preferred) or short-acting regular insulin.

correct hyperglycemia and/or ketosis (Table 18.25). The child who has a gastrointestinal illness with nausea, vomiting or diarrhea and low, normal or near-normal blood glucose concentrations is a special case because there is an increased risk of hypoglycemia. The dose of insulin may have to be temporarily reduced and "mini" doses of glucagon can be used to prevent or treat mild hypoglycemia in a child with nausea or vomiting who is unable or unwilling to eat or drink (Table 18.25) [102]. Ketosis with blood glucose concentrations normal or near-normal usually signifies starvation but must be distinguished from "euglycemic ketoacidosis." βOHB does not usually exceed 3 mmol/L in starvation ketosis.

Fluid requirements increase as a result of osmotic diuresis and increased insensible fluid losses due to fever; dehydration can develop rapidly if fluid intake is insufficient. The child should be encouraged to drink at least 2–4 mL/kg body weight/h (or a minimum of 1500 mL/m^2/24 h, the usual maintenance fluid requirement) with fluids that provide sodium, glucose and potassium to replace the urinary losses of these electrolytes that occur with metabolic decompensation (Table 18.26).

Fluids suitable for sick days are water, broth or bouillon (high content of salt), carbonated beverages (Coca Cola, ginger ale), sports drinks such as Gatorade, electrolyte mixtures and fruit juices. Sugar-free fluids are recommended if the child is able to

Table 18.26 Fluids used for oral hydration with sick day management.

Product	Carbohydrate (g/100 mL)	Na$^+$ (mmol/L)	K$^+$ (mmol/L)
Coca-Cola	10.9	4.3	0.1
Ginger ale	9.0	3.5	0.1
Apple juice	11.9	0.4	26
Orange juice	10.4	0.2	49
Gatorade	5.9	21	2.5
Pedialyte	2.5	45	20
Milk	4.9	22	36
Broth/bouillon	0	129–149	~8

continue to follow his/her meal plan and/or blood glucose is >11 mmol/L (200 mg/dL). However, when the child is unable to eat solid foods and the blood glucose is <11 mmol/L (200 mg/dL), the liquids should contain a source of glucose. Weight loss is a reliable sign of dehydration and, if a bathroom scale is available, the child should be carefully weighed several times each day.

Blood glucose concentration should be measured every 2–4 h throughout the day and night and urine ketone concentrations checked each time the child urinates. If the blood glucose concentration is <4.5 mmol/L (80 mg/dL), measurements should be

Table 18.27 Signs the sick child with diabetes mellitus must receive urgent medical attention.

The nature of the underlying condition is unclear
Signs of dehydration: dry mouth or tongue, cracked lips, sunken eyes, dry flushed skin, decreased urine output, weight loss
Inability to consume the recommended amount of fluid or carbohydrate
Vomiting for more than 2 h (particularly in young children)
Symptoms suggestive of DKA: nausea, abdominal pain, hyperventilation, confusion, drowsiness
Blood glucose increases or >14 mmol/L (250 mg/dL) despite extra insulin
Inability to maintain blood glucose >4.5 mmol/L (80 mg/dL)
Persistent or increasing ketonuria or blood ketones >1–1.5 mmol/L
Care providers are exhausted
Language barriers make it difficult to communicate with care providers

DKA, diabetic ketoacidosis.

repeated hourly until it is >4.5 mmol/L (80 mg/dL). Cotton balls placed in the diaper can be used to obtain urine for ketone testing in infants and toddlers. Alternatively, blood β-OHB concentration can be measured directly in capillary blood with a meter (Precision Xtra®). Normal concentrations are <0.5 mmol/L. During starvation or illness or when insulin delivery is insufficient for any reason, the blood ketone concentration rapidly increases and a level of ≥3.0 mmol/L together with hyperglycemia indicates DKA.

The blood glucose concentrations and severity of ketonuria or ketonemia is used to guide the administration of supplemental insulin (Table 18.25). Rapid-acting insulin (lispro or insulin aspart) may be given every 2–3 h or short-acting (regular) insulin every 3–4 h until blood glucose is less than 11 mmol/L (200 mg/dL) and ketonuria has been reduced to negative or trace or blood β-OHB <0.5 mmol/L.

Evidence that continued management of the child at home may no longer be safe and the child requires urgent medical attention are listed in Table 18.27. Assiduous attention to these guidelines enables most intercurrent childhood illnesses to be managed successfully at home.

Illness in the child managed with an insulin pump

The child using an insulin pump requires specific attention during sick day management. Patients on pumps use only rapid- or short-acting insulin and do not have a depot of long-acting insulin so DKA can develop rapidly. Nausea and vomiting may be the earliest manifestations of interrupted insulin delivery and impending ketoacidosis but the patient may incorrectly assume that the symptoms are caused by a viral illness and not recognize the insulin deficient state.

The patient who experiences nausea or vomiting must immediately check blood or urine for ketones. Ketosis is evidence of a potential impending medical emergency; when insulin delivery is interrupted, DKA can develop within 4–6 h. Rapid-acting insulin must immediately be given SC with a syringe or pen, not with the pump because malfunction may be the cause of ketosis.

The dose may be based on the child's usual "correction factor" to reduce the blood glucose concentration to 6 mmol/L. Alternatively, the guidelines for supplemental insulin in Table 18.25 may be used. The infusion set should be replaced and the pump carefully examined to look for possible causes of failure, which include battery or mechanical failure, an empty insulin reservoir, leakage at the site where the catheter connects to the syringe, occlusion of the catheter and withdrawal of the catheter from its SC insertion site on the skin. A temporary 25% increase in the basal insulin infusion rate may be required during illness [103].

Side effects of treatment

Weight gain

Intensively treated subjects in the DCCT had a considerably increased risk of becoming overweight [104], which was greatest in individuals with higher baseline HbA1c concentrations. Weight gain is attributable to reduced glycosuria and daily energy expenditure. Frequent symptomatic hypoglycemia necessitating snacks to restore normoglycemia also contributes to the tendency to gain weight in some intensively managed individuals.

It is possible that intermittent hyperinsulinemia and lack of amylin to regulate appetite may underlie the propensity to weight gain in type 1 diabetes but, because longitudinal studies have found a J-shaped curve relating body mass index (BMI) to mortality in type 1 diabetes, with the highest relative all-cause mortality in those with the lowest BMI, it is generally accepted that the long-term benefits of intensive glycemic control greatly outweigh the adverse effects of weight gain.

Children and adolescents who adopt basal-bolus insulin therapy may be tempted to eat more liberally and increase their calorie consumption and this issue should be addressed in advance. The highly motivated patient can take advantage of the flexibility of a basal-bolus regimen to balance insulin replacement with calorie intake to avoid obesity or even lose weight.

Local effects of insulin

Lipohypertrophy refers to the accumulation of excess adipose tissue at the sites of SC insulin injection. It is the most common cutaneous side effect of insulin administration, occurring in 25–50% of individuals. Rotation of injection sites, thereby avoiding repeated insulin injections in a single area, prevents lipohypertrophy. In addition to its undesirable cosmetic appearance, it is important to avoid lipohypertrophy because it causes erratic absorption of insulin.

Lipoatrophy and insulin allergy are much less common with use of human insulin preparations. Rotation of the site of insulin injections may decrease the risk of lipoatrophy. Insulin absorption from lipoatrophic areas may also be erratic. Lipoatrophy may resolve by carefully injecting insulin into the perimeter of the affected area. In severe cases, topical glucocorticoid injection into and around the site may be helpful. If the patient is using an animal-source insulin, switching to human insulin may prevent further atrophy and lead to gradual filling in of the atrophic area.

Insulin allergy may result in local or systemic effects, with acute redness, itching, burning, hives or chronic reactions. Generalized urticaria and anaphylaxis, are extremely rare. Switching to synthetic human insulin may prevent further allergic reactions and should be done after preliminary skin testing in a supervised setting. Insulin delivery by pump has been reported to stop local reactions in some cases. In rare instances, insulin desensitization may be necessary.

Cellulitis or abscess may occur at the injection site but is rare when patients use sterile disposable syringes and needles hygienically. Injection through clothing is strongly discouraged. Insulin pump therapy is associated with increased rates of cellulitis, abscess and local scarring at the sites of subcutaneous catheter insertion. It is essential to replace the catheter every 2–3 days and remove a catheter if the site becomes red or painful.

Hypoglycemia

Hypoglycemia is the most common acute complication of the treatment of diabetes mellitus and concern about hypoglycemia is a central issue in treating children. It is the principal factor limiting attempts to achieve near-normal glycemic control [105]. Patients, parents and the diabetes team have to balance the risks of hypoglycemia against those of long-term hyperglycemia. After an episode of severe hypoglycemia, the confidence of the patient and parents is often shaken, and fear of a recurrence may induce the patient or parents to change their diabetes management to prevent a recurrence. Altered patient behaviors may include overeating and/or deliberate selection of inadequate doses of insulin to maintain higher blood glucose concentrations perceived as being safe, resulting in deterioration of glycemic control [106]. Concern about nocturnal hypoglycemia causes more anxiety for some parents than any other aspect of diabetes, including the fear of long-term complications. Some parents believe that an episode of severe hypoglycemia during the nighttime may go undetected or not be treated in a timely fashion and lead to permanent brain damage or death [107].

The glucagon response to hypoglycemia is lost early in the course of the disease and patients with type 1 diabetes depend on sympathoadrenal responses to prevent or correct hypoglycemia [108]. Mild hypoglycemia itself reduces epinephrine responses and symptomatic awareness of subsequent episodes of hypoglycemia. Little is known about counter-regulatory responses in preschool-age children.

Symptoms and signs of hypoglycemia

Symptoms of hypoglycemia are caused by neuronal deprivation of glucose and have been categorized into autonomic (sweating, palpitations, shaking, hunger), neuroglycopenic (confusion, drowsiness, odd behavior, speech difficulty, incoordination) and non-specific malaise (hunger and headache) [109]. The most common signs and symptoms of hypoglycemia in children with

diabetes are pallor, weakness, tremor, hunger, fatigue, drowsiness, sweating and headache. Autonomic symptoms are less common in children less than 6 years old whose symptoms are more often neuroglycopenic or non-specific in nature. Behavioral changes are often the primary manifestation of hypoglycemia in young children and this difference has important implications for parent education on hypoglycemia.

In contrast to adult patients, who are usually able to distinguish between autonomic and neuroglycopenic symptoms, children and their parents report that symptoms tend to cluster [110]. The coalescence of autonomic and neuroglycopenic symptoms in children may indicate that both types of symptoms are generated at similar glycemic thresholds.

Hypoglycemia is classified as mild, moderate or severe. Most episodes are mild and cognitive impairment does not occur: older children are able to treat themselves. Mild symptoms abate within about 15 min after treatment with rapidly absorbed carbohydrate. Moderate hypoglycemia has neuroglycopenic and adrenergic symptoms causing mood changes, irritability, decreased attentiveness, drowsiness and behavior change. Young children typically require assistance with treatment because they are often confused and have impaired judgment and weakness and poor coordination may make self-treatment difficult. Moderate hypoglycemia causes more protracted symptoms and may require a second treatment with oral carbohydrate. Severe hypoglycemia is characterized by unresponsiveness, unconsciousness or convulsions and requires emergency treatment with parenteral glucagon or intravenous glucose.

Children who have had diabetes for several years may describe a change in symptomatology over time with less severe autonomic symptoms occurring less frequently and neuroglycopenic symptoms more common. Patients must learn to recognize the change in symptoms to prevent severe episodes. The blood glucose concentration at which symptoms occur varies between patients and the threshold may vary in the same individual in parallel with antecedent glycemic control. Children with poorly controlled diabetes experience symptoms of hypoglycemia at higher blood glucose concentrations than those with good glycemic control.

Impact of hypoglycemia on the child's brain

Numerous studies have documented cognitive impairments in children and adolescents diagnosed with type 1 diabetes in early childhood [111,112]. Global intellectual deficits have been described as well as specific neurocognitive impairments in memory, visuospatial skills and attention. Neuropsychological complications have been detected within 2 years of onset of diabetes [113]. Children with long-term diabetes, especially those who developed the disease before age 6 years, appear to be at the greatest risk. However, it is difficult to dissect the contributions of metabolic disturbances (hyperglycemia and hypoglycemia) from the psychosocial effects of chronic disease [114]. There is evidence linking episodes of hypoglycemia to the neuropsychological defects [115] but others have found no evidence of an association with severe episodes and postulate that asymptomatic hypoglycemia may be more important [116]. Cognitive impairments in children with early onset diabetes mellitus may result from severe hypoglycemia, recurrent asymptomatic hypoglycemia, psychosocial effects of chronic illness and chronic hyperglycemia [114,117]. The neurocognitive sequelae of intensive diabetes management in children whose brains are still developing are unknown. Preliminary findings suggest poorer memory skills, presumably the consequence of recurrent and severe hypoglycemia [118].

Even in the absence of typical symptoms, cognitive function deteriorates at low blood glucose concentrations [119]. Moderate and severe hypoglycemia is disabling, affects school performance and makes driving a car or operating dangerous machinery hazardous and the utmost effort should be made to avoid such events. Repeated or prolonged severe hyperinsulinemic hypoglycemia can cause permanent central nervous system damage, especially in very young children but hypoglycemia is a rare cause of death in diabetic children [120].

Frequency of hypoglycemia

The true frequency of mild (self-treated) symptomatic hypoglycemia is almost impossible to ascertain because mild episodes are quickly forgotten and/or are not recorded.

The literature is replete with reports of the frequency of severe hypoglycemia in children and adolescents with diabetes but the various methods of collecting data, variability among clinic populations and therapeutic methods and definitions of severe hypo-

glycemia, make comparisons among the reports and interpretation of the data difficult [114]. Recent prospective studies with strict definitions of hypoglycemic events and well-described populations continue to show disturbingly high rates of severe hypoglycemia; younger children and patients with tight glycemic control are at greatest risk (Table 18.28) [114].

Many, but not all, studies have found an increased frequency of severe hypoglycemia in younger children and in association with lower HbA1c concentrations. Other factors associated with a higher risk of moderate and severe hypoglycemia are a prior history of severe hypoglycemia, relatively higher doses of insulin and low C-peptide secretion, longer duration of diabetes, male gender, psychiatric disorders, treatment at small diabetes centers and lack of health insurance [121,122].

Causes of hypoglycemia in diabetes mellitus

Patients with type 1 diabetes mellitus are susceptible to hypoglycemia for many reasons (Table 18.29). Patient errors relating to insulin dosage, decreased food intake or unplanned exercise account for 50–85% of episodes of hypoglycemia in children and adolescents. After years of living with diabetes, some patients and/or their parents become cavalier about diabetes without thought for the balance of insulin, food and exercise.

Newer and improved methods of replacing insulin (CSII and multiple dose regimens with insulin analogs) combined with education specifically informing subjects about hypoglycemia [123], behavioral educational approaches such as blood glucose awareness training and intermittent continuous glucose monitoring, may enable patients to achieve improved glycemic control with

Table 18.28 Incidence of severe hypoglycemia in children and adolescents. Severe hypoglycemia is variably defined in these studies as coma, seizure, treatment with glucagon, intravenous dextrose, treatment in an emergency department or admission to hospital.

Study Author, year	Age group (years)	No. of patients	Definition of severe hypoglycemia	Incidence*	Mean or median HbA1c (%)	Methodology
DCCT 1994	13–17	195	Coma, seizure			Prospective randomized clinical trial
intensive therapy				26.7	8.06	
conventional therapy				9.7	9.76	
Nordfeldt 1997	1–18	146	Coma, seizure	15–19	8.1–6.9	Prospective
Mortensen 1997	1–18	2873	Coma, seizure	22	8.6	Cross-sectional international
Rosilio 1998	1–19	2579	Coma, seizure, glucagon	45	8.97	Cross-sectional national
Davis 1998	0–18	709	Coma, seizure	15.6	8.6	Prospective population based
Tupola 1998	1–24	329	Coma, seizure, glucagon	3.6	9.1–9.6	Retrospective
Tupola 1998	1–24	287	Coma, seizure, glucagon	3.1	9.0–9.1	Prospective
Thomsett 1999	1–19	268	Coma, seizure	25	8.6	Retrospective
Nordfeldt 1999	1–18	139	Unconsciousness	17.0	6.9†	Prospective
Levine 2001	7–16	300	Coma, seizure, glucagon, IV dextrose	8	8.7–8.9	Prospective
Rewers 2002	0–19	1243	Coma, seizure, admission	19	8.8–9.0‡	Prospective
Bulsara 2004	0–18	801	Coma, seizure	16.6	8.1	Prospective
Svoren 2007	8–16	152	Coma, seizure, glucagon, IV dextrose	10.9	8.6	Prospective

*Events per 100 patient years.

†Median value, normal range 3.6–5.4%.

‡Range of median values. Adapted from data in [121].

Table 18.29 Causes of hypoglycemia in children and adolescents with diabetes mellitus.

Insulin errors (inadvertent or deliberate)
Reversal of morning and evening dose
Reversal of short- or rapid-acting insulin and intermediate-acting insulin
Improper timing of insulin in relation to food
Excessive insulin dosage
Surreptitious insulin administration, suicide gesture or attempt

Erratic or altered absorption
Inadvertent intramuscular injection
More rapid absorption from exercising limbs
Unpredictable absorption from lipohypertrophy at injection sites
More rapid absorption after sauna, hot bath, sunbathing

Diet
Omission or reduced size of meals or snacks
Delayed snacks or meals
Eating disorders
Gastroparesis
Malabsorption, e.g. gluten enteropathy

Exercise
Unplanned physical activity
Prolonged duration and/or increased intensity of physical activity
Failure to reduce the dose of basal insulin to combat the "lag effect" of exercise

Alcohol and/or drugs
Impaired gluconeogenesis from excessive consumption of ethanol
Impaired cognition from use of ethanol, marijuana, cocaine, other recreational drugs

Hypoglycemia-associated autonomic failure
Hypoglycemia unawareness
Defective glucose counter-regulation

Miscellaneous uncommon causes of hypoglycemia
Adrenocortical insufficiency
Hypothyroidism
Growth hormone deficiency
Renal failure
Decreased insulin requirement in first trimester of pregnancy
Insulin antibodies

less risk of severe hypoglycemia than was previously possible [72,124].

Several reports have shown that insulin pump therapy is associated with fewer hypoglycemic events despite improved glycemic control. This may be because CSII permits lower (and adjustable) rates of basal insulin delivery compared with injection therapy, especially at night when hypoglycemia is most common. Rapid-acting acting insulin analogs decrease the frequency of hypoglycemia and insulin glargine together with pre-meal insulin lispro decreases the incidence of nocturnal hypoglycemia in adolescents when compared with NPH combined with regular insulin [59].

Nocturnal hypoglycemia

Hypoglycemia, often asymptomatic, frequently occurs during sleep. Moderate and severe hypoglycemia are more common during the night and early morning (before breakfast) than during the daytime [125]. In the DCCT, 55% of severe hypoglycemia events occurred during sleep and 43% occurred between midnight and 8 a.m. [125,126]. In children, up to 75% of severe hypoglycemia occurred during the night-time hours [127].

Both children and adults with diabetes studied, either in hospital or at home with frequent intermittent or continuous blood glucose measurements during the night, show a high incidence of asymptomatic hypoglycemia [128,129]. Episodes of hypoglycemia during sleep often exceed 4 h in duration and up to half of these episodes may be undetected because the subject does not awaken from sleep. The incidence of hypoglycemia on any given night may be affected by numerous factors, including the insulin regimen, the timing and content of meals and snacks and antecedent physical activity [130]. Long after strenuous exercise has ended, there is a sustained increase in insulin action on muscle and liver and blunting of the counter-regulatory response to hypoglycemia [131]. The highest frequency of asymptomatic nocturnal hypoglycemia occurs in children less than 10 years old. Low blood glucose concentrations in the early morning (before breakfast) are associated with a higher frequency of preceding nocturnal hypoglycemia. Knowledge of this fact is useful in counseling patients to modify the evening insulin regimen and bedtime snack to prevent more severe nocturnal hypoglycemia.

Sleep impairs counter-regulatory hormone responses to hypoglycemia in normal subjects and in patients with diabetes mellitus [132]. Because a rise in plasma epinephrine is normally the main hormonal defense against hypoglycemia in patients with diabetes, impaired counter-regulatory hormone responses to hypoglycemia explain the increased susceptibility to hypoglycemia during sleep. Furthermore, asymptomatic nocturnal hypoglycemia may impair counter-regulatory hormone responses. Thus, impaired defenses against hypoglycemia during sleep may contribute to the vicious cycle of hypoglycemia, impaired counter-regulatory responses and unawareness of hypoglycemia either awake or asleep. Recurrent asymptomatic nocturnal hypoglycemia is an important cause of hypoglycemia unawareness, which leads to more frequent and severe hypoglycemia because of failure to experience autonomic warning symptoms before the onset of neuroglycopenia [133].

Treatment

Except in preschool-age children, most episodes of symptomatic hypoglycemia are self-treated. Glucose tablets raise blood glucose concentrations more rapidly than orange juice or milk and are the treatment of choice for children old enough to chew and safely swallow large tablets. The recommended dose is 5–15 g oral fast-acting carbohydrate or 0.3 g glucose/kg body weight (Table 18.30). Blood glucose should be remeasured 15 min after treatment and if the concentration does not exceed 3.9–4.4 mmol/L (70–80 mg/dL), treatment should be repeated. The glycemic

SINGLETON HOSPITAL
STAFF LIBRARY

Table 18.30 Sources of carbohydrate.

The following all have approximately 15 g carbohydrate:
  Apple juice 4 oz or ½ cup, unsweetened apple sauce ½ cup
  Grape juice 3 oz or 1/3 cup
  Orange juice 4 oz or ½ cup
  Coca-Cola and ginger ale 5 oz (~2/3 cup)
  Twin Popsicle (1)
  Regular jello ½ cup
  Regular ice cream ½ cup
  Honey 1 tablespoon
  Cake frosting 4 teaspoons
  Table sugar 1 tablespoon
  Glucose tablets 3 (each contains 5 g)
  Lifesavers® 6
  Saltines 6

response to oral glucose usually lasts less than 2 h so, after treatment with oral glucose, unless a scheduled meal or snack is due within an hour, the patient should be given either a snack or a meal containing carbohydrate and protein.

Hypoglycemia frequently occurs when a child with diabetes is unable to consume or absorb oral carbohydrate because of nausea and vomiting associated with an intercurrent illness (e.g. gastroenteritis) or food refusal. To maintain blood glucose concentrations in a safe range, parents either seek emergency medical attention or attempt to force-feed oral carbohydrate in an ill child, which often leads to more vomiting. Mini-dose glucagon raises blood glucose by 3.3–5 mmol/L (60–90 mg/dL) within 30 min and its effect lasts approximately 1 h. Using a U100 insulin syringe and after dissolving 1 mg glucagon in 1 mL diluent, children ≤2 years receive 2 "units" (20 μg) of glucagon SC and children older than 2 years receive 1 unit (10 μg) per year of age up to 15 units (150 μg). If the blood glucose concentration does not increase within 30 min, double the initial dosage should be administered [102,134].

Severe reactions (unresponsiveness, unconsciousness or convulsions) require emergency treatment with parenteral glucagon (IM or SC). The usual recommended dose is 0.5 mg if less than 5 years and 1 mg if older than 5 years. Glucagon raises blood glucose concentrations within 5–15 min and usually relieves symptoms of hypoglycemia. In children with diabetes and in healthy adults there are no important difference between the effects of glucagon injected either SC or IM. The plasma glucagon concentrations attained are higher than those in peripheral venous or portal blood of healthy adults during insulin-induced hypoglycemia and are probably higher than necessary for maximal effect. The increase in blood glucose concentration after glucagon administration is sustained for at least 30 min so it is not necessary to repeat the dose or force the child to eat or drink for at least 30 min. Intranasal glucagon has a similar effect.

In an emergency department or hospital, the preferred treatment is intravenous glucose (0.3 g/kg). Because the glycemic response is transient after bolus administration of glucose, intravenous glucose infusion should be continued until the patient is able to swallow safely. If severe hypoglycemia was prolonged and the patient had a seizure, complete recovery of mental and neurologic function may take many hours despite restoration of normal blood glucose concentrations. Permanent hemiparesis or other neurologic sequelae are rare but the post-ictal period may be complicated by headache, lethargy, nausea, vomiting and muscle ache.

Driving a motor vehicle

Hypoglycemia increases the rate of driving mishaps among adults with type 1 diabetes. Factors associated with an increased risk of accidents are failure to measure the blood glucose before driving and a too low blood glucose level at which subjects choose not to drive [135]. Driving is impaired at plasma glucose concentrations of ≤3.3 mol/L (60 mg/dL) [136]. Adolescents with diabetes should measure blood glucose before driving and not drive unless the concentration is >4 mmol/L (70 mg/dL). The glove compartment should be stocked with a source of rapidly absorbed carbohydrate and non-perishable snacks to take when symptoms of hypoglycemia are detected.

Dead in bed

Sudden unexplained deaths during sleep have been described in adolescents with type 1 diabetes. These events are rare. Young adult males are at highest risk. Lethal cardiac arrhythmias triggered by hypoglycemia may be responsible for some cases and severe hypoglycemia related to recreational drug abuse may account for others.

Chronic complications of type 1 diabetes

Non-vascular complications of diabetes
Cataracts

Cataracts rarely occur in children with diabetes but when present at the time of diagnosis may regress after treatment of diabetes has been instituted.

Limited joint mobility

Limited joint mobility (LJM), also referred to as cheiroarthropathy, is caused by glycosylation of collagen in the connective tissue of skin and tendons. It manifests as inability to extend the fingers and/or wrists because of loss of skin elasticity and contraction of tendons. LJM is a sign of chronic poor glycemic control and associated with increased risk of microvascular complications.

Growth

Growth failure in children with diabetes is uncommon even with only "average" glycemic control. Nonetheless, abnormality of the GH–IGF-1 axis is common. With average blood glucose control, GH secretion is increased and serum concentrations of IGF-1 and

IGFBP-3 tend to be reduced. Delayed puberty and growth failure typically occur when a child or adolescent experiences chronic, very poor glycemic control (Mauriac syndrome). It is thought to be caused by recurrent cycles of adequate insulinemia alternating with inadequate insulinemia.

Skin

Necrobiosis lipoidica diabeticorum is an uncommon poorly understood complication which causes unsightly lesions that usually appear in the pretibial area. Intralesional injection of corticosteroids often results in improvement.

Disordered eating and eating disorders

Adolescent females with type 1 diabetes have a twofold increased risk of developing an eating disorder compared to their peers without diabetes [137]. Eating disorders in adolescents with type 1 diabetes are associated with poor metabolic control and earlier onset and progression of microvascular complications. The problem should be suspected in adolescent females who are unable to achieve and maintain blood glucose targets or who have unexplained weight loss or deterioration of metabolic control [138]. Screening should be conducted by asking non-judgmental questions about weight and shape concerns, dieting, episodes of binge eating and insulin omission for the purpose of controlling weight [137]. Patients with identified eating disorders or deliberate misuse of insulin are at extremely high risk for morbidity and mortality [139] and should receive intensive multidisciplinary care that includes a mental health professional with expertise in eating disorders. Use of a basal-bolus insulin regimen allows increased meal flexibility.

Vascular complications

The vascular complications of diabetes are either microvasacular (retinopathy, nephropathy and neuropathy) or macrovascular, which includes coronary artery, peripheral and cerebral vascular disease. The microvascular complications can develop within 5 years of the onset of type 1 diabetes mellitus but rarely develop before the onset of puberty. Clinically significant macrovascular complications are very rare until adulthood.

Intensive glycemic control decreases the risk of both microvascular and macrovascular disease [140] but several other modifiable risk factors in addition to hyperglycemia contribute to and influence the risk of vascular complications. Use of tobacco considerably increases the risk of onset and progression of nephropathy and macrovascular disease. Hypertension is associated with increased risk and rate of progression of retinopathy, nephropathy and macrovascular disease. Dyslipidemia contributes to the risk of macrovascular disease, nephropathy and retinopathy. A family history of hypertension or nephropathy increases the risk of nephropathy.

Retinopathy

Diabetic retinopathy damages the microvasculature of the retina and is the most common cause of acquired blindness in developed countries. Although improvement in glycemic control delays the onset of retinopathy and retards its progression, nearly all individuals with diabetes eventually develop mild non-proliferative retinopathy. This may progress to moderate or severe non-proliferative retinopathy, characterized by abnormal blood flow in the retinal microvasculature. Proliferative retinopathy, characterized by growth of new vessels, carries a high risk of visual loss from hemorrhage or retinal detachment. Macular edema may occur at any stage of retinopathy and threaten visual acuity. Screening detects early disease and leads to effective treatment with laser retinal photocoagulation before vision is impaired.

Nephropathy

Diabetic nephropathy is the most common cause of end-stage renal disease in Western countries and eventually occurs in 30–40% of persons with type 1 diabetes. Improving glycemic control and treatment of hypertension, if present, delays the onset of nephropathy and slows its progression. Microalbuminuria, defined as ≥30 mg/day or ≥20 µg/min albumin in the urine, is the earliest stage of clinical nephropathy. Sustained microalbuminuria is highly predictive of progression to overt nephropathy (clinical albuminuria) defined as ≥300 mg/24 h or ≥200 µg/min albumin in the urine but microalbuminuria may be less predictive in adolescents during the first decade of diabetes. Overt albuminuria is accompanied by systemic hypertension and progressive impairment of glomerular filtration and typically precedes the development of end-stage renal disease by 10 years. Progression of nephropathy can be delayed by improving glycemic control, controlling hypertension and by treatment with an angiotensin-converting enzyme (ACE) inhibitor. If an ACE inhibitor is used, it is important to monitor for hyperkalemia.

Neuropathy

Clinically significant diabetic neuropathy is rare in children. Early signs include loss of ankle reflexes and decreased vibration sense or touch sensation to monofilament in the great toe. Although cardiovascular testing may detect subtle autonomic abnormalities in some adolescents with diabetes, they tend to be transient and their clinical importance is unknown. Improvements in HbA1c decrease the risk of onset of neuropathy.

Macrovascular

Men and women whose diabetes commences in childhood are at high risk for macrovascular disease and women lose the protective effect of their gender. Although the absolute risk is low before age 30 years, macrovascular events are the most common cause of death in persons with type 1 diabetes. Individuals with renal complications have an especially high risk. Other predictors of macrovascular risk and/or progression include dyslipidemia, hypertension and smoking. Strategies to reduce lifetime risk of macrovascular disease in children with diabetes include avoiding tobacco, early and vigorous treatment of hypertension and dyslipidemia (Table 18.31) and intensive glycemic control.

Screening for long-term complications

Diabetic complications can usually be detected years before the patient has symptoms or organ function is impaired when intervention to arrest, reverse or retard the disease process will have the greatest impact [141]. Diabetic retinopathy is rare before puberty or in patients who have had diabetes for less than 5 years:

Table 18.31 Principles of management of hypertension and dyslipidemia in youth with diabetes. After [78,144,145].

Hypertension

Measure blood pressure at each physical examination and compare to normative data for age, gender and height

Elevated values should be confirmed with a second measurement

Exclude causes of hypertension unrelated to diabetes

High-normal blood pressure (systolic or diastolic blood pressure >90th percentile):

- Lifestyle intervention: eliminate excess dietary sodium, encourage physical exercise, weight reduction if appropriate
- Initiate pharmacologic treatment if target blood pressure is not reached within 3–6 months of lifestyle intervention

Hypertension (systolic or diastolic blood pressure >95th percentile or consistently >130/80 mmHg):

- Pharmacologic treatment: ACE inhibitors are the agents of choice
- Titrate dose to achieve blood pressure consistently <130/80 mmHg or below the 90th percentile
- If target blood pressure is not achieved, consider adding second agent
- ACE inhibitors are contraindicated during pregnancy

Dyslipidemia

Screening:

- Fasting lipid profile after glycemic control has been achieved
- Type 2 diabetes: Screen at diagnosis and every 2 years thereafter
- Type 1 diabetes:
  Age < 12: Screen only if family history of hypercholesterolemia, cardiovascular event prior to age 55 or family history is unknown
  Repeat screening every 5 years
  Age ≥ 12: Screen at diagnosis and every 2 years thereafter

Goals:

- LDL < 100 mg/dL
- HDL > 35 mg/dL
- Triglycerides < 150 mg/dL

Treatment if goals are not met:

- Initial therapy
  AHA step 2 diet (dietary cholesterol < 200 mg/day and saturated fat <7% of total calories)
  Maximize glycemic control and reduce weight if indicated
- Pharmacologic therapy:
  Statins ± bile acid sequestrants
  Recommended if LDL-cholesterol remains ≥160 mg/dL and age > 10
  Consider if LDL-cholesterol remains 130–159 mg/dL, especially if other cardiovascular risk factors are present
  Statins are potent teratogens
  Fibric acid derivatives if triglycerides > 1000 mg/dL

ACE, angiotensin-converting enzyme; AHA, American Heart Association; HDL, high density lipoprotein; LDL, low density lipoprotein;

an annual dilated retinal examination should begin 3–5 years after diagnosis and when the child is aged 10 years or older [142]. Temporary rapid progression of retinopathy may occur when metabolic control improves drastically and, in these circumstances, retinal examinations should be performed more frequently.

After 5 years, screening of urine albumin and creatinine concentrations should be performed annually to detect microalbuminuria [142]. The preferred method is to measure the albumin:creatinine ratio in a random spot urine specimen. First-void collections in the morning avoid the confounding effect of increased albumin excretion induced by upright posture. Timed collections (24 h or overnight) are more accurate but less convenient than spot samples. Standard assays for urinary protein are insufficiently sensitive and measurement should be performed by an assay that specifically detects microalbuminuria. Albumin excretion is transiently elevated by hyperglycemia, exercise and febrile illness. Because of marked day-to-day variability in albumin excretion, microalbuminuria should be confirmed in at least two of three collections over a 3- to 6-month period to establish the diagnosis of diabetic nephropathy before instituting treatment. Circulatory and neurologic complications of diabetes are seldom clinically significant during childhood and adolescence.

Co-morbidities and complications of type 2 diabetes

Co-morbid conditions are prevalent in children with type 2 diabetes (Table 18.32) [143] and screening for them should begin at diagnosis. Several of these co-morbidities are attributable to insulin resistance rather than to hyperglycemia and may antedate

Table 18.32 Co-morbidities at diagnosis of youth with type 2 diabetes mellitus.

Characteristic	Average prevalence*
Related to insulin resistance	
Hypertension	33% (10–59)
PCOS	21% (18–23)
Dyslipidemia	23% (4–40)
NAFLD†	48%
Related to obesity	
Sleep apnea	6%
Multifactorial	
Known psychiatric illness	19%
Psychotropic medication	12%

NAFLD, non-alcoholic fatty liver disease; PCOS, polycystic ovarian syndrome.
*Mean of the averages reported by each study, with the range of reported averages shown in parentheses.
†NAFLD as evidenced by elevated alanine aminotransferase.

the clinical onset of diabetes. Dyslipidemia and hypertension should be treated according to current guidelines (Table 18.29) [144,145].

Management of type 2 diabetes should include routine assessment for hepatomegaly and measurement of serum aminotransferase concentrations [143]. Elevations of alanine aminotransferase (ALT) are common in children with type 2 diabetes, often because of non-alcoholic fatty liver disease (NAFLD) [146], which is characterized by two- to fivefold elevations above the upper limit of normal in ALT and aspartate aminotransferase (AST) concentrations, with ALT greater than AST. NAFLD often has an indolent course but inflammation can progress to chronic liver disease and cirrhosis. Elevated concentrations of AST and ALT typical of NAFLD can be managed conservatively by ruling out other common causes of hepatitis, promoting gradual weight loss, improving glycemic control and remeasuring ALT concentrations. Mild elevations of ALT associated with NAFLD are not a contraindication to the use of metformin. Higher elevations of ALT or ALT unresponsive to conservative management should be referred to an appropriate specialist.

It is not uncommon for psychiatric disease to complicate type 2 diabetes, although the underlying reasons for this association are incompletely understood and are probably multifactorial. Optimal treatment should include evaluation by a mental health specialist when psychiatric disease is suspected. Atypical antipsychotic medications are associated with excess weight gain and insulin resistance and thus a child receiving an atypical antipsychotic will occasionally present with type 2 diabetes The treating psychiatrist should consider discontinuing or switching the atypical antipsychotic but these agents are often required for their potent effect on the psychiatric disease.

The prevalence of microalbuminuria at diagnosis of type 2 diabetes in young persons is 7–22% and 8–28% at 0–5 years of diabetes duration. After 5–10 years, macroalbuminuria occurs in 7–17% of patients. From the time of diagnosis, the incidence curves for nephropathy are similar between child- and adult-onset type 2 diabetes. Patients with type 2 diabetes are more likely to have microalbuminuria even with lower HbA1c concentrations and shorter duration of diabetes than patients with type 1. The prevalence of retinopathy after 0–5 years duration of youth-onset type 2 diabetes is 0–4%. For these reasons, in contrast to type 1 diabetes in children, screening for microvascular complications should commence shortly after diagnosis and be repeated annually. Among Pima Indians aged 25–50 years diagnosed with type 2 diabetes in youth, the age- and sex-adjusted mortality was three time higher as compared to their non-diabetic peers, with the excess mortality accounted for by nephropathy, infections and cardiovascular disease.

Transition from pediatric to adult care

Emerging adulthood (18–25 years) poses many challenges for the diabetic [147]. The transition from a pediatric to an adult service should be planned carefully at an age varying according to the maturity of the adolescent and the availability of appropriate services for the young person in an adult clinic. It may be determined by hospital and clinic facilities and local regulations.

Young people value continuity of care by diabetes team members whom they trust [148] and, regardless of the age of transfer from the pediatric clinic, patients often have concerns about potential differences in style and approach to care. The change from the family-based pediatric clinic to the adult clinic can lead to anxiety and patients may become lost in the process and cease regular attendance at the specialized service [149]. This is likely to be associated with poor adherence to treatment, increased risk of acute and long-term complications and increased mortality. The British Diabetes Association Cohort Study found that mortality in the 20–29-year age group is increased threefold in men and sixfold in women compared to the general population [150]. Poor clinic attendance post-transfer has been observed particularly among individuals with high HbA1c values before transfer [149]. Several strategies have been devised to address this problem, including establishment of joint clinics staffed by pediatric and adult physicians or young adult clinics staffed by adult physicians but run separately from the main adult clinic [149]. A major imperative is to ensure that the young adult patient continues to have regular follow-up.

The goal of transition is to provide developmentally appropriate health care services that continue uninterrupted as the individual moves from adolescence to adulthood [151]. To manage the transition process, the ISPAD Clinical Practice Consensus Guidelines offers the following recommendations [152]:

• Identify an adult service able and willing to provide for the needs of young adults with diabetes.

• Provide a joint adolescent or young adult clinic with members of both professional teams working together to facilitate the transition process.

• Establish a liaison (transition coordinator) between the pediatric and adult services. This should be a specific person (e.g. a specialist nurse) able to move between services and facilitate the transition process by working with the patient and family to link them to clinical and educational resources.

• Commence discussion with the adolescent/young adult and parent well in advance to determine the best time for transfer based on the patient's preference and readiness but also considering the availability of services and, in some countries, the dictates of hospital policies and health insurance requirements.

• Develop a clear transition plan in collaboration with the young adult and provide a comprehensive summary of the patient's medical history.

• Ensure there is no significant gap in care between leaving the pediatric service and entering the adult service.

• The diabetes service should have a mechanism to identify and locate young people who fail to attend follow-up.

Conclusions

In 1993, the DCCT recommended that children and adolescents with diabetes should receive intensive therapy. Technological innovations since then have made it possible to achieve tighter blood glucose control with reduced risk of severe hypoglycemia. Increased use of more physiologic and flexible insulin regimens together with frequent blood glucose monitoring, carbohydrate counting and patient empowerment has made it possible to ensure normal growth and development and to achieve concentrations of blood glucose control that were previously unattainable.

The benefits of sustained improvement in glycemic control should prevent or, at least, delay the appearance of the chronic complications of diabetes. Epidemiologic data provide evidence that this is the case [153] but the arduous and unceasing task of controlling blood glucose is difficult and frustrating and the risk of hypoglycemia is always present. The resources of a multidisciplinary health care team in collaboration with the child's primary care physician are essential for the successful management of childhood diabetes but type 2 diabetes has emerged as a major new challenge.

References

1 Diagnosis and classification of diabetes mellitus. *Diabetes Care* 2008; **31** (Suppl 1): S55–60.

2 Pugliese A, Gianani R, Moromisato R, Awdeh ZL, Alper CA, Erlich HA, *et al.* HLA-DQB1*0602 is associated with dominant protection from diabetes even among islet cell antibody-positive first-degree relatives of patients with IDDM. *Diabetes* 1995; **44**: 608–613.

3 Komulainen J, Kulmala P, Savola K, Lounamaa R, Ilonen J, Reijonen H, *et al.* Clinical, autoimmune and genetic characteristics of very young children with type 1 diabetes. Childhood Diabetes in Finland (DiMe) Study Group. *Diabetes Care* 1999; **22**: 1950–1955.

4 Pearson ER, Starkey BJ, Powell RJ, Gribble FM, Clark PM, Hattersley AT. Genetic cause of hyperglycaemia and response to treatment in diabetes. *Lancet* 2003; **362**: 1275–1281.

5 Maassen JA. Mitochondrial diabetes: pathophysiology, clinical presentation and genetic analysis. *Am J Med Genet* 2002; **115**: 66–70.

6 Pearson ER, Flechtner I, Njolstad PR, Malecki MT, Flanagan SE, Larkin B, *et al.* Switching from insulin to oral sulfonylureas in patients with diabetes due to Kir6.2 mutations. *N Engl J Med* 2006; **355**: 467–477.

7 Moran A, Hardin D, Rodman D, Allen HF, Beall RJ, Borowitz D, *et al.* Diagnosis, screening and management of cystic fibrosis related diabetes mellitus: a consensus conference report. *Diabetes Res Clin Pract* 1999; **45**: 61–73.

8 Luna B, Feinglos M. Drug-induced hyperglycemia. *JAMA* 2001; **286**: 1945–1948.

9 Incidence and trends of childhood type 1 diabetes worldwide 1990–1999. *Diabet Med* 2006; **23**: 857–866.

10 Gale EA. The rise of childhood type 1 diabetes in the 20th century. *Diabetes* 2002; **51**: 3353–3361.

11 Atkinson MA, Eisenbarth GS. Type 1 diabetes: new perspectives on disease pathogenesis and treatment. *Lancet* 2001; **358**: 221–229.

12 Redondo MJ, Eisenbarth GS. Genetic control of autoimmunity in type I diabetes and associated disorders. *Diabetologia* 2002; **45**: 605–622.

13 Knip M, Veijola R, Virtanen SM, Hyoty H, Vaarala O, Akerblom HK. Environmental triggers and determinants of type 1 diabetes. *Diabetes* 2005; **54** (Suppl 2): S125–136.

14 Skyler JS. Prediction and prevention of type 1 diabetes: progress, problems and prospects. *Clin Pharmacol Ther* 2007; **81**: 768–771.

15 Verge CF, Gianani R, Kawasaki E, Yu L, Pietropaolo M, Jackson RA, *et al.* Prediction of type I diabetes in first-degree relatives using a combination of insulin, GAD and ICA512bdc/IA-2 autoantibodies. *Diabetes* 1996; **45**: 926–933.

16 Diabetes Prevention Trial – Type 1 Diabetes Study Group. Effects of insulin in relatives of patients with type 1 diabetes mellitus. *N Engl J Med* 2002; **346**: 1685–1691.

17 Chase HP, Cuthbertson DD, Dolan LM, Kaufman F, Krischer JP, Schatz DA, *et al.* First-phase insulin release during the intravenous glucose tolerance test as a risk factor for type 1 diabetes. *J Pediatr* 2001; **138**: 244–249.

18 Sosenko JM, Palmer JP, Greenbaum CJ, Mahon J, Cowie C, Krischer JP, *et al.* Patterns of metabolic progression to type 1 diabetes in the Diabetes Prevention Trial – Type 1. *Diabetes Care* 2006; **29**: 643–649.

19 Skyler JS, Krischer JP, Wolfsdorf J, Cowie C, Palmer JP, Greenbaum C, *et al.* Effects of oral insulin in relatives of patients with type 1 diabetes: The Diabetes Prevention Trial – Type 1. *Diabetes Care* 2005; **28**: 1068–1076.

20 Gale EA, Bingley PJ, Emmett CL, Collier T. European Nicotinamide Diabetes Intervention Trial (ENDIT): a randomised controlled trial of intervention before the onset of type 1 diabetes. *Lancet* 2004; **363**: 925–931.

21 Diabetes Control and Complications Trial Research Group. Effect of intensive therapy on residual beta-cell function in patients with type 1 diabetes in the diabetes control and complications trial: a randomized, controlled trial. *Ann Intern Med* 1998; **128**: 517–523.

22 Raz I, Elias D, Avron A, Tamir M, Metzger M, Cohen IR. Beta-cell function in new-onset type 1 diabetes and immunomodulation with a heat-shock protein peptide (DiaPep277): a randomised, double-blind, phase II trial. *Lancet* 2001; **358**: 1749–1753.

23 Agardh CD, Cilio CM, Lethagen A, Lynch K, Leslie RD, Palmer M, *et al.* Clinical evidence for the safety of GAD65 immunomodulation in adult-onset autoimmune diabetes. *J Diabetes Complications* 2005; **19**: 238–246.

24 Herold KC, Hagopian W, Auger JA, Poumian-Ruiz E, Taylor L, Donaldson D, *et al.* Anti-CD3 monoclonal antibody in new-onset type 1 diabetes mellitus. *N Engl J Med* 2002; **346**: 1692–1698.

25 Keymeulen B, Vandemeulebroucke E, Ziegler AG, Mathieu C, Kaufman L, Hale G, *et al.* Insulin needs after CD3-antibody therapy in new-onset type 1 diabetes. *N Engl J Med* 2005; **352**: 2598–2608.

26 Study design of the Trial to Reduce IDDM in the Genetically at Risk (TRIGR). *Pediatr Diabetes* 2007; **8**: 117–137.

27 Kordonouri O, Klinghammer A, Lang EB, Gruters-Kieslich A, Grabert M, Holl RW. Thyroid autoimmunity in children and adolescents with type 1 diabetes: a multicenter survey. *Diabetes Care* 2002; **25**: 1346–1350.

28 Freemark M, Levitsky LL. Screening for celiac disease in children with type 1 diabetes: two views of the controversy. *Diabetes Care* 2003; **26**: 1932–1939.

29 Devendra D, Eisenbarth GS. 17. Immunologic endocrine disorders. *J Allergy Clin Immunol* 2003; **111** (Suppl): S624–636.

30 Frayling TM. Genome-wide association studies provide new insights into type 2 diabetes aetiology. *Nat Rev Genet* 2007; **8**: 657–662.

31 Franks PW, Hanson RL, Knowler WC, Moffett C, Enos G, Infante AM, et al. Childhood predictors of young-onset type 2 diabetes. *Diabetes* 2007; **56**: 2964–2972.

32 Couper J, Donaghue K. Phases of diabetes. *Pediatr Diabetes* 2007; **8**: 44–47.

33 Wolfsdorf J, Glaser N, Sperling MA. Diabetic ketoacidosis in infants, children and adolescents: a consensus statement from the American Diabetes Association. *Diabetes Care* 2006; **29**: 1150–1159.

34 Majaliwa ES, Munubhi E, Ramaiya K, Mpembeni R, Sanyiwa A, Mohn A, et al. Survey on acute and chronic complications in children and adolescents with type 1 diabetes at Muhimbili National Hospital in Dar es Salaam, Tanzania. *Diabetes Care* 2007; **30**: 2187–2192.

35 Barker JM, Goehrig SH, Barriga K, Hoffman M, Slover R, Eisenbarth GS, et al. Clinical characteristics of children diagnosed with type 1 diabetes through intensive screening and follow-up. *Diabetes Care* 2004; **27**: 1399–1404.

36 Libman IM, Pietropaolo M, Arslanian SA, LaPorte RE, Becker DJ. Evidence for heterogeneous pathogenesis of insulin-treated diabetes in black and white children. *Diabetes Care* 2003; **26**: 2876–2882.

37 Katz LE, Jawad AF, Ganesh J, Abraham M, Murphy K, Lipman TH. Fasting c-peptide and insulin-like growth factor-binding protein-1 concentrations help to distinguish childhood type 1 and type 2 diabetes at diagnosis. *Pediatr Diabetes* 2007; **8**: 53–59.

38 Herskowitz-Dumont R, Wolfsdorf JI, Jackson RA, Eisenbarth GS. Distinction between transient hyperglycemia and early insulin-dependent diabetes mellitus in childhood: a prospective study of incidence and prognostic factors. *J Pediatr* 1993; **123**: 347–354.

39 Dunger DB, Sperling MA, Acerini CL, Bohn DJ, Daneman D, Danne TP, et al. ESPE/LWPES consensus statement on diabetic ketoacidosis in children and adolescents. *Arch Dis Child* 2004; **89**: 188–194.

40 Anderson BJ, Wolfsdorf JI, Jacobson AM. Psychosocial adjustment in children with type 1 diabetes. In: Lebovitz HE, ed. *Therapy for Diabetes Mellitus and Related Disorders*, 4th edn. Alexandria, Virginia: American Diabetes Association; 2004: 75–81.

41 Cameron FJ, Northam EA, Ambler GR, Daneman D. Routine psychological screening in youth with type 1 diabetes and their parents: a notion whose time has come? *Diabetes Care* 2007; **30**: 2716–2724.

42 Swift PG. Diabetes education. ISPAD clinical practice consensus guidelines 2006–2007. *Pediatr Diabetes* 2007; **8**: 103–109.

43 Diabetes Control and Complications Trial Research Group. The effect of intensive treatment of diabetes on the development and progression of long-term complications in insulin-dependent diabetes mellitus [see comments]. *N Engl J Med* 1993; **329**: 977–986.

44 Diabetes Control and Complications Trial Research Group. Effect of intensive diabetes treatment on the development and progression of long-term complications in adolescents with insulin-dependent diabetes mellitus: Diabetes Control and Complications Trial [see comments]. *J Pediatrics* 1994; **125**: 177–188.

45 Reichard P, Nilsson BY, Rosenqvist U. The effect of long-term intensified insulin treatment on the development of microvascular complications of diabetes mellitus [see comments]. *N Engl J Med* 1993; **329**: 304–309.

46 UK Prospective Diabetes Study (UKPDS) Group. Intensive blood-glucose control with sulphonylureas or insulin compared with conventional treatment and risk of complications in patients with type 2 diabetes (UKPDS 33). *Lancet* 1998; **352**: 837–853.

47 Effect of intensive blood-glucose control with metformin on complications in overweight patients with type 2 diabetes (UKPDS 34). UK Prospective Diabetes Study (UKPDS) Group [see comments] *Lancet* 1998; **352**: 854–865. [Published erratum appears in *Lancet* 1998; **352**: 1557.]

48 Nathan DM, Cleary PA, Backlund JY, Genuth SM, Lachin JM, Orchard TJ, et al. Intensive diabetes treatment and cardiovascular disease in patients with type 1 diabetes. *N Engl J Med* 2005; **353**: 2643–2653.

49 Diabetes Control and Complications Trial/Epidemiology of Diabetes Interventions and Complications Research Group. Retinopathy and nephropathy in patients with type 1 diabetes four years after a trial of intensive therapy. *N Engl J Med* 2000; **342**: 381–389.

50 Diabetes Control and Complications Trial/Epidemiology of Diabetes Interventions and Complications Research Group. Effect of intensive therapy on the microvascular complications of type 1 diabetes mellitus. *JAMA* 2002; **287**: 2563–2569.

51 Donaghue KC, Fairchild JM, Craig ME, Chan AK, Hing S, Cutler LR, et al. Do all prepubertal years of diabetes duration contribute equally to diabetes complications? *Diabetes Care* 2003; **26**: 1224–1229.

52 Rewers M, Pihoker C, Donaghue K, Hanas R, Swift P, Klingensmith GJ. Assessment and monitoring of glycemic control in children and adolescents with diabetes. *Pediatr Diabetes* 2007; **8**: 408–418.

53 Krolewski AS, Laffel LM, Krolewski M, Quinn M, Warram JH. Glycosylated hemoglobin and the risk of microalbuminuria in patients with insulin-dependent diabetes mellitus [see comments]. *N Engl J Med* 1995; **332**: 1251–1255.

54 Holl RW, Swift PG, Mortensen HB, Lynggaard H, Hougaard P, Aanstoot HJ, et al. Insulin injection regimens and metabolic control in an international survey of adolescents with type 1 diabetes over 3 years: results from the Hvidore study group. *Eur J Pediatr* 2003; **162**: 22–29.

55 de Beaufort CE, Swift PG, Skinner CT, Aanstoot HJ, Aman J, Cameron F, et al. Continuing stability of center differences in pediatric diabetes care: do advances in diabetes treatment improve outcome? The Hvidoere Study Group on Childhood Diabetes. *Diabetes Care* 2007; **30**: 2245–2250.

56 Fanelli CG, Pampanelli S, Porcellati F, Rossetti P, Brunetti P, Bolli GB. Administration of neutral protamine Hagedorn insulin at bedtime versus with dinner in type 1 diabetes mellitus to avoid nocturnal hypoglycemia and improve control: a randomized, controlled trial. *Ann Intern Med* 2002; **136**: 504–514.

57 Schober E, Schoenle E, Van Dyk J, Wernicke-Panten K. Comparative trial between insulin glargine and NPH insulin in children and adolescents with type 1 diabetes. *Diabetes Care* 2001; **24**: 2005–2006.

58 Lepore M, Pampanelli S, Fanelli C, Porcellati F, Bartocci L, Di Vincenzo A, et al. Pharmacokinetics and pharmacodynamics of subcutaneous injection of long-acting human insulin analog glargine,

NPH insulin and ultralente human insulin and continuous subcutaneous infusion of insulin lispro. *Diabetes* 2000; **49**: 2142–2148.

59 Murphy NP, Keane SM, Ong KK, Ford-Adams M, Edge JA, Acerini CL, *et al*. Randomized cross-over trial of insulin glargine plus lispro or NPH insulin plus regular human insulin in adolescents with type 1 diabetes on intensive insulin regimens. *Diabetes Care* 2003; **26**: 799–804.

60 Chase HP, Dixon B, Pearson J, Fiallo-Scharer R, Walravens P, Klingensmith G, *et al*. Reduced hypoglycemic episodes and improved glycemic control in children with type 1 diabetes using insulin glargine and neutral protamine hagedorn insulin. *J Pediatr* 2003; **143**: 737–740.

61 Robertson KJ, Schoenle E, Gucev Z, Mordhorst L, Gall MA, Ludvigsson J. Insulin detemir compared with NPH insulin in children and adolescents with type 1 diabetes. *Diabet Med* 2007; **24**: 27–34.

62 Porcellati F, Rossetti P, Busciantella NR, Marzotti S, Lucidi P, Lizio S, *et al*. Comparison of pharmacokinetics and dynamics of the long-acting insulin analogs glargine and detemir at steady state in type 1 diabetes. *Diabetes Care* 2007; **30**: 1261–1263.

63 Phillip M, Battelino T, Rodriguez H, Danne T, Kaufman F. Use of insulin pump therapy in the pediatric age-group: Consensus statement from the European Society for Paediatric Endocrinology, the Lawson Wilkins Pediatric Endocrine Society and the International Society for Pediatric and Adolescent Diabetes, endorsed by the American Diabetes Association and the European Association for the Study of Diabetes. *Diabetes Care* 2007; **30**: 1653–1662.

64 Pickup J, Mattock M, Kerry S. Glycaemic control with continuous subcutaneous insulin infusion compared with intensive insulin injections in patients with type 1 diabetes: meta-analysis of randomised controlled trials. *Br Med J* 2002; **324**: 705.

65 Weissberg-Benchell J, Antisdel-Lomaglio J, Seshadri R. Insulin pump therapy: a meta-analysis. *Diabetes Care* 2003; **26**: 1079–1087.

66 Amiel SA, Caprio S, Sherwin RS, Plewe G, Haymond MW, Tamborlane WV. Insulin resistance of puberty: a defect restricted to peripheral glucose metabolism. *J Clin Endocrinol Metab* 1991; **72**: 277–282.

67 Mortensen HB, Robertson KJ, Aanstoot HJ, Danne T, Holl RW, Hougaard P, *et al*. Insulin management and metabolic control of type 1 diabetes mellitus in childhood and adolescence in 18 countries. Hvidore Study Group on Childhood Diabetes. *Diabet Med* 1998; **15**: 752–759.

68 Danne T, Mortensen HB, Hougaard P, Lynggaard H, Aanstoot HJ, Chiarelli F, *et al*. Persistent differences among centers over 3 years in glycemic control and hypoglycemia in a study of 3,805 children and adolescents with type 1 diabetes from the Hvidore Study Group. *Diabetes Care* 2001; **24**: 1342–1347.

69 Rosilio M, Cotton JB, Wieliczko MC, Gendrault B, Carel JC, Couvaras O, *et al*. Factors associated with glycemic control. A cross-sectional nationwide study in 2,579 French children with type 1 diabetes. The French Pediatric Diabetes Group [see comments]. *Diabetes Care* 1998; **21**: 1146–1153.

70 Scottish Study Group for the Care of the Young Diabetic. Factors influencing glycemic control in young people with type 1 diabetes in Scotland: a population-based study (DIABAUD2). *Diabetes Care* 2001; **24**: 239–244.

71 Knerr I, Hofer SE, Holterhus PM, Nake A, Rosenbauer J, Weitzel D, *et al*. Prevailing therapeutic regimes and predictive factors for

prandial insulin substitution in 26 687 children and adolescents with type 1 diabetes in Germany and Austria. *Diabet Med* 2007; **24**: 1478–1481.

72 Bulsara MK, Holman CD, Davis EA, Jones TW. The impact of a decade of changing treatment on rates of severe hypoglycemia in a population-based cohort of children with type 1 diabetes. *Diabetes Care* 2004; **27**: 2293–2298.

73 Jones KL, Arslanian S, Peterokova VA, Park JS, Tomlinson MJ. Effect of metformin in pediatric patients with type 2 diabetes: a randomized controlled trial. *Diabetes Care* 2002; **25**: 89–94.

74 Effect of intensive blood-glucose control with metformin on complications in overweight patients with type 2 diabetes (UKPDS 34). UK Prospective Diabetes Study (UKPDS) Group. *Lancet* 1998; **352**: 854–865.

75 Eppens MC, Craig ME, Jones TW, Silink M, Ong S, Ping YJ. Type 2 diabetes in youth from the Western Pacific region: glycaemic control, diabetes care and complications. *Curr Med Res Opin* 2006; **22**: 1013–1020.

76 Alemzadeh R, Ellis J, Calhoun M, Kichler J. Predictors of metabolic control at one year in a population of pediatric patients with type 2 diabetes mellitus: a retrospective study. *J Pediatr Endocrinol Metab* 2006; **19**: 1141–1149.

77 Wolfsdorf J, Quinn M, Warman K. Diabetes mellitus. In: Walker W, Watkins J, Duggan C, eds. *Nutrition in Pediatrics: Basic Science and Clinical Applications*, 4th edn. Hamilton, Ontario: BC Decker, Inc., 2008: 617–630.

78 American Diabetes Association Standards of medical care in diabetes – 2008. *Diabetes Care* 2008; **31** (Suppl 1): S12–54.

79 Knowler WC, Barrett-Connor E, Fowler SE, Hamman RF, Lachin JM, Walker EA, *et al*. Reduction in the incidence of type 2 diabetes with lifestyle intervention or metformin. *N Engl J Med* 2002; **346**: 393–403.

80 Franz MJ, Bantle JP, Beebe CA, Brunzell JD, Chiasson JL, Garg A, *et al*. Evidence-based nutrition principles and recommendations for the treatment and prevention of diabetes and related complications. *Diabetes Care* 2002; **25**: 148–198.

81 Brand-Miller J, Hayne S, Petocz P, Colagiuri S. Low-glycemic index diets in the management of diabetes: a meta-analysis of randomized controlled trials. *Diabetes Care* 2003; **26**: 2261–2267.

82 Overby NC, Margeirsdottir HD, Brunborg C, Andersen LF, Dahl-Jorgensen K. The influence of dietary intake and meal pattern on blood glucose control in children and adolescents using intensive insulin treatment. *Diabetologia* 2007; **50**: 2044–2051.

83 American Diabetes Association. Management of dyslipidemia in children and adolescents with diabetes. *Diabetes Care* 2003; **26**: 2194–2197.

84 Kavey RE, Allada V, Daniels SR, Hayman LL, McCrindle BW, Newburger JW, *et al*. Cardiovascular risk reduction in high-risk pediatric patients: a scientific statement from the American Heart Association Expert Panel on Population and Prevention Science; the Councils on Cardiovascular Disease in the Young, Epidemiology and Prevention, Nutrition, Physical Activity and Metabolism, High Blood Pressure Research, Cardiovascular Nursing and the Kidney in Heart Disease; and the Interdisciplinary Working Group on Quality of Care and Outcomes Research: endorsed by the American Academy of Pediatrics. *Circulation* 2006; **114**: 2710–2738.

85 Riddell MC, Iscoe KE. Physical activity, sport and pediatric diabetes. *Pediatr Diabetes* 2006; **7**: 60–70.

86 Temple MY, Bar-Or O, Riddell MC. The reliability and repeatability of the blood glucose response to prolonged exercise in adolescent boys with IDDM. *Diabetes Care* 1995; **18**: 326–332.

87 Guelfi KJ, Jones TW, Fournier PA. The decline in blood glucose concentrations is less with intermittent high-intensity compared with moderate exercise in individuals with type 1 diabetes. *Diabetes Care* 2005; **28**: 1289–1294.

88 Schiffrin A, Belmonte M. Multiple daily self-glucose monitoring: its essential role in long-term glucose control in insulin-dependent diabetic patients treated with pump and multiple subcutaneous injections. *Diabetes Care* 1982; **5**: 479–484.

89 Levine B, Anderson B, Butler D, Antisdel J, Brackett J, Laffel L. Predictors of glycemic control and short-term adverse outcomes in youth with type 1 diabetes. *J Pediatr* 2001; **139**: 197–203.

90 Weinzimer S, Xing D, Tansey M, Fiallo-Scharer R, Mauras N, Wysocki T, *et al.* FreeStyle navigator continuous glucose monitoring system use in children with type 1 diabetes using glargine-based multiple daily dose regimens: results of a pilot trial Diabetes Research in Children Network (DirecNet) Study Group. *Diabetes Care* 2008; **31**: 525–527.

91 Rewers A, McFann K, Chase HP. Bedside monitoring of blood beta-hydroxybutyrate concentrations in the management of diabetic ketoacidosis in children. *Diabetes Technol Ther* 2006; **8**: 671–676.

92 Laffel LM, Wentzell K, Loughlin C, Tovar A, Moltz K, Brink S. Sick day management using blood 3-hydroxybutyrate (3-OHB) compared with urine ketone monitoring reduces hospital visits in young people with T1DM: a randomized clinical trial. *Diabet Med* 2006; **23**: 278–284.

93 Sacks DB, Bruns DE, Goldstein DE, Maclaren NK, McDonald JM, Parrott M. Guidelines and recommendations for laboratory analysis in the diagnosis and management of diabetes mellitus. *Clin Chem* 2002; **48**: 436–472.

94 Mosca A, Goodall I, Hoshino T, Jeppsson JO, John WG, Little RR, *et al.* Global standardization of glycated hemoglobin measurement: the position of the IFCC Working Group. *Clin Chem Lab Med* 2007; **45**: 1077–1080.

95 Nathan DM, Kuenen J, Borg R, Zheng H, Schoenfeld D, Heine RJ. Translating the A1C assay in to estimated average glucose values. *Diabetes Care* 2008; **31**: 1–6.

96 Wolfsdorf J, Craig ME, Daneman D, Dunger D, Edge J, Lee WR, *et al.* Diabetic ketoacidosis. *Pediatr Diabetes* 2007; **8**: 28–43.

97 Edge JA, Jakes RW, Roy Y, Hawkins M, Winter D, Ford-Adams ME, *et al.* The UK case–control study of cerebral oedema complicating diabetic ketoacidosis in children. *Diabetologia* 2006; **49**: 2002–2009.

98 Glaser N, Barnett P, McCaslin I, Nelson D, Trainor J, Louie J, *et al.* Risk factors for cerebral edema in children with diabetic ketoacidosis. The Pediatric Emergency Medicine Collaborative Research Committee of the American Academy of Pediatrics. *N Engl J Med* 2001; **344**: 264–269.

99 Muir AB, Quisling RG, Yang MC, Rosenbloom AL. Cerebral edema in childhood diabetic ketoacidosis: natural history, radiographic findings and early identification. *Diabetes Care* 2004; **27**: 1541–1546.

100 Glaser N. New perspectives on the pathogenesis of cerebral edema complicating diabetic ketoacidosis in children. *Pediatr Endocrinol Rev* 2006; **3**: 379–386.

101 Marcin JP, Glaser N, Barnett P, McCaslin I, Nelson D, Trainor J, *et al.* Factors associated with adverse outcomes in children with diabetic ketoacidosis-related cerebral edema. *J Pediatr* 2002; **141**: 793–797.

102 Haymond MW, Schreiner B. Mini-dose glucagon rescue for hypoglycemia in children with type 1 diabetes. *Diabetes Care* 2001; **24**: 643–645.

103 Brink S, Laffel L, Likitmaskul S, Liu L, Maguire AM, Olsen B, *et al.* Sick day management in children and adolescents with diabetes. *Pediatr Diabetes* 2007; **8**: 401–407.

104 The DCCT Research Group. Weight gain associated with intensive therapy in the Diabetes Control and Complications Trial. *Diabetes Care* 1988; **11**: 567–573.

105 Cryer PE. Banting Lecture. Hypoglycemia: the limiting factor in the management of IDDM. *Diabetes* 1994; **43**: 1378–1389.

106 Clarke WL, Gonder-Frederick A, Snyder AL, Cox DJ. Maternal fear of hypoglycemia in their children with insulin dependent diabetes mellitus. *J Pediatr Endocrinol Metab* 1998; **11** (Suppl 1): 189–194.

107 Santiago JV. Nocturnal hypoglycemia in children with diabetes: an important problem revisited [editorial; comment]. *J Pediatr* 1997; **131** (1 Pt 1): 2–4.

108 Cryer PE, Davis SN, Shamoon H. Hypoglycemia in diabetes. *Diabetes Care* 2003; **26**: 1902–1912.

109 Hepburn DA, Deary IJ, Frier BM, Patrick AW, Quinn JD, Fisher BM. Symptoms of acute insulin-induced hypoglycemia in humans with and without IDDM: factor-analysis approach. *Diabetes Care* 1991; **14**: 949–957.

110 McCrimmon RJ, Gold AE, Deary IJ, Kelnar CJ, Frier BM. Symptoms of hypoglycemia in children with IDDM. *Diabetes Care* 1995; **18**: 858–861.

111 Kaufman FR, Epport K, Engilman R, Halvorson M. Neurocognitive functioning in children diagnosed with diabetes before age 10 years. *J Diabetes Complications* 1999; **13**: 31–38.

112 Hershey T, Craft S, Bhargava N, White NH. Memory and insulin dependent diabetes mellitus (IDDM): effects of childhood onset and severe hypoglycemia. *J Int Neuropsychol Soc* 1997; **3**: 509–520.

113 Northam EA, Anderson PJ, Jacobs R, Hughes M, Warne GL, Werther GA. Neuropsychological profiles of children with type 1 diabetes 6 years after disease onset. *Diabetes Care* 2001; **24**: 1541–1546.

114 Jones T, Davis E. Hypoglycemia in children with type 1 diabetes: current issues and controversies. *Pediatric Diabetes* 2003; **4**: 143–150.

115 Rovet JF, Ehrlich RM. The effect of hypoglycemic seizures on cognitive function in children with diabetes: a 7-year prospective study [see comments]. *J Pediatr* 1999; **134**: 503–506.

116 Schoenle EJ, Schoenle D, Molinari L, Largo RH. Impaired intellectual development in children with type I diabetes: association with HbA(1c), age at diagnosis and sex. *Diabetologia* 2002; **45**: 108–114.

117 Ryan CM. Why is cognitive dysfunction associated with the development of diabetes early in life? The diathesis hypothesis. *Pediatr Diabetes* 2006; **7**: 289–297.

118 Hershey T, Bhargava N, Sadler M, White NH, Craft S. Conventional versus intensive diabetes therapy in children with type 1 diabetes: effects on memory and motor speed [see comments]. *Diabetes Care* 1999; **22**: 1318–1324.

119 Ryan CM, Becker DJ. Hypoglycemia in children with type 1 diabetes mellitus: risk factors, cognitive function and management. *Endocrinol Metab Clin North Am* 1999; **28**: 883–900.

120 Edge JA, Ford-Adams ME, Dunger DB. Causes of death in children with insulin dependent diabetes 1990–96. *Arch Dis Child* 1999; **81**: 318–323.

121 Rewers A, Chase HP, Mackenzie T, Walravens P, Roback M, Rewers M, *et al.* Predictors of acute complications in children with type 1 diabetes. *JAMA* 2002; **287**: 2511–2518.

122 Wagner VM, Grabert M, Holl RW. Severe hypoglycaemia, metabolic control and diabetes management in children with type 1 diabetes in the decade after the Diabetes Control and Complications Trial: a large-scale multicentre study. *Eur J Pediatr* 2005; **164**: 73–79.

123 Nordfeldt S, Johansson C, Carlsson E, Hammersjo JA. Prevention of severe hypoglycaemia in type I diabetes: a randomised controlled population study. *Arch Dis Child* 2003; **88**: 240–245.

124 Svoren BM, Volkening LK, Butler DA, Moreland EC, Anderson BJ, Laffel LM. Temporal trends in the treatment of pediatric type 1 diabetes and impact on acute outcomes. *J Pediatr* 2007; **150**: 279–285.

125 The Diabetes Control and Complications Trial Research Group. Epidemiology of severe hypoglycemia in the Diabetes Control and Complications Trial. The DCCT Research Group [see comments]. *Am J Med* 1991; **90**: 450–459.

126 The Diabetes Control and Complications Trial Research Group. Hypoglycemia in the Diabetes Control and Complications Trial. *Diabetes* 1997; **46**: 271–286.

127 Davis EA, Keating B, Byrne GC, Russell M, Jones TW. Hypoglycemia: incidence and clinical predictors in a large population-based sample of children and adolescents with IDDM. *Diabetes Care* 1997; **20**: 22–25.

128 Bode BW, Schwartz S, Stubbs HA, Block JE. Glycemic characteristics in continuously monitored patients with type 1 and type 2 diabetes: normative values. *Diabetes Care* 2005; **28**: 2361–2366.

129 Raju B, Arbelaez AM, Breckenridge SM, Cryer PE. Nocturnal hypoglycemia in type 1 diabetes: an assessment of preventive bedtime treatments. *J Clin Endocrinol Metab* 2006; **91**: 2087–2092.

130 Tsalikian E, Mauras N, Beck RW, Tamborlane WV, Janz KF, Chase HP, *et al.* Impact of exercise on overnight glycemic control in children with type 1 diabetes mellitus. *J Pediatr* 2005; **147**: 528–534.

131 Sandoval DA, Guy DL, Richardson MA, Ertl AC, Davis SN. Effects of low and moderate antecedent exercise on counterregulatory responses to subsequent hypoglycemia in type 1 diabetes. *Diabetes* 2004; **53**: 1798–1806.

132 Jones TW, Porter P, Sherwin RS, Davis EA, O'Leary P, Frazer F, *et al.* Decreased epinephrine responses to hypoglycemia during sleep. *N Engl J Med* 1998; **338**: 1657–1662.

133 Cryer PE. Diverse causes of hypoglycemia-associated autonomic failure in diabetes. *N Engl J Med* 2004; **350**: 2272–2279.

134 Hartley M, Thomsett MJ, Cotterill AM. Mini-dose glucagon rescue for mild hypoglycaemia in children with type 1 diabetes: the Brisbane experience. *J Paediatr Child Health* 2006; **42**: 108–111.

135 Cox DJ, Penberthy JK, Zrebiec J, Weinger K, Aikens JE, Frier B, *et al.* Diabetes and driving mishaps: frequency and correlations from a multinational survey. *Diabetes Care* 2003; **26**: 2329–2334.

136 Weinger K, Kinsley BT, Levy CJ, Bajaj M, Simonson DC, Cox DJ, *et al.* The perception of safe driving ability during hypoglycemia in patients with type 1 diabetes mellitus. *Am J Med* 1999; **107**: 246–253.

137 Jones JM, Lawson ML, Daneman D, Olmsted MP, Rodin G. Eating disorders in adolescent females with and without type 1 diabetes: cross-sectional study. *Br Med J* 2000; **320**: 1563–1566.

138 Rydall AC, Rodin GM, Olmsted MP, Devenyi RG, Daneman D. Disordered eating behavior and microvascular complications in young women with insulin-dependent diabetes mellitus. *N Engl J Med* 1997; **336**: 1849–1854.

139 Goebel-Fabbri AE, Fikkan J, Franko DL, Pearson K, Anderson BJ, Weinger K. Insulin restriction and associated morbidity and mortality in women with type 1 diabetes. *Diabetes Care* 2008; **31**: 415–419.

140 Stettler C, Allemann S, Juni P, Cull CA, Holman RR, Egger M, *et al.* Glycemic control and macrovascular disease in types 1 and 2 diabetes mellitus: Meta-analysis of randomized trials. *Am Heart J* 2006; **152**: 27–38.

141 Sochett E, Daneman D. Early diabetes-related complications in children and adolescents with type 1 diabetes. Implications for screening and intervention. *Endocrinol Metab Clin North Am* 1999; **28**: 865–882.

142 American Diabetes Association. Standards of medical care in diabetes. *Diabetes Care* 2009; **32** (Suppl 1): 513–561.

143 Norris AW, Svoren BM. Complications and comorbidities of type 2 diabetes. *Pediatr Ann* 2005; **34**: 710–718.

144 Silverstein J, Klingensmith G, Copeland K, Plotnick L, Kaufman F, Laffel L, *et al.* Care of children and adolescents with type 1 diabetes: a statement of the American Diabetes Association. *Diabetes Care* 2005; **28**: 186–212.

145 Management of dyslipidemia in children and adolescents with diabetes. *Diabetes Care* 2003; **26**: 2194–2197.

146 Nadeau KJ, Klingensmith G, Zeitler P. Type 2 diabetes in children is frequently associated with elevated alanine aminotransferase. *J Pediatr Gastroenterol Nutr* 2005; **41**: 94–98.

147 Weissberg-Benchell J, Wolpert H, Anderson BJ. Transitioning from pediatric to adult care: a new approach to the post-adolescent young person with type 1 diabetes. *Diabetes Care* 2007; **30**: 2441–2446.

148 Court JM. Issues of transition to adult care. *J Paediatr Child Health* 1993; **29** (Suppl 1): S53–55.

149 Kipps S, Bahu T, Ong K, Ackland FM, Brown RS, Fox CT, *et al.* Current methods of transfer of young people with type 1 diabetes to adult services. *Diabet Med* 2002; **19**: 649–654.

150 Laing SP, Swerdlow AJ, Slater SD, Botha JL, Burden AC, Waugh NR, *et al.* The British Diabetic Association Cohort Study. I. All-cause mortality in patients with insulin-treated diabetes mellitus. *Diabet Med* 1999; **16**: 459–465.

151 A consensus statement on health care transitions for young adults with special health care needs. *Pediatrics* 2002; **110** (6 Pt 2): 1304–1306.

152 Court J, Cameron F, Swift P. Diabetes in adolescence. *Pediatr Diabetes* 2008; **9**: 255–262.

153 Bojestig M, Arnqvist HJ, Hermansson G, Karlberg BE, Ludvigsson J. Declining incidence of nephropathy in insulin-dependent diabetes mellitus. *N Engl J Med* 1994; **330**: 15–18. [Published erratum appears in *N Engl J Med* 1994; **330**: 584.]

154 Kaplan W, Rodriguez LM, Smith OE, Haymond MW, Heptulla RA. Effects of mixing glargine and short-acting insulin analogs on glucose control. *Diabetes Care* 2004; **27**: 2739–2740.

155 Fiallo-Scharer R, Horner B, McFann K, Walravens P, Chase HP. Mixing rapid-acting insulin analogues with insulin glargine in children with type 1 diabetes mellitus. *J Pediatr* 2006; **148**: 481–484.

156 Plank J, Wutte A, Brunner G, Siebenhofer A, Semlitsch B, Sommer R, *et al*. A direct comparison of insulin aspart and insulin lispro in patients with type 1 diabetes. *Diabetes Care* 2002; **25**: 2053–2057.

157 Danne T, Lupke K, Walte K, Von Schuetz W, Gall MA. Insulin detemir is characterized by a consistent pharmacokinetic profile across age-groups in children, adolescents and adults with type 1 diabetes. *Diabetes Care* 2003; **26**: 3087–3092.

158 Franz MJ, Bantle JP, Beebe CA, Brunzell JD, Chiasson JL, Garg A, et al. Nutrition principles and recommendations in diabetes. *Diabetes Care* 2004; **27** (Suppl 1): S36–46.

159 Bantle JP, Wylie-Rosett J, Albright AL, Apovian CM, Clark NG, Franz MJ, *et al*. Nutrition recommendations and interventions for diabetes – 2006: a position statement of the American Diabetes Association. *Diabetes Care* 2006; **29**: 2140–2157.

160 Gale EA. The rise of childhood type 1 diabetes in the 20th Century. *Diabetes* 2002; 51: 3353–3361.

161 Mortensen HB, Hougaard P. Comparison of metabolic control in a cross-sectional study of 2873 children and adolescents with IDDM from 18 countries. The Hvidore Study Group on Childhood Diabetes. *Diabetes Care* 1997; **20**: 714–720. [Published erratum appears in *Diabetes Care* 1997; **20**: 1216.]

19 Hypoglycemia: Assessment and Management

Andrew Cotterill[1], David Cowley[2] & Ristan Greer[1]

[1] Department of Paediatric Endocrinology, Mater Children's Hospital, Brisbane, Queensland, Australia
[2] Mater Health Services Brisbane Ltd, Brisbane, Queensland, Australia

Hypoglycemia is a medical emergency which carries serious short and long-term consequences from incorrect management. It is unfortunate that the point of crisis is often the best time to make the diagnosis by taking the correct or "critical" blood and urine samples. Delay in management may precipitate complications but intervention without the diagnostic samples delays the diagnosis until either another similar event takes place or hypoglycemia can be reproduced during a planned elective fasting study. The most practical course is to take samples at the first opportunity and institute treatment without delay.

In neonates in developed countries, the most common cause of hypoglycemia is related to diabetes-affected pregnancy, whereas it relates to intra-uterine growth retardation and lack of breast milk in developing countries. In children, the most common cause of hypoglycemia in developed countries relates to treatment of type 1 diabetes, whereas, in developing countries, it is likely to be associated with lack of nutrition or starvation due to exhausted liver glycogen stores. Even after excluding these causes, hypoglycemia is a common metabolic and endocrine abnormality in infancy and childhood and yet there has been controversy about its definition and management [1].

Hypoglycemia results in reduced supply of glucose to vital organs, particularly those without the ability for glycogen storage, such as the brain, which is almost entirely dependent on a continuous supply of glucose to maintain normal function and therefore most vulnerable to hypoglycemic events. Recurrent and persistent hypoglycemia can cause morbidity and sudden death due to damage to brain tissue deprived of glucose supply. The prevention of morbidity and mortality is central to management for which the key is making the correct diagnosis at the time of hypoglycemia.

The incidence of the causes of hypoglycemia varies with age but can be classified into five groups:

1 Excess insulin (or insulin-like factors) for the given circumstances;

2 Lack of one or more of the counter-regulatory hormones (particularly cortisol, growth hormone);

3 Disturbance of intermediate metabolism causing impairment of gluconeogenesis and/or glycogenolysis;

4 Disturbance of fat breakdown or ketone body formation or utilization; or

5 Lack of nutrient sufficient for current energy demands.

Definition

Hypoglycemia with or without the associated symptoms and signs is defined by a blood glucose concentration <2.6 mmol/L (45 mg/dL) when impairment of cognitive function is observed [2]. Cognitive function is not impaired above this concentration in most adults and neonates but may be impaired in some. Glucose homeostatic mechanisms are designed to maintain blood glucose concentrations >2.6 mmol/L in order to allow continuation of normal cognitive function.

If blood glucose concentrations are >2.6 mmol/L but below the lower limit of the normal laboratory range, the patient may experience symptoms that may resolve with glucose but it is difficult to make a confident diagnosis of the underlying cause until failure of glucose homeostasis has taken place. The diagnosis of hypoglycemia has previously been made using the criteria of Whipple's triad (symptoms consistent with hypoglycemia, low blood glucose concentration and resolution of symptoms with correction of hypoglycemia) developed to assist in the diagnosis of insulinoma in adult patients [1]. In children, particularly the very young, it is not possible to consider symptoms as part of the diagnosis.

Using the biochemical definition of hypoglycemia, 20% of normal asymptomatic full-term infants have a low blood glucose concentration (<2.6 mmol/L) and concurrent high ketone concentrations in the first 48 h of life [3]. It is assumed that if the period of hypoglycemia is short and alternative fuels are available, impairment of neuronal function is reversible. After the first day

Brook's Clinical Pediatric Endocrinology, 6th edition. Edited by C. Brook, P. Clayton, R. Brown. © 2009 Blackwell Publishing, ISBN: 978-1-4051-8080-1.

of life, hypoglycemia is uncommon and the duration of the period of hypoglycemia that would cause permanent damage is not known. It is presumed to depend on the degree and frequency of hypoglycemia and the concurrent circumstances, such as the availability of alternative fuels and the presence or absence of factors such as infection, trauma and hypoxia and the degree of resilience of the brain tissue to periodic loss of energy supply.

Measurement of glucose concentrations depends on many factors independent of the "true" glucose concentration. The point of access used for the sampling of blood, capillary, arterial or venous and the hematocrit lead to slight but significant variations in the glucose concentration because of differing rates of consumption of the glucose by the tissues before sampling. Glucose concentrations vary slightly due to the preparation of the sample after it has been obtained and whether whole blood or plasma is used in the assay, particularly if the hematocrit is high. Finally, the glucose concentration recorded depends on the biochemical method, such as point-of-care blood gas machine, central blood gas analyzer, biochemistry laboratory multiple biochemical analyzer, hand-held glucometers or continuous glucose monitoring systems.

A false low blood glucose can result from continued glucose breakdown by red blood cells after the sample has been taken, particularly if the sample is left for more than 30 min before processing. When the sample is to be transported to a central laboratory, a fluoride oxalate collection tube should always be used to block post-sampling glucose metabolism. It is therefore important to discuss the glucose results with the laboratory to confirm the validity of the results to avoid unnecessary investigation and concern.

Clinical assessment

Despite the urgent requirement to treat hypoglycemia, an initial assessment of history, examination and the collection of critical blood and urine samples is vital. Treatment should proceed with oral or intravenous glucose. Hypoglycemia is often overlooked because the history and signs may be vague and nonspecific, particularly in the neonate and infant. A high level of suspicion is required in a neonate presenting with apnoeic events, twitches or other subtle signs but many hypoglycemia infants are asymptomatic, which has led to routine screening in at-risk infants, such as infants of a diabetic mother, babies born with extreme intra-uterine growth retardation and babies with hypothermia.

Studies in adults have clearly defined the progressive development of symptoms and signs of hypoglycemia using hyperinsulinemic-induced hypoglycemia. As the blood glucose concentrations are artificially lowered, there is a classic progression from hunger and food-seeking to onset of sympathetic nervous system activation with the associated features of sweating, tremor and tachycardia. As the glucose concentrations fall further, impairment of cognitive function occurs with confusion,

mental slowness, inappropriate behavior, loss of consciousness, generalized convulsions and death (Table 19.1).

The history should focus on the presence of repeated episodes of hypoglycemia, the timing of such events in relation to nutrient supply and the presence of predisposing and associated factors. The time from the last meal to the onset of hypoglycemia is important in determining the possible underlying causes. Early onset of hypoglycemia (within 2–3 h of the last meal) suggests increased utilization of glucose because of high insulin concentrations, e.g. congenital hyperinsulinism of infancy (CHI). Conditions associated with onset of symptoms >4 h after the last meal are those that involve defects in glycogenolysis, gluconeogenesis, production of free fatty acids and ketone bodies or lack of counter-regulatory hormones. Rare conditions, such as mitochondrial disorders linked with intracellular energy deprivation, may present with symptoms of hypoglycemia with a normal plasma glucose concentration (pseudohypoglycemia).

Age of onset

Severe neonatal hypoglycemia suggests a congenital defect in insulin release, whereas hypoglycemia on day 1 and 2 of life managed with increased feeds would be typical of a baby born with deficiency of counter-regulatory hormones such as cortisol or growth hormone. Presentation of the first episode of hypoglycemia in infancy after weaning and prolongation of fasting to 8 h raises the possibility of defects in the gluconeogenic or fat metabolism pathways. Children presenting for the first time with hypoglycemia in mid-childhood raise questions of common disorders, such as ingestion of alcohol, or extremely rare conditions, such as insulinomas or exercise-induced hypoglycemia.

Past history

A critical review may reveal missed events that suggest the duration of hypoglycemia may be more prolonged than first thought. The child may often be sweaty, shaky, cold and clammy early in the morning and mood and general cognition improves after breakfast. The diagnosis of idiopathic epilepsy may need to be revised with the discovery of hypoglycemia.

Table 19.1 Symptoms and signs of hypoglycemia.

System	Symptom
Adrenergic	Sweating, trembling, tachycardia, anxiety, weakness, nausea, vomiting, hunger
Neuroglycopenic	Headaches, visual disturbances, lethargy, irritability, confusion, affected speech, motor and sensory neurological signs, personality and behavioral changes, seizures, loss of consciousness, permanent neurological damage
	Neonates/infants: cyanosis, apnea, hypothermia, "respiratory distress," feeding difficulties, jitteriness, irritability

Pregnancy, birth and neonatal history

Premature infants have an increased frequency of hypoglycemia compared to term infants, as do babies born small for gestational age. Pregnancy affected by diabetes of any type, particularly if glucose control was suboptimal, leads to increased risk of neonatal hypoglycemia and of macrosomia, perhaps leading to a difficult or prolonged delivery. Babies born by a traumatic and/or difficult delivery associated with hypoxia are at risk of hypoglycemia. Polycythemia in the neonatal period is associated with hypoglycemia and often resolves with exchange transfusion. In the neonatal period, symptoms and signs of hypoglycemia are vague and non-specific, such as jitteriness, apnea, cyanosis, floppiness and jaundice.

Family history

In some populations, there is an increase in the prevalence of inherited causes of hypoglycemia. Predisposing factors, such as adrenal dysfunction, can also be inherited and need to be noted.

Dietary and drug history

The relationship between hypoglycemia and timing of the last meal is important. Hypoglycemia may be triggered by certain types of food, such as high protein load, high fructose content, toxin of tropical fruit after consumption of unripe ackee fruit (as seen in Jamaican vomiting sickness) and high glycemic index foods, which may lead to rebound hypoglycemia. A number of drugs and chemicals (e.g. alcohol, aspirin, oral hypoglycemic agents, insulin injected, beta-blockers and quinine) may interrupt intermediate metabolism leading to episodes of hypoglycemia.

Examination

The initial examination should record height, weight, body mass index and, in the neonate, features suggesting macrosomia, small for gestational age and prematurity. Dysmorphic features may suggest inborn errors of metabolism, midline defects, such as cleft lip/palate, linking with hypopituitarism and organomegaly may be associated with Beckwith–Wiedemann syndrome. Other relevant findings are hyperventilation, suggesting metabolic acidosis linked with metabolic disorders, hyperpigmentation associated with adrenocorticotropic hormone (ACTH) excess and, in the neonate, ambiguous genitalia linked with cortisol deficiency. Liver enlargement is a clue to some disorders of glycogen storage.

The child presenting late with hypoglycemia may demonstrate evidence of the deleterious effects of previous episodes of hypoglycemia, such as delayed development, behavioral disorders, hemiplegia or blindness.

Urgent investigations

Because 20% of healthy term infants have an abnormally low blood glucose in the first 2 days of life as part of the normal switch from maternal nutrient supply, which corrects with no adverse consequences, most babies do not need blood sampling, assuming that the plasma glucose concentration returns to and remains normal with feeding. When hypoglycemia occurs in a large for gestational age infant born to a mother with poorly controlled diabetes, the cause for the hypoglycemia is almost certainly transient hyperinsulinism. When the cause of hypoglycemia is obvious, the need for full investigation will depend on the age of the child, whether a diagnosis is certain, whether a diagnosis is required, the frequency, duration and intractability of the hypoglycemia and, most importantly, clinical judgment.

Despite these reservations it is appropriate to investigate almost all situations in which hypoglycemia occurs. The presence or absence of ketonuria and/or ketonemia is central to the systematic approach to assessment and management. Some investigations are indicated only if ketones are absent (Fig. 19.1) but hyperinsulinism can coexist with high ketones in the first 2 days of life. In these circumstances, it is likely that the ketones are of maternal origin and have crossed the placenta during hyperketosis of labor. Whether all blood and urine samples (Table 19.2) should be taken at the time of hypoglycemia or whether a staged approach should be taken is debatable. Given the vital nature of the investigations at the time of hypoglycemia, it is easier to take all samples and review the results to decide further analysis of stored samples. In elucidating a cause for hypoglycemia, the measurement of hormones and metabolites during an episode of confirmed hypoglycemia (the "critical sample") is of enormous value. The information provided from the sample is often not able to be replicated during a formal fasting study because of the limited ability to reproduce hypoglycemia in controlled circumstances, particularly if the period of fasting is limited to 24 h. A 72-h fast may produce a result but is difficult to conduct.

Pediatric laboratories should be able to provide all these tests on 1 mL blood collected into fluoride oxalate (unless glucose is measured on a point of care blood gas analyzer), 1.5 mL blood collected into lithium heparin and 2.5 mL clotted blood, preferably collected into neonatal microcollection tubes to maximize the yield of plasma and serum. Samples should be forwarded to the laboratory immediately on ice. A 5-mL urine sample should also be collected from the first urine passed after the event. If additional blood is available, samples for measurement of urea and electrolytes, liver function, C-peptide, ACTH and transferrin isoforms could also be sent to the laboratory. Of these tests, only C-peptide and ACTH need to be collected before giving glucose. Transferrin isoforms are not informative in the first month of life.

A "hypoglycemic kit" may therefore be developed for neonatal and hospital emergency units. Obtaining the required blood volume is difficult at times of crisis and an order of priority in the samples so that maximum information can be obtained should be formulated. Extended newborn screening programs available in some countries should identify a number of patients likely to be affected by hypoglycemia soon after birth, e.g. medium-chain acyl coenzyme A dehydrogenase deficiency

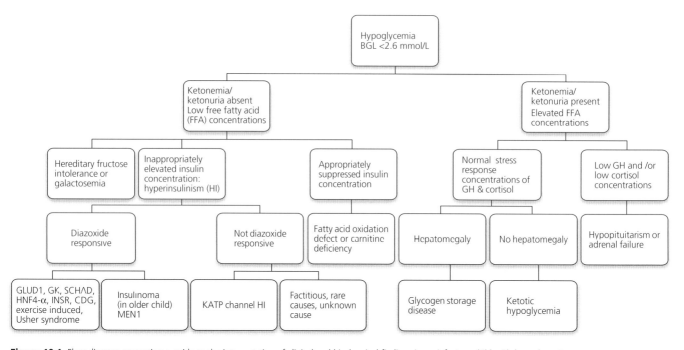

Figure 19.1 Flow diagram presenting a guide to the interpretation of clinical and biochemical findings in an infant or child with hypoglycemia.

Table 19.2 The critical samples that should be taken during hypoglycemia.

Assays required	Assays desirable if sufficient blood available
Glucose	Urea & electrolytes
Insulin	C-peptide
Growth hormone	Ammonia
Cortisol	ACTH
β-Hydroxybutyrate	Lactate
Plasma acylcarnitine profile	Plasma amino acids
Urine ketones	Free fatty acids
Urine metabolic screen incl. organic acids	Transferrin isoforms

ACTH, adenocorticotropic hormone.

(MCAD). Despite the usefulness of these neonatal screening programs, false-negative results may occur, particularly because the first episode of hypoglycemia may occur before the complete results of the screening program are available.

Management

The emergency treatment of hypoglycemia involves rapid clinical assessment and institution of standard resuscitation procedures. Intravenous access should be obtained and, providing the immediate circumstances allow, the critical blood and urine samples should be taken. In some instances of hypoglycemia, there is impairment of brain function leading to apnea, unconsciousness, unprotected airway and generalized convulsions.

If the infant or child is conscious and cooperative, carbohydrate should be offered in an appropriate form such as milk or a glucose drink. The patient should respond with an increase in glucose over the next 5–10 min with decrease in associated symptoms. If the patient has impaired consciousness or is uncooperative, a glucose infusion can be administered with an initial bolus of 0.25 g/kg and an infusion of glucose 3–6 mg/kg/min varying according to weight. The dose of glucose should be adjusted to maintain blood glucose at >3.6 mmol/L (65 mg/dL).

When an intravenous glucose infusion is not possible, glucagon can be given either by nasal spray (1.0 mg for children), subcutaneous injection (0.02–0.15 mg for conscious infants to adolescents and 0.30–1.0 mg for unconscious infants to adolescents) or intramuscular injection (0.50–1.0 mg for unconscious infants to adolescents). In most cases the plasma glucose will respond within 15 min with an increase of 2.0–5.0 mmol/L. Vomiting is often a side effect of a large dose of glucagon which precludes further oral intake of carbohydrate so it is appropriate to titrate the dose of glucagon unless the circumstances demand immediate restoration of normal glucose concentrations. If the hypoglycemia recurs soon after initial attempts at resuscitation, a longer term strategy is required to maintain plasma glucose to prevent damage to the CNS which depends on the circumstances, the age of the child and the severity of the persisting hypoglycemia and, most importantly, the underlying diagnosis.

Newborn infants with persistent hypoglycemia may respond simply to feed supplementation until breast milk is available or to increased frequency of feeds or fortification of feeds. Clear instructions are required as to the glucose concentration at which intervention should be instituted and the frequency that glucose concentrations should be assessed.

At some stage a re-evaluation is required to determine whether the hypoglycemia is transient or persistent and whether the condition is mild, moderate or severe. This evaluation will influence the next steps and repeated attempts should be made to determine the diagnosis and institute specific treatment.

Before discharging the patient from hospital, the family will need an emergency plan as to how long the child should be allowed to sleep, the feed frequency and what changes to this regimen should be made if the child is unwell. The clinician will need to decide on whether to teach the family how to monitor glucose concentrations at home and how they should be interpreted. In some conditions, ongoing feed supplementation is required to maintain glucose concentrations overnight. Corn starch can be used as a "slow release" form of glucose so that the child and the family can sleep through the night. This may not be effective in young infants because of low concentrations of pancreatic amylase and pancreatic enzyme supplements can be used in these circumstances. Specific diets may be needed to care for the children with protein sensitivity.

In some neonates, increased feeds and fortification of feeds is insufficient to maintain plasma glucose concentrations in the normal range. The next step to consider is continuous glucose infusion. In some instances, this may be an obvious decision; in others, this may be decided by the fact that the infant cannot tolerate increased feed volume and osmotic load. The amount of glucose infused should be titrated to maintain plasma glucose concentrations within the normal range. The amount of glucose required to achieve this may help define the diagnosis. Glucose requirements <10 mg/kg/min suggest the diagnosis is lack of substrate or failure of counter-regulatory hormones. A requirement >10 mg/kg/min points to increased glucose utilization driven by insulin. In these circumstances, venous access often becomes an issue because veins, particularly in neonates, cannot tolerate 10–15% glucose infusions and extravasation causes tissue damage. Long or central lines are required to deliver high concentration glucose solutions and, in this circumstance, clinical judgment has to decide how long the condition is likely to last. If it appears transient (likely to resolve within 5 days), the high glucose requirement may be managed by a peripheral long line.

Alternative methods of maintaining plasma glucose over a short-term period of 5 days include the use of a glucagon infusion or hydrocortisone administered orally or intravenously. Glucagon is infused at a starting dose of 1.0 µg/kg/h to normalize glucose concentrations while allowing reintroduction of oral feeding. The dose is titrated to maintain glucose concentrations while other supports are weaned. Hydrocortisone (10–30 mg/m^2/day) can be used to induce gluconeogenesis and insulin resistance. In premature infants, there appears to be an underlying dysfunction of the adrenal cortex with impaired cortisol production so that hydrocortisone may be a more appropriate therapy in this setting. Hydrocortisone may also be the first-line treatment in situations when adrenal failure is likely as when the patient presents with hyperpigmentation.

If the hypoglycemia appears to be lasting more than 5 days, other therapies should be considered. If the diagnosis is likely to be hyperinsulinism, diazoxide 5.0–20 mg/kg/day should be considered; a thiazide diuretic should be added when the diazoxide dose is above 5 mg/kg/day. Oral diazoxide may be preferable to allow early discharge of the infant if plasma glucose concentrations are stable and the patient can tolerate a limited period of fasting, i.e. 6 h. If diazoxide at a dose of 15 mg/kg/day does not easily control plasma glucose concentrations, additional therapy is required and the diagnosis would appear to be CHI. Such a child should be referred to a unit able to manage these extremely rare, vulnerable and difficult patients.

Interpretation of results

The interpretation of results must take into account the clinical circumstances, the sample preparation, preservation and transportation, the sensitivity and limitations of the biochemical assays used, the pattern of results and the response of the patient to therapeutic intervention. The first principle of data interpretation is whether hypoglycemia has been confirmed by reliable laboratory methods.

Low plasma ketone and free fatty acid concentrations

Assuming the plasma glucose concentration is <2.6 mmol/L, the diagnosis can be approached by determining the presence or absence of ketones and the plasma free fatty acid concentrations. If both are undetectable or low, this suggests that they are suppressed by an abnormality in insulin secretion or, more rarely, a defect in fatty acid metabolism. If insulin concentrations are detectable (>1.0–3.0 mU/L; see below for insulin assay interpretation), the diagnosis is likely to be inappropriate insulin release.

High plasma ketone and free fatty acid concentrations

If ketone and free fatty acid concentrations are high and insulin concentrations are low or undetectable, the likely diagnosis is either an abnormality in counter-regulatory hormone release or an abnormality in glucose release from stores. In the presence of hypoglycemia, the counter-regulatory hormones, particularly growth hormone (GH) and cortisol, should be elevated (GH >10 mU/L, cortisol >500 nmol/L, 18 µg/dL). If they are low (GH <10 mU/L and/or cortisol <500 nmol/L), the likely diagnosis is either hypopituitarism (both low) or adrenal failure (cortisol low and confirmed by an significant elevation of ACTH concentrations).

There is occasionally difficulty in distinguishing excess insulin or lack of cortisol, particularly in the neonate in whom cortisol responses to insulin-induced hypoglycemia are sometimes much lower than seen in children or adults. This difficulty usually occurs only in the mild or transient forms of hyperinsulinism because the insulin concentrations are unmistakably high in the severe forms in the presence of profound hypoglycemia. The diagnosis in less severe situations is more likely to be mild transient hyperinsulinism if ketones and free fatty acids are absent.

When concentrations of ketones and free fatty acids are high, insulin suppressed and the counter-regulatory hormone responses high, the diagnosis is likely to be idiopathic ketotic hypoglycemia or, more rarely, an inborn error of metabolism. The former should be considered as the diagnosis of exclusion. If the child presents with recurrent episodes of what appears to be "ketotic hypoglycemia" after a minimal period of starvation, at an older than expected age or associated with significant neurological impairment, the diagnosis of idiopathic ketotic hypoglycemia should be reviewed.

Sensitivity of insulin assays

The biochemical methods used in the analysis of insulin and the lower limit of the detection for insulin are important in the interpretation of results. An insensitive insulin assay may not detect low but inappropriate insulin concentrations in hypoglycemic children, thereby masking a diagnosis of hyperinsulinism; conversely, an ultra-sensitive insulin assay may detect the presence of some residual insulin in patients with ketotic hypoglycemia when the presence of ketones suggests that functional insulin activity is suppressed. In general in the investigation of hypoglycemic children, the assay used should have a sensitivity of at least 1 mU/L (6 pmol/L) and a lower limit of detection of 0.1 U/L (0.6 pmol/L). A profile of results that includes free fatty acids, β-hydroxybutyrate, proinsulin, C-peptide and insulin-like growth factor binding protein 1 (IGFBP-1) may be helpful rather than relying solely on the measurement of insulin, particularly if an insensitive insulin assay is used.

Furthermore, the issue needs to be addressed as to whether insulin secretion is as adequately suppressed as would normally be expected in the presence of hypoglycemia. Some laboratories report that the insulin concentration detected is within the range of "normal fasting insulin concentrations" but this range is based on insulin concentrations seen in normoglycemic subjects after an overnight fast. While such normal ranges are helpful in the context of diagnosing peripheral insulin resistance in hyperglycemic or obese subjects, the comment is inappropriate for the interpretation of results from samples taken from a hypoglycemic patient.

Further investigations

Fasting study

If the hypoglycemic event takes place and is treated before the critical blood samples can be taken, it is usually necessary to try to reproduce a hypoglycemic event in a controlled situation. There must be a 24-h laboratory service to process the samples and provide urgent results. The fast may be dangerous because it could trigger an emergency.

The child should be admitted to hospital and remain until fully recovered from the fast, having tolerated a substantial meal without vomiting and demonstrated normal post-prandial blood glucose concentrations. The duration of the fast should be determined by the age of the child, the normal duration of fasting for the child when at home (e.g. 2 h between frequent feeds or 12 h overnight from an early evening meal). Venous access should be established throughout the fast. The timing of the start of the fast is defined as the commencement of the last meal or feed. The child can drink water but should have no other intake until the final blood samples are taken. Exercise is permitted.

The completion of the fast will be at a point agreed before the start of fasting either with the development of hypoglycemia or at the completion of the planned duration of fasting, whichever is the sooner. The critical blood and urine samples are taken following the confirmation of the low blood glucose concentration by the biochemistry department, unless the child has impaired consciousness in which case intervention with oral or intravenous glucose should proceed as soon as the samples have been taken. The blood samples should be taken with a urine sample, even if no hypoglycemic event has taken place, because these results may give some clues to a diagnosis, even if the child is not hypoglycemic. Interpretation of results of fasting tests is similar to those stated above for the critical blood and urine samples.

Glucagon stimulation

At the completion of the fast or during an episode of hypoglycemia, a glucagon stimulation test can be performed. This is designed to determine the extent of glycogen available for release of glucose at this time. Glucagon 0.03 mg/kg is administered intravenously or intramuscularly and the change in glucose concentrations is monitored from before (0 min) and 10, 20 and 30 min after the injection. A positive response, an increase in glucose concentrations of at least 1 mmol/L (18 mg/dL), suggests there has been a previous failure to increase glucose from glycogen stores because of a failure of release of glucose due to hyperinsulinism.

Glucose tolerance

A standard glucose tolerance test (GTT) may help because it will clarify the lactate and insulin response to a glucose load. This is key in the investigation of possible glycogen synthase deficiency [glycogen storage disease type 0 (GSD0)]. Success of the GTT requires the administration of the glucose in a timely (within 5 min) and well-tolerated fashion. A glucose polymer preparation is often better tolerated than glucose and usually causes an appropriate rise in plasma glucose concentrations although this depends on the production of amylase to breakdown the polymer into glucose. The dose of glucose has been standardized to 1.75 g/kg to a maximum of 75 g. In the setting of hypoglycemia, the GTT is most useful in examining the lactate response to a glucose load. In subjects with GSD0, there is an exaggerated rise in lactate because of the diversion of glucose away from glycogen storage to the glycolytic pathway and release of lactate from the liver because of saturation of the Krebs cycle.

GTTs have been used previously to investigate rebound hypoglycemia. Interpretation of results was made simpler when the adult dose of glucose administered was reduced from 100 g glucose to the current 75 g dose because the incidence of rebound hypoglycemia has been significantly reduced. Rebound hypoglycemia is still seen in certain circumstances such as after gastric bypass surgery in the dumping syndrome. This is caused in part by the failure to suppress insulin secretion quickly enough after the clearance of glucose from the circulation and perhaps because of decreasing IGFBP-1 concentration increasing "free" IGF-I concentrations (and hence increased insulin-like activity) after glucose.

Protein load

A standard protein load after a period of fasting may induce hyperinsulinemic hypoglycemia in subjects affected by glutamate dehydrogenase deficiency or protein sensitivity. Fourtner *et al.* [4] suggest a standard protocol of 1.0–1.5 g/kg protein given as an amino acid hydrolysate drink. It is important to avoid giving carbohydrate with the protein load because this can confound interpretation of the results. Plasma glucose, ammonia and insulin concentrations are measured at −15, 0, 15, 30, 45, 60, 90, 120, 150 and 180 min or until the blood glucose falls to <2.6 mmol/L (45 mg/dL). When or if the patient is symptomatic, he/she should be fed and observed to ensure that the post-prandial plasma glucose concentration returns to pretest concentrations before the patient is discharged. The normal response is a minimal change in glucose concentrations. An abnormal response is recognized as a fall in glucose because of a rise in insulin concentrations induced by the protein or, more particularly, by leucine or glutamate. Glutamate dehydrogenase deficiency induces similar changes in glucose and insulin to other cases of protein sensitivity but is also accompanied by a rise in plasma ammonia concentrations.

Genetic investigations

The genetic causes of some types of hypoglycemia have now been sufficiently characterized to consider routine genetic analysis as part of the diagnostic work-up for glucokinase, glutamate dehydrogenase, ABCC8 (SUR), KCNJ11 (KIR) and MODY1 defects in insulin secretion, 21-hydroxylase in CAH, DAX-1 in congenital adrenal hypoplasia, the gene for AAA syndrome and the gene for aldolase B deficiency in adrenal insufficiency. Analysis of the two genes involved in severe congenital hyperinsulinism, ABCC8 and KCNJ11, may be extended further by analysis of gene copy number. The value of a certain diagnosis from the genetic studies needs to be weighed against the cost and chances of a positive result.

Consequences of hypoglycemia

Immediate

The effects of hypoglycemia are initially to trigger the glucose homeostatic mechanisms. Thus, the early events encountered during an episode of hypoglycemia are those associated with increased adrenergic activity (Table 19.1). In some individuals who have experienced repeated episodes of hypoglycemia, the adrenergic response is blunted and these patients often do not encounter the classic symptoms of hypoglycemia. This is dangerous because one of the normal protective mechanisms has been lost. Neonates also appear to have impaired counter-regulatory responses and do not show signs of increased adrenergic activity. It is not clear whether this is a normal neonatal response, because of immaturity or accommodation to previous hypoglycemic events.

The brain requires a constant supply of high-energy nutrients either as glucose or ketones. If neither is available, the brain ceases to function and permanent damage ensues over a variable time course, the severity depending on the concentration of glucose, the rapidity of the fall in glucose and the energy demands of the particular part of the brain.

The features of immediate or short-term neurological impairment are often seen in subjects with type 1 diabetes. These range from impaired consciousness to loss of consciousness and generalized convulsions. Signs of focal neurological impairment, such as blurred vision, amblyopia, hemiparesis, paralysis and amnesia sometimes occur. Studies using positron emission tomography (PET) scanning and magnetic resonance spectroscopy (MRS) have demonstrated changes in the CNS during these episodes with high energy-requiring areas showing changes in metabolism.

After recovery of blood glucose into the normal range, neurological impairment recovers over a time period of minutes to hours, often associated with headache and amnesia. If episodes are frequent, periods of amnesia may be such that their memory loss renders patients unemployable. In adults, it appears that, despite the severity of these episodes, the subjects usually recover completely, although those with amnesia associated with hypounawareness may recover only following islet cell transplantation. Thus, the neurological impairment seen in an adult appears not to be permanent. However, hypoglycemia can and does lead to death either from the consequences of an unprotected airway during a hypoglycemic event leading to aspiration and asphyxia or the complication "dead in bed" syndrome reported in young adults with type 1 diabetes.

Long-term outcome

Children under the age of 5 years appear to be much more sensitive to the effects of hypoglycemia than adults. The reasons are not clear but may relate to the higher energy requirements and immaturity of the homeostatic mechanisms in the brain. In children with type 1 diabetes undergoing repeated episodes of hypoglycemia, there are conflicting reports whether reduced IQ, impaired behavior and developmental delay occur more frequently in those subjects. The younger the infant affected and the more profound the hypoglycemia, the more significant are the effects so that the rates of severe neurological impairment remain as high as 20–50% of some form of permanent neurological impairment in patients with CHI. The link between mild transient hypoglycemia in the neonatal period and later permanent neurological sequelae has been harder to establish mainly because of the heterogeneous nature of the population studied and the confounding events that occur in such infants. The effects of hypoglycemia obviously need to be separated from the effects of the underlying condition, such as seen in glycosylation defects.

Glucose is the major energy substrate for normal brain function [5]. The entry of glucose into the brain and brain glucose metabolism are not insulin-sensitive [6]. The maturation and density of the glucose transporter GLUT-1 (located at the blood–brain barrier) and GLUT-3 (at the neuronal membrane) parallel the development of cerebral glucose utilization. Certain parts of the brain (e.g. the cortex) seem to be more susceptible to hypoglycemic damage than others (e.g. the cerebellum). There are regional differences in cerebral metabolic capacity [7]. PET has shown minute-to-minute regional changes in cerebral glucose consumption and blood flow during a variety of sensory and motor activities in humans. In newborn dogs, the brain can alter regional blood flow to ensure that brainstem structures continue to receive adequate glucose compared with other regions [8]. Similar increases in cerebral blood flow have been documented in human preterm infants during hypoglycemia [9].

During moderate acute hypoglycemia in adults, there are no changes in cerebral functional activity; cerebral glucose utilization decreases and blood flow increases only when hypoglycemia is severe (<2 mmol/L) [10]. During chronic hypoglycemia, the brain adapts to the low circulating concentrations of glucose by increasing the number of glucose transporter sites and decreasing cerebral glucose utilization. Neuronal damage brought about by severe and prolonged hypoglycemia occurs mainly in the cerebral cortex, hippocampus and caudate putamen. Neurochemical changes include an arrest of protein synthesis, a shift of brain redox equilibria toward oxidation, loss of ion homeostasis and cellular calcium influx [11,12].

Ketones produced in the liver from the oxidation of fatty acids are exported to peripheral tissues as an alternative energy source during fasting. Ketones are particularly important for the brain, which has no other substantial non-glucose-derived energy source. Ketones can replace glucose as the predominant fuel for nervous tissue, thereby reducing the obligatory glucose requirement of the brain [13]. In healthy adults infused with β-hydroxybutyrate during insulin-induced hypoglycemia, the threshold for the counter-regulatory hormonal response to hypoglycemia is lowered [14]. The uptake of ketones by the brain is proportional to the circulating concentration and uptake is higher in neonates than in adults. Adults show a gradual increase in plasma concentrations of free fatty acids, glycerol and ketones during starvation; in contrast to this, children demonstrate a more rapid rise suggesting that they convert to fat-based fuel more rapidly [15,16]. Oral supplementation of DL sodium β-hydroxybutyrate may be a means of reducing the high rates of brain damage in susceptible children by providing an alternative energy supply to brain tissue [17,18].

Glucose homeostasis in the fed and fasted infant and child

In utero
The growing fetus is supplied with glucose at a steady rate to allow smooth growth and development. Excess glucose stimulates growth by an increase in insulin (the main fetal anabolic hormone) secretion from the fetus produced to maintain euglycemia. The fetus relying on maternal supplies is never without glucose and does not express the key enzymes in the gluconeogenic pathway. If nutrient supply is limited, growth is restricted and the baby is born small for gestational age (SGA). Babies born either large or small for gestational age are at risk of hypoglycemia, the former because of continued excess insulin secretion from islet hyperplasia and the latter because of lack of available glycogen for breakdown during periods between feeds, although some SGA infants are also affected by excess insulin secretion.

At birth
With the cutting of the umbilical cord, the baby is separated from the continuous supply of nutrients and a crisis occurs with a fall of plasma glucose during the first 4 h of life. This stimulates a counter-regulatory response with increases in plasma glucagon, catecholamines, GH and cortisol within minutes to hours of birth. These hormones induce glycogenolysis, lipolysis and proteolysis and the induction of the gluconeogenic enzyme pathway and, as the milk supply is often delayed, the baby is dependent on these homeostatic mechanisms for some time. The transition to a fed–fasted cycle is accomplished with little consequence in the normal term infant but the transition is often compromised in the premature or SGA infant.

Adaptation to fasting
Babies adapt from continuous nutrient supply *in utero* to fed–fasted cycle with induction of the glycogenolytic and gluconeogenic pathways and changes in the regulation of insulin secretion. It is not clear how the latter occurs but the role of SUR/KIR potassium channel in newborns must change with the introduction of the fed–fasted cycle. The primary role of glucose is as a major energy supply molecule. The maintenance of a normal blood glucose concentration is therefore crucial to energy supply to the body.

Plasma glucose concentration is tightly controlled by a balance between glucose production and utilization. The homeostatic mechanisms involve a complex interaction between plasma glucose, insulin and the counter-regulatory hormones. Insulin decreases glucose production and increases glucose utilization. Glucagon stimulates the controlled release of glucose from liver glycogen. Cortisol and GH have permissive roles in setting the sensitivity of the peripheral tissues to glucagon and insulin.

Circulating glucose is available from food ingestion and digestion of carbohydrate, from the breakdown of glycogen (glycogenolysis) and from *de novo* manufacture from amino acid or fat (gluconeogenesis) from the liver and, to a small extent, the kidneys, the only two organs with glucose-6-phosphatase able to release glucose into the circulation.

Glucose supply

After the ingestion and digestion of carbohydrate, glucose is taken up from the intestine into the splanchnic circulation. In the absorptive phase, maintenance of normal glucose homeostasis is controlled by insulin secretion from the β cells stimulated in response to hyperglycemia and the stimuli from neurogenic and enteroinsular axes, glucose removal from the circulation by uptake to the tissues is stimulated by the combination of hyperglycemia and hyperinsulinemia and hepatic glucose production inhibited primarily by insulin [19]. Following the ingestion of a meal, plasma glucose concentration increases within 15 min, peaks at around 30–60 min and declines until absorption is complete, usually about 4–5 h later, with plasma insulin concentrations following a similar time course [20]. In the fasting or post-absorptive state, the fasting plasma glucose concentration is maintained within a narrow range, 3.6–5.8 mmol/L (65–105 mg/dL). During the post-absorptive phase, breakdown of stored glycogen to glucose (glycogenolysis) and de novo glucose production (gluconeogenesis) are required to maintain stable blood glucose concentrations.

Glycogenolysis occurs as a result of the actions of several enzymes: glycogen phosphorylase initiates glycogen breakdown by cleaving the 1,4 straight chain linkages in glycogen releasing glucose-1-phosphate, which is converted to glucose-6-phosphate by the enzyme phosphoglucomutase. The alpha 1,6 linkages at the branch points of the glycogen structure are broken by the debrancher enzyme. The metabolism of glycogen is predominantly controlled by the activities of glycogen synthase and phosphorylase and insulin and glucagon are the major hormones controlling these enzymes.

Gluconeogenesis involves the synthesis of glucose from lactate and alanine via the Cori cycle and also from glutamine, glycerol and pyruvate. The first step in gluconeogenesis involves the conversion of pyruvate to oxaloacetate to phosphoenolpyruvate by pyruvate carboxylase and phosphoenolpyruvate carboxykinase. Pyruvate carboxylase is regulated by the mitochondrial acetyl CoA and ADP concentrations and is induced by alterations in plasma insulin, glucagon and cortisol concentrations during the postnatal starvation soon after birth. The next reaction in gluconeogenesis is catalyzed by fructose-1,6-bisphosphatase, which converts fructose-1,6-biphosphate to fructose-6-phosphate, the rate-limiting step for the process of gluconeogenesis [21]. Both glycogenolysis and gluconeogenesis result in the production of glucose-6-phosphate which is hydrolyzed by glucose-6-phosphatase to glucose which is able to enter the extracellular space and the circulation.

In adults, the normal metabolic adaptation to fasting results from hormonal changes, principally decreased secretion of insulin and increased production of counter-regulatory hormones (Table 19.3; Fig. 19.2). This process is similar in children but there is a

Table 19.3 Normal sequence of metabolic changes in fasting.

Metabolic process	Metabolic effect
Glycogenolysis	Acute provision of glucose from hepatic glycogen stores. In infants, this may provide only 4 h of glucose
Gluconeogenesis	Muscle breakdown to provide substrates (e.g. alanine) Ongoing glucose supply for glucose dependent tissues during prolonged fasting
Lipolysis Fatty acid oxidation Ketogenesis	Ketones are used as an alternative fuel allowing a reduction in glucose utilization particularly by the brain. Lipolysis also provides glycerol for gluconeogenesis. In infants, ketones usually appear after 12–18 h of fasting

more rapid decline in glucose concentration and a more rapid increase in ketone concentrations. As the period of fast lengthens, hepatic glucose output is reduced. Glucagon secretion with reduced insulin allows stored fats to be converted to glycerol and fatty acids and proteins to be converted to amino acids for gluconeogenesis. The liberated free fatty acids are bound to albumin and transported to the liver where they undergo beta oxidation in the mitochondria to yield ketones. Muscle and other tissues become progressively more dependent on free fatty acids and ketone bodies for their continued energy requirements as the period of the fast is prolonged.

Infants from 1 week to 1 year of age can usually tolerate 15–18 h of fasting and this increases to 24 h between 1 and 5 years. Children develop hypoglycemia after 36 h, whereas adults can survive without food for a number of weeks. This is because of the glucose-sparing effect of ketones and free fatty acids, which allow the limited capacity of gluconeogenesis to provide glucose for glucose-dependent tissues (brain, red blood cells and renal tubules) and preserve muscle mass, which is the source of gluconeogenic substrate (amino acids) (Table 19.3).

Glucose utilization

The basal rate of glucose uptake is precisely equaled by an equivalent rate of glucose output by the liver and kidney. The tissues responsible for the removal of glucose from the circulation include the liver, small intestine, brain, muscle and adipose tissue. The magnitude of glucose uptake by the insulin-dependent tissues is determined largely by the plasma insulin concentration. Glucose uptake by the insulin-independent tissues, such as the brain and splanchnic organs, is determined by the plasma glucose concentration, the tissue requirement for glucose and availability of alternative substrates. This accounts for 80% of total body glucose utilization under fasting conditions, mainly by the brain (50% of the total) [22]. Muscle, an insulin-dependent tissue, is

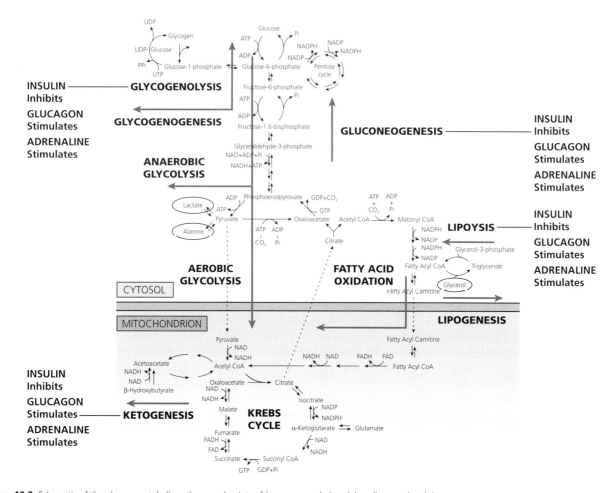

Figure 19.2 Schematic of the glucose metabolic pathway and points of hormone regulation. Adrenaline = epinephrine.

responsible for most of the remaining glucose utilization in the fasting state. As fasting progresses, tissue glucose utilization decreases while utilization of free fatty acids and ketone bodies increases.

Children have higher glucose production rates to meet increased metabolic demands than adults. Brain size is the principal determinant of factors that regulate hepatic glucose output throughout life [23]. Glucose requirements change as the child grows because the relative weight of brain mass to body mass changes and fasting newborn and young children demonstrate a high glucose utilization rate per kilogram body weight relative to adults [24,25]. In younger children, the high glucose requirements of the brain and the relative weight of the brain to the body mean that the child will more rapidly consume the available glucose and develop hypoglycemia (Table 19.4).

The transport of glucose into tissues is by facilitated diffusion and depends on the specific glucose transporters, GLUT-1–5. GLUT-1 (insulin independent) is found in all cells and is responsible for glucose transport across the blood–brain barrier. In human β cells, GLUT-1 is the major glucose transporter but GLUT-2 (insulin independent) is also present, being important

Table 19.4 Typical glucose utilization rates brain [mg/kg (% of total)] and body [mg/kg (% of total)] at various ages together with total glucose utilization rates expressed as mg/kg/min.

	Glucose utilization rates		
	Brain (mg/min)	Body (mg/min)	Total (mg/kg/min)
Neonate (3 kg)	16 (80%)	4 (20%)	6.3
Infant (10 kg)	36 (60%)	24 (40%)	6
Child (30 kg)	52 (40%)	78 (60%)	4.3
Adult (70 kg)	48 (30%)	112 (70%)	2.2

because of its low affinity for glucose and therefore not easily saturated, even at high plasma glucose concentrations, so that the β cells can "sense" major increases in plasma glucose. GLUT-3 (insulin independent) is distributed in the central nervous system and has the highest affinity for glucose. GLUT-4 (insulin dependent) is the glucose transporter in muscle and adipose tissue. GLUT-5 is primarily expressed in the jejunal brush border and is mainly a fructose transporter.

The interaction of insulin and its cell surface receptor initiates a variety of biochemical functions as well as endocytosis of insulin and its degradation or transcellular transport. Insulin regulates the steady-state concentration of the insulin-dependent transporters by promoting synthesis and mobilization of these transporters to the cell membrane when the plasma glucose concentration increases. Uptake of glucose by cells leads to storage, oxidization or conversion to lactate. The fate of intracellular glucose is determined by the relative concentrations of insulin and the counter-regulatory hormones and the general metabolic state. The breakdown of glucose by oxidation generates adenosine triphosphate (ATP) by glycolysis (conversion of glucose to pyruvate) and oxidative phosphorylation (Krebs cycle) by mitochondria (conversion of pyruvate to carbon dioxide and water) [22].

The pancreas

The pancreas is a combined exocrine and endocrine gland that is highly specialized in its ability to synthesize and secrete a wide variety of specific proteins. It weighs 70–140 g in adults and extends from the duodenum to the hilum of the spleen. In the fetus, exocrine cells and islets are derived from a common pool of precursor endodermal cells from the dorsal and ventral portions of the embryonic midgut. The dorsal and ventral primordia fuse during development in the seventh week of gestation, with the ventral area forming the inferior and posterior parts of the head of the pancreas and the dorsal area forming the remainder of the head, body and tail of the pancreas [26]. The boundary between the head and body is marked by the axis of the aorta and superior mesenteric vessels. The pancreatic duct system drains the digestive enzymes produced by the acinar cells via ductules that join to form intralobular ducts and join interlobular ducts, finally draining into the main pancreatic duct into the duodenum.

The exocrine pancreas is composed of acinar and ductal cells. More than 80% of the gland consists of acinar cells and the duct system constitutes 2–4% of cells. The volume of the endocrine tissue, the islets of Langerhans, varies with age. Islets comprise 20% of the pancreatic tissue in newborns, 7.5% in children (1.5–11 years) and 1% in adults. There are four islet cell types: β, (insulin); α, (glucagon); δ (somatostatin); and PP (pancreatic polypeptide) [27]. There is a consistent pattern of organization within islets, with the δ, α or PP cells occurring as a discontinuous mantle 1–3 cells thick, around a central core of β cells [27]. There are distinct regional differences in the distribution of the islet hormone cells, with a PP-rich glucagon-poor region in the posterior part of the head of the pancreas. The islets of the developing pancreas are generated from the pancreatic ductal epithelium by neogenesis and mature by a process that involves a balance of proliferation and apoptosis [28]. After partial removal of the pancreas, islands of islet tissue regenerate from stem cells that also appear to reside in the ductules.

Islet development

Endocrine cells can be detected in 9–10 week human embryos in the order of insulin, somatostatin, glucagon and PP cells [29]. Around 13 weeks' gestation, formation of the islets of Langerhans commences with the appearance of duct-associated non-vascularized buds that separate to form the mantle type of vascularized islets characterized by a central mass of insulin-producing cells surrounded by several layers of non-β-cells. Between 21 and 26 weeks' gestation, non-β-cells appear in peripheral and central parts of the islets and the adult type of islets are formed. Islet formation continues during intra-uterine life and, by the neonatal period, both the fetal and adult types of islets are observed [26,30,31]. The adult islet consists of β cells (48–59% of the islet cell population), α cells (33–46%) and δ cells (8–12%) [32]. In the neonatal period and infancy, there is a markedly higher relative incidence (about 20 times) of δ cells (about 30%) in the pancreatic islets (in the non-PP-rich parts) than in those of the adult.

A large number of factors regulate islet development including differentiation factors [sonic hedgehog signaling protein, activin, follistatin, transforming growth factor a (TGF-α)], transcriptional factors (PDX-1, Islet-1, Pax4, Pax6, Nkx2.2 and Nkx6.1, BETA2/NeuroD1, hepatocyte nuclear factors), growth factors (epidermal growth factors, hepatocyte growth factor, IGF-I, IGF-II, regulatory gene protein, INGAP, PDGF, FGF, VEGF, NGF), hormones (insulin, GH, parathyroid hormone related protein, thyrotropin releasing hormone, gastrin) and cell adhesion molecules (N-CAM and cadherins) [33]. This process has been studied most carefully in the mouse [34].

Regulation of insulin production and secretion

Insulin is the major peptide hormone synthesized by β cells of the pancreatic islets. A single copy of the insulin gene is located on the short arm of chromosome 11 in band p15. Insulin contains two separate polypeptide chains, the A chain containing 21 amino acid residues and the B chain containing 30 residues, which are linked to each other by a pair of disulfide bonds. Insulin is first synthesized as preproinsulin, which is processed into proinsulin in the rough endoplasmic reticulum and transported via a regulated secretory pathway to storage granules, where it is cleaved to yield insulin and a 31-residue fragment called the C-peptide. A small amount of proinsulin (0.5–2%) escapes from this route and is released through a constitutive unregulated pathway.

Insulin and C-peptide are stored in the secretory granules, along with small amounts of residual proinsulin and partially cleaved intermediate forms. The biological function of the C-peptide is uncertain but it is useful as a peripheral marker of insulin secretion because it is secreted in equimolar concentration with insulin and does not undergo the significant hepatic extraction that insulin does [35–37].

Glucose rapidly stimulates insulin biosynthesis through stimulation of insulin messenger RNA (mRNA) translation. The rate of transcription of insulin mRNA is also upregulated by cyclic adenosine monophosphate (cAMP), partly through phosphorylation of PDX-1, the homeodomain protein that binds to regulatory elements of the insulin gene promotor. Insulin mRNA has a half-life of 30 h under normal conditions but hypoglycemia leads to rapid declines in insulin mRNA and hyperglycemia increases its half-life dramatically. Glucose also regulates the turnover of insulin stores within β cells.

Insulin and/or proinsulin release occurs predominantly through calcium-dependent exocytosis of preformed storage granules. There is also a small amount of "unregulated" or constitutive release of insulin (1–2% of the total). Insulin secretagogues may be divided into initiators and potentiators [38]. Initiators can stimulate insulin release on their own and include nutrients metabolized by the β cell. Glucose is the most important physiological substance regulating insulin release. Amino acids stimulate insulin release in the absence of glucose, with the essential amino acids, leucine, arginine and lysine, being the most potent secretagogues. The effects of the amino acids, while independent of glucose, are potentiated by glucose. The amino acid metabolites, phenylpyruvate, α-ketoisocaproate, α-keto-β-methylvalerate and α-ketocaproate are also potent stimulators of insulin release, most potent in the absence of glucose. Various lipids and their metabolites appear to have minor effects on insulin release.

Potentiators of insulin secretion require the presence of a sub-stimulatory concentration of an initiator. The "incretin effect" refers to the enhanced insulin response to oral glucose versus intravenous glucose. Following exposure to glucose post-prandially, intestinal endocrine cells release a number of gastrointestinal hormones into the bloodstream, including glucose-dependent insulinotropic peptide (GIP), cholecystokinin (CKK) and glucagon-like peptide (GLP-1). These act through second messengers in the β cells to increase their sensitivity to glucose and their effects are evident only in the presence of hyperglycemia. Vasoactive intestinal peptide (VIP), secretin and gastrin may also modify the post-prandial insulin response in a similar manner. Inhibitors of insulin release include somatostatin and epinephrine [38].

Glucose causes a dose-dependent increase in insulin and C-peptide concentrations after oral and intravenous glucose loads. The relationship of glucose concentration to the rate of insulin release is sigmoidal, with the steep portion of the dose–response curve corresponding to the range of glucose concentrations normally seen post-prandially. Insulin release is biphasic with an early rapid insulin peak (first phase response) followed by a more gradual rise.

The first phase insulin response may reflect a compartment of readily releasable insulin within the β cell or may represent the transient rise and fall of a metabolic signal for insulin secretion. The second phase response is related directly to the elevation in glucose concentration (Fig. 19.2). Glucose enters the β cell via GLUT-1 and GLUT-2. It is metabolized by glucokinase and and increases the intracellular concentration of ATP, changing the ATP:ADP ratio, which triggers closure of the KATP channel by the glycolytic and oxidative phosphorylation pathways. The KATP channel consists of an octameric complex constituted by four SUR1 proteins which surround four Kir6.2 proteins, through which the potassium ions are conducted across the cell membrane (Figs 19.3 & 19.4). The cessation of this efflux by closure of the KATP channel results in depolarization of the β-cell membrane, which leads to the influx of calcium through voltage-gated channels triggering insulin exocytosis [39,40]. The exocytosis of insulin involves an intricate pathway of the storage granule membrane fusing with the cell membrane and extracellular release of the contents. A number of proteins are involved in this process, some of which are the SNARE proteins [41], which also interact with the SUR protein of the KATP channel. Defects in any part of this pathway may lead to disorders of insulin secretion predisposing to either hyperinsulinism or diabetes.

Drugs interact with the insulin secretory pathway: sulfonylureas interact with the KATP channel to enhance insulin release; diazoxide inhibits insulin release by a similar process. Quinine may also increase insulin release by an unknown process.

Basal release of insulin accounts for approximately 50% of insulin secreted by the pancreas in a 24-h period. The remainder is secreted in response to meals, with the maximum response after breakfast and diminished responses to afternoon and evening meals. Diurnal differences are also seen in responses to oral and intravenous GTTs.

Insulin is released in a pulsatile manner with rapid oscillations, occurring every 8–15 min, superimposed on slower oscillations occurring at a periodicity of 80–150 min. The oscillations are thought to reflect the activity of an intrinsic pancreatic pacemaker likely to be modulated by neural factors. The rapid oscillations are of small amplitude in the systemic circulation but of greater amplitude in the portal circulation because of extraction of insulin by the liver. The slower oscillations are of much larger amplitude in the peripheral circulation, being present under basal conditions and amplified post-prandially. The slower oscillations appear to be synchronous with pulses of similar period in glucose and may be the product of the insulin–glucose feedback mechanism.

Specific causes of hypoglycemia

In neonatal practice, hypoglycemia is common but its duration is usually short and can be classified as transient when lasting up to 5 days (maximum 10 days). If hypoglycemia persists longer than 10 days, the most common cause is hyperinsulinism. The various diagnoses made in those in whom the hypoglycemia lasts >4 h, which is approximately 5 in 1000 deliveries, are shown in Table 19.5. The most common causes in childhood are due to excess insulin in a type 1 diabetic, ketotic hypoglycemia and Addison disease followed by many rare conditions.

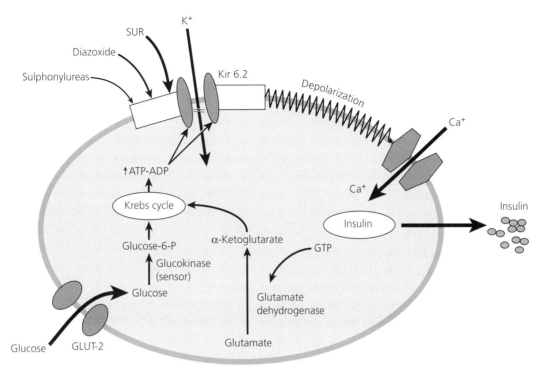

Figure 19.3 The major pathways controlling glucose regulated insulin secretion. Glucose entry is mediated by the transporter GLUT-2, resulting in an increase in ATP:ADP ratio. This causes the K_{ATP} to close, depolarizing the plasma membrane and opening the Ca^+ channel. Increased Ca^+ stimulates insulin secretion [114].

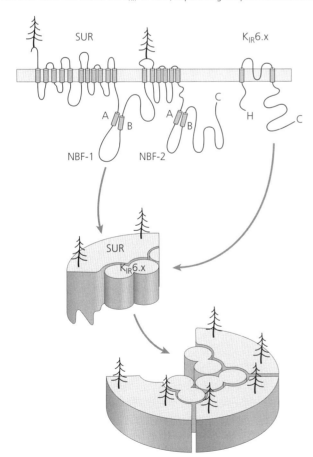

Figure 19.4 A schematic representation of the topology and structure of K_{ATP}. N and C represent the N- and C-termini. Trees represent known glycosylation sites. This illustration does not represent the actual shape or conformation of K_{ATP} [115].

Table 19.5 Diagnoses associated with neonatal hypoglycemia in a tertiary level maternity unit.

Diagnosis	Number identified with hypoglycemia lasting more than 4 h over 5-year audit period	Cases (%)
Total	122	100
Infant of diabetic mother	32	26
Hypopituitarism	3	2.5
BWS	2	1.5
CHI	1	0.8
<30 weeks' gestation	14	11
SGA	21	17
LGA (no GDM on testing)	5	4
Unknown cause	44	36

BWS, Beckwith–Wiedemann syndrome; CHI, congenital hyperinsulinism of infancy; GDM, gestational diabetes mellitus; LGA, large for gestational age; SGA, small for gestational age.

Hyperinsulinism

Hyperinsulinism of infancy (HI), which covers a spectrum of conditions, is the most common cause of recurrent and severe hypoglycemia [42]. It is characterized by excessive and inappropriate secretion of insulin in relation to the prevailing blood glucose concentration and can be transient or persistent.

Transient hyperinsulinemic hypoglycemia

The transient form is associated with maternal diabetes mellitus, intra-uterine growth retardation, perinatal asphyxia, erythroblastosis fetalis, Beckwith–Wiedemann syndrome, administration of some drugs (e.g. sulfonylureas) to the mother and after intravenous maternal glucose infusions during labor. There appears to be an association between high lactate concentrations and severe transient neonatal hyperinsulinism in non-asphyxiated infants [43]. Iatrogenic hyperinsulinism may occur because of a malpositioned umbilical artery catheter [44], but in most cases the cause is unknown [45]. Despite this, a large number of infants require intensive monitoring during this period of potential hypoglycemia and a number require diazoxide therapy to allow discharge from hospital with the therapy weaned within the first few months of life. Some of these infants may have abnormalities in MODY1.

Maternal diabetes

Transient HI is seen most commonly in the infant born to a mother with poorly controlled diabetes. Excess glucose crosses the placenta by facilitated diffusion, which stimulates increased secretion of insulin *in utero*. The infant of a diabetic mother (IDM) is often macrosomic, which is attributed to the anabolic effects fetal hyperinsulinemia [46]. The organomegaly is selective in the liver and heart and length is increased in proportion to weight but brain size is not increased relative to gestational age so the head may appear disproportionately small. Congenital anomalies in IDM, which include anencephaly, meningomyelocele, holoprosencephaly, sacral agenesis and the small left colon syndrome, occur two to four times more frequently than in the general population. The cause of diabetic embryopathy is not understood. There are a number of structural abnormalities of the heart but hypertrophic cardiomyopathy is transient.

The continued increased secretory capacity of the islets resulting from hyperplasia and hypertrophy developed *in utero* leads to transient asymptomatic hypoglycemia in the first 1–4 h of life but some infants have more prolonged and severe hypoglycemia. All regain normal blood glucose control within the 10 days of birth.

Plasma glucose concentrations should be monitored 2–4 hourly before feeds for 6–12 h after birth and more frequently if low concentrations are detected. Sick infants unable to tolerate enteral feeding or those who remain hypoglycemic despite full enteral feeds should receive an intravenous infusion of glucose at a rate of 4–6 mg/kg/min which should be withdrawn slowly to prevent reactive hypoglycemia for which a single injection of glucagon (0.03–0.1 mg/kg) may be appropriate.

Beckwith–Wiedemann syndrome

Beckwith–Wiedemann syndrome (BWS) is a congenital clinically and genetically heterogeneous overgrowth syndrome. Phenotypically, it is associated with pre- and postnatal overgrowth organomegaly, hemihypertrophy, omphalocele, ear lobe anomalies and renal tract abnormalities with increased risk of embryonal tumours (liver and kidney). Genetically, BWS is a multigenic disorder caused by dysregulation of imprinted growth regulatory genes within the 11p15 region [47]. At this location, genetic imprinting with loss of maternally expressed tumor and/or growth suppressor genes (p57KIP2 and H19) or duplications and uniparental disomy of paternally expressed growth promoter genes (IGFII) have been implicated in the pathogenesis of BWS. About 20% of patients with BWS have paternal uniparental disomy for 11p15 [48].

The incidence of hyperinsulinemic hypoglycemia in children with BWS is about 50% [49]. It can be transient or prolonged and is asymptomatic in the majority of infants, resolving within 3 days of life. About 5% of infants with BWS have hyperinsulinemic hypoglycemia beyond the neonatal period requiring either continuous feeding or a partial pancreatectomy. Milder forms respond to diazoxide and somatostatin analogs [50].

Congenital hyperinsulinism of infancy

Congenital hyperinsulinism of infancy (CHI) is by far the most difficult cause to manage. It is associated with a high (14–44%) incidence of neurological handicap [51], which has not changed over the last 20 years. A number of genetic causes for CHI have been identified (Table 19.6), although up to 50% of patients remain undiagnosed.

ABCC8 and KCNJ11 mutations

CHI associated with ABCC8 or KCNJ11 genes is the most severe form of HI. It has been assigned a variety of terms, including idiopathic hypoglycemia of infancy, neonatal insulinoma, microadenomatosis, focal hyperplasia, nesidioblastosis and persistent hyperinsulinemic hypoglycemia of infancy (PHHI) [45]. Leucine-sensitive hypoglycemia is caused by mutations in the GLUD1 gene. Initially described as "idiopathic hypoglycemia of infancy" [52], CHI was later called "nesidioblastosis," until it was shown that budding of islet cells from pancreatic ducts is a normal developmental phase of the pancreas in early infancy [53].

Mutations in ABCC8 or KCNJ11 cause defects in the inwardly rectifying potassium channel (KATP channel) situated in the β-cell membrane. Reduced or absent function of the channel results in unregulated insulin release, even in the presence of low glucose concentration. Class I mutations result in failure of protein trafficking to the membrane, complete loss of channel function and severe disease. Class II mutations result in generation of nonfunctional or partially functional channels which reach the plasma membrane and may retain some residual function resulting in

Table 19.6 Genes associated with congenital hyperinsulinism of infancy. OMIM numbers refer to Online Mendelian Inheritance in Man [113].

Causes of congenital hyperinsulinism	Basis of disease	Disease characteristics	Age group	Mode of inheritance
Mutation in ABCC8 encoding for SUR1 (OMIM 256450, HHF1) chr 11p15.1	DIFFUSE defect in β cell membrane KATP channel throughout the pancreas FOCAL Paternal inherited defect with maternal gene silenced leading focal area of islet clonal expansion	Severe hypoglycemia, variable, usually poor response to diazoxide	Neonatal–infant	Usually autosomal recessive, homozogous or compound heterozygous; rarely *de novo* mutation or autosomal dominant Sporadic
Loss-of-function mutation in KCNJ11 encoding for Kir6.2 (OMIM 601820, HHF2), chr 11p15.1	Defect in β cell membrane KATP channel	Severe hypoglycemia, variable, usually poor response to diazoxide	Neonatal–infant	Usually autosomal recessive, homozygous or compound heterozygous
Gain-of-function mutation in glucokinase (GK) gene encoding for the enzyme glucokinase (OMIM 602485, HHF3), chr 7p15–p13	Defect in rate-limiting step of β cell glucose metabolism	Diazoxide responsive, variable severity	Variable age of onset from neonatal onwards	Autosomal dominant
Loss-of-function mutation in the HADHSC gene encoding short-chain 3-hydroxylacyl-CoA dehydrogenase (SCHAD) (OMIM 609975, HHF4), chr 4q22–q26	Defect in mitochondrial fatty acid oxidation	Diazoxide responsive	Neonatal–infant	Autosomal recessive
Mutation in INS encoding for the insulin receptor (OMIM 609968, HHF5) chr 19p13.2			Reported from 3 years of age onwards	Autosomal dominant
Gain-of-function mutation in glutamate dehydrogenase (GLUD1) gene (hyperinsulinemic hyperammonemic hyperinsulinism, HI/HA) (OMIM 606762, HHF6) chr10q23.3	Loss of inhibition of glutamate dehydogenase by GTP (and ATP) and uninhibited protein (leucine) stimulated insulin release	Diazoxide responsive	Infant	Autosomal dominant or *de novo*
Congenital disorders of glycosylation (CDG) (genetically heterogeneous)	A range of disorders of glycosylation, basis of hypoglycemia not known	Diazoxide responsive	Infant–toddler	Autosomal recessive
Mutation in HNF4-α gene (OMIM 600281) chr 20q12–13.1		Diazoxide responsive, hypoglycemia often mild or transient in infant progressing to diabetes in adolescence (MODY1), family history of diabetes	Infant	Autosomal dominant
Usher syndrome type 1C (OMIM 276904) chr 11p15.1	Usher type 1C maps to the region containing the genes ABCC8 and KCNJ11	Severe hypoglycemia, diazoxide insensitive, sensorineural deafness, pigmentary retinopathy	Infant	Autosomal recessive

milder disease [54]. Some mutations result in channels which reach the membrane but are at a lower density than normal.

Inappropriately high concentrations of insulin cause hypoglycemia primarily as a result of increased glucose disposal and a decreased rate of endogenous glucose production. The incidence of CHI has been estimated at rates from 1 per 40 000 live births to as high as 1 in 2500 live births in communities with high levels of consanguinity [55,56]. The age at presentation varies from the newborn period or during the first few months of life after birth in term and preterm neonates [57]. Many neonates strikingly resemble an IDM but do not have the same profile as congenital abnormalities.

Biochemical and metabolic features

The characteristic metabolic and endocrine profile at the time of hypoglycemia is a measurable insulin concentration in the presence of hypoglycemia with low ketones, β-hydroxybutyrate and fatty acids with high C-peptide plasma concentrations [45]. Intravenous infusion rates >10 mg/kg/min to maintain a blood glucose concentration >3.6 mmol/L (65 mg/dL) are also suggestive as are increased glucose concentrations after administration of glucagon. Hypoglycemic neonates with HI fail to generate an adequate serum cortisol counter-regulatory hormonal response, which appears to be related to inappropriately low plasma ACTH [58].

Pharmacologic management

Glucose sufficient to maintain blood glucose concentrations >3.6 mmol/L is required and infusion rates >4–6 mg/kg/min, even >20 mg/kg/min, may be necessary. Diazoxide and a thiazide diuretic should be given concurrently to decrease the tendency of diazoxide to cause fluid retention and to capitalize on the fact that the drugs have synergistic effects in increasing blood glucose concentration [39]. A suitable starting dose of diazoxide is 5–10 mg/kg/day in three 8-hourly aliquots, increasing to a maximum of 20 mg/kg/day. Toxic effects include cardiac or cardiopulmonary failure, fluid retention and electrolyte imbalance [59–61]. For a child who is unresponsive to diazoxide, some centers opt for management with a long-term combined continuous subcutaneous infusion of glucagon and/or octreotide and strategies such as day and continuous nocturnal gastrostomy feeding which may be supplemented with raw cornstarch [51].

Intravenous octreotide (a synthetic octapeptide that mimics somatostatin) may be effective in suppressing insulin secretion and controlling the hypoglycemia but care must be taken if the infusion is interrupted because this may result in a sudden fall in blood glucose concentrations [51]. Calcium channel blockers such as nifedipine, which suppresses insulin secretion downstream of the defect in the KATP channel, have been successful in the management of a small proportion of patients [62,63]. Glucagon given by continuous infusion (starting dose 1.0 µg/kg/h) concurrently with octreotide may confer substantial benefit [64].

Surgical resection of the pancreas is considered following the failure of medical therapy. Partial pancreatectomy is not a procedure to be undertaken lightly. The operation most commonly performed is a 95% pancreatectomy but some children remain hypoglycemic and a further attempt can be made to control the procedure with diazoxide. In infants with diffuse HI, a total pancreatectomy may be necessary to control hyperinsulinism, which may be exacerbated by regeneration of the pancreatic remnant [65]. CHI has been classified into diffuse and focal disease (Plate 19.1) and attempts to diagnose focal disease are important because surgical resection of the focal area is curative. Preoperative detection is desirable to avoid extending the time in surgery.

Diagnosis of diffuse and focal disease

Neither magnetic resonance imaging (MRI) nor computed tomography (CT) scan are able to detect focal lesions. Functional techniques to identify focal lesions include pancreatic venous sampling (PVS) with the withdrawal of multiple blood samples to identify local increases in insulin secretion, sometimes combined with arterial calcium stimulation, have been used with some success but these techniques are invasive and not without risk. PET using fluro-dopa with CT or MRI scan is a non-invasive accurate modality, which is able to detect most focal cases [66,67]. PET scanning is also able to detect ectopic focal lesions that would not be found at surgery [68]. Rapid-frozen sections can be used to identify areas of focal hyperplasia at surgery, which are resected.

Diffuse disease is usually caused by the presence of two mutations in ABCC8 or (rarely) KCNJ11, and inherited in an autosomal recessive fashion. Dominant mutations and *de novo* mutations have been reported. Diffuse disease is characterized by the presence of enlarged islet cell nuclei with abnormal architecture throughout the pancreas but "atypical" histology has been described with departures from normal in terms of islet and acinar architecture but no evidence of enlarged islet cell nuclei.

Focal disease is caused by a focal clonal expansion of β cells lacking the maternal 11p15.1 allele because of loss of maternal chromosome 11p material. When these cells have a paternal mutation in the ABCC8 gene, a clone of β cells unable to express the inwardly rectifying potassium channel KATP channel results. As the clone increases in size, unregulated insulin secretion causes hypoglycemia. Focal disease is characterized by expansion of the islet cells within the lobule such that >40% of the area is occupied by islet tissue, with the acinar elements being pushed to the periphery of the lobule. Focal disease has been termed focal hyperplasia or microadenomatosis.

The difficulties of management of infants with CHI should not be underestimated and these patients should be managed in a tertiary facility with experience in the condition [45]. Insulin and glucose concentrations are extremely labile and the aim of early management is to protect the brain. Secure intravenous access is mandatory and, even with high rates of glucose infusion and pharmacological therapy, it may be difficult or impossible to maintain blood glucose concentrations >2.6 mmol/L. The aim should be to maintain concentrations >3.6 mmol/L to allow a margin of error. Infants may be asymptomatic in the presence of low blood glucose but there is no evidence that absence of symptoms equates with neurological safety. Macrosomia can hamper venous access and a central line may be considered.

Feeding difficulties, which occur in a substantial proportion of infants with CHI, compound the problem of maintaining blood glucose at a safe concentration. Determined food refusal, reflux and poorly understood foregut dysmotility [69] make a regimen of frequent feeding difficult or impossible. Many centers use percutaneous gastrostomy feeding to circumvent some of these issues. Oral raw cornstarch has been described as a useful adjunct to therapy [51,70]. A low protein diet, which avoids normal protein-stimulated insulin secretion, may aid management in infants with HI associated with KATP channelopathies. Intravenous glucose may produce a more stable blood glucose profile as oral feeds may promote hypoglycemia because they augment insulin secretion by stimulating the GIP and GLP-1 to enhance insulin secretion via the enteroinsular axis.

Long-term outcome

Most infants who have undergone pancreatectomy develop diabetes. Older age at surgery, greater extent of resection and previous pancreatectomy increase the risk of insulin dependence immediately following pancreatectomy [71,72]. Many infants, even those who undergo 95–98% resection, require a second or even third operation to control blood glucose and continuing medical therapy with diazoxide and/or octreotide may be required. Most pancreatectomized patients develop diabetes around puberty [72–74] but non-pancreatectomized infants with HI resulting from ABCC8 mutations have also been reported to develop impaired glucose tolerance and diabetes in childhood or young adulthood [75].

The proportion of infants who sustain neurologic impairment ranges from 10% to 44% [72,74,76,77]. Commonly reported problems include poor motor skills, seizures or epilepsy, speech problems, cerebral palsy, eye problems (notably strabismus) and learning difficulties. Children with mild dysfunction may benefit from early preschool intervention.

Hyperinsulinism/hyperammonemia syndrome

Abnormal activation of glutamate dehydrogenase leads to increased intracellular concentrations of ATP which trigger insulin secretion in the absence of any defect in membrane polarization. Infants with hyperinsulinism/hyperammonemia syndrome (HI/HA) have an activating mutation in the gene encoding glutamate dehydrogenase, with a mild persistent hyperammonemia which does not have any clinical signs. Most mutations occur *de novo* but families with dominant modes of transmission have been reported. Fasting or post-prandial hypoglycemia resulting from inappropriate insulin concentration may occur because of the stimulatory effects of ingested protein. The hypoglycemia may be intermittent and milder than in infants with ABCC8 or KCNJ11 mutations, often leading to delay in recognition of signs and presentation at a few months of age. It responds well to diazoxide but lifelong therapy is usually required [78].

Activating glucokinase mutations

Abnormal activation of glucokinase increases intracellular concentration of ATP and activates insulin secretion. Glucokinase gene mutations have been reported in a small number of families and are transmitted in an autosomal dominant pattern resulting in gain of function, increased affinity of glucokinase for glucose and inappropriate insulin secretion. The hypoglycemia is mild and of variable severity within families. It may be controlled with food or diazoxide if necessary [79,80].

HADH

This form of hyperinsulinism is caused by a mutation in the HADH gene encoding the enzyme short chain 3-hydroxyacyl-CoA dehydrogenase (SCHAD) involved in mitochondrial fatty acid metabolism, which has reduced activity in affected patients. Mutations are inherited in an autosomal recessive mode. Disease varies from mild to severe forms. Patients present in the neonatal or infant period and the hypoglycemia is diazoxide-responsive [81,82]. The presence of 3-hydroxyglutaric acid in urine, raised plasma concentrations of 3-hydroxybutyryl-carnitine and diazoxide responsiveness may aid diagnostic evaluation [82].

Congenital disorders of glycosylation

Congenital disorders of glycosylation (CDG) comprises a large family of genetic diseases that result from defects in glycan metabolism, associated with a wide variety of different clinical presentations, such as hypoglycemia, neurological impairment, gastrointestinal problems, hypertrophic cardiomyopathy, seizures, short stature and physical dysmorphisms. Over 27 types have been described but new types arise frequently and some have a characteristic physical or biochemical profile [83–85]. Hyperinsulinemic hypoglycemia has been reported as the presenting feature of CDG in the absence of other signs. Abnormal serum transferrin isoforms are a screening test for CDG but should be delayed until the infant is over 1 month of age because the test is unreliable before this. A positive transferrin test should be followed by enzyme assay in cultured fibroblasts to confirm the type of CDG, which will guide prognosis and clinical management. CDG associated HI is responsive to diazoxide. CDG type Ib caused by a deficiency in phosphomannose isomerase is the only treatable type, being responsive to oral mannose supplementation [83,86–88].

Hepatocyte nuclear factor 4α

Mutations in the gene encoding hepatocyte nuclear factor 4α (HNF-4α) cause maturity onset diabetes of the young type 1 (MODY1). Infants with these mutations may present with severe hypoglycemia and macrosomia. The mode of inheritance is autosomal dominant. The hypoglycemia may be transient or persistent and is responsive to diazoxide. The natural history of the disease is hyperinsulinemic hypoglycemia in infancy, progressing to impaired insulin secretion and diabetes in adolescence or young adulthood. Thus, infants who present with macrosomia and HI and a family history of young onset diabetes should be screened for HNF-4 mutations [86–89].

Rare causes of hypoglycemia caused by excess insulin or insulin-like activity

Usher syndrome caused by mutations in the gene region contiguous with ABCC8 and KCNJ11 results in infants presenting with sensorineural deafness and retinopathy [90,91]. Mutations in the INSR gene encoding for insulin have been associated with HI but reported only in adults [92]. Exercise-induced hypoglycemia associated with abnormalities of the monocarboxylate pathway have also only been reported in adults [93–95]. HI can be caused by surreptitious administration of sulfonylurea drugs causing a rise in endogenous insulin secretion together with high concentrations of C-peptide or insulin injection, which will be associated with inappropriately low concentrations of C-peptide.

HI presenting for the first time in children over 5 years of age may be because of an insulinoma which is likely to be associated with the overall diagnosis of multiple endocrine neoplasia type 1 (MEN1). Genetic studies of the MEN1 gene (OMIM 131100) should be performed in child and family. Non-islet cell tumor hypoglycemia, caused by abnormal insulin-like activity due to the production of prepro-IGF-II by the tumour that does not bind to the IGF binding proteins and hence is "free" acting via the IGF receptor rather than the insulin receptor, is another rare syndrome presenting with persistent hypoglycemia, low ketone, free fatty acid and insulin concentrations [96]. Hirata disease, a rare syndrome seen in Japan, where it is the third most common cause of hypoglycemia in adults, is brought about by the presence of high concentrations of insulin autoantibodies which possibly sequester insulin for later release during fasting. This syndrome is also associated with persistent hypoglycemia with high insulin antibody titres and low concentrations of ketones, free fatty acids and insulin. There is an human leukocyte antigen (HLA) linkage in this condition [97].

Failure of counter-regulatory hormones

Deficiency of the counter-regulatory hormones can cause hypoglycemia. Deficiency of glucagon or epinephrine, the two hormones important for the immediate restoration of the blood glucose concentration, is rare. More common is hypoglycemia brought about by GH and/or cortisol deficiency. The hypoglycemia results from a combination of factors that include reduced gluconeogenic substrate availability (decreased mobilization of fats and proteins) and increased glucose utilization because of increased insulin sensitivity of tissues in the absence of GH and cortisol. The threshold for the release of GH and cortisol in adults lies within or just below the physiological blood glucose concentration [98], implying that GH and cortisol start to rise in response to blood glucose concentrations within the normoglycemic range and that these increases are probably inversely proportional to the nadir in blood glucose [99]. GH and cortisol respond differ-

ently to spontaneous hypoglycemia compared with that induced by insulin infusion (insulin tolerance test) [100]. This may be related to the rate of fall of the blood glucose concentration, which is why a low GH value at the time of spontaneous hypoglycemia may not necessarily indicate GH deficiency.

Pituitary disorders

Growth hormone and cortisol deficiencies are seen in combination in congenital or acquired disorders of pituitary function. Congenital hypopituitarism may present with life-threatening hypoglycemia, abnormal serum sodium concentrations, shock, microphallus and growth failure later. The incidence of hypoglycemia from panhypopituitarism can be as high as 20% and hypoglycemia associated with hypopituitarism may be a cause of sudden death [101]. Standard replacement doses of hydrocortisone and GH prevent further hypoglycemia, although the dose of hydrocortisone will need to be increased during stress. The causes of congenital hypopituitarism are shown in Table 19.7 together with the possible genetic associations. Acquired hypopituitarism may result from tumors (most commonly craniopharyngioma), radiation, infection, hydrocephalus, vascular anomalies and trauma.

Adrenal disorders

Adrenal disorders should be considered where the patient describes a recent increase in pigmentation and are confirmed by the presence of low cortisol concentrations with a significantly increased ACTH concentration. Hyperinsulinemic infants may mount a suboptimal cortisol response to hypoglycemia, which can cause difficulty in interpretation; a short synacthen test with basal ACTH concentration can be useful in these circumstances. Adrenal disorders can be classified into adrenal dysgenesis, impaired steroidogenesis and adrenal destruction (Fig. 19.5; Table 19.8) [102].

Adrenal dysgenesis or hypoplasia

The clinical forms of adrenal dysgenesis or hypoplasia causing adrenal insufficiency include a sporadic form associated with pituitary hypoplasia, an autosomal recessive form, an X-linked form and a number of forms caused by ACTH resistance. These disorders are likely to present in the first few months of life. Deficiency of steroidogenic factor-1 (SF-1) (OMIM 184757) on chromosome 9q 33 can lead to adrenal failure with complete XY sex reversal due to testicular dysgenesis. In females, the ovaries may be spared. Congenital X-linked adrenal hypoplasia (OMIM 300200) is caused by mutations in the dosage-sensitive sex reversal-adrenal hypoplasia gene 1 (DAX-1) (OMIM 300473) which can present in males in the first few months of life as the fetal adrenal cortex atrophies. The gene on Xp21.3 encodes a nuclear hormone receptor and expression of DAX-1 is important for development of gonads, adrenal cortex, hypothalamus and pituitary. The condition is associated with hypogonadotrophic hypogonadism. Loss of this gene maybe part of a contiguous gene syndrome with DAX-1, glycerol kinase deficiency and occasionally Duchenne muscular dystrophy. Familial glucocorticoid

Table 19.7 Causes of congential hypopituitarism.

Disorder	Presentation	Genetic association
Septo-optic dysplasia	Optic nerve hypoplasia Anterior pituitary hormone deficiency Diabetes insipidus	HESX1 (OMIM 182230)
Midline syndromes	Optic nerve hypoplasia Anterior pituitary hormone deficiency Diabetes insipidus Major CNS disruption and/or cervical spine defects	LHX3 (OMIM 600577) and LHX4 (OMIM 602146)
Anterior pituitary dysfunction	Deficiency of GH, TSH, prolactin	Pit-1 (OMIM 173110)
Anterior pituitary dysfunction	Deficiency of GH, TSH, prolactin and ACTH	PROP-I (OMIM 601538)
Anterior pituitary dysfunction	Deficiency of GH, TSH, prolactin, LH, FSH and ACTH	Unknown

ACTH, adenocorticotropic hormone; FSH, follicle stimulating hormone; GH, growth hormone; LH, luteinizing hormone; TSH, thyrotropin stimulating hormone.

Table 19.8 Presentation with adrenal insufficiency according to underlying diagnosis over 15 years [excluding congenital adrenal hypoplasia (CAH)] [102].

	Total	Male	Female
Diagnosis	29	16	13
Autoimmune	16 (55%)	6 (38%)	10 (77%)
Congenital hypoplasia	6 (21%)	6 (38%)	
AAA syndrome	4 (14%)	1 (6%)	3 (23%)
ALD	3 (10%)	3 (19%)	

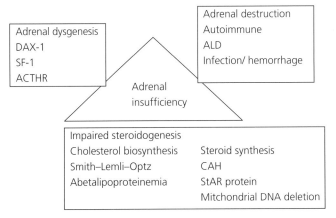

Figure 19.5 Schematic representation of the three main causes of adrenal insufficiency in childhood. ACTHR, adrenocorticotropic hormone resistance; ALD, adrenoleukodystropy; CAH, congenital adrenal hyperplasia.

deficiency (FGD) is a rare autosomal recessive syndrome characterized by a failure of cortisol production because of adrenal ACTH resistance (OMIM 607397). AAA syndrome (OMIM 231550) occurs in males and females and should be considered when glucocorticoid deficiency occurs with other features including achalasia, alacrima and autonomic neuropathy in association with hyperpigmentation.

Table 19.9 Types of autoimmune polyglandular syndromes (APS) associated with adrenal insufficiency.

APS-1 (OMIM 240300)	APS-2 (OMIM 269200)
Mucocutaneous candidiasis	Autoimmune thyroid disease
Hypoparathyroidism	Type 1 diabetes
Adrenal insufficiency	Adrenal insufficiency

Impaired steroidogenesis

Congenital adrenal hyperplasia (CAH) caused by 21-hydroxylase deficiency (OMIM 201901) is one of the most common autosomal recessive disorders in humans. 21-Hydroxylase is encoded by CYP21 and the estimated carrier frequency of deleterious CYP21 mutations is 1 in 50. The CAH phenotype reflects the degree of 21-hydroxylase enzyme deficiency. Complete enzyme deficiency, with impairment of both cortisol and aldosterone synthesis, results in the salt-wasting form characterized by prenatal virilization in females and salt-wasting crises in the neonatal period. Partial enzyme deficiency leads to simple virilizing CAH characterized only by prenatal virilization in females and pseudo-precocious puberty in males and females. The incidence of CAH is 1 in 15 000 live births. The first clue to the condition in a male infant may be collapse in the first 1–8 weeks of life with hypoglycemia, hypotension and hyperkalemia. Other causes of impaired steroidogenesis are much less common.

Adrenal destruction

Secondary adrenal failure is of autoimmune origin in approximately 50% of cases and can be associated with failure of other endocrine organs in the polyglandular syndromes. Adrenoleukodystrophy (OMIM 300100) can be confirmed in males by measurement of plasma long-chain fatty acids. Adrenal destruction from hemorrhage or ischemia can occur in the context of a severe systemic illness, such as neonatal hypoxia or meningococcal septicemia (Table 19.9).

Metabolic causes of hypoglycemia

Defects in hepatic glycogen release/storage

Glucose is stored as glycogen mainly in the liver but also in the muscle and kidneys. Defects in the storage or release of hepatic glycogen can cause hypoglycemia (Table 19.10). Glucose-6-phosphatase deficiency [glycogen storage disease type 1, von Gierke disease (OMIM 232200)] is the most common glycogen storage disease. Glycogen is broken down to glucose-6-phosphate and the deficiency of glucose-6-phosphatase results in the inability to release free glucose from the glucose-6-phosphate, with resultant hepatomegaly due to stored glycogen. Glucose-6-phosphate is also the penultimate product of gluconeogenesis which is also blocked resulting in lactic acidosis, hyperuricemia and hyperlipidemia. Blockage of both these pathways of glucose homeostasis results in recurrent hypoglycemia The aim of treatment is to prevent hypoglycemia using a combination of continuous nasogastric drip feeding and cornstarch.

The two other glycogen storage diseases causing hypoglycemia result from deficiencies of the enzymes amylo-1,6-glucosidase [glycogen storage disease type III, GSDIII (OMIM 232400)] and liver phosphorylase [glycogen storage disease VI (OMIM 232700)]. The clinical and biochemical features of GSDIII subjects are quite heterogeneous: the clinical manifestations are hepatomegaly, hypoglycemia, hyperlipidemia, short stature and, in a number of subjects, cardiomyopathy and myopathy. Glycogen storage disease type VI (GSDVI) presents with mild clinical manifestations and

Table 19.10 Metabolic causes of recurrent hypoglycemia.

Defect	Diagnostic clues
Defects in hepatic glycogen release/storage	
Glucose-6-phosphatase deficiency	Fasting hypoglycemia with hepatomegaly. Fasting lactic acidosis as well in glucose-6-phosphatase deficiency
Amylo-1,6-glucosidase deficiency	
Liver phosphorylase deficiency	
Liver phosphorylase kinase deficiency	
Hepatic glycogen synthase deficiency	Fasting hypoglycemia with post-prandial hyperglycemia and lactic acidosis
Defects in gluconeogenesis	
Glucose-6-phosphatase deficiency	Fasting hypoglycemia with lactic acidosis. Lactic acidosis may be the presenting problem in the early blocks
Fructose-1,6-bisphosphatase deficiency	
Phosphoenolpyruvate carboxykinase (PEPCK) deficiency	
Pyruvate carboxylase deficiency	
Defects of fatty acid oxidation and carnitine metabolism	
Very-long-chain acyl CoA dehydrogenase (VLCAD) deficiency	Fasting hypoglycemia with characteristic abnormalities in plasma acylcarnitine profiles and often in urine organic acid profiles. Total and free plasma carnitine are low in carnitine deficiency
Medium-chain acyl CoA dehydrogenase (MCAD) deficiency	
Short-chain acyl CoA dehydrogenase (SCAD) deficiency	
Long-/short-chain L 3 hydroxy acyl CoA (L/SCHAD) deficiency	
Carnitine deficiency (primary and secondary)	
Carnitine palmitoyltransferase deficiency (CPT 1 and 2)	
Defects in ketone body synthesis/utilization	
Mitochondrial HMG CoA synthase deficiency	Hypoketotic hypoglycemia with elevated plasma free fatty acids and characteristic abnormalities in urine organic acid profiles
HMG CoA lyase deficiency	
Succinyl CoA:3 oxoacid CoA transferase (SCOT) deficiency	Intermittent ketoacidotic crises with persistent ketonemia
Metabolic conditions (relatively common ones)	
Organic acidemias (propionic/methylmalonic)	Characteristic abnormalities in plasma amino acid and/or acylcarnitine profiles and urine organic acid profiles
Maple syrup urine disease	
Tyrosinemia	
Glutaric aciduria type 2	
Galactosemia	Positive neonatal screen if performed. Galactose present in urine sugar chromatography, absent RBC galactose-1-phosphate uridylyltransferase activity
Hereditary fructose intolerance	History of proximate sucrose intake or aversion, fructose present in urine sugar chromatography

RBC, red blood cell.

follows a benign course. Patients have prominent hepatomegaly, growth retardation and variable but mild episodes of fasting hypoglycemia and hyperketosis during childhood. High plasma concentrations of lactate and uric acid are characteristically absent. These clinical features and biochemical abnormalities generally resolve by puberty.

Deficiency of liver phosporylase kinase [GSDIXa (OMIM 306000)], which is required to activate liver phosphorylase, results in variable hypoglycemia with hepatomegaly, growth retardation, mildly elevated transaminases, hyperlipidemia and fasting ketosis. Symptoms become milder with age. The condition is inherited in X-linked manner.

Glycogen synthase (OMIM 240600) has an important role in the storage of glycogen in the liver and deficiency of it is a rare cause of hypoglycemia in childhood [103]. The characteristic features include fasting hypoglycemia with high ketone concentrations but with normal plasma lactate concentration. Mutations in the hepatic isomer of glycogen synthase (GYS2 – encoded on 12p12.2) result in an inability to form α-1,4-linkages between glucose molecules to form glycogen. A lack of glycogen stores results in fasting hypoglycemia. Post-prandial hyperglycemia occurs following a carbohydrate-rich meal and shunting of glucose into the glycolytic pathways results in elevated lactate and triglyceride concentrations. Affected individuals are asymptomatic during the neonatal and early infancy periods but have difficulties weaning from overnight feeds with fasting ketotic hypoglycemia or irritability occurring before breakfast. There is a paucity of symptoms even at blood glucose concentrations of 1.6–2.4 mmol/L (30–45 mg/dL) because of the availability of alternative fuels. Fasting is better tolerated with increasing age but this is not a universal feature. Overnight fasting is achieved at around 7 years of age. Hypoglycemia remains a problem in adulthood in the setting of increased metabolic requirements. Mutation analysis is available but diagnoses made on liver biopsy have been made in the absence of an identifiable mutation.

Defects in gluconeogenesis

Gluconeogenesis, the formation of glucose from lactate/pyruvate, glycerol, glutamine and alanine, has an essential role in the maintenance of normoglycemia during fasting. Gluconeogenesis can be viewed as a reversal of glycolysis but four of the reactions in the glycolytic pathway are irreversible and different enzymes perform the reverse reaction in gluconeogenesis. Inborn deficiencies of each of the four unique enzymes of the gluconeogenic pathway that insure a unidirectional flux from pyruvate to glucose [pyruvate carboxylase (OMIM 608786), phosphoenolpyruvate carboxykinase (PEPCK) (OMIM 261650), fructose-1,6-bisphosphatase (OMIM 229700) and glucose-6-phosphatase] are known [104]. Patients with defects in gluconeogenesis present with fasting hypoglycemia and lactic acidosis. Pyruvate carboxylase deficiency may lead to a more widespread clinical presentation with lactic acidosis, severe mental and developmental retardation and proximal renal tubular acidosis [105].

Disorders of carnitine metabolism and defects of fatty acid oxidation

Primary carnitine deficiency (OMIM 212140) is an autosomal recessive disorder of fatty acid oxidation that can present at different ages with low ketone concentrations hypoglycemia and cardiomyopathy and/or skeletal myopathy. This disease is suspected by reduced concentrations of carnitine in plasma and confirmed by measurement of carnitine transport in the patient's fibroblasts. Carnitine transport is markedly reduced (usually <5% of normal) in fibroblasts from patients with primary carnitine deficiency.

The "hepatic" carnitine palmitoyl transferase 1 (CPT1 isoform) is expressed in liver, kidney and fibroblasts and at low concentrations in the heart, while the other isoform (muscle) occurs in skeletal muscle and is the predominant form in the heart. Patients with hepatic CPT1 isoform deficiency (OMIM 255120) present with low ketone concentrations, hypoglycemia, hepatomegaly with raised transaminases, renal tubular acidosis, transient hyperlipidemia and, paradoxically, myopathy with elevated creatinine kinase or cardiac involvement and seizures and coma in the neonatal period [106]. The typical biochemical finding in the urine organic acids is a dicarboxylic aciduria of chain lengths C6–C10.

CPT2 deficiency has several clinical presentations. The "benign" adult form (OMIM 255110) is characterized by episodes of rhabdomyolysis triggered by prolonged exercise. The infantile type CPT2 deficiency (OMIM 600649) presents as severe attacks of hypoglycemia with low ketone concentrations hypoglycemia despite high plasma free fatty acids and occasionally with cardiac damage commonly responsible for sudden death before 1 year of age [106]. In addition to these symptoms, features of brain and kidney dysorganogenesis are frequently seen in neonatal onset CPT2 deficiency (OMIM 608836), which is almost always lethal during the first month of life. Treatment is based upon avoidance of fasting and/or exercise and a low fat diet enriched with medium chain triglycerides and carnitine ("severe" CPT2 deficiency). Laboratory findings may include a long-chain dicarboxylic aciduria and decreased serum and tissue total and free carnitine and increased serum and tissue long-chain acylcarnitines.

The most common disorder of fatty acid beta oxidation is MCAD (OMIM 201450). This autosomal recessive condition is characterized by intolerance to prolonged fasting, recurrent episodes of hypoglycemic coma with medium-chain dicarboxylicaciduria and increased hexanoyl and suberylglycine excretion on urine organic acids and increased octanylcarnitine on the plasma acylcarnitine profile, impaired ketogenesis and low plasma and tissue carnitine concentrations [107]. The disorder may be severe and even fatal in young patients. Other defects of beta oxidation [very-long-chain acyl CoA dehydrogenase (VLCAD) (OMIM 201475) and long-chain acyl CoA dehydrogenase (LCHAD) (OMIM 609016)] may present with hypoglycemia-associated low ketone concentrations and with neurological (hypotonia) and cardiovascular complications (cardiomyopathy). The pattern of dicarboxylicaciduria accumulation and abnormal plasma acylcarnitines is characteristic for each enzymatic defect of the beta oxidation spiral. Short-chain hydroxy acyl CoA dehydrogenase (SCHAD) (OMIM 601609) is unusual being associated with hyperinsulinism and increased 3-hydroxyglutarate in the urine organic acid profile. Diagnosis can be confirmed by enzyme assay of cultured fibroblasts.

Defects in ketone body synthesis/utilization

Ketone bodies are an alternative form of fuel to glucose for the brain. Each ketone body is synthesized from the combination of acetyl CoA and acetoacetyl CoA by liver mitochondrial HMG CoA synthase to form hydroxymethylglutaryl CoA (HMG CoA). This is split by HMG CoA lyase to yield acetoacetate in the liver, which is converted to beta hydroxybutyrate. In the peripheral tissues, acetoacetate is activated back to acetoacetyl CoA by succinyl CoA:3 oxoacid CoA transferase (SCOT). Hypoglycemia may occur as a result of defects in either the synthesis or the utilization of ketone bodies.

Hereditary deficiency of mitochondrial HMG CoA synthase (OMIM 600234) can cause episodes of severe hypoglycemia with low ketone concentrations. Typical findings include low ketones concentrations, elevated free fatty acids, normal acylcarnitines and massive dicarboxylic aciduria without adequate ketonuria during acute episodes by urinary organic acid analysis [108].

HMG CoA lyase deficiency (OMIM 246450) presents with recurrent hypoglycemia with low ketone concentrations which can be complicated on occasions with a Reye-like syndrome and acute pancreatitis. The urine organic acids are characteristic showing increased 3-hydroxy-3-methylglutarate, 3-methylglutaconate, 3-methylglutarate, 3-hydroxyisovalerate and 3-methylglutarylcarnitine [109].

A rare cause of hypoglycemia caused by the inability to utilize ketone bodies is deficiency of SCOT (OMIM 245050) [110], which is characterized by intermittent ketoacidotic crises and persistent ketosis.

Miscellaneous metabolic and toxic causes of hypoglycemia

Hypoglycemia can occur as a result of a number of metabolic conditions including galactosemia, hereditary fructose intolerance, tyrosinemia, organic acidemias, maple syrup urine disease, glutaric aciduria type 11 and in mitochondrial respiratory chain defects [111].

Hereditary fructose intolerance (OMIM 229600), caused by catalytic deficiency of aldolase B (fructose-1,6-bisphosphonate aldolase), is a recessively inherited condition in which affected homozygotes develop hypoglycemia, vomiting and severe abdominal symptoms after taking foods containing fructose or sucrose and quickly learn to avoid foods containing these sugars. Continued ingestion of noxious sugars leads to hepatic and renal injury and growth retardation. The presence of positive reducing substances with the presence of fructose and/or glucose on urine sugar chromatography may provide a clue in the critical urine

sample. Most cases (95%) can be confirmed by screening for mutations in the aldolase B gene.

Where neonatal screening for galactosemia (OMIM 606999) is not performed, patients present in the first weeks of life with poor feeding and weight loss, vomiting, diarrhea, lethargy, hypotonia, liver dysfunction and bleeding tendencies. Urine-reducing substances may be positive if the child is ingesting milk and urine sugar chromatography may show increased glucose and galactose. The deficiency of galactose-1-phosphate uridylyltransferase can be readily demonstrated in red blood cells confirming the diagnosis.

The diagnosis of organic acidemias is evident from plasma amino acid and/or acylcarnitine profiles and urine organic acid results. A greatly increased urine methylmalonate is indicative of methylmalonic aciduria (OMIM 251000), increased urine 3-hydroxypropionate, propionylglycine, methylcitrate and tiglylglycine are seen in propionic acidemia (OMIM 606054), increased urine ethylmalonate, adipate, glutarate, 2-hydroxyglutarate, hexanoyl and suberylglycine and abnormal plasma acylcarnitines are seen in glutaric aciduria type 2 (OMIM 231680), increased 2-hydroxyisovalerate and plasma branched chain amino acids and alloisoleucine are seen in maple syrup urine disease (OMIM 248600) and an increased urine succinylacetone is seen in tyrosinemia (OMIM 276700).

Hypoglycemia may be triggered after certain types of food such as high protein load, high fructose content, toxin of unripe ackee fruit and high glycemia index foods (which may lead to rebound hypoglycemia). There are a number of drugs and chemicals that if ingested or administered can lead to episodes of hypoglycemia via interruption of the intermediate metabolism. They include alcohol, aspirin, oral hypoglycemic agents, insulin, injected beta-blockers and quinine.

Idiopathic ketotic hypoglycemia

Ketotic hypoglycemia is also referred to as accelerated starvation, idiopathic hypoglycemia or substrate-limited hypoglycemia. It is a diagnosis of exclusion but, although it is common [112], the pathogenesis is not understood. The differential diagnosis includes various inborn errors of metabolism. There is an association with low birthweight, poor weight gain and male gender. The typical age of presentation is between 18 months and 5 years. The age of spontaneous resolution is usually around 8–9 years of age.

The typical history is of a child who may miss a meal and develop hypoglycemia unpredictably, usually following an upper respiratory tract infection. The hypoglycemia is associated with raised ketones and free fatty acids with suppressed insulin concentrations. The theory of decreased availability or impaired mobilization of muscle amino acids (and other substrates) for gluconeogenesis is thought to be unlikely because their contribution is small except in the acidotic state. An alternative explanation is the imbalance between the limited rate of hepatic glucose production and insufficient suppression of glucose utilization in the brain by ketone bodies and free fatty acids. This is supported by the observation that the age of spontaneous resolution of ketotic hypoglycemia coincides with the age at which both the brain:body weight ratio is decreasing and endogenous substrate availability is increasing. Ketotic hypoglycemia may also be seen in various situations of lack of substrate and increased metabolic demands in which there is an obvious cause such as severe illness, sepsis, malaria and liver disease. Teenage girls prone to eating disorders may also present with low blood glucose concentrations particularly after ingestion of small amounts of alcohol and carbohydrate.

References

1 Cornblath M, et al. Controversies regarding definition of neonatal hypoglycemia: suggested operational thresholds. *Pediatrics* 2000; **105**: 1141–1145.

2 Koh TH, et al. Neural dysfunction during hypoglycemia. *Arch Dis Child* 1988; **63**: 1353–1358.

3 Hawdon JM. Hypoglycemia and the neonatal brain. *Eur J Pediatr* 1999; **158** (Suppl 1): S9–S12.

4 Fourtner SH, Stanley CA, Kelly A. Protein-sensitive hypoglycemia without leucine sensitivity in hyperinsulinism caused by K(ATP) channel mutations. *J Pediatr* 2006; **149**: 47–52.

5 Cryer PE. Regulation of glucose metabolism in man. *J Intern Med Suppl* 1991; **735**: 31–39.

6 Cranston I, et al. Regional differences in cerebral blood flow and glucose utilization in diabetic man: the effect of insulin. *J Cereb Blood Flow Metab* 1998; **18**: 130–140.

7 Frackowiak RS, Jones T. PET scanning. *Br Med J* 1989; **298**: 693–694.

8 Anwar M, Vannucci RC. Autoradiographic determination of regional cerebral blood flow during hypoglycemia in newborn dogs. *Pediatr Res* 1988; **24**: 41–45.

9 Skov L, Pryds O. Capillary recruitment for preservation of cerebral glucose influx in hypoglycemic, preterm newborns: evidence for a glucose sensor? *Pediatrics* 1992; **90**: 193–195.

10 Nehlig A. Cerebral energy metabolism, glucose transport and blood flow: changes with maturation and adaptation to hypoglycemia. *Diabetes Metab* 1997; **23**: 18–29.

11 Auer RN. Hypoglycemic brain damage. *Metab Brain Dis* 2004; **19**: 169–175.

12 Ballesteros JR, Mishra OP, McGowan JE. Alterations in cerebral mitochondria during acute hypoglycemia. *Biol Neonate* 2003; **84**: 159–163.

13 Patel MS, et al. The metabolism of ketone bodies in developing human brain: development of ketone-body-utilizing enzymes and ketone bodies as precursors for lipid synthesis. *J Neurochem* 1975; **25**: 905–908.

14 Amiel SA, et al. Ketone infusion lowers hormonal responses to hypoglycemia: evidence for acute cerebral utilization of a non-glucose fuel. *Clin Sci (Lond)* 1991; **81**: 189–194.

15 Cahill GF Jr. Fuel metabolism in starvation. *Annu Rev Nutr* 2006; **26**: 1–22.

16 Mitchell GA, et al. Medical aspects of ketone body metabolism. *Clin Invest Med* 1995; **18**: 193–216.

17 Plecko B, et al. Oral beta-hydroxybutyrate supplementation in two patients with hyperinsulinemic hypoglycemia: monitoring of beta-hydroxybutyrate concentrations in blood and cerebrospinal fluid and in the brain by in vivo magnetic resonance spectroscopy. *Pediatr Res* 2002; **52**: 301–306.

18 Haymond MW, et al. Differences in circulating gluconeogenic substrates during short-term fasting in men, women and children. *Metabolism* 1982; **31**: 33–42.

19 Mitrakou A, et al. Role of reduced suppression of glucose production and diminished early insulin release in impaired glucose tolerance. *N Engl J Med* 1992; **326**: 22–29.

20 Mitrakou A, et al. Contribution of abnormal muscle and liver glucose metabolism to postprandial hyperglycemia in NIDDM. *Diabetes* 1990; **39**: 1381–1390.

21 Jitrapakdee S, Wallace JC. Structure, function and regulation of pyruvate carboxylase. *Biochem J* 1999; **340**: 1–16.

22 Bolli GB, Fanelli CG. Physiology of glucose counterregulation to hypoglycemia. *Endocrinol Metab Clin North Am* 1999; **28**: 467–493, v.

23 Bier DM, et al. Measurement of "true" glucose production rates in infancy and childhood with 6,6-dideuteroglucose. *Diabetes* 1977; **26**: 1016–1023.

24 Haymond MW, et al. Effects of ketosis on glucose flux in children and adults. *Am J Physiol* 1983; **245**: E373–378.

25 Hsu A, et al. Larger mass of high-metabolic-rate organs does not explain higher resting energy expenditure in children. *Am J Clin Nutr* 2003; **77**: 1506–1511.

26 Peters J, Jurgensen A, Kloppel G. Ontogeny, differentiation and growth of the endocrine pancreas. *Virchows Arch* 2000; **436**: 527–538.

27 Bonner-Weir S. Morphology of the endocrine pancreas. In: Becker KL, ed. *Principles and Practice of Endocrinology and Metabolism.* Philadelphia: Lippincott Williams & Wilkins, 2001; 1292–1295.

28 Slack JM. Developmental biology of the pancreas. *Development* 1995; **121**: 1569–1580.

29 Van Noorden S, Falkmer S. Gut-islet endocrinology: some evolutionary aspects. *Invest Cell Pathol* 1980; **3**: 21–35.

30 Madsen OD. Pancreas phylogeny and ontogeny in relation to a 'pancreatic stem cell'. *C R Biol* 2007; **330**: 534–537.

31 Edlund H. Developmental biology of the pancreas. *Diabetes* 2001; **50** (Suppl 1): 5–9.

32 Cabrera O, et al. The unique cytoarchitecture of human pancreatic islets has implications for islet cell function. *Proc Natl Acad Sci U S A* 2006; **103**: 2334–2339.

33 Yamaoka T, Itakura M. Development of pancreatic islets (review). *Int J Mol Med* 1999; **3**: 247–261.

34 Jorgensen MC, et al. An illustrated review of early pancreas development in the mouse. *Endocr Rev* 2007; **28**: 685–705.

35 Steiner DF, James DE. Cellular and molecular biology of the beta cell. *Diabetologia* 1992; **35** (Suppl 2): S41–48.

36 Steiner DF. New aspects of proinsulin physiology and pathophysiology. *J Pediatr Endocrinol Metab* 2000; **13**: 229–239.

37 Steiner DF. The proinsulin C-peptide: a multirole model. *Exp Diabesity Res* 2004; **5**: 7–14.

38 Ashcroft FM, Rorsman P. Electrophysiology of the pancreatic beta-cell. *Prog Biophys Mol Biol* 1989; **54**: 87–143.

39 Dunne MJ, et al. Hyperinsulinism in infancy: from basic science to clinical disease. *Physiol Rev* 2004; **84**: 239–275.

40 De Leon DD, Stanley CA. Mechanisms of disease: advances in diagnosis and treatment of hyperinsulinism in neonates. *Nat Clin Pract Endocrinol Metab* 2007; **3**: 57–68.

41 Leung YM, *et al.* SNAREing voltage-gated K$^+$ and ATP-sensitive K$^+$ channels: tuning beta-cell excitability with syntaxin-1A and other exocytotic proteins. *Endocr Rev* 2007; **28**: 653–663.

42 Stanley CA. Hypoglycemia in the neonate. *Pediatr Endocrinol Rev* 2006; **4** (Suppl 1): 76–81.

43 Hussain K, Aynsley-Green A. Management of hyperinsulinism in infancy and childhood. *Ann Med* 2000; **32**: 544–551.

44 Malik M, Wilson P. Umbilical artery catheterization: a potential cause of regractory hypoglycemia. *Clin Pediatr (Phila)* 1987; **26**: 181–12.

45 Aynsley-Green A, *et al.* Practical management of hyperinsulinism in infancy. *Arch Dis Child Fetal Neonatal Ed* 2000; **82**: F98–107.

46 Carrapato MR, Marcelino F. The infant of the diabetic mother: the critical developmental windows. *Early Pregnancy* 2001; **5**: 57–58.

47 Li M, Squire JA. Molecular biology of Beckwith–Wiedemann syndrome. *Curr Opin Pediatr* 1996; **9**: 623–629.

48 Slatter RE, *et al.* Mosaic uniparental disomy in Beckwith–Wiedemann syndrome. *J Med Genet* 1994; **3**: 749–753.

49 DeBaun MR, King AA, White N. Hyperinsulinism in Beckwith–Wiedemann syndrome. *Semin Perinatol* 2000; **24**: 164–171.

50 Munns CF, Batch JA. Hyperinsulinism and Beckwith–Wiedemann syndrome. *Arch Dis Child Fetal Neonatal Ed* 2001; **84**: F67–69.

51 Mazor-Aronovitch K, *et al.* Long-term neurodevelopmental outcome in conservatively treated congenital hyperinsulinism. *Eur J Endocrinol* 2007; **157**: 491–497.

52 McQuarrie I. Idiopathic spontaneously occurring hypoglycemia in infants: clinical significance of problem and treatment. *Am J Dis Child* 1954; **87**: 399–428.

53 Rahier J, Guiot Y, Sempoux C. Persistent hyperinsulinaemic hypoglycemia of infancy: a heterogeneous syndrome unrelated to nesidioblastosis. *Arch Dis Child Fetal Neonatal Ed* 2000; **82**: F108–112.

54 Ashcroft FM. ATP-sensitive potassium channelopathies: focus on insulin secretion. *J Clin Invest* 2005; **115**: 2047–2058.

55 Dekelbab BH, Sperling MA. Recent advances in hyperinsulinemic hypoglycemia of infancy. *Acta Paediatr* 2006; **95**: 1157–1164.

56 Mathew PM, *et al.* Persistent neonatal hyperinsulinism. *Clin Pediatr (Phila)* 1988; **27**: 148–151.

57 Hussain K, Aynsley-Green A. Hyperinsulinaemic hypoglycemia in preterm neonates. *Arch Dis Child Fetal Neonatal Ed* 2004; **89**: F65–67.

58 Hussain K, Hindmarsh P, Aynsley-Green A. Neonates with symptomatic hyperinsulinemic hypoglycemia generate inappropriately low serum cortisol counterregulatory hormonal responses. *J Clin Endocrinol Metab* 2003; **88**: 4342–4347.

59 Nebesio TD, *et al.* Development of pulmonary hypertension in an infant treated with diazoxide. *J Pediatr Endocrinol Metab* 2007; **20**: 939–944.

60 Silvani P, *et al.* A case of severe diazoxide toxicity. *Paediatr Anaesth* 2004; **14**: 607–609.

61 Abu-Osba YK, Manasra KB, Mathew PM. Complications of diazoxide treatment in persistent neonatal hyperinsulinism. *Arch Dis Child* 1989; **64**: 1496–1500.

62 Bas F, *et al.* Successful therapy with calcium channel blocker (nifedipine) in persistent neonatal hyperinsulinemic hypoglycemia of infancy. *J Pediatr Endocrinol Metab* 1999; **12**: 873–878.

63 Eichmann D, *et al.* Treatment of hyperinsulinaemic hypoglycemia with nifedipine. *Eur J Pediatr* 1999; **158**: 204–206.

64 Hussain K, Aynsley-Green A, Stanley CA. Medications used in the treatment of hypoglycemia due to congenital hyperinsulinism of infancy (HI). *Pediatr Endocrinol Rev* 2004; **2** (Suppl 1): 163–167.

65 Greer RM, *et al.* Genotype–phenotype associations in patients with severe hyperinsulinism of infancy. *Pediatr Dev Pathol* 2007; **10**: 25–34.

66 Hardy OT, *et al.* Diagnosis and localization of focal congenital hyperinsulinism by 18F-fluorodopa PET scan. *J Pediatr* 2007; **150**: 140–145.

67 Ribeiro MJ, *et al.* Functional imaging of the pancreas: the role of [18F]fluoro-L-DOPA PET in the diagnosis of hyperinsulinism of infancy. *Endocr Dev* 2007; **12**: 55–66.

68 Peranteau WH, *et al.* Multiple ectopic lesions of focal islet adenomatosis identified by positron emission tomography scan in an infant with congenital hyperinsulinism. *J Pediatr Surg* 2007; **42**: 188–192.

69 Cade A, *et al.* Foregut dysmotility complicating persistent hyperinsulinaemic hypoglycemia of infancy. *J Pediatr Gastroenterol Nutr* 1998; **27**: 355–358.

70 Glaser B, Hirsch HJ, Landau H. Persistent hyperinsulinemic hypoglycemia of infancy: long-term octreotide treatment without pancreatectomy. *J Pediatr* 1993; **123**: 644–650.

71 Palladino AA, Bennett MJ, Stanley CA. Hyperinsulinism in infancy and childhood: when an insulin concentration is not always enough. *Clin Chem* 2008; **54**: 256–263.

72 Jack MM, *et al.* The outcome in Australian children with hyperinsulinism of infancy: early extensive surgery in severe cases lowers risk of diabetes. *Clin Endocrinol (Oxf)* 2003; **58**: 355–364.

73 Leibowitz G, *et al.* Hyperinsulinemic hypoglycemia of infancy (nesidioblastosis) in clinical remission: high incidence of diabetes mellitus and persistent beta-cell dysfunction at long-term follow-up. *J Clin Endocrinol Metab* 1995; **80**: 386–392.

74 Cherian MP, Abduljabbar MA. Persistent hyperinsulinemic hypoglycemia of infancy (PHHI): long-term outcome following 95% pancreatectomy. *J Pediatr Endocrinol Metab* 2005; **18**: 1441–1448.

75 Gussinyer M, *et al.* Glucose intolerance and diabetes are observed in the long-term follow-up of non-pancreatectomized patients with persistent hyperinsulinemic hypoglycemia of infancy due to mutations in the ABCC8 gene. *Diabetes Care*, 2008; **31**: 1257–1259.

76 Steinkrauss L, *et al.* Effects of hypoglycemia on developmental outcome in children with congenital hyperinsulinism. *J Pediatr Nurs* 2005; **20**: 109–118.

77 Meissner T, *et al.* Long-term follow-up of 114 patients with congenital hyperinsulinism. *Eur J Endocrinol* 2003; **149**: 43–51.

78 Stanley CA. Hyperinsulism/hyperammonemia syndrome: insights into the regulatory role of glutamate dehydrogenase in ammonia metabolism. *Mol Genet Metab* 2004; **81** (Suppl 1): S45–51.

79 Dullaart RP, *et al.* Family with autosomal dominant hyperinsulinism associated with A456V mutation in the glucokinase gene. *J Intern Med* 2004; **255**: 143–145.

80 Giurgea I, *et al.* Molecular mechanisms of neonatal hyperinsulinism. *Horm Res* 2006; **66**: 289–296.

81 Clayton PT, *et al.* Hyperinsulinism in short-chain L-3-hydroxyacyl-CoA dehydrogenase deficiency reveals the importance of beta-oxidation in insulin secretion. *J Clin Invest* 2001; **108**: 457–465.

82 Molven A, et al. Familial hyperinsulinemic hypoglycemia caused by a defect in the SCHAD enzyme of mitochondrial fatty acid oxidation. *Diabetes* 2004; **53**: 221–227.

83 Eklund EA, Freeze HH. The congenital disorders of glycosylation: a multifaceted group of syndromes. *NeuroRx* 2006; **3**: 254–263.

84 Freeze HH. Congenital disorders of glycosylation: CDG-I, CDG-II and beyond. *Curr Mol Med* 2007; **7**: 389–396.

85 Jaeken J, Matthijs G. Congenital disorders of glycosylation: a rapidly expanding disease family. *Annu Rev Genomics Hum Genet* 2007; **8**: 261–278.

86 Kapoor RR, et al. Persistent hyperinsulinaemic hypoglycemia and maturity onset diabetes of the young (MODY) due to heterozygous HNF4A mutations. *Diabetes* 2008; **57**: 1659–1663.

87 Fajans SS, Bell GI. Macrosomia and neonatal hypoglycemia in RW pedigree subjects with a mutation (Q268X) in the gene encoding hepatocyte nuclear factor 4alpha (HNF4A). *Diabetologia* 2007; **50**: 2600–2601.

88 Pearson ER, et al. Sensitivity to sulphonylureas in patients with hepatocyte nuclear factor-1alpha gene mutations: evidence for pharmacogenetics in diabetes. *Diabet Med* 2000; **17**: 543–545.

89 Pearson ER, et al. Macrosomia and hyperinsulinaemic hypoglycemia in patients with heterozygous mutations in the HNF4A gene. *PLoS Med* 2007; **4**: e118.

90 Hussain K, et al. Infantile hyperinsulinism associated with enteropathy, deafness and renal tubulopathy: clinical manifestations of a syndrome caused by a contiguous gene deletion located on chromosome 11p. *J Pediatr Endocrinol Metab* 2004; **17**: 1613–1621.

91 Bitner-Glindzicz M, et al. A recessive contiguous gene deletion causing infantile hyperinsulinism, enteropathy and deafness identifies the Usher type 1C gene. *Nat Genet* 2000; **26**: 56–60.

92 Hojlund K, et al. A novel syndrome of autosomal-dominant hyperinsulinemic hypoglycemia linked to a mutation in the human insulin receptor gene. *Diabetes* 2004; **53**: 1592–1598.

93 Otonkoski T, et al. Physical exercise-induced hypoglycemia caused by failed silencing of monocarboxylate transporter 1 in pancreatic beta cells. *Am J Hum Genet* 2007; **81**: 467–474.

94 Otonkoski T, et al. Physical exercise-induced hyperinsulinemic hypoglycemia is an autosomal-dominant trait characterized by abnormal pyruvate-induced insulin release. *Diabetes* 2003; **52**: 199–204.

95 Meissner T, et al. Exercise induced hypoglycaemic hyperinsulinism. *Arch Dis Child* 2001; **84**: 254–257.

96 de Groot JW, et al. Non-islet cell tumour-induced hypoglycemia: a review of the literature including two new cases. *Endocr Relat Cancer* 2007; **14**: 979–993.

97 Fineberg SE, et al. Immunological responses to exogenous insulin. *Endocr Rev* 2007; **28**: 625–652.

98 Schwartz NS, et al. Glycemic thresholds for activation of glucose counterregulatory systems are higher than the threshold for symptoms. *J Clin Invest* 1987; **79**: 777–781.

99 Santiago JV, et al. Epinephrine, norepinephrine, glucagon and growth hormone release in association with physiological decrements in the plasma glucose concentration in normal and diabetic man. *J Clin Endocrinol Metab* 1980; **51**: 877–883.

100 Hussain K, Hindmarsh P, Aynsley-Green A. Spontaneous hypoglycemia in childhood is accompanied by paradoxically low serum growth hormone and appropriate cortisol counterregulatory hormonal responses. *J Clin Endocrinol Metab* 2003; **88**: 3715–3723.

101 Nanao K, Anzo M, Hasegawa Y. Morning hypoglycemia leading to death in a child with congenital hypopituitarism. *Acta Paediatr* 1999; **88**: 1173.

102 Gazarian M, et al. The "4A" syndrome: adrenocortical insufficiency associated with achalasia, alacrima, autonomic and other neurological abnormalities. *Eur J Pediatr* 1995; **154**: 18–23.

103 Aynsley-Green A, Williamson DH, Gitzelmann R. Asymptomatic hepatic glycogen-synthetase deficiency. *Lancet* 1978; **1**: 147–148.

104 van den Berghe G. Disorders of gluconeogenesis. *J Inherit Metab Dis* 1996; **19**: 470–477.

105 Atkin BM, et al. Pyruvate carboxylase deficiency and lactic acidosis in a retarded child without Leigh's disease. *Pediatr Res* 1979; **13**: 109–116.

106 Olpin SE, et al. Features of carnitine palmitoyltransferase type I deficiency. *J Inherit Metab Dis* 2001; **24**: 35–42.

107 Clayton PT, et al. Screening for medium chain acyl-CoA dehydrogenase deficiency using electrospray ionisation tandem mass spectrometry. *Arch Dis Child* 1998; **79**: 109–115.

108 Aledo R, et al. Genetic basis of mitochondrial HMG-CoA synthase deficiency. *Hum Genet* 2001; **109**: 19–23.

109 Gibson KM, Breuer J, Nyhan WL. 3-Hydroxy-3-methylglutaryl-coenzyme A lyase deficiency: review of 18 reported patients. *Eur J Pediatr* 1988; **148**: 180–186.

110 Berry GT, et al. Neonatal hypoglycemia in severe succinyl-CoA: 3-oxoacid CoA-transferase deficiency. *J Inherit Metab Dis* 2001; **24**: 587–595.

111 Saudubray JM, et al. Clinical approach to inherited metabolic disorders in neonates. *Biol Neonate* 1990; **58** (Suppl 1): 44–53.

112 Daly LP, Osterhoudt KC, Weinzimer SA. Presenting features of idiopathic ketotic hypoglycemia. *J Emerg Med* 2003; **25**: 39–43.

113 Online Mendelian Inheritance in Man (OMIM), Johns Hopkins University, Baltimore, MD. www.ncbi.nlm.nih.gov/omim

114 Glaser B, et al. Intragenic single nucleotide polymorphism haplotype analysis of SUR1 mutations in familial hyperinsulinism. *Hum Mutat* 1999; **14**: 23–29.

115 Babenko AP, Aguilar-Bryan L, Bryan J. A view of sur/KIR6.X, KATP channels. *Annu Rev Physiol* 1998; **60**: 667–687.

20 Childhood Obesity

Michael Freemark

Division of Pediatric Endocrinology and Diabetes, Duke University Medical Center, Durham, NC, USA

The prevalence of obesity in young people has increased dramatically during the past generation; the problem now impacts developing as well as industrialized nations and exacts an enormous toll on medical, social and financial communities [1–3]. The causes of this obesity epidemic include changes in food intake, composition, availability and cost, as well as modifications of lifestyle that affect energy expenditure.

Obesity in children predisposes to subsequent adult obesity and to metabolic co-morbidities including insulin resistance and type 2 diabetes, dyslipidemia, hypertension, hepatic steatosis/steatohepatitis, focal glomerulosclerosis, ovarian hyperandrogenism, gynecomastia, cholecystitis, pancreatitis, pseudotumor cerebri and obstructive sleep apnea. Long-standing obesity and insulin resistance in children and adults increase the risks of subsequent cardiovascular disease and some malignancies.

The treatment of obesity aims to:

1 Reduce body mass index (BMI) and fat mass;

2 Normalize glucose tolerance, plasma lipid concentrations, hepatic and renal function and blood pressure; and

3 Prevent or reverse acute and chronic co-morbidities.

These objectives can sometimes be achieved through lifestyle intervention (caloric restriction and exercise). Pharmacologic agents or surgical intervention may reinforce the effects of diet and exercise and reduce the risk of, or even reverse, complications. In all cases, the social milieu functions as a critical determinant of therapeutic success.

Fat deposition in health and illness

The accumulation of fat in normal weight individuals follows a predictable pattern. Body fat content is low in the fetus until 30 weeks' gestation but then increases markedly to a peak of 14–15% at birth. Fat increases after birth to 25% at 6 months of age,

Brook's Clinical Pediatric Endocrinology, 6th edition. Edited by C. Brook, P. Clayton, R. Brown. © 2009 Blackwell Publishing, ISBN: 978-1-4051-8080-1.

declining thereafter to age 5–8 years before rising again. Adiposity rebound is of greater magnitude and occurs earlier in children destined to become obese in later childhood and adolescence [4–8]. Before and during the early puberty, fat mass increases in both boys and girls; after mid-puberty, body fat content continues to rise in girls but declines in boys in parallel with a sharp increase in lean body mass.

Excess fat deposition in childhood or adulthood reflects an imbalance (Fig. 20.1) between energy intake (food ingestion and gastrointestinal absorption) and energy expenditure, which comprises basal (resting) metabolism (determined largely by lean body mass), physical activity (purposeful and otherwise) and the thermogenic responses to feeding and cold exposure (which account for approximately 10% of total daily energy expenditure). An increase in energy intake and/or a decline in energy expenditure limit lipolysis and stimulate lipogenesis, thereby promoting fat storage (Fig. 20.2). The effects of chronic energy surfeit are mediated partly by increases in insulin production but a fall in growth hormone secretion may contribute. Nutrients may also have direct metabolic actions that promote weight gain: in the presence of carbohydrate, saturated fat limits triglyceride breakdown; concentrated glucose and fructose on the other hand are lipogenic.

Defining obesity

Obesity means an excess of fat relative to lean body mass. In the absence of standardized measures of body fatness, BMI (weight in kilograms divided by the square of the height in meters) serves as a useful surrogate, is easily obtained in clinic settings and correlates strongly with percent body fat and risks of co-morbidities in obese subjects. Age- and gender-dependent BMI (e.g. www.cdc.gov/nccdphp/dnpa/bmi/calc-bmi.htm) and BMI Z standards (http://stokes.chop.edu/web/zscore/) are now widely available. Children with BMI in the 85–95th centiles for age and gender are considered overweight, while those with BMI exceeding 30 kg/m^2 >95th centile for age and gender are termed obese. Increases in lean body muscle mass in adolescent boys may raise BMI without an increase in fat deposition but virtually all children and teenagers considered obese by BMI standards have excess fat. Weight-for-recumbent length centiles are used for infants and toddlers; those with values over 95th centile are considered overweight.

The relationship between BMI and body fat varies with race and ethnicity so that, at any given BMI, Mexican-American and Asian children have relatively more fat and African-American children less fat than White children [9,10]. These differences may have important implications for the risk of type 2 diabetes and cardiovascular disease.

Measures other than BMI may correlate as well or better with percent body fat and co-morbidities. For example, skinfold

thickness correlates with total body fat and with blood pressure, lipid concentrations and insulin sensitivity. Measuring skinfolds is not easy and impossible in the very obese. Waist circumference measurements in children correlate with systolic and diastolic blood pressure, fasting insulin and markers of dyslipidemia and are related inversely to adiponectin concentrations and insulin sensitivity [11]. Waist circumference, which provides an estimate of visceral fat mass and varies with age, gender and ethnicity (Fig. 20.3) [12], may be a better predictor of childhood blood pressure, high density lipoprotein (HDL) and low density lipoprotein (LDL) concentrations than BMI [13]. BMI and skinfold thickness are better measures of subcutaneous adipose tissue stores.

Causes of obesity

Roles of genetics and environment
Genetic factors contribute to the risk of childhood obesity [14–17] and a number of deactivating genetic mutations have been identified in children with early-onset progressive weight gain. These monogenic obesity syndromes are described in detail in Chapter 22 but a variety of other complex genetic syndromes are associated with weight gain in early or mid-childhood (Table 20.1).

The roles of genetic variation in the development of non-syndromic "exogenous" or polygenic obesity in childhood are poorly understood. Family congruence and racial or ethnic differences in weight gain are often assumed to reflect inborn genetic traits; the high rates of overweight and obesity among African-American, Latino and American-Indian children are well documented [18] but work with the Pima Indians in Mexico and the USA suggests that the development of obesity and type 2 diabetes in genetically prone populations are determined, at least partly, by environmental factors [19]. Obesity is 10 times more common

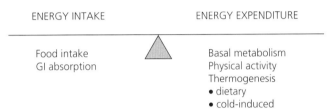

Figure 20.1 Energy balance. GI, gastrointestinal.

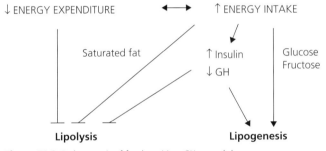

Figure 20.2 Pathogenesis of fat deposition. GH, growth hormone.

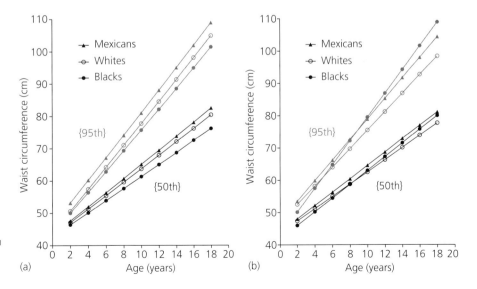

Figure 20.3 Waist circumference measurements in various ethnic groups. (a) Boys. (b) Girls. Redrawn from Fernandez *et al.* [12] with permission.

Table 20.1 Complex syndromes associated with obesity [18–20].

Syndrome	Characteristics of obesity	Key clinical features	Genetic marker
Prader–Willi syndrome	Early childhood onset (6 months to 6 years), voracious appetite	Neonatal hypotonia and failure to thrive, mental retardation, developmental delay, short stature, cryptorchidism, hypogonadism, obsessive compulsive behavior, paradoxical hyperghrelinemia, relative hyperadiponectinemia	Paternally derived 15q11–q13 deletion or maternal UPD 15 (OMIM 176270)
Albright hereditary osteodystrophy	Moderate obesity	Short stature, mental deficiency, short metacarpals and metatarsals, variable hypocalcemia and hyperphosphatemia with elevated PTH levels, primary hypothyroidism and hypogonadism	Mutations GNAS1 at 20q13.2, autosomal dominant (OMIM 103580)
Fragile X syndrome	Early onset	Moderate to severe mental retardation, macroorchidism, macrocephaly, prominent jaw, high-pitched jocular speech	FMR1 gene (OMIM 309550)
Lawrence–Moon–Bardet–Biedl	Obesity beginning toddler or late childhood	Mental deficiency (mild to moderate), retinal dystrophy, polydactyly, renal cysts/disease, hypogonadism, anosmia	Multiple loci, recessive transmission (OMIM 245880/209900)
Alström	Mild truncal obesity develops in childhood	Retinopathy, sensorineural hearing loss, type 2 diabetes mellitus, nephropathy, dilated cardiomyopathy, late-onset short stature, variable hypothyroidism, hypogonadism, and hepatic fibrosis	Autosomal recessive ALMS1 at 2p13 (OMIM 203800)
WAGR	Early onset, persistent hyperphagia	Wilms tumour, aniridia, genitourinary anomalies, mental retardation, obesity in patients with BDNF haploinsufficiency	Heterozygous deletions of 11p13 with haploinsufficiency of WT1, PAX6; 11p14 deletions lead to BDNF haploinsufficiency
Borjeson–Forssman–Lehman	School-age onset, moderate obesity	Hypotonia, developmental delay, mental deficiency, short stature, large ears, hypogonadism and gynecomastia	Mutations PHF6 at Xq26–27 (OMIM 301900)
Killian/Teschler–Nicola syndrome (Pallister Killian syndrome)	Postnatal obesity	Mental retardation, seizures, hypotonia	Tetrasomy 12p, mosaic isochromosome 12p syndrome (OMIM 601803)
Cohen syndrome	Mild truncal obesity mid-childhood onset	Hypotonia, short stature, prominent incisors, microcephaly, mild psychomotor retardation, joint laxity, variable neutropenia, retinochoroidal dystrophy	Autosomal recessive, COH1 at 8q22–q23 (OMIM 216550)
Carpenter syndrome	Late childhood onset obesity	Acrocephaly, syndactyly, polydactyly, mental retardation, hypogonadism	Autosomal recessive (OMIM 201000)
SIM 1 deficiency	Early onset	Hyperphagia and increased linear growth	SIM 1 deletion resulting translocation of 1p22.1 and 6q16.2
Down syndrome	Increased weight, particularly in adolescence	Hypotonia, mental retardation, developmental delay	Trisomy 21 (OMIM 190685)

BDNF, brain-induced neurotropic factor; OMIM, Online Mendelian Inheritance in Man (available at: http://www.ncbi.nlm.nih.gov/omim/); PTH, parathyroid hormone.

in US Pima men and three times more frequent in US Pima women than in their Mexican counterparts, even though the Mexican and American Pima populations are genetically similar (as determined by tree analysis of 309 DNA markers). Type 2 diabetes is five times more common in US Pima Indians than in Mexican Pima Indians.

A study in monozygotic and dizygotic twins suggested that household environment accounts for 50% of the variation in adolescent overweight while genetic effects account for 32% [15]. A few genetic variants have been reproducibly associated with non-syndromic obesity or treatment response: for example, single nucleotide polymorphisms in the FTO (fat mass and obesity associated or "fatso") gene were associated with obesity (odds ratio 1.20–1.67) and fat deposition in Caucasian and African-American children and adults although not in children of Chinese or Oceanic origin [20–22].

The FTO gene is expressed in adipose tissue and in the arcuate nucleus and is downregulated by fasting and exposure to cold. A deletion of the chromosomal region containing the FTO gene was accompanied by obesity, mental retardation and digital anomalies in a single individual. This and other genetic associations explain only some of the variation in rates of childhood obesity or co-morbidities [23]. More importantly, the worldwide increase in childhood obesity during the past generation cannot be ascribed to genetic factors alone. It is clear that environmental influences interact powerfully with genetic factors in the development of childhood and adult obesity and its complications.

Roles of environmental and perinatal influences

A variety of societal and environmental factors have contributed to the rise in childhood obesity in the general population:
1 Widespread availability of low-cost energy-dense fast food and sugary drinks and the relatively high cost of nutrient-dense (protein/vitamin) "healthy" foods;
2 Increasing adoption of sedentary lifestyles associated with higher screen (television, computer, cell phone) times, cutbacks on school physical activity, reductions in outdoor play (resulting from concerns about neighborhood safety) and the "professionalization" of childhood sports; and

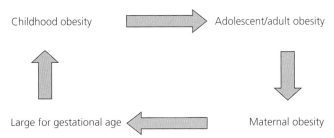

Figure 20.4 A transgenerational cycle of obesity in women.

3 Stress and/or time constraints on parents and children with family/meal disruption and reductions in sleep duration, which correlate with obesity rates [24,25].

There is also increasing evidence that the metabolic milieu of pregnancy and the perinatal period plays a critical part in the pathogenesis of childhood obesity and its complications. Children born to obese mothers or to women with gestational diabetes have two- to threefold increased risks for developing obesity and type 2 diabetes in adolescence and adulthood [26–30]. This facilitates a vicious cycle among women in which obesity and type 2 diabetes can be transmitted across generations (Fig. 20.4).

Children born prematurely or growth retarded *in utero* also have increased risks of obesity and type 2 diabetes if they show rapid and excessive catch-up growth during early childhood [4–8, 31–33]. Pathogenic mechanisms in the latter case (Fig. 20.5) include precocious induction of hepatic gluconeogenesis (GNG), inadequate muscle development and β-cell hypoplasia.

A number of environmental influences preferentially target high-risk racial or ethnic groups (Table 20.2) [26–30,33–47]: disproportionate rates of poverty and educational failure, high rates of maternal obesity and gestational diabetes, premature birth and intra-uterine growth failure, low rates of breastfeeding, excessive intake of fast food and higher rates of sleep deprivation. Thus, race and ethnicity may sometimes serve as markers for environmental or socio-economic status rather than for biologic or genetic risk.

Metabolic and hormonal disorders

Hormonal disorders commonly associated with weight gain and increases in the ratio of fat to lean body mass (Fig. 20.6) include growth hormone (GH) deficiency, hypothyroidism,

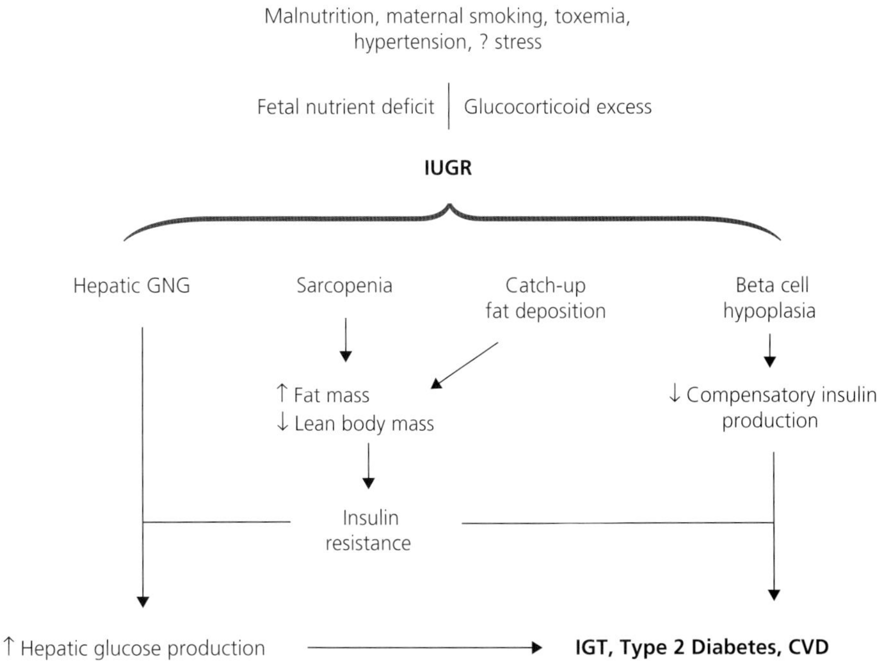

Malnutrition, maternal smoking, toxemia, hypertension, ? stress

Fetal nutrient deficit | Glucocorticoid excess

IUGR

Hepatic GNG   Sarcopenia   Catch-up fat deposition   Beta cell hypoplasia

↑ Fat mass
↓ Lean body mass

↓ Compensatory insulin production

Insulin resistance

↑ Hepatic glucose production ⟶ **IGT, Type 2 Diabetes, CVD**

Figure 20.5 Pathogenesis of glucose intolerance and cardiovascular disease in subjects born small for gestational age. CVD, cardiovascular disease; GNG, gluconeogenesis; IGT, impaired glucose tolerance; IUGR, intra-uterine growth retardation.

Table 20.2 Socio-economic and "environmental" risk factors that may contribute to racial/ethnic differences in rates of childhood obesity.

Factor	Racial difference
Socio-economic status (SES)/ income and educational attainment [34,35]	Poverty and low educational status predict overweight and obesity in Westernized countries. The strength of this correlation in adolescents varies among races, particularly in girls. Conversely, among adult females in developing nations, rates of overweight correlate positively with SES
	In the USA the prevalence of overweight decreases with increasing SES/educational level among White (−19.5%) and Latina (−14.2%) females. Prevalence decreases in African-American girls with increasing SES/educational level (−5.9%), but still exceeds that of Caucasian and Hispanic females of the same SES. Obesity rates do not decline with increasing SES in Latino (+2.1%) or African-American males (+5.8%)
Maternal obesity [27–29,36–38]	Maternal obesity increases by 2.5- to 5-fold the rate of GDM and by 3-fold the rate of childhood overweight by age 7. 63% of obese pregnant women are Latino, 23% African-American and 14% White
Maternal gestational diabetes mellitus (GDM) [26,30,36–38]	Maternal GDM increases by 3-fold the risk of being overweight in adolescence and increases sharply the risk of type 2 diabetes in adolescence and adulthood. African-American (OR 1.17), Latino (OR 1.44), and Asian/Pacific Islander (OR 2.05) women are more likely to develop GDM than White women
Prematurity/low birthweight [27,33,40]	Low birthweight with rapid catch-up growth increases risks for obesity and type 2 diabetes. Rates of preterm birth and low birthweight are higher in African-Americans (12.6–15.3%) than in Whites (6.3–8.4%). Mean birthweight in subcontinental Indian children is only 2700 g, reflecting their mothers' low caloric intake and body fat content
Breastfeeding [41–43]	Breastfeeding may protect against childhood obesity. 60% of White, 54% of Latino, and 26% of African-American children are ever breastfed. African-Americans have consistently lower breastfeeding rates than Whites, regardless of SES (difference of 17.6–30.7% depending on education/income)
Diet quality [44,45]	Low cost diets are typically energy dense and nutrient poor; protein/micronutrient/vitamin-rich diets are expensive. Low income in Western countries favors intake of low-cost fast foods, snacks and sweets. African-American teens have the highest consumption of energy-dense diets
Sleep duration [24,25,46]	Sleep duration may vary inversely with the risk of childhood obesity. Mean sleep duration is ~3 h/week less in African-American children than in White children
Neighborhood safety [47]	Parental perception of home neighborhood as unsafe was associated with an increased risk of overweight at the age of 7 years. African-American parents more likely than Whites to describe home neighborhoods as unsafe

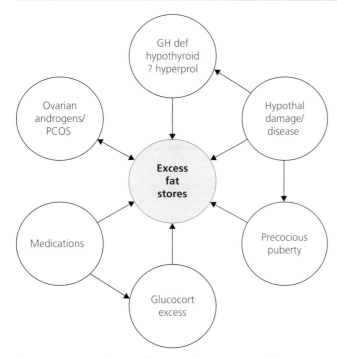

Figure 20.6 Hormonal causes of excess weight gain. GH, growth hormone; Glucort, glucocorticoid; Hyperprol, hyperprolactinemia; Hypothal, hypothalamic; PCOS, polycystic ovary syndrome.

glucocorticoid excess and the polycystic ovarian syndrome (PCOS). Pathogenic mechanisms (Table 20.3) include hyperphagia, increased rates of lipogenesis and decreased lipolysis (owing in part to increases in insulin production and adipose insulin sensitivity), sarcopenia and/or reductions in total body energy expenditure. Ovarian hyperandrogenism may be a consequence rather than a cause of obesity, given the ability of insulin to stimulate ovarian androgen production (see below). Obesity also reduces GH secretion but does not cause true GH deficiency because linear growth is preserved and in some cases enhanced. Centripetal weight gain is often but not always marked in glucocorticoid excess but abdominal fat increase is also noted in hypothyroidism, PCOS and GH deficiency. The latter may be related in part to induction of 11β-hydroxysteroid dehydrogenase 1 in visceral or abdominal fat, resulting in local overproduction of cortisol [48].

Hyperprolactinemia has been associated with weight gain in men and women with prolactinomas [49]; hypogonadism probably plays an important part but direct effects of prolactin on food intake and adipogenesis may also contribute. The relation between prolactin and weight gain in children is less clear but,

Table 20.3 Mechanisms of weight gain in hormonal disorders.

Hormonal disorder	Major mechanisms
GH deficiency	Increased insulin sensitivity
	Increased lipogenesis, decreased lipolysis
	Increased 11β-HSD-1 in abdominal/viceral fat
	Sarcopenia and decreased resting energy expenditure
Hypothyroidism	Reduced resting energy expenditure
	Decreased exercise
	? Sarcopenia
Glucocorticoid excess	Hyperphagia
	Increased adipogenesis
	Sarcopenia
PCOS/ovarian hyperandrogenism	? Hyperinsulinemia
Hyperprolactinemia (variable)	Hypogonadism
	? Increased food intake
	? Increased adipogenesis
"Hypothalamic obesity"	Central leptin resistance with hyperphagia
	Heightened vagal tone with hyperinsulinemia
	GH deficiency, hypothyroidism, +/− precocious puberty
	Glucocorticoid excess (surgical and postop periods)

GH, growth hormone; HSD, hydroxysteroid dehydrogenase; PCOS, polycystic ovarian syndrome.

Table 20.4 Medications commonly associated with weight gain and/or dyslipidemia [62].

Weight gain
Atypical antipsychotics
Glucocorticoids (including high-dose inhaled)
Sex steroids: medroxyprogesterone, oral contraceptives
Hypoglycemic agents: insulin, sulfonylureas and thiazolidinediones
Tricyclic antidepressants
Anti-epileptics: valproate, gabapentin

Dyslipidemia

Medication	Triglycerides	HDL
Estrogens	Increased	Increased
Androgens	Increased	Decreased
Progestins	Decreased	Decreased
Glucocorticoids	Increased	Increased
Thiazides	Increased	Decreased
Beta-blockers	Increased	Decreased
Valproic acid	Increased	Decreased
Isotretinoin	Increased	Decreased
Ciclosporin	Increased	Increased
Tacrolimus	Increased	Increased
Protease inhibitors	Increased	–

among 50 pediatric patients with prolactinomas, 50% were overweight and 4% were obese [56].

Hyperprolactinemia may result from hypothalamic damage or disease. Damage to the ventromedial hypothalamus following surgery for craniopharynigioma often produces insatiable appetite and progressive weight gain [51–55]. Reductions in basal metabolic rate and physical activity contribute to hypothalamic obesity [55]. These in turn predispose to glucose intolerance and hepatic steatohepatitis, which in some cases progresses to cirrhosis. Deficiencies of GH, thyroid hormone and glucocorticoids are common in this setting; many patients have diabetes insipidus and some have precocious puberty, which can promote fat deposition, particularly in girls. The insatiable appetite and obesity probably result from central leptin resistance and heightened vagal tone with hyperinsulinemia. Associated hormonal abnormalities, as well as the use of high dose glucocorticoids around surgery facilitate the weight gain.

Role of drugs and medications

Many medications are associated with weight gain and dyslipidemia (Table 20.4) [56]. Clinicians should begin aggressive lifestyle intervention before or immediately after surgery when hypothalamic damage or long-term use of glucocorticoids or other high-risk medications are anticipated.

Screening for genetic and hormonal causes

Genetic screening should be considered for children with excessive weight gain beginning in infancy and for obese children with dysmorphic features and/or developmental delay. Commercial screening is now available for measurements of plasma leptin and for detection of mutations in the melanocortin 4 receptor and GNAS 1 genes and deletions or methylation abnormalities of chromosome 15 characteristic of Prader–Willi syndrome. With the very rare exception of primary leptin deficiency, there is currently no specific therapy for the hyperphagia characteristic of these disorders. Nevertheless, the identification of genetic mutations provides an explanation for the child's phenotype and insight into the probable course of the disease. The family may benefit from advice regarding risks in current and future family members.

The medical history, physical examination and growth chart should provide important clues regarding the likelihood of a hormonal or neurologic disorder which might explain the child's weight gain. In general, hormonal disorders are less likely. Bone age X-rays must be interpreted with caution because marked weight gain alone will advance bone maturation; conversely, bone age may not be advanced or delayed in children whose hormonal disorders are of recent onset.

Metabolic adaptations to weight gain and the development of insulin resistance

Clinical investigations and studies in experimental animals suggest that excess energy intake and fat deposition are accompanied in the short term by increases in plasma insulin, leptin and triiodothyronine (T3) and reductions in insulin sensitivity and plasma ghrelin, an orexigenic hormone produced by the stomach. These adaptations serve to attenuate food intake and increase energy expenditure, thereby limiting the rate of weight gain (Fig. 20.7). However, in the face of chronic caloric excess and obesity, the effects of insulin and leptin on appetite appear to be blunted although not abolished [57–60].

In peripheral tissues, leptin and adiponectin increase insulin sensitivity so the development of leptin resistance and the fall in

plasma adiponectin concentrations contribute to the development of insulin resistance in obesity. The pathogenesis of the condition is complex (Fig. 20.8) [61–63].

A critical role is postulated for adipokines [interleukin 6 (IL-6), plasminogen activator inhibitor-1 (PAI-1), retinol binding protein-4 (RBP-4) and monocyte chemoattractant protein-1 (MCP-1)] and inflammatory cytokines [tumor necrosis factor α (TNF-α) and resistin] produced by white adipose tissue and infiltrating macrophages. In concert with hypoadiponectinemia and leptin resistance, the adipokines and inflammatory cytokines attenuate fatty acid oxidation in liver and skeletal muscle, thereby promoting the accumulation of diacylglycerol, ceramides and triglyceride in myocytes and hepatocytes.

These in turn impair mitochondrial function and endoplasmic reticulum protein-processing and raise the intracellular concentrations of reactive oxygen species, which in combination activate serine kinases that induce serine phosphorylation of insulin receptor substrate 1 (IRS-1), a major intracellular mediator of insulin action. The resulting resistance to insulin action impairs hepatic insulin clearance, increases hepatic glucose production, reduces skeletal muscle glucose and amino acid uptake and utilization and increases lipolysis in white adipose tissue. These in turn raise peripheral concentrations of glucose, free fatty acids and branched chain amino acids, thereby completing a vicious cycle.

In blocking the lipogenic effects of insulin in adipose tissue, the emergence of insulin resistance may limit further weight gain but insulin resistance has deleterious effects on metabolic function.

Metabolic complications

Impaired glucose tolerance and type 2 diabetes mellitus

Type 2 diabetes, which was nearly unknown in children 20 years ago, now accounts for 15% or more of all cases of diabetes in

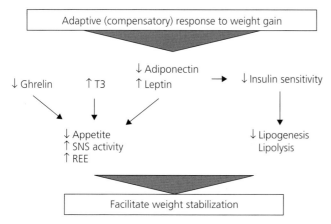

Figure 20.7 Adaptive response to weight gain. REE, resting energy expenditure; SNS, sympathetic nervous system; T3, triiodothyronine.

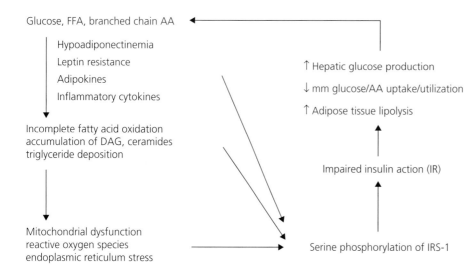

Figure 20.8 Pathogenesis of insulin resistance in obesity. AA, amino acids; DAG, diacylglycerol; FFA, free fatty acids; IRS-1, insulin receptor substrate 1.

American children aged 10–19 years [64]. The great majority of children with type 2 diabetes are obese but poorly defined familial/racial/genetic factors also have important roles in diabetogenesis. The disease occurs more commonly in African-Americans, Hispanic-Americans, American-Indians, Pacific Islanders and South Asians than in Caucasians (relative incidence per 100 000 person-years: American-Indian children 25.3 in 10- to 14-year-olds, 49.4 in 15- to 19-year-olds; African-American 22.3; 19.4; Asian/Pacific Islander 11.8; 22.7; Hispanic 8.9; 17.0; Whites 3.0; 5.6) and is far more prevalent in those with a family history [65–68]. The prevalence of diabetes increases markedly after the onset of puberty, owing to growth hormone- and sex steroid-antagonism of insulin action.

Risk is modified by events that occur before or immediately after birth: the disease occurs more frequently in children whose mothers were obese or diabetic during pregnancy [26–30,68] and in children born small for gestational age, particularly if there is rapid catch-up growth in early childhood [31–33,69–71]. Rates of type 2 diabetes mellitus are higher in girls (1.7-fold) than boys. Teenage girls and young women with ovarian hyperandrogenism or PCOS are at high risk; prepubertal girls with adrenarche also appear to be vulnerable as they develop [72,73].

The pathogenesis of glucose intolerance is complex and controversial [61–63,74–76]. Most evidence suggests that metabolic dysfunction commences with resistance to insulin action (Fig. 20.9). Accumulation of abdominal subcutaneous and visceral fat, which appear to have heightened sensitivity to the lipolytic effects of catecholamines, associates strongly with insulin resistance, while insulin sensitivity correlates less well with stores of femoral and gluteal subcutaneous fat [75–76]. Plasma insulin concentrations are elevated, a consequence of nutrient, hormone and vagal dependent increases in insulin synthesis and secretion and reduced hepatic insulin clearance. The acute insulin secretory response to glucose may be blunted in those destined to develop glucose intolerance.

Progression from insulin resistance with hyperinsulinemia to impaired fasting glucose (IFG) and impaired glucose tolerance (IGT or prediabetes) is modulated by genetic, perinatal, nutritional and inflammatory factors, which induce β-cell mitochondrial dysfunction and oxidative and endoplasmic reticulum stress in susceptible people. Cellular function is further compromised by toxic effects exerted by free fatty acids in the presence of hyperglycemia (glucolipotoxicity), islet inflammation and O-linked glycosylation of proteins. These factors together cause β-cell dysfunction and apoptosis with dysregulation of basal insulin secretion, loss of first-phase glucose-dependent insulin secretion and altered insulin processing, revealed as an increase in the circulating ratio of proinsulin to insulin [63].

Overt glucose intolerance and type 2 diabetes are characterized by a decline in total insulin production, relative or absolute hypoinsulinemia, a reduction in β-cell mass and, in some but not all cases, deposition of amyloid in the pancreatic islets.

Various auxologic and metabolic factors predict the risk of type 2 diabetes in adolescents and children. Longitudinal studies [66,77,78] in the Pima Indians found that the strongest predictors of diabetes before the age of 30 years were intra-uterine exposure to diabetes (5.9-fold increase), parental history of diabetes (3.6-fold increase), childhood waist circumference, BMI and the 2-h glucose concentration during an oral glucose tolerance test. Lower plasma HDL concentrations and higher fasting glucose and insulin concentrations also predicted diabetes risk. A website that employs these findings can be used to assess (imperfectly) a child's risk of developing type 2 diabetes (http://intramural.niddk.nih.gov/research/T2Diabetescalc/startPage.shtml).

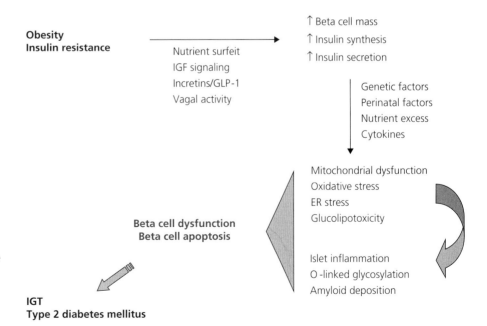

Figure 20.9 Pathogenesis of glucose intolerance in obesity and insulin resistance. ER, endoplasmic reticulum; GLP-1, glucagons-like peptide 1; IGF, insulin-like growth factor; IGT, impaired glucose tolerance.

In a mixed ethnic group of markedly obese adolescents followed for 20 months, the best predictors of type 2 diabetes were pre-existing impaired glucose tolerance, BMI Z score, rate of weight gain, disposition index (a measure of insulin secretion relative to insulin sensitivity) and ethnicity; African-American children were at highest risk [79]. Their predilection to childhood type 2 diabetes is thought to reflect a lower hepatic insulin sensitivity and an inadequate insulin secretory response to insulin resistance [80–82]. When matched for BMI and total body fat, obese African-American children and adolescents have more severe insulin resistance despite lesser visceral and hepatic adipose stores than obese Caucasian children [80,82]. It is currently unclear if racial or ethnic differences in fat distribution and diabetes prevalence reflect genetic variations or environmental influences such as diet, physical activity, stress or the intra-uterine milieu.

Dyslipidemia

Abnormalities in plasma lipids [reductions in plasma HDL concentrations and increases in plasma very low density lipoprotein (VLDL) cholesterol] are detected in 12–17% of overweight and obese children [83–87]. Triglyceride (TG) concentrations are elevated more commonly in obese White than in obese African-American children and adolescents. The reduction in plasma HDL results from exchange of VLDL-TG for cholesterol esters in HDL which increases renal HDL clearance. Hypertriglyceridemia reflects impaired TG clearance because of downregulation of lipoprotein lipase as well as heightened hepatic VLDL-TG production. Serum cholesterol and LDL are usually normal or moderately increased.

The lipid profile changes with sexual maturation: plasma cholesterol and LDL concentrations in normal weight subjects decline approximately 15% in boys and 5% in girls during puberty, while TG concentrations rise. Conversely, HDL concentrations fall in pubertal boys but not girls. In obese boys, puberty reduces total cholesterol, LDL and HDL concentrations but not TG concentrations. Similar changes of lesser magnitude are noted in pubertal girls.

Hepatic steatosis/steatohepatitis

Severe obesity in adults and children predisposes to liver fat deposition (steatosis), hepatic inflammation (steatohepatitis) and elevations in serum alanine and aspartate aminotransferase (ALT and AST) concentrations [88–93]. A subset of adults and children with fatty liver disease progresses to hepatic fibrosis and cirrhosis, which increase the long-term risks of hepatocellular carcinoma and hepatic failure [94,95].

The pathogenesis of hepatocellular dysfunction in obesity is beginning to emerge [96,97]. Free fatty acids (FFA) diverted or released in excess (as a consequence of insulin resistance) from visceral and subcutaneous fat are utilized for triglyceride synthesis, begetting the fatty liver common in obese subjects. Dietary fructose and fat and de novo lipogenesis may also contribute to hepatic fat accumulation. Lipid storage is facilitated by a resistance to or a relative deficiency of leptin and adiponectin, which

normally stimulate tissue fatty acid oxidation and inhibit lipogenesis [61,62]. In combination with inflammatory cytokines including TNF-α, MCP-1, IL-1β and IL-6, which block hepatic fatty acid oxidation, the accumulation of FFA and lipid metabolites may impair mitochondrial function, leading to oxidative and endoplasmic reticulum stress, hepatic inflammation and hepatocyte necrosis.

In severe cases, hepatic fibrosis may be facilitated by fibrogenic factors released by inflammatory cells and by leptin and angiotensin II, which promote fibrogenesis. Hepatic insulin resistance derives from induction of serine kinases that phosphorylate insulin signaling molecules like IRS-1. This explains why hepatic steatosis and increases in serum aminotransferase concentrations are commonly accompanied by insulin resistance and glucose intolerance [88–93]. Hypertension, dyslipidemia and increases in carotid intimal medial thickness are more common in obese adolescents with fatty liver disease than in obese adolescents without hepatic steatosis.

Factors predisposing to hepatic steatosis, aminotransferase elevations, steatohepatitis and cirrhosis in adults include visceral adiposity and insulin resistance, type 2 diabetes, excessive alcohol intake, increasing age, male gender and Hispanic or Asian ethnicity. Insulin resistance and type 2 diabetes predispose to hepatic steatosis in children as well as adults: among 127 obese adolescents with mean BMI 35.2, 23% had serum ALT concentrations exceeding 40 U/L [89,90].

An autopsy study [90] of 742 children between 2 and 19 years of age found that 38% of obese subjects had fatty liver. ALT concentrations and rates of hepatic fat accumulation are higher in obese boys than in girls and in Hispanics and Caucasians than in African-Americans. For example, elevated ALT concentrations (>40 U/L) were detected 50% more frequently in Caucasian teenagers and 2.5 times more frequently in Hispanic teenagers than in African-American teens and fatty liver disease was five times more common in Hispanics and 2.7 times more common in Caucasian children than in African-American children [88,89].

Hypertension

Systolic hypertension is 3.3 times more common in obese children than in normal weight children; 30–50% of obese teenagers are affected, boys more frequently than girls [98]. Diastolic hypertension is less common than systolic hypertension. The disorder may manifest first as a loss of the normal blood pressure decline during sleep. Subsequently, the rise in pressure is detected throughout the day. Hypertension in obesity appears to result from vasoconstriction and sodium and water retention (Fig. 20.10) [99–101]. These are the consequence of:

1 Leptin-dependent activation of the sympathetic nervous system (SNS), which induces vasoconstriction through catecholamine secretion;

2 Hypoadiponectinemia, which reduces insulin sensitivity and endothelial nitric oxide synthesis and thereby limits vasodilatation; and

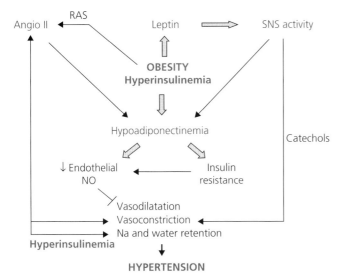

Figure 20.10 Pathogenesis of hypertension in obesity. Angio, angiotensin; NO, nitrous oxide; RAS, renin-angiotensin system; SNS, sympathetic nervous system.

3 Activation of the renin-angiotensin system and a rise in angiotensin II production, which reduces adiponectin secretion, promotes vasoconstriction, enhances aldosterone production and, in combination with hyperinsulinemia, increases salt and water retention.

Metabolic syndrome

The constellation of abdominal adiposity, dyslipidemia, glucose intolerance and hypertension has been termed the metabolic syndrome. Many but not all studies suggest that the combination of factors identifies individuals at high risk of type 2 diabetes and cardiovascular disease more effectively than any of the individual factors alone [68,102–105].

An expert task force of the International Diabetes Federation [106] proposed the following criteria for metabolic syndrome in children aged 10–16 years:

- Abdominal adiposity manifest as waist circumference >90th centile (alternatively, many investigators have used BMI >95th centile) for age, gender and ethnicity, plus two or more of the following:
- Triglycerides ≥1.7 mmol (150 mg%);
- HDL <1.03 mmol (40 mg%);
- Blood pressure ≥130 mmHg systolic or ≥85 mmHg diastolic;
- Fasting glucose ≥5.6 mmol (100 mg%) or known type 2 diabetes.

For adolescents over the age of 16 years the task force recommended use of the existing adult criteria, which specify absolute gender- and ethnicity-dependent waist circumference measurements as well as a cutoff of 50 mg% for HDL in women.

Studies in mixed groups of obese White, Black and Latino children and adolescents report the prevalence of the metabolic syndrome increasing markedly with the severity of obesity; in one study, each 0.5 unit increase in BMI Z score was associated with a 55% increase in risk [102]. A 25–30 year follow-up study of Black (28%) and White (72%) Americans found that the metabolic syndrome in childhood (age 5–19 years) predicts a 9.4-fold increase in the odds of metabolic syndrome and an 11.5-fold increased risk of type 2 diabetes in adulthood [105].

Linear growth and bone maturation

Rates of linear growth and bone maturation are often increased in obese prepubertal children despite marked reductions in basal and stimulated GH concentrations and a reduction in circulating GH half-life [107]. The reduction in GH secretion has been ascribed to negative feedback by FFA, a reduction in plasma ghrelin (a GH secretagog) and nutrient-stimulated increases in IGF-1 production.

Total IGF-1 and IGF binding protein 3 (IGFBP-3) concentrations in obese subjects are typically normal or only mildly elevated; this may reflect in part the production of IGF-1 and IGFBP-3 by white adipose tissue [108,109] and/or an increase in hepatic GH sensitivity resulting from induction of hepatic GH receptors by hyperinsulinemia. Induction of GH receptor expression in obesity is suggested by an increase in concentrations of GH binding protein [110], the circulating form of the extracellular GH receptor domain, and by heightened production of IGF-1 following a single dose of GH [111].

Total IGF-2 concentrations were elevated in obese adults in two studies but were normal in a study of obese adolescents [112]. In some investigations, serum IGFBP-1 and IGFBP-2 concentrations are reduced. This is postulated to increase the bioavailability of IGF-1, which may thereby maintain or increase linear growth in obesity despite diminished GH secretion. Free IGF-1 concentrations have been found to be elevated in some studies of obese adults [113,114] but technical difficulties with the assay currently limit the applicability of free IGF measurements.

By promoting IGF action, a reduction in plasma IGFBP-1 or IGFBP-2 concentrations in obese subjects may facilitate further weight gain. Overexpression of IGFBP-1 or IGFBP-2 in transgenic mice reduces adipogenesis and prevents diet-induced obesity. IGFBP-1 excess reduces insulin sensitivity but IGFBP-2 excess improves glucose tolerance [115,116].

The effects of IGF-1 on growth and bone maturation in obese subjects may be potentiated by hyperleptinemia. Circulating leptin concentrations rise in proportion to body (particularly subcutaneous) fat stores and are higher in girls than in boys. Leptin stimulates proliferation of isolated mouse and rat osteoblasts and increases the width of the chondroprogenitor zone of the mouse mandible *in vivo*. In leptin-deficient ob/ob mice, leptin increases femoral length, bone area and bone mineral content [117]. The effects of leptin may be exerted in concert with IGF-1 because leptin increases IGF-1 receptor expression in mouse chondrocytes [118]. Nevertheless, linear growth is normal in patients with congenital deficiencies of leptin or the leptin receptor [119,120].

Thyroid function

Plasma T4 and TSH concentrations generally fall within the normal range in obese subjects but T3 concentrations are mildly elevated, a consequence of nutrient-dependent thyroxine (T4) to T3 conversion [107]. The elevation of T3 increases resting energy expenditure and may thereby limit further weight gain. Caloric restriction and weight loss, on the other hand, decrease total and free T4 and T3 concentrations, reducing energy expenditure and thereby facilitating weight regain.

Gonadal function and pubertal development, ovarian hyperandrogenism and gynecomastia

Obesity in early childhood (age 36–54 months) and excessive weight gain between 3 and 9 years of age increases the risks of precocious thelarche and may reduce the age of menarche [121]. Because leptin promotes gonadotropin secretion and rises transiently before the onset of puberty in normal weight children, it is possible that the hyperleptinemia of obesity promotes early sexual maturation, at least in girls.

More commonly, obese girls and boys develop precocious adrenarche without true puberty and teenage obese girls are prone to ovarian hyperandrogenism with mild hirsutism, acne, anovulation and menstrual irregularity.

The pathogenesis of ovarian hyperandrogenism remains poorly understood but insulin and IGF-1 in excess act in synergy with adrenocorticotropic hormone (ACTH) and luteinizing hormone (LH) to stimulate the production of androgens from adrenocortical cells and ovarian theca cells, respectively. These effects are mediated through induction of P450c 17α-hydroxylase activity. The biologic availability of ovarian and adrenal androgens is increased because insulin suppresses hepatic sex hormone binding globulin (SHBG) expression and reduces plasma SHBG concentrations. Free androgens increase the frequency of gonadotropin-releasing hormone (GnRH) pulses and the ratio of LH to follicle-stimulating hormone (FSH), thereby exacerbating thecal androgen production. The increase in free androgens may induce precocious adrenarche in prepubertal girls and boys and may cause anovulation and hirsutism in adolescent girls and young women (Fig. 20.11) [122,123].

Free and total testosterone concentrations are generally normal in obese boys but may decline with dramatic weight gain in association with a fall in gonadotropin concentrations. These changes can reverse with weight loss. Aromatization of androstenedione in adipose tissue increases plasma estrone concentrations, causing gynecomastia in adolescent boys.

In rare cases, the gynecomastia and ovarian hyperandrogenism in obese children derives from hyperprolactinemia. Prolactin concentrations are typically normal or low in obese children or adults but hyperprolactinemia deriving from a pituitary tumor may be associated with weight gain in children as well as in adults [49,50].

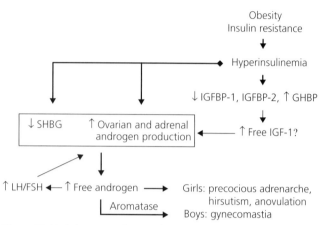

Figure 20.11 Pathogenesis of ovarian hyperandrogenism and gynecomastia in obesity. FSH, follicle stimulating hormone; GHBP, growth hormone binding protein; IGFBP, insulin-like growth factor binding protein; LH, lutenizing hormone; SHBG, sex hormone binding globulin.

Adrenal function

The abdominal weight gain, striae, hirsutism and menstrual irregularity that may accompany obesity are often confused with Cushing syndrome. In contrast to exogenous obesity, Cushing syndrome is typically associated with linear growth failure and delayed bone maturation (unless a primary adrenal tumor produces excess androgens as well as glucocorticoids) as well as hemorrhagic or violaceous, rather than pink, striae. Basal plasma, salivary and urinary free cortisol concentrations and basal ACTH concentrations in obese non-Cushingoid children generally fall within the normal range and diurnal variation and the response to dexamethasone are maintained [124]. However, body fat mass correlates with total excretion of glucocorticoid metabolites, suggesting that obesity is accompanied by increased cortisol secretion and turnover.

Changes in tissue glucocorticoid metabolism may modulate fat distribution and peripheral insulin sensitivity [125]. For example, polymorphisms in the glucocorticoid receptor have been associated with obesity, hypertension and insulin resistance in some studies in adults. Additional investigations suggest that overexpression of 11β-hydroxysteroid dehydrogenase type 1 (11βHSD₁) in visceral adipose tissue may exacerbate weight gain by increasing local production of cortisol from inactive cortisone. In contrast, other studies find lower expression of 11βHSD₁ in pre-adipocytes of obese non-diabetic adults [126]; the expected reduction in tissue cortisol concentrations is postulated to counteract the insulin resistance and weight gain in obese patients. An increase in 11βHSD₁ expression after weight loss may facilitate adipose cortisol production, adipogenesis and weight rebound.

Calcium homeostasis and bone mineralization

Adolescents and adults with severe obesity, particularly those with dark skin, may have reduced 25-hydroxyvitamin D (25-OHD) concentrations and secondary hyperparathyroidism [127];

1,25-dihydroxy vitamin D concentrations have been elevated in obese subjects in some studies and reduced in others. These abnormalities might be explained by a reduction in cutaneous synthesis of vitamin D3 or by decreased bioavailability of vitamin D3 owing to deposition in adipose tissue; they are reversed with weight loss.

Some studies show variable decreases in bone mineral content in obese subjects; others find that overweight and obese children have normal or increased bone mass compared with lean children. Physical activity probably plays a determining part; highly active adolescents accrue more bone than their inactive counterparts.

Renal dysfunction

Renal effects of obesity include increased renal blood flow and glomerular filtration rate, renal hypertrophy and proteinuria. Microalbuminuria, detected in 10% of obese insulin-resistant adolescents [128], correlates with the degree of insulin resistance and 2-h glucose concentrations. Renal biopsies in obese subjects may demonstrate histological features of focal segmental glomerulosclerosis, mesangial proliferation and hypertrophy and glomerulomegaly [129,130]. The glomerulopathy associated with obesity differs in some ways from idiopathic focal segmental glomerulosclerosis, which is more commonly associated with nephrotic syndrome and progression to end-stage renal disease. Factors contributing to obesity-related glomerulopathy include hypertension, hyperinsulinemia, hyperlipidemia and, possibly, increases in free IGF-1 concentrations.

Cholecystitis, pancreatitis and pseudotumor cerebri

Cholecystitis, pancreatitis and pseudotumor cerebri occur more frequently in obese than in normal weight children. Among 123 children (mean age 7.8 years) with cholelithiasis, 12 were obese and four had hypercholesterolemia. In another study, gallstones were found in 2% of obese children and only 0.6% of non-obese children [131]. Gallstone formation is thought to result from an increased rate of biliary cholesterol excretion relative to that of bile acid or phospholipids. Interestingly, rapid weight loss also predisposes to gallbladder disease.

Obesity may place teenage girls at higher risk of idiopathic pancreatitis. The hypertriglyceridemia of obesity/insulin resistance probably has a pathogenic role.

Overweight and obesity increase by 15-fold the risk of pseudotumor cerebri [132]. The pathogenesis of pseudotumor in obesity remains obscure. Increases in intra-abdominal pressure may increase central venous and intrathoracic pressures and thereby raise intracranial pressure.

Obstructive sleep apnea and sleep deprivation

Obstructive sleep apnea is characterized by recurrent episodes of upper airway obstruction accompanied by intermittent hypoxemia and hypercapnia. The disorder is caused by narrowing of the upper airway during sleep; in young children this results most commonly from upper airway inflammation and tonsillar hyper-

trophy; in older adolescents and adults the obstruction appears to result from excessive adipose deposition in the neck and parapharyngeal fat pads. Thus, the risk of obstructive sleep apnea correlates more strongly with obesity in adolescents and adults than in prepubertal children; rates of sleep apnea are increased four- to ninefold in obese teenagers [133]. African-American and Hispanic children are at particularly high risk and Asians may have higher rates at any given BMI.

Sleep apnea is associated with sleep deprivation, cognitive dysfunction, behavioral disorders, hypertension and the panoply of biochemical changes associated with the metabolic syndrome. It is currently unclear whether the latter are caused by the sleep apnea or the obesity that underlies the condition and it is not known whether sleep deprivation, which is associated with daytime sleepiness and childhood weight gain, is a cause as well as a consequence of obesity. Studies in adults [134,135] suggest that sleep deprivation may reduce plasma leptin (anorexigenic) and increase plasma ghrelin (orexigenic) and thereby increase daytime food intake.

The usual treatment of obstructive sleep apnea in children is tonsillectomy and adenoidectomy. Although this may improve mood and cognitive function in theory, the reversal of airway obstruction may reduce the energy costs of breathing and facilitate food intake and may thereby increase body weight [136].

Identification and screening for metabolic complications

The goals of metabolic screening are:

1 To identify (and treat) existing co-morbidities not apparent from clinical history and physical examination; and
2 To identify patients who are at particularly high risk for co-morbidities and who could therefore benefit most from intensive intervention.

For example, most children and adolescents with impaired glucose tolerance and a subset of those with established type 2 diabetes lack classic symptoms such as polyuria and polydipsia. Moreover, dyslipidemia and hepatic and renal dysfunction would go undetected without investigation.

Patients with marked weight gain, abdominal adiposity, severe insulin resistance and strong family histories of type 2 diabetes, gestational diabetes and/or cardiovascular disease are at highest risk for co-morbidities. Thus, metabolic screening of obese children and of overweight children who have one or more of the risk factors listed in Table 20.5 is recommended. Given the strong association of PCOS with insulin resistance, all girls with ovarian hyperandrogenism should be screened, regardless of BMI.

Minimal screening should include measurements of blood pressure, fasting glucose, insulin, lipids and ALT, as well as HbA1c and/or plasma glucose and insulin concentrations following oral glucose or a mixed meal. Urinalysis should be performed to detect glycosuria or microalbuminuria. Measurements of serum leptin and adiponectin may also prove clinically useful.

Table 20.5 Screening for glucose intolerance and metabolic complications in obese children and adolescents.

Populations to be screened

1 Obese children and adolescents with BMI ≥95th percentile for age and gender or waist circumference >90th percentile for age, gender or ethnicity

2 Overweight children (BMI 85–95th percentile) *with one or more of the following:*

  (a) Acanthosis nigricans (a marker of insulin resistance in Whites, Latinos and Asians and of obesity and/or insulin resistance in Blacks); and/or

  (b) Hypertension; and/or

  (c) Precocious adrenarche; and/or

  (d) Membership in a high-risk ethnic group and /or family history of type 2 diabetes, gestational diabetes, or early (age <50 years) cardiovascular disease

3 Teenage girls with ovarian hyperandrogenism with or without obesity

Screening procedures

1 Blood pressure

2 Fasting glucose, insulin, lipids, and alanine aminotransferase

3 HbA1c and/or glucose and insulin concentrations following oral glucose (OGTT) or mixed meal

4 Urinalysis and urine microalbumin and creatinine

BMI, body mass index; OGTT, oral glucose tolerance test.

Analysis of insulin sensitivity and secretion

Insulin sensitivity has generally been assessed using hyperinsulinemic, euglycemic clamps or intravenous infusion of glucose with frequent blood sampling for plasma insulin and glucose concentrations ("minimal model"). These techniques have been applied successfully in research studies but have little use clinically. Estimates of insulin sensitivity based on glucose and insulin concentrations obtained under fasting conditions or following the administration of glucose or a mixed meal correlate reasonably well with clamp and minimal model studies and are therefore clinically useful. Several calculated values have been applied in a variety of clinical investigations; these include:

1 The homeostasis model of insulin resistance (HOMA-IR), calculated as the fasting glucose (in mg%) multiplied by the fasting insulin concentration (in μU/mL) divided by 405 or [fasting glucose (mmol) × insulin (μU/mL)/22.5]

2 QUICKI = 1/[log fasting insulin (μU/mL) + log fasting glucose (mg%)]

3 Modified QUICKI = 1/[log fasting insulin (μU/mL) + log fasting glucose (mg%) + log free fatty acids (mmol)], which may be more useful for detection of insulin resistance in non-obese subjects.

4 Whole body insulin sensitivity index [141] (WBISI, Matsuda index) = 10000 divided by the square root of [fasting glucose × fasting insulin × mean fasting glucose × mean fasting insulin concentrations obtained during an oral glucose tolerance test]. Multiplication of the square root of the WBISI by the "insulinogenic index" (the ratio of increments in insulin and glucose concentrations during the first 30 minutes after glucose ingestion)

provides a disposition index, which provides a measure of insulin secretion at a given level of insulin sensitivity.

Insulin action in normal weight and obese subjects is modulated by GH, glucocorticoids and sex steroids. Consequently, the metabolic response to insulin is gender-dependent and changes with age and state of sexual maturation. Insulin sensitivity declines during mid to late puberty, reflecting an increase in growth hormone secretion and, in girls, progesterone production and the accumulation of body fat. Insulin sensitivity increases thereafter but falls again during aging.

No single insulin assay has been standardized and adopted for general use. Consequently, measurements of insulin sensitivity obtained in one laboratory may not replicate measurements obtained at a different site. Nevertheless, a broad-based study of insulin sensitivity (assessed with an insulin radioimmunoassay) in 4092 American adolescents [138] found that the 97.5th centile for HOMA-IR values was 4.39; at this level, 52% of obese, 16% of overweight and 3–4% of normal-weight adolescents would be considered insulin-resistant. Fasting insulin concentrations exceeding 24.1 μU/ml and HOMA-IR values greater than 5.63 exceeded the 95th centile for all obese adolescents, suggesting that these concentrations indicate severe insulin resistance. Children with severe insulin resistance are at the highest risk for metabolic complications and warrant additional investigation, intervention and follow-up. Marked elevations in serum ALT and/or plasma lipids should prompt consultations with other pediatric subspecialists.

Long-term risks

Adult obesity

Childhood obesity predisposes to obesity in adolescence and adulthood. In general, the correlation between childhood and adult obesity increases with the age of the child; the probability that an obese child will be obese at age 35 years increases from 0.15–0.24 at age 3 years to 0.98–0.99 at age 20 years (Fig. 20.12) [139]; until age 17, the risk for obese girls exceeds the risk for obese boys. The odds that an obese child will remain obese as a young adult increase from 1.3 at the age of 1–2 years to 20.3 at the age of 15–17 years [17]. The persistence of obesity into adulthood has ominous implications; severe obesity increases 40 times the rates of type 2 diabetes in adult women and by 2–3 times the risks of gestational diabetes. Microvascular complications, including neuropathy, retinopathy and microalbuminuria, all occur with increased frequency in adults with impaired glucose tolerance as well as diabetes and rates of myocardial infarction and stroke are increased two- to fivefold [140–143].

Cardiovascular disease

Childhood obesity itself appears to predispose to development and progression of cardiovascular disease even early in life. Severe obesity in 9- to 11-year-old children is associated with increased stiffness of the carotid arteries and obesity, hypoadiponectinemia, and insulin resistance. Impaired glucose tolerance in adolescence is associated with increases in carotid intimal media thickness [144–146], which may be reduced in adult life by weight loss.

Among 93 subjects who underwent autopsy at age 2–39 years, the prevalence of fatty streaks and fibrous plaques in the aorta and coronary arteries increased with age and correlated positively with standard deviation (Z) scores for BMI, serum triglycerides, cholesterol and blood pressure [151]. The combination of multiple risk factors increased exponentially the extent of arterial intimal surface involvement. Postmortem analysis of more than 3000 subjects who died of natural causes at 15–34 years of age (Pathological Determinants of Atherosclerosis in Youth [148]) showed that obesity and impaired glucose tolerance were associated with progression of atheromatous lesions in adolescents and young adults. In young men, BMI and abdominal fat mass correlated with the number and size of fatty streaks and raised lesions in the right and left anterior descending coronary arteries. In both women and men, the extent of fatty streaks correlated with glycated hemoglobin concentrations.

In a study of 276 385 subjects followed from 7–13 years of age to 25–60 years, a one unit increase in BMI Z score (BMI + 1 SDS, equivalent to the 88th centile in American BMI charts) at age 13 years was associated with a 12–17% increase in the risk of fatal and non-fatal cardiac events resulting from coronary heart disease (Fig. 20.13) [149], so even modest increases in body fat deposition during the early years of life have grave implications for adult cardiovascular health.

Malignancy

The prevalence of endometrial cancer, cervical cancer and renal cell carcinoma in women increases in proportion to BMI, while rates of liver cancer (and to a lesser extent gastrointestinal malignancies) are increased markedly in obese men (Fig. 20.14) [150,151]. It is not known whether childhood obesity predisposes to childhood or adult malignancy, although a retrospective study

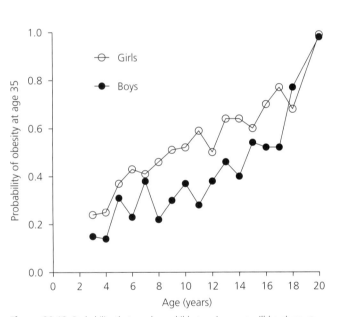

Figure 20.12 Probability that an obese child at a given age will be obese at age 35 years. Redrawn from Guo *et al.* [143] with permission.

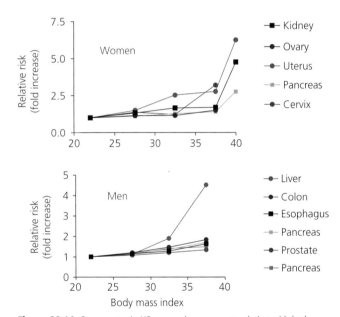

Figure 20.14 Cancer rates in US men and women – correlation with body mass index (BMI). Adapted from Calle *et al.* [154] with permission.

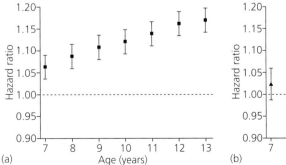

Figure 20.13 A one unit increase in BMI Z score in childhood increases the risk of adult coronary heart disease. (a) Boys. (b) Girls. Reprinted from Calle *et al.* [154] with permission.

[152] revealed a 9.1 times (range 1.1–77.5) increase in the incidence of colon cancer among elderly men (not women) who had been obese as adolescents.

Management of obesity and its co-morbidities

Lifestyle intervention
General considerations
The overall success of lifestyle intervention in children and adolescents has been limited and variable. Intervention has been most successful in homogeneous populations of prepubertal children whose mothers have received intensive dietary and behavioral counseling. Parental counseling alone may be as or more effective than counseling of the young child and parent(s).

Behavior modification forms the basis of current clinical practice. Ten-year outcome data show that 34% of participants decreased percentage overweight by 20% or more and 30% were no longer obese [153]. No racial breakdown for participants has been provided but the great majority of subjects were Caucasian. All were pre-adolescent (6–12 years old at study onset), of middle to high socio-economic status and none was massively obese. The intervention had little or no effect in children with at least one obese parent, which limits the generalizability of these studies.

However, some investigations do shed light on the efficacy of lifestyle intervention in ethnically diverse groups of children. A mixed group of 7- to 12-year-old African-Americans, Whites and Latinos was studied to assess the effects of weight maintenance behavioral therapy delivered for 4 months after the completion of a structured weight loss program focusing on diet, activity and self-monitoring [154]. Those who received maintenance therapy had a mean decrease in BMI Z score of 0.04 compared with an increase of 0.05 in the control group but treatment efficacy declined over the subsequent 2-year follow-up. The study did not control for frequency of health-care contacts or pubertal stage and severely overweight children were excluded.

The success of lifestyle intervention in adolescence has been disappointing but a year-long intensive family-based intervention [155], which employed nutrition education, behavior modification and supervised exercise sessions, reduced BMI by 1.7 kg/m^2 and improved insulin sensitivity in a mixed ethnic group of American teenagers, although only 53% of the participants completed the study. Drop-out rate was even higher (83%) in a substudy that recommended a structured meal plan.

Dietary intervention: macro- and micronutrients
Mild caloric restriction can be safe and effective when obese children and their families are highly motivated and encouraged to change feeding behaviors. Significant reductions in weight are unusual and often transient unless caloric restriction is accompanied by increased energy expenditure. Diets severely restricted in calories produce more dramatic weight loss but cannot be sustained under free-living conditions. Very-low-calorie low-protein diets are potentially dangerous and may precipitate recurrent and futile cycles of dieting and binge eating.

The role of dietary macronutrients in the pathogenesis of obesity, insulin resistance and type 2 diabetes is highly controversial. The majority of studies in humans and animals suggest that insulin sensitivity correlates inversely with the saturated fat content of the diet [156,157]. Replacement of saturated fat with polyunsaturated fat and long-chain omega-3 fatty acid can reduce total energy intake, improve insulin sensitivity and, in combination with exercise, reduce the risks of type 2 diabetes and cardiovascular disease in adults with IGT.

Nevertheless, obese men and women lost more weight during short-term trials (6 months) and had more significant reductions in plasma TG concentrations on low-carbohydrate diets than on conventional low-fat diets [158,159]. The relative benefits of a low carbohydrate diet were lost by 12 months and long-term compliance with the regimen was variable [160,161].

It is possible that the nature or quality of ingested carbohydrate may modulate weight gain. The insulin-secretory response to foods containing rapidly absorbed, concentrated carbohydrates (high glycemic index) exceeds the response to foods containing protein, fat and fiber. The rapid rise and subsequent fall in blood glucose following ingestion of sucrose may precipitate hunger and fructose is lipogenic and delays the oxidation of fatty acids, facilitating fat storage [162,163]. Substitution of low for high glycemic carbohydrates had no effect on energy intake or body weight in overweight or obese women [164].

Studies of the effects of glycemic index on weight gain in children are inconclusive. A 19-month study of school children found a positive correlation between BMI and the consumption of sugar-sweetened drinks: a modified low-glycemic diet (45–50% carbohydrate, 30–35% fat) reduced BMI Z score and fat mass in a pilot study of seven obese adolescents [165]. However, a systematic review [166] concluded that caloric restriction is as or more effective in reducing BMI than selective restriction of fat or carbohydrate. Anecdotal evidence suggests that elimination of concentrated soft drinks and reduction of high density starches can reduce caloric intake in some obese adolescents by as much as 500–1000 kcal/day and thereby facilitate weight reduction.

Other macronutrients, vitamins and trace elements may contribute to the risk of diabetes. Intake of fiber, particularly whole grains and cereal, correlates inversely with the risks of type 2 diabetes and cardiovascular disease [167]. Insoluble and soluble fiber may limit fat absorption and thereby improve glucose tolerance. The intake of magnesium from whole grains, nuts and green leafy vegetables and dairy products containing vitamin D and calcium may also correlate inversely with diabetes risk in young adults [168,169].

Exercise
A sedentary lifestyle increases the risk of diabetes, while exercise, in combination with caloric and fat restriction, reduces the rate

of progression to diabetes in adults with IGT. Lifestyle intervention can reduce the rate of progression to diabetes in adults with IGT between 63% [170] and 36% [171].

The Finnish Diabetes Prevention Study [172] randomized individuals with IGT and BMI >25 kg/m^2 to a control or to an intervention group counseled to reduce total and saturated fat intake, increase fiber intake, reduce body weight and increase physical activity. No subjects who achieved target goals developed diabetes but one-third of those who failed to reach a single target developed diabetes. The primary determinant of diabetes prevention was an increase in insulin sensitivity associated with weight loss. The Diabetes Prevention Program (DPP) [173] compared intensive with standard lifestyle recommendations. Intensive lifestyle changes, which included weight reduction, a decrease in saturated fat intake and regular exercise (150 min/week), were accompanied by a 58% relative risk reduction in the prevalence of diabetes during a 3-year period.

The mechanisms by which exercise improves insulin sensitivity and glucose tolerance are complex, involving metabolic adaptations in adipose tissue, liver and skeletal muscle (Fig. 20.15) [174]. Exercise has beneficial effects on fat storage and distribution, with losses of visceral fat depots exceeding those of subcutaneous fat stores. Lean body mass increases, thereby augmenting resting energy expenditure. A reduction in visceral fat mass increases adipose tissue sensitivity to insulin which partly explains the reductions in fasting and post-prandial FFA, LDL and TG concentrations and the increase in plasma HDL concentrations in adults who adhere to a rigorous diet and exercise regimen. The effect of exercise on plasma TG is mediated through induction of lipoprotein lipase and reduction in TG production.

Exercise increases hepatic glucose uptake and glycogen synthesis and decreases hepatic glucose production, thereby reducing fasting glucose and insulin concentrations. In skeletal muscle, exercise stimulates insulin-dependent glucose uptake and thereby reduces post-prandial glucose concentrations; this action is mediated by increases in muscle GLUT-4 synthesis and induction of GLUT-4 translocation from intra-cellular pools to the plasma membrane [178]. The induction of GLUT-4 activity may be mediated in turn by an increase in cellular concentrations of AMP-activated protein kinase (AMPK) [175]. Activation of AMPK promotes increased cycling of existing GLUT-4 transporters in skeletal muscle as well as enhanced expression of hexokinase II and mitochondrial enzymes.

Several studies suggest that insulin action is related to the oxidative capacity of skeletal muscle. Insulin-resistant individuals, including those with type 2 diabetes, have reduced activities of muscle oxidative enzymes; aerobic training increases muscle oxidative enzyme activity and improves insulin sensitivity by 26–46%. The effect of exercise on oxidative enzyme activity may reflect in part an increase in mitochondrial size [176]. Weight loss alone may improve insulin sensitivity but does not alter fasting rates of lipid oxidation, while weight loss coupled with exercise increases fat oxidation.

Few studies have assessed the effects of exercise on insulin resistance in children. A randomized modified cross-over study of 79 obese children (aged 7–11 years) demonstrated that 4 months of exercise training (40 min of activity on 5 days a week) decreased fasting insulin (10%), TG (17%) concentrations and percentage body fat (5%), even in the absence of dietary intervention [177]. The effects on plasma insulin and body fat were reversed when training was discontinued.

An 8-week trial of cycle ergometry and resistance training in obese adolescents reduced abdominal (7.0%) and trunk (3.7%) fat mass and normalized flow-mediated dilation of the brachial artery [178,179].

Although preliminary, these findings suggest that exercise has beneficial effects in obese children as well as adults but exercise alone is unlikely to induce weight loss in obese patients in the absence of caloric restriction [180]. The capacity for voluntary exercise declines as BMI rises so it is critical to begin regular exercise before the child becomes morbidly obese and functionally immobile.

Benefits from lifestyle intervention are most likely when diet and exercise programs are coordinated with individual and family

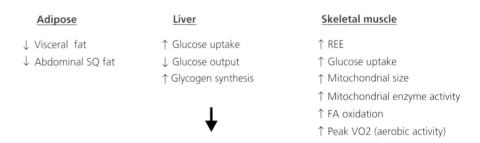

Adipose	Liver	Skeletal muscle
↓ Visceral fat	↑ Glucose uptake	↑ REE
↓ Abdominal SQ fat	↓ Glucose output	↑ Glucose uptake
	↑ Glycogen synthesis	↑ Mitochondrial size
		↑ Mitochondrial enzyme activity
		↑ FA oxidation
		↑ Peak VO2 (aerobic activity)

Decreased FFA and TG, increased HDL, increased insulin sensitivity, improved glucose tolerance

Reduced risks of type 2 diabetes and cardiovascular disease

Figure 20.15 Metabolic benefits of exercise. FFA, free fatty acids; HDL, high density lipoprotein cholesterol; REE, resting energy expenditure; SQ, subcutaneous; TG, triglycerides.

counseling and behavior modification. School-based programs, supported by community groups and by state and federal agencies, may assist families and reduce the child's sense of isolation, frustration and guilt. Pilot investigations suggest that school-based physical education programs may reduce body fat and blood pressure in children and young teenagers but have negligible effects on BMI [180]; such findings might implicate increases in lean body mass, which in theory may improve long-term cardiovascular health.

The long-term success of lifestyle intervention alone has been disappointing. Rates of obesity and insulin resistance in children and adults continue to increase, despite widespread recognition of the dangers of dietary indiscretion and a sedentary existence. This may reflect the resistance of complex feeding and activity behaviors to change as well as the power of social and economic forces that shape lifestyles. Metabolic and hormonal adaptations to initial weight loss may also create barriers to long-term success; for example, reductions in food intake and body weight decrease the circulating concentrations of T3 and leptin and increase circulating concentrations of adiponectin and ghrelin (Fig. 20.16) [181]. The fall in T3 and leptin concentrations limits energy expenditure and sympathetic nervous system activity and may facilitate rebound food intake. Hunger may be intensified by the rise in plasma ghrelin and adiponectin, which stimulate food intake [182,183]. Food restriction also causes a secondary resistance to GH action, which in combination with a rise in insulin sensitivity may reduce rates of lipolysis and fat breakdown [124,181]. These adaptations facilitate weight regain, the major barrier to long-term treatment success [184].

Pharmacotherapy

The obstacles to success with lifestyle intervention have stimulated interest in pharmacologic approaches to the treatment of obesity and the prevention of diabetes and other metabolic complications.

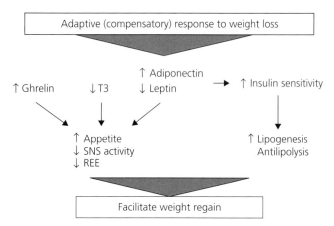

Figure 20.16 Adaptive response to weight loss. REE, resting energy expenditure; SNS, sympathetic nervous system; T3, triiodothyronine. Reprinted from Freemark [181] with permission.

Anorectic agents

Among pharmacologic agents used for weight loss, anorectic drugs are the most powerful [181]. Unfortunately, many of these drugs initially considered safe for the treatment of obesity (e.g. amphetamines, diethylpropion, fenfluramine, ephedra and phenylpropanolamine) have been withdrawn because of life-threatening complications. The only anorexic agent currently approved for use in obese adolescents (>age 16 years) is sibutramine, a non-selective inhibitor of neuronal reuptake of serotonin, norepinephrine and dopamine.

This drug reduces hunger, increases satiety and promotes thermogenesis in brown adipose tissue, increasing energy expenditure (Fig. 20.17) [182]. In combination with caloric restriction and a comprehensive family-based behavioral program [185,186], sibutramine reduced BMI by 8.5 ± 6.8% in 43 obese adolescents during an initial 6-month period; 39 placebo-treated subjects had a 4.0 ± 5.4% reduction in BMI. No additional weight loss occurred during a subsequent 6 months of therapy. There were no changes in fasting glucose, insulin or lipid concentrations.

Nineteen of the 43 subjects developed mild hypertension and tachycardia, necessitating reduction in drug dosage and five had sustained elevations in blood pressure that required discontinuation of the drug. A subsequent randomized controlled trial excluded subjects with baseline blood pressure >130/85 mmHg and/or pulse >95 and, following a 12-month period, sibutramine and behavior therapy combined reduced BMI (−2.9 kg/m², 9.4%), waist circumference, triglycerides (−24 mg/dL), insulin (−7.6 µU/mL) and HOMA-IR. Blood pressure and pulse rate were marginally higher in treated subjects.

Other potential adverse effects of the drug include insomnia, anxiety, headache and depression. There is a heightened risk of the serotonin syndrome [187] if sibutramine is used in combination with monoamine oxidase inhibitors, buspirone, lithium, meperidine) or selective serotonin reuptake inhibitors (such as fluoxetine), triptans, dextromethorphan, ergot alkaloids or fentanyl.

Rimonabant is a specific inhibitor of cannabinoid receptor 1. It reduces food intake through actions on the hypothalamus, mesolimbic system and vagus nerve and stimulates directly the expression of adiponectin in white adipose tissue [181]. Its effects have not been studied in children but the drug reduced BMI with a potency comparable to that of sibutramine in obese adults and, with higher doses, increased HDL and reduced TG. Unfortunately, it also caused an excess (5.6%) of "psychiatric and nervous system disorders" including anxiety, depression and insomnia [181]. Such findings are of concern given the prevalence of eating and mood disorders in severely obese children.

Anorectic agents should complement and never replace a diet and exercise program. Responses to treatment vary considerably among individuals: most weight loss is achieved within the first 4–6 months and regain of weight is the norm unless drug therapy is maintained. Close monitoring for adverse effects is essential.

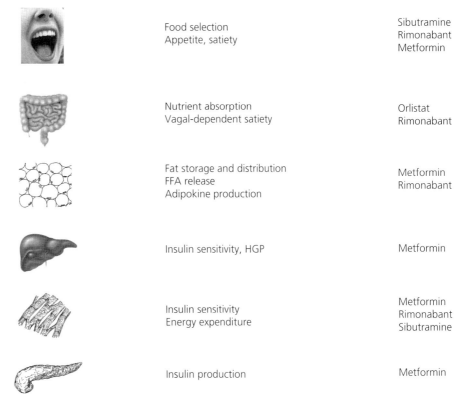

Figure 20.17 Mechanisms of action of pharmacologic agents used in the treatment of obesity. FFA, free fatty acids; HGP, hepatic glucose production. The relative size of the drug name correlates with the magnitude of its effect. Reprinted from Freemark [181] with permission.

Drugs that limit absorption

Orlistat (approved for treatment of obese children over the age of 12 years) inhibits pancreatic lipase and thereby increases fecal losses of TG. The drug reduces body weight and total and LDL cholesterol concentrations and reduces the risk of type 2 diabetes in adults with IGT (Fig. 20.18) [188]. Serum cholesterol and LDL concentrations are also reduced in adults and the LDL:HDL ratio declines slightly. In a year-long study of obese adolescents, orlistat reduced weight by 2.6 kg and BMI by 0.86 kg/m² but had no effect on blood glucose, insulin or lipid concentrations [189]. There was considerable variability in response and the high drop-out rates (33% or more) suggest that long-term fat restriction is a problem for teenagers; dietary non-compliance results in flatulence and diarrhea that ultimately prove unacceptable.

Side effects are tolerable as long as subjects reduce fat intake but vitamin A, D and E concentrations may decline and a multivitamin may help to prevent osteopenia. Seven of 357 children who took orlistat for a single year developed new gallbladder disease [189], of whom one required cholecystectomy. Among the 182 placebo-treated patients, only one developed new gallbladder disease. Because cholecystitis occurs more commonly even in untreated obese people [124,131], it is unclear if orlistat increases the risk of gallbladder disease or if long-term use of the drug should be discouraged for patients with pre-existing gallstones.

Insulin suppressors and sensitizers

The synthesis and storage of TG in adipose tissue is stimulated by insulin so increases in nutrient-dependent insulin production

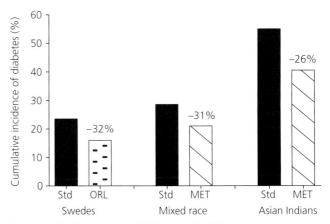

Figure 20.18 Effects of orlistat (ORL), metformin (MET) or standard therapy (STD) on rates of type 2 diabetes in major randomized controlled trials. From Freemark [181] with permission. Orlistat data are from Torgersen et al. [188]; metformin data are from Knowler et al. [173] and Ramachandran et al. [202].

and/or fasting hyperinsulinemia may contribute to fat storage and limit fat mobilization. By reducing fasting or post-prandial insulin concentrations, pharmacologic agents may be useful for the treatment of obese children and adults.

Metformin is a bisubstituted, short-chain hydrophilic guanidine derivative. Its major site of action is the liver: through activation of AMP protein kinase [190], the drug increases hepatic glucose uptake and fatty acid oxidation, decreases gluconeogenesis and reduces hepatic glucose production [181]. Metformin increases insulin receptor binding but has variable effects on peripheral insulin sensitivity; in contrast to the thizolidinediones, there is no induction of skeletal muscle glucose uptake or plasma adiponectin concentrations [191,192].

Major advantages of the medication include reductions in food intake and fat deposition (subcutaneous > visceral) and improved lipid profiles [181,193,194]. A meta-analysis [195] of 31 trials with 4570 high-risk subjects followed for a total of 8267 patient-years showed that metformin reduces BMI (−5.3%), fasting insulin concentrations (−14.4%), calculated insulin resistance (−22.6%), triglycerides (−5.3%) and LDL (−5.6%) and raises HDL concentrations (+5%). The drug reduced the incidence of new-onset diabetes by 40% (odds ratio 0.6) during a mean of 1.8 years [195] and may limit cardiovascular morbidity and mortality in diabetic adults [196].

There have been at least six randomized double-blind placebo-controlled studies of metformin in obese adolescents with insulin resistance and normal glucose tolerance. In the first trial ($n = 29$), which lasted 6 months, metformin reduced BMI Z score 0.12 SDS (−3.6% relative to placebo controls), plasma leptin and fasting glucose (−9.8 mg%) and insulin (−12 μU/mL) concentrations, even in the absence of dietary intervention [197]. Because increases in BMI and fasting glucose and insulin concentrations predict the development of type 2 diabetes in target populations, these findings suggested that metformin might prove useful in the prevention of glucose intolerance in high-risk adolescents.

Subsequent studies [198–200] confirmed these findings: in each case metformin caused small but significant reductions in BMI (0.9–1.26 kg/m^2) and fasting insulin concentrations and increased insulin sensitivity. Stores of deep abdominal subcutaneous fat, which may function metabolically like visceral fat, were selectively reduced [199,200].

A 3-month trial ($n = 24$) found that the combination of a low-calorie diet (1500–1800 calories/day for girls and boys, respectively) and metformin reduced weight by 6.5%; diet alone caused a 3.8% weight loss [198]. Patients treated with metformin had greater decline in body fat (−6% versus −2.7% in the placebo group), a decrease in plasma leptin concentrations, a 50% decrease in plasma insulin concentrations and increased insulin sensitivity as determined by fasting and 2-h glucose and insulin concentrations. Plasma cholesterol and TG concentrations also declined by 22% and 39%, respectively. These findings suggested that metformin and diet may act synergistically to limit weight gain and increase glucose tolerance in obese insulin-resistant adolescents. Finally, metformin prevented weight gain and increased insulin sensitivity in children treated for 4 months with atypical antipsychotic agents [201].

Effects on long-term metabolic complications have been demonstrated most convincingly in studies of adults with IGT. The DPP [173] and the Indian Diabetes Prevention Programme [202] showed that metformin decreased body weight and reduced the rates of type 2 diabetes in high-risk adults by 26–31%

(Fig. 20.18). Intensive lifestyle intervention was more potent (58% reduction in diabetes rates) than metformin alone but the drug was as effective as lifestyle change in the youngest patients studied and in those with highest BMI. After the first year of the study, fasting blood glucose concentrations, HbA1c concentrations and rates of diabetes increased in both the intensive lifestyle and the metformin groups in parallel with those in the placebo group (standard lifestyle counseling). This suggests that the interventions may delay rather than prevent the development of type 2 diabetes [203].

No studies have examined the effects of lifestyle intervention or pharmacotherapy on rates of type 2 diabetes in obese adolescents but metformin has been shown to reduce rates of other complications in high-risk teenagers. For example, it reduces central obesity, free testosterone concentrations and hirsutism scores and increases ovulation rates in adolescents and adults with PCOS [195,204–206], most of whom are overweight or obese. Preliminary evidence suggests that it may also reduce the serum concentrations of ALT, a marker of hepatic dysfunction, in obese insulinresistant adolescents [207,208].

Heart rate recovery after submaximal exercise, which may predict cardiovascular mortality in adults, may be improved in obese adolescents by metformin [200]. Two studies suggest that it may reduce the rates of cardiovascular disease in high risk adults: in the UKPDS study of adults with new onset type 2 diabetes, metformin reduced the incidence of various diabetes-related endpoints including death by 32–42% [196]. In adults with type 2 diabetes and coronary artery disease, metformin reduced the rates of myocardial infarction and deaths by 28% compared with patients treated with sulfonylureas or insulin [209]. There are no comparable data on sibutramine or orlistat.

The thiazolidinedione (TZD) rosiglitazone may be more potent in reducing rates of development of type 2 diabetes in obese adults with IGT than metformin [210,211]. Pioglitazone reduces liver fat stores and hepatic inflammation in glucose-intolerant and diabetic adults with non-alcoholic steatohepatitis [212]. TZDs may cause weight gain, edema, heart failure and bone loss and are therefore less suitable for treatment of obese adolescents [213].

Metformin is generally well tolerated by the majority of subjects, although many have transient abdominal discomfort which can be minimized by taking the medication with food. A reduction in dosage may also relieve gastrointestinal distress. Reversible hepatic dysfunction with cholestasis can develop in rare cases. The drug should not be administered to patients with acute or chronic organ failure and should be discontinued for radiologic contrast studies. Because metformin reduces absorption of B vitamins, a daily vitamin supplement containing vitamins B_6 and B_{12} should be included during treatment.

Octreotide binds to the somatostatin-5 receptor and thereby impairs closure of the β-cell calcium channel, reducing glucose-dependent insulin secretion. Unfortunately, the cost of the medication, the need for parenteral administration and the drug's side effects, which include gastrointestinal distress, edema, gallstones, suppression of GH and TSH secretion and cardiac dysfunction, limit its potential applicability to patients with intractable obesity from hypothalamic injury [214].

Selection of pediatric candidates for pharmacotherapy

The use of pharmacologic agents in the treatment of obese children is highly controversial. It can be warranted in carefully selected subjects, at the proper time and with appropriate safeguards. In general, pharmacotherapy should be reserved for obese, rather than overweight, children. Pharmacologic agents *may* (not necessarily *should*) be considered when obesity and co-morbidities persist despite formal counseling and a good faith effort at diet and exercise. Relevant co-morbidities include:

• Impaired fasting glucose (≥100 mg%), IGT (random or 2-h glucose 140–199 mg%) or HbA1c >5.9%;
• Severe insulin resistance manifested by:
  ○ Plasma triglycerides >150 mg% and/or blood pressure 2 SD above the mean for age and sex;
  ○ HDL concentrations <40 mg%;
  ○ Fasting insulin >24 μU/mL or HOMA-IR >5.6 (both >95th centile for obese adolescents, NHANES 1999–2002 [138]);
  ○ Increased serum ALT (in absence of liver disease other than fatty liver);
• Ovarian hyperandrogenism/PCOS.

The case for pharmacologic intervention is strengthened by the persistence of more than one of these co-morbidities, particularly if there is a strong family history of type 2 diabetes or early cardiovascular disease. Prominent abdominal adiposity warrants special concern.

Timing of pharmacologic intervention

If pharmacotherapy is initiated early in the course of obesity, it may be possible to prevent severe weight gain and metabolic complications but early intervention inevitably results in some unnecessary treatment, raises the rate of side effects and increases costs. If medication is begun later, it is possible to treat existing complications but this approach runs the risk of run-away weight gain and long-term morbidity.

A way to reconcile these difficulties is to act aggressively with lifestyle intervention to prevent severe obesity and to consider pharmacotherapy when the risk of complications is extremely high or soon after complications have begun to emerge (dotted line in Fig. 20.19). Therapy could be started slightly sooner if the family history for a major co-morbidity, say type 2 diabetes, is particularly strong but lifestyle intervention should always precede pharmacotherapy and be maintained during it.

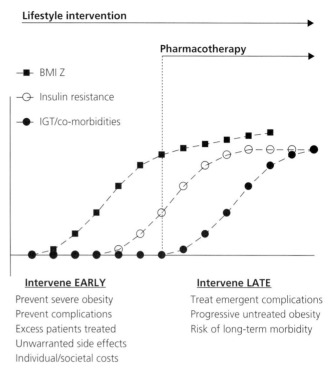

Figure 20.19 Approach to lifestyle intervention and pharmacotherapy in obese children. From Freemark [181] with permission.

Medication selection and therapeutic objectives

Drug selection should be tailored to the individual patient, with strong attention paid to the family history. The goal of preventing or treating complications supersedes the goal of reducing body weight per se. The benefits of any drug used to treat childhood obesity should clearly outweigh its risks.

Metformin is a valuable adjunct to the treatment of obese adolescents with severe insulin resistance, IFG, IGT or PCOS. Dyslipidemic patients might also benefit from orlistat or metformin, which reduce LDL concentrations and the LDL:HDL ratio in adults.

Sibutramine remains an experimental approach for the treatment of obesity in children because of its tendency to raise blood pressure and pulse and the lack of information regarding its long-term safety. It should not be used in children with poorly controlled hypertension or cardiovascular disease of any sort and neither sibutramine nor rimonabant should be used in children with a history of psychiatric disease or mood disorders.

The goals of pharmacological treatment are similar to those of lifestyle intervention: reduction in BMI Z score (≥10%) and prevention and/or treatment of co-morbidities with normalization of blood pressure, plasma lipids and hepatic and renal function. Additional goals in PCOS include reduction in hirsutism scores and restoration of ovulatory menses.

Duration of pharmacologic treatment

In the Rimonabant In Obesity-North America (RIO-NA) trial [215], discontinuation of the drug was associated with nearly complete regain of weight lost within 1 year. Likewise, withdrawal of metformin in the DPP [203] partly reversed its protective effects on the development of diabetes. Thus, adults may require long-term pharmacotherapy for long-lasting benefit.

It is not clear if this is true for children. If therapeutic goals are achieved, it may be possible to reduce the dosage of the medication or discontinue the drug entirely. Nevertheless, it is essential that lifestyle intervention be maintained throughout or a rebound in body weight and a relapse of co-morbidities is inevitable. If co-morbidities such as glucose intolerance persist despite compliance with the medical/pharmacologic regimen, it may be necessary to intensify lifestyle intervention and/or to increase the dosage of medication. If glucose tolerance declines or the patient develops overt diabetes, it may be necessary to add insulin or another pharmacologic agent to the therapeutic regimen.

Bariatric surgery
General considerations

Lifestyle intervention and pharmacotherapy in subjects with severe (or "morbid") obesity has been disappointing. Marked weight loss is unusual and rarely sustained, and metabolic and vascular complications are common, although not invariable. Bariatric surgery may be indicated in selected subjects with extreme obesity and serious co-morbidities.

A prospective controlled trial demonstrated that surgical intervention (gastric banding, vertical banded gastroplasty and gastric bypass) reduced body weight in obese adults by 23.4% at 2 years follow-up and 16.1% at 10 years, whereas body weight increased 1.6% in matched controls [216]. Bariatric surgery reduced energy intake, increased physical activity and reduced significantly the prevalence of diabetes, hypertension, hypertriglyceridemia, HDL cholesterol and hyperuricemia. Another randomized controlled trial showed that laparoscopic adjustable gastric banding reduced body weight by 20% and reversed type 2 diabetes in 73% of obese adults during a 2-year follow-up period; remission was achieved in only 13% of a matched group using conventional diabetic therapy [217].

Bariatric surgery is now employed increasingly in older adolescents with severe obesity and co-morbidities using either the laparoscopic gastric banding procedure or the Roux-en-Y gastric bypass.

Laparoscopic adjustable gastric banding

This procedure utilizes a prosthetic band to encircle the proximal stomach (Fig. 20.20). The ability to adjust band tension as stomach volume changes and the reversibility of the procedure provide important theoretical advantages. A meta-analysis (http://www.hta.hca.wa.gov/past_materials.html) of treatment of 179 adolescents with pretreatment mean BMI ranging 45.2–50.5 kg/

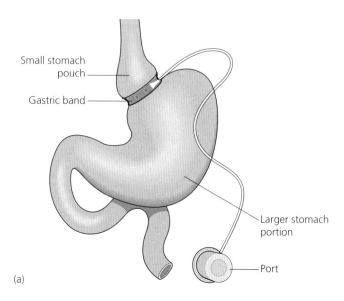

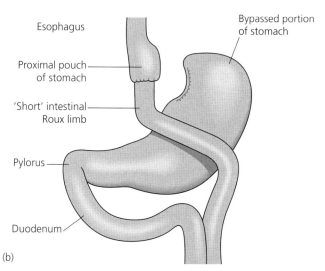

Figure 20.20 (a) Laparoscopic gastric banding and (b) Roux-en-Y bypass surgical procedures.

m² found that laparoscopic adjustable gastric banding (LAGB) reduced BMI by 8.3–14 kg/m² during a 1.7–3.3 year follow-up period, eliminated diabetes in 8 of 12 patients and hypertension and sleep apnea in the majority with pre-existing disease. No deaths were reported, the major complication being band slippage, necessitating re-operation in 7.9% of subjects. Gastric banding may also cause esophageal dilatation, achalasia and exacerbate gastroesophageal reflux. Other potential complications include port-site malfunction, balloon rupture and infection. Weight regain over time is common because high caloric intake can be maintained by ingestion of sugary drinks.

Roux-en-Y gastric bypass

Roux-en-Y gastric bypass (RYGB) involves the creation of a small stomach pouch into which a distal segment of jejunum is inserted

(Fig. 20.20). This combines the restrictive nature of gastrectomy with the consequences of dumping physiology as a negative conditioning response when high-calorie liquid meals are ingested. Food intake may decline as stomach-derived ghrelin concentrations fall [218].

Pilot studies report favorable results in morbidly obese adolescents who failed to respond to lifestyle intervention and/or pharmacotherapy. In a total of 125 patients (BMI range 47–56.5), some of whom had Prader–Willi syndrome, gastric bypass reduced BMI by 15–24 kg/m² during follow-up periods ranging 1–6.3 years. Diabetes was reversed in three of six patients and hypertension and sleep apnea in most of those with pre-existing disease (http://www.hta.hca.wa.gov/past_materials.html). The relatively low rates of type 2 diabetes in this population probably reflect the predominance of Caucasian patients.

Overall mortality rates for RYGB in adults range 0.5–2%, mostly from pulmonary embolus, sepsis and *Clostridium difficile* colitis [219]. Risk factors include older age, higher BMI, pre-existing co-morbidities and hypoventilation. Mortality rates are lower (0.35%) in specialized centers with experienced surgeons and a multispecialty team approach. One postoperative death of a child was reported 9 months following gastric bypass. Other complications include iron deficiency anemia (50%), folate deficiency (30%), cholecystitis (20%), wound infections and dehiscence (10%), small bowel or stomach obstruction (5–10%), atelectasis and pneumonia (12%) and incisional hernia (10%). Prophylactic tracheostomy may be required to maintain airway patency and to correct preoperative hypercapnia. Other possible complications include leaks at the junction of stomach and small intestine requiring re-anastomosis, acute gastric dilatation, which may arise spontaneously or secondary to intestinal obstruction or narrowing of the stoma, and dumping syndrome.

Deficiencies of vitamin B$_{12}$, iron, calcium and thiamine are common following bypass surgery. It is recommended that subjects receive a multivitamin containing ≥400 U vitamin D and 400–1000 µg folate, as well as supplements of vitamin B$_{12}$ (500 µg) and calcium citrate (1200–1500 mg) [220]. Menstruating girls also require iron supplements and are expected to use contraception for at least 12–18 months postoperatively. The diet should consist of frequent small meals containing fiber but no simple sugars, fruit juices or sugary drinks. Fish is preferred to red meat.

Selection of pediatric patients

Bariatric surgery should be *considered* for late-pubertal or post-pubertal adolescents with BMI >40 when severe obesity and co-morbidities persist despite a formal program of lifestyle modification and/or pharmacotherapy. Given its reversibility and lower incidence of severe complications, gastric banding is preferred to gastric bypass in children. An experienced surgeon is mandatory and psychological evaluation must confirm the stability and competence of the family unit. A multidisciplinary team of specialists in pediatric endocrinology, gastroenterology and nutrition, cardiology, pulmonology and orthopedics is essential.

Presurgical assessment of psychological function and postoperative psychological and nutritional counseling of the surgical patient are obligatory. The patient and family should demonstrate the ability (or at least the willingness) to adhere to the principles of healthy dietary and activity habits before surgery so bariatric surgery is not favored for patients with unresolved eating disorders, untreated psychiatric disorders, substance abuse or Prader–Willi syndrome.

Prevention of complications

The major causes of death in adults with IGT and type 2 diabetes are myocardial infarction and stroke. Although cardiovascular risk in patients with IGT and type 2 diabetes varies with glycemic control, other factors have equal or more important roles. These include obesity, hypertension, smoking, dyslipidemia, ethnic background and family history. In theory, aggressive lifestyle intervention in children and adolescents must include smoking avoidance, treatment of hypertension, microalbuminuria and dyslipidemia, as well as reduction in BMI Z score.

A combined approach of dietary counseling, statins, angiotensin-converting enzyme inhibitors and low-dose aspirin reduced the long-term (8 year) risks of nephropathy, retinopathy, autonomic neuropathy and cardiovascular endpoints (myocardial disease and stroke and amputation) in diabetic adults with microalbuminuria by 50–60% [221]. Such an approach may be necessary in the management of obese, insulin-resistant and glucose-intolerant adolescents, who are commonly hypertensive and hyperlipidemic. The timing and intensity of intervention will depend upon the family history of cardiovascular disease and the severity of the teenager's metabolic disease.

Prevention of childhood obesity

Obesity can be prevented, even in those genetically prone to weight gain, by the adoption of a nutritious diet and regular exercise. The first step in this process is breastfeeding, which some but not all studies suggest may limit weight gain in children and reduce the risk of type 2 diabetes [222–224].

The stability and consistency of the home environment, the selection of food for meals and snacks and the modeling behavior of the parents have central roles in preventing adiposity in childhood and adolescence; peer interactions are also highly relevant [225].

Later in life the health of a woman before, during and after pregnancy assumes critical importance in reducing the risk of obesity in her child.

From a global perspective, the epidemic of obesity derives from the widespread availability of low-cost energy-dense fast food, the high cost of nutrient-dense (protein and vitamin) healthy foods, the increasing adoption of sedentary lifestyles and the stress and time constraints of modern life. In these respects, the prevention

Table 20.6 Foods that are nutrient-rich, low in energy content, and affordable [44].

Carrots
Cabbage
Dried fruits
Legumes
Powdered milk
Nuts
Canned fish
Liver
Offal

of obesity necessitates collaboration between the medical and lay communities to address societal conditions that nurture and sustain childhood weight gain and the development of type 2 diabetes.

For example, ongoing efforts to eliminate soda and candy from school cafeterias and vending machines should be supported enthusiastically. Schools should require periods of exercise for children of all ages, with facilities to make that exercise participatory and exciting. Communities should expand opportunities for exercise and energy expenditure through development of bike and hiking trails, open and park space, pedestrian walkways and public transportation.

Thus far, attempts to prevent obesity through such community initiatives have been only marginally successful; a meta-analysis of informational, cognitive, behavioral and environmental interventions showed small but statistically significant reductions in sedentary and unhealthy dietary behaviors but no effect on BMI [186]. A major barrier to success is probably the cost of nutritious food [226] and children at highest risk for obesity tend to come from low income communities.

Economic incentives to healthy eating, including subsidization of the costs of fruits, vegetables, nuts, low fat meats and milk should be considered (Table 20.6) [44]. This effort should coincide with federal and local public relation campaigns that publicize the risks of type 2 diabetes in minority populations, the hazards of excessive weight gain in childhood and the short- and long-term benefits of breastfeeding and daily exercise.

References

1 Wang Y, Lobstein T. Worldwide trends in childhood overweight and obesity. *Int J Pediatr Obes* 2006; **1**: 11–25.

2 Kelishadi R. Childhood overweight, obesity, and the metabolic syndrome in developing countries. *Epidemiol Rev* 2007; **29**: 62–76.

3 Sturm R. The effects of obesity, smoking and problem drinking on chronic medical problems and health care costs. *Health Affairs* 2002; **21**: 245–253.

4 Ezzahir N, Alberti C, Deghmoun S, Zaccaria I, Czernichow P, Lévy-Marchal C, *et al.* Time course of catch-up in adiposity influences adult anthropometry in individuals who were born small for gestational age. *Pediatr Res* 2005; **58**: 243–247.

5 Eriksson JG, Forsén T, Tuomilehto J, Osmond C, Barker DJ. Early adiposity rebound in childhood and risk of Type 2 diabetes in adult life. *Diabetologia* 2003; **46**: 190–194.

6 Stettler N, Kumanyika SK, Katz SH, Zemel BS, Stallings VA. Rapid weight gain during infancy and obesity in young adulthood in a cohort of African Americans. *Am J Clin Nutr* 2003; **77**: 1374–1378.

7 Ekelund U, Ong K, Linné Y, Neovius M, Brage S, Dunger DB, *et al.* Upward weight percentile crossing in infancy and early childhood independently predicts fat mass in young adults: the Stockholm Weight Development Study (SWEDES). *Am J Clin Nutr* 2006; **83**: 324–330.

8 Dennison BA, Edmunds LS, Stratton HH, Pruzek RM. Rapid infant weight gain predicts childhood overweight. *Obesity (Silver Spring)* 2006; **14**: 491–499.

9 Ehtisham S, Crabtree N, Clark P, Shaw N, Barrett T. Ethnic differences in insulin resistance and body composition in United Kingdom adolescents. *J Clin Endocrinol Metab* 2005; **90**: 3963–3969.

10 Yajnik CS. Obesity epidemic in India: intrauterine origins? *Proc Nutr Soc* 2004; **63**: 387–396.

11 Lee S, Bacha F, Gungor N, Arslanian SA. Waist circumference is an independent predictor of insulin resistance in black and white youths. *J Pediatr* 2006; **148**: 188–194.

12 Fernandez JR, Redden DT, Pietrobelli A, Allison DB. Waist circumference percentiles in nationally representative samples of African-American, European-American, and Mexican-American children and adolescents. *J Pediatr* 2004; **145**: 439–444.

13 Savva SC, Tornaritis M, Savva ME, Kourides Y, Panagi A, Silikiotou N, *et al.* Waist circumference and waist-to-height ratio are better predictors of cardiovascular disease risk factors in children than body mass index. *Int J Obes* 2000; **24**: 1453–1458.

14 Loos and Rankinen. Gene-diet interactions on body weight changes. *J Am Diet Assoc* 2005; **105**: S29–S34.

15 Nelson MC, Gordon-Larsen P, North KE, Adair LS. Body mass index gain, fast food, and physical activity: effects of shared environments over time. *Obesity* 2006; **14**: 701–709.

16 Malis C, Rasmussen EL, Poulsen P, Petersen I, Christensen K, Beck-Nielsen H, *et al.* Total and regional fat distribution is strongly influenced by genetic factors in young and elderly twins. *Obesity Res* 2005; **13**: 2139–2145.

17 Whitaker RC, Wright JA, Pepe MS, Seidel KD, Dietz WH. Predicting obesity in young adulthood from childhood and parental obesity. *N Engl J Med* 1997; **337**: 869–873.

18 Freedman D, Khan L, Serdula M, Ogden C, Dietz W. Racial and ethnic differences in secular trends for childhood BMI, weight, and height. *Obesity (Silver Spring)* 2006; **14**: 301–308.

19 Schulz L, Bennett P, Ravussin E, Kidd J, Kidd K, Esparza J, *et al.* Effects of traditional and western environments on prevalence of type 2 diabetes in Pima Indians in Mexico and the US. *Diabetes Care* 2006; **29**: 1866–1871.

20 Dina C, Meyre D, Gallina S, Durand E, Körner A, Jacobson P, *et al.* Variation in FTO contributes to childhood obesity and severe adult obesity. *Nat Genet* 2007; **39**: 724–726.

21 Grant SF, Li M, Bradfield JP, Kim CE, Annaiah K, Santa E, *et al.* Association analysis of the FTO gene with obesity in children of Caucasian and African ancestry reveals a common tagging SNP. *PLoS ONE* 2008: e1746.

22 Stratigopoulos G, Padilla SL, LeDuc CA, Watson E, Hattersley AT, McCarthy MI, *et al.* Regulation of Fto/Ftm gene expression in mice

and humans. *Am J Physiol Regul Integr Comp Physiol* 2008; **294**: R1185–1196.

23 Dahlman I, Arner P. Obesity and polymorphisms in genes regulating human adipose tissue. *Int J Obes (Lond)* 2007; **31**: 1629–1641.

24 Chaput JP, Brunet M, Tremblay A. Relationship between short sleeping hours and childhood overweight/obesity: results from the 'Quebec en Forme' project. *Int J Obes (Lond)* 2006; **30**: 1080–1085.

25 Lumeng JC, Somashekar D, Appugliese D, Kaciroti N, Corwyn RF, Bradley RH. Shorter sleep duration is associated with increased risk for being overweight at ages 9 to 12 years. *Pediatrics* 2007; **120**: 1020–1029.

26 Dabelea D. The predisposition to obesity and diabetes in offspring of diabetic mothers. *Diabetes Care* 2007; **30**: S169–S174.

27 Reece EA. Perspectives on obesity, pregnancy and birth outcomes in the United States: the scope of the problem. *Am J Obstet Gynecol* 2008; **198**: 23–27.

28 Gordon-Larsen, Adair L, Suchindran C. Maternal obesity is associated with younger age at obesity onset in US adolescent offspring followed into adulthood. *Obesity* 2007; **15**: 2790–2796.

29 Hedderson MM, Williams MA, Holt VL, Weiss NS, Ferrara A. Body mass index and weight gain prior to pregnancy and risk of gestational diabetes mellitus. *Am J Obstet Gynecol* 2008; **198**: 409.

30 Silverman BL, Rizzo TA, Cho NH, Metzger BE, Long-term effects of the intrauterine environment: the Northwestern University Diabetes in Pregnancy Center. *Diabetes Care* 1998; **21** (Suppl 2): 142–149.

31 Eriksson JG, Osmond C, Kajantie E, Forsén TJ, Barker DJ. Patterns of growth among children who later develop type 2 diabetes or its risk factors. *Diabetologia* 2006; **49**: 2853–2858.

32 Dunger DB, Salgin B, Ong KK. Session 7: Early nutrition and later health early developmental pathways of obesity and diabetes risk. *Proc Nutr Soc* 2007; **66**: 451–457.

33 Yeung MY. Postnatal growth, neurodevelopment and altered adiposity after preterm birth: from a clinical nutrition perspective. *Acta Paediatrica* 2006; **95**: 909–917.

34 Tanumihardjo S, Anderson C, Kauger-Horwitz M, Emenaker N, Haqq A, Satia J, et al. Poverty, obesity, and malnutrition: an international perspective recognizing the paradox. *J Am Diet Assoc* 2007; **107**: 1966–1972.

35 Gordon-Larsen P, Adair L, Popkin B. The relationship of ethnicity, socioeconomic factors, and overweight in US adolescents. *Obes Res* 2003; **11**: 121–129.

36 Saldana TM, Siega-Riz AM, Adair LS, Suchindran C. The relationship between pregnancy weight gain and glucose tolerance status among black and white women in central North Carolina. *Am J Obstet Gynecol* 2006; **195**: 1629–1635.

37 Steinfeld J, Valentine S, Lerer T, Ingardia C, Wax J, Curry S. Obesity-related complications of pregnancy vary by race. *J Matern Fetal Med* 2000; **9**: 238–241.

38 Shen J, Tymkow C, MacMullen N. Disparities in maternal outcomes among four ethnic populations. *Ethn Dis* 2005; **15**: 492–497.

39 Hillier TA, Pedula KL, Schmidt MM, Mullen JA, Charles MA, Pettitt DJ. Childhood obesity and metabolic imprinting: the ongoing effects of maternal hyperglycemia. *Diabetes Care* 2007; **30**: 2287–2292.

40 Branum A, Schoendorg K. Changing patterns of low birthweight and preterm birth in the United States, 1981–98. *Paediatr Perinat Epidemiol* 2002; **16**: 8–15.

41 Toschke AM, Martin RM, von Kries R, Wells J, Smith GD, Ness AR. Infant feeding method and obesity: body mass index and dual energy X-ray absorptiometry measurements at 9–10 y of age from the Avon Longitudinal Study of Parents and Children (ALSPAC). *Am J Clin Nutr* 2007; **85**: 1578–1585.

42 Li R, Grummer-Strawn L. Racial and ethnic disparities in breast-feeding among United States infants: Third National Health and Nutrition Examination Survey, 1988–1994. *Birth* 2002; **29**: 251–257.

43 Woo JG, Dolan LM, Morrow AL, Geraghty SR, Goodman E. Breast-feeding helps explain racial and socioeconomic status disparities in adolescent adiposity. *Pediatrics* 2008; **121**: e458–465.

44 Andrieu E, Darmon N, Drewnowski A. Low-cost diets: more energy, fewer nutrients. *Eur J Clin Nutr* 2006; **60**: 434–436.

45 Mendoza JA, Drewnowski A, Cheadle A, Christakis DA. Dietary energy density is associated with selected predictors of obesity in US children. *J Nutr* 2006; **136**: 1318–1322.

46 Adam EK, Snell EK, Pendry P. Sleep timing and quantity in ecological and family context: a nationally representative time-diary study. *J Fam Psychol* 2007; **21**: 4–19.

47 Lumeng JC, Appugliese D, Cabral HJ, Bradley RH, Zuckerman B. Neighborhood safety and overweight status in children. *Arch Pediatr Adolesc Med* 2006; **160**: 25–31.

48 Agha A, Monson JP. Modulation of glucocorticoid metabolism by the growth hormone: IGF-1 axis. *Clin Endocrinol (Oxf)* 2007; **66**: 459–465.

49 Colao A, Sarno AD, Cappabianca P, Briganti F, Pivonello R, Somma CD, et al. Gender differences in the prevalence, clinical features and response to cabergoline in hyperprolactinemia. *Eur J Endocrinol* 2003; **148**: 325–331.

50 Gillam MP, Molitch ME, Lombardi G, Colao A. Advances in the treatment of prolactinomas. *Endocr Rev* 2006; **27**: 485–534.

51 Ahmet A, Blaser S, Stephens D, Guger S, Rutkas JT, Hamilton J. Weight gain in craniopharyngioma: a model for hypothalamic obesity. *J Pediatr Endocrinol Metab* 2006; **19**: 121–127.

52 Di Battista E, Naselli A, Queirolo S, Gallarotti F, Garré ML, Milanaccio C, Cama A. Endocrine and growth features in childhood craniopharyngioma: a mono-institutional study. *J Pediatr Endocrinol Metab* 2006; **19** (Suppl 1): 431–437.

53 Srinivasan S, Ogle GD, Garnett SP, Briody JN, Lee JW, Cowell CT. Features of the metabolic syndrome after childhood craniopharyngioma. *J Clin Endocrinol Metab* 2004; **89**: 81–86.

54 Adams LA, Feldstein A, Lindor KD, Angulo P. Nonalcoholic fatty liver disease among patients with hypothalamic and pituitary dysfunction. *Hepatology* 2004; **39**: 909–914.

55 Shaikh MG, Grundy RG, Kirk JMW. Reductions in basal metabolic rate and physical activity contribute to hypothalamic obesity. *J Clin Endocrinol Metab* 2008; **93**: 2588–2593.

56 Brunzell JD. Hypertriglyceridemia. *N Engl J Med* 2007; **357**: 1009–1017.

57 El-Haschimi K, Pierroz DD, Hileman SM, Bjørbaek C, Flier JS. Two defects contribute to hypothalamic leptin resistance in mice with diet-induced obesity. *J Clin Invest* 2000; **105**: 1827–1832.

58 Howard JK, Flier JS. Attenuation of leptin and insulin signaling by SOCS proteins. *Trends Endocrinol Metab* 2006; **1**: 365–371.

59 Irani BG, Dunn-Meynell AA, Levin BE. Altered hypothalamic leptin, insulin, and melanocortin binding associated with moderate-fat diet and predisposition to obesity. *Endocrinology* 2007; **148**: 310–316.

60 Martin TL, Alquier T, Asakura K, Furukawa N, Preitner F, Kahn BB. Diet-induced obesity alters AMP kinase activity in hypothalamus and skeletal muscle. *J Biol Chem* 2006; **281**: 18933–18941.

61 Qatanani M, Lazar MA. Mechanisms of obesity-associated insulin resistance: many choices on the menu. *Genes Dev* 2007; **21**: 1443–1455.

62 Després JP, Lemieux I. Abdominal obesity and metabolic syndrome. *Nature* 2006; **444**: 881–887.

63 Prentki M, Nolan CJ. Islet β cell failure in type 2 diabetes. *J Clin Invest* 2006; **116**: 1802–1812.

64 Liese AD. SEARCH for Diabetes in Youth Study Group. The burden of diabetes mellitus amojng US youth: prevalence estimates from the SEARCH for Diabetes in Youth Study. *Pediatrics* 2006; **118**: 1510–1518.

65 Dabelea D, Bell R, D'Agostino R, Imperatore G, Hohansen J, Linder B et al Incidence of diabetes in youth in the United States. *JAMA* 2007; **297**: 2716–2724.

66 Bergman RN, Finegood DT, Kahn SE. The evolution of β-cell dysfunction and insulin resistance in type 2 diabetes. *Eur J Clin Invest* 2002; **32**: 35–45.

67 Goldfine AB, Bouche C, Parker RA, *et al.* Insulin resistance is a poor predictor of type 2 diabetes in individuals with no family history of disease. *Proc Natl Acad Sci U S A* 2003; **100**: 2724–2729.

68 Franks PW, Hanson RL, Knowler WC, Moffett C, Enos G, Infante AM, *et al.* Childhood predictors of young-onset type 2 diabetes. *Diabetes* 2007; **56**: 2964–2972.

69 Veening MA, van Weissenbruch MM, Heine RJ, Delemarre-van de Waa HA. Beta-cell capacity and insulin sensitivity in prepubertal children born small for gestational age: influence of body size during childhood. *Diabetes* 2003; **52**: 1756–1760.

70 Hypponen E, Power C, Smith GD. Prenatal growth, BMI and risk of type 2 diabetes by early midlife. *Diabetes Care* 2003; **26**: 2512–2517.

71 Pettitt DJ, Jovanovic L. Low birth weight as a risk factor for gestational diabetes, diabetes, and impaired glucose tolerance during pregnancy. *Diabetes Care* 2007; **30** (Suppl 2): S147–S149.

72 Silfen ME, Manibo AM, McMahon DJ, Levine LS, Murphy AR, Oberfield SE. Comparison of simple measures of insulin sensitivity in young girls with premature adrenarche: the fasting glucose to insulin ratio may be a simple and useful measure. *J Clin Endocrinol Metab* 2001; **86**: 2863–2868.

73 Utriainen P, Jääskeläinen J, Romppanen J, Voutilainen R. Childhood metabolic syndrome and its components in premature adrenarche. *J Clin Endocrinol Metab* 2007; **92**: 4282–4285.

74 Boden G, Shulman GI. Free fatty acids in obesity and type 2 diabetes: defining their role in the development of insulin resistance and β-cell dysfunction. *Eur J Clin Invest* 2002; **32**: 14–23.

75 Taksali SE, Caprio S, Dziura J, Dufour S, Calí AM, Goodman TR, *et al.* High visceral and low abdominal subcutaneous fat stores in the obese adolescent: a determinant of an adverse metabolic phenotype. *Diabetes* 2008; **57**: 367–371.

76 Petersen KF, Dufour S, Befroy D, Garcia R, Shulman GI. Impaired mitochondrial activity in the insulin-resistant offspring of patients with type 2 diabetes. *N Engl J Med* 2004; **350**: 664–671.

77 McCance DR, Pettitt DJ, Hanson RL, Jacobsson LTH, Bennett PH, Knowler WC. Glucose, insulin concentrations and obesity in childhood and adolescence as predictors of NIDDM. *Diabetologia* 1994; **37**: 617–623.

78 Martin BC, Warram JH, Krolewski AS, Bergman RN, Soeldner JS, Kahn CR. Role of glucose and insulin resistance in development of type 2 diabetes mellitus: results of a 25 year follow-up study. *Lancet* 1992; **340**: 925–929.

79 Weiss R, Taksall SE, Tamborlane WV, Burgert TS, Savoye M, Caprio S. Predictors of changes in glucose tolerance status in obese youth. *Diabetes Care* 2005; **28**: 902–909.

80 Arslanian SA. Metabolic differences between Caucasian and African-American children and the relationship to type 2 diabetes mellitus. *J Pediatr Endocrinol Metab* 2002; **15** (Suppl 1): 509–517.

81 Weiss R, Dziura JD, Burgert TS, Taksali SE, Tamborlane WV, Caprio S. Ethnic differences in beta cell adaptation to insulin resistance in obese children and adolescents. *Diabetologia* 2006; **49**: 571–579.

82 Liska D, Dufour S, Zern TL, Taksali S, Cali AMG, Dziura J, *et al.* Interethnic differences in muscle, liver and abdominal fat partitioning in obese adolescents. *PLoS ONE* 2007; e569–576.

83 Jago R, Harrell JS, McMurray RG, Edelstein S, El Ghormli L, Bassin S. Prevalence of abnormal lipid and blood pressure values among an ethnically diverse population of eighth-grade adolescents and screening implications. *Pediatrics* 2006; **117**: 2065–2073.

84 Freedman DS, Dietz WH, Srinivasan SR, Berenson GS. The relation of overweight to cardiovascular risk factors among children and adolescents: the Bogalusa Heart Study. *Pediatrics* 1999; **103**: 1175–1182.

85 Herd SL, Gower BA, Dashti N, Goran MI. Body fat, fat distribution and serum lipids, lipoproteins and apolipoproteins in African-American and Caucasian-American prepubertal children. *Int J Obes* 2001; **25**: 198–204.

86 Bacha F, Saad R, Gungor N, Janosky J, Arslanian SA. Obesity, regional fat distribution, and syndrome X in obese black versus white adolescents: race differential in diabetogenic and atherogenic risk factors. *J Clin Endocrinol Metab* 2003; **88**: 2534–2540.

87 Pinhas-Hamiel O, Lerner-Geva L, Copperman NM, Jacobson MS. Lipid and insulin levels in obese children: changes with age and puberty. *Obesity (Silver Spring)* 2007; **15**: 2825–2831.

88 Schwimmer JB, McGreal N, Deutsch R, Finegold MJ, Lavine JE. Influence of gender, race and ethnicity on suspected fatty liver in obese adolescents. *Pediatrics* 2005; **115**: 561–565.

89 Schwimmer JB, Deutsch R, Kahen T, Lavine JE, Stanley C, Behling C. Prevalence of fatty liver in children and adolescents. *Pediatrics* 2006; **118**: 1388–1393.

90 Schwimmer JB, Behling C, Newbury R, Duetsch R, Nievergelt C, Schork NJ, *et al.* Histopathology of pediatric nonalcoholic fatty liver disease. *Hepatology* 2005; **42**: 641–649.

91 Burgert TS, Taksali SE, Dziura J, Goodman TR, Yeckel CW, Papademetris X, *et al.* Alanine aminotransferase levels and fatty liver in childhood obesity: associations with insulin resistance, adiponectin, and visceral fat. *J Clin Endocrinol Metab* 2006; **91**: 4287–4294.

92 Schwimmer JB, Pardee PE, Lavine JE, Blumkin AK, Cook S. Cardiovascular risk factors and the metabolic syndrome in pediatric nonalcoholic fatty liver disease. *Circulation* 2008; **118**: 277–283.

93   Pacifico L, Cantisani V, Ricci P, Osborn JF, Schiavo E, Anania C, et al. Nonalcoholic fatty liver disease and carotid atherosclerosis in children. *Pediatr Res* 2008; **63**: 423–427.

94   Marrero J. Hepatocellular carcinoma. *Curr Opin Gastroenterol* 2006; **22**: 248–53.

95   Smedile A, Bugianesi E. Steatosis and hepatocellular carcinoma risk. *Eur Rev Med Pharmacol Sci* 2005; **9**: 291–293.

96   Marra F, Gastaldelli A, Svegliati Baroni G, Tell G, Tiribelli C. Molecular basis and mechanisms of progression of non-alcoholic steatohepatitis. *Trends Mol Med* 2008; **14**: 72–81.

97   Ouyang X, Cirillo P, Sautin Y, McCall S, Bruchette JL, Diehl AM, et al. Fructose consumption as a risk factor for non-alcoholic fatty liver disease. *J Hepatol* 2008; **48**: 993–999.

98   Koenigsberg J, Boyd GS, Gidding SS, Hassink SG, Falkner B. Association of age and sex with cardiovascular risk factors and insulin sensitivity in overweight children and adolescents. *J Cardiometabolic Synd* 2006; **1**: 253–258.

99   Wang ZV, Scherer PE. Adiponectin, cardiovascular function, and hypertension. *Hypertension* 2008; **51**: 8–14.

100   Yang R, Barouch LA. Grassi. G. Leptin signaling and obesity: cardiovascular consequences. *Circ Res* 2007; **101**: 545–559.

101   Grassi, G. Sympathetic overdrive and cardiovascular risk in the metabolic syndrome. *Hypertens Res* 2006; **29**: 839–847.

102   Weiss R, Dziura J, Burgert TS, Tamborlane WV, Taksali SE, Yeckel CW, et al. Obesity and the metabolic syndrome in children and adolescents. *N Engl J Med* 2004; **350**: 2362–2374.

103   Lee S, Bacha F, Gungor N, Arslanian S. Comparison of different definitions of pediatric metabolic syndrome: relation to abdominal adiposity, insulin resistance, adiponectin, and inflammatory biomarkers. *J Pediatr* 2008; **152**: 177–184.

104   Shaibi GQ, Cruz ML, Weigensberg MJ, Toledo-Corral CM, Lane CJ, Kelly LA, et al. Adiponectin independently predicts metabolic syndrome in overweight Latino youth. *J Clin Endocrinol Metab* 2007; **92**: 1809–1813.

105   Morrison JA, Friedman LA, Wang P, Glueck CJ. Metabolic syndrome in childhood predicts adult metabolic syndrome and type 2 diabetes mellitus 25 to 30 years later. *J Pediatr* 2008; **152**: 201–206.

106   Alberti KGMM, Zimmet PZ, Shaw JE. The metabolic syndrome in children and adolescents. *Lancet* 2007; **369**: 2059–2061.

107   Douyon L, Schteingart DE. Effect of obesity and starvation on thyroid hormone, growth hormone and cortisol secretion. *Endocrinol Metab Clin North Am* 2002; **31**: 173–189.

108   Wabitsch M, Heinze E, Debatin KM, Blum WF. IGF-I- and IGFBP-3-expression in cultured human preadipocytes and adipocytes. *Horm Met Res* 2000; **32**: 555–559.

109   Peter MA, Winterhalter KH, Boni-Schnetzler M, Froesch ER, Zapf J. Regulation of insulin-like growth factor-I (IGF-I) and IGF-binding proteins by growth hormone in rat white adipose tissue. *Endocrinology* 1993; **133**: 2624–2631.

110   Kratzsch J, Dehmel B, Pulzer F, et al. Increased serum GHBP levels in obese pubertal children and adolescents: relationship to body composition, leptin and indicators of metabolic disturbances. *Int J Obes* 1997; **21**: 1130–1136.

111   Gleeson HK, Lissett CA, Shalet SM. Insulin-like growth factor-I response to a single bolus of growth hormone is increased in obesity. *J Clin Endocrinol Metab* 2005; **90**: 1061–1067.

112   Wabitsch M, Blum WF, Muche R, Heinze E, Haug C, Mayer H, et al. Insulin-like growth factors and their binding proteins before and after weight loss and their associations with hormonal and metabolic parameters in obese adolescent girls. *Int J Obes Relat Metab Disord* 1996; **20**: 1073–1080.

113   Frystyk J, Skjaerbaek C, Vestbo E, Fisker S, Orskov H. Circulating levels of free insulin-like growth factors in obese subjects: the impact of type 2 diabetes. *Diabetes Metab Res Rev* 1999; **15**: 314–322.

114   Rasmussen MH, Juul A, Kjems LL, Hilsted J. Effects of short-term caloric restriction on circulating free IGF-I, acid-labile subunit, IGF-binding proteins (IGFBPs)-1-4, and IGFBPs-1-3 protease activity in obese subjects. *Eur J Endocrinol* 2006; **155**: 575–581.

115   Rajkumar K, Modric T, Murphy LJ. Impaired adipogenesis in insulin-like growth factor binding protein-1 transgenic mice. *J Endocrinol* 1999; **162**: 457–465.

116   Wheatcroft SB, Kearney MT, Shah AM, Ezzat VA, Miell JR, Modo M, et al. IGF-binding protein-2 protects against the development of obesity and insulin resistance. *Diabetes* 2007; **56**: 285–294.

117   Steppan CM, Crawford DT, Chidsey-Frink KL, Ke H, Swick AG. Leptin is a potent stimulator of bone growth in ob/ob mice. *Regul Pept* 2000; **92**: 73–78.

118   Maor G, Rochwerger M, Segev Y, Phillip M. Leptin acts as a growth factor on the chondrocytes of skeletal growth centers. *J Bone Miner Res* 2002; **17**: 1034–1043.

119   Montague CT, Farooqi IS, Whitehead JP, Soos MA, Rau H, Wareham NJ, et al. Congenital leptin deficiency is associated with severe early-onset obesity in humans. *Nature* 1997; **387**: 903–908.

120   Farooqi IS, Wangensteen T, Collins S, Kimber W, Matarese G, Keogh JM, et al. Clinical and molecular genetic spectrum of congenital deficiency of the leptin receptor. *N Engl J Med* 2007; **356**: 237–247.

121   Lee JM, Appugliese D, Kaciroti N, Corwyn RF, Bradley RH, Lumeng JC. Weight status in young girls and the onset of puberty. *Pediatrics* 2007; **119**: e624–630.

122   Sam S, Dunaif A. Polycystic ovary syndrome: syndrome XX? *Trends Endocrinol Metab* 2003; **14**: 365–370.

123   Chang RJ. The reproductive phenotype in polycystic ovary syndrome. *Nat Clin Pract Endocrinol Metab* 2007; **3**: 688–695.

124   Artz E, Haqq A, Freemark M. Hormonal and metabolic consequences of childhood obesity. *Endocrinol Metab Clin North Am* 2005; **34**: 643–658.

125   Wake DJ, Rask E, Livingstone DEW, Soderberg S, Olsson T, Walker BR. Local and systemic impact of transcriptional up-regulation of 11β-hydroxysteroid dehydrogenase type 1 in adipose tissue in human obesity. *J Clin Endocrinol Metab* 2003; **88**: 3983–3988.

126   Tomlinson JW, Moore JS, Clark PM, Holder G, Shakespeare L, Stewart PM. Weight loss increases 11β-hydroxysteroid dehydrogenase type 1 expression in human adipose tissue. *J Clin Endocrinol Metab* 2004; **89**: 2711–2716.

127   Zamboni G, Soffiati M, Giavarina D, Tato L. Mineral metabolism in obese children. *Acta Paediatr Scand* 1988; **77**: 741–746.

128   Burgert TS, Dziura J, Yeckel C, Taksali SE, Weiss R, Tamborlane W, et al. Microalbuminuria in pediatric obesity: prevalence and relation to other cardiovascular risk factors. *Int J Obes (Lond)* 2006; **30**: 273–280.

129   Kaambham N, Markowitz GS, Valeri AM, Lin J, D'Agati VD. Obesity-related glomerulopathy: an emerging epidemic. *Kidney Int* 2001; **59**: 1498–1509.

130 Adelman RD, Restaino IG, Alon US, Blowey DL. Proteinuria and focal segmental glomerulosclerosis in severely obese adolescents. *J Pediatr* 2001; **138**: 481–485.

131 Ruibal FJ, Aleo LE, Alvarez MA, Pinero ME, Gomez CR. Childhood cholelithiasis: analysis of 24 patients diagnosed in our department and review of 123 cases published in Spain. *Ann Esp Pediatr* 2001; **54**: 120–125.

132 Balcer LJ, Liu GT, Forman S, *et al*. Idiopathic intracranial hypertension: relation of age and obesity in children. *Neurology* 1999; **52**: 870–872.

133 Ievers-Landis CE, Redline S. Pediatric sleep apnea: implications of the epidemic of childhood ooverweight. *Am J Resp Crit Care* 2007; **175**: 436–441.

134 Van Cauter E, Holmback U, Knutson K, Leproult R, Miller A, Nedeltcheva A, *et al*. Impact of sleep and sleep loss on neuroendocrine and metabolic function. *Horm Res* 2007; **67** (Suppl 1): 2–9.

135 Knutson KL, Spiegel K, Penev P, Van Cauter E. The metabolic consequences of sleep deprivation. *Sleep Med Rev* 2007; **11**: 163–178.

136 Soultan Z, Wadowski S, Rao M, Kravath RE. Effect of treating obstructive sleep apnea by tonsillectomy and/or adenoidectomy on obesity in children. *Arch Pediatr Adolesc Med* 1999; **153**: 33–37.

137 Matsuda M, DeFronzo RA. Insulin sensitivity indices obtained from oral glucose tolerance testing: comparison with the euglycemic insulin clamp. *Diabetes Care* 1999; **22**: 1462–1470.

138 Lee JM, Okumura MJ, Davis MM, Herman WH, Gurney JG. Prevalence and determinants of insulin resistance among US adolescents: a population-based study. *Diabetes Care* 2006; **29**: 2427–2432.

139 Guo SS, Wu W, Chumlea WC, Roche AF. Predicting overweight and obesity in adulthood from body mass index values in childhood and adolescence. *Am J Clin Nutr* 2004; **76**: 653–658.

140 Singleton JR, Smith AG, Russell JW, Feldman EL. Microvascular complications of impaired glucose tolerance. *Diabetes* 2003; **52**: 2867–2873.

141 Kuller LH, Velentgas P, Barzilay J, Beauchamp NJ, O'Leary DH, Savage PJ. Diabetes mellitus: subclinical cardiovascular disease and risk of incident cardiovascular disease and all-cause mortality. *Arterioscler Thromb Vasc Biol* 2000; **20**: 823–829.

142 Haffner SM, Lehto S, Ronnemaa T, Pyorala K, Laasko M. Mortality from coronary heart disease in subjects with type 2 diabetes and in nondiabetic subjects with and without prior myocardial infarction. *N Engl J Med* 1998; **339**: 229–234.

143 Bonora E, Kiechl S, Willeit J, *et al*. Carotid atherosclerosis and coronary heart disease in the metabolic syndrome: prospective data from the Bruneck Study. *Diabetes Care* 2003; **26**: 1251–1257.

144 Atabek ME, Pirgon O, Kivrak AS. Evidence for association between insulin resistance and premature carotid atherosclerosis in childhood obesity. *Pediatr Res* 2007; **61**: 345–349.

145 Beauloye V, Zech F, Tran HT, Clapuyt P, Maes M, Brichard SM. Determinants of early atherosclerosis in obese children and adolescents. *J Clin Endocrinol Metab* 2007; **92**: 3025–3032.

146 Reinehr T, Wunsch R, de Sousa G, Toschke AM. Relationship between metabolic syndrome definitions for children and adolescents and intima-media thickness. *Atherosclerosis* 2008; **199**: 193–200.

147 Berenson GS, Srinivasan SR, Bao W, Newman WP III, Tracy RE, Wattigney WA. Association between multiple cardiovascular risk factors and atherosclerosis in children and young adults. *N Engl J Med* 1998; **338**: 1650–1656.

148 McGill HC Jr, McMahan CA, Herderick EE, *et al*. Pathological Determinants of Atherosclerosis in Youth (PDAY) Research Group. Obesity accelerates the progression of coronary atherosclerosis in young men. *Circulation* 2002; **105**: 2712–2718.

149 Baker JL, Olsen LW, Sørensen TIA. Childhood body-mass index and the risk of coronary heart disease in adulthood. *N Engl J Med* 2007; **357**: 2329–2337.

150 Calle EE, Rodriguez C, Walker-Thurmond K, Thun MJ. Overweight, obesity and mortality from cancer in a prospectively studied cohort of US adults. *N Engl J Med* 2003; **348**: 1625–1638.

151 Renehan AG, Tyson M, Egger M, Heller RF, Zwahlen M. Body mass index and incidence of cancer: a systematic review and meta-analysis of prospective observational studies. *Lancet* 2008; **371**: 569–578.

152 Must A, Jacques PF, Dallal GE, Bajema CJ, Dietz WH. Long-term morbidity and mortality of overweight adolescents: a follow-up of the Harvard Growth Study of 1922 to 1935. *N Engl J Med* 1992; **327**: 1350–1355.

153 Epstein L, Valoski A, Wing R, McCurley J. Ten-year outcomes of behavioral family-based treatment for childhood obesity. *Health Psychol* 1994; **13**: 373–383.

154 Wilfley D, Stein R, Saelens B, Mockus D, Matt G, Hayden-Wade H, *et al*. Efficacy of maintenance treatment approached for childhood overweight: a randomized controlled trial. *JAMA* 2007; **298**: 1661–1673.

155 Savoye M, Shaw M, Dziura J, Tamborlane W, Rose P, Guandalini C, *et al*. Effects of a weight management program on body composition and metabolic parameters in overweight children: a randomized controlled trial. *JAMA* 2007; **297**: 2697–2704.

156 Lovejoy JC. The influence of dietary fat on insulin resistance. *Curr Diab Rep* 2002; **2**: 435–440.

157 Johnson L, Mander AP, Jones LR, Emmett PM, Jebb SA. Energy-dense, low-fiber, high-fat dietary pattern is associated with increased fatness in childhood. *Am J Clin Nutr* 2008; **87**: 846–854.

158 Samaha FF, Iqbal N, Seshadri P, *et al*. Low-carbohydrate as compared with a low-fat diet in severe obesity. *N Engl J Med* 2003; **348**: 2074–2081.

159 Foster GD, Wyatt HR, Hill JO, *et al*. A randomized trial of a low-carbohydrate diet for obesity. *N Engl J Med* 2003; **348**: 2082–2090.

160 Bravata DM, Sanders L, Huang J, Krumholz HM, Olkin I, Gardner CD. Efficacy and safety of low-carbohydrate diets: a systematic review. *JAMA* 2003; **289**: 1837–1850.

161 Gardner CD, Kiazand A, Alhassan S, Kim S, Stafford RS, Balise RR, *et al*. Comparison of the Atkins, Zone, Ornish, and LEARN diets for change in weight and related risk factors among overweight premenopausal women: the A TO Z Weight Loss Study: a randomized trial. *JAMA* 2007; **297**: 969–977.

162 Warren JM, Henry CJ, Simonite V. Low glycemic index breakfasts and reduced food intake in preadolescent children. *Pediatrics* 2003; **112**: e414.

163 Elliott SS, Keim NL, Stern JS, Teff K, Havel PJ. Fructose, weight gain and the insulin resistance syndrome. *Am J Clin Nutr* 2002; **76**: 911–922.

164 Aston LM, Stokes CS, Jebb SA. No effect of a diet with a reduced glycaemic index on satiety, energy intake and body weight in overweight and obese women. *Int J Obes* 2008; **32**: 160–165.

165 Ebbeling CB, Leidig MM, Sinclair KB, Hangen JB, Ludwig DS. A reduced glycemic load diet in the treatment of adolescent obesity. *Arch Pediatr Adolesc Med* 2003; **157**: 773–779.

166 Gibson LJ, Peto J, Warren JM, dos Santos Silva I. Lack of evidence on diets for obesity for children: a systematic review. *Int J Epidemiol* 2006; **35**: 1544–1552.

167 Montonen J, Knekt P, Jarvinene R, Aromaa A, Reunanen A. Whole-grain and fiber intake and the incidence of type 2 diabetes. *Am J Clin Nutr* 2003; **77**: 622–629.

168 Pereira MA, Jacobs DR, Van Horn L, Slattery ML, Kartashov AI, Ludwig DS. Dairy consumption, obesity and the insulin resistance syndrome in young adults: the CARDIA Study. *JAMA* 2002; **287**: 2081–2089.

169 Rodriguez-Moran M, Guerrero-Romero F. Oral magnesium supplementation improves insulin sensitivity and metabolic control in type 2 diabetic subjects: a randomized double-blind controlled trial. *Diabetes Care* 2003; **26**: 1147–1152.

170 Eriksson KF, Lingarde F. Prevention of type 2 (non-insulin dependent) diabetes mellitus by diet and physical exercise: the 6-year Malmo feasibility study. *Diabetologia* 1991; **34**: 891–898.

171 Pan XR, Li GW, Hu YH, *et al*. The Da Qing IGT and Diabetes Study: effects of diet and exercise in preventing NIDDM in people with impaired glucose tolerance. *Diabetes Care* 1997; **20**: 537–544.

172 Uusitupa M, Lindi V, Louheranta A, Salopuro T, Lindstrom J, Tuomilehto J. Long-term improvement in insulin sensitivity by changing lifestyles of people with impaired glucose tolerance. 4-year results from the Finnish Diabetes Prevention Study. *Diabetes* 2003; **52**: 2532–2538.

173 Knowler WC, Barrett-Connor E, Fowler SE, *et al*. Reduction in the incidence of type 2 diabetes with lifestyle intervention or metformin. *N Engl J Med* 2002; **346**: 393–403.

174 Spriet LL, Watt MJ. Regulatory mechanisms in the interaction between carbohydrate and lipid oxidation during exercise. *Acta Physiol Scand* 2003; **178**: 443–452.

175 McGee SL, Howlett KF, Starkie RL, Cameron-Smith D, Kemp BE, Hargreaves M. Exercise increases nuclear AMPK in human skeletal muscle. *Diabetes* 2003; **52**: 926–928.

176 Santoro C, Cosmas A, Forman D, *et al*. Exercise training alters skeletal muscle mitochondrial morphometry in heart failure patients. *J Cardiovasc Risk* 2002; **9**: 377–381.

177 Ferguson MA, Gutin B, Le NA, *et al*. Effects of exercise training and its cessation on components of the insulin resistance syndrome in obese children. *Int J Obes* 1999; **22**: 889–895.

178 Watts K, Beye P, Siafarikas A, *et al*. Exercise training normalizes vascular dysfunction and improves central adiposity in obese adolescents. *J Am Coll Cardiol* 2004; **43**: 1823–1827.

179 Watts K, Beye P, Siafarikas A, O'Driscoll G, Jones TW, Davis EA, *et al*. Effects of exercise training on vascular function in obese children. *J Pediatr* 2004; **144**: 620–625.

180 Sharma M. School-based interventions for childhood and adolescent obesity. *Obes Rev* 2006; **7**: 261–269.

181 Freemark M. Pharmacotherapy of childhood obesity: an evidence-based, conceptual approach. *Diabetes Care* 2007; **30**: 395–402.

182 Coll AP, Farooqi IS, O'Rahilly S. The hormonal control of food intake. *Cell* 2007; **129**: 251–262.

183 Higgins SC, Gueorguiev M, Korbonits M. Ghrelin, the peripheral hunger hormone. *Ann Med* 2007; **39**: 116–136.

184 Rolland-Cachera MF, Thibault H, Souberbielle JC, Soulié D, Carbonel P, Deheeger M, *et al*. Massive obesity in adolescents: dietary interventions and behaviours associated with weight regain at 2 y follow-up. *Int J Obes Relat Metab Disord* 2004; **28**: 514–519.

185 Berkowitz RI, Fujioka K, Daniels SR, Hoppin AG, Owen S, Perry AC, *et al*. Sibutramine Adolescent Study Group. Effects of sibutramine treatment in obese adolescents: a randomized trial. *Ann Intern Med* 2006; **145**: 81–90.

186 Berkowitz RI, Wadden TA, Tershakovec AM, Cronquist JL. Behavior therapy and sibutramine for the treatment of adolescent obesity. *JAMA* 2003; **289**: 1805–1812.

187 Mason PJ, Morris VA, Balcezak TJ. Serotonin syndrome. Presentation of 2 cases and review of the literature. *Medicine* 2000; **79**: 201–209.

188 Torgersen JS, Hauptman J, Boldrin MN, Sjostrom L. XENical in the prevention of Diabetes in Obese Subjects (XENDOS) Study: a randomized study of orlistat as an adjunct to lifestyle changes for the prevention of type 2 diabetes in obese patients. *Diabetes Care* 2004; **27**: 155–161.

189 Chanoine J-P, Hampl S, Jensen C, Boldrin, M, Hauptman J: Effects of orlistat on weight and body composition in obese adolescents: a randomized controlled trial. *JAMA* 2005; **293**: 2873–2883.

190 Zhou G, Myers R, Li Y, *et al*. Role of AMP-activated protein kinase in mechanism of metformin action. *J Clin Invest* 2001; **108**: 1167–1174.

191 Hallsten K, Virtanen KA, Lonnqvist F, *et al*. Rosiglitazone but not metformin enhances insulin- and exercise-stimulated skeletal muscle glucose uptake in patients with newly diagnosed type 2 diabetes. *Diabetes* 2002; **51**: 3479–3485.

192 Virtanen KA, Hallsten K, Parkkola R, *et al*. Differential effects of rosiglitazone and metformin on adipose tissue distribution and glucose uptake in type 2 diabetic subjects. *Diabetes* 2003; **52**: 283–290.

193 Paolisso G, Amato L, Eccellente R, *et al*. Effect of metformin on food intake in obese subjects. *Eur J Clin Invest* 1998; **28**: 441–446.

194 Glueck CJ, Fontaine RN, Wang P, *et al*. Metformin reduces weight, centripetal obesity, insulin, leptin and low-density lipoprotein cholesterol in nondiabetic, morbidly obese subjects with body mass index greater than 30. *Metabolism* 2001; **50**: 856–861.

195 Salpeter SR, Buckley NS, Kahn JA, Salpeter EE. Meta analysis: metformin treatment in persons at risk for diabetes mellitus. *Am J Med* 2008; **121**: 149–157.

196 UK Prospective Diabetes Study (UKPDS) Group. Effect of intensive blood-glucose control with metformin on complications in overweight patients with type 2 diabetes (UKPDS 34). *Lancet* 1998; **352**: 854–865.

197 Freemark M, Bursey D. The effects of metformin on body mass index and glucose tolerance in obese adolescents with fasting hyperinsulinemia and a family history of type 2 diabetes. *Pediatrics* 2001; **107**: e55–e61.

198 Kay JP, Alemzadeh R, Langley G, D'Angelo L, Smith P, Holshouser S. Beneficial effects of metformin in normoglycemic morbidly obese adolescents. *Metabolism* 2001; **50**: 1457–1461.

199 Srinivasan S, Ambler GR, Baur LA, Garnett SP, Tepsa M, Yap F, *et al*. Randomized, controlled trial of metformin for obesity and insulin resistance in children and adolescents: improvement in body composition and fasting insulin. *J Clin Endocrinol Metab* 2006; **91**: 2074–2080.

200 Burgert T, Duran E, Goldberg-Gell R, Dziura J, Yeckel C, Katz S, *et al*. Short-term metabolic and cardiovascular effects of metformin in markedly obese adolescents with normal glucose tolerance. *Pediatr Diabetes*, 2008; **9**: 567–576.

201 Klein DJ, Cottingham EM, Sorter M, Barton BA, Morrison JA. A randomized, double-blind, placebo-controlled trial of metformin treatment of weight gain associated with initiation of atypical antipsychotic therapy in children and adolescents. *Am J Psychiatry* 2006; **163**: 2072–2079.

202 Ramachandran A, Snehalatha C, Mary S, Mukesh B, Bhaskar AD, Vijay V. The Indian Diabetes Prevention Programme shows that lifestyle modification and metformin prevent type 2 diabetes in Asian Indian subjects with impaired glucose tolerance (IDPP-1). *Diabetologia* 2006; **49**: 289–297.

203 Diabetes Prevention Program Research Group. Effects of withdrawal from metformin on the development of diabetes in the diabetes prevention program. *Diabetes Care* 2003; **26**: 977–980.

204 Allen HF, Mazzoni C, Heptulla RA, Murray MA, Miller N, Koenigs L, *et al.* Randomized controlled trial evaluating response to metformin versus standard therapy in the treatment of adolescents with polycystic ovary syndrome. *J Pediatr Endocrinol Metab* 2005; **18**: 761–768.

205 Ibáñez L, Valls C, Marcos MV, Ong K, Dunger DB, De Zegher F. Insulin sensitization for girls with precocious pubarche and with risk for polycystic ovary syndrome: effects of prepubertal initiation and postpubertal discontinuation of metformin treatment. *J Clin Endocrinol Metab* 2004; **89**: 4331–4337.

206 Hoeger K, Davidson K, Kochman L, *et al.* The impact of metformin on oral contraceptives and lifestyle modification on PCOS in obese adolescent women. *J Clin Endocrinol Metab* 2008; **93**: 4299–4306.

207 Freemark M. Liver dysfunction in paediatric obesity: a randomized, controlled trial of metformin. *Acta Paediatrica* 2007; **96**: 1326–1332.

208 Schwimmer JB, Middleton MS, Deutsch R, Lavine JE. A phase 2 clinical trial of metformin as a treatment for non-diabetic paediatric non-alcoholic steatohepatitis. *Aliment Pharmacol Ther* 2005; **21**: 871–879.

209 Kao J, Tobis J, McClelland RL, Heaton MR, Davis BR, Holmes DR Jr, *et al.* the Investigators in the Prevention of Restenosis With Tranilast and Its Outcomes Trial: Relation of metformin treatment to clinical events in diabetic patients undergoing percutaneous intervention. *Am J Cardiol* 2004; **93**: 1347–1350.

210 Gerstein HC, Yusuf S, Bosch J, Pogue J, Sheridan P, Dinccag N, *et al.* The DREAM (Diabetes REduction Assessment with ramipril and rosiglitazone Medication) Trial Investigators: Effect of rosiglitazone on the frequency of diabetes in patients with impaired glucose tolerance or impaired fasting glucose: a randomized controlled trial. *Lancet* 2006; **368**: 1096–1105.

211 Xiang AH, Peters RK, Kjos SL, Marroquin A, Goico J, Ochoa C, *et al.* Effect of pioglitazone on pancreatic beta-cell function and diabetes risk in Hispanic women with prior gestational diabetes. *Diabetes* 2006; **55**: 517–522.

212 Belfort R, Harrison SA, Brown K, Darland C, Finch J, Hardies J, *et al.* A placebo-controlled trial of pioglitazone in subjects with nonalcoholic steatohepatitis. *N Engl J Med* 2006; **355**: 2297–2307.

213 Bolen S, Feldman L, Vassy J, Wilson L, Yeh HC, Marinopoulos S, *et al.* Systematic review: comparative effectiveness and safety of oral medications for type 2 diabetes mellitus. *Ann Intern Med* 2007; **147**: 386–399.

214 Lustig RH, Hinds PS, Ringwald-Smith K, Christensen RK, Kaste SC, Schreiber RE, *et al.* Octreotide therapy of pediatric hypothalamic obesity: a double-blind, placebo-controlled trial. *J Clin Endocrinol Metab* 2003; **88**: 2586–2592.

215 Pi-Sunyer F, Aronne LJ, Heshmati HM, Devin J, Rosenstock J. Effect of rimonabant, a cannabinoid-1 receptor blocker, on weight and cardiometabolic risk factors in overweight or obese patients: RIONorth America. *JAMA* 2006; **295**: 761–775.

216 Sjöström L, Lindroos AK, Peltonen M, Torgerson J, Bouchard C, Carlsson B, *et al.* Swedish Obese Subjects Study Scientific Group. Lifestyle, diabetes, and cardiovascular risk factors 10 years after bariatric surgery. *N Engl J Med* 2004; **351**: 2683–2693.

217 Dixon JB, O'Brien PE, Playfair J, Chapman L, Schachter LM, Skinner S, *et al.* Adjustable gastric banding and conventional therapy for type 2 diabetes: a randomized controlled trial. *JAMA* 2008; **299**: 316–323.

218 Leonetti F, Silecchia G, Iacobellis G, *et al.* Different plasma ghrelin levels after laparoscopic gastric bypass and adjustable gastric banding in morbid obese subjects. *J Clin Endocrinol Metab* 2003; **88**: 4227–4231.

219 Buchwald H, Estok R, Fahrbach K, Banel D, Sledge I. Trends in mortality in bariatric surgery: a systematic review and meta-analysis. *Surgery* 2007; **142**: 621–632.

220 Favretti F, O'Brien PE, Dixon JB. Patient management after LAP-BAND placement. *Am J Surg* 2002; **184**: 38S–41S.

221 Gaede P, Vedel P, Larsen N, Jensen GV, Parving HH, Pedersen O. Multifactorial intervention and cardiovascular disease in patients with type 2 diabetes. *N Engl J Med* 2003; **348**: 383–393.

222 Hawkins SS, Law C. A review of risk factors for overweight in preschool children: a policy perspective. *Int J Pediatr Obes* 2006; **1**: 195–209.

223 Wells JC, Chomtho S, Fewtrell MS. Programming of body composition by early growth and nutrition. *Proc Nutr Soc* 2007; **66**: 423–434.

224 Mayer-Davis EJ, Dabelea D, Lamichhane AP, D'Agostino RB Jr, Liese AD, Thomas J, *et al.* Breast feeding and type 2 diabetes in youth of three ethnic droups: the SEARCH for Diabetes in Youth case–control study. *Diabetes Care* 2008; **31**: 470–475.

225 Christakis NA, Fowler JH. The spread of obesity in a large social network over 32 years. *N Engl J Med* 2007; **357**: 370–379.

226 Monsivais P, Drewnowski A. The rising cost of low-energy-density foods. *J Am Diet Assoc* 2007; **107**: 2071–2076.

21 Polycystic Ovarian Syndrome

M. Isabel Hernandez & Verónica Mericq

Institute of Maternal and Child Research, Faculty of Medicine, University of Chile, Santiago, Chile

Polycystic ovarian syndrome (PCOS) is one of the most common endocrinopathies, affecting 6–10% of women of reproductive age [1]. Its pathogenesis is unknown. A heterogeneous disorder, its definition remains controversial. It is characterized by clinical and/or biochemical hyperandrogenism of ovarian and usually also adrenal origins, menstrual irregularities, variable insulin resistance and polycystic ovaries. PCOS, a lifelong disorder, often presents during late adolescence but manifests itself in some cases with signs of adrenarche [2].

PCOS appears to be inherited but many factors are associated with its development, including androgen exposure *in utero*, possibly low birthweight and, later, exogenous insulin. Because the symptoms emerge insidiously and are coincident with changes that accompany normal puberty, early subtle features may be missed, which delays treatment. Identifying girls at risk for PCOS and implementing treatment early may prevent some of the long-term complications.

Normal menstrual cycles

Menarche occurs 2–3 years after thelarche, at Tanner stage IV of breast development at a median age of 12–13 years, which has remained stable over the past 30 years. Although Black girls start to mature earlier than non-Hispanic White and Hispanic girls, US females complete secondary sexual development at approximately the same age. An increased body mass index (BMI) during childhood is related to earlier onset of puberty which may affect the age of menarche.

Early postmenarcheal menstrual cycles are often irregular and anovulatory. The frequency of ovulation is related to the time since menarche and the age at menarche, which means that early menarche is associated with earlier onset of ovulatory cycles. Girls

Brook's Clinical Pediatric Endocrinology, 6th edition. Edited by C. Brook, P. Clayton, R. Brown. © 2009 Blackwell Publishing, ISBN: 978-1-4051-8080-1.

with later onset menarche may take 8–12 years to attain ovulatory cycles.

The length of a menstrual cycle ranges from 21 to 45 days. An individual's cycle length is established around the sixth year after menarche, if it started within the normal age range. During the early postmenarcheal years, cycles may be long because of anovulation.

Definitions

PCOS is the most frequent cause of oligo-ovulatory infertility [3] but a precise and universal definition of the syndrome is lacking. A relatively invariable characteristic is androgen excess [4] and two other features, often considered fundamental to diagnosis, are ovulatory dysfunction and polycystic ovarian morphology. There are three major consensuses of the diagnostic criteria (Table 21.1).

1 **National Institutes of Health (NIH) 1990** criteria [5] included:

  (a) Hyperandrogenism and/or hyperandrogenemia;

  (b) Oligo-anovulation; and

  (c) Exclusion of related known disorders such as hyperprolactinemia, thyroid disorders, congenital adrenal hyperplasia (CAH) and Cushing syndrome.

The ultrasound demonstration of polycystic ovaries was considered suggestive but not diagnostic.

2 The **Rotterdam 2003** consensus required two of the following criteria:

  (a) Oligo- or anovulation;

  (b) Clinical and/or biochemical signs of hyperandrogenism; and

  (c) Polycystic ovaries on ultrasound [6,7]).

The Rotterdam criteria are relatively vague in adolescents [8].

3 Based on the previous considerations, the **Androgen Excess Society** (AES) charged a taskforce to review all available data and recommend an evidence-based definition for PCOS. The AES 2006 conclusion was that PCOS should be considered a disorder

Table 21.1 Diagnostic criteria for the diagnosis of polycystic ovarian syndrome (PCOS).

NIH 1990 (NICDH)	Rotterdam Criteria 2003 (ESHRE/ASRM)	Androgen Excess Society 2006 (AES)
Oligo-ovulation	Oligo-or anovulation	Clinical and/or biochemical hyperandrogenism
Clinical and/or biochemical hyperandrogenism	Clinical and/or biochemical hyperandrogenism	Ovarian dysfunction: oligoanovulation and/or Polycystic
	Polycystic ovaries (US)	ovaries (US)
Both criteria must be present	Two of the three criteria must be present	Both criteria must be present
Exclusion		
Congenital adrenal hyperplasia	Congenital adrenal hyperplasia, Androgen secreting	Congenital adrenal hyperplasia, Androgen-secreting
Androgen-secreting tumors	tumors, Cushing syndrome	tumors, Androgenic/anabolic drug
Cushing syndrome		Cushing syndrome
Hyperprolactinemia		Syndromes of severe insulin resistance
		Thyroid dysfunction
		Hyperprolactinemia

of androgen excess or hyperandrogenism. The absence of hyperandrogenism makes a diagnosis of PCOS less certain [9]. The AES agreed there should be acceptance of the NIH criteria with some modifications expressed in the Rotterdam conference. The AES criteria for the diagnosis of PCOS should include the following criteria:

(a) Hyperandrogenism (hirsutism and/or hyperandrogenemia);

(b) Ovarian dysfunction (oligo-anovulation and/or polycystic ovaries); and

(c) Exclusion of other androgen excess or related disorders.

The inclusion of ovulatory dysfunction, hirsutism, hyperandrogenemia and polycystic ovaries resulted in the taskforce identifying nine different phenotypes as being included in a diagnosis of PCOS. The presence of obesity, insulin resistance, hyperinsulinism and increased luteinizing hormone (LH) concentrations, although observed in many patients, should not be considered as part of the definition of PCOS [9].

Epidemiology

The prevalence of PCOS has been studied in different populations, as has the incidence of metabolic consequences in PCOS women, but clearly the prevalence of PCOS depends on the criteria used to define the disorder, the population studied and the selection bias [1,10]. Studies in different populations have suggested prevalence of 6–8% in reproductive-age women using the 1990 NIH criteria.

In 277 unselected women (148 Black and 129 White) of reproductive age examined at the time of their pre-employment physical examination at a university in the south-eastern USA, the overall prevalence of PCOS diagnosed by the NIH 1990 criteria was 4.0% (3.4% among Black and 4.7% among White, NS) [11]. The same investigators repeated the evaluation in a group of 400 unselected women seeking a pre-employment physical at the University of Alabama at Birmingham, USA. The estimated prevalence was 6.6% (Black 8.0% and White 4.8%, NS).

Table 21.2 Predisposing factors to develop polycystic ovarian syndrome (PCOS).

1 Prenatal exposure to androgens
  Non-controlled congenital adrenal hyperplasia
  PCOS
  Drugs
  Tumors
2 Low birthweight?
3 Premature pubarche
4 Epilepsy and anti-epileptic drugs (valproate)
5 Type 1 diabetes mellitus
6 Obesity – insulin resistance
7 Heritability

Among the diagnosed patients, 86% of women presenting with menstrual dysfunction and hirsutism had PCOS, 75% were hirsute and 42% were obese [1]). This rate is very similar to those reported from Greece, the UK and Spain [12–14], although in the UK study the prevalence of PCOS using the NIH criteria was 8% but rose to 26% using the Rotterdam criteria [13].

Predisposing factors

Several conditions have been associated with an increased prevalence of PCOS, including obesity, insulin resistance and the metabolic syndrome, although the last two conditions may be complications associated with the development of PCOS (Table 21.2) [3,15].

Other predisposing factors
Prenatal exposure to androgens
PCOS may originate very early in development: according to this hypothesis, fetal exposure to androgen excess can induce changes

in differentiating tissues leading to PCOS phenotype in adult life [16]. Experiments in rats and sheep provide evidence that exposure to androgen excess may cause anovulatory sterility and polycystic ovaries [17,18]. Prenatally androgenized female rhesus monkeys exhibit all three main features required for the diagnosis of PCOS [16,19].

Pregnant PCOS women have slightly higher concentrations of androgens than pregnant women without PCOS. The origin of the androgen excess is uncertain but higher concentrations of insulin may inhibit aromatase activity in humans and stimulate 3β-hydroxysteroid dehydrogenase activity [20,21]. Increased androgen concentration during pregnancy has been also associated with lower birthweight of offspring [20].

Low birthweight

This is associated with an increased risk of developing the metabolic syndrome, comprising central obesity, insulin resistance, type 2 diabetes and hypertension and this has been associated with an increased risk in the development of a pattern of ovarian function resembling PCOS, fertility problems and other metabolic diseases. It should be noted that these observations have been made only in a selected population [22,23].

The generally accepted hypothesis explaining the development of these long-term alterations relates to an adaptive response to intra-uterine malnutrition, developmental plasticity. This hypothesis includes the additional contribution of growth patterns and environmental factors in infancy and childhood. The adaptation of the fetus to conditions of undernutrition *in utero* involves an alteration in the endocrine setpoint of insulin, insulin-like growth factor, growth hormone pathways and probably the pituitary–gonadal axes. Transition from low birthweight to normal or increased weight during childhood is commonly associated with the development of precocious pubarche, exaggerated adrenarche and an increased risk for subsequent PCOS and hyperinsulinemia [24]. A common path to the abnormal ovarian function reported in these girls is decreased insulin sensitivity, which has been documented in children with a history of low birthweight [25]. These findings have not been confirmed by others.

In a preliminary report from a sample of lean healthy girls, studied at the age of puberty, recruited from the community born either small for gestational age (SGA) or appropriate for gestational age (AGA) at the beginning of puberty, no differences in the presence of pubic hair, axillary hair or apocrine odor were found. Androgen concentrations were within the normal range and the groups of girls did not show differences in the concentrations of dehydroepiandrosterone sulfate (DHEAS) [26]. However, after 2 years, low birthweight girls displayed a different gonadotropin pattern with higher LH : FSH ratio and higher estradiol and 17-OH progesterone (17-OHP) than AGA girls. These differences may allow a faster transition throughout puberty and an androgenic gonadal steroid pattern later. Follow-up of these girls has not been completed so definitive conclusions may be premature [27]. At this time, there are too few data to support ovarian dysfunction, reduced fertility or early menopause in girls born SGA.

Premature pubarche

This indicates the appearance of pubic hair, which may be accompanied by axillary hair. This process is considered premature if it occurs before age 8 years in girls. Pubertal girls with a history of premature pubarche have been reported to show a distinct pattern of ovarian maturation characterized by increased ovarian androgen synthesis throughout puberty, based on both peak after gonadotropin releasing hormone (GnRH) test and incremental increases of 17-pregnenolone and DHEA throughout puberty and of 17-OHP and androstenedione in late puberty which were significantly higher in premature pubarche girls than in controls in a selected population [28].

The same team studying the postpubertal outcome in 35 girls diagnosed with premature pubarche during childhood found hirsutism, acne and PCOS as a form of functional ovarian hyperandrogenism in 45% of the girls. It was proposed that precocious pubarche in childhood is followed after puberty by functional ovarian hyperandrogenism, together with the metabolic syndrome [29]. Another study failed to demonstrate evidence of ovarian hyperandrogenism in prepubertal girls with precocious pubarche but found an association with functional adrenal hyperandrogenism [30].

In a study in Turkey of 16 patients with a history of premature pubarche, 40.7% had evidence of ovarian hyperandrogenism in response to a GnRH test, three also had PCO morphology on pelvic ultrasound examination [31]. Therefore, premature pubarche may be a risk factor for the development of PCOS in the latest stages of puberty and later in life.

Epilepsy and anti-epileptic drugs

Epileptic seizures have been associated with the development of PCOS and hypersecretion of LH and reproductive endocrine disorders such as PCOS, hypothalamic amenorrhea, premature menopause and hyperprolactinemia. All have been reported to be more common in women with epilepsy than in the general female population [32]. The prevalence reported by different authors in women with temporal lobe epilepsy is 20–25% and the syndrome has been observed in women not treated with anti-epileptic drugs. PCOS was associated with predominantly left-sided lateralization of inter-ictal epileptic discharges [33].

In 15% of women with primary generalized epilepsy, epilepsy itself has been suggested to be responsible for the development of reproductive endocrine disorders.

In addition to epilepsy, anti-epileptic drugs can alter endocrine function. Therapy with valproate affects both metabolic and endocrine function and has been related to weight gain during treatment [34]. PCOS and hyperandrogenism have been observed in 60% of women receiving valproate as a monotherapy and were particularly common if the treatment was started before 20 years of age [35,36]. It was suggested that obesity, hyerinsulinemia and low serum insulin-like growth factor binding protein 1 (IGFBP-1) concentrations may have a role in the development of PCOS. Replacement of valproate with lamotrigine resulted in normalization of endocrine function. Carbamazepine has not been related with the development of PCOS and could be considered a safe drug in women with epilepsy and hyperandrogenism because it is associated with low serum testosterone concentrations and low free androgen index.

Type 1 diabetes mellitus

After insulin became widely available for the treatment of type 1 diabetes mellitus (DM), it became apparent that menstrual disturbances were common, irrespective of metabolic control, and that increased serum androgen concentrations found in some of these women could play a part in these abnormalities. The reported prevalence of PCOS in adult women with type 1 DM is 12–18% using NIH criteria and 31–40% using the Rotterdam criteria [14,36]. Mild hirsutism and biochemical hyperandrogenism are present in 30% and 20%, respectively, in some populations, but in less than 10% in others [14,36,37]. Menstrual abnormalities are observed in 20% of adult women with type 1 DM and polycystic ovarian morphology has been reported in up to 50% [36,37].

Puberty is a critical period for women with DM and it seems to be involved in the pathogenesis of hyperandrogenism. The onset of type 1 DM before menarche in an adolescent receiving intensive insulin therapy has been found as the only factor associated with the development of PCOS [37]. It has been suggested that exogenous hyperinsulinism at the onset of ovarian function during puberty reprograms ovarian function towards increased androgen secretion, leading to hyperandrogenism [38].

Obesity and insulin resistance

The association between PCOS and type 2 DM has long been recognized. Obesity in children and adolescents is well known to be associated with high androgenic activity, increased androgen production, precocious puberty and accelerated bone age with relatively tall stature and also with premature adrenarche and PCOS [39]. Obese women with increased androgens are more prone to metabolic syndrome. Studies in prepubertal and pubertal obese girls reported higher concentrations of testosterone and also DHEAS than in lean girls [40]. Moreover, studies in obese prepubertal and adolescents girls and also in obese women have shown a normalization of hyperandrogenemia and metabolic disturbances after weight loss [40]. In obese individuals with insulin resistance, hyperinsulinemia acts in conjunction with LH to increase androgen production by ovarian theca cells: additionally, insulin suppresses hepatic production of sexual hormone binding globulin (SHBG) leading to a marked elevation of free or unbound plasma testosterone [41]. The marked increase in obesity in adolescent girls is associated with increased hyperandrogenemia that could be a genetic marker for the propensity to develop PCOS [42].

Genetics of PCOS

PCOS is a complex genetic disorder with a multifactorial etiology, in which a variety of predisposing genes interact with environ-

mental factors to produce elements characteristic of the disease. Family studies demonstrate that PCOS is significantly more prevalent among family members than in the general population.

Heritability

The first genetic study in 1968 reported the families of 18 Caucasian patients with Stein–Leventhal syndrome compared with the families of 18 paired control women. The incidence of oligomenorrhea, hirsutism and enlarged ovaries was much more common in sisters of affected subjects than in sisters of controls [43].

Subsequently, a series of 81 families with patients presenting with hirsutism and either polycystic or bilaterally enlarged ovaries were studied, indicating that PCOS could be inherited in an X-linked dominant fashion with familial aggregation of hyperandrogenic symptoms and metabolic disorders [44]. In a study of first-degree relatives of 381 patients with hirsutism, with or without enlarged ovaries and/or oligomenorrhea, patients had a higher prevalence of oligomenorrhea and infertility and their first-degree relatives had higher incidence of hirsutism than a control group of 179 women [45]. Among first- degree relatives with hirsutism and enlarged ovaries, the presence of oligomenorrhea and infertility was more prevalent than in first-degree relatives lacking these characteristics. Similar data demonstrating that the prevalence of PCOS among female relatives (mothers and sisters) of PCOS patients is significantly higher than in the general population have been published [46–49].

Not only is PCOS itself an heritable condition, insulin resistance, insulin secretion and metabolic syndrome appear also to be under genetic control. In a study of families of 15 patients with PCOS, 73% of sisters had polycystic ovaries on ultrasound and 87% had elevated testosterone concentrations. Hyperinsulinemia was present in 69% and hypertriglyceridemia in 56% of family members, making hyperinsulinemia a genetic marker for subjects who may be carriers of a familial tendency for PCOS [50].

In 115 sisters of 80 women with PCOS following the NIH criteria, 22% had the criteria for PCOS, 24% had hyperandrogenemia plus regular menstrual cycles and their sisters with PCOS or hyperandrogenemia had elevated serum LH concentrations compared to control women [51]. Of these sisters of women with PCOS, those with PCOS or hyperandrogenism had significantly elevated fasting insulin concentrations and decreased fasting insulin:glucose ratio suggestive of insulin resistance. Markers of insulin resistance were associated with hyperandrogenemia but not with menstrual irregularity. PCOS sisters also demonstrate decreased concentrations of SHBG and higher incidence of obesity [52].

Relatives may be at higher risk for type 2 diabetes, glucose intolerance and insulin resistance [53–56]. Metabolic syndrome has also been associated with the PCOS phenotype: in an evaluation of parents of girls with PCOS, a higher prevalence of metabolic syndrome was found, particularly in fathers (79%) [57].

Studies of daughters of PCOS women are scarce. In a study of 53 prepubertal and 22 pubertal daughters of PCOS women, higher concentrations of insulin and lower concentrations of adiponectin were observed in prepubertal girls than in controls. During mid-puberty, higher concentrations of testosterone, 2-h insulin and triglycerides were detected. SHBG was lower in both groups of daughter from PCOS women, suggesting some of the metabolic features of PCOS may be present in daughters of PCOS women before the onset of hyperandrogenism [58].

In a cohort of 40 girls (8–14 years) who have at least one female first-degree relative with PCOS, significant changes in insulin sensitivity during maturation from Tanner stage 1 to 3 have been demonstrated. These changes appear dependent on both the glucose tolerance of the PCOS proband and the relationship between proband and subject (daughters versus younger sisters). Subjects whose PCOS proband is glucose tolerant are more insulin-sensitive at Tanner stage 1 than subjects whose PCOS proband is glucose intolerant, both in cross-sectional and longitudinal analyses. These data suggest that the family history of PCOS-associated glucose intolerance may exert a significant effect on the flux of insulin sensitivity during pubertal maturation and the ability of the female first-degree relative to resolve pubertal insulin resistance [59].

There are a few data regarding PCOS in twins [60,61].

Finally, premature balding and increased hirsutism in male relatives were found in 19.7% of PCOS relatives of patients compared with only 6.5% of control relatives. Abnormalities in plasma LH and DHEAS concentrations in PCOS brothers, insulin resistance in PCOS fathers and brothers and different responses to leuprolide test in PCOS brothers have also been shown.

Candidate genes

The genetic mechanisms underlying PCOS remain largely unknown. The elucidation of the molecular genetic basis has been complicated by the heterogeneity in the diagnostic criteria to define PCOS and, despite many positive results, no gene or genes have clearly emerged as most important. Candidate genes evaluated so far were selected from pathways affecting single components of PCOS and to date no genome-wide analysis has been published for PCOS.

Candidate genes (Table 21.3) [42] have generally targeted loci regulating:

1 Androgen biosynthesis, transport and action;
2 Regulation of androgen biosynthesis (gonadotropic action);
3 Insulin secretion and action and associated disorders;
4 Proinflammatory genotypes; and
5 Others.

Phenotypes and special characteristic in adolescent girls

Most women with PCOS date the onset of symptoms to the peripubertal or early adolescent periods. Symptoms of PCOS emerge insidiously contemporaneously with normal pubertal development (Figs 21.1 & 21.2).

Hirsutism and hyperandrogenism

"Hyperandrogenism" is a term used to describe the most common clinical signs in women with higher concentrations of androgens and comprise hirsutism, acne and alopecia. "Hirsutism" is defined as excessive hair growth in women in anatomic areas where the hair follicles are most androgen-sensitive. About 60% of PCOS women have hirsutism and this sign is considered the most characteristic clinical feature [9] but there are important inter-racial and inter-individual differences in the appearance of hirsutism which seem to be caused by individual variability in pilosebaceous unit sensitivity to androgens. East Asians tend to be less hairy than Euro-Americans, even with the same concentrations of testosterone.

In girls, increased hair (especially facial) is noted at or soon after puberty. The appearance of hair is difficult at first to distinguish from hair growth resulting from normal adrenarche. Initially, the hair is lightly pigmented and thin but, in the presence of persistent elevated concentrations of androgens, it becomes more abundant, darkly pigmented and thick and is localized in a male pattern.

Table 21.3 Candidate genes for polycystic ovarian syndrome (PCOS).

Androgen biosynthesis transport and action	Gonadotropic action and regulation	Insulin secretion, metabolism and associated disorders	Proinflammatory genotypes	Others
CYP17	LH-β subunit	Insulin receptor gene	TNF-α	Follistatine
CYP11B2	FSH-β subunit*	IRS 1 and 2	TNFRSF1B	Microsomal epoxide hydrolase
CYP11A	Dopamine D3 receptor*	Insulin	IL-6	Bone morphogenetic proteins
CYP21*		IGF-2	gp130	
CYP19*		IGF-1R	IL-6Rα*	
SHBG		PPAR-γ2	Paraoxane*	
Androgen receptor		PON1	Pal-1	
H6PD (Hexose-6-phosphate dehydrogenase)*		SORBS1	Matrix metalloproteinase-1*	
		Calpain-10	Factor V*	
			Adiponectine	

*Positive result only one report.

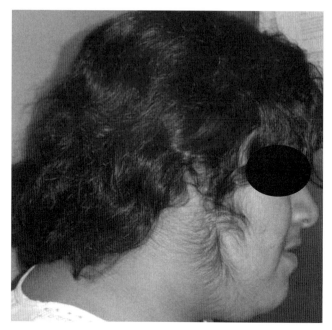

Figure 21.1 A 16-year-old girl diagnosed with polycystic ovarian syndrome (PCOS): history of hirsutism and menstrual irregularities.

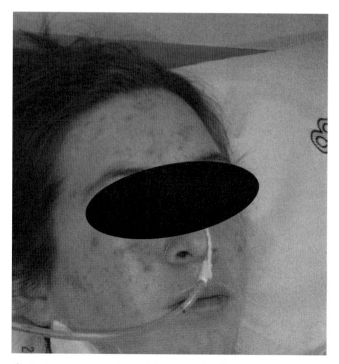

Figure 21.2 Severe acne in an adolescent with insulinoma.

Hirsutism is commonly graded according to the Ferriman–Gallwey system in which a score <8 is considered normal in adults. The degree of facial and body terminal hair growth in women represents a continuum and most investigators have used the 95th centile of controls as the upper limit, which corresponds to a score of 6–8 in the White or Black population [62].

Other signs of hyperandrogenism include acne, seborrhea and alopecia, which typically begins in the frontoparietal area and is fairly diffuse compared to males. The AES task force noted that these clinical signs could not be used as reliable indicators of hyperandrogenism in the diagnosis of PCOS [9]. Rapid onset of hirsutism and very high androgen concentrations should alert the clinician to the possibility of an adrenal or ovarian neoplasm.

Menstrual irregularities

In a large series of patients diagnosed with PCOS, 75% have clinically evident menstrual dysfunction [9]. In adolescents with PCOS, menstrual irregularity is found in about two-thirds [63] but, because the duration of the menstrual cycle and the physiologic irregularity that accompanies normal puberty may be variable, the irregular bleeding patterns among adolescent girls with PCOS and postmenarcheal girls are indistinguishable and the diagnosis of PCOS based purely on menstrual history is not advisable in young girls. Most early postmenarcheal cycles are anovulatory but the diagnosis of PCOS may be suspected in girls, especially those 2 years after menarche, who present with:

1 *Oligomenorrhea*: menstrual bleeding that occurs at intervals over 40 days or fewer than 9 periods per year.

2 *Primary amenorrhea*: absence of menarche by 16 years of age.

3 *Secondary amenorrhea*: absence of menses for at least 3 months.

4 *Dysfunctional uterine bleeding*: excessive and irregular vaginal bleeding.

The diagnosis of PCOS can be made after ruling out the differential diagnosis of menstrual disturbances (Fig. 21.3).

In a study of 58 adolescents with regular menstrual cycles, 50 with irregular menstrual cycles and 29 with oligomenorrhea, the prevalence of polycystic ovaries (PCO) increased significantly with the irregularity of the menstrual cycle pattern (45% in oligomenorrheic girls compared with 9% and 28% in girls with regular cycles and irregular cycles, respectively). Higher concentrations of LH and androgens in the PCO group were also reported [64].

Ovarian morphology

The relevance of adult polycystic ovary criteria to adolescents is unclear. Polycystic ovaries detected by transvaginal ultrasonography may be found in approximately 75% of women with a clinical diagnosis of PCOS. The most common criteria to define PCOS include 12 or more follicles measuring 2–9 mm in diameter or increased ovarian volume (>10 cm^3) (Fig. 21.4) [65].

The usefulness of ultrasonography in young girls is commonly limited by the necessity of abdominal scanning and the difficulty of getting adequate imaging in obese girls. In addition, the number of large antral follicles is at its maximum around the time of menarche [66] and it is suggested that polycystic ovarian morphology in asymptomatic adolescents may be a normal variant [67]. Ovarian morphology in adolescent girls must be interpreted

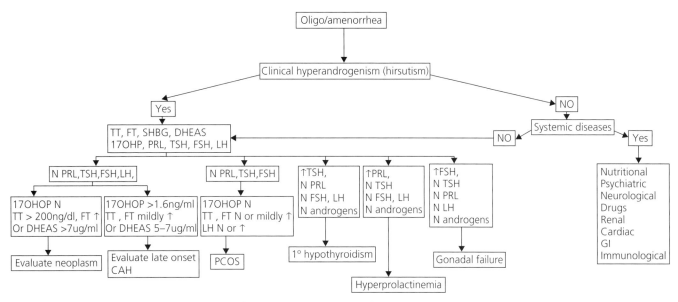

Figure 21.3 Flow diagram for the laboratory evaluation of oligo-/amenorrhea and hyperandrogenism.

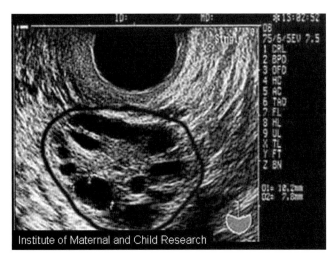

Figure 21.4 Ultrasound with polycystic ovarian (PCO) morphology.

with caution because of the limitations exposed above and the normal maturation of the reproductive axis.

Insulin resistance, obesity and metabolic syndrome

The National Health and Nutritional Examination Survey (NHANES) indicates a marked increase in obesity over the past 30 years in children and adolescents (Fig. 21.5). Coincident with the increase in obesity, there has also been a marked increase in the recognition of the prevalence of type 2 DM and metabolic syndrome in this age group [68]. The prevalence of obesity in PCOS adult women is approximately 50–70%, with a fat distribution characterized by increased central adiposity. A 43% prevalence of metabolic syndrome in PCOS women, nearly twofold higher than that reported for age-matched women in the general population has been reported [68].

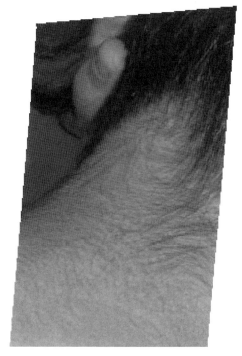

Figure 21.5 The same girl as shown in Fig. 21.4: severe obesity and acanthosis nigricans.

Studies in adolescents with PCOS, both lean and obese, have demonstrated increased risk for impaired glucose tolerance and DM which was attributed to the presence of a defect in insulin action and pancreatic β-cell dysfunction.

In 36 PCOS girls aged 12–19 years, a 27.8% prevalence of metabolic syndrome was found, threefold greater than expected for obesity status [57] and a prevalence of 37% of metabolic syndrome in 49 adolescent girls compared with 5% of NHANES girls has been reported; in this group, hyperandrogenemia was a risk factor independent of obesity and insulin resistance [69].

A high prevalence of early asymptomatic coronary atherosclerosis in young obese women with PCOS compared with obese controls has been reported and it is suggested that this increased risk is independent of traditional cardiovascular risk factors [70]. The AES considers that, although obesity, insulin resistance and hyperinsulinism are observed in a significant fraction of patients and are important features in the follow-up of these patients, they should not be used as a part of the definition of PCOS [9], although others disagree [71].

Approaches to the diagnosis of PCOS in adolescents

PCOS should be suspected in adolescents with signs of hyperandrogenism with or without menstrual irregularities and early recognition is important. The following points are relevant to consider:

1 *Family history* Infertility, menstrual disorders and hirsutism in female relatives. Early baldness in male relatives. History of metabolic syndrome in the family.

2 *Past medical history* History of maternal androgen excess during pregnancy, low birthweight or a high birthweight, precocious pubarche/adrenarche, epilepsy and anti-epileptic drugs. Obesity or metabolic disorders.

3 *Physical examination* Severity and distribution of hirsutism according to Ferriman–Gallwey score. Weight, BMI, general body habitus (gynecoid versus android), fat distribution, presence of acanthosis nigricans and blood pressure that suggest the presence of metabolic syndrome. Genital examination to assess Tanner stage and signs of virilization. The presence of severe virilization should alert to the possibility of a virilizing tumor or CAH. Purple striae with a decreased muscle mass suggest Cushing syndrome.

Endocrine evaluation

Blood should be drawn during the early follicular phase and must exclude other conditions that may increase androgens, alter menstrual cycle or induce anovulation (Table 21.4). The following observations may be relevant.

• Total testosterone concentrations higher than 90 ng/dL (3120 pmol/L) are clear evidence of androgen excess and concentrations above 200 ng/dL (6935 pmol/L) suggest tumor. Most of manual and automated immunoassays tests lack accuracy to measure total testosterone in females and prepubertal children, except in certain situations when testosterone concentrations are elevated.

• Free testosterone measurement by equilibrium dialysis is considered the gold standard; a plasma free testosterone level above the normal adult range, as determined by a reliable laboratory, is the preferred screening test. However, because it is technically

Table 21.4 Expected hormonal profile in adolescents suspicious of polycystic ovarian syndrome (PCOS).

Laboratory test	Expected
Total testosterone	↑
Free testosterone	↑
SHBG	↓
Androstenedione	↑ or normal
DHEAS	↑ slightly
LH	↑ or normal
FSH	Normal
Insulin	↑ or normal
Glicemia	↑ or normal
IGFBP-1	↓ or normal

DHEAS, dehydroepiandrosterone sulfate; FSH, follicle stimulating hormone; IGFBP-1, insulin-like growth factor binding protein-1; LH, luteizing hormone; SHBG, sexual hormone binding globulin.

more demanding, time-consuming and expensive, these assays are not used by most clinical laboratories, although available from reference laboratories. The most widely used assays for measurement of free T in clinical laboratories are direct radio immunoassay tests performed either manually or on automated platforms. Alternatively, some laboratories and investigators have measured total T and SHBG and used the ratio T:SHBG, the so-called free androgen index (FAI), as a surrogate or estimate for free T. Both free and bioavailable T may be calculated by measuring total T, SHBG and albumin concentrations and using the equilibrium binding constants of T to the latter binding proteins in published equations. It is important to note that calculated free and bioavailable testosterone concentrations using less sensitive and precise direct immunoassays would be inaccurate in women and children. An FAI > 4.5 suggests hyperandrogenemia.

• Sex hormone binding globulin

• Androstenedione. Recently published guidelines for the diagnosis of PCOS consider that the value of measuring androstenedione is unclear but it may increase the number of subjects identified as hyperandrogenism by approximately 10% [9].

• 17-OHP basal and after adrenocorticotropic hormone (ACTH) test. A basal value of 17-OHP above 1.6 ng/mL (4841 pmol/L) suggests adrenal hyperandrogenism.

• DHEAS.

• FSH:LH.

• Prolactin.

• Thyroid function.

• Urinary free cortisol (if suggested by history and physical examination).

• Oral glucose tolerance test to rule out glucose intolerance or DM.

• IGFBP-1 as a marker of insulin resistance.

• Lipid profile.

Imaging

There is no agreement on the necessity of obtaining pelvic ultrasound unless a tumor is suspected.

Treatment

The goals of the treatment in PCOS are:

1 Reduce hyperandrogenism in order to improve hirsutism and acne;

2 Restore regular ovulatory cycles; and

3 Correct the metabolic syndrome.

Several treatment options are available and also combined therapies but the treatment depends on the severity of the symptoms and the specific goals to be achieved.

Treatment of clinical hyperandrogenism

Cosmetic and dermatologic

Usually includes depilation (e.g. shaving or chemical depilatories), epilation (e.g. waxing), inhibition of local hair growth (e.g. eflornithine hydrochloride cream, Vaniqua®). Consider that hair grows back after discontinuation of these treatments. Laser treatment was approved by the Food and Drug administration (FDA) for permanent hair reduction.

Oral contraceptive pill

The oral contraceptive pill (OCP) is the first-line endocrine treatment for adolescents with regular sexual activity with dermatological or menstrual abnormalities of PCOS. Oral contraceptives with non-androgenic progestin to suppress ovarian function restore regular menstrual cycles and normalize androgen concentrations by suppressing plasma androgens, particularly free testosterone, within the first month of therapy. They also raise SHBG and modestly lower DHEAS concentrations. The fourth-generation OCP ethinyl estradiol/drospirenone (Yasmin®) has a particularly anti-androgenic progesterone component. It is similar in structure to spironolactone, and has some antimineralocorticoid properties. Benefits or risks in terms of metabolic derangement or embolism have been recently assessed and appear not to be increased [72]. Patients should be reviewed every 3 months of therapy to assess the efficacy of the treatment and the normalization of androgen concentrations. OCP therapy should be continued until gynecological maturity is reached (5 years postmenarche) or substantial loss of weight is achieved. After that period it is recommended to withhold treatment for a few months and assess the function of the pituitary–gonadal axis again.

Anti-androgens

These agents are used to improve the hirsutism score. They act as competitive antagonist of steroid binding to the androgen receptor and reverse the androgen-induced transformation of vellus to terminal hair. Sexual hair follicles have long growth cycles therefore the effect of anti-androgens is appreciated usually after 9–12 months of treatment. They must be used in combination with OCP because of the risk of feminization of the male fetus.

The following anti-androgens are available:

• *Spironolactone*, an aldosterone agonist, is most commonly used in adolescents in the USA. It is recommended to start with 100 mg twice a day until the maximal effect has been achieved and then to reduce to 50 mg twice a day for maintenance therapy. Electrolytes should be monitored. The anti-androgenic effect of spironolactone includes an additional effect of inhibition of ovarian and adrenal androgen production, blockade of dihydrotestosterone binding to skin androgen receptors, elevation of SHBG concentrations, increased testosterone clearance and decreased 5α-reductase activity.

• *Flutamide* is a potent non-steroidal anti-androgen that blocks androgen binding at the level of the nuclear receptor. It use has been limited by the potential risk for hepatocellular toxicity which in low doses appears to be minimal. The recommended dose is 62.5–250 mg once a day.

• *Cyproterone acetate* is a progestin with anti-androgen activity competitively inhibiting binding of testosterone and 5α-dihydrotestosterone to the androgen receptor. It also has weak antiglucocorticoid effects. It is not available in the USA but is available in Europe and Canada as a combination oral contraceptive containing ethinyl estradiol. There are controversies with regard to worsening triglyceride concentrations and an increased risk of venous thrombosis, although this is disputed [72].

• *Finasteride*, a type 1 5α-reductase inhibitor, is less effective than other anti-androgens to treat hirsutism.

Treatment of menstrual irregularities

The options include cyclic progestins, OCPs and insulin-lowering agents.

• *Progestin* induces withdrawal bleeding in most patients, permitting the emergence of normal menstrual cyclicity. The effective dose with micronized progestin is 100–200 mg/day at bedtime for 7–10 days a month. Some progestins have more androgenic activity than others. Desogestrel, gestodene and norgestimate are considered to have low androgenic potential and are preferred by pediatric endocrinologists. Levonorgestrel and norgestrel have high androgenic activity. Perimenarcheal girls who respond well to therapy can be maintained at 6-week cycles to permit the detection of spontaneous menses.

• *Oral contraceptives* were discussed in the preceding section and are useful in dysfunctional uterine bleeding. OCPs should be used with caution and with the lowest possible dose of estrogen in patients with migraine. OCPs are not curative for PCOS and the long-term consequences on fertility are unknown.

Treatment of obesity and insulin resistance

Treatment of obesity improves ovulation and hyperandrogenism in PCOS women who have this feature.

Lifestyle modification

Although no studies have isolated the effect of therapeutic lifestyle on PCOS adolescents, this is the first line of treatment for obese adolescents with PCOS. Unfortunately, it is hardest for patients to get a good compliance and maintain it. In obese adult women with PCOS, a 5–10% weight reduction yielded lower biochemical and clinical hyperandrogenism, lower fasting insulinemia and improved ovulation.

Insulin sensitizers

Because of the important role of insulin resistance in PCOS, insulin-sensitizing drugs have emerged as the first-choice therapy in obese insulin-resistant adolescents. Insulin sensitizers include metformin and thiazolinediones. They should be used as an adjuvant to general lifestyle improvement and do not replace them. There are no large-scale double-blind placebo-controlled studies in the adolescent age group using metformin. Studies in adult women with PCOS show promising results. Metformin acts by inhibiting hepatic glucose output and increasing insulin sensitivity in peripheral tissues. Decreased insulin concentrations lead to increased SHBG concentrations, lower free testosterone, improved androgen excess and ovulation [73,74]. Therefore, this therapy has been linked to improvement in insulin concentrations and regularization of the menstrual cycles [75]. The recommended starting dose is 500 mg with dinner, with an increase in the dosage by 500 mg/week, if needed, to a maximal dose of 2000 mg/day as tolerated. A rare complication is lactic acidosis. The presence of renal failure is a contraindication. Thiazolinediones act by improving insulin action and glucose utilization and are potentially effective in treatment of PCOS.

References

1 Azziz R, Woods KS, Reyna R, Key TJ, Knochenhauer ES, Yildiz BO. The prevalence and features of the polycystic ovary syndrome in an unselected population. *J Clin Endocrinol Metab* 2004; **89**: 2745–2749.

2 Meas T, Chevenne D, Thibaud E, Léger J, Cabrol S, Czernichow P, *et al*. Endocrine consequences of premature pubarche in postpubertal Caucasian girls. *Clin Endocrinol (Oxf)* 2002; **57**: 101–106.

3 Dunaif A, Segal KR, Futterweit W, Dobrjansky A. Profound peripheral insulin resistance, independent of obesity, in polycystic ovary syndrome. *Diabetes* 1989; **38**: 1165–1174.

4 Azziz R. Androgen excess is the key element in polycystic ovary syndrome. *Fertil Steril* 2003; **80**: 252–254.

5 Zawadzki JK, Dunaif A. Diagnostic criteria for polycystic ovary syndrome: towards a rational approach. In: Dunaif A, Givens JR, Haseltine F, Merriam GR, eds. *Polycystic Ovary Syndrome*. Boston: Blackwell Scientific Publications, 1992: 377–384.

6 Rotterdam ESHRE/ASRM-Sponsored PCOS Consensus Workshop Group. Revised 2003 consensus on diagnostic criteria and long-term health risks related to polycystic ovary syndrome. *Fertil Steril* 2004; **81**: 19–25.

7 Rotterdam ESHRE/ASRM-Sponsored PCOS Consensus Workshop Group. Revised 2003 consensus on diagnostic criteria and long-term health risks related to polycystic ovary syndrome (PCOS). *Hum Reprod* 2004; **19**: 41–47.

8 Azziz R. Controversy in clinical endocrinology: diagnosis of polycystic ovarian syndrome: the Rotterdam criteria are premature. *J Clin Endocrinol Metab* 2006; **91**: 781–785.

9 Azziz R, Carmina E, Dewailly D, Diamanti-Kandarakis E, Escobar-Morreale HF, Futterweit W, *et al*. Androgen Excess Society Position Statement. Criteria for defining polycystic ovary syndrome as a predominantly hyperandrogenic syndrome: an Androgen Excess Society guideline. *J Clin Endocrinol Metab* 2006; **91**: 4237–4245.

10 Carmina E, Azziz R. Diagnosis, phenotype, and prevalence of polycystic ovary syndrome. *Fertil Steril* 2006; **86** (Suppl 1): S7–8

11 Knochenhauer ES, Key TJ, Kahsar-Miller M, Waggoner W, Boots LR, Azziz R. Prevalence of the polycystic ovary syndrome in unselected black and white women of the southeastern United States: a prospective study. *J Clin Endocrinol Metab* 1998; **83**: 3078–3082.

12 Diamanti-Kandarakis E, Kouli CR, Bergiele AT, Filandra FA, Tsianateli TC, Spina GG, *et al*. A survey of the polycystic ovary syndrome in the Greek island of Lesbos: hormonal and metabolic profile. *J Clin Endocrinol Metab* 1999; **84**: 4006–4011.

13 Michelmore KF, Balen AH, Dunger DB, Vessey MP. Polycystic ovaries and associated clinical and biochemical features in young women. *Clin Endocrinol (Oxf)* 1999; **51**: 779–786.

14 Asunción M, Calvo RM, San Millán JL, Sancho J, Avila S, Escobar-Morreale HF. A prospective study of the prevalence of the polycystic ovary syndrome in unselected Caucasian women from Spain. *J Clin Endocrinol Metab* 2000; **85**: 2434–2438.

15 Littlejohn EE, Weiss RE, Deplewski D, Edidin DV, Rosenfield R. Intractable early childhood obesity as the initial sign of insulin resistant hyperinsulinism and precursor of polycystic ovary syndrome. *J Pediatr Endocrinol Metab* 2007; **20**: 41–51.

16 Abbott DH, Barnett DK, Bruns CM, Dumesic DA. Androgen excess fetal programming of female reproduction: a developmental aetiology for polycystic ovary syndrome? *Hum Reprod Update* 2005; **11**: 357–374.

17 Vom Saal FS, Bronson FH. Sexual characteristics of adult female mice are correlated with their blood testosterone levels during prenatal development. *Science* 1980; **208**: 597–599.

18 Robinson JE, Forsdike RA, Taylor JA. *In utero* exposure of female lambs to testosterone reduces the sensitivity of the gonadotropin-releasing hormone neuronal network to inhibition by progesterone. *Endocrinology* 1999; **140**: 5797–5805.

19 Zhou R, Bird IM, Dumesic DA, Abbott DH. Adrenal hyperandrogenism is induced by fetal androgen excess in a rhesus monkey model of polycystic ovary syndrome. *J Clin Endocrinol Metab* 2005; **90**: 6630–6637.

20 Sir-Petermann T, Maliqueo M, Angel B, Lara HE, Pérez-Bravo F, Recabarren SE. Maternal serum androgens in pregnant women with polycystic ovarian syndrome: possible implications in prenatal androgenization. *Hum Reprod* 2002; **17**: 2573–2579.

21 Nestler JE. Insulin and insulin-like growth factor-I stimulate the 3 beta-hydroxysteroid dehydrogenase activity of human placental cytotrophoblasts. *Endocrinology* 1989; **125**: 2127–2133.

22 Ibáñez L, de Zegher F. Puberty after prenatal growth restraint. *Horm Res* 2006; **65** (Suppl 3): 112–115.

23 Ibáñez L, Potau N, Enriquez G, Marcos MV, de Zegher F. Hypergonadotrophinaemia with reduced uterine and ovarian size in women born small-for-gestational-age. *Hum Reprod* 2003; **18**: 1565–1569.

24 Ibáñez L, Potau N, Francois I, de Zegher F. Precocious pubarche, hyperinsulinism, and ovarian hyperandrogenism in girls: relation to reduced fetal growth. *J Clin Endocrinol Metab* 1998; **83**: 3558–3562.

25 Hofman PL, Cutfield WS, Robinson EM, *et al.* Insulin resistance in short children with intrauterine growth retardation. *J Clin Endocrinol Metab* 1997; **82**: 402–406.

26 Hernández MI, Martínez A, Capurro T, Peña V, Trejo L, Avila A, *et al.* Comparison of clinical, ultrasonographic, and biochemical differences at the beginning of puberty in healthy girls born either small for gestational age or appropriate for gestational age: preliminary results. *J Clin Endocrinol Metab* 2006; **91**: 3377–3381.

27 Hernandez MI, Iniguez G, Marinez A, *et al.* Serum levels of anti-Müllerian hormone (AMH) and gonadal function during puberty in girls born with low birth weight (LBW) and appropriate for gestational age (AGA). Toronto: 89th Annual Meeting Endocrine Society, 2007.

28 Ibáñez L, Potau N, Zampolli M, Street ME, Carrascosa A. Girls diagnosed with premature pubarche show an exaggerated ovarian androgen synthesis from the early stages of puberty: evidence from gonadotropin-releasing hormone agonist testing. *Fertil Steril* 1997; **67**: 849–855.

29 Ibañez L, Potau N, Virdis R, Zampolli M, Terzi C, Gussinyé M, *et al.* Postpubertal outcome in girls diagnosed of premature pubarche during childhood: increased frequency of functional ovarian hyperandrogenism. *J Clin Endocrinol Metab* 1993; **76**: 1599–1603.

30 Mathew RP, Najjar JL, Lorenz RA, Mayes DE, Russell WE. Premature pubarche in girls is associated with functional adrenal but not ovarian hyperandrogenism. *J Pediatr* 2002; **141**: 91–98.

31 Siklar Z, Oçal G, Adiyaman P, Ergur A, Berbero lu M. Functional ovarian hyperandrogenism and polycystic ovary syndrome in prepubertal girls with obesity and/or premature pubarche. *J Pediatr Endocrinol Metab* 2007; **20**: 475–481.

32 Isojärvi JI. Reproductive dysfunction in women with epilepsy. *Neurology* 2003; **61**(Suppl 2): S27–34.

33 Herzog AG, Seibel MM, Schomer DL, Vaitukaitis JL, Geschwind N. Reproductive endocrine disorders in women with partial seizures of temporal lobe origin. *Arch Neurol* 1986; **43**: 341–346.

34 Isojärvi JI, Laatikainen TJ, Pakarinen AJ, Juntunen KT, Myllylä VV. Polycystic ovaries and hyperandrogenism in women taking valproate for epilepsy. *N Engl J Med* 1993; **329**: 1383–1388.

35 Mikkonen K, Vainionpää LK, Pakarinen AJ, Knip M, Järvelä IY, Tapanainen JS, *et al.* Long-term reproductive endocrine health in young women with epilepsy during puberty. *Neurology* 2004; **62**: 445–450.

36 Codner E, Soto N, Lopez P, Trejo L, Avila A, Eyzaguirre FC, *et al.* Diagnostic criteria for polycystic ovary syndrome and ovarian morphology in women with type 1 diabetes mellitus. *J Clin Endocrinol Metab* 2006; **91**: 2250–2256.

37 Escobar-Morreale HF, Roldan B, Barrio R, Alonso M, Sancho J, de la Calle H, *et al.* High prevalence of the polycystic ovary syndrome and hirsutism in women with type 1 diabetes mellitus. *J Clin Endocrinol Metab* 2000; **85**: 4182–4187.

38 Codner E, Escobar-Morreale HF. Clinical review: Hyperandrogenism and polycystic ovary syndrome in women with type 1 diabetes mellitus. *J Clin Endocrinol Metab* 2007; **92**: 1209–1216.

39 Saenger P, Dimartino-Nardi J. Premature adrenarche. *J Endocrinol Invest* 2001; **24**: 724–733.

40 Reinehr T, de Sousa G, Roth CL, Andler W. Androgens before and after weight loss in obese children. *J Clin Endocrinol Metab* 2005; **90**: 5588–5595.

41 Dunkel L, Sorva R, Voutilainen R. Low levels of sex hormone-binding globulin in obese children. *J Pediatr* 1985; **107**: 95–97.

42 Escobar-Morreale HF, Luque-Ramírez M, San Millán JL. The molecular-genetic basis of functional hyperandrogenism and the polycystic ovary syndrome. *Endocr Rev* 2005; **26**: 251–282.

43 Cooper HE, Spellacy WN, Prem KA, Cohen WD. Hereditary factors in the Stein–Leventhal syndrome. *Am J Obstet Gynecol* 1968; **100**: 371–387.

44 Givens JR. Familial polycystic ovarian disease. *Endocrinol Metab Clin North Am* 1988; **17**: 771–783.

45 Ferriman D, Purdie AW. The inheritance of polycystic ovarian disease and a possible relationship to premature balding. *Clin Endocrinol (Oxf)* 1979; **11**: 291–300.

46 Hague WM, Adams J, Reeders ST, Peto TE, Jacobs HS. Familial polycystic ovaries: a genetic disease? *Clin Endocrinol (Oxf)* 1988; **29**: 593–605.

47 Kahsar-Miller MD, Nixon C, Boots LR, Go RC, Azziz R. Prevalence of polycystic ovary syndrome (PCOS) in first-degree relatives of patients with PCOS. *Fertil Steril* 2001; **75**: 53–58.

48 Sir-Petermann T, Codner E, Maliqueo M, Echiburú B, Hitschfeld C, Crisosto N, *et al.* Increased anti-Müllerian hormone serum concentrations in prepubertal daughters of women with polycystic ovary syndrome. *J Clin Endocrinol Metab* 2006; **91**: 3105–3109.

49 Crisosto N, Codner E, Maliqueo M, Echiburú B, Sánchez F, Cassorla F, *et al.* Anti-Müllerian hormone levels in peripubertal daughters of women with polycystic ovary syndrome. *J Clin Endocrinol Metab* 2007; **92**: 2739–2743.

50 Norman RJ, Masters S, Hague W. Hyperinsulinemia is common in family members of women with polycystic ovary syndrome. *Fertil Steril* 1996; **66**: 942–947.

51 Legro RS, Driscoll D, Strauss JF 3rd, Fox J, Dunaif A. Evidence for a genetic basis for hyperandrogenemia in polycystic ovary syndrome. *Proc Natl Acad Sci U S A* 1998; **95**: 14956–14960.

52 Legro RS, Bentley-Lewis R, Driscoll D, Wang SC, Dunaif A. Insulin resistance in the sisters of women with polycystic ovary syndrome: association with hyperandrogenemia rather than menstrual irregularity. *J Clin Endocrinol Metab* 2002; **87**: 2128–2133.

53 Yildiz BO, Yarali H, Oguz H, Bayraktar M. Glucose intolerance, insulin resistance, and hyperandrogenemia in first degree relatives of women with polycystic ovary syndrome. *J Clin Endocrinol Metab* 2003; **88**: 2031–2036.

54 Sir-Petermann T, Angel B, Maliqueo M, Carvajal F, Santos JL, Pérez-Bravo F. Prevalence of type II diabetes mellitus and insulin resistance in parents of women with polycystic ovary syndrome. *Diabetologia* 2002; **45**: 959–964.

55 Kaushal R, Parchure N, Bano G, Kaski JC, Nussey SS. Insulin resistance and endothelial dysfunction in the brothers of Indian subcontinent Asian women with polycystic ovaries. *Clin Endocrinol (Oxf)* 2004; **60**: 322–328.

56 Colilla S, Cox NJ, Ehrmann DA. Heritability of insulin secretion and insulin action in women with polycystic ovary syndrome and their first degree relatives. *J Clin Endocrinol Metab* 2001; **86**: 2027–2031.

57 Leibel NI, Baumann EE, Kocherginsky M, Rosenfield RL. Relationship of adolescent polycystic ovary syndrome to parental metabolic syndrome. *J Clin Endocrinol Metab* 2006; **91**: 1275–1283.

58 Sir-Petermann T, Maliqueo M, Codner E, Echiburú B, Crisosto N, Pérez V, et al. Early metabolic derangements in daughters of women with polycystic ovary syndrome. *J Clin Endocrinol Metab* 2007; **92**: 4637–4642.

59 Geller DH, Oberfield SE, Leibel N, Ten S, Hernandez MI, Codner E, et al. Insulin sensitivity (SI) of adolescents at high risk for polcystic ovary syndrome (PCOS). Toronto, Ontario, Canada: Pediatric Academic Societies Annual Meeting (Abstract 158), 2007.

60 Jahanfar S, Eden JA, Nguyen T, Wang XL, Wilcken DE. A twin study of polycystic ovary syndrome and lipids. *Gynecol Endocrinol* 1997; **11**: 111–117.

61 Vink JM, Sadrzadeh S, Lambalk CB, Boomsma DI. Heritability of polycystic ovary syndrome in a Dutch twin-family study. *J Clin Endocrinol Metab* 2006; **91**: 2100–2104.

62 DeUgarte CM, Woods KS, Bartolucci AA, Azziz R. Degree of facial and body terminal hair growth in unselected black and white women: toward a populational definition of hirsutism. *J Clin Endocrinol Metab* 2006; **91**: 1345–1350.

63 Treloar AE, Boynton RE, Behn BG, Brown BW. Variation of human menstrual cycle through reproductive life. *Int J Fertil* 1967; **12**: 77.

64 Van Hooff MH, Voorhorst FJ, Kaptein MB, Hirasing RA, Koppenaal C, Schoemaker J. Polycystic ovaries in adolescents and the relationship with menstrual cycle patterns, luteinizing hormone, androgens, and insulin. *Fertil Steril* 2000; **74**: 49–58.

65 Jonard S, Robert Y, Cortet-Rudelli C, Pigny P, Decanter C, Dewailly D. Ultrasound examination of polycystic ovaries: is it worth counting the follicles? *Hum Reprod* 2003; **18**: 598–603.

66 Mortensen M, Rosenfield RL, Littlejohn E. Functional significance of polycystic-size ovaries in healthy adolescents. *J Clin Endocrinol Metab* 2006; **91**: 3786–3790.

67 Rosenfield RL, Ghai K, Ehrmann DA, Barnes RB. Diagnosis of polycystic ovary syndrome in adolescence. Comparison of adolescent and adult hyperandrogenism. *J Pediatr Endocrinol Metab* 2000; **13**: 1285.

68 Apridonidze T, Essah PA, Iuorno MJ, Nestler JE. Prevalence and characteristics of the metabolic syndrome in women with polycystic ovary syndrome. *J Clin Endocrinol Metab* 2005; **90**: 1929–1935.

69 Coviello AD, Legro RS, Dunaif A. Adolescent girls with polycystic ovary syndrome have an increased risk of the metabolic syndrome associated with increasing androgen levels independent of obesity and insulin resistance. *J Clin Endocrinol Metab* 2006; **91**: 492–497.

70 Shroff R, Kerchner A, Maifeld M, Van Beek EJ, Jagasia D, Dokras A. Young obese women with polycystic ovary syndrome have evidence of early coronary atherosclerosis. *J Clin Endocrinol Metab* 2007; **92**: 4609–4614.

71 Sultan C, Paris F. Clinical expression of polycystic ovary syndrome in adolescent girls. *Fertil Steril* 2006; **86** (Suppl 1): S6.

72 Luque-Ramírez M, Alvarez-Blasco F, Botella-Carretero JI, Martínez-Bermejo E, Lasunción MA, Escobar-Morreale HF. Comparison of ethinyl-estradiol plus cyproterone acetate versus metformin effects on classic metabolic cardiovascular risk factors in women with the polycystic ovary syndrome. *J Clin Endocrinol Metab* 2007; **92**: 2453–2461.

73 Arslanian SA, Lewy V, Danadian K, Saad R. Metformin therapy in obese adolescents with polycystic ovary syndrome and impaired glucose tolerance: amelioration of exaggerated adrenal response to adrenocorticotropin with reduction of insulinemia/insulin resistance. *J Clin Endocrinol Metab* 2002; **87**: 1555–1559.

74 Loverro G, Lorusso F, De Pergola G, Nicolardi V, Mei L, Selvaggi L. Clinical and endocrinological effects of 6 months of metformin treatment in young hyperinsulinemic patients affected by polycystic ovary syndrome. *Gynecol Endocrinol* 2002; **16**: 217–224.

75 Glueck CJ, Wang P, Fontaine R, Tracy T, Sieve-Smith L. Metformin to restore normal menses in oligo-amenorrheic teenage girls with polycystic ovary syndrome (PCOS). *J Adolesc Health* 2001; **29**: 160–169.

22 Weight Regulation and Monogenic Obesity

I. Sadaf Farooqi

University of Cambridge Metabolic Research Laboratories, Addenbrooke's Hospital, Cambridge, UK

The prevalence of obesity in children is difficult to determine because there is no definition of pathological adiposity. A range of methods that estimate total body fat is available but none is easily applicable to the clinical situation. Body weight is reasonably well correlated with body fat but also highly correlated with height, so children of the same weight but different heights can have widely differing amounts of fat. Body mass index [BMI: weight (kg) divided by height^2 (m^2)] in adults correlates reasonably well with more specific measurements of body fat but centile charts relating BMI to age are needed to relate BMI to body fat in children.

In the 10 years between the National Health and Nutrition Examination Survey (NHANES) II (1976–1980) and NHANES III (1988–1991), the prevalence of overweight in the USA, based on BMI corrected for age and sex, has increased by approximately 40%, to 11% in the 6- to 11-year age group [1]. Thus, childhood obesity is emerging as a global problem. Its immediate adverse effects include orthopedic complications, sleep apnea and psychosocial disorders. Because obese children are more likely to become obese adults, we can expect profound public health consequences as a result of the emergence in later life of associated co-morbidities, such as type 2 diabetes mellitus, ischemic heart disease and stroke.

Genetic and environmental factors

The rising prevalence of obesity can be explained partly by the availability of an unlimited supply of convenient, palatable, energy-dense foods, coupled with a lifestyle typified by low physical activity but obesity is a multifactorial disease arising from a complex mix of behavioral, environmental and genetic factors

that influence individual responses to diet and physical activity. The relative importance of particular etiological factors is likely to be different when considering mild overweight versus morbid obesity so interventions that may make a clinically significant impact on the overweight may have negligible effects in a morbidly obese person.

Weight, like height, is a heritable trait [2] and data from twin and adoption studies are consistent with a genetic contribution to the variance of BMI of between 40 and 70% [3]. In 2007, the first common genetic variant associated with an increased risk of obesity was identified: individuals who are homozygous for the high-risk allele of FTO (fat mass and obesity associated gene) weigh on average 3 kg more than those with two low-risk alleles, with heterozygotes having an intermediate risk [4]. This has been replicated in multiple studies and it seems likely that intronic variation in the FTO gene influences obesity through its effects on some brain process relevant to energy balance. Other common variants associated with obesity risk are emerging [5].

Clinical approach

Obesity is a complex phenotype and clinical assessment should be directed at screening for potentially treatable endocrine conditions and identifying genetic conditions so that appropriate genetic counseling and, in some cases, treatment can be instituted (Table 22.1).

Patients affected by obesity syndromes have been identified as a result of their association with mental retardation, dysmorphic features and/or other developmental abnormalities and several monogenic disorders have been identified. Obesity is often the predominant presenting feature but is often accompanied by neuroendocrine dysfunction so it remains useful to categorize the genetic obesity syndromes as those with and without associated developmental delay (Figs 22.1 & 22.2).

Brook's Clinical Pediatric Endocrinology, 6th edition. Edited by C. Brook, P. Clayton, R. Brown. © 2009 Blackwell Publishing, ISBN: 978-1-4051-8080-1.

Table 22.1 Assessment of the obese child/adult.

History

- Age of onset – use of growth charts and family photographs. Early onset (<5 years of age) suggests a genetic cause

- Duration of obesity – short history suggests endocrine or central cause

- A history of damage to the CNS (e.g. infection, trauma, hemorrhage, radiation therapy, seizures) suggests hypothalamic obesity with or without pituitary growth hormone deficiency or pituitary hypothyroidism. A history of morning headaches, vomiting, visual disturbances and excessive urination or drinking also suggests that the obesity may be caused by a tumor or mass in the hypothalamus

- A history of dry skin, constipation, intolerance to cold or fatigue suggests hypothyroidism. Mood disturbance and central obesity suggests Cushing syndrome. Frequent infections and fatigue may suggest ACTH deficiency resulting from POMC mutations

- Hyperphagia – often denied but sympathetic approach needed and specific questions, such as waking at night to eat and/or demanding food very soon after a meal, suggest hyperphagia. If severe, especially in children, suggests a genetic cause for obesity

- Developmental delay – milestones, educational history, behavioral disorders. Consider craniopharyngioma or structural causes (often relatively short history) and genetic causes

- Visual impairment and deafness suggest genetic causes

- Onset and tempo of pubertal development – onset can be early or delayed in children and adolescents. Primary hypogonadotropic hypogonadism or hypogenitalism associated with some genetic disorders

- Family history – consanguineous relationships, other children affected, family photographs useful. Severity may differ as a result of environmental effects

- Treatment with certain drugs or medications. Glucocorticoids, sulfonylureas, MAOIs, oral contraceptives, risperidone, clozapine

Examination

- Document weight and height compared with normal centiles. Calculate BMI and WHR (in adults). In children, obtain parental heights and weights where possible

- Head circumference if clinically suggestive

- Short stature or a reduced rate of linear growth in a child with obesity suggests the possibility of growth hormone deficiency, hypothyroidism, cortisol excess, pseudohypoparathyroidism or a genetic syndrome such as Prader–Willi syndrome

- Obese children and adolescents are often tall (on the upper centiles), however, accelerated linear growth (height SDS >2) is a feature of MC4R deficiency

- Body fat distribution – central distribution with purple striae suggests Cushing syndrome. Selective fat deposition (60%) is a feature of leptin and leptin receptor deficiency

- Dysmorphic features or skeletal dysplasia

- Hair color – red hair (if not familial) may suggest mutations in POMC in white Caucasians

- Pubertal development/secondary sexual characteristics. Most obese adolescents grow at a normal or excessive rate and enter puberty at the appropriate age; many mature more quickly than children with normal weight and bone age is commonly advanced. In contrast, growth rate and pubertal development are diminished or delayed in growth hormone deficiency, hypothyroidism, cortisol excess and a variety of genetic syndromes. Conversely, growth rate and pubertal development are accelerated in precocious puberty and in some girls with PCOS

- Acanthosis nigricans

- Valgus deformities in severe childhood obesity

Investigations

- Fasting and 2-h post glucose and insulin levels. Proinsulin if PC1 deficiency considered

- Fasting lipid panel for detection of dyslipidemia

- Thyroid function tests

- Serum leptin if indicated

- Karyotype

- DNA for molecular diagnosis

- Bone age

- Growth hormone secretion and function tests, when indicated

- Assessment of reproductive hormones, when indicated

- Serum calcium, phosphorus and parathyroid hormone levels to evaluate for suspected pseudohypoparathyroidism

- MRI scan of the brain with focus on the hypothalamus and pituitary, when clinically indicated

---

ACTH, adrenocorticotropic hormone; BMI, body mass index; MAOI, monoamine oxidase inhibitor; MRI, magnetic resonance imaging; POMC, pro-opiomelanocortin; PCOS, polycystic ovarian syndrome; SDS, standard deviation score; WHR, weight:height ratio.

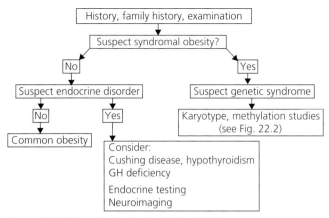

Figure 22.1 Diagnostic algorithm for childhood obesity.

Pleiotrophic obesity syndromes

Obesity runs in families, although the majority of cases do not segregate with a clear Mendelian pattern of inheritance. There are about 30 Mendelian disorders with obesity as a clinical feature, frequently associated with mental retardation, dysmorphic features and organ-specific developmental abnormalities (i.e. pleiotrophic syndromes). A number of families with these rare syndromes have been studied by linkage analysis and the known chromosomal loci for obesity syndromes are summarized in Table 22.2. In a number of cases, mutations in genes have been identified by positional cloning and the mechanism underlying the development of obesity is becoming clear in some instances [6].

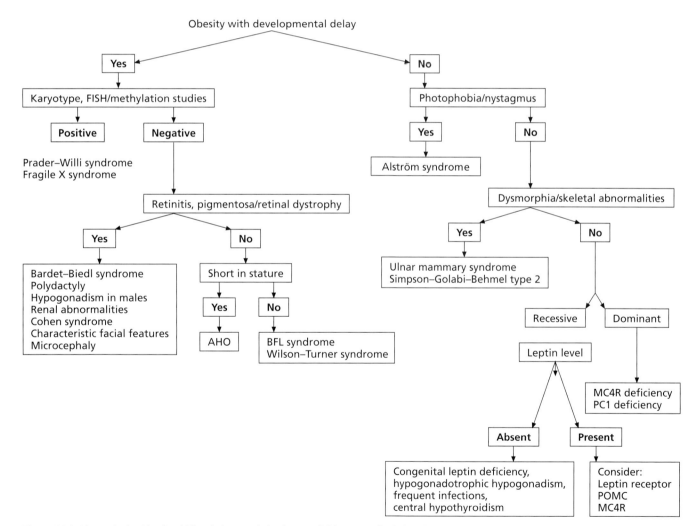

Figure 22.2 Diagnostic algorithm for childhood obesity with developmental delay. AHO, Albright hereditary osteodystrophy; BFL, Börjesen–Forssman–Lehmann.

Table 22.2 Obesity syndromes.

Syndrome	Additional clinical features	Locus
Autosomal dominant		
Prader–Willi syndrome	Hypotonia, mental retardation, short stature hypergonadotrophic hypogonadism	Lack of the paternal segment 15q11.2–q12
Albright hereditary osteodystrophy	Short stature, skeletal defects and impaired olfaction	20q13.2
Ulnar–mammary syndrome	Ulnar defects, delayed puberty, hypoplastic nipples	12q24.1
Autosomal recessive		
Bardet–Biedl syndrome	Mental retardation, dysmorphic extremities, retinal dystrophy, or pigmentary retinopathy, hypogonadism and structural abnormalities of the kidney or functional renal impairment	11q13 (BBS1) 16q21 (BBS2) 3p13 (BBS3) 15q22 (BBS4) 2q31 (BBS5) 20p12 (BBS6) 4q27 (BBS7) 14q32 (BBS8)
Alström syndrome	Retinal dystrophy, neurosensory deafness, diabetes	2p13
Cohen syndrome	Prominent central incisors, ophthalmopathy, microcephaly	8q22
X-linked		
Fragile X syndrome	Mental retardation, hyperkinetic behavior, macroorchidism, large ears, prominent jaw, high-pitched jocular speech	Xq27.3
Börjeson–Forssman–Lehmann syndrome	Mental retardation, hypogonadism, large ears	Xq26
Mehmo syndrome	Mental retardation, epilepsy, hypogonadism, microcephaly	Xp22.13
Simpson–Golabi–Behmel syndrome type 2	Craniofacial defects, skeletal and visceral abnormalities	Xp22
Wilson–Turner syndrome	Mental retardation, tapering fingers, gynecomastia	Xp21.2

Molecular mechanisms involved in energy homeostasis

In the 1990s, the genes responsible for a number of obesity syndromes in rodents were identified, mostly by positional cloning techniques. These observations have given substantial insight into the physiological disturbances that can lead to obesity, the metabolic and endocrine abnormalities associated with the obese phenotype and the more detailed anatomical and neurochemical pathways that regulate energy intake and energy expenditure [7]. They provide the framework upon which the understanding of the more complex mechanisms in humans can be built.

Leptin–melanocortin pathway

Initial observations in this field were made as a result of positional cloning strategies in two strains of severely obese mice (ob/ob and db/db). ob/ob mice were found to harbor mutations in the ob gene resulting in a complete lack of its protein product leptin [8]. Administration of recombinant leptin reduced the food intake and body weight of leptin-deficient ob/ob mice and corrected all their neuroendocrine and metabolic abnormalities [6]. The signaling form of the leptin receptor is deleted in db/db mice, which are consequently unresponsive to endogenous or exogenous leptin [9]. The identification of these two proteins established the first components of a nutritional feedback loop from adipose tissue to the brain. The physiological role of leptin in humans and rodents might be to act as a signal for starvation because, as fat mass increases, further rises in leptin have a limited ability to suppress food intake and prevent obesity [10].

Considerable attention has focused on deciphering the hypothalamic pathways that coordinate the behavioral and metabolic effects downstream of leptin. The first-order neuronal targets of leptin action in the brain are anorectic (reducing food intake), pro-opiomelanocortin (POMC) and orexigenic (increasing food intake) neuropeptide-Y/Agouti-related protein (NPY/AgRP) neurons in the hypothalamic arcuate nucleus, where the signaling isoform of the leptin receptor is highly expressed. Forty percent of POMC neurons in the arcuate nucleus express the mRNA for the long form of the leptin receptor and POMC expression is positively regulated by leptin. POMC is sequentially cleaved by prohormone convertases to yield peptides, including α-melanocyte-stimulating hormone (MSH), that have been shown to have a role in feeding behavior. There is clear evidence in rodents that α-MSH acts as a suppressor of feeding behavior, probably through the melanocortin 4 receptor (MC4R). Targeted disruption of MC4R in rodents leads to increased food intake, obesity, severe early hyperinsulinemia and increased linear growth; heterozygotes have an intermediate phenotype compared with homozygotes and wild-type mice [11].

Mutations in all the main components of this pathway have been found to result in obesity in humans. The phenotypic characterization of patients has informed the physiological role of the pathway and its interaction with neuroendocrine function.

Human monogenic obesity syndromes

Congenital leptin deficiency

In 1997, we reported two severely obese children (an 8-year-old girl weighing 86 kg and her 2-year-old cousin weighing 29 kg) from a highly consanguineous family of Pakistani origin [12]. These children had normal developmental milestones, no dysmorphic features and a normal karyotype. Despite their severe obesity, both children had undetectable concentrations of serum leptin and were homozygous for a frameshift mutation in the ob gene (ΔG133), which resulted in a truncated protein that was not secreted.

We have since identified four further affected individuals from three other families who are also homozygous for the same mutation in the ob gene. All the families are of Pakistani origin but not known to be related over five generations. A large consanguineous Turkish family that carries a homozygous missense mutation has also been described [13]. All the subjects had intense hyperphagia after weaning, waking at night to seek food and demanding food immediately after a meal.

The disabling obesity of leptin deficiency is characterized by the selective deposition of fat: children often develop valgus deformities of the knees by the age of 5–6 years, sleep apnea and high rates of childhood infection and atopic disease resulting from abnormalities of T-cell number and function. An advanced bone age is a recognized feature with failure to undergo pubertal development because of hypogonadotrophic hypogonadism.

Response to leptin therapy

Congenital leptin deficiency, although rare, is amenable to therapy [14,15]. Patients treated with once-daily subcutaneous injections of recombinant human leptin all lost weight (specifically fat), often with dramatic clinical benefit (Fig. 22.3). The major effect of leptin was on appetite, with normalization of hyperphagia. The administration of leptin permits progression of appropriately timed pubertal development and does not cause the early onset of puberty.

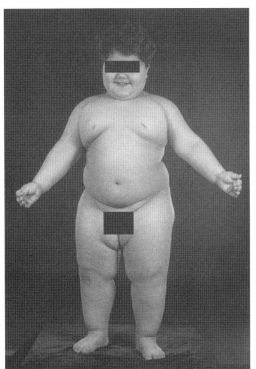
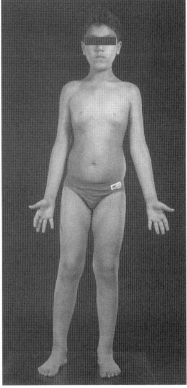

Figure 22.3 Response to leptin therapy in a child with leptin deficiency. (a) Before therapy. (b) After therapy.

(a)

(b)

Free thyroxine and thyroid-stimulating hormone (TSH) concentrations, although usually in the normal range before treatment, had consistently increased at the earliest post-treatment time point and subsequently stabilized at this elevated level. These findings are consistent with evidence from animal models that leptin influences thyrotrophin-releasing hormone (TRH) release from the hypothalamus and from studies illustrating the effect of leptin deficiency on TSH pulsatility in humans.

After approximately 6 weeks of leptin therapy, all subjects developed antileptin antibodies, which interfered with interpretation of serum leptin concentrations and, in some cases, were capable of neutralizing leptin in a bioassay and were the likely cause of refractory periods occurring during therapy. The fluctuating nature of the antibodies probably reflects the fact that leptin deficiency is itself an immunodeficient state. Administration of leptin leads to a change from the secretion of predominantly Th2 to Th1 cytokines, which may directly influence antibody production. Thus far, we have been able to regain control of weight loss by increasing the dose of leptin.

Although congenital leptin deficiency is an autosomal recessive condition, heterozygotes or carriers for the ob mutation have a partial deficiency that is associated with an increase in body fat.

Leptin receptor deficiency

Leptin receptor-deficient subjects were of normal birthweight but exhibited rapid weight gain in the first few months of life, with severe hyperphagia and aggressive behavior when food was denied, as in leptin deficiency. Basal temperature and resting metabolic rate were normal, cortisol concentrations were in the normal range and all individuals were normoglycemic with mildly elevated plasma insulin concentrations similar to leptin-deficient subjects. Serum leptin levels were not elevated. Several mutations in the leptin receptor gene have been reported [16].

Pro-opiomelanocortin (POMC) deficiency

In 1998, Krude *et al.* reported two unrelated obese German children homozygous or compound heterozygous for mutations in POMC and another five children have been reported [17]. Because POMC is a precursor of adrenocorticotropic hormone (ACTH) in the pituitary, presentation is in the neonatal period with adrenal crisis brought about by ACTH deficiency. The children require long-term corticosteroid replacement. They have pale skin and red hair because of the lack of MSH function at melanocortin 1 receptors in the skin, although this may be less obvious in children from different ethnic backgrounds. POMC deficiency results in hyperphagia and early-onset obesity because of loss of melanocortin signaling at the MC4R. Although trials of treatment have not been performed, selective MC4R agonists may become available in the near future.

Prohormone convertase 1 (PC1) deficiency

In 1997, we identified a defect in prohormone processing in a 47-year-old woman with severe childhood obesity, abnormal glucose homeostasis, very low plasma insulin with elevated concentrations of proinsulin, hypogonadotrophic hypogonadism and hypocortisolemia associated with increased concentrations of POMC. She was found to be a compound heterozygote for mutations in prohormone convertase 1 enzyme, which cleaves prohormones at pairs of basic amino acids leaving C-terminal basic residues that are excised by carboxypeptidase E (CPE) [18].

We have recently identified a second child with severe early-onset obesity who was compound heterozygote for complete loss-of-function mutations in PC1 [19]. As well as a failure to process a number of prohormones, such as preprogonadotropin-releasing hormone (GnRH), preproTRH and POMC, this patient had a small bowel enteropathy, possibly resulting from a failure to process gut-derived neuropeptides. Although the inability to cleave POMC is a probable mechanism for obesity in these patients, PC1 cleaves a number of other neuropeptides in the hypothalamus, including glucagon-like peptide 1, which may influence feeding behavior.

MC4R deficiency

In 1998, two groups in the UK and France reported a dominantly inherited obesity from heterozygous mutations in the MC4 receptor [20,21]. Since then, heterozygous mutations in MC4R have been reported in obese humans from various ethnic groups with an estimated prevalence of 0.5–1% in obese patients, increasing to 6% in our cohort of severe early-onset obesity [22]. Thus, MC4R deficiency represents the most common known monogenic cause of human obesity. While we found 100% penetrance of early-onset obesity in heterozygous probands, others have described obligate carriers who were not obese. The maintenance of this reasonably high disease frequency is likely to be caused, at least partly, by the fact that obesity is expressed in heterozygotes and there is no evidence of an effect of the mutations on reproductive function.

Given the large number of potential influences on body weight, it is perhaps not surprising that genetic and environmental modifiers have important effects in some pedigrees. Indeed, we have now studied six families in whom the probands were homozygotes and they were all more obese than heterozygotes, some of whom were not obese. This may reflect ethnic-specific effects because all these families were of Indo origin. Taking account of all these observations, co-dominance, with modulation of expressivity and penetrance of the phenotype, is the most appropriate description of the mode of inheritance.

We have defined the phenotype in a large series of patients with MC4R deficiency [23]. Affected subjects were hyperphagic but this was not as severe as that seen in leptin deficiency, although it often started in the first year of life. The severity of receptor dysfunction seen in *in vitro* assays predicts the amount of food ingested at a test meal by the subject harboring that particular mutation. As well as the increase in fat mass, MC4R-deficient subjects have an increase in lean mass not seen in leptin deficiency and an increase in bone mineral density. Thus, they often appear "big-boned." Linear growth is striking, with affected children having a height standard deviation score (SDS) of +2, whereas the mean height SDS of other obese children in our cohort is +0.5. MC4R-deficient subjects have higher concentrations of fasting insulin than age-, sex- and BMI SDS-matched children. The accelerated linear growth does not appear to be a result of dysfunction of the growth hormone (GH) axis and may be a consequence of the disproportionate early hyperinsulinemia and impaired suppression of GH secretion compared to that seen in common obesity.

Conclusions

Although monogenic obesity syndromes are rare, understanding the nature of the inherited component of severe obesity has undoubted medical benefits and helps dispel the notion that obesity represents an individual defect in behavior with no biological basis. For individuals at highest risk of the complications of severe obesity, such findings provide a starting point for rational mechanism-based therapies, as has successfully been achieved for congenital leptin deficiency.

References

1 Farooqi IS, O'Rahilly S. Monogenic obesity in humans. *Annu Rev Med* 2005; **56**: 443–458.

2 Barsh GS, Farooqi IS, O'Rahilly S. Genetics of body-weight regulation. *Nature* 2000; **404**: 644–651.

3 Stunkard AJ, Harris JR, Pedersen NL, McClearn GE. The body-mass index of twins who have been reared apart. *N Engl J Med* 1990; **322**: 1483–1487.

4 Frayling TM, Timpson NJ, Weedon MN, Zeggini E, Freathy RM, Lindgren CM, *et al*. A common variant in the FTO gene is associated with body mass index and predisposes to childhood and adult obesity. *Science* 2007; **316**: 889–894.

5 Loos RJ, Lindgren CM, Li S, Wheeler E, Zhao JH, Prokopenko I, *et al*. Common variants near MC4R are associated with fat mass, weight and risk of obesity. *Nat Genet* 2008; **40**: 768–775.

6 Halaas JL, Gajiwala KS, Maffei M, Cohen SL, Chait BT, Rabinowitz D, *et al*. Weight-reducing effects of the plasma protein encoded by the obese gene. *Science* 1995; **269**: 543–546.

7 Schwartz MW, Woods SC, Porte D Jr, Seeley RJ, Baskin DG. Central nervous system control of food intake. *Nature* 2000; **404**: 661–671.

8 Zhang Y, Proenca R, Maffei M, Barone M, Leopold L, Friedman JM. Positional cloning of the mouse obese gene and its human homologue. *Nature* 1994; **372**: 425–432.

9 Chen H, Charlat O, Tartaglia LA, Woolf EA, Weng X, Ellis SJ, *et al*. Evidence that the diabetes gene encodes the leptin receptor: identification of a mutation in the leptin receptor gene in db/db mice. *Cell* 1996; **84**: 491–495.

10 Flier JS. Clinical review 94: What's in a name? In search of leptin's physiologic role. *J Clin Endocrinol Metab* 1998; **83**: 1407–1413.

11 Huszar D, Lynch CA, Fairchild-Huntress V, Dunmore JH, Fang Q, Berkemeier LR, *et al*. Targeted disruption of the melanocortin-4 receptor results in obesity in mice. *Cell* 1997; **88**: 131–141.

12 Montague CT, Farooqi IS, Whitehead JP, Soos MA, Rau H, Wareham NJ, *et al*. Congenital leptin deficiency is associated with severe early-onset obesity in humans. *Nature* 1997; **387**: 903–908.

13 Ozata M, Ozdemir IC, Licinio J. Human leptin deficiency caused by a missense mutation: multiple endocrine defects, decreased sympathetic tone and immune system dysfunction indicate new targets for leptin action, greater central than peripheral resistance to the effects of leptin and spontaneous correction of leptin-mediated defects. *J Clin Endocrinol Metab* 1999; **84**: 3686–3695.

14 Farooqi IS, Jebb SA, Langmack G, Lawrence E, Cheetham CH, Prentice AM, *et al*. Effects of recombinant leptin therapy in a child with congenital leptin deficiency. *N Engl J Med* 1999; **341**: 879–884.

15 Farooqi IS, Matarese G, Lord GM, Keogh JM, Lawrence E, Agwu C, *et al*. Beneficial effects of leptin on obesity, T cell hyporesponsiveness and neuroendocrine/metabolic dysfunction of human congenital leptin deficiency. *J Clin Invest* 2002; **110**: 1093–1103.

16 Farooqi IS, Wangensteen T, Collins S, Kimber W, Matarese G, Keogh JM, *et al*. Clinical and molecular genetic spectrum of congenital deficiency of the leptin receptor. *N Engl J Med* 2007; **356**: 237–247.

17 Krude H, Biebermann H, Schnabel D, Tansek MZ, Theunissen P, Mullis PE, *et al*. Obesity due to proopiomelanocortin deficiency: three new cases and treatment trials with thyroid hormone and ACTH4-10. *J Clin Endocrinol Metab* 2003; **88**: 4633–4640.

18 Jackson RS, Creemers JW, Ohagi S, Raffin-Sanson ML, Sanders L, Montague CT, *et al*. Obesity and impaired prohormone processing associated with mutations in the human prohormone convertase 1 gene [see comments]. *Nat Genet* 1997; **16**: 303–306.

19 Jackson RS, Creemers JW, Farooqi IS, Raffin-Sanson ML, Varro A, Dockray GJ, *et al*. Small-intestinal dysfunction accompanies the complex endocrinopathy of human proprotein convertase 1 deficiency. *J Clin Invest* 2003; **112**: 1550–1560.

20 Yeo GS, Farooqi IS, Aminian S, Halsall DJ, Stanhope RG, O'Rahilly S. A frameshift mutation in MC4R associated with dominantly inherited human obesity. *Nat Genet* 1998; **20**: 111–112.

21 Vaisse C, Clement K, Guy-Grand B, Froguel P. A frameshift mutation in human MC4R is associated with a dominant form of obesity. *Nat Genet* 1998; **20**: 113–114.

22 Farooqi IS, Yeo GS, Keogh JM, Aminian S, Jebb SA, Butler G, *et al*. Dominant and recessive inheritance of morbid obesity associated with melanocortin 4 receptor deficiency. *J Clin Invest* 2000; **106**: 271–279.

23 Farooqi IS, Keogh JM, Yeo GS, Lank EJ, Cheetham T, O'Rahilly S. Clinical spectrum of obesity and mutations in the melanocortin 4 receptor gene. *N Engl J Med* 2003; **348**: 1085–1095.

23 Ethical Issues in Clinical Pediatric Endocrinology

Leena Patel[1] & Peter E. Clayton[2]

[1] Department of Paediatric Endocrinology, Royal Manchester Children's Hospital, Manchester, UK
[2] Endocrine Science Research Group, University of Manchester, Manchester, UK

The responsibility to do good and to do no harm and to respect autonomy, truth telling, disclosure, confidentiality and informed consent constitute the ethical principles that underpin clinical practice. Pediatric endocrinology presents many challenging ethical issues, which may include human biological processes, such as decisions about the sex of rearing of a child, interventions to manipulate growth in a child without a defined endocrinopathy or puberty in a disabled young person. Special consideration of such issues is vital to protect patients, guide appropriate decision-making, justify actions, support good practice, recognize limitations and ensure professional liability. In this chapter, three examples have been taken to highlight their individual ethical dilemmas.

Disorders of sex development in early life

Disorders of sex development (DSD) include anomalies of the sex chromosomes, gonads, reproductive organs and genitalia [1,2]. Individuals may present with ambiguous genitalia or a lack of congruence between chromosomal and physical aspects. The decision about gender assignment requires examination and investigations to delineate genital anatomy, hormone physiology, karyotype, diagnosis and likely cosmetic and functional outcome as well as honest and sensitive discussion with the family.

The process of gender assignment or reassignment in DSD and variations in management of such infants over the years has generated criticism from dissatisfied patients and dissent among professionals. Prompt assignment of gender by the medical team coupled with surgery in early life has been standard practice but this approach has been questioned.

Brook's Clinical Pediatric Endocrinology, 6th edition. Edited by C. Brook, P. Clayton, R. Brown. © 2009 Blackwell Publishing,
ISBN: 978-1-4051-8080-1.

Gender assignment

A newborn baby is identified as a girl or a boy from the appearance of the external genitalia. The situation is far from simple for infants with DSD. Understanding which gender is the best option for an infant with DSD requires careful consideration of genotype, phenotype and other issues.

Gender options

Society conforms to the two gender rule and adults with or without unusual genital anatomy do not identify with an alternative gender ("neutral," "middle," "third") [3–6]. Although more likely in some DSDs than others, a small minority of individuals choose to change gender in later life. Therefore, once assigned, gender should not be considered immutable. Failure to assign gender can make individuals feel confused, isolated, imperfect and ashamed; deferring until the child is old enough to decide is difficult to justify.

Appearance of the external genitalia

Normal variations in the appearance of external genitalia and physiological changes throughout childhood occur, as with all physical attributes [7,8]. Conceptualizing male and female appearance as a bimodal distribution along a continuum and with an overlapping region highlights that biological gender is not distinct and permits acceptance of unusual morphology within the realms of normal variation (Fig. 23.1) [9].

Knowledge about outcome in some DSD provides helpful guidance. Classic congenital adrenal hyperplasia (CAH) is the most common cause of 46XX DSD and assignment of female gender is recommended by the Joint European Society for Pediatric Endocrinology (ESPE)/Lawson Wilkins Pediatric Endocrine Society (LWPES) CAH Working Group [10]. Most patients adjust well to being raised as females despite varying degrees of virilization, the probability of imprinting of the brain with androgens and masculinized gender role behavior, [11–13]. Rarely do they change gender in later life [14,15].

A small penis in an infant is generally defined as stretched length <2.5 cm [16] but 1.5 cm has also been accepted [17] and

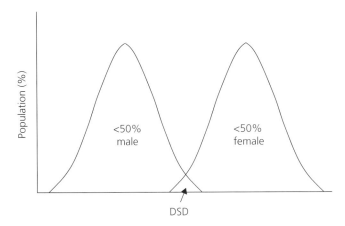

Quantitative and functional variability in
external genitalia, internal structures,
gonads, chromosomes and hormones

Figure 23.1 Bimodal distribution of male and female morphology along a
continuum with an overlapping region representing disorders of sex development
(DSD) [9]. (Reproduced with permission from Wiley-Liss, Inc. Blackless M,
Charuvastra A, Derryck A, Fausto-Sterling A, Lauzanne K, Lee E. How sexually
dimorphic are we? Review and Synthesis. *Am J Hum Biol* 2000; **12**: 151–166.

does not preclude normal male behavior and sexual function
[18]. There is now consensus that a small or absent penis alone
does not justify gender reassignment from male to female, and
that males with micropenis or cloacal exstrophy and 46XY karyotype should be raised as males [19].

Cases of complete androgen insensitivity syndrome (CAIS)
generally accept female gender. In contrast, individuals with
partial androgen insensitivity syndrome (PAIS), whether raised
as male or female, might prefer a different identity in later life to
the one initially assigned [20].

Determinants of gender identity and psychosexual orientation

Gender identity is defined as an individual's self-image as a male
or female. Psychosexual orientation, preferring hetero-, homo- or
bisexuality, develops through an individual's life and is a component of gender identity [21]. Interactions between biological
factors, particularly hormonal milieu and genetic factors (nature),
as well as the social and cultural environment in which a child is
brought up (nurture) contribute to the development of gender
identity [6,19,22–24], but neither can predict stable gender identity or variations in its outcome for psychosexual orientation
[3,5,25–29].

Development of gender identity does not require gender-
typical appearance of external genitalia nor does the latter ensure
that corresponding gender identity will develop [18,30]. The
majority of children with ambiguous genitalia are capable of
adopting stable gender identity and are not at greater risk for
psychosocial problems [18]. Therefore, the traditional view, that
nurture is more important and that a child can be raised as a girl

or a boy, provided there is concordance with external genital
appearance, has been questioned [2].

Biological factors, including the Y chromosome, specific genes,
testes and phallus, are also not considered to be sufficient on their
own to determine male identity, as illustrated by individuals
with CAIS. Although an influence of prenatal androgen exposure
on brain masculinization is recognized, the majority of girls
with CAH have female-typical gender identity despite moderate
levels of androgen exposure [31]. A small number have gender
dysphoria and identify as males and, contrary to expectation, this
is more likely to occur in simple-virilizing than in salt-wasting
CAH [32,33]. Because there is no clear association between
disease severity, degree of virilization and gender identity
[34–36], gender assignment should not be based on probable
imprinting of the brain by androgens or genital appearance
[11,30].

Potential for endocrine, sexual and reproductive function

The potential for endocrine, sexual and reproductive function,
whether inherent or amenable to hormonal and surgical interventions, vary according to the nature of the DSD and are important outcomes to consider when deciding the appropriate gender.
Thus, for example, all three aspects are well preserved in 46XX
CAH babies raised as females but some compromise occurs if
raised as males. A 46XY individual with a small penis raised as a
boy may develop when exposed to testosterone and retain potential for normal sexual and reproductive function but function is
compromised if raised as a girl. Individuals will have different
preferences and priorities about potential functional capacity and
should be empowered to discuss them.

Surgical interventions to support gender assignment

Surgical interventions do not assign gender but offer the opportunity to align anatomy with the chosen gender. The timing of
surgery in infancy rather than later in life has generated considerable debate.

Traditional practice of early genital surgery and its undesirable consequences

A mismatch between the appearance of the external genitalia and
assigned gender is distressing for parents and the child, was
believed to hinder appropriate rearing of the child and considered
incompatible with establishing heterosexual relationships and
adult sexual function [37]. Cosmetic surgery was intended to
"normalize" anatomy and foster optimal gender outcome and
was therefore performed early. Psychological trauma associated
with the procedure (anesthetic and surgery) was thought to be
minimal in infancy [38–41]. It was also believed that possession
of a phallus was more important than of a vagina, an organ for
accommodating a normal erectile penis, and that making genitalia resemble a normal female was easier than constructing a functioning penis [42,43]. Thus, even an otherwise normal boy with
a small phallus (micropenis) was likely to be subjected to feminizing surgery and raised as a girl.

Reconstructed genitalia may appear abnormal owing to variable cosmetic results of surgery, and further interventions are frequently required [44,45]. If surgery is undertaken early, for instance in the 46XX virilized female with CAH, short-term success is dependent on the expertise of the surgeon. Complications associated with feminizing surgery include disruption in urinary function, vaginal stenosis, chronic pain, repeated infections, loss of sensation, poorer sexual function and less sexual satisfaction [46]. Surgical procedures are also associated with psychological trauma, described by affected individuals as mutilating, embarrassing, humiliating, degrading and feeling of failure.

The phenotype of the underlying condition and nature of surgery frequently necessitates compromising some aspect of cosmetic appearance, potential endocrine function, fertility or psychosexual well-being. Non-operative management with psychological support can have the same effect as surgery in relieving the family's distress but has no irrevocable effects and permits deferring major decisions until the patient is old enough to participate in choosing the nature and timing of surgery. Potentially normal gonadal tissue should be removed only with informed consent and provided there are good indications, such as high tumor risk.

Undue emphasis on the genital abnormality that early surgery is attempting to alter is itself an undesirable consequence [47,48]. Many professionals and patient groups advocate that early surgery is justified only in life-threatening situations, e.g. absent urethral opening. They recommend a judicious approach to all other genital surgery not imminently essential which can be deferred without risk [2,49]. Parents and patients should be informed about the meagre evidence for long-term outcomes and the risks and undesirable consequences of surgery so that they can balance these against the benefits [47].

Informed consent and respect for autonomy

Information pertaining to DSD is difficult for parents and patients to comprehend. The duty to respect the autonomy of children and parents and give informed consent requires the presentation of information clearly and repeatedly, reviewing understanding, enabling active participation in decisions and supporting them throughout (Tables 23.1–23.3) [27,50,51].

Informed consent and "proxy consent"

Parents have the authority to consent for infants and young children. This is "proxy consent" because it is influenced by parents' personal values and preferences, which may differ from the child's

Table 23.1 The elements of informed consent [48].

Informed consent comprises:
1 Provision of information
2 Assessment of parents' and patient's understanding
3 Assessment of parents' and patient's capacity to make decisions
4 Assurance that parents and patient have the freedom to choose treatment without coercion or manipulation

[52]. A competent individual, including a child, can give informed consent if the decision about elective surgery is deferred to a time when the child has sufficient maturity and ability to understand the treatment and its implications. Evaluation of the child's

Table 23.2 What parents need to understand in order to actively participate in decisions and give informed consent [1,2].

Moral obligations of professionals
Parents will be kept fully informed and involved in any decisions
Confidentiality and privacy assured
The truth – prioritized and selected appropriately
Areas of uncertainty acknowledged

Information about DSD
Unusual appearance of external genitalia compared to what is normally expected
Such unusual appearance is not uncommon and they are not alone
How this came about
The process of diagnosis and management, and anticipated duration
Implications for their baby in the short- and long-term
Treatment options, and potential benefits and risks

Involvement of professionals
Experience and roles of the professionals involved
A need to consult various professionals with expertise

Other support for the family
Sources of reliable information
Local peer support from families who have faced the same situation

DSD, disorders of sex development.

Table 23.3 How information should be conveyed to parents [1,2].

At the time of diagnosis, ongoing and repeated according to the family's needs
With assistance from trained interpreters if professionals do not know parents' primary language
An atmosphere that fosters mutuality and respect, and strengthens doctor–patient and parent relationships
Interactive process in which information and values are shared
Awareness of parents' positive and negative feelings, and social, cultural and religious beliefs
Attend to emotions and behavior as well as facts and physical aspects
Presence of friends and family, if parents wish
Promote active participation by parents
A calm, supportive and appropriately reassuring manner
Sensitive, thoughtful and non-judgmental approach
Frank, honest and open discussion
Questions invited and answered
Undue anxiety and panic avoided
Stigmatizing labels and terms avoided
Embarrassment, shame, guilt and humiliation avoided and allayed
Conflict, confusion and misunderstanding avoided
Complexity needs to be presented clearly and in a way in which it is understood using appropriate language, e.g. in small chunks, repeated and clarified, with diagrams or models
Verbally and supplemented with educational material, e.g. written and audiovisual information

SINGLETON HOSPITAL
STAFF LIBRARY

cognitive ability is a prerequisite to informed consent. Although this is generally carried out by pediatricians, a more detailed assessment by a clinical psychologist may be required for the complex decisions surrounding DSD. In exceptional situations when conflict arises, professionals have a duty to provide care to the child based on what is in the child's best interest and not what parents desire. A clinical ethicist can help decide what constitutes the child's best interest [2].

Assent

Children without the capacity to consent but developmentally appropriate should be involved in their management and empowered (Table 23.4). This includes obtaining consent for physical examination and diagnostic procedures. Ongoing education about the DSD needs to be provided so that the child can be encouraged to assume responsibility for his/her health and well-being over time.

Truth and information disclosure

Deception, withholding information and selective telling of the truth undermines the patient's autonomy and invalidates consent [53,54]. Reasoning that the lack of disclosure is intended to protect patients because the truth would cause unnecessary distress and would be too confusing for patients is not justified and can be harmful [55,56]. No matter how upsetting, telling the truth takes precedence over beneficence. Personal experiences of adults with DSD indicate that ignorance and betrayal of trust is psychologically more harmful than knowing the truth [48,54,57]. Silence, secrecy and ignorance does not erase an individual's experiences about being different nor about the treatment to which they were subjected through life [48]. On the contrary, it is counterproductive and reinforces a lack of identity and being "freakish," leading to stigma, fear, isolation and shame instead of alleviating it [20,58,59]. Inadvertent discovery and fragmented information about DSD can be upsetting and may be misconstrued as a terrible illness such as cancer [48]. The desire for self-knowledge can force individuals to seek information from parents, professionals, medical records and libraries but knowledge obtained and shared with others with similar problems is likely to bring relief and dignity [48].

Table 23.4 The elements of assent [48].

Assent comprises the following elements:

1 Assisting the child to know about his/her condition at a level appropriate for age and developmental maturity

2 Telling the child about physical examination, tests and treatment he/she requires

3 Assessing the child's understanding and views in response to this

4 Identifying the child's willingness to have physical examination, tests and treatment

5 Clarifying any physical procedures, tests or treatments which the child requires despite his/her objection

---

Voices of powerful advocates

Adults with DSD with their wealth of personal experience are a valuable source of information for patients and professionals. They can offer support, advocacy, a social network and individual and community empowerment through various organizations [e.g. Intersex Society of North America (http://www.isna.org/)]. Close collaboration between patient support groups and health professionals avoids biased opinions and has resulted in consensus guidelines for the diagnosis and management of DSD [1,2]. The emphasis on patient-centered care is grounded in ethical practice and focuses on the physical, psychological and sexual well-being of patients.

Involvement of patients with DSD in medical education

Patients should be respected as individuals and not viewed as medical disorders, fascinations or oddities. Whether patients with DSD should be involved in medical education requires consideration about who needs to learn about DSD, what the learner needs to know and whether this requires the direct involvement of a patient. Without supervision, the educational benefit of a learning session is questionable and the supervising professional should be responsible for obtaining consent.

Informed consent is specific and a patient's consent for one procedure does not imply consent for other interventions nor for medical education. The need for informed consent also applies to learning from examining patients when they are asleep or anesthetized: consent must have been obtained when the patient is conscious so that confidentiality, privacy and respect for dignity are assured.

Professionals need to be aware that patients may consent to teaching sessions or repeated unpleasant examination because they feel obliged or cannot decline. Language used in the presence of the patient, discussion, demonstration, repeated examination, measurements of external genitalia and medical photographs can inadvertently arouse distress and heighten negative feelings [60,61].

Role of research

While the focus of this chapter has been on the ethical viewpoints regarding early surgery, the alternative to assign gender in early life and defer elective surgery until the child is older, is not yet evidence-based. Anecdotal reports provide insight about crucial issues but cannot be generalized. Research is required to support robust decisions. Knowledge about a number of the DSD conditions offers helpful guidance but more needs to be known about the long-term outcomes of psychological, medical and surgical interventions regarding gender assignment, gender identity, psychosexual orientation, sexual function, reproductive ability and quality of life. Psychosocial adaptation needs to be considered in the context of a changing society where attitudes have evolved, and which is much more liberal and tolerant about atypical attributes.

Summary

Ethical standards are the same for all individuals and those with DSD are no exception. Gender-typical appearance of external genitalia is not a prerequisite for development of gender identity and it is influenced by nature and nurture. Gender assignment in infants with DSD requires evaluation, discussion with the family and a sensitive approach. Past practices, such as the obsession and urgency to normalize anatomy with surgery in early life, doctors withholding information and professionals making decisions for patients, are not ethically justified. Meagre evidence of long-term outcomes raises considerable uncertainty and what prevails now will be subject to future scrutiny. It is essential that beliefs and practices are repeatedly and openly questioned and modified on the basis of new and changing knowledge.

Growth hormone treatment for idiopathic short stature

The availability of unlimited supplies of growth hormone (GH) through recombinant technology extended its use from children with growth hormone deficiency (GHD) to other non-GHD short stature conditions. GH has been used in children with GHD, Turner syndrome (TS), Prader–Willi syndrome, chronic renal failure (CRF) and infants born small for gestational age (SGA). The use of GH in children with idiopathic short stature (ISS) who are GH replete has not been licensed in Europe but was approved in the USA by the Food and Drug Administration (FDA) in 2003 [62].

In the UK, a 1988 audit estimated that 19.8/100 000 children under the age of 16 years were receiving GH and 22% of these were for unlicensed indications [63], including SGA, skeletal dysplasias and Noonan syndrome, in addition to "short normals." Another audit found a comparable proportion of children treated for unlicensed indications (20%) and no escalating trends in GH prescribing in 1990–1999 [64]. Following FDA approval in 2003, a US survey has revealed that 82% of pediatric endocrinologists use GH for ISS [65]. Increasing numbers of otherwise healthy children now present to pediatricians because they are short. Whether they should be treated with GH raises important ethical issues [66–73].

Evaluation of children with idiopathic short stature in clinical practice

An understanding of different ethical perspectives requires uniform clinical evaluation which includes:
- Clinical assessment to exclude growth hormone deficiency and other recognized causes of short stature;
- Assessing the child's height in comparison to parents and the variations in height in the normal population;
- Identifying the physical and psychosocial cost of short stature on the child as experienced or perceived by the child and parents;

- Exploring the motives of child and parents for treatment, perceptions about a treatment that entails daily injections for several years and expectations about likely outcomes;
- Benefits of GH treatment on stature;
- Benefits of GH treatment on alleviating or preventing psychosocial problems;
- Risks to the child; and
- Financial cost.

Motives for treatment and expectations

Children with ISS and their parents may seek GH treatment for varied reasons, such as to:
- Enhance final height;
- Enhance growth in height during a specific period in life (e.g. before starting senior school);
- Prevent and/or ameliorate potential emotional and psychosocial problems related to short stature;
- Ameliorate emotional and psychosocial dysfunction related to short stature;
- Optimize future prospects in life for education, career and relationships.
- Parental perceptions are frequently at odds with the child's, and while they tend to be especially concerned about psychosocial dysfunction and future opportunities, children are more likely to focus on current height [74]. These motives and expectations of treatment provide a starting point to initiate discussion and guidance toward realistic decisions. Wide discrepancies between expectations and what might be achieved can be disappointing and detrimental to quality of life [75].

The ethical debate

The ethical debate for and against the use of GH in ISS can be considered according to the rationale for treatment and probable outcomes.

Idiopathic short stature is not a disease

If the aim of health care is to restore health and prevent ill health, children with ISS do not require treatment: they are healthy and do not have a disease. Short stature (height <2 SD below the mean) is one extreme of normal variation. Treatment with GH medicalizes such children, labels them as patients and imposes the burden of daily injections and hospital visits for many years [72,73]. If the aim of GH in ISS is to enhance physical appearance, cosmetic treatment is not essential for health [72].

Counter to this is the argument that children with ISS are a heterogeneous group and may have pathology that has not yet been identified [66,72]. Although the majority are GH replete and have normal or high GH concentrations to stimulation tests, 25% have low insulin-like growth factor 1 (IGF-1) levels suggestive of GH resistance [76]. Future work on the GH–IGF axis is likely to unravel the etiology of the short stature in some of these children so they cannot strictly be categorized as being healthy and treatment is indicated to restore health [68].

The value of stature in society

In favor of GH treatment are the physical disability and negative impact on psychosocial adjustment in short children, independent of underlying pathology. The physical handicap affects daily life and necessitates bespoke modifications, such as adjustments to furniture and car pedal extensions.

Predisposition to problems of psychosocial functioning can arise from the short child's experiences, such as problematic peer relationships, bullying, juvenilization and discrimination [77,78]. Others are secondary to parental anxiety and perceptions, because short children are perceived to be more vulnerable and prone to over-protection [79]. Preoccupation with this can itself be detrimental for parents and the child. Because height gain has the potential to improve quality of life, GH treatment is a therapeutic intervention to correct a physical abnormality and prevent or alleviate psychosocial problems [68,73].

Evaluation of the relationship between adult height in the general UK population and aspects of quality of life that affect health [health-related quality of life (HRQoL)] shows that height is a significant predictor of HRQoL in those who are the shortest (height −2.0 SDS or less) [80]. A small increase in height among the shortest individuals but not among those with normal height is associated with better HRQoL and lends support to the potential benefit of growth-promoting treatment in those with the most marked short stature.

However, the majority of children who are short experience no significant disadvantage on physical functioning [77], perception about their appearance, self-esteem, emotional adjustment, social functioning (friendship, popularity, reputation), cognitive development or academic achievement [66,81–85]. Because parental expectation about the change in the child's appearance and behavior may not be achieved, what they desire may not be in the best interests of the child [70]. The burden of treatment and disappointment if treatment expectations are not met can itself have a detrimental effect on psychosocial functioning [66,73].

Despite numerous trials on the effects of treatment on height, there is paucity of data about the quality of life benefits of GH treatment and gain in height does not necessarily imply better psychosocial function [77,85–88]. Emotional and psychosocial adaptation are more strongly related to a child's satisfaction with height and perceived height than actual height or growth itself [88]. Some improvement in behavior can occur during GH treatment in children who have significant problems initially but this is likely to be a small group referred for specialist treatment [89].

Alternative interventions, such as psychological support during growth and development, are safer than GH [73]. Many negative experiences that children and adults have because of their short stature are caused by public prejudices and stereotypes; changing this requires enlightening society [69,73]. A focus on height overvalues it compared to other characteristics such as personality.

Benefits of growth hormone on stature

Treatment with GH results in short- and long-term improvements in height [90,91] ranging from 0.6–1.6 SDS over 1 year to up to 1.1–2.2 SDS over 2–3 years of treatment. A good initial response will generally set the scene for good growth in subsequent years. For children treated to near-final height, GH regimens of 0.22–0.3 mg/kg/week over 2–10 years result in a modest increase in adult height SDS compared to those not treated (−1.8 to −1.5 SDS), in estimated gain compared to predicted adult height of 3–9 cm and in estimated gain compared to untreated controls (2–9 cm) [92–94]. Higher doses (up to 0.4 mg/kg/week) result in greater increase in height but the risk of adverse effects is also increased [95].

The arguments against GH treatment include the variable growth response from no gain in height to a gain of several centimeters in final height. Not all treated children benefit and it is not possible to predict who will gain the most [72,92,93]. How much height gain is required to prevent or relieve physical disability and psychosocial problems is not known. Even in children who do respond, treatment rarely results in adult height above the 50th centile and does not improve quality of life for the majority [66,70]. Factors contributing to poor response include non-compliance, inadequate dosage and inherent biological influences on GH sensitivity. There is also a view that treatment cannot be considered beneficial to society as a whole because the increase in height of a GH treated child means that another individual will be relatively disadvantaged [66].

Risks of growth hormone treatment

In support of treatment is the wide safety margin demonstrated by worldwide pharmaco-surveillance since the availability of recombinant GH in 1985. Side effects are infrequent and there is reassuring evidence against risk of malignancy. Opposing this is that much of this evidence for adverse effects comes from children with GHD or the non-licensed indications rather than large numbers of children with ISS. Additionally, ongoing monitoring is recommended for all children treated with GH to identify unknown long-term consequences [96] and the benefit of treatment does not outweigh the potential risks and burden of daily injections [70].

Financial cost of GH treatment

A point to support GH treatment is that children with ISS who seek treatment are, like all individuals in society, entitled to it but GH is expensive and its use needs to be considered from the perspective of distributive justice, equable distribution of health resources and offering treatments to those most in need [66,70]. Children with ISS are neither most in need nor do they have a life-threatening condition. No cost–utility analysis that includes quality of life outcome has yet been performed for GH treatment in ISS. An economic evaluation in 2002 estimated the incremental cost for every centimeter gained in final height to be 9400–18 930 euro [97]. More recently, the incremental cost-effectiveness of treatment compared with no treatment in prepubertal boys with ISS has been estimated at $52 000 per 2.54 cm [72]. Cost-effectiveness is better for a subset of exceptionally short children who have a good growth response to GH treatment, and more so if physical, mental and psychosocial well-being improves with the gain in final height. Such cases are a minority, and it is difficult to conclude that GH treatment for the majority of children with ISS is cost-effective.

Role (if any) of regulatory authorities and consensus statements

Before the era of recombinant human GH, 1978–1985, the Health Services Human Growth Hormone Committee was responsible for recommending, approving and allocating pituitary GH to patients in the UK [98]. The committee regulated not only supply and demand, but also maintained a database of all treated patients. Since the availability of recombinant GH, there has been no such central regulatory authority in the UK, treatment decisions rest with pediatricians or pediatric endocrinologists and prescriptions are provided by general practitioners. For any pediatrician, whose foremost duty is to the individual child, consensus guidelines from reputed organizations [e.g. National Institute for Health and Clinical Excellence (NICE), ESPE, LWPES, American Academy of Pediatrics (AAP), Growth Hormone Research Society (GRS)] offer reasoned recommendations to support better and consistent management decisions while at the same time safeguarding the interests of the public [72,99].

Summary

An understanding of the ethical arguments for and against GH treatment is essential for clinicians involved in managing children with ISS. These are otherwise healthy children for whom short stature will not be a handicap for the majority. Discussion about parental anxieties and request for GH treatment, about lack of tangible benefits and limitations of treatment helps reframe unrealistic perceptions. The decision to treat must be individualized and reached after detailed discussion with the child and parents. Children with ISS are generally old enough to express views about their height as well as treatment, and these must be respected. A select group of children who are exceptionally short and at greatest risk of physical and psychosocial dysfunction are likely to be those for whom a growth-promoting treatment would be justified. However, evidence to support this is required to justify the high cost of GH treatment.

Manipulating puberty in girls with severe learning difficulties

The onset of puberty and anticipated menarche in girls with severe learning difficulties (SLD) frequently raises anxiety in families and caregivers [100]. A number of treatments are available for suppressing and manipulating pubertal development and their use in children with precocious puberty can be justified. The problem is not so straightforward when pediatricians are

approached with a request to manipulate normal puberty in girls with SLD. There is a lack of evidence about the level of burden imposed on carers of girls with SLD and the benefits and risks of interventions to manipulate puberty. Practice is therefore based on personal experience, anecdotal reports and extrapolation from studies in healthy girls. Ethical evaluation requires consideration of what is in the best interest of the child and of the caregivers who have a pivotal role in the child's well-being.

Clinical approach

Manipulating puberty, particularly halting relatively early or normal puberty, requires consideration of:
• Cognitive and physical abilities of the child;
• Level of support required from caregivers;
• Impact of pubertal development on the patient and the carers;
• Reasons for seeking treatment;
• Intervention options to manipulate puberty;
• Benefits of interventions to the patient and carers;
• Risks of intervention;
• When interventions might be justified; and
• Who makes the decisions.

Intellectual and physical abilities of the child

Children with severe and profound learning difficulty can be defined by intelligence quotients (IQ) <70 and 55, respectively: they frequently have difficulties with mobility, coordination and communication. Cognitive and physical potential can vary from some ability to understand and acquire self-help skills to no verbal communication and total dependence on caregivers for all basic needs. Caregivers may view their ward as a perpetual child and not expect them to grow, mature physically or become sexually active.

Impact of puberty in a girl with SLD

The onset of puberty, age at menarche and frequency of menstrual abnormalities are no different in girls with SLD from healthy peers [101,102] but there is a predisposition to early development because of a number of co-morbidities and their treatments. Obesity is associated with earlier menarche [103] and girls with SLD have an increased tendency to gain excessive weight [104–106]. Other problems, such as hypo- and hyperthyroidism in Down syndrome [107] and hyperprolactinemia secondary to treatment with neuroleptics may contribute to menstrual irregularities.

The main impact of puberty on a girl with SLD is menstrual hygiene, menstrual abnormalities and effects on mood and behavior; less frequently carers worry about the child's vulnerability to sexual abuse and unwanted pregnancy. Periods compound the burden of personal care at home and at school for patients who have an inability to self-care, physical disability, bowel and bladder incontinence and other coexisting medical problems. Irregular, prolonged and heavy periods can disrupt the schedule for other essential needs such as feeding, physiotherapy and education [100,108]. Cyclic changes and dysmenorrhea can adversely affect mood, behavior, sleep and seizure control. Time, effort and patience required to look after the child, lack of control and uncertainties about the future contribute to the stress on caregivers [109]. Even before menarche, carers anticipate an inability to cope and worry about the possibility of not being able to continue caring for their child. In reality, it is likely that, with support and advice, carers will be able adequately to handle the problems that unfold as puberty occurs.

Interventions to manipulate puberty: benefits and risks

Puberty can be manipulated by a range of medical and surgical options but should generally be indefinitely postponed because of side effects of intervention (Table 23.5) [100,102,108,110–112]. The potential benefits of suppressing puberty and menses include easing the burden of care, freeing time to attend to essential needs, allowing families to continue caring for the child at home,

relieving stress and anxiety in carers, and positive effects on the carer and the child's quality of life [100].

Medical treatments are reversible and relatively non-invasive but carry significant adverse effects if used long term. They include loss of bone mineral density and fracture risk with use of depot medroxyprogesterone acetate (Depo-Provera) for >2 years [113], venous thromboembolism with oral contraceptives and weight gain with gonadotrophin-releasing hormone analogs. Girls with SLD and problems with weight-bearing and mobility, fits and falls are likely to be at greater risk from these adverse effects. Interactions between anticonvulsants and estrogen–progesterone preparations can reduce efficacy of treatment.

Surgical procedures are considered in exceptional situations and as a last resort when menstruation significantly impacts on the quality of life of the patient and caregiver [108,112,114]. They are invasive, require anesthesia and have substantial immediate risks but, set against the adverse effects of hormonal treatment,

Table 23.5 Interventions to manipulate puberty in girls with severe learning difficulties [100,102,108,110–112].

Intervention	Method	Benefits	Risks
Non-steroidal anti-inflammatory drugs (e.g. mefenamic acid)	Oral tablets, capsules	Relieves dysmenorrhea May reduce menstrual flow	Gastrointestinal bleeding
GnRH analogs	Injection every 3–12 weeks	Suppresses pubertal development and menstruation Contraceptive effect	Impaired BMD with long-term use
Continuous combined oral contraceptives	Oral tablet taken daily for 9 weeks followed by 7-day withdrawal period or continuous until breakthrough bleeding followed by 7 day withdrawal period Supervision required	Reduce frequency of menstruation and flow Relieve dysmenorrhea Contraceptive effect	Efficacy affected by anticonvulsants or antibiotics Thromboembolism especially in immobile girls Increased risk of breast and cervical cancer
Depot medroxyprogesterone acetate	Injection every 10–12 weeks	Menstruation suppressed Contraceptive effect	Impaired BMD with long-term use Weight gain
Levonorgestrel intra-uterine system	Requires sedation or anesthetic Procedure performed by an experienced professional Uterine size must be adequate (minimum cavity of 5–6 cm); therefore not suitable in petite girls and requires preplacement assessment with ultrasound	Reduce menstrual flow within 3–6 months Suppress menstruation Contraceptive effect Effect lasts up to 5 years	Device expulsion Mastalgia and mood changes for initial few months Functional ovarian cysts which are usually asymptomatic and resolve spontaneously
Endometrial ablation	Requires anesthetic Procedure performed by a competent professional Necessitates cervical dilatation which can be difficult in nulliparous girls	Reduce menstrual flow Suppress menstruation	Possible need to repeat the procedure Risks lower than hysterectomy
Hysterectomy, vaginal or abdominal	Informed consent required Requires anesthetic Procedure performed by a competent professional	Relieve intractable menstrual problems Definitive option for menstrual problems but not perimenstrual syndrome	Irreversible Intra-operative and postoperative risks

BMD, bone mineral density.

especially if used long term, the irreversible nature of surgical intervention can be advantageous. Surgical procedures can be justified ethically for girls with profound cognitive impairment and high support needs who are unable to express an interest or consent to sexual intercourse, are incapable of choosing to become pregnant and cannot mother a child [108].

Thorough discussion about treatment options and surgical procedures should be carried out by expert professionals. Clinicians unfamiliar with the pubertal problems of girls with SLD should refer to appropriate specialists.

Who decides?

Children with SLD require individual evaluation when carers seek treatment to manipulate puberty. Mental and physical impairment, cognition, medical problems and social context of each child will be different. Multidisciplinary assessment by neurodisability specialists and pediatric or adolescent endocrinologists or gynecologists together with carers is essential.

Exhaustion, stress and burnout in caregivers threaten the welfare of the child and their anxieties must be respected and discussed. Advice about coping strategies, social support and respite care for the child are essential. It is the unknown and lack of control that frequently overwhelms carers and having information about possible options if life became too stressful is reassuring. Information about intervention must include the modes of administration, potential benefits and adverse effects. The duration of treatment and limitations to how long hormonal treatment might safely be continued require explicit clarification.

The child's ability to contribute to decision-making must be maximized. Parents and legal guardians are appropriate surrogates for making shared decisions when the child lacks this capacity but they should act in the best interests of the child and the clinician's duty is to ensure this. Hospital clinical ethics committees can help in situations when carers' and professionals' views differ and, exceptionally, approval may need to be sought from the Courts.

Summary

While what is in the best interest of the child should be foremost, the pivotal role of caregivers in the well-being of girls with SLD and high support needs cannot be overlooked. Puberty and menstruation can interfere adversely with quality of life of some carers as well as some girls with SLD. Each case requires individual consideration. Carers may sometimes have disparate views and may disregard professional advice. In addressing carer's concerns about the impact of puberty and menses on the patient's health, level of care offered and quality of life, benefits of treatment must outweigh risks, limitations and lack of research evidence. Safer alternatives, such as education, counseling and social support, should precede medical or surgical intervention. Carers' perceptions about dealing with problems of puberty are frequently disproportionate to their actual ability to cope. Instead of treating in anticipation, deferring decisions about intervention until after the onset of puberty means that treatment is reserved for those

who have real problems. Any potential the child has to contribute to decisions must be maximized. The interest of the child is best safeguarded by multidisciplinary evaluation and shared decision-making with carers.

References

1 Hughes IA, Houk C, Ahmed SF, Lee PA; LWPES/ESPE Consensus Group. Consensus statement on management of intersex disorders. *Arch Dis Child* 2006; **91**: 554–563.

2 Intersex Society of North America. *Consortium on the Management of Disorders of Sex Development: Handbook for Parents*. Rohnert Park. California: Intersex Society of North America, 2006. Available online at www.dsdguidelines.org.

3 Dessens A, Slijper F, Drop S. Gender dysphoria and gender change in chromosomal females with congenital adrenal hyperplasia. *Arch Sex Behav* 2005; **34**: 389–397.

4 Fausto-Sterling A. The five sexes: why male and female are not enough. *Sciences* 1993; **33**: 20–25.

5 Mazur T. Gender dysphoria and gender change in androgen insensitivity or micropenis. *Arch Sex Behav* 2005; **34**: 411–421.

6 Meyer-Bahlburg H. Gender identity outcome in female-raised 46,XY persons with penile agenesis, cloacal exstrophy of the bladder, or penile ablation. *Arch Sex Behav* 2005; **34**: 423–438.

7 Camurdan AD, Oz MO, Ilhan MN, Camurdan OM, Sahin F, Beyazova U. Current stretched penile length: cross-sectional study of 1040 healthy Turkish children aged 0 to 5 years. *Urology* 2007; **70**: 572–575.

8 Verkauf BS, Von Thron J, O'Brien WF. Clitoral size in normal women. *Obstet Gynecol* 1992; **80**: 41–44.

9 Blackless M, Charuvastra A, Derryck A, Fausto-Sterling A, Lauzanne K, Lee E. How sexually dimorphic are we? Review and synthesis. *Am J Hum Biol* 2000; **12**: 151–166.

10 Clayton PE, Miller WL, Oberfield SE, Ritzén EM, Sippell WG, Speiser PW; ESPE/LWPES CAH Working Group. Consenus statement on 21-hydroxylase deficiency from the European Society for Pediatric Endocrinology and the Lawson Wilkins Pediatric Endocrine Society. *Horm Res* 2002; **58**: 188–195.

11 Berenbaum SA, Bailey JM. Effects of gender identity of prenatal androgens and genital appearance: evidence from girls with congenital adrenal hyperplasia. *J Clin Endocrinol Metab* 2003; **88**: 1102–1106.

12 Kuhnle U, Bullinger M, Schwarz HP. The quality of life in adult female patients with congenital adrenal hyperplasia: a comprehensive study of the impact of genital malformations. *Eur J Pediatr* 1995; **154**: 708–716.

13 Meyer-Bahlburg HFL. Gender and sexuality in classical congenital adrenal hyperplasia. *Endocrinol Metab Clin North Am* 2001; **30**: 155–171.

14 Ehrhardt AA, Meyer-Bahlburg HFL. Effects of prenatal sex hormones on gender related behaviour. *Science* 1981; **211**: 1312–1318.

15 Mosley M, Bidder R, Hughes I. Sex role behaviour and self-image in young patients with congenital adrenal hyperplasia. *Br J Sexual Med* 1989; **16**: 72–75.

16 Shah R, Woolley MM, Costin G. Testicular feminization: the androgen insensitivity syndrome. *J Pediatr Surg* 1992; **27**: 757–760.

17 Donahoe PK. The diagnosis and treatment of infants with intersex abnormalities. *Pediatr Clin North Am* 1987; **34**: 1333–1348.

18 Reilly JM, Woodhouse CR. Small penis and the male sexual role. *J Urol* 1989; **142**: 569–571.

19 Reiner W, Gearhart J. Discordant sexual identity in some genetic males with cloacal exstrophy assigned to female sex at birth. *N Engl J Med* 2004; **350**: 333–341.

20 Brinkmann I, Schuetzmann K, Richter-Appelt H. Gender assignment and medical history of individuals with different forms of intersexuality: evaluation of medical records and the patients' perspective. *J Sex Med* 2007; **4**: 964–980.

21 McCullough LB. A framework for the ethically justified clinical management of intersex conditions. In: Zderic SA, Canning DA, Carr MC, Snyder HM, eds. *Pediatric Gender Assignment: A Critical Reappraisal*. New York: Kluwer Academic/Plenum, 2002: 149–173.

22 Cohen-Kettenis P. Gender change in 46,XY persons with 5alpha-reductase-2 deficiency and 17beta-hydroxysteroid dehydrogenase-3 deficiency. *Arch Sex Behav* 2005; **34**: 399–410.

23 Dittmann R, Kappes M, Kappes M, *et al.* Congenital adrenal hyperplasia. I: Gender-related behavior and attitudes in female patients and sisters. *Psychoneuroendocrinology* 1990; **15**: 401–420.

24 Reiner W. Assignment of sex in neonates with ambiguous genitalia. *Curr Opin Pediatr* 1999; **11**: 363–365

25 Meyer-Bahlburg H, Migeon C, Berkovitz G, Gearhart J, Dolezal C, Wisniewski A. Attitudes of adult 46,XY intersex persons to clinical management policies. *J Urol* 2004; **171**: 1615–1619.

26 Reiner W. Case study: sex reassignment in a teenage girl. *J Am Acad Child Adolesc Psychiatry* 1996; **35**: 799–803.

27 Wisniewski A, Migeon C, Meyer-Bahlburg H, *et al.* Complete androgen insensitivity syndrome: long-term medical, surgical, and psychosexual outcome. *J Clin Endocrinol Metab* 2000; **85**: 2664–2669.

28 Wisniewski AB, Migeon C, Gearhart JP, *et al.* Congenital micropenis: long-term medical, surgical and psychosexual follow-up of individuals raised male or female. *Horm Res* 2001; **56**: 3–11.

29 Zucker KJ. Intersexuality and gender identity differentiation. *Annu Rev Sex Res* 1999; **10**: 1–69.

30 Diamond M, Sigmundson HK. Sex reassignment at birth: long-term review and clinical implications. *Arch Pediatr Adolesc Med* 1997; **15**: 298–304.

31 Berenbaum S, Sandberg D. Sex determination, differentiation, and identity. *N Engl J Med* 2004; **350**: 2204–2206.

32 Speiser P. Congenital adrenal hyperplasia owing to 21-hydroxylase deficiency. *Endocrinol Metab Clin North Am* 2001; **30**: 31–59.

33 Wedell A, Thilen A, Ritzen E, Stengler B, Luthman H. Mutational spectrum of the steroid 21-hydroxylase gene in Sweden: implications for genetic diagnosis and association with disease manifestation. *J Clin Endocrinol Metab* 1994; **78**: 1145–1152.

34 Meyer-Bahlburg HFL, Gruen RS, New MI, *et al.* Gender change from female to male in classical congenital adrenal hyperplasia. *Horm Behav* 1996; **30**: 319–332.

35 Sripathi V, Ahmed S, Sakati N, al-Ashwal A. Gender reversal in 46XX congenital virilizing adrenal hyperplasia. *Br J Urol* 1997; **79**: 785–789.

36 Zucker KJ, Bradley SJ, Oliver G, Blake J, Fleming S, Hood J. Psychosexual development of women with congenital adrenal hyperplasia. *Horm Behav* 1996; **30**: 300–318.

37 Crouch N, Creighton S. Minimal surgical intervention in the management of intersex conditions. *J Pediatr Endocrinol Metab* 2004; **17**: 1591–1596.

38 American Academy of Pediatrics, Section on Urology. Timing of elective surgery on the genitalia of male children with particular reference to the risks, benefits, and psychological effects of surgery and anesthesia. *Pediatrics* 1996; **97**: 590–594.

39 Money J, Hampson J, Hampson J. Hermaphroditism: recommendations concerning assignment of sex, change of sex and psychologic management. *Bull Johns Hopkins Hosp* 1955; **97**: 284–300.

40 Money J, Ehrhardt A. *Man & Woman Boy & Girl: The Differentiation and Dimorphism of Gender Identity from Conception to Maturity*. Baltimore: Johns Hopkins University Press, 1972.

41 Glassberg K. The intersex infant: early gender assignment and surgical reconstruction. *J Pediatr Adolesc Gynecol* 1998; **11**: 151–154.

42 Bailez MM, Gearhart JP, Migeon C, Rock J. Vaginal reconstruction after initial construction of the external genitalia in girls with salt-wasting adrenal hyperplasia. *J Urol* 1992; **148**: 680–684.

43 Schober JM. Long-term outcomes and changing attitudes to intersexuality. *BJU Int* 1999; **83**: 39–50.

44 Migeon CJ, Wisniewski AB, Gearhart JP, *et al.* Ambiguous genitalia with perineoscrotal hypospadias in 46,XY individuals: long-term medical, surgical, and psychosexual outcome. *Pediatrics* 2002; **110**: e31.

45 Migeon CJ, Wisniewski AB, Brown TR, *et al.* 46,XY intersex individuals: phenotypic and etiologic classification, knowledge of condition, and satisfaction with knowledge in adulthood. *Pediatrics* 2002; **110**: e32.

46 Creighton SM, Liao L-M. Changing attitudes to sex assignment in intersex. *BJU Int* 2004; **93**: 659–664.

47 Newman K, Randolph J, Anderson K. The surgical management of infants and children with ambiguous genitalia. *Ann Surg* 1992; **215**: 644–653.

48 Preves SE. For the sake of children: destigmatizing intersexuality. *J Clin Ethics* 1998; **9**: 411–420.

49 Diamond M, Beh HG. Changes in the management of children with intersex conditions. *Nat Clin Pract Endocrinol Metabol* 2008; **4**: 4–5.

50 American Academy of Pediatrics Committee on Bioethics. Informed consent, parental permission, and assent in pediatric practice. *Pediatrics* 1995; **95**: 314–317.

51 Daaboul J, Frader J. Ethics and the management of the patient with intersex: a middle way. *J Pediatr Endocrinol Metab* 2001; **14**: 1575–1583.

52 Greenberg JA. International legal developments protecting the autonomy rights of sexual minorities: who should decide the appropriate treatment for an intersex child? In: Sytsma SE, ed. *Ethics and Intersex*. Dordrecht: Springer, 2006: 87–101.

53 Elias S, Annas GJ. The whole truth and nothing but the truth? *Hastings Center Rep* 1988; **18**: 35–36.

54 Groveman SA. Sex, lies and androgen insensitivity syndrome. Letter to the editor. *Can Med Assoc J* 1996; **154**: 1829–1832.

55 Beh HG, Pietsch JH. Legal implications surrounding adolescent health care decision-making in matters of sex, reproduction, and gender. *Child Adolesc Psychiatr Clin N Am* 2004; **13**: 675–693.

56 Minogue BP, Taraszewski R. The whole truth and nothing but the truth? *Hastings Center Rep* 1988: **18**: 34–35.

57 Kemp BD. Sex, lies and androgen insensitivity syndrome. Letter to the editor. *Can Med Assoc J* 1996; **154**: 1829–1832.

58 Anonymous. Be open and honest with sufferers. *Br Med J* 1994; **308**: 1041–1042.

59 Coventry M. Finding the words. *Chrysalis: J Transgres Gender Ident* 1997; **2**: 27–30.

60 Creighton S, Alderson J, Brown S, Minto CL. Medical photography: ethics, consent, and the intersex patient. *BJU Int* 2002; **89**: 67–71.

61 Lee P. A perspective on the approach to the intersex child born with genital ambiguity. *J Pediatr Endocrinol Metab* 2004; **17**: 133–140.

62 Food and Drug Administration: FDA approves Humatrope for short stature. FDA Talk paper. July 25, 2003. Available at: www.fda.gov/bbs/topics/ANSWERS/2003/ANS01242.html.

63 Hilken J, for the British Society for Paediatric Endocrinology and Diabetes Clinical Trials/Audit Group. UK audit of childhood growth hormone prescription 1998. *Arch Dis Child* 2001; **84**: 387–389.

64 Paterson WF, Donaldson MD, Greene SA, Kelnar CJ, Smail PJ. The boom that never was: results of a 10 year audit of paediatric growth hormone prescribing in Scotland. *Health Bull (Edinb)* 2000; **58**: 457–466.

65 Hardin DS, Woo J, Butsch R, Huett B. Current prescribing practices and opinions about growth hormone therapy: results of a nationwide survey of paediatric endocrinologists. *Clin Endocrinol* 2007; **66**: 85–94.

66 Allen DB, Fost N. hGH for short stature: ethical issues raised by expanded access. *J Pediatr* 2004; **144**: 648–652.

67 Allen DB. Growth hormone therapy for short stature: is the benefit worth the burden? *Pediatrics* 2006; **118**: 343–348.

68 Bolt LLE, Mul D. Growth hormone in short children: beyond medicine? *Acta Pædiatr* 2001; **90**: 69–73.

69 Freemark M. [Editorial] Growth hormone treatment of "Idiopathic short stature": not so fast. *J Clin Endocrinol Metab* 2004; **89**: 3138–3139.

70 Gill DG. Anything you can do, I can do bigger? The ethics and the equity of growth hormone for small normal children. *Arch Dis Child* 2006; **91**: 270–272.

71 Haverkamp F, Ranke MB. The ethical dilemma of growth hormone treatment of short stature: a scientific theoretical approach. *Horm Res* 1999; **51**: 301–304.

72 Lee JM, Davis MM, Clark SJ, Hofer TP, Kemper AR. Estimated cost-effectiveness of growth hormone therapy for idiopathic short stature. *Arch Pediatr Adolesc Med* 2006; **160**: 263–269.

73 Verweij M, Kortmann F. Moral assessment of growth hormone therapy for children with idiopathic short stature. *J Med Ethics* 1997; **23**: 305–309.

74 Visser-van Balen H, Geenen R, Kamp GA, Huisman J, Wit JM, Sinnema G. Motives for choosing growth-enhancing hormone treatment in adolescents with idiopathic short stature: a questionnaire and structured interview study. *BMC Pediatrics* 2005; **5**: 15.

75 Calman KC. Quality of life in cancer patients: an hypothesis. *J Med Ethics* 1984; **10**: 124–127.

76 Rosenfeld RG. The molecular basis of idiopathic short stature. *Growth Horm IGF Res* 2005; **15**: S3–S5.

77 Wheeler PG, Bresnahan K, Shephard BA, Lau J, Balk EM. Short stature and functional impairment: a systematic review. *Arch Pediatr Adolesc Med* 2004; **158**: 236–243.

78 Voss LD, Mulligan J. (2000) Bullying in school: are short pupils at risk? Questionnaire study in a cohort. *Br Med J* 2000; **320**: 612–613.

79 Molinari E, Sartori A, Ceccarelli A, Marchi S. Psychological and emotional development, intellectual capabilities, and body image in short normal children. *J Endocrinol Invest* 2002; **25**: 321–328.

80 Christenson TL, Djurhuus CB, Clayton P, Christiansen JS. An evaluation of the relationship between adult height and health-related quality of life in the general UK population. *Clin Endocrinol* 2007; **67**: 407–412.

81 Busschbach JJ, Rikken B, Grobbee DE, De Charro FT, Wit JM. Quality of life in short adults. *Horm Res* 1998; **49**: 32–38.

82 Downie AB, Mulligan J, Stratford RJ, Betts PR, Voss LD. Are short normal children at a disadvantage? The Wessex Growth Study. *Br Med J* 1997; **314**: 97–100.

83 Kranzler JH, Rosenbloom AL, Proctor B, Diamond FB Jr, Watson M. Is short stature a handicap? A comparison of the psychosocial functioning of referred and nonreferred children with normal short stature and children with normal stature. *J Pediatr* 2000; **136**: 96–102.

84 Sandberg DE, Bukowski WM, Fung CM, Noll RB. Height and social adjustment: are extremes a cause for concern and action? *Pediatrics* 2004; **114**: 744–750.

85 Sandberg DE, Colsman M. Growth hormone treatment of short stature: status of the quality of life rationale. *Horm Res* 2005; **63**: 275–283.

86 Downie AB, Mulligan J, McCaughey E, Stratford RJ, Betts PR, Voss LD. Psychological response to growth hormone treatment in short normal children. *Arch Dis Child* 1996; **75**: 32–35.

87 Ross JL, Sandberg DE, Rose SR, *et al.* Psychological adaptation in children with idiopathic short stature treated with growth hormone or placebo. *J Clin Endocrinol Metab* 2004; **89**: 4873–4878.

88 Theunissen NC, Kamp GA, Koopman HM, Zwinderman KA, Vogels T, Wit JM. Quality of life and self-esteem in children treated for idiopathic short stature. *J Pediatr* 2002; **140**: 507–515.

89 Stabler B, Siegel PT, Clopper RR, Stoppani CE, Compton PG, Underwood LE. Behavior change after growth hormone treatment of children with short stature. *J Pediatr* 1998; **133**: 366–373.

90 Bryant J, Baxter L, Cave CB, Milne R. Recombinant growth hormone for idiopathic short stature in children and adolescents. *Cochrane Database Syst Rev* 2007; **3**: CD004440.

91 Finkelstein BS, Imperiale TF, Speroff T, Marrero U, Radcliffe DJ, Cuttler L. Effect of growth hormone therapy on height in children with idiopathic short stature: a meta-analysis. *Arch Pediatr Adolesc Med* 2002; **156**: 230–240.

92 Buchlis JG, Irizarry L, Crotzer BC, Shine BJ, Allen L, Macgillivray MH. Comparison of final heights of growth hormone-treated vs untreated children with idiopathic growth failure. *J Clin Endocrinol Metab* 1998; **83**: 1075–1079.

93 Hintz RL, Attie KM, Baptista J, Roche A. Effect of growth hormone treatment on adult height of children with idiopathic short stature. Genentech Collaborative Group. *N Engl J Med* 1999; **340**: 502–507.

94 Leschek EW, Rose SR, Yanovski JA, *et al.* Effects of growth hormone treatment on adult height in peripubertal children with idiopathic short stature: a randomized, double-blind, placebo-controlled trial. *J Clin Endocrinol Metab* 2004; **89**: 3140–3148.

95 Rekers-Mombarg LTM, Busschbach JJV, Massa GG, Dicke J, Wit JM. Quality of life of young adults with idiopathic short stature: effect of growth hormone treatment. *Acta Paediatr* 1998; **87**: 865–870.

96 Wilson TA, Rose SR, Cohen P, *et al*. Update of guidelines for the use of growth hormone in children: the Lawson Wilkins Pediatric Endocrinology Society Drug and Therapeutics Committee. *J Pediatr* 2003; **143**: 415–421.

97 Bryant J, Loveman E, Chase D, *et al*. Clinical effectiveness and cost-effectiveness of growth hormone in adults in relation to impact on quality of life: a systematic review and economic evaluation. *Health Technol Assess* 2002; **6**: 1–106.

98 Department of Health and Social Security. *Arrangements for treatment of children with growth hormone deficiency*. London: Department of Health and Social Security, 1977 (Health Circular **77**: 21).

99 National Institute for Clinical Excellence (NICE). *TA42 Growth Hormone Deficiency (Children) – Human Growth Hormone: Guidance*. NICE, 2002. Available at: http://www.nice.org.uk/

100 Dizon CD, Allen LM, Ornstein MP. Menstrual and contraceptive issues among young women with developmental delay: a retrospective review of cases at the Hospital for Sick Children, Toronto. *J Pediatr Adolesc Gynecol* 2005; **18**: 157–162.

101 Lindgren GW, Katoda H. Maturational rate of Tokyo children with and without mental retardation. *Am J Ment Retard* 1993; **98**: 128–134.

102 Quint EH. The conservative management of abnormal bleeding in teenagers with developmental disabilities. *J Pediatr Adolesc Gynecol* 2003; **16**: 54–56.

103 Kaplowitz PB. Link between body fat and the timing of puberty. *Pediatrics* 2008; **121** (Suppl 3): S208–217.

104 Bandini LG, Curtin C, Hamad C, Tybor DJ, Must A. Prevalence of overweight in children with developmental disorders in the continuous national health and nutrition examination survey (NHANES) 1999–2002. *J Pediatr* 2005; **146**: 738–743.

105 McKinlay I, Ferguson A, Jolly C. Ability and dependency in adolescents with severe learning disabilities. *Dev Med Child Neurol* 1996; **38**: 48–58.

106 Takano T, Takaki H, Kawano H, Nonaka K. Early menarche in Japanese Down syndrome. *Pediatrics* 1999; **103**: 854–855.

107 Karlsson B, Gustafsson J, Hedov G, Ivarsson SA, Annerén G. Thyroid dysfunction in Down's syndrome: relation to age and thyroid autoimmunity. *Arch Dis Child* 1998; **79**: 242–245.

108 Paransky OI, Zurawin RK. Management of menstrual problems and contraception in adolescents with mental retardation: a medical, legal, and ethical review with new suggested guidelines. *J Pediatr Adolesc Gynecol* 2003; **16**: 223–235.

109 Murphy NA, Christian B, Caplin DA, Young PC. The health of caregivers for children with disabilities: caregiver perspectives. *Child Care Health Dev* 2006; **33**: 180–187.

110 Albanese A, Hopper NW. Suppression of menstruation in adolescents with severe learning disabilities. *Arch Dis Child* 2007; **92**: 629–632.

111 Atkinson E, Bennett MJ, Dudley J, *et al*; Australian Society of Paediatric and Adolescent Gynaecology Working Party. Consensus statement: Menstrual and contraceptive management in women with an intellectual disability. *Aust N Z J Obstet Gynaecol* 2003; **43**: 109–110.

112 Zurawin RK, Paransky OI. The role of surgical techniques in the treatment of menstrual problems and as contraception in adolescents with disabilities. *J Pediatr Adolesc Gynecol* 2003; **16**: 51–53.

113 Cromer BA, Scholes D, Berenson A, Cundy T, Clark MK, Kaunitz AM. Depot medroxyprogesterone acetate and bone mineral density in adolescents – the Black Box warning: a position paper of the Society for Adolescent Medicine. *J Adolesc Health* 2006; **39**: 296–301.

114 Grover SR. Menstrual and contraceptive management in women with an intellectual disability. *Med J Aust* 2002; **176**: 108–110.

Appendix: Syndrome-specific Growth Charts

Growth charts for specific growth disorders are depicted here.

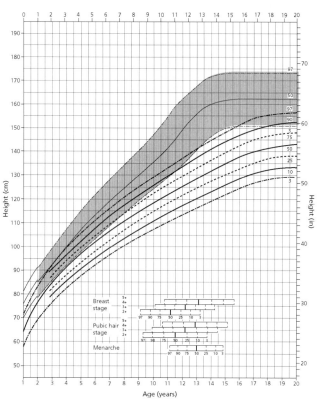

Figure A.1 Height centiles for girls with untreated Turner syndrome aged 1–20 years. The gray-shaded area represents the 3rd to 97th centiles for normal girls. Pubertal staging is for normal girls. Adapted from Lyon A, Preece M, Grant D. Growth curves for girls with Turner syndrome. *Arch Dis Child* 1985; 60: 932–935.

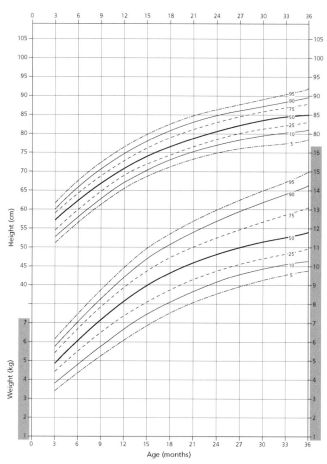

Figure A.2 Height and weight centiles for boys with trisomy 21 syndrome aged 3–36 months. Adapted from Cronk C, Crocker A, Peuschel S *et al.* Growth charts for children with Down syndrome. *Pediatrics* 1988; 81: 102–10.

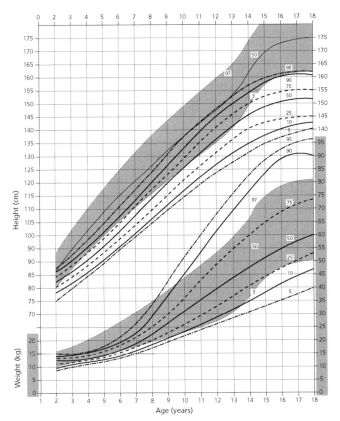

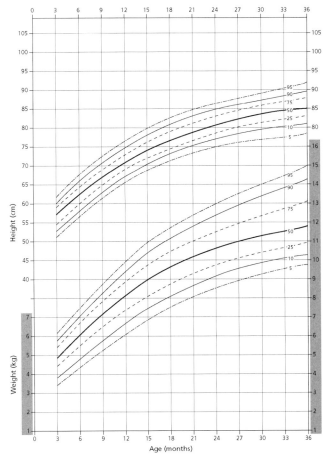

Figure A.3 Height and weight centiles for boys with trisomy 21 syndrome aged 2–18 years. The gray-shaded areas represent the comparable values for the 3rd to 97th centiles for normal children. Adapted from Cronk C, Crocker A, Peuschel S *et al*. Growth charts for children with Down syndrome. *Pediatrics* 1988; 81: 102–10.

Figure A.4 Height and weight centiles for girls with trisomy 21 syndrome aged 3–36 months. Adapted from Cronk C, Crocker A, Peuschel S *et al*. Growth charts for children with Down syndrome. *Pediatrics* 1988; 81: 102–10.

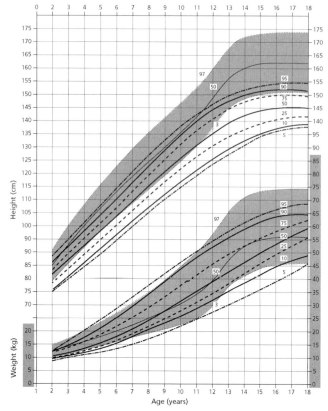

Figure A.5 Height and weight centiles for girls with trisomy 21 syndrome aged 2–18 years. The gray-shaded areas represent the comparable values for the 3rd to 97th centiles for normal children. Adapted from Cronk C, Crocker A, Peuschel S *et al*. Growth charts for children with Down syndrome. *Pediatrics* 1988; 81: 102–10.

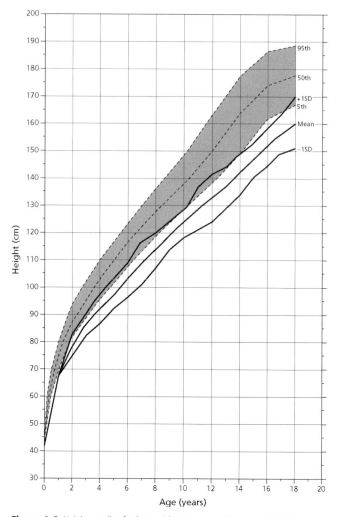

Figure A.6 Height centiles for boys with Noonan syndrome aged 0–18 years compared with normal values (dashed lines). The data were obtained from 64 Noonan syndrome males in a collaborative retrospective review. Adapted from Witt D, Keena B, Hall J *et al*. Growth curves for height in Noonan syndrome. *Clin Genet* 1986; 30: 150–3.

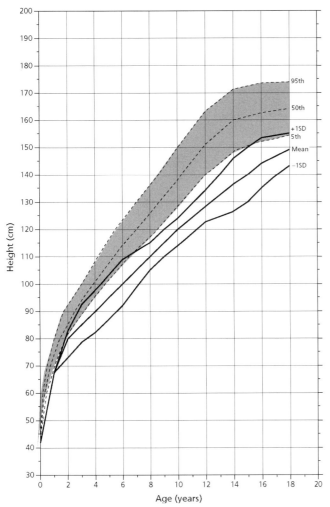

Figure A.7 Height centiles for girls with Noonan syndrome aged 0–18 years compared with normal values (dashed lines). The data were obtained from 48 Noonan syndrome females in a collaborative retrospective review. Adapted from Witt D, Keena B, Hall J *et al*. Growth curves for height in Noonan syndrome. *Clin Genet* 1986; 30: 150–3.

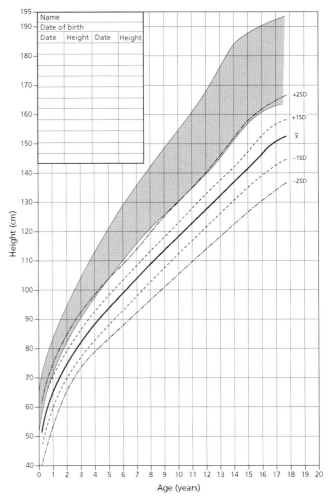

Figure A.8 Height centiles for boys with Silver–Russell syndrome. The gray-shaded area indicates normal boys ±2 standard deviations (SD). Adapted from Wollman H, Kirchner T, Enders H *et al*. Growth and symptoms in Silver–Russell syndrome: review on the basis of 386 patients. *Eur J Pediatr* 1995; 154: 958–68.

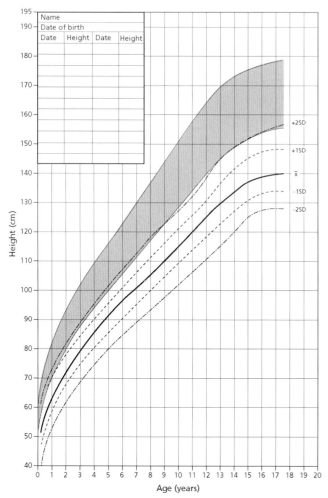

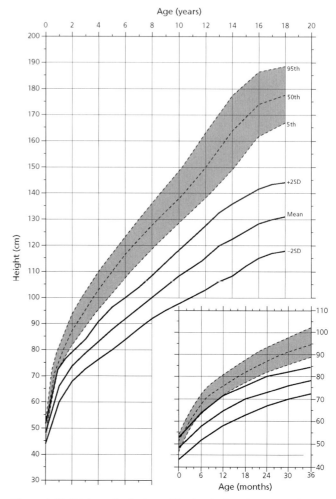

Figure A.9 Height centiles for girls with Silver–Russell syndrome. The gray-shaded area indicates normal girls ±2 standard deviations (SD). Adapted from Wollman H, Kirchner T, Enders H *et al.* Growth and symptoms in Silver–Russell syndrome: review on the basis of 386 patients. *Eur J Pediatr* 1995; 154: 958–68.

Figure A.10 Height centiles for boys with achondroplasia (mean ± 2 SD) compared with normal standard curves (dashed lines). Data derived from 189 males. Adapted from Horton W, Rotter J, Rimoin D *et al.* Standard growth curves for achondroplasia. *J Pediatr* 1978; 93: 435–8.

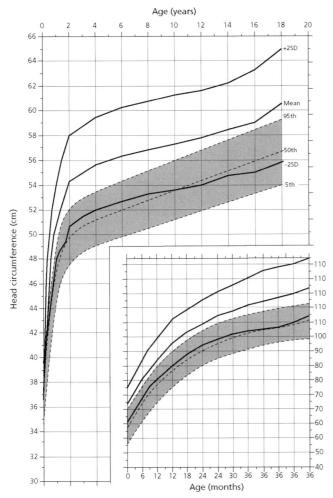

Figure A.11 Head circumference centiles for boys with achondroplasia compared with normal curves (dashed lines). Data derived from 114 males. Adapted from Horton W, Rotter J, Rimoin D *et al*. Standard growth curves for achondroplasia. *J Pediatr* 1978; 93: 435–8.

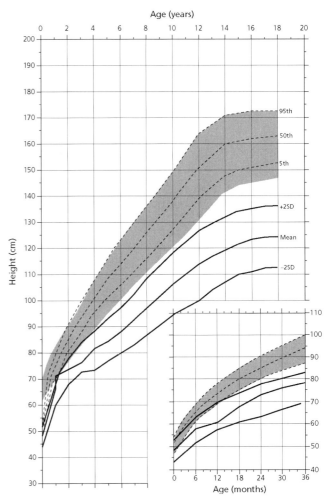

Figure A.12 Height centiles for girls with achondroplasia (mean ± 2 SD) compared with normal standard curves (dashed lines). Data derived from 214 females. Adapted from Horton W, Rotter J, Rimoin D *et al*. Standard growth curves for achondroplasia. *J Pediatr* 1978; 93: 435–8.

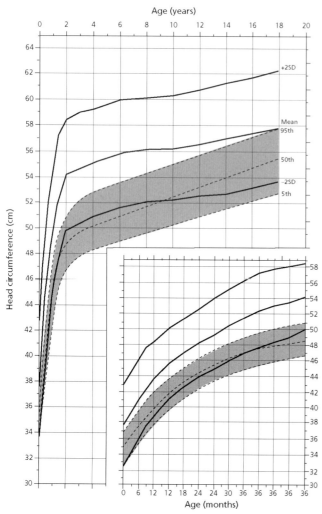

Figure A.13 Head circumference centiles for girls with achondroplasia compared with normal curves (dashed lines). Data derived from 145 females. Adapted from Horton W, Rotter J, Rimoin D *et al.* Standard growth curves for achondroplasia. *J Pediatr* 1978; 93: 435–8.

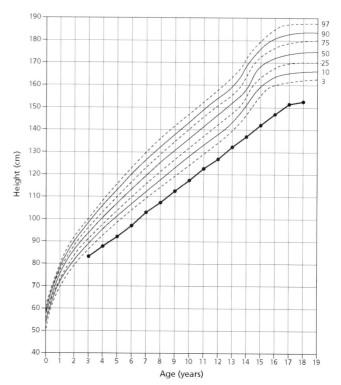

Figure A.14 Linear growth in hypocondroplasic boys (solid line). Adapted from Appan S, Laurent S, Chapman M *et al.* Growth and growth hormone therapy in hypochondroplasia. *Acta Paediatr Scand* 1990; 79: 796–803.

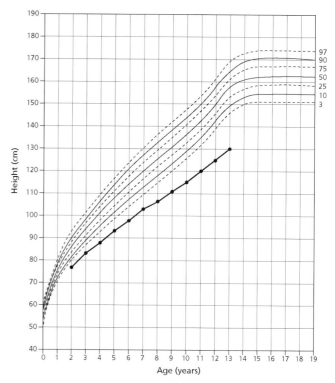

Figure A.15 Linear growth in hypocondroplasic girls (solid line). Adapted from Appan S, Laurent S, Chapman M *et al.* Growth and growth hormone therapy in hypochondroplasia. *Acta Paediatr Scand* 1990; 79: 796–803.

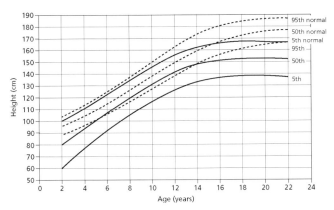

Figure A.16 Standardized curves for height in Prader–Willi syndrome (PWS) in male patients (solid line) and healthy individuals (broken line). Adapted from Butler MG, Brunschwig A, Miller LK *et al*. Standards for selected anthropometric measurements in Prader–Willi syndrome. *Pediatrics* 1991; 88: 853–60.

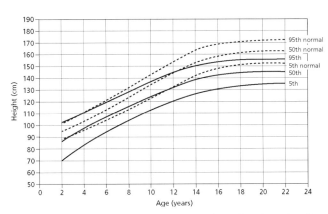

Figure A.17 Standardized curves for height in Prader–Willi syndrome (PWS) in female patients (solid line) and healthy individuals (broken line). Adapted from Butler MG, Brunschwig A, Miller LK *et al*. Standards for selected anthropometric measurements in Prader–Willi syndrome. *Pediatrics* 1991; 88: 853–60.

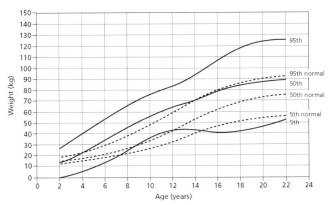

Figure A.18 Standardized curves for weight in Prader–Willi syndrome (PWS) in male patients (solid line) and healthy individuals (broken line). Adapted from Butler MG, Brunschwig A, Miller LK *et al*. Standards for selected anthropometric measurements in Prader–Willi syndrome. *Pediatrics* 1991; 88: 853–60.

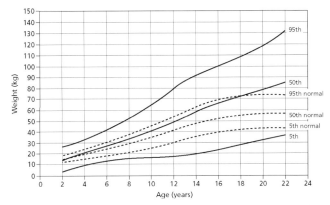

Figure A.19 Standardized curves for weight in Prader–Willi syndrome (PWS) in female patients (solid line) and healthy individuals (broken line). Adapted from Butler MG, Brunschwig A, Miller LK *et al*. Standards for selected anthropometric measurements in Prader–Willi syndrome. *Pediatrics* 1991; 88: 853–60.

Index

SINGLETON HOSPITAL
STAFF LIBRARY